world
databases
in

MEDICINE

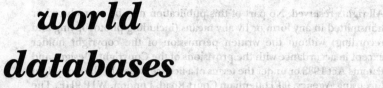

world databases in MEDICINE

volume

② 2

edited by

C. J. ARMSTRONG

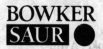

BOWKER SAUR ●

London · Melbourne · Munich · New Jersey

British Library Cataloguing in Publication Data

A catalogue record for this book is available from the British Library

Library of Congress Cataloging-in-Publication Data

A catalog record for this book is available from the Library of Congress

Published by Bowker-Saur
60 Grosvenor Street, London W1X 9DA
Tel: +44 (0)71 493 5841 Fax: +44 (0)71 580 4089

Bowker-Saur is a division of REED REFERENCE PUBLISHING

ISBN 0-86291-613-5

Cover design by John Cole
Phototypesetting by Florencetype Ltd, Kewstoke, Avon
Printed on acid-free paper
Printed and bound in Great Britain by BPCC Wheatons Ltd, Exeter

INTRODUCTION

World Databases in Medicine is the first in a series of directories whose overall aim is to map the databases in twenty-three clearly defined subject disciplines – twenty-three disciplines which encompass all of mankind's knowledge. As its name implies, this directory like the others to follow, is attempting worldwide coverage and includes databases from Australasia, CIS, Europe, Scandinavia and the Far East as well as from UK and North America. *Not* explicit in the name, is the degree of detail which has been built into the directory: not only are the databases described in as much detail as possible but wherever possible, third-party, evaluative and review extracts are included in the descriptions making this unique as an evaluative directory. The *World Databases Series* aims to become the *de facto* authority on electronically published databases with details of content, size, access and pricing as well as expert commentary on the major databases. With so much discussion in the professional press on quality and Total Quality Management, it is incumbent on us to include such qualitative information as is available. *World Databases* seeks to identify those databases in which users and reviewers have the greatest confidence by including extracts from reviews. As review material and critical commentaries are received they are added to the database so that a database commentary archive is gradually being built up and the master database represents a comparative knowledge base covering most of the world's larger databases and database vendors (hosts).

Based on our major database of databases, the directories are the product of extensive desk research. Their aim is to enable location of any database and to make explicit its links with other similar databases: thus if a CD-ROM marketed as **WONDERmed** is in fact a subset of **MEDLINE** this will be clear from the directory where the CD-ROM will appear as a part of the **MEDLINE** family of databases. *World Databases* has taken the database rather than the product as the baseline so that links between various information providers should be explicit; a database or service which is a merged file combining two databases available separately elsewhere will be shown as such.

For each unique database there is a master record which describes in as much detail as possible the database as it is produced by the information provider or publisher; this record contains the most detailed subject and content description possible. Following the master record will be one or more smaller records giving details of each implementation of the database – on the various online hosts, as one or more CD-ROMs, as tapes, as diskettes and so on. On many online hosts databases are broken up into chronological divisions, for instance, 1966–1976, 1977–1986 and 1987–present day, and in these cases each file is given a separate entry/reference in the directory. This complete cluster of records detailing each and every version of a database available we have referred to as a family. Where a database has been available on an online host and subsequently been with-

drawn, this fact will be noted immediately below the master record if the departure is recent. Where a CD-ROM publisher has developed and marketed a CD-ROM which contains subsets of more than one database, this has been given a family of its own. This family will comprise a master record describing the CD-ROM product and a *see* reference pointing users to the details of the constituent databases. In order to give adequate detail, databases which comprise a series of newsletters, journals and trade or industry newsletters (for example, the **PTS Newsletter Database**) have each of their constituent publications listed at the end of the family so that users may locate records for each newsletter. Although a particular newsletter (say, *Medical Scan*) may not be available in its own right as a database, it will have a master record giving the details of the publication itself, such records for online or CD-ROM versions of the newsletter if available (where the newsletter is the complete database) and a reference, 'This database can (also) be found on:' directing users to the compilation databases such as **PTS Newsletter Database** on which the newsletter can be found. On the Mead Data Central **LEXIS** service, each publication is given a separate family.

In all of the directories, the definition of subject matter which is used to determine a database's relevance will be the broadest possible and databases which are deemed to have even slight relevance will be added. While this means that some databases will turn up regularly in many of the directories, it does ensure that searchers will not miss any potentially helpful sources. On the other hand, databases which are truly multi-disciplinary – such as library catalogues – will not feature in each subject directory.

This directory is divided into twenty sections – starting with General Medicine, moving through more specific areas of health care and ending with a section on topics not covered elsewhere. Details of these sections are given below. In an attempt to make the directory easy to use, databases which have relevance to more than one of these divisions within medicine have their families repeated in their entirety in each section. While large, general, all-embracing databases such as **MEDLINE** or **EMBASE** can be found in the first, general section, these frequently also have subsets specific to a particular illness or topic available as separate databases and where this is the case the master record for the parent database is repeated above the subset in its appropriate section. An example of this is Aries System Corporation's **PathLine** which is a subset of **MEDLINE** covering pathology.

Classification areas

The directory is divided into twenty sections which are in turn followed by the addresses of information providers, producers, hosts and CD-ROM publishers and then the indexes. The twenty sections in the body of the directory are as follows.

Section 1 – General medicine

In this section are included the databases which carry a range of records, data or information relevant across the whole spectrum of health care with no specific emphasis. Generally, these databases will not appear in any of the following sections unless a subset of the database particularly relevant to that area is available as a seperate file. In this case the master record will appear followed only by the subset for that area.

Section 2 – Specific illnesses

A number of databases relate specifically to a particular illness or disease and these can be found in this section. Examples are AIDS, cancer, cardiovascular disease, and gastroenterology.

Section 3 – Reproduction/Child care

This section includes databases dealing with the following areas: abortion, adolescent fertility, adolescent pregnancy, ante-natal health care, birth defects, birth rate, contraception, family planning, fertility, gifted children, gynaecology, hormone disorders, human sexuality, infertility, maternity care, neonatal medicine, obstetrics, paediatrics, parenthood, perinatal illness and care, pregnancy, reproduction, sexual dysfunction, sexually-transmitted disease and women's health.

Section 4 – Handicapped/Social medicine

Although much of this section will cover material also to be found in the future directory dealing with the Social Sciences, much has a medical slant. Areas covered include alcohol and drug abuse, autism, child abuse, counselling, the disabled, gifted children, handicapped, hearing and visual impairment, learning disorders, mental retardation, motor disorders, rehabilitation, speech therapy and vocational education.

Section 5 – Gerontology

Covers all areas to do with aging, death, mortality and the old.

Section 6 – Psychiatry

Includes child psychiatry, criminology, developmentally disabled, dyslexia, mental health, mentally handicapped and rehabilitation. Also includes neurology, neurological disorders, neuroscience and neuromuscular disease.

Section 7 – Psychology

Includes child psychology, educational psychology, linguistics, neuropsychology, psychometrics, psychotherapy, psychopharmacology and special education.

Section 8 – Dentistry

Includes dental systems development, oral epidemiology, oral hygiene, periodontal diseases and stomatology.

Section 9 – Nutrition/Dietetics/Food science

The section also includes food additives and food hygiene.

Section 10 – Health and safety

One of the larger sections, Health and safety has considerable potential for overlap with the following Health hazards section and several databases will be found in both; in making a division between the two in order to make access easier, the intention has been to separate general and home-based health care from that associated with external sources and the workplace. Health and safety includes databases covering alternative medicine, ante-natal care, beauty care and cosmetics, community health, family medicine, family welfare, first aid, health, health aids, health services, home health care, hygiene, maternity leave, nursing homes, oral health, parenthood, personal health care, physical fitness, primary health, public health, social medicine, sports medicine and travel medicine.

Section 11 – Health hazards and pollution

Although for comprehensive coverage both this and the previous section should be used, Health hazards and pollution covers databases with material more relevant to external sources; these include: accident prevention, asbestosis, asthma, carcinogens, chemical hazards, dangerous or hazardous chemicals, environmental health, environmental hygiene, fire safety, hazardous materials, hazardous waste, industrial accidents, industrial health and safety, occupational health and safety, occupational hygiene, occupational medicine, occupational therapy, personal injury, pollution, Repetitive Strain Injury, safety education, toxic substances and toxicology.

Section 12 – Genetics

Covers such topics as amino acids, bioengineering, chromosome abnormalities, DNA sequences, enzymology, genetic engineering, genetic intervention, genetic manipulation, genetic research, MRNA, nucleic acids, RNA sequences, viral genetics and viruses.

Section 13 – Ethics

Includes consumer protection, euthanasia, genetic intervention, medical codes, medical malpractice, practice management.

Section 14 – Drugs and pharmacy

This section includes alcohol abuse, alternative medicine, drug abuse, drug consumption, drug therapy, drug treatment, pharmacology, smoking, substance abuse, therapeutic drugs and therapeutic medicine.

Section 15 – Forensic science

The section also covers anatomy, forensic medicine and pathology.

Section 16 – Hospital administration

Includes emergency health care, health education, health care administration, health care costs, health care management, health care marketing, health care services, hospital facilities, hospital hygiene, medical insurance, medical librarianship, medical records, Medicare, nursing homes, patient management, practice management, and public service administration.

Section 17 – Nursing

Including medical social work, paramedicine, surgical nursing and therapy (various).

Section 18 – Medical devices

Includes biomedical engineering, dental equipment, ergonomics, laboratory technology, magnetic resonance imaging, medical equipment, medical textiles, ophthalmic instuments, pharmaceutical products and radiography.

Section 19 – Veterinary medicine

Covers such topics as animal breeding, animal diseases, animal health care products, animal husbandry, ichthyology, regulatory agencies – veterinary medicine, veterinary drugs, veterinary entomology and veterinary mycology.

Section 20 – Other topics

This section includes those databases which are not so broad as to encompass the whole of medicine and health care but which do not fit into one of the above eighteen sections on specific aspects of health care.

Many of the master records have descriptors included; these are chiefly an extention of the descriptive material and, as printed, are not necessarily exhaustive or comprehensive. In some cases where it was felt that the simple subject code used to mark the record for inclusion in a particular section of the directory was sufficient, no additional descriptors were allocated.

Within each section the database families are ordered alphabetically by database name. Because of the enormous variation in database types, media and hosts a further ordering was necessary within each family. Following the master record are the records devoted to the various versions of the database available on online hosts, CD-ROM, diskette, etc; first for the full database and then for subsets (that is, topical subsets or subject files rather than those simply divided by a timespan; these are not treated as subsets if they cover the entire subject span of the database). These records are first ordered by medium and then by the online host or CD-ROM producers. The media are ordered as follows (although, of course, in any database family only a few are likely to be present):

1   Online
2   CD-ROM
3   CD-ROM 8cm
4   Diskette
5   Fixed disk
6   Tape
7   Videotex
8   E-mail
9   CDTV, CD-I, CD-ROM XA, DVI, Videodisc
10 Printout
11 Bernouilli box cartridge

Thus, schematically a full family might have elements or entries such as those shown in Figure 1.

A typical family is shown in Figure 2 (see over). The master record describing the database-as-produced can be seen at the head of the family group followed by a number of host records. At the end of the family are notes indicating where else this database can be found – this points to composite CD-ROMs which carry several individual databases or to databases which contain records sourced from this database – and indicating the names of databases which contribute to this product. In both cases it is possible that the databases referred to may not be found in the same section of the directory.

Indexes

Following the Addresses section are the indexes. As it is thought that the primary access route for users will be subject based, the indexes have been divided into the same twenty sections as the body of the directory so that there are, for example four Section 1 indexes, four Section 2 indexes and so on. All the indexes are brought together at the end of the volume and follow the order of the main sections. Finally there is a master Database Name Index which contains references to databases in all twenty sections. For each of the twenty sections there is a producer index, a host index, a medium index (online, CD-ROM, tape, etc) and a database type (bibliographic, factual, statistical, etc) index.

The indexes refer to item numbers rather than page numbers so that a reference to 2:100 means the

```
Master record
  Full database:
    Online – Hosts (A to Z)
      Host Aaaa
        Database1 – 1966 – 1976
        Database2 – 1977 – 1986
        Database3 – 1987 –
      Host Bbbb
        Complete Database
      •
      •
      Host Zzzz
        Complete Database
        Current Month Database
    CD-ROM – Publishers (A to Z)
      Publisher Cccc
        Database – most recent six years
      Publisher Dddd
        Complete Database
      •
      •
      Publisher Xxxx
        Database – most recent two years
        Complete Database
    Diskette – Publishers (A to Z)
    Videotex – Hosts (A to Z)
  Database subsets
    Online – Hosts (A to Z)
      Host Aaaa
        Database1a – Subject subset archive file
        Database1b – Subject subset current file
      •
      •
      Host Yyyy
        Complete Database Subset
    CD-ROM – Publishers (A to Z)
    CD-ROM 8cm – Publishers (A to Z)
    Tape – Producers (A to Z)
  Links to other databases (either from which
  material is drawn or which contain some or all
  of this database).
```

Figure 1: Schematic representation of a database family

Population File of ESCAP Bibliographic Information System
ESCAP. Population Division

[Master record]

10:1027. Master record

Alternative name(s)	EBIS/POPFILE
Database type	Bibliographic
Number of journals	
Sources	
Start year	1982
Language	English
Coverage	Asia and the Pacific
Number of records	301,000
Update size	—
Update period	Monthly
Thesaurus	POPIN Thesaurus

Keywords

Contraception; Demography; Family Planning; Fertility; Mortality; Population; Regional Studies

Description

A database of citations to Asia-Pacific and worldwide literature on population topics, including demography, family planning, fertility, migration mortality, population policy, programmes and projections.

Available to UN system organisations; also to external users with restrictions. The database is available also as a printout.

Indexing terms are drawn from the *POPIN thesaurus*.

10:1028. Diskette   ESCAP

File name	Population File of ESCAP Bibliographic Information System
Alternative name(s)	EBIS/POPFILE
Format notes	NEC
Software	IRS-4
Start year	1982
Number of records	301,000
Update period	Monthly

10:1029. Tape   ESCAP

File name	Population File of ESCAP Bibliographic Information System
Alternative name(s)	EBIS/POPFILE
Format notes	NEC
Software	IRS-4
Start year	1982
Number of records	301,000
Update period	Monthly

[Factual Information]

Product Alert
Marketing Intelligence Service Ltd

10:1030. Master record

Database type	Textual
Number of journals	1
Sources	
Start year	1988
Language	English
Coverage	USA
Number of records	16,00
Update size	—
Update period	Daily added

Keywords

Beauty Care; Consumer Products; Health Care Products; Marketing Catalogues

[Details of databases (not necessarily in this section) containing this database, or records drawn from it.]

Description

A weekly newslette consumer products introduced in North America. Covers packaged foods and beverages, household products, pet products and health and beauty aids. Includes product description, key ingredients, retail price, packaging information and manufacturer's name and location.

Corresponds to *Product Alert* weekly newsletter. On CORIS, DIALOG and Data-Star, this newsletter is available as part of the PTS Newsletter Database, supplied by Predicast.

This database can be found on:
PTS Newsletter Database

[Database and information provider/publisher]

PRODUCTSCAN
Marketing Intelligence Service Ltd

10:1032. Master record

Database type	Textual
Number of journals	1
Sources	Press releases, Trade journals, Periodicals, Evaluation studies and Consumer reports
Start year	1980
Language	English
Coverage	International, North America, Europe, Scandinavia, South Africa, Australia and New Zealand
Number of records	175,000
Update size	—
Update period	Weekly

Keywords

Beauty Care; Consur Products; Pets

[General description of database]

Description

Descriptions of new consumer products introduced in eighteen markets across the world: North America, Europe, South Africa, Australia and New Zealand. Covers over 170 product categories in food and drink, household products, pet products and health and beauty aids. Gives manufacturer's name and address, description of the product, its packaging, merchandising and positioning, target market and the producer's innovation rating.

Notes

On CORIS, DIALOG and Data-Star, this newsletter is made available as part of the PTS Newsletter Database.

10:1033. Online   Infomart Online News$ource

File name	PRODUCTSCAN
Start year	1980
Number of records	175,000
Update period	Weekly

[Record for first online host]

10:1034. Online   Marketing Intelligence Service Ltd

File name	PTS Newsletter Database
Start year	1980

[Index reference number: 1033rd record in the tenth section]

Figure 2: A typical database family

hundredth record/reference in Section 2. An item is a particular version of a database so that a reference in the Database Name index which will be to a family of databases is given as 2:100 – 2:136.

The rest of the World Databases series

World Databases in Medicine is the first in a series of ten directories covering twenty-three subject areas and encompassing the entire corpus of electronic information in every area of human knowledge and enterprise. The subsequent directories will be:

Business;
Science, Patents, Geography, Geology;
Agriculture and Chemistry;
Humanities and Social Sciences;
Energy, Electronics, Environment and Engineering;
Computing and Library and Information Science;
Government and Law;
Biosciences and Pharmacology; and finally
Leisure, Education and News/Current Affairs.

Where a title includes more than one discipline, these will be treated as separate directories within the single

volume; the subject contents will not be merged.

We hope that you find *World Databases in Medicine* useful and informative.

C J Armstrong
Editor

How to use this directory

The design of the directory is based upon the premise that the majority of use will be subject based – that is, users will be trying to locate databases relevant to Dentistry or Psychology, for example. For these users, it should be sufficient to turn to the relevant section and work through the contents. Users should, however, bear in mind that the first section contains general databases which will also have material of use to them.

The indexes for each section allow the bringing together of databases from the same producer, on the same host, on the same medium or of the same type. This may be useful in locating other databases of interest. Finally, the master index, by showing in which other sections a particular database figures, may highlight other areas worthy of attention.

ACKNOWLEDGEMENTS

The editor and publishers would like to acknowledge the help gained from other directories of databases and CD-ROMs, particularly those published by Cuadra/Gale and TFPL.

Some database records in this directory have been added from *I'M-GUIDE, the Directory of the European* *Electronic Information Services Market*, produced by the European Commission's DG XIII/E, and some as the result of cooperation with the China Cooperative Library and Information Science Linkage Project (CINFOLINK), Canada.

Disclaimer

While the editor and publishers have made every attempt to maintain the very highest levels of detail and accuracy, this is a very fast moving industry and users should be aware that databases, host services and information providers may have changed during the time the directory was at press. We are aware, for instance, that all the compact disc titles published by Compact Cambridge are now being produced, marketed, distributed and supported by SilverPlatter while Cambridge Scientific Abstracts have made a strategic decision to concentrate on database compilation – that is concentrating on the content rather than the distribution of databases. Similarly, the online host, ESA-IRS, has withdrawn some forty databases from its stable having decided to concentrate on those databases which are relevant to technical and scientific information in aerospace and its applications. Although the databases were in fact withdrawn in January 1993, no official announcement was made and ESA-IRS has only made a public announcement recently. Considerable disquiet has been voiced by users at this sudden loss of databases and at least two databases have since been reinstated. Unfortunately the timing of all these changes was such as to make it impossible to make corrections to the body of the directory.

The databases removed from ESA-IRS are as follows (as of June 1993):

- Acid Rain (File 109)
- Artificial Intelligence (File 106)
- BIIPAM (File 71)
- Biobusiness (File 137)
- Business Software (File 89)
- CAD/CAM (File 107)
- Canadiana (File 226)
- Chemical Engineering and Biotechnology Abstracts (File 85)
- Chemical Safety Newsbase (File 90)
- Conference Papars Index (File 36)
- Current Biotechnology Abstracts (File 95)
- Delft Hydro (File 91)
- ENEL (File 60)
- Energyline (File 19)
- Finlandiana (File 227)
- INSPEC Information Science (File 31)
- Intime (File 79)
- International Pharmaceutical Abstracts (File 102)
- ISMEC (File 10)
- Masslit (File 86)
- Merlin Tech (File 65)
- NSA (File 44)
- Robomatix (File 84)
- Siderdoc (File 194)
- Telecom Abstracts (File 108)
- Telegen (File 49)
- Training ABI/Inform (File 113)
- Training BIOSIS (File 209)
- Training CAB (File 112)
- Training Chemabs (File 38)
- Training Compendex (File 81)
- Training Metadex (File 189)
- Training Pascal (File 37)
- Ulrich Periodicals (File 103) and
- VITIS/FSTA (File 133)

With Pergamon Financial Data Service's (PFDS) demise in 1992, DIALOG's acquisition of Data-Star and CompuServe's acquisition of DIALOG's Knowledge Index service, it is obvious that changes are afoot in the information industry. I am certainly not the only observer to be concerned by what seems to be a near-monopoly situation in the generalist online database sector – generalist, that is, as opposed to hosts specialising in patents, marketing or company information, for example. Although all of the hosts concerned profess to having the needs of their users very much at heart, it is difficult not to worry when databases accessible only on a single host are unceremoniously removed and, on the other side of the world, a single company is responsible for nearly 700 databases – many of these not available online elsewhere.

While every care is taken, neither the publishers nor the printers can admit liability for any loss incurred through misprint or other circumstances.

CONTENTS

GENETICS

Abstracts in BioCommerce
BioCommerce Data Ltd

12:1. Master record

Alternative name(s)	BioCommerce Abstracts and Directory
Database type	Bibliographic, Directory
Number of journals	100+
Sources	Journals, Newsletters, Newspapers and Trade journals
Start year	1981
Language	English
Coverage	UK (primarily), USA (primarily) and International (some)
Number of records	180,000+
Update size	—
Update period	Every two weeks
Index unit	Articles
Database aids	Major Journals Abstracted for ABC, Slough, BioCommerce Data Ltd., quarterly

Keywords
Immunology

Description

This database indexes and abstracts news items concerned with the business aspects of biotechnology and the commercial applications of biological sciences. The database covers the biotechnologies of: biological control, biotransformation, cell hybridisation, DNA probes, fermentation, genetic engineering, immuno-diagnostics, industrial enzymes, monoclonal antibodies, protein engineering, recombinant DNA, tissue culture and the commercial aspects of: biochemistry, genetics, immunology, microbiology, molecular biology and their applications in: agriculture, animal production, brewing, chemical manufacture, crop protection, diagnostic tests, energy production, food technology, health care, horticulture, medicine, pesticides, veterinary sciences and waste treatment. The database provides up-to-date abstracts (55,000+ abstracts referencing over 250,000 articles and 1,700+ directory entries with multiple citations of source journals to prevent duplication of facts, and each record is fully indexed under the organisations mentioned in each article. Other subjects covered by the database include: industry news, reports of corporate financial developments, research and development projects, personnel changes and relevant legislation. The database can be used for competitor monitoring, business planning, investment analysis, identifying product licensing opportunities, science and policy studies and monitoring legislation and case law. The database also contains directory-style company profile records on many of the organisations mentioned in the abstracted articles containing addresses, contact names and profiles of their activities. Sources include more than 100 trade publicatins, newsletters and newspapers.

The database corresponds to *Abstracts in BioCommerce (ABC)* – print and online, and *UK Biotechnology Handbook*, with additional data available online.

Articles sourced in *Abstracts in BioCommerce* are taken from over 100 English language specialist and popular media sources, mainly published in the USA and United Kingdom. Each abstract may cite several sources where the articles contain substantially the same information and typically, at least three sources are given. Directory entries are copiled from questionnaires, updated from abstracted articles and verified regularly.

12:2. Online   Data-Star

File name	CELL
Alternative name(s)	BioCommerce Abstracts and Directory
Start year	1981
Number of records	55,000+ abstracts referencing over 250,000 articles and 1,700+ directory entries
Update period	Twice monthly
Database aids	Data-Star Business Manual and Data-Star Online Manual (search for NEWS-CELL in NEWS)
Price/Charges	Subscription: SFr80.00
	Connect time: SFr179.20
	Online print: SFr0.00–1.33
	Offline print: SFr0.26–1.28
	SDI charge: SFr6.80

Downloading is allowed

Notes

To search for specific bibliographic documents the search terms should be qualified by using the data field Source (SO). To search for directory documents use the quick code AT=P. To search for bibliographic documents use the quick code AT=A. For bibliographic documents there are six different abstract types currently available in CELL: 1. Company information, 2. Institution information, 3. National and International information, 4. (Not used in Data-Star), 5. Peripheral information not in hardcopy ABC, 6. Diagnostics information not in hardcopy ABC, 7. Review articles.

From June 1993 Data-Star have introduced an annual fee/subscription per contract (that is, not per password) of SFr 80.00 (c.UK£ 32.00) payable every June. For North American customers billed in dollars who also use DIALOG, the DIALOG fee also covers access to Data-Star. Academic customers, 'commitment' customers and customers currently billed in dollars are exempt.

Record composition

Abstract text (Bibliographic documents only) AB; Accession number and update code AN; Address AD; Alternative name AL; Business area descriptors DE; Company name and code CO; Company name CX; Country CN; Document type AT; Entry date ED; Location LO; Management MM; Organisation type OT; Note NT; Profile text (Directory documents only) TX; Source SO; Street ST; Telephone, telex, fax TL; Update code UP and Year YR

12:3. Online   DIALOG

File name   File 286
Alternative name(s)   BioCommerce Abstracts and
                         Directory
Start year   1981
Number of records   76,000+ abstracts referencing
                         300,000 articles and 1,900+
                         directory entries
Update period   Twice a month
Price/Charges   Connect time: US$105.00
                         Online print: US$0.70
                         Offline print: US$0.70
                         SDI charge: US$6.95

Downloading is allowed

Notes

DIALOG also provides profiles of over 1,000 organisations involved in biotechnology.

12:4. Diskette   BioCommerce Data Ltd

File name
Alternative name(s)   BioCommerce Abstracts and
                         Directory
Start year   1981
Number of records   130,000+
Update period   Every two weeks
Price/Charges   Subscription: UK£780

Aneuploidy
Oak Ridge National Laboratory, Environmental Teratology Information Centre

12:5. Master record

Database type   Bibliographic
Number of journals
Sources   Journals
Start year   1970
Language   English
Coverage   International
Number of records   3,600
Update size   —
Update period   Semiannually

Keywords

Aneuploidy; Chromosome Abnormalities

Description

Contains citations to literature on research in aneuploidy (numerical chromosome abnormalities) in humans and experimental systems. Citations are classified into one of the following groups:

(1) population studies covering spontaneous incidence of aneuploidy in human populations;

(2) screening studies covering the testing of chemicals or physical agents for the induction of aneuploidy; and

(3) general studies that do not fit into the other categories.

Only available as part of TOXLINE.

This database can be found on:
PolTox I: NLM, CSA, IFIS
TOXLINE
TOXLINE Plus

Applied Genetics News
Business Communications Company (BCC)

12:8. Master record

Database type   Textual
Number of journals   1
Sources   Newsletter
Start year   1989
Language   English
Coverage   International
Number of records
Update size   —
Update period   Daily

Keywords

Biotechnology; Genetic Engineering; Patents

Description

Contains the full text of the monthly newsletter *Applied Genetics News*. Monitors the business and technology of biotechnology, with information on individuals, companies, new products and technology, patents, contracts, research and field testing in areas such as agriculture, health care, chemicals and waste treatment.

Correspond to *Applied Genetics News* monthly. On CORIS, DIALOG and Data-Star this database is available as part of the PTS Newsletter Database, supplied by Predicast.

12:9. Online   NewsNet Inc

File name
Start year   1989
Number of records
Update period   Daily

This database can also be found on:
PTS Newsletter Database

BioBusiness
BIOSIS

12:11. Master record

Database type   Bibliographic
Number of journals   500
Sources   Conference proceedings, journals,
                         monographs, newsletters, research
                         reports and patents (US)
Start year   1985
Language   English
Coverage   International
Number of records   480,000
Update size   42,000
Update period   Monthly
Database aids   BioBusiness Search Guide,
                         Philadelphia, BIOSIS, How to
                         search BioBusiness,Philadelphia,
                         BIOSIS and Newsletters:
                         BioSearch, BioScene.

Keywords

Cosmetics; Fishing; Forestry; Genetic Engineering; Immunology

Description

BioBusiness is a bibliographic database which focuses specifically on the business applications of biomedical research. It contains citations, with abstracts, to the worldwide periodical literature on business applications of biological and biomedical research. Subjects covered include: agriculture and forestry, animal production, biomass conversion, crop production, diet and nutrition, fermentation, food technology, cosmetics, genetic engineering, health care, industrial microbiology, pharmaceutical products, medical technology, medical diagnostics, medical instrumentation, occupational health, pesticides, pharmaceuticals, protein production, toxicology, veterinary science, waste treatment, energy and the environment, and other industries affected by biotechnological developments. Also covers patents in such areas as immunological testing, food processes, and fishing. For each patent record, includes inventor's name and address, patent title and number, patent classes, date granted, and assignee. BioBusiness can be used to discover: the latest legislation and regulatory controls affecting implementation of biotechnology research; the impact of economic fluctuations on price and production forecasts for agricultural commodities; the financial effects of recycling programs on business; the increased use of natural ingredients in cosmetic and personal care products; the applications of bioengineering in pharmaceuticals; trends in the development and marketing of food products; etc.

A broad spectrum of life science, business and management journals are scanned. Abstracts are included for approximately 55–60% of the records.

Both controlled and uncontrolled terms are used for indexing. The concept codes used are different from the BIOSIS concept codes.

12:12. Online — BIOSIS Life Science Network

File name	
Start year	1985
Number of records	480,000
Update period	Monthly
Price/Charges	Connect time: US$9.00
	Online print: US$6.00 per 10; 2.25 per abstract; 3.50 per full text article

Downloading is allowed
Also available via the Internet by telnetting to LSN.COM.

Notes

On Life Science Network users can search this database or they can scan a group of subject-related databases. There is a charge of $2.00 per scan of subject-related databases. To search one database and display up to ten citations costs $6.00. Most charges are for information retrieved. There are no charges if there are no results and no charge to transfer results to a printer or diskette. Articles may also be ordered via an online document delivery request. A telecommunications software package is also available, costing $12.95, providing an automatic connection to Life Science Network for heavy users of the service, with capability to transfer to print or disk and customised colour options.

12:13. Online — BRS

File name	BBUS
Start year	1985
Number of records	480,000
Update period	Weekly

Price/Charges	Connect time: UK£88.00/98.00
	Online print: UK£0.46/0.54
	Offline print: UK£0.52
Downloading is allowed	

12:14. Online — CISTI, Canadian Online Enquiry Service CAN/OLE

File name	
Start year	1985
Number of records	480,000
Update period	Monthly
Downloading is allowed	

12:15. Online — Data-Star

File name	BBUS
Start year	1985
Number of records	277,972
Update period	Weekly
Database aids	Data-Star Business Manual and Online manual (search NEWS-BBUS in NEWS)
Price/Charges	Subscription: UK£32.00
	Connect time: UK£63.60
	Online print: UK£0.41
	Offline print: UK£0.36
	SDI charge: UK£3.94

Downloading is allowed

Notes

From June 1993 Data-Star have introduced an annual fee/subscription per contract (that is, not per password) of SFr 80.00 (c.UK£ 32.00) payable every June. For North American customers billed in dollars who also use DIALOG, the DIALOG fee also covers access to Data-Star. Academic customers, 'commitment' customers and customers currently billed in dollars are exempt.

Record composition

Abstract AB; Accession Number and Update Code AN; Author AU; Author Affliation IN; Company Name CO; Concept Codes CC; Descriptors DE; Language of Article LG; Named Person(s) NA; Publication Details PU; Source SO; Title TI; Update Codes UP and Year of Publication YR

12:16. Online — DIALOG

File name	File 285
Start year	1985
Number of records	371,575
Update period	Weekly
Price/Charges	Connect time: US$126.00
	Online print: US$0.85
	Offline print: US$0.85
	SDI charge: US$10.50

Downloading is allowed

Notes

DIALINDEX Categories: AGRIBUS, BIOBUS, BIOTECH, PHARMINA.

12:17. Online — ESA-IRS

File name	File 137
Start year	1985
Number of records	372,000 (October 1991)
Update period	Weekly
Price/Charges	Subscription: UK£70.29
	Database entry fee: UK£3.49
	Online print: UK£0.74
	Offline print: UK£0.79
	SDI charge: UK£3.49

Downloading is allowed

Notes

The default supplier of original document is British Library Documentation Supply Centre.

From 1993 ESA-IRS are charging an annual fee of 100 Accounting Units (c.UK£ 70.29) to all users. This is equivalent to the fee for full documentation and will not be charged to customers already paying for documentation.

Record composition

Abstract /AB; Additional Source Information NT; Author AU; Concept Code CC; Concept Code Name CN; Corporate Source CS; ISBN BN; Journal Name JN; Language LA; Named Company NM; Named Person SP; Native Number NN; Patent Assignee PH; Patent Number PN; Publication Year PY; Subfile (1) SF; Title /TI; Uncontrolled Terms /UT and US Patent Classification PC

12:18. Online   STN

File name	BIOBUS
Start year	1985
Number of records	480,000
Update period	Weekly
Downloading is allowed	

12:19. Tape   BIOSIS

File name	
Format notes	9-track, 800, 1600 or 6250 bpi, variable length records, variable block size.
Start year	1985
Number of records	480,000
Update period	Monthly

Notes

Corresponds to the BioBusiness online database. Annual lease price is $2,350 plus additional usage charges; contact BIOSIS for archival tape prices.

BIOCAS
BIOSIS
Chemical Abstracts Service

12:20. Master record

Alternative name(s)	BIOSIS/CAS Registry Number Concordance
Database type	Directory
Number of journals	
Sources	
Start year	1969–1985
Language	English
Coverage	International
Number of records	1.2 million
Update size	—
Update period	Quarterly

Keywords

Animal Sciences; Bioengineering; Biophysics; Fishing; Immunology; Patents; Plant Sciences

Description

Contains references to citations common to both CA Search and BIOSIS Previews. Each record currently includes the BIOSIS Document Number, the equivalent CA Search Abstract Number and, for approximately 78 percent of the references, CAS Registry

Numbers (see Registry Nomenclature and Structure Service). In subsequent updates, CAS Registry Numbers will be available for the remaining BIOSIS citations.

12:21. Online   STN

File name	BIOCAS
Alternative name(s)	BIOSIS/CAS Registry Number Concordance
Start year	
Number of records	
Update period	

Biochemistry and Biophysics Citation Index
Institute for Scientific Information

12:22. Master record

Database type	Bibliographic, Citation
Number of journals	7,250
Sources	
Start year	
Language	English
Coverage	International
Number of records	100,000
Update size	100,000
Update period	Six times per year

Keywords

Biochemistry; Biophysics

Description

Abstracted citation index, with abstracts, offering complete coverage of significant published literature in biochemistry or biophysics. Covers an estimated 90,000 to 100,000 articles and proceedings per year. Includes full coverage of over 250 journals, with every significant item in these journals included (letters, notes, editorials, corrections, reviews). In addition to the over 250 journals related to the topics of biochemistry and biophysics, selected relevant articles from another 7,000 journals from the entire ISI database are included. The primary advantages in this repackaging are the abstracts included in all records and the greater precision in subject searching. The disc offers full bibliographic information, abstracts and cited references.

All ISI databases have a linked service known as The Genuine Article which can deliver the full text of located articles by mail, facsimile transmission or courier. Orders can be placed via the host service in use, mail, facsimile transmission, telephone or telex. Diskette products have a single-keystroke order information facility.

The minimum charge is US$ 11.25 within USA and Canada and US$ 12.20 elsewhere.

12:23. CD-ROM   Institute for Scientific Information

File name	Biochemistry and Biophysics Citation Index
Format notes	IBM, Mac, NEC
Start year	
Number of records	
Update period	Six times per year
Price/Charges	Subscription: US$1,950

Notes

A particular feature of the CD-ROM is ISI's unique Related Records search facility which provides access to records with cited references in common, allowing documents on similar subjects to be easily retrieved and browsed.

Each issue is a year-to-date cumulation ending with the final annual cumulation. Back years are available to 1991.

Bioethicsline

Kennedy Institute of Ethics,
Georgetown University
National Library of Medicine

12:24. Master record

Database type	Bibliographic
Number of journals	2,000
Sources	A-V material, Grey literature, Journals, Laws/regulations, Legal papers, Newspapers and Monographs
Start year	1973
Language	English
Coverage	International, English-speaking countries especially USA (primarily) and International
Number of records	35,000
Update size	2,400
Update period	Every two months
Index unit	Articles (selected) and Book chapters
Abstract details	Database producer
Thesaurus	Bioethics Thesaurus – devised by Kennedy Institute of Ethics, new editions annually; Medical Subject Headings (MeSH)

Keywords

Philosophy; Abortion; HIV; Euthanasia; Genetic Intervention

Description

Bioethicsline is a cross-disciplinary database containing references to documents which deal with ethical, legal and public policy issues of medicine, health care and biomedical research. It contains citations to the literature on abortion; AIDS; euthanasia; genetic intervention; human and animal experimentation; medical confidentiality; new reproductive technologies; surrogate motherhood; organ tissue donation and transplantation; patients' rights; in-vitro fertilization; professional ethics; resource allocation in health care; torture. Covers literature of many disciplines including religion, law, behavioural science and philosophy.

Corresponds to the annual *Bibliography of Bioethics*. About fifty of the ninety journals covered are also indexed in MEDLINE. Abstracts have been added to about twenty per cent of records from fifteen Core Journals since 1982 and from court decisions since 1984. Contains information mainly from English speaking countries, especially the USA. Relevant citations from Catline, Popline and MEDLINE are transferred to Bioethicsline; the overlap between Bioethicsline and MEDLINE is approximately fifty per cent. Unlike NLM databases, multiword source names are not abbreviated. Relevant articles have been drawn from 65 indexes, more than seventy journals and newspapers, four online databases and selected other tools. Journals represent sixty-eight per cent of all citations; monographs and book chapters nineteen per cent; newspapers seven per cent; court decisions five per cent and unpublished documents/audiovisual material two per cent.

The Kennedy Institute of Ethics developed its own thesaurus with approximately 600 descriptors; about eighty per cent of which are identical to *MeSH* descriptors. Documents are indexed with both vocabularies. Following the application of Index Terms, *MeSH* descriptors (CT) are added automatically so that there is a double indexing using the two vocabularies. No *MeSH* Supplemental Chemical Records, Gene Symbols or Qualifiers are used. From December 1982, one of thirteen section codes have been added to each record as a coarse classification. The section codes are: BE – Bioethics and professional ethics; BR – Biomedical and behavioral research; CL – Clinical approach; DE – Death, euthanasia and the prolongation of life; GR – Genetics, reproduction and abortion; HP – Health care and health care policy; LE – Legal approach; MH – Mental health therapies and behavior control; PH – Philosophical approach; PO – Popular approach; PP – Professional patient relationship; RE – Religious approach; and XX – Miscellaneous.

12:25. Online
BLAISE-LINK

File name	BIOETHICS
Start year	1973
Number of records	
Update period	Quarterly

12:26. Online
CISTI MEDLARS

File name	Bioethicsline
Start year	1973
Number of records	35,000
Update period	Twice per month

12:27. Online
Data-Star

File name	ETHI
Start year	1973
Number of records	34,000
Update period	Every two months
Database aids	Biomedical Manual and Online Guide (search NEWS-ETHI in NEWS)

Downloading is allowed
Thesaurus is online

Notes

The command 'AB=AB' will locate documents which contain abstracts. Publication types (JOURNAL.PT.) are: Analytic; Audiovisual-material; Bill; Court-decision; Journal-article; Law; Monograph; Newspaper-article; and Unpublished-document. Index month (IM>9210) can be used to locate documents added recently.

From June 1993 Data-Star have introduced an annual fee/subscription per contract (that is, not per password) of SFr 80.00 (c.UK£ 32.00) payable every June. For North American customers billed in dollars who also use DIALOG, the DIALOG fee also covers access to Data-Star. Academic customers, 'commitment' customers and customers currently billed in dollars are exempt.

Record composition

Accession Number AN; Author AU; Title TI; Source SO; Language LG; Publication Type PT; Descriptors (MeSH) DE; Keywords (Bioethics Thesaurus) KW; Subject Captions SC; Abstract AB; Publication Year

YR; Index Month IM; Corporate Name CN and General Notes NT

Keywords (.KW.) are controlled vocabulary terms taken from the Bioethics Thesaurus: multiword terms are double posted and searchable hyphenated or as a word fragment, thus STERILIZATION.KW. and INVOLUNTARY-STERILIZATION.KW. will both work. MeSH descriptors (.DE.) are also double posted: EUTHANASIA.DE. retrieves both EUTHANASIA and EUTHANASIA as a MeSH fragment of EUTHANASIA-PASSIVE. The command '.MESH term' will display the thesaurus terms.

12:28. Online   DIMDI

File name	BE73
Software	GRIPS
Start year	1973
Number of records	34,300
Update period	Every two months
SDI period	Bimonthly
Database aids	Memocard
Price/Charges	Connect time: UK£5.84–10.58
	Online print: UK£0.17–0.35
	Offline print: UK£0.09–0.15

Downloading is allowed
Thesaurus is online

Notes

The overlap between Bioethicsline and MEDLINE is approximately fifty per cent, however, citations originating in MEDLINE are not marked as in Aidsline, Health or Cancerlit. Document supply is from the British Library Document Supply Centre, Boston Spa, England; Harkers Information Retrieval System, Sydney, Australia; Intituto de Informacion y Documentacion en Ciencia y Tecnologia, Madrid, Spain and Zentralbibliotehk der Medizin, Köln, Germany.

Record composition

Abstract AB; Abstract Source AS (Display only); Author AU; Book Title BTI; Classification Code CC; Corporate Source CS; Controlled Term CT; Document Type DT; Entry Date ED (Find only); Entry Month EM (Display only); Freetext (Basic Index) FT; Index Term IT; Journal Title JT; Language LA; Number of Document ND; Notes NO (Display only); Publication Place PL; Publisher PU (Display only); Publication Year PY; Number of References RN (Display only); ISBN SB; Section Code SC; Series Title SE; Source SO (Display only); ISSN SS; Title TI and Uncontrolled Terms UT

Bioethics Thesaurus descriptors are hierarchically arranged to three levels in the printed version of the thesaurus only. Index terms covering the main aspect of the document are weighted in the same way as MeSH terms (shown by '*' in the record). Uncontrolled Terms contain uncontrolled nouns, personal/corporate names, geographics etc that previously were part of the datafield Index Terms (IT). With the retrospective introduction of Uncontrolled Terms, the Index Terms at DIMDI now only contain the approximately 600 descriptors of the *Bioethics Thesaurus* and other descriptors, proposed for a later integration into the *Bioethics Thesaurus*. Uncontrolled Terms are, like Index Terms, directly and freetext searcheable.

12:29. Online   National Library of Medicine

File name	Bioethicsline
Start year	
Number of records	
Update period	

12:30. Online   Questel

File name	BIOETHICS
Start year	1973
Number of records	33,000
Update period	

12:31. CD-ROM   SilverPlatter

File name	Bioethicsline
Format notes	IBM
Software	SPIRS
Start year	1973
Number of records	35,000
Update period	Every two months
Price/Charges	
Downloading is allowed	

12:32. Videotex   Minitel
                                               Questel
                                               INSERM

File name	BIOETHICS 36290036
Start year	1973
Number of records	33,000
Update period	
Database aids	User Guide

Notes

Accessible via Minitel at either direct dial (kiosk) or subscription rates. Menu-guided searching in either French or English allow five choices of access: French keywords, English keywords, English title or abstract terms, author or journal name. Citations can be displayed or printed with or without abstracts and offline prints as well as photocopies of the original article may be ordered. Direct dial access requires no subscription and no password and charging is for connect time only with a maximum of fifteen citations sent free of charge. Subscription charging requires a password and an identity code and has three charging parameters: connection time, citations displayed and citations sent by post.

For more details of constituent databases, see:
MEDLINE
Popline
CATLINE

This database can also be found on:
AIDSLINE

BIOLIS
Informationzentrum für Biologie am Forschungsinstitut Senckenberg

12:35. Master record

Alternative name(s)	Biologische Literaturinformation Senckenberg
Database type	Bibliographic
Number of journals	
Sources	Periodicals and serials
Start year	1970
Language	German and English
Coverage	Germany, Switzerland and Austria
Number of records	53,3532,214
Update size	6,000
Update period	Every two months
Index unit	Articles

Keywords

Animal Sciences; Bioengineering; Biophysics; Fishing; Immunology; Patents; Plant Sciences

Description

BIOLIS is a bilingual (German/English) database in the field of biology. It is intended as a supplement to the American database BIOSIS PREVIEWS. Subjects covered include: biology; botany; zoology; ecology; environmental protection and paleontology. Each record contains details of authors, title and other bibliographic data as well as free key words and the codes and terms of the BIOSIS classification system.

Sources are publications in the Federal Republic of Germany, Switzerland or Austria which are not listed in BIOSIS PREVIEWS.

Articles from serials and periodicals which are published in the Federal Republic of Germany, Switzerland and Austria.

12:36. Online   DIMDI

File name	BS70
Alternative name(s)	Biologische Literaturinformation Senckenberg
Start year	1970
Number of records	53,353
Update period	Every two months
SDI period	2 months
Price/Charges	Connect time: UK£10.55–13.39
	Online print: UK£0.30–0.48
	Offline print: UK£0.23–0.30

Downloading is allowed

Notes

Suppliers of online documents: British Library Document Supply Centre, Boston Spa, England; Harkers Information Retrieval System, Sydney, Australia.

The unit record contains information about author(s), title, and other bibliographic data as well as free key words and the codes and terms of the BIOSIS classification system. At present there are no abstracts. Searches are possible from January 1970. The English biosystematic names in BIOLIS are associated to the Latin biosystematic names in BIOSIS Previews. BIOLIS is the only database into which Latin biosystematic names have been introduced.

Biological and Agricultural Index
HW Wilson Company

12:37. Master record

Alternative name(s)	BAI; Wilson Biological and Agricultural Index
Database type	Bibliographic
Number of journals	200+
Sources	Journals
Start year	1983 (July)
Language	English
Coverage	International
Number of records	184,000
Update size	54,000
Update period	Twice per week
Index unit	Articles, Book reviews, Symposia, Conference papers and Letters to the editor (selected)

Keywords

Plant Sciences; Physiology; Horticulture; Forestry; Animal Sciences; Agricultural Economics; Agrochemicals; Agricultural Engineering

Description

Indexing of 226 key periodicals in the life sciences; A separate index of current book reviews. The major areas covered include: Agriculture; Agricultural chemistry, economics, engineering and research; Animal husbandry; Biochemistry; Biology; Botany; Cytology; Ecology; Entomology; Environmental sciences; Food science; Forestry; Genetics; Horticulture; Marine biology and limnology; Microbiology; Nutrition; Physiology; Plant pathology; Soil science; Veterinary medicine; Zoology.

Corresponds to *Biological & Agricultural Index.*

English-language periodicals on biology and agriculture.

Articles indexed under specific, accessible subject headings in a single alphabet; Extensive cross referencing; Title enhancement for titles with ambiguous titles; Complete bibliographic data on each article indexed.

12:38. Online   OCLC EPIC; OCLC FirstSearch

File name	
Alternative name(s)	BAI
Start year	
Number of records	
Update period	

12:39. Online   WilsonLine

File name	
Alternative name(s)	BAI; Wilson Biological and Agricultural Index
Start year	1983 (July)
Number of records	
Update period	Twice per week

12:40. CD-ROM   Wilsondisc

File name	
Alternative name(s)	BAI; Wilson Biological and Agricultural Index
Format notes	IBM
Software	WilsonDisc
Start year	1983 (July)
Number of records	
Update period	Quarterly
Price/Charges	Subscription: US$1,495

Notes

Subscription fee includes unlimited online access to BAI file through WilsonLine.

Biosis Previews Vocabulary
BIOSIS

12:41. Master record

Database type	Factual, Directory, Thesaurus
Number of journals	
Sources	
Start year	
Language	English
Coverage	
Number of records	
Update size	—
Update period	Irregular

Keywords

Immunology; Fishing; Animal Sciences; Plant Sciences; Bioengineering; Biophysics; Patents

Description

Contains the meaning of the numeric code in natural language.

Corresponds to the *Alphabetic Directory of Concept Headings*.

12:42. Online   Data-Star

File name	BVOC
Start year	
Number of records	
Update period	
Price/Charges	Subscription: SFr80.00
	Connect time: SFr147.00
	Online print: SFr0.00
	Offline print: SFr0.83

Notes

From June 1993 Data-Star have introduced an annual fee/subscription per contract (that is, not per password) of SFr 80.00 (c.UK£ 32.00) payable every June. For North American customers billed in dollars who also use DIALOG, the DIALOG fee also covers access to Data-Star. Academic customers, 'commitment' customers and customers currently billed in dollars are exempt.

BIOSIS Previews
BIOSIS

12:43. Master record

Alternative name(s)	Biological Abstracts
Database type	Bibliographic
Number of journals	9,300
Sources	Bibliographies, conference proceedings, government documents, journals, letters, meeting abstracts, monographs, notes, patents, reviews, reports, research communications, symposia and theses
Start year	1969
Language	English
Coverage	International
Number of records	7,826,768
Update size	535,000
Update period	Weekly
Index unit	Articles, book chapters, letters, meeting abstracts, reports and reviews
Database aids	BIOSIS Previews Search Guide, BIOSCENE BIOSEARCH, BIOSIS Previews Search Guide Master Index and Discovering BIOSIS Previews: An Interactive Disk (IBM-compatible CAL software US$ 45.00)

Keywords

Animal Sciences; Bioengineering; Biophysics; Fishing; Immunology; Patents; Plant Sciences

Description

BIOSIS Previews, the world's largest English language indexing and abstracting service for biology and biomedicine, contains citations, with abstracts, to the worldwide literature on research in the life sciences: microbiology; plant and animal science; experimental medicine; agriculture; pharmacology; ecology; biochemistry; bioengineering; biophysics; including the basic biological disciplines of zoology, genetics, botany; related interdisciplinary fields including food science, veterinary medicine and research medicine, and associated areas of life sciences such as instrumentation.

It covers original research reports, reviews of original research, history and philosophy of biology and biomedicine, and documentation and retrieval of biological information, including references to accounts of field, laboratory, clinical, experimental and theoretical work. The database presents research findings and literature references on all living things and emphasizes their identification (taxonomy), their life processes, environments and applications. From 1986 to 1989 the database covers selective US patents in such areas as immunological testing, food processes, and fishing. For each patent record, the database includes the inventor's name and address, patent title and number, patent classes, date granted, and assignee.

The database corresponds in coverage to *Biological Abstracts (BA)* (1969+) and *Biological Abstracts/RRM (Reports, Reviews, Meetings) (BA/RRM)* (1980+) and *BioResearch Index (BioI)*, the major publications of BIOSIS (BA/RRM is the successor to BioI beginning in 1980). *Biological Abstracts* includes approximately 275,000 accounts of original research yearly and *Biological Abstracts/RRM* includes 260,000 citations yearly. As to the origin or sources, approximately fifty per cent of the items in the database originate from Europe and Middle East, twenty six per cent from North America, fifteen per cent from Asia and Australia, six per cent from Central and South America and three per cent from Africa. Approximately forty-five per cent of database records relate to non-journal literature which means that of the leading bioscience databases, BIOSIS offers the most extensive coverage of this type of literature, EMBASE and MEDLINE both having ceased coverage of non-journal literature in 1980 and 1981 respectively. The references to non-journal literature do not contain abstracts but title keywords augmented by natural language descriptors provide access to scientific communications not found in many other life science databases. Approximately eighty-six per cent of records contain citations to English language sources. This compares to seventy five per cent in EMBASE, seventy-four per cent in MEDLINE and eighty-eight per cent in SciSearch. In addition fifty-four per cent of records contain abstracts (from 1986 onwards). This compares with sixty-five per cent of records in MEDLINE and sixty per cent in EMBASE. The other leading bioscience database, SciSearch, now does contain abstracts. In BIOSIS sixty-seven per cent of records with non-English sources contain English-language abstracts online. This compares with thirty- seven per cent on EMBASE and twenty six per cent on MEDLINE (since 1980). In the UK, the Royal Society of Chemistry operates an SDI service against the tapes of the latest two weeks of BIOSIS and Chemical Abstracts under the name of BIOSCAN. Results are mailed on diskette ready for use with most PC-based searching packages. Printed output is also available. Abstracts from July 1976 to date (from BA on Tape) are available online through BRS, Data-Star, DIALOG, DIMDI, ESA-IRS, and STN International. Abstracts from 1982 to date are available through CISTI.

Most BIOSIS PREVIEWS descriptors are natural language terms added by editors to enrich or claify information provided in titles, identifying such factors as: specific scientific or common names or organisms discussed in a source if not included in the citationtitle; virus names; organ systems or tissues used or affected; diseases discussed; geographic location, if pertinent and instrumentation, apparatus methodology. Three data elements are indexed: Keywords, Cross Codes and Biosystematic Codes. The free-text file comprises two data fields: title and added keywords or uncontrolled terms. The added keywords are a data element of indexing whereas the title is a bibliographic data element and is taken from the original publication. The following categories of keywords are added to explain or supplement the title: Descriptors describing the type of the work, for example, Review, Book, Letter, Abstract; Organisms; Virus-affiliation terms; organs, tracts, tissues; geographic terms; drugs and their affiliation terms; chemical substances and their affiliation terms; enzymes; instrumentation, apparatus, methods; diseases; topics and purposes of a publication. Organisms: each organism is indexed twice – by a keyword and by a Biosystematic code. Categories of keywords used for organism-related concepts include scientific and/or colloquial names, depending on how they appear in the article; abbreviations which characterise the taxonomical classification of an organism (for example SP for species, VAR for variety); pathogenic organisms as causes of diseases and keywords characterising the sex and/or age groups for human beings and animals. Drugs and their affiliation terms: the name of a drug is taken from the publication in the form in which it is given, that is as a commercial or generic name. For each drug mentioned in the title or in the added keywords one or more drug affiliation terms are indexed. Chemical substances and their affiliation terms: for every chemical substance mentioned in the title or added to the title as a keyword, BIOSIS indexes an affiliation term if the effect of the substance is described in the article (herbicide, insecticide). Enzymes: are only indexed with their Enzyme Commission Number (EC) when the EC-number is mentioned in the article. Spelling: prior to 1985 BIOSIS used word segmentation for some biological, anatomical, chemical and enzyme terms in title and added descriptors. This segmentation was dropped from January 1985 to standardise spelling in the freetext sections. Hyphenated words: in the title and added keywords field the words which form a logical unit are linked by a hypen. This spelling is not used in the abstract. Concept Headings: there are more than 500 concept headings used to index according to broader concepts. These are hierarchically ordered with the section names in the hierarchy corresponding to the section headings in the printed issues. The Concept Headings are weighted into three categories according to the emphasis of an aspect of an article: primary level for the main aspect of an article, secondary level for important aspects and tertiary level for incidental aspects.

The availability of weighted indexing is useful as it provides a method for reducing output while maintainin high precision. Biosystematic Codes are also used to denote concept terms and groups of organisms which removes the need to list individually all the items and their synonyms within a group and automatically produces a context of further, more specific queries within that category. Strategy Recommendations (See References) are also given as part of the scope notes on concept codes, providing pointers towards other areas of possibly fruitful examination. The Biosystematic Codes group organisms by accepted taxonomic rules which make it possible to search references to large taxonomic groupings. New Biosystematic Codes for bacteria, based primarily on Bergey's *Manual of Systematic Bacteriology*, were effective from the first update of 1992. 140 new Biosystematic Codes (BCs) for bacteria replaced the 81 codes in use up to the end of 1991. To avoid incorrect use the names of the respective BCs have been supplemented with the years of their validity, for example BS:RHODOSPIRILLACEAE (1979–91). As there was a comparable change with viruses in 1979 respective in 1981, these BCs have been supplemented in the same way, for example BS: COMOVIRUS (1979–). The group known as the blue-green algae or Cyanophyta or Cyanobacteria, indexed till the end of 1991 as algae (BS: CYANOPHYTA, BC : 13900) will now be indexed as bacteria (BS: CYANOBACTERIA (1992–), BC: 09200). Entering the new text version of Biosystematic Codes for viruses and bacteria may cause errors and the use of the numeric version of BC is therefore recommended.

According to Snow in Chapter Five of the *Manual of Online Search Strategies* (2nd Ed. Aldershot: Ashgate, 1992) the Master Index in the *Biosis Previews Search Guide* should not be regarded as an authority list or thesaurus, since it does not include all words or concepts that are searchable as indexer-added keywords in the online database. Snow also points out the value of controlled vocabulary when searching for topics where a subject population has been specified. Relatively few bioscience databases provide consistent indexing for subject populations (for example humans or specific test animals) and related characteristics commonly requested such as age groups, gender, occupation and racial or ethnic groups. BIOSIS provides consistent indexing for the identification of humans and test animals with less consistent indexing of occupational groups and racial/ethnic groups and uses a natural language approach for the identification of gender. She also notes that American spellings are used as standard. In most bioscience files a form of pharmaceutical nomenclature exists. For BIOSIS the preferred terminology consists of generic names, classification by use/action and CAS Registry Numbers although certain restrictions apply to the latter (for example date, subfile or vendor restrictions). The use of enzyme commission number, investigational code, chemical name or trade name is inconsistent and it is recommended that alternative names should be used in search strategies. In addition retrospective searching may require entry of other names used for the same substance at earlier stages in its development life cycle.

Review articles can be retrieved by adding the word 'review', restricted to title and added keywords, to a search strategy.

12:44. Online — BRS, Morning Search, BRS/Colleague

File name	BIOL
Alternative name(s)	Biological Abstracts
Start year	1976
Number of records	
Update period	Monthly
Price/Charges	Connect time: US$53.00/83.00
	Online print: US$0.44/0.52
	Offline print: US$0.52
	SDI charge: US$10.75

Notes

Users can search in BIOZ, the merged file for both the current file BIOL and the back file BIOB. Abstracts from July 1976 to date are available.

12:45. Online — BRS, Morning Search, BRS/Colleague

File name	BIOB
Alternative name(s)	Biological Abstracts
Start year	1976

Number of records
Update period   Monthly
Price/Charges   Connect time: US$53.00/83
                       Online print: US$0.44/0.52
                       Offline print: US$0.52
                       SDI charge: US$10.75

Notes

Users can search in BIOZ, the merged file for both the current file BIOL and the back file BIOB. Abstracts from July 1976 to date are available.

12:46. Online   BRS, Morning Search, BRS/Colleague

File name   BIOZ
Alternative name(s)   Biological Abstracts
Start year   1976
Number of records
Update period   Monthly
Price/Charges   Connect time: US$53.00/83
                       Online print: US$0.44/0.52
                       Offline print: US$0.52
                       SDI charge: US$10.75

Notes

Users can search in BIOZ, the merged file for both the current file BIOL and the back file BIOB. Abstracts from July 1976 to date are available.

12:47. Online   CISTI, Canadian Online Enquiry Service CAN/OLE

File name   BA69
Alternative name(s)   Biological Abstracts
Start year   1969–1984
Number of records   4,267,300
Update period   Closed File
Price/Charges   Connect time: Canadian $40.00
                       Online print: Canadian $0.275 – 0.33
                       Offline print: Canadian $0.275 – 0.33

Notes

Abstracts from 1982 to date are available. CISTI is accessible only in Canada.

12:48. Online   CISTI, Canadian Online Enquiry Service CAN/OLE

File name   BA85
Alternative name(s)   Biological Abstracts
Start year   1985–1991
Number of records   3,532,472
Update period   Closed File
Price/Charges   Connect time: Canadian $40.00
                       Online print: Canadian $0.275 – 0.33
                       Offline print: Canadian $0.275 – 0.33

Notes

Abstracts from 1982 to date are available. CISTI is accessible only in Canada.

12:49. Online   CISTI, Canadian Online Enquiry Service CAN/OLE

File name   BA92
Alternative name(s)   Biological Abstracts
Start year   1992
Number of records   185,400
Update period   48 per year

Price/Charges   Connect time: Canadian $40.00
                       Online print: Canadian $0.275 – 0.33
                       Offline print: Canadian $0.275 – 0.33

Notes

Abstracts from 1982 to date are available. CISTI is accessible only in Canada.

12:50. Online   CompuServe Information Service

File name   IQUEST File 1182
Alternative name(s)   Biological Abstracts
Start year   1969
Number of records   7,713,784
Update period   Twice per month
Price/Charges   Subscription: US$8.95 per month
                       Database entry fee: US$9/search;
                       some databases carry a surcharge
                       ($2–75)
                       Online print: US$10 references free;
                       then $9 per ten; abstracts $3 each
Downloading is allowed

Notes

Accessed via IQUEST or IQMEDICAL, this database is offered by a DIALOG gateway. IQUEST can either search across all databases, a database of the user's choice or selected multiple databases.

12:51. Online   Council of Scientific Research

File name
Alternative name(s)   Biological Abstracts
Start year
Number of records
Update period

12:52. Online   Data-Star

File name   BIOL
Alternative name(s)   Biological Abstracts
Start year   1985
Number of records   6,000,000
Update period   Fortnightly
Database aids   Data-Star Biomedical Manual and
                       Data-Star Online Manual (search
                       for NEWS-BIOL in NEWS)
Price/Charges   Subscription: SFr80.00
                       Connect time: SFr147.00
                       Online print: SFr0.40–1.03
                       Offline print: SFr0.90
                       SDI charge: SFr4.94

Notes

Abstracts are provided for about two-thirds of the database.

From June 1993 Data-Star have introduced an annual fee/subscription per contract (that is, not per password) of SFr 80.00 (c.UK£ 32.00) payable every June. For North American customers billed in dollars who also use DIALOG, the DIALOG fee also covers access to Data-Star. Academic customers, 'commitment' customers and customers currently billed in dollars are exempt.

Record composition

Abstract AB; Accession Number or and Update Code AN; Authors AU; Author Affiliation IN; Biosystematic Codes BC; Coden CD; Concept Codes CC; Keywords KW; Language LG; Supertaxa ST; Source SO; Title TI and Year of Publication YR

12:53. Online Data-Star

File name	BI84
Alternative name(s)	Biological Abstracts
Start year	1970–1984
Number of records	
Update period	
Database aids	Data-Star Biomedical Manual and Data-Star Online Manual (search NEWS-BIOL in NEWS)
Price/Charges	Subscription: SFr80.00
	Connect time: SFr147.00
	Online print: SFr0.40–1.03
	Offline print: SFr0.90
	SDI charge: SFr4.94

Notes

Abstracts from July 1976 are available.

From June 1993 Data-Star have introduced an annual fee/subscription per contract (that is, not per password) of SFr 80.00 (c.UK£ 32.00) payable every June. For North American customers billed in dollars who also use DIALOG, the DIALOG fee also covers access to Data-Star. Academic customers, 'commitment' customers and customers currently billed in dollars are exempt.

Record composition

Abstract AB; Accession Number or and Update Code AN; Authors AU; Author Affiliation IN; Biosystematic Codes BC; Coden CD; Concept Codes CC; Keywords KW; Language LG; Supertaxa ST; Source SO; Title TI and Year of Publication YR

12:54. Online Data-Star

File name	BIZZ
Alternative name(s)	Biological Abstracts
Start year	1970+
Number of records	6 million
Update period	Every two weeks
Database aids	Data-Star Biomedical Manual and Data-Star Online Manual
Price/Charges	Subscription: SFr80.00
	Connect time: SFr147.00
	Online print: SFr0.40–1.03
	Offline print: SFr0.90
	SDI charge: SFr4.94

Notes

Abstracts from July 1976 to date are available. Abstracts are provided for about two-thirds of the database.

From June 1993 Data-Star have introduced an annual fee/subscription per contract (that is, not per password) of SFr 80.00 (c.UK£ 32.00) payable every June. For North American customers billed in dollars who also use DIALOG, the DIALOG fee also covers access to Data-Star. Academic customers, 'commitment' customers and customers currently billed in dollars are exempt.

Record composition

Abstract AB; Accession Number or and Update Code AN; Authors AU; Author Affiliation IN; Biosystematic Codes BC; Coden CD; Concept Codes CC; Keywords KW; Language LG; Supertaxa ST; Source SO; Title TI and Year of Publication YR

12:55. Online DIALOG

File name	File 5
Alternative name(s)	Biological Abstracts
Start year	1969
Number of records	7,713,784 Files 5, 55
Update period	Weekly

Price/Charges	Connect time: US$90.00
	Online print: US$0.75
	Offline print: US$0.75
	SDI charge: US$10.50 (biweekly)/14.95 (monthly)

Notes

Abstracts from July 1976 to date are available and for book synopses in BA/RRM from 1985. Most BA/RRM records do not contain abstracts; no Biol records contain abstracts. On DIALOG there are two files – File 5 covers 1969 to the present, File 55 1985 to the present.

DIALINDEX categories: AGRI, BIOCHEM, BIOSCI, BIOTECH, ENRION, FOODSCI, MARINE, MEDENG, MEDICINE, NUTRIT, PHARM, PHARMR, SAFETY, TOXICOL, VETSCI.

12:56. Online DIALOG

File name	File 55
Alternative name(s)	Biological Abstracts
Start year	1985
Number of records	
Update period	
Price/Charges	Connect time: US$90.00
	Online print: US$0.75
	Offline print: US$0.75
	SDI charge: US$10.50 (biweekly)/14.95 (monthly)

Notes

Abstracts from July 1976 to date are available and for book synopses in BA/RRM from 1985. Most BA/RRM records do not contain abstracts and no Biol records contain abstracts. On DIALOG there are two files – File 5 covers 1969 to the present, File 55 1985 to the present.

DIALINDEX categories: AGRI, BIOCHEM, BIOSCI, BIOTECH, ENRION, FOODSCI, MARINE, MEDENG, MEDICINE, NUTRIT, PHARM, PHARMR, SAFETY, TOXICOL, VETSCI.

12:57. Online DIMDI

File name	BA70
Alternative name(s)	Biological Abstracts
Software	GRIPS
Start year	1970–1982
Number of records	8,033,918
Update period	Monthly
Database aids	User Manual BIOSIS Previews and Memocard Biosis Previews
Price/Charges	Connect time: UK£23.42–32.18
	Online print: UK£0.37–0.55
	Offline print: UK£0.29–0.36
Downloading is allowed	
Thesaurus is online	

Notes

Abstracts (52% of the records) are available from July 1976 to date. Searches are possible from January 1970. The Basic Index includes the data fields: Title, Abstract, Uncontrolled Terms. Suppliers of online documents: British Library Document Supply Centre, Boston Spa, England; Bayerishe Staatsbibliothek München, München, Germany; Harkers Information Retrieval System, Sydney, Australia; Koninklijke Nederlandse Akademie van Wetenschapen, Amsterdam, The Netherlands.

Record composition

Abstract AB; Author AU; Biosystematic Code BC; Biosystematic Code-New /NEW; Biosystematic Heading BS; Biosystematic Heading-New /NEW; Coden CD; Corporate Source CS; Entry Date ED;

Free Text FT; Index Term IT; Journal Title JT; Language LA; Document Number ND; Publication Year PY; Subject Code SC; Subject Heading SH; Source SO; Title TI and Uncontrolled Terms UT

12:58. Online   DIMDI

File name	BA83
Alternative name(s)	Biological Abstracts
Software	GRIPS
Start year	1983
Number of records	4,681,303
Update period	Monthly
SDI period	1 month
Database aids	User Manual BIOSIS Previews and Memocard Biosis Previews
Price/Charges	Connect time: UK£23.42–32.18
	Online print: UK£0.37–0.55
	Offline print: UK£0.29–0.36

Downloading is allowed
Thesaurus is online

Notes

Abstracts are available from July 1976 to date. The Basic Index includes the data fields: Title, Abstract, Uncontrolled Terms. Suppliers of online documents: British Library Document Supply Centre, Boston Spa, England; Bayerishe Staatsbibliothek München, München, Germany; Harkers Information Retrieval System, Sydney, Australia; Koninklijke Nederlandse Akademie van Wetenschapen, Amsterdam, The Netherlands.

Record composition

Abstract AB; Author AU; Biosystematic Code BC; Biosystematic Code-New /NEW; Biosystematic Heading BS; Biosystematic Heading-New /NEW; Coden CD; Corporate Source CS; Entry Date ED; Free Text FT; Index Term IT; Journal Title JT; Language LA; Document Number ND; Publication Year PY; Subject Code SC; Subject Heading SH; Source SO; Title TI and Uncontrolled Terms UT

12:59. Online   ESA-IRS

File name	File 7
Alternative name(s)	Biological Abstracts
Start year	1970
Number of records	7,517,000 (October 1991)
Update period	Every two weeks

Downloading is allowed

Notes

From 1973–84 the records contain terms physically split into their components for example PHOSPHO and LIPID (not PHOSPHOLIPID). From 1984 the splitting has been interrupted by the Biosis producer. Abstracts from July 1976 to date are available. BIOSIS on ESA-IRS from February 1992 includes new biosystematic codes.

From 1993 ESA-IRS are charging an annual fee of 100 Accounting Units (c.UK£ 70.29) to all users. This is equivalent to the fee for full documentation and will not be charged to customers already paying for documentation.

Record composition

Author AU; Biosystematic Codes BC; Biosystematic Code Name BN; CODEN CO; Concept Codes CC; Concept Code Name CN; Descriptors /UT; Journal Name JN and Title /TI

12:60. Online   Japan Information Center of Science and Technology (JICST)

File name	BIOSIS
Alternative name(s)	Biological Abstracts
Start year	1969
Number of records	6,800,000
Update period	
SDI period	Monthly/bi-weekly
Database aids	Thesaurus Translation List:
	Japanese-English 1987:
	English-Japanese 1987.
Price/Charges	Connect time: US$85.00
	Online print: US$0.32
	Offline print: US$0.38
	SDI charge: US$6.10

12:61. Online   OCLC EPIC; OCLC FirstSearch

File name	BIOSIS Previews
Alternative name(s)	Biological Abstracts
Start year	1976
Number of records	
Update period	

12:62. Online   STN

File name	BIOSIS Previews/RN
Alternative name(s)	Biological Abstracts
Start year	1969
Number of records	8,334,568
Update period	Weekly
Price/Charges	Connect time: DM139.00
	Online print: DM1.32
	Offline print: DM1.40
	SDI charge: DM10.70

Downloading is allowed

Notes

Abstracts from July 1976 to date are available.

CAS Registry Numbers, derived from a computer check for chemical names in the title and added keyword fields are present for citations from July 1980 onwards. There is an online thesaurus for for the Biosystematic Code Superterms (/BC) field.

12:63. Online   University of Tsukuba

File name	
Alternative name(s)	Biological Abstracts
Start year	
Number of records	
Update period	

Notes

Access through University of Tsukuba is limited to affiliates of the University of Japan.

12:64. Tape   BIOSIS

File name	BIOSIS Previews
Alternative name(s)	Biological Abstracts
Start year	1969
Number of records	7,826,768
Update period	4 times a month
Price/Charges	Subscription: US$9,125

Notes

Two tapes correspond to *Biological Abstracts* and two tapes correspond to *Biological Abstracts/Reports, Reviews, Meeting Literature (BA/RRM)*. Corresponds in coverage to *Biological Abstracts (BA)* and *Biological*

Abstracts/RRM (BA/RRM) (formerly *BioResearch Index*), and to the BIOSIS Previews online database. Annual licence fee is $9,125 plus additional usage charges; contact BIOSIS for archival tape prices.

12:65. Database subset

Online **CISTI, Canadian Online Enquiry Service CAN/OLE**

File name	ABC3
Alternative name(s)	Biological Abstracts
Start year	1989
Number of records	47,138
Update period	Closed File

Notes

Static training file for BIOSIS Previews enabling users to practice searching using free-text terms, Concept Codes, Biosystematic Codes, Super Taxonomic Codes and bibliographic information.

12:66. Database subset

Online **Data-Star**

File name	TRBI – Biosis Training File
Alternative name(s)	Biological Abstracts
Start year	1984
Number of records	100,000
Update period	Fortnightly
Database aids	Data-Star Biomedical Manual and Data-Star Online Manual (search for NEWS-BIOL in NEWS)
Price/Charges	Connect time: Free

Notes

Static training file for BIOSIS Previews enabling users to practice searching using free-text terms, Concept Codes, Biosystematic Codes, Super Taxonomic Codes and bibliographic information. Records are taken from 1984, 1990 and 1992 from both the *Biological Abstracts* and the *Biological Abstracts/RRM* subfiles of the database.

Record composition

Abstract AB; Accession Number or and Update Code AN; Authors AU; Author Affiliation IN; Biosystematic Codes BC; Coden CD; Concept Codes CC; Keywords KW; Language LG; Supertaxa ST; Source SO; Title TI and Year of Publication YR

12:67. Database subset

Online **DIALOG**

File name	File 205 – ONTAP BIOSIS Previews Training File
Alternative name(s)	Biological Abstracts
Start year	January 1986 updates to File 5, BIOSIS Previews
Number of records	43,406
Update period	Closed File
Price/Charges	Connect time: US$15.00

Notes

The training file from the January updates of File 5, the main BIOSIS Preview file on DIALOG. It includes records from both Biological Abstracts and Biological Abstracts/Reports, Reviews, Meetings. Allows for low-cost practice using the BISOIS biosystematic and concept codes for searching. Offline prints are not available in ONTAP files.

12:68. Database subset

Online **ESA-IRS**

File name	File 209 – Training Biosis
Alternative name(s)	Biological Abstracts

Start year	References from 1970, 1980, 1986
Number of records	40,000
Update period	Not updated

Notes

A fixed subset of the main BIOSIS database (File 7), enabling the user to practise ESA-QUEST at low cost. Services such as offline prints, auomatic current awareness and document ordering are not available.

Record composition

Author AU; Biosystematic Codes BC; Biosystematic Code Name BN; CODEN CO; Concept Codes CC; Concept Code Name CN; Descriptors /UT; Journal Name JN and Title /TI

12:69. Database subset

CD-ROM **SilverPlatter**

File name	BA on CD
Alternative name(s)	Biological Abstracts
Format notes	Mac, IBM
Software	SPIRS v.2.0/MacSPIRS
Start year	1985
Number of records	280,000
Update period	Quarterly
Database aids	The SilverPlatter Users' Manual and Quick Reference Card
Price/Charges	Subscription: UK£1,647 – 6,762

Notes

When combined with BA/RRM on CD, BA on CD forms the equivalent of the online database BIOSIS Previews, incorporating the concept codes, biosystematic codes and super taxonomical codes used by searchers of the online database. On its own this CD-ROM version includes only *Biological Abstracts* whereas BIOSIS online includes *Biological Abstracts* and *Biological Abstract/RRM (Reports, Reviews, Meetings)*. This version only provides initials to authors' first and middle names. According to Condic (Condic, K.S. *CD-ROM Librarian* 6(3) 1991 29–33) each year of the database will appear on a separate CD-ROM, making searching cumbersome for multiple-year access.

In early 1993, SilverPlatter prices for BA on CD were: regular subscriptions UK£5,880 for single users, £6,762 for 2–8 networked users. Prices for those who subscribe to the print or microfilm version – for single users £1,489 and £3,797 for 2–8 networked users. For subscribers to the cumulative index £1,647 for single users and £2,529. For the collection starting with the calendar year 1993 (1985–88, 1989, 1990, 1991 and 1992) prices vary, depending on the user's current subscriptions – prices on application. There are now available back files to 1985. BA on CD requires a signed subscription and licence agreement.

Record composition

Abreviated Journal Title AJ; Abstract AB; Author AU; Biosystematic Codes; Coden CO; Concept Codes CC; Corporate Source CS; Descriptors DE; Journal Anouncement JA; Language of Article LA; Language of Summary LS; Major Concept Codes MJCC; Minor Concept Codes MNCC; Publication Year PY; Source Journal SO; Super Taxa ST; Title TI and Update Code UD

Subject access is via concept codes, biosystematic codes, super taxonomic groups and descriptors. The disc contains over 600 concept codes from the BIOSIS Search Guides. Articles have from one to ten codes assigned to them which are divided into major and minor categories resembling major or minor descriptors found in other databases. Most articles also have one to twelve biosystematic codes assigned to them. Supertaxonomic groups consist of related groups of biosystematic codes which search the English names of groups of animals. Descriptors consist of natural language or controlled vocabulary terms.

12:70. Database subset

CD-ROM   **SilverPlatter**

File name	BA/RRM on CD
Alternative name(s)	Biological Abstracts
Format notes	IBM, Mac
Software	SPIRS
Start year	1989
Number of records	260,000
Update period	Quarterly
Database aids	Software Manual, Database Manual and Quick Reference Cards
Price/Charges	Subscription: UK£841 – 6,762

Notes

Most records in this database do not contain abstracts as abstracts are included only in the form of book sysnopses. Equivalent to the printed *Biological Abstracts/RRM (Reports, Reviews and Meetings)*, previously entitled *BioResearch Index*. Records in the database cover notes, short communications, technical reports, bibliographies and taxonomic keys. Books are also included as are abstracts from meetings. When combined with BA on CD, forms the equivalent of the online database BIOSIS Previews. According to Shirley Cousin's review (*CD-ROM Information Products: The Evaluative Guide* 1993 4(1) p.1–12), the majority of records are from Europe and the Middle East (48%) with a further 28 per cent from North America, 16 per cent from Asia and Australia, 6 per cent from South and Central American and the final 2 per cent from Africa.

Pricing, as of January 1993 is: for regular subscribers, single user UK£3,021, and for 2–8 networked users £3,903; Discounts are available for subscribers to the print or microfilm versions of BA – £1,480 for single users, £2,362 for 2–8 networked users; for cumulative index subscribers prices are £841 for single users and £1,723 for 2–8 networked users. For the collection starting with the calendar year 1993 (1985–88, 1989, 1990, 1991 and 1992) prices vary, depending on the user's current subscriptions – prices on application. BA on CD requires a signed subscription and licence agreement.

12:71. Database subset

Tape   **BIOSIS**

File name	BAT – Biological Abstracts on Tape
Alternative name(s)	Biological Abstracts
Format notes	9-track, 800, 1600, or 6250 bpi, variable length record, variable block size.
Start year	1976
Number of records	
Update period	Twice a month
Price/Charges	Subscription: US$11,000

Notes

Contains abstracts of the worldwide literature on research in the life sciences. Covers articles from over 9,000 periodicals cited in BIOSIS Previews. Corresponds to the abstracts appearing in *Biological Abstracts*, and in part to the BIOSIS Previews online database.

Annual licence fee $11,000 plus additional usage charges; contact BIOSIS for archival tape prices.

This database can also be found on:
TOXLIT
BA/RRM on CD
Foods Intelligence on CD
Toxline Plus

Biotechnologie Informations Knoten für Europa
Gesellschaft für Biotechnologische Forschung mbH

12:73. Master record

Alternative name(s)	BIKE
Database type	Bibliographic, Factual, Directory
Number of journals	
Sources	Questionnaires, Conferences, Direct contacts and Meetings
Start year	1987
Language	German
Coverage	Germany, Switzerland and Austria
Number of records	4,000
Update size	–
Update period	Quarterly
Thesaurus	BIKE-Thesaurus, Braunschweig, GBF mbH, 1989

Keywords

Bioengineering

Description

BIKE (Biotechnologie-Informationsknoten für Europa) is a German language factual database which answers questions like 'who does what and where in biotechology' for the German language countries (Federal Republic of Germany, Switzerland and Austria). It covers the whole field of biotechnology from bioprocess technology to genetic engineering. It contains profiles of organisations, institutes and companies involved with biotechnological research and production. These include industrial companies, universities, research institutes, associations, unions, authorities, technology transfer organizations, consultants, organism collections and government bodies in Germany, Switzerland and Austria. Every document profile contains a comprehensive description of the biotechnological activities and includes, for industrial companies, for example, the contact persons, details of products, company structure, address, number of employees and amount of sales. For research organizations there are given the names of leading scientists, subjects of research and cooperative partners. All data are derived from questionnaires disseminated by the database producer.

Information is obtained by direct contact with the organizations concerned, and by questionnaire, meetings and conferences, as well as from published sources.

BIKE is a free-text database which is indexed by a hierarchically structured thesaurus. All subject related fields are freetext searchable. The umlauts of the German language are converted for searching the database.

12:74. Online — Data-Star

File name	BIKE
Alternative name(s)	BIKE
Start year	1987
Number of records	4,000
Update period	Quarterly
Database aids	Data-Star Biomedical Manual, Berne, 1989 and Online manual (search for NEWS-BIKE in NEWS)
Price/Charges	Subscription: SFr80.00
	Connect time: SFr175.00
	Online print: SFr1.28
	Offline print: SFr1.50

Notes

From June 1993 Data-Star have introduced an annual fee/subscription per contract (that is, not per password) of SFr 80.00 (c.UK£ 32.00) payable every June. For North American customers billed in dollars who also use DIALOG, the DIALOG fee also covers access to Data-Star. Academic customers, 'commitment' customers and customers currently billed in dollars are exempt.

12:75. Online — DIMDI

File name	BK00
Alternative name(s)	BIKE
Start year	1987
Number of records	2,370
Update period	Quarterly reloads
Price/Charges	Connect time: UK£50.29–53.13
	Online print: UK£0.43–0.60
	Offline print: UK£0.36–0.43

Downloading is allowed

Record composition

Corporate code CCD; City CI; Corporate Name CNA; Cooperation Partners COOP; Controlled Terms CT; Controlled Terms in Context CTX; Corporate Type CTYP; Country CY; Entry Day EDY; Foundation Year FY; Number of Document ND; Notes NOTE; Products PRO; Sales Biotechnological SLB; Sales General SLG; State STATE; Staff Biotechnological STB; Staff Biotechnological Research STBR; Staff General STG; Street STR; Telefon, Telex, Telefax TEL; Update Status US and Zip Code ZP

The documents are indexed by descriptors taken from the thesaurus, and they appear in the documents in two fields: as directly searchable single descriptors (example: F CT=monoklonal AND CT=antikoerper), where the thesaurus structure can also be used (example: F CT DOWN enzym AND CT=produktion); or as freetext desxcriptors which are arranged in sentences, where every sentence contains those descriptors which describe closely related concepts (field CTX). Therefore all freetext searches in this field should be limited to 'the same sentence' (example: F monoklonal,? antikoerper./CTX). The freetext search 'in the same sentence' will usually give more specific search results; there is, however, the disadvantage that the thesaurus structure cannot be used with freetext searches. The field NOTES contains for research institutes a rough description of the fields of research, then the specific subjects of research and leading scientists. For industrial companies it contains the fields of trade, subjects of research and development, contact persons and further general information. The field PRODUCT shows the products of a company, but also pure sale activities. Trade names are not entered in BIKE. Information on services are to be found in this field also. The field CTYP can be used especially for search limitation. It contains ten codes which describe the type of documented institution, for example, AUT: AUTHORITIES, UNI: UNIVERSITIES.

Biotechnology Abstracts
Derwent Publications Ltd

12:76. Master record

Database type	Bibliographic
Number of journals	1,200
Sources	Journals, Patents and Conference proceedings
Start year	1982 (June)
Language	English
Coverage	International
Number of records	110,000
Update size	15,000
Update period	Monthly

Keywords

Biochemical Engineering; Genetic Engineering; Waste Management

Description

Contains citations, with abstracts and indexing, to the worldwide journal and patent literature on biotechnology. It covers all aspects of biotechnology, including genetic engineering, biochemical engineering, fermentation, cell culture, microbiology, down-stream processing, pharmaceuticals, industrial uses of microorganisms, plant breeding, cell hybridization, and industrial waste management.

Each record in the database comprises a detailed abstract of up to 200 words together with controlled-language indexing. Literature records also include complete bibliographic information, and patent documents include patent number, patentee, and publication details. Approximately 27% of the records are patent records.

Corresponds to *Biotechnology Abstracts*.

Differential charges for subscribers and non-subscribers to *Biotechnology Abstracts*.

12:77. Online — DIALOG

File name	File 357
Start year	1982
Number of records	123,404
Update period	Monthly
Price/Charges	Subscription: US$96.00 – 155.00
	Online print: US$0.27 – 0.70
	Offline print: US$0.49 – 0.75
	SDI charge: US$9.75

Notes

Differential pricing for subscribers and non-subscribers.

12:78. Online — ORBIT

File name	BIOT – Biotechnology Abstracts
Start year	1982 (July)
Number of records	110,000
Update period	Monthly
Database aids	Quick Reference Guide (9/88) Free (single copy)

Notes

Differential charges for subscribers and non-subscribers to *Biotechnology Abstracts*. Electronic SDI service is now available within two hours on ORBIT. They can be downloaded and reformatted on a word processor. Results are retrieved in the low cost PRINTS file, $15 per connect hour.

12:79. CD-ROM   SilverPlatter

File name	Biotechnology Abstracts
Format notes	IBM, Mac
Software	SPIRS/MacSPIRS
Start year	1982
Number of records	140,000
Update period	Quarterly
Price/Charges	Subscription: UK£1,000 – 2,800

Notes

Data can be displayed in individual fields: title; abstract; journal; classification; etc. There is a discount for academics – subscription cost is £1,000 for single users, £2,000 for 2–8 networked users. The regular subscription is £ 1,400 for single users, £2,800 for 2–8 networked users. Requires a signed subscription and licence agreement.

Biotechnology Citation Index
Institute for Scientific Information

12:80. Master record

Database type	Bibliographic, Citation
Number of journals	7,250
Sources	
Start year	
Language	English
Coverage	International
Number of records	50,000
Update size	50,000
Update period	Six times per year

Description

Citation index, with abstracts, offering complete coverage of significant published literature in biotechnology. Spans all aspects from genetic cloning, molecular biology and microbiology to new applications in agriculture, medicine, industry and the environment.

Includes full coverage of over 250 journals, with every significant item in these journals included (letters, notes, editorials, corrections, reviews). In addition to the over 250 journals related to the topics of biotechnology, selected relevant articles from another 7,000 journals from the entire ISI database are included. The primary advantages in this repackaging are the abstracts included in all records and the greater precision in subject searching. Katie Clark (Discipline Specific Citation Indexes From ISI. *CD-ROM Professional* 6(1) 1993 p.135–138) noted that the biotechnology core journal list includes 174 titles. 'Sixty-three percent (110) of these core titles are also indexed by MEDLINE, although 43 were indexed only selectively. Sixty-six percent (115) of the core titles are indexed by BIOSIS and 39 percent (68) are also indexed by Agricola. Only three of the core biotechnology titles were not indexed by either MEDLINE, BIOSIS, or Agricola. According to Ulrich's International Periodicals Directory, seventeen of the core biotechnology titles are not indexed in any other sources. The core list of titles is truly 'core'; almost all the titles are indexed by other standard sources. It is important to note that even the core titles are not

indexed cover-to-cover. Only items relevant to biotechnology are included.' Initially sceptical about the ISI discipline-specific databases on the grounds that no complete list of journal titles is available and that even the core journals are not indexed cover-to-cover, her comparison of Biotechnology Citation Index with MEDLINE was not entirely unfavourable and ended by admitting that they may solve a problem for specific users.

All ISI databases have a linked service known as The Genuine Article which can deliver the full text of located articles by mail, facsimile transmission or courier. Orders can be placed via the host service in use, mail, facsimile transmission, telephone or telex. Diskette products have a single-keystroke order information facility. The minimum charge is US$ 11.25 within USA and Canada and US$ 12.20 elsewhere.

12:81. CD-ROM   Institute for Scientific Information

File name	Biotechnology Citation Index
Format notes	IBM, Mac
Start year	
Number of records	
Update period	Six times per year
Price/Charges	Subscription: US$1,950

Notes

A particular feature of the CD-ROM is ISI's unique Related Records search facility which provides access to records with cited references in common, allowing documents on similar subjects to be easily retrieved and browsed. The software for this repackaged subset of Science Citation Index also gives the ability to search the basic index or all fields at once. An initially negative reviewer, Frederick Gilmore (*CD-ROM Librarian* 7(10) p51–54) found himself pleased with the performance and the manageability of the data and preferred the Biotechnology Citation Index to its parent as it includes full-text searchable abstracts and keywords.

Each issue is a year-to-date cumulation ending with the final annual cumulation. Back years are available to 1991.

Biotechnology Investment Opportunities
High Tech Publishing Company

12:82. Master record

Database type	Textual
Number of journals	1
Sources	Newsletter
Start year	Current and previous years
Language	English
Coverage	International
Number of records	
Update size	—
Update period	Monthly

Keywords

Genetic Engineering; Investment

Description

A newsletter on investment opportunities in genetic engineering, covering initial public stock offerings, company profiles and activities, current research, markets and applications, industry trends and government policies and activities.

Equivalent to *Biotechnology Investment Opportunities* monthly.

12:83. Online — CompuServe Information Service

File name	IQUEST File 1768
Start year	Current year
Number of records	
Update period	Monthly
Price/Charges	Subscription: US$8.95 per month
	Database entry fee: US$9/search; some databases carry a surcharge ($2–75)
	Online print: US$10 references free; then $9 per ten; abstracts $3 each
Downloading is allowed	

Notes

Accessed via IQUEST or IQMEDICAL, this database is offered by a NewsNet gateway. IQUEST can either search across all databases, a database of the user's choice or selected multiple databases.

12:84. Online — NewsNet Inc

File name	
Start year	Current and previous years
Number of records	
Update period	Monthly

Notes

Monthly subscription to NewsNet required; differential charges for subscribers and non-subscribers to the print version.

BISANCE CD

European Molecular Biology Laboratory (EMBL)
CITIS Ltd

12:85. Master record
CD-ROM — CITIS Ltd

Database type	Bibliographic
Number of journals	
Sources	
Start year	1990
Language	English
Coverage	Europe
Number of records	
Update size	—
Update period	Twice a month

Keywords

DNA Sequences; RNA Sequences; MRNA; Bacteriophages; Biotechnology; Genetics; Microbiology; Molecular Biology; Nucleotides; Viruses

Description

Contains the EMBL Nucleotide Sequence online database, European databank of nucleic acids and proteins. Information is provided on most published DNA and RNA chains.

For more details of constituent databases, see:
BISANCE
EMBL Nucleotide Sequence Database

BISANCE

Universite de Lyon I, Institut d'Evolution Moleculaire

12:87. Master record

Alternative name(s)	Base Informatique sur les Sequences de Biomolecules pour les Chercheurs Europeens
Database type	Factual, Bibliographic, Chemical structures/DNA sequences
Number of journals	75
Sources	Journals
Start year	Current Information
Language	English (primarily) and French (Bibliographie en biotechnologie)
Coverage	International
Number of records	
Update size	—
Update period	Every two months

Keywords

DNA Sequences; RNA Sequences; MRNA; Bacteriophages; Biotechnology; Genetics; Microbiology; Molecular Biology; Nucleotides; Viruses

Description

Contains six databases on molecular biology.

Banque de Sequences d'Acides Nucleiques de l'EMBL (EMBL Nucleotide Sequence database);
GenBank: descriptions of RNA and DNA sequences with 50+ nucleotide bases;
Banque de Proteines (NBRF-NIH);
Banque de Proteines (GENPRO);
Banque de Coordonnees Cristallographiques;
Bibliographie en biotechnologie: 90,000 citations, with abstracts, to articles in biotechnology journals.

12:88. Online — Universite de Paris V, CITI

File name	BISANCE
Alternative name(s)	Base Informatique sur les Sequences de Biomolecules pour les Chercheurs Europeens
Start year	Current Information
Number of records	
Update period	Every two months

For more details of constituent databases, see:
Banque de Sequences d'Acides Nucleiques de l'EMBL (EMBL Nucleotide Sequence Database
GenBank
Banque de Proteines (NBRF-NIH)
Banque de Proteines (GENPRO)
Banque de Coordonnees Cristallographiques
Bibliographie en biotechnologie

CAB Abstracts
CAB International

12:90. Master record

Database type	Bibliographic
Number of journals	14,000
Sources	Books, company reports, conference proceedings, dissertations, grey literature, journals, monographs, patents, research reports, standards and theses
Start year	1972
Language	English (original language titles)
Coverage	International

Number of records	2,800,000
Update size	150,000
Update period	Monthly
Abstract details	CAB's own indexers write detailed informative English-language summaries for each record.
Thesaurus	CAB Abstracts Thesaurus
Database aids	CAB Abstracts Online Manual, CAB Serials Checklist, CAB Section Code Lists, CAB International Database News. and IULAS (International Union List of Agricultural Serials)

Keywords

Agricultural Economics; Agrochemicals; Anatomy; Animal Breeding; Animal Diseases; Bioagriculture; Crop Protection; Diet; Entomology; Environmental Health; Forestry; Horticulture; Immunology; Medical Entomology; Medical Immunology; Medical Mycology; Medical Parasitology; Mycology; Nutrition; Paper and Packaging; Pathology; Pest Management; Physiology; Plant Diseases; Plant Genetics; Pollution; Public Health; Rural Sociology; Soil Management; Sport; Tourism; Travel; Veterinary Entomology; Veterinary Mycology; Water Management

Description

Contains citations, with abstracts, to the worldwide literature in the agricultural sciences and related areas of applied biology. Subjects covered include agricultural engineering; agricultural entomology; animal breeding; biocontrol; biodeterioration and biodegradation; biotechnology; crop protection; dairy science and technology; economics; engineering; environment; forestry and forest products; genetics; herbicides; helminthology; horticulture; irrigation; leisure, recreation and tourism; medical and veterinary entomology; microbiology; mycology; nutrition (human and animal); parasitology (human and animal); plant breeding and pathology; protozoology; rural development and sociology; soil science and fertilizers and arid lands (1980 to 1982). Coverage of veterinary medicine begins in 1972. Also contains useful material on rural development in third world countries. Animal breeding and production, animal nutrition & dairy science and technology, covers: animals including farm mammals of economic or domestic importance; laboratory mammals; poultry, game and other birds of economic importance; fish, molluscs and crustacea; and certain invertebrates used in genetic studies. Subjects covered include performance traits and products; breeding and genetics; biotechnology; reproduction; nutrition; the dairy industry; housing and equipment for livestock and in aquaculture; and nongenetic effects on animals. Crop protection and pests covers: entomology; plant pathology; nematology and weed science for the full ranges of agricultural, horticultural, plantation and forestry crops. Covers areas of pest taxonomy; biology; ecology; management; and economic and social impact. Environmental health and toxicology covers: environmental agrochemicals (insecticides, fungicides, pesticides, fertilisers); groundwater contamination, runoff and leaching; heavy metals in soil, crops and animals; reclamation and re-vegetation of polluted sites; environmental impact of farming; waste management, treatment and disposal; toxicology (toxic plants, wastes, food poisoning, carcinogens); and steroids and hormones in animals. Forestry covers: silviculture and forestry management; tree biology; forest pests and their control; forest land use; wood properties; timber extrac-

tion, conversion and management; wood products; marketing and trade; agroforestry systems and related land use; plant and animal species for agroforestry; environmental and service aspects of agroforestry systems; and sociological, cultural and economic aspects of agroforestry systems. Horticulture covers: literature on temperate tree fruits and nuts; small fruits; viticulture; vegetables; temperate, tropical and greenhouse; ornamental plants; minor industrial crops; subtropical and tropical fruits and plantation crops. Leisure, recreation and tourism covers: leisure industries, travel and transport, marketing of services and products, natural resources and environmental issues, facility management and planning, sport, and leisure and tourism policies. Plant genetics covers: material on breeding; genetic resources; varieties; molecular and general genetics; in vitro culture; cytology and ploidy; reproductive behaviour; evolution and taxonomy; stress tolerance; disease and pest resistance; and quality and yield components. Soil science covers: soil management; crop management; fertilisers and amendments; agricultural meteorology; pollution; land reclamation; irrigation and drainage; plant nutrition and plant water relations. Veterinary science covers: animals including farm animals; pets; game animals; all animals of economic importance, including farmed fish and shellfish; commercially important wild fish; zoo animals and wild animals. Subjects include viral and bacterial diseases; protozoology; mycology; helminthology; arthropod parasites; toxicology; immunology; pharmacology and therapeutics; physiology; biochemistry and anatomy; zootechny, hygiene and food inspection, and related areas. About 85% of items are abstracted in English with each abstract containing 80–100 words. Sources are published in 74 languages.

Corresponds to the fifty main journals and specialised journals published by the Commonwealth Agricultural Bureaux (CAB) International, an international, intergovernmental organisation registered with the United Nations. Membership is open to all governments wishing to participate. The International Union List of Agricultural Serials, a compilation of the serials indexed in AGRICOLA, AGRIS and CAB lists which database indexes a given title. Several hosts have separate subfiles by subject. On all BRS services four subsets are available separately; on agricultural economics, rural development and sociology; on human nutrition; on leisure, recreation and tourism; and on medical and veterinary sciences. On Data-Star, three subsets are available separately: on human nutrition, on human parasitology and mycology; and on medical and veterinary sciences. On DIMDI there are eleven subsets available separately: Animal; Animal Production; Economics; Engineering; Forestry; Human; Nutrition; Plant; Plant Protection; Tourism; and Veterinary Science.

From 1972 to 1983 the Controlled Terms take the form of subject index entries and additional index entries. The number of controlled terms allocated varies from one item/abstract to another. Various collections of uncontrolled, semi-controlled and controlled terms and phrases (keyword units) were used. The Controlled Terms vary between abstract journals. The most strictly controlled list of terms are used in Index Veterinarius, which from 1972 to 1976 used 'Veterinary Subject Headings' (CAB, 1972) and from 1977 the Veterinary Multilingual Thesaurus (there is about 60% agreement between them). The Controlled Terms are the subject index entries used to generate the printed subject indices of the abstract journals, while the additional index entries, where present are used to facilitate retrieval. No hierarchical structure is available for controlled terms. The controlled terms comprise various categories of descriptors and names of organisms are in Latin or in English. Various systems of chemical notation and geographical terms are also used. From 1984 onwards controlled indexing terms are allocated from the *CAB Thesaurus*. A cumulative, alphabetic list of all Controlled Terms, including the descriptors from 1972/83 plus the descriptors of the CAB thesaurus can be accessed by the DISPLAY-command. Almost every abstract is accompanied by a Section Code except the title-only items in *Index Veterinarius*. Usually the Section Codes are structured hierarchically corresponding to the sections and subsections of the CABI abstract journals. Two types of Section Codes are in use: Primary Sequencing Codes and Cross Reference Codes. Primary Sequencing Codes describe the main topic of an article and place an abstract within a given section of an abstract journal. These sections are often subdivided into several subsections; accordingly the assigned Primary Sequencing Codes are taken from the lower levels of the hierarchy. One to two Primary Sequencing Codes are allocated to each abstract.

Cross Reference Codes, which do not occur in every abstract, cover the secondary aspects of an article and refer to another relevant journal section. Where allocated, they are taken from the higher levels of the hierarchy. Four to five Cross Reference Codes may be assigned to an abstract. The Section Codes are up to ten characters long, prefixed by a two character abstract journal code. Different codes and headings are used in each abstract journal so two different codes may be allocated. Section Headings refer to chapter headings and are broader terms to the Section Codes which makes it possible to use them for coarse subdivisions of a subject. (See CAB Abstracts Online for further advice).

12:91. Online   BIS

File name	CABA
Start year	
Number of records	
Update period	

12:92. Online   BRS, Morning Search, BRS/Colleague

File name	
Start year	
Number of records	
Update period	Monthly
Price/Charges	Connect time: US$62.00/72.00
	Online print: US$0.47/0.55
	Offline print: US$0.55
	SDI charge: US$12.50

Downloading is allowed

Notes

Indexing is detailed and comprehensive using a controlled vocabulary.

12:93. Online   CISTI, Canadian Online Enquiry Service CAN/OLE

File name	CAB
Start year	
Number of records	
Update period	
Price/Charges	Connect time: Canadian $40.00
	Online print: Canadian $0.45
	Offline print: Canadian $0.45

Notes

CISTI accessible only in Canada. US$ 26.50 royalty per connect hour; print charges in US dollars

12:94. Online   Data-Star

File name	CABI
Start year	1984
Number of records	1,000,000
Update period	Monthly
Database aids	Data-Star Biomedical, Business and Chemical Manuals. and Online manual (search NEWS-CABI in NEWS)
Price	SFr1.04
	Subscription: SFr80.00
	Connect time: SFr50.80
	Online print: SFr127.00
	Offline print: SFr1.01
	SDI charge: SFr12.40

Downloading is allowed
Thesaurus is online

Notes

From June 1993 Data-Star have introduced an annual fee/subscription per contract (that is, not per password) of SFr 80.00 (c.UK£ 32.00) payable every June. For North American customers billed in dollars who also use DIALOG, the DIALOG fee also covers access to Data-Star. Academic customers, 'commitment' customers and customers currently billed in dollars are exempt.

Record composition

Abstract AB; Accession Number and Update Code AN; Article Type AT; Author(s) AU; Author Affiliation IN; Descriptors DE; Foreign Title TT; Geographic Descriptor CN; ISBN Number IS; Language of summary in original LS; Original Language LG; Publication Year YR; References AV; Section heading(s) SC; Source SO; Title TI; Update Code UP and Updated Code UD

12:95. Online   DIALOG, Knowledge Index

File name	File 50
Start year	1972 – 1983
Number of records	13,000
Update period	Monthly
Price/Charges	Connect time: US$54.00
	Online print: US$0.90
	Offline print: US$0.90
	SDI charge: US$15.00

Downloading is allowed
Thesaurus is online

Notes

This database is also available to home users during evenings and weekends at a reduced rate on the Knowledge Index service of DIALOG – file name in this case is CAB ABSTRACTS, and searches are made with simplified commands or menus.

DIALINDEX Categories: AGRI, BIOTECH, CAB, ENVIRON, FOODSCI, LEISURE, NUTRIT, VETSCI. The One-Search facility enables the two files of AGRICOLA, the one file of AGRIS and the two files of CAB to be searched simultaneously.

12:96. Online   DIALOG, Knowledge Index

File name	File 53
Start year	1984
Number of records	2,500,000
Update period	Monthly
Price/Charges	Connect time: US$54.00
	Online print: US$0.90
	Offline print: US$0.90

Downloading is allowed

Notes

This database is also available to home users during evenings and weekends at a reduced rate on the Knowledge Index service of DIALOG – file name in this case is CAB ABSTRACTS, and searches are made with simplified commands or menus.

DIALINDEX Categories: AGRI, BIOTECH, CAB, ENVIRON, FOODSCI, LEISURE, NUTRIT, VETSCI.

12:97. Online   DIMDI

File name	CV72
Software	GRIPS
Start year	1972
Number of records	2,842,569
Update period	Monthly
SDI period	1 month
Database aids	Memocard CAB ABSTRACTS and User Manual CAB ABSTRACTS
Price/Charges	Connect time: UK£18.74–22.53
	Online print: UK£0.40–0.58
	Offline print: UK£0.33–0.40

Downloading is allowed
Thesaurus is online

Notes

Contains all citations included in the abstract journals of the CAB. Abstracted records are 82% of the total. The unit record contains information about author(s), title and other bibliographic data as well as institutions, keywords, subunit(s) and abstracts (eighty-four per cent). More complex subjects or clearly defined subject areas are represented in the following DIMDI subfiles consisting of one or several subunits which can be used like individual databases: CAB Ado; CAB Animal; CAB Animal Products; CAB Economics; CAB Engineering; CAB Forestry; CAB Human; CAB Nutrition; CAB Plant; CAB Plant Protection; CAB Leisure Recreation Tourism; CAB Veterinary Science. Suppliers of online documents: British Library Document Supply Centre, Boston Spa, England; Harkers Information Retrieval System, Sydney, Australia; Instituto de Informacion y Documentacion en Ciencia y Tecnologia, Madrid, Spain; Universitätsbibliothek und TIB, Hannover, Germany; Zentralbibliothek der Landbauwissenschaft, Bonn, Germany.

Record composition

Additional Author AA; Abstract AB; Abstractor's Initials AI; Abstract Language AL; Author AU; Author's Variants AV; Classification Code CC; Corporate Author CA; Corporate Source CS; Controlled Terms CT; Decimal Code DC; Document Type DT; Entry Date ED; Entry Month EM; Free Text FT; Geographical Codes GC; Geographical Heading GH; Journal Title JT; Language LA; Abstract Number NA; Document Number ND; Cross Reference Number NX; Original Field OF; Order Number OD; Publisher's Name PU; Preprocessed Searches PPS; Publication Year PY; ISBN SB; Section Code SC; Subfile SF; Section Headings SH; Source SO; Secondary Journal Source SSO; Subunit SU and Title TI

The Basic Index includes the data fields: Title, Abstract, Controlled Term, Section Heading, Geographical Heading. Controlled Terms from 1984 correspond to the polyhierarchic structured CAB thesaurus; prior to 1984: mixture of terms. Access points with Producer's equivalent name in brackets: Subunits (SU) (Abstract Journals); Section Codes (SC) (Sequencing Code Numbers); Section Headings (SH) (Section Headings); Decimal Codes (DC) (Decimal Codes); Geographical Codes (GC) (Geographical Codes); Controlled Terms (CT) Subject Index Entries; Geographical Headings (GH) Countries.

12:98. Online   ESA-IRS

File name	File 16
Start year	1972–1985
Number of records	1,900,000
Update period	Closed File
Price/Charges	Subscription: UK£70.29
	Database entry fee: UK£3.51
	Online print: UK£0.07 – 0.60
	Offline print: UK£0.64
	SDI charge: UK£2.46

Downloading is allowed
Thesaurus is online

Notes

From 1993 ESA-IRS are charging an annual fee of 100 Accounting Units (c.UK£ 70.29) to all users. This is equivalent to the fee for full documentation and will not be charged to customers already paying for documentation.

Record composition

Abstract /AB; Abstract Journal AJ; Author AU; Bureau Bees Decimal Code (1) BD; CAB Record No. NR; Classification Code CC; Classification Name CN; Controlled Terms /CT; Corporate Source CS; Fertilizer Decimal Code (1) SD; Journal Announcement (Updates) UP; Journal Name JN; Language LA; Native Number NN; Publication Year PY; Publisher PB; Summary Language SL; Title /TI and UDC Number UC

12:99. Online   ESA-IRS

File name	File 124
Start year	1986+
Number of records	760,000
Update period	Monthly
Price/Charges	Subscription: UK£70.29
	Database entry fee: UK£3.51
	Online print: UK£0.07 – 0.60
	Offline print: UK£0.64
	SDI charge: UK£2.46

Downloading is allowed
Thesaurus is online

Notes

From 1993 ESA-IRS are charging an annual fee of 100 Accounting Units (c.UK£ 70.29) to all users. This is equivalent to the fee for full documentation and will not be charged to customers already paying for documentation.

Record composition

Abstract /AB; Abstract Journal AJ; Author AU; Bureau Bees Decimal Code (1) BD; CAB Record No. NR; Classification Code CC; Classification Name CN; Controlled Terms /CT; Corporate Source CS; Fertilizer Decimal Code (1) SD; Journal Announcement (Updates) UP; Journal Name JN; Language LA; Native Number NN; Publication Year PY; Publisher PB; Summary Language SL; Title /TI and UDC Number UC

12:100. Online   ESA-IRS

File name	File 132
Start year	1972+
Number of records	2,600,000
Update period	Monthly

Price/Charges

Subscription: UK£70.29
Database entry fee: UK£3.51
Online print: UK£0.07 – 0.60
Offline print: UK£0.64
SDI charge: UK£2.46

Downloading is allowed
Thesaurus is online

Notes

From 1993 ESA-IRS are charging an annual fee of 100 Accounting Units (c.UK£ 70.29) to all users. This is equivalent to the fee for full documentation and will not be charged to customers already paying for documentation.

Record composition

Abstract /AB; Abstract Journal AJ; Author AU; Bureau Bees Decimal Code (1) BD; CAB Record No. NR; Classification Code CC; Classification Name CN; Controlled Terms /CT; Corporate Source CS; Fertilizer Decimal Code (1) SD; Journal Announcement (Updates) UP; Journal Name JN; Language LA; Native Number NN; Publication Year PY; Publisher PB; Summary Language SL; Title /TI and UDC Number UC

12:101. Online — Japan Information Center of Science and Technology (JICST)

File name: CABA
Start year: 1979
Number of records: 1,590,000
Update period: Monthly
Price/Charges:
Connect time: US$55.00
Online print: US$0.20
Offline print: US$0.20
SDI charge: US$11.48

Downloading is allowed

Record composition

Abstract AB; Accession Number AN; Author AU; Broader Terms BT; Classification Codes CC; Controlled Terms CT; Corporate Source CS; Country of Publication CY; Document Type DT; Language LA; Source SO and Title TI

12:102. Online — STN

File name: CABA
Start year: 1979
Number of records: 1,900,000
Update period: Monthly
Price/Charges:
Connect time: DM85.00
Online print: DM1.34
Offline print: DM1.42
SDI charge: DM17.57

Also available on JICST.

12:103. Online — University of Tsukuba

File name: CAB Abstracts
Start year:
Number of records:
Update period:

Notes

Access through University of Tsukuba limited to affiliates of the University of Japan.

12:104. CD-ROM — SilverPlatter

File name: CABCD Vol.1 1984–86
Format notes: IBM, Mac, NEC
Software: SPIRS
Start year: 1984–1986

Number of records:
Update period: Annually
Database aids: Silverplatter CAB User Manual, Quick Reference Cards and SPIRS User Manual
Price/Charges: Subscription: UK£1,425–2,850
Thesaurus is online

Notes

Nearly sixty-five per cent of the records are drawn from English language sources, the remainder from articles in over 75 languages. Approximately ninety-five per cent of records have an English language abstract. CABCD has 930,000 records in total, with 130,000 records being added each year. It is available in separate discs as four volumes to date, dating from 1984 through to 1995. There are various price ranges depending on number of volumes purchased. Vol.1, 1984–1986, costs UK£ 1,425 for single users, £2,850 for 2–8 networked users.

Record composition

English language title; foreign language title (where appropriate); author; author's address; source title; citation details; publication year; publication type; language of original document; summary language; abstract; subject index terms; geographic index terms and subfile codes (CABI Abstract Journal code)

The Index command can be used to provide access to a list of all words, descriptors and hyphenated phrases which have been indexed in the free-text fields. The index excludes information present in the limit fields, such as language and date. The index is arranged alphabetically word by word, and can be browsed and terms selected which are then searched for automatically using the OR operator.

12:105. CD-ROM — SilverPlatter

File name: CABCD Vol.2 1987–89
Format notes: IBM, Mac, NEC
Software: SPIRS
Start year: 1987–1989
Number of records:
Update period: Annually
Database aids: Silverplatter CAB User Manual, Quick Reference Cards and SPIRS User Manual
Price/Charges: Subscription: UK£2,850 5,700
Thesaurus is online

Notes

Nearly sixty-five per cent of the records are drawn from English language sources, the remainder from articles in over 75 languages. Approximately ninety-five per cent of records have an English language abstract. This is the second volume of CABCD. CABCD has 930,000 records in total, with 130,000 records being added each year. It is available in separate discs as four volumes to date, dating from 1984 through to 1995. There are various price ranges depending on number of volumes purchased: Vol.2, 1987–1989, £2,850 for single users, £5,700 for 2–8 networked users.

Record composition

English language title; foreign language title (where appropriate); author; author's address; source title; citation details; publication year; publication type; language of original document; summary language; abstract; subject index terms; geographic index terms and subfile codes (CABI Abstract Journal code)

The Index command can be used to provide access to a list of all words, descriptors and hyphenated phrases which have been indexed in the free-text fields. The index excludes information present in the limit fields, such as language and date. The index is arranged alphabetically word by word, and can be browsed and terms selected which are then searched for automatically using the OR operator.

12:106. CD-ROM   SilverPlatter

File name	CABCD Vol.3 1990–92
Format notes	IBM, Mac, NEC
Software	SPIRS
Start year	1990–92
Number of records	
Update period	Annually
Database aids	Silverplatter CAB User Manual, Quick Reference Cards and SPIRS User Manual
Price/Charges	Subscription: UK£1,710–9,000
Thesaurus is online	

Notes

Nearly sixty-five per cent of the records are drawn from English language sources, the remainder from articles in over 75 languages. Approximately ninety-five per cent of records have an English language abstract. CABCD has 930,000 records in total, with 130,000 records being added each year. This is the third volume of CABCD. It is available in separate discs as four volumes to date, dating from 1984 through to 1995. There are various price ranges depending on number of volumes purchased: Vol.3, 1990–1992, £3,845 for single users, £7,690 for 2–8 networked users; Vol.3 1992 renewal purchase £1,710 for single users, £3,420 for 2–8 networked users.

Record composition

English language title; foreign language title (where appropriate); author; author's address; source title; citation details; publication year; publication type; language of original document; summary language; abstract; subject index terms; geographic index terms and subfile codes (CABI Abstract Journal code)

The Index command can be used to provide access to a list of all words, descriptors and hyphenated phrases which have been indexed in the free-text fields. The index excludes information present in the limit fields, such as language and date. The index is arranged alphabetically word by word, and can be browsed and terms selected which are then searched for automatically using the OR operator.

12:107. CD-ROM   SilverPlatter

File name	CABCD Vol.4 1993–95
Format notes	IBM, Mac, NEC
Software	SPIRS
Start year	1993–95
Number of records	
Update period	Annually
Database aids	Silverplatter CAB User Manual, Quick Reference Cards and SPIRS User Manual
Price/Charges	Subscription: UK£4,500 – 9,000
Thesaurus is online	

Notes

Nearly sixty-five per cent of the records are drawn from English language sources, the remainder from articles in over 75 languages. Approximately ninety-five per cent of records have an English language abstract. This is the prospective fourth volume of CABCD. CABCD has 930,000 records in total, with 130,000 records being added each year. It is available

in separate discs as four volumes to date, dating from 1984 through to 1995. There are various price ranges depending on number of volumes purchased: Vol.4 1993–1995 £4,500 for single users, £9,000 for 2–8 networked users. Prices on application for purchase of Vol.4 1993.

Record composition

English language title; foreign language title (where appropriate); author; author's address; source title; citation details; publication year; publication type; language of original document; summary language; abstract; subject index terms; geographic index terms and subfile codes (CABI Abstract Journal code)

The Index command can be used to provide access to a list of all words, descriptors and hyphenated phrases which have been indexed in the free-text fields. The index excludes information present in the limit fields, such as language and date. The index is arranged alphabetically word by word, and can be browsed and terms selected which are then searched for automatically using the OR operator.

12:108. Diskette   CAB International

File name	CABI Abstract Journals on Floppy Disk
Format notes	IBM
Start year	
Number of records	
Update period	Same as for printed journal
Price/Charges	

Notes

Any one of the CAB International Abstract Journals may be received on floppy disk, according to the purchaser's requirements. Update frequency is the same as for the particular printed journal (monthly, bimonthly or quarterly). Price is double the cost of the equivalent printed journal. The diskettes are supplied without retrieval software, but the subscriber has the choice of three formats – comma delimited, CDS-ISIS or Pro-Cite – to enable use with most commercial database management software, with Micro CDS-ISIS or with Pro-Cite.

12:109. Database subset

Online   Data-Star

File name	VETS – CAB: Veterinary Science/Medicine
Start year	1984
Number of records	150,000
Update period	Monthly
Database aids	Data-Star Biomedical Manual
Price/Charges	Subscription: SFr80.00
	Connect time: SFr127.00
	Online print: SFr1.01
	Offline print: SFr1.04
	SDI charge: SFr12.40
Downloading is allowed	
Thesaurus is online	

Notes

A bibliographic source of information on all aspects of veterinary science and medicine. Documents comprising bibliographic details with or without an abstract are included for literature on all aspects of veterinary medicine. Subjects covered include: diseases of livestock, poultry, pets, laboratory animals, zoo animals, farmed fish and shellfish and certain wild animals; anatomy, physiology, biochemistry, pharmacology, surgery, radiography, toxicology, immunology and immunogenetics of domestic animals; bacteriology, virology, mycology, protozoology, helminthology and entomology related to animal diseases; zoonoses; meat inspection and economics of animal diseases.

Abstracts sources include: Veterinary Bulletin, *Index Veterinarius* and *Small Animal Abstracts* and, in part, *Helminthological Abstracts, Review of Medical and Veterinary Entomology; Protozoological Abstracts, Review of Medical and Veterinary Mycology, Animal Breeding Abstrats, Dairy Science Abstracts* and *Nutrition Abstracts and Reviews Series B, Livestock Feeds and Feeding.*

From June 1993 Data-Star have introduced an annual fee/subscription per contract (that is, not per password) of SFr 80.00 (c.UK£ 32.00) payable every June. For North American customers billed in dollars who also use DIALOG, the DIALOG fee also covers access to Data-Star. Academic customers, 'commitment' customers and customers currently billed in dollars are exempt.

Record composition
Abstract AB; Accession Number and Update Code AN; Article Type AT; Author AU; Author Affiliation IN; Description DE; Foreign Title TT; Geographic Descriptor CN; ISBN Number IS; Language of Original Summary; Original Language LG; Publication Year YR; Section code and heading SC; Source SO; Title TI and Update Code UP

12:110. Database subset

Online   **DIALOG, Knowledge Index**

File name	File 250 – ONTAP CAB Abstracts Training File
Start year	January – March 1985
Number of records	34,388
Update period	Closed File
Price/Charges	Connect time: US$15.00

Notes
The low-cost training file containing records from the January to March 1985 updates to File 50, the main CAB Abstracts file on DIALOG. Offline prints are not available in ONTAP files.

12:111. Database subset

Online   **DIMDI**

File name	C980 – CAB ADO
Alternative name(s)	Animal Disease Occurrence
Start year	1980
Number of records	
Update period	Twice a year
Price/Charges	Connect time: UK£18.74–22.53
	Online print: UK£0.40–0.58
	Offline print: UK£0.33–0.40

Downloading is allowed

Notes
Equivalent to the printed: *Animal Disease Occurrence.* Covers epidemiology of animal diseases. Contains records on the incidence of animal diseases worldwide. Data include the country of occurrence, number of animals affected, duration of the disease, number of deaths, and economic effects. Each record includes a citation to the source publication. All documents have abstracts. Approximately ninety per cent of the ADO documents are also published in the *Veterinary Bulletin* but without additional factual data.

12:112. Database subset

Online   **DIMDI**

File name	CX72 – CAB ANIMAL
Start year	1972
Number of records	1,629,488
Update period	Monthly
SDI period	1 month

Price/Charges	Connect time: UK£18.74–22.53
	Online print: UK£0.40–0.58
	Offline print: UK£0.33–0.40

Downloading is allowed

Notes
Contains the animal-relevant documents of CAB Abstracts. Journals referenced: *Animal Breeding Abstracts; Apicultural Abstracts; Dairy Science Abstracts; Helminthological Abstracts (A. Animal and Human); Index Veterinarius; Review of Applied Entomology (B. Medical and Veterinary); Review of Applied Entomology (B. Medical and Veterinary); Review of Medical and Veterinary Mycology; Nutrition Abstracts and Reviews (A. Human and Experimental)* (from 1977); *World Agricultural Economics and Rural Sociology Abstracts; Nutrition Abstracts and Reviews (A.Human and Experimental); Veterinary Bulletin; Protozoological Abstracts* (from 1977); *Nutrition Abstracts* (1973–1976); *Rural Extension, Education and Training Abstracts* (from 1978); *Rural Development Abstracts; Animal Disease Occurence; Leisure, Recreation and Tourism Abstracts; Poultry Abstracts; Pig News and Information; Biocontrol News and Information; Biodeterioration Abstracts; Small Animal Abstracts; Agricultural Engineering Abstracts.* Searches are possible from January 1972. 70% of the records have abstracts.

12:113. Database subset

Online   **DIMDI**

File name	C773 – CAB ANIMAL PROD
Start year	1972
Number of records	541,364
Update period	Monthly
SDI period	1 month
Price/Charges	Connect time: UK£18.74–22.53
	Online print: UK£0.40–0.58
	Offline print: UK£0.33–0.40

Downloading is allowed

Notes
Contains the relevant citations on animal breeding and production from CAB Abstracts. Journals referenced: *Animal Breeding Abstracts; Dairy Science Abstracts; Nutrition Abstracts and Reviews (B. Livestock Feeds and Feeding); Nutrition Abstracts* (1973–1976); *Poultry Abstracts; Pig News and Information.* Searches are possible from January 1973. 95% of thte records have abstracts.

CAB ANIMAL PROD is defined as subfile to CAB ABASTRACTS with: FIND SU=(0A;0D;0N;1N;2N; 7A;7D).

12:114. Database subset

Online   **DIMDI**

File name	C872 – CAB VET SCIENCE
Start year	1972
Number of records	678,064
Update period	Monthly
SDI period	1 month
Price/Charges	Connect time: UK£18.74–22.53
	Online print: UK£0.40–0.58
	Offline print: UK£0.33–0.40

Downloading is allowed

Notes
Contains citations on veterinary science from CAB Abstracts. Journals referenced: *Helminothological Abstracts (A. Animal and Human); Index Veterinarius; Review of Applied Entomology (B. Medical and Veterinary); Review of Medical and Veterinary Mycology; Veterinary Bulletin; Protozoological*

Abstracts (from 1977); *Animal Disease Occurrence* (from 1980); *Small Animal Abstracts* (from 1984). Searches are possible from January 1972. 95% of the records have abstracts.

CAB VET SCIENCE is defined as subfile to CAB ABSTRACTS with: FIND SU= (0H;0I;0L;0V;0Y; 2V;7V).

12:115. Database subset

Online	ESA-IRS
File name	File 112 – Training CAB Abstracts
Start year	1984/5
Number of records	28,000
Update period	None
Thesaurus is online	

Notes

Training file and subset of the full CAB Abstracts file which has the file numbers 16 (1972–1985), 124 (1986 to date) and 132 (1972 to date). It is available at a low access fee for user training. Services such as offline prints, automatic current awareness and document ordering are not available with the training file.

Record composition

Abstract /AB; Abstract Journal AJ; Author AU; CAB Record Number NR; Classification Codes CC; Classification Names CN; Controlled Terms /CT; Corporate Source CS; Journal Announcement (Updates) UP; Journal Name JN; Language LA; Native Accession Number NN; Publication Year PY; Publisher PB; Summary Language SL; Title /TI and UDC Numbers UC

12:116. Database subset

CD-ROM	SilverPlatter
File name	BeastCD (CAB Spectrum series)
Alternative name(s)	CABBeastCD (CAB Spectrum series)
Format notes	IBM, Mac, NEC
Software	SPIRS/MacSPIRS
Start year	1973
Number of records	340,000
Update period	Annually
Price	UK£2,890 – 5,780
	Subscription: UK£910 – 1,820

Notes

Subset of CAB Abstracts database covering: animal breeding and production, animal nutrition, dairy science and technology; management and biotechnology of economically valuable animals and of laboratory species relevant to agriculture. Contains all records published in *Animal Breeding Abstracts* (1983–), *Nutrition Abstracts and Reviews-Series B: Livestock Feeds and Feeding* (1931–) and relevant records from *Dairy Science Abstracts* (1939–), *Pig News and Information, Poultry Abstracts* and *AgBiotech News and Information*. Animals covered include farm mammals of economic importance; laboratory mammals; poultry; game and other birds of economic importance; fish, molluscs, and crustaceans; and certain invertebrates used in genetic studies. Subjects covered include performance traits and products; breeding and genetics; biotechnology; reproduction; nutrition; the dairy industry; housing and equipment for livestock and in aquaculture; and non-genetic effects on animals and traits.

A full set of archival discs covering 1973–1991 is available for outright purchase at UK£ 2,890 for single user, £5,780 for 2–8 networked users (member country). Annual renewal costs are £910 for single users, £1,820 for 2–8 networked users (member country). There are various journals options and print/updates prices on application to CAB or SilverPLatter. There is also a VETCD/BEASTCD combined set available: full set £5,495 for single users, £10,990 for 2–8 networked users; annual renewal £1,655 for single users, £3,310 for 2–8 networked users.

In-depth indexing, using controlled terms from the *CAB Thesaurus*

This database can also be found on:
Human Nutrition on CD-ROM

Cambridge Scientific Abstracts Engineering
Cambridge Information Group

12:118. Master record

Alternative name(s)	CSAE; Hard Sciences
Database type	Bibliographic, Factual
Number of journals	
Sources	Journals, Monographs, Conference proceedings, Technical reports, Patents, Theses and Dissertations
Start year	1981
Language	English
Coverage	International
Number of records	450,000
Update size	–
Update period	Monthly

Keywords

Computer Science; Health and Safety; Mechanical Engineering; Safety; Occupational Health and Safety

Description

A superfile, comprising five subfiles, providing access to the following abstracting services:

Electronics and Communications Abstracts;
ISMEC: Mechanical Engineering Abstracts;
Computer and Information Systems Abstracts;
Solid State/Superconductivity Abstracts;
Health and Safety Science Abstracts.

It includes references selected from a wide range of worldwide literature including journals, government reports, technical reports, conference proceedings, dissertations, theses and patents. Subject coverage includes: communications, telecommunications, information and computer sciences, electronics, medicine, health and safety and mechanical engineering.

12:119. Online

	BRS
File name	Cambridge Scientific Abstracts Engineering
Alternative name(s)	CSAE; Hard Sciences
Start year	
Number of records	
Update period	Monthly

12:120. Online

	ESA-IRS
File name	Hard Sciences
Alternative name(s)	Cambridge Scientific Abstracts Engineering; CSAE
Start year	1981
Number of records	454,000 (October 1991)
Update period	Monthly

Notes

Comprises five subfiles corresponding to the following:
ISMEC: Mechanical Engineering Abstracts;
Solid State/Superconductivity Abstracts;

Electronics and Communications Abstracts;
Computer and Information Systems Abstracts; and
Health and Safety Science Abstracts.

From 1993 ESA-IRS are charging an annual fee of
100 Accounting Units (c.UK£ 70.29) to all users. This
is equivalent to the fee for full documentation and will
not be charged to customers already paying for
documentation.

For more details of constituent databases, see:
Electronics and Communications Abstracts
ISMEC: Mechanical Engineering Abstracts
Computer and Information Systems Abstracts
Solid State/Superconductivity Abstracts
Health and Safety Science Abstracts

Cambridge Scientific Abstracts Life Sciences
Cambridge Scientific Abstracts

12:122. Master record

Alternative name(s)	CSAL
Database type	Bibliographic
Number of journals	
Sources	Journals, Books, Conference papers, Technical reports, Patents, Theses and Dissertations
Start year	1978
Language	English
Coverage	International
Number of records	1,164,810
Update size	–
Update period	Monthly

Keywords

Acute Poisoning; Aging; Air Pollution; Algology;
Amino-Acids; Anatomy; Antibiotics; Aquaculture;
Atmospheric Science; Bacteriology; Behavioural
Ecology; Bioengineering; Biological Membranes;
Biotechnology; Bone Disease; Calcium Metabolism;
Chemoreception; Chronic Poisoning; Clinical
Medicine; Clinical Toxicology; DNA; Drugs; Ecology;
Ecosystems; Endocrinology; Entomology –
Agricultural; Entomology – Applied; Entomology –
Human; Entomology – Veterinary; Environmental
Biology; Ethology; Genetic Engineering; Hazardous
Substances; HIV; Histology; Human Ecology;
Immune Disorders; Immunology; Infectious
Diseases; Land Pollution; Marine Biotechnology;
Marine Engineering; Microbiology; Molecular Biology;
Molecular Neurobiology; Mycology; Naval
Engineering; Noise Pollution; Oceanography;
Neurology; Neuropharmacology; Neurophysiology –
Animal; Neuroscience; Nucleic Acids; Nutrition;
Oncology; Occupational Health and Safety;
Osteoporosis; Osteomalacia; Pathology; Peptides;
Pharmaceuticals; Pheromones; Physiology;
Pollution; Proteins; Protozoology; Psychophysics;
Public Health; Radiation; Rhinology; RNA; Sleep;
Smoking; Substance Abuse; Taste Perception;
Thermal Pollution; Viral Genetics; Water; Water
Pollution

Description

A superfile providing access to the following abstracting services:

Life Sciences Collection;
Aquatic Sciences and Fisheries Abstracts;

Oceanic Abstracts;
Pollution Abstracts.

Covers the worldwide technical literature on medical
and biological disciplines from journals, books, conference papers, technical reports, patents, theses and
dissertations.

12:123. Online   BRS

File name	Cambridge Scientific Abstracts Life Sciences
Alternative name(s)	CSAL
Start year	1978
Number of records	1,164,810
Update period	Monthly

Notes

A superfile providing access to the following abstracting services: the Life Science Collection, Aquatic
Sciences and Fisheries Abstracts, Oceanic Abstracts
and Pollution Abstracts.

For more details of constituent databases, see:
Life Sciences Collection
Aquatic Sciences and Fisheries Abstracts
Oceanic Abstracts
Pollution Abstracts

Cancerlit
National Cancer Institute, US National Institutes of Health

12:125. Master record

Alternative name(s)	Cancer Literature Online
Database type	Bibliographic
Number of journals	3,500+
Sources	Conference proceedings, dissertations, government publications, journals, meeting abstracts, monographs, reports, symposia, technical reports and theses
Start year	1963
Language	English
Coverage	International
Number of records	778,000+
Update size	100,000
Update period	Monthly
Index unit	Articles
Abstract details	Authors
Thesaurus	Medical Subject Headings (MeSH) (from 1980); annual editions
Database aids	MeSH Tree Structures; annual editions, MeSH Permuted Terms; annual editions and Gene Symbols (from 1991)

Keywords

Cancer; Oncology; Immunology; Pathology

Description

Contains citations, with abstracts, to the worldwide
literature on oncological epidemiology, pathology,
treatment, and research. The database covers the
treatment of cancer as well as information on epidemiology, pathogenesis and immunology. Another important aspect is chemical, physical and viral
carcinogenesis. Subject coverage within oncology:
biochemistry, biology, carcinogenesis (viral, chemical,
other), epidemiology, genetics, growth factors, im-

munology, mutagents – mutagenicity, pathology, physiology, physiopathology, pathogenesis and prevention. Approximately eighty per cent of references are stored with an English abstract, all documents between 1963 and 1983 having abstracts. Since 1977 proceedings of meetings, mongraphs, theses and Government and symposia reports have been included. The database contains information from approximately seventy countries.

References are included from: *Cancer Therapy Abstracts* (formerly *Cancer Chemotherapy Abstracts* 1967–80) and *Carcinogenesis Abstracts* from 1963–1976. From 1977 citations are taken only from primary publications. From June 1983 all citations from MEDLINE with an oncological content are automatically transferred to CANCERLIT. They are marked in the data field SEC with SEC=MEDL and SEC =L. From June 1983 85% of the citations are from MEDLINE. As the rate of abstracts is approximately 60% in MEDLINE, a decline in the rate of abstracts is expected. All non-MEDLINE-derived documents still have 100% English abstracts. Databases providing citations: MEDLINE; Carcinogenesis Abstracts – CARC (only up to 1979); Cancer Therapy Abstracts (only up to 1979); Herner & Company (as from 1982 – some meeting abstracts) International Cancer Research Data Bank Program (most non-MEDLINE derived records). *Oncology Abstracts*, the print equivalent has been available since 1986. Biomedical journals account for approximately eighty-six per cent of sources, reports twelve per cent, monographs one per cent and these one per cent. Cancerlit contains documents in about forty languages.

Before 1980 documents were not indexed with any vocabulary. From 1980, *MeSH* is used for indexing and the hierarchical structure of *MeSH* makes it possible to search for a whole group of related descriptors in one step. Since January 1985 new records have been indexed with chemical names and CAS Registry/EC numbers. Corresponds in part to the printed *Index Medicus*.

12:126. Online   BLAISE-LINK

File name	CANCERLIT
Alternative name(s)	Cancer Literature On-Line
Start year	1963
Number of records	
Update period	Monthly

12:127. Online   BRS, BRS After Dark, BRS/Colleague

File name	CANR
Alternative name(s)	Cancer Literature On-Line
Start year	
Number of records	
Update period	Monthly
Price/Charges	Connect time: US$26.00/36.00
	Online print: US$0.07/0.15
	Offline print: US$0.20
	SDI charge: US$5.60

12:128. Online   CISTI MEDLARS

File name	CANCERLIT
Alternative name(s)	Cancer Literature On-Line
Start year	1963
Number of records	625,000+
Update period	Monthly

12:129. Online   CompuServe Information Service

File name	IQUEST File 1931
Alternative name(s)	Cancer Literature On-Line
Start year	1980
Number of records	
Update period	Monthly
Price/Charges	Subscription: US$8.95 per month
	Database entry fee: US$9/search; some databases carry a surcharge ($2–75)
	Online print: US$10 references free; then $9 per ten; abstracts $3 each

Downloading is allowed

Notes
Accessed via IQUEST or IQMEDICAL, this database is offered by a BRS gateway. IQUEST can either search across all databases, a database of the user's choice or selected multiple databases.

12:130. Online   Data-Star

File name	CANC
Alternative name(s)	Cancer Literature On-Line
Start year	1983+
Number of records	
Update period	Monthly
Database aids	Data-Star Biomedical Manual and Online manual (search NEWS-CANC in NEWS)
Price/Charges	Subscription: SFr80.00
	Connect time: SFr78.00
	Online print: SFr0.00–0.18
	Offline print: SFr0.21–0.24
	SDI charge: SFr6.80

Downloading is allowed
Thesaurus is online

Notes
From June 1993 Data-Star have introduced an annual fee/subscription per contract (that is, not per password) of SFr 80.00 (c.UK£ 32.00) payable every June. For North American customers billed in dollars who also use DIALOG, the DIALOG fee also covers access to Data-Star. Academic customers, 'commitment' customers and customers currently billed in dollars are exempt.

Record composition
Abstract AB; Accession Number AN; Author(s) AU; Author Affiliation IN; CAS Registry Number or Enzyme Commission Number RN; Comment CM; Descriptors DE; Entry Month EM; Gene symbol GE; Journal Code JC; Journal Subset SB; Language of Original LG; Original Language Title TT; Publication Type PT; Secondary Source Identifier SI; Source SO; Title TI and Year of Publication YR

12:131. Online   Data-Star

File name	CAZZ
Alternative name(s)	Cancer Literature On-Line
Start year	1963
Number of records	778,662
Update period	Monthly
Database aids	Data-Star Biomedical Manual and Online manual (search NEWS-CANC in NEWS)
Price/Charges	Subscription: SFr80.00
	Connect time: SFr78.00
	Online print: SFr0.00–0.18
	Offline print: SFr0.21–0.24
	SDI charge: SFr6.80

Downloading is allowed
Thesaurus is online

Notes
From June 1993 Data-Star have introduced an annual fee/subscription per contract (that is, not per password) of SFr 80.00 (c.UK£ 32.00) payable every June. For North American customers billed in dollars who

also use DIALOG, the DIALOG fee also covers access to Data-Star. Academic customers, 'commitment' customers and customers currently billed in dollars are exempt.

Record composition

Abstract AB; Accession Number AN; Author(s) AU; Author Affiliation IN; CAS Registry Number or Enzyme Commission Number RN; Comment CM; Descriptors DE; Entry Month EM; Gene symbol GE; Journal Code JC; Journal Subset SB; Language of Original LG; Original Language Title TT; Publication Type PT; Secondary Source Identifier SI; Source SO; Title TI and Year of Publication YR

12:132. Online   Data-Star

File name	CANX
Alternative name(s)	Cancer Literature On-Line
Start year	Latest month
Number of records	
Update period	Monthly
Database aids	Data-Star Biomedical Manual
Price/Charges	Subscription: SFr80.00
	Connect time: SFr78.00
	Online print: SFr0.00–0.18
	Offline print: SFr0.21–0.24
	SDI charge: SFr6.80

Downloading is allowed
Thesaurus is online

Notes

From June 1993 Data-Star have introduced an annual fee/subscription per contract (that is, not per password) of SFr 80.00 (c.UK£ 32.00) payable every June. For North American customers billed in dollars who also use DIALOG, the DIALOG fee also covers access to Data-Star. Academic customers, 'commitment' customers and customers currently billed in dollars are exempt.

Record composition

Abstract AB; Accession Number AN; Author(s) AU; Author Affiliation IN; CAS Registry Number or Enzyme Commission Number RN; Comment CM; Descriptors DE; Entry Month EM; Gene symbol GE; Journal Code JC; Journal Subset SB; Language of Original LG; Original Language Title TT; Publication Type PT; Secondary Source Identifier SI; Source SO; Title TI and Year of Publication YR

12:133. Online   DIALOG, Knowledge Index

File name	File 159
Alternative name(s)	Cancer Literature On-Line
Start year	1963
Number of records	823,103
Update period	Monthly
Price/Charges	Connect time: US$36.00
	Online print: US$0.12
	Offline print: US$0.12
	SDI charge: US$5.25

Notes

This database is also available to home users during evenings and weekends at a reduced rate on the Knowledge Index service of DIALOG – file name in this case is Cancerlit, and searches are made with simplified commands or menus.

DIALINDEX Categories: MEDICINE, RNMED

12:134. Online   DIMDI

File name	CL80
Alternative name(s)	Cancer Literature On-Line
Software	GRIPS
Start year	1980
Number of records	786,183
Update period	Monthly
SDI period	1 month
Database aids	Memocard CANCERLIT and User Manual MEDLINE, AIDSLINE, BIOETHICSLINE, CANCERLIT, HEALTH
Price/Charges	Connect time: UK£5.84–10.58
	Online print: UK£0.17–0.35
	Offline print: UK£0.09–0.15

Downloading is allowed
Thesaurus is online

Notes

File CL80 covers the period 1980 to date. Suppliers of online documents: British Library Document Supply Centre, Boston Spa, England; Bayerische Statts-bibliothek München, München, Germany; Harkers Information Retrieval System, Sydney, Australia; Institute for Scientific Information, Philadelphia, USA; Koninklijke Nederlandse Akademie van Wetenschapen, Amsterdam, The Nederlands; Zentralbibliothek der Medizin, Köln, Germany.

German author names with a dipthong (ä,ö,ü) are treated differently from MEDLINE (in MEDLINE ae;oe;ue). In CANCERLIT the 'e' of the umlaut is usually deleted and it is recommended to use the truncation symbol (#). For example, Alfred Müller (F AU=MULLER A OR AU = MUELLER A, or F AU = MU#LLER (preferable). Deviating from MEDLINE, the numerical code carries a prefix in CANCERLIT indicating the secondary source of a citation. The Number of Report is the Cancergram identification number, available from 1978. Cancergrams are monthly current awareness publications of the National Cancer Institute with over 60 different subject related bulletins. Articles are selected by scientists. The first four characters identify the Cancergram series and the last four digits identify the publication month and year of the particular Cancergram issue. Approximately one-third of records carry one or more Cancergram Numbers which are assigned to records annually in January. The Secondary Source Identifier is the secondary supplier or source of a citation. Deviating from MEDLINE, AIDSLINE and HEALTH, only the following abbreviations without numerical codes are used in CANCERLIT: CARTH – Carcinogenesis Abstracts; CATH – Cancer Therapy Abstracts; HERN – Herner & Company; ICDB – International Cancer Research Data Bank Program.

Record composition

Abstract AB; Abstract Source AS; Author AU; Classification Code CC; CAS-Reg.No. CR; Corporate Source CS; Controlled Term CT; Document Type DT; Entry Date ED; Enzyme Code EZ; Gene Symbol GE; ITTRI/Franklin Number IF; Journal Title Code JC; Journal Title JT; Language LA; Last Revision Date LR; Number of Contract NC; Number of Document ND; Notes NO; Number of Report NR; Publication Year PY; Qualifier QF; Secondary Source Identifier SEC; Source SO; ISSN SS; Terminology TE and Title Ti

12:135. Online   DIMDI

File name	CL63
Alternative name(s)	Cancer Literature On-Line
Software	GRIPS

Start year	1963–1979
Number of records	194,832
Update period	Not updated
SDI period	1 month
Database aids	Memocard CANCERLIT and User Manual MEDLINE, AIDSLINE, BIOETHICSLINE, CANCERLIT, HEALTH
Price/Charges	Connect time: UK£5.84–10.58
	Online print: UK£0.17–0.35
	Offline print: UK£0.09–0.15

Downloading is allowed
Thesaurus is online

Notes

File CL 63 covers records for the period 1963–1979. 100% of the records have abstracts. Suppliers of online documents: British Library Document Supply Centre, Boston Spa, England; Bayerische Statts-bibliothek München, München, Germany; Harkers Information Retrieval System, Sydney, Australia; Institute for Scientific Information, Philadelphia, USA; Koninklikjke Nederlandse Akademie van Weten-schapen, Amsterdam, The Nederlands; Zentral-bibliothek der Medizin, Köln, Germany.

German author names with a dipthong (ä,ö,ü) are treated differently from MEDLINE (in MEDLINE ae;oe;ue). In CANCERLIT the 'e' of the umlaut is usually deleted and it is recommended to use the truncation symbol (#). For example Alfred Müller (F AU=MULLER A OR AU = MUELLER A, or F AU = MU#LLER (preferable). For Number of Document, from June 1983 the three letter standardised NLM-codes for journals are used. Prior to June 1983, five letter codes were used. Deviating from MEDLINE, the numerical code carries a prefix in CANCERLIT indicating the secondary source of a citation. The Number of Report is the Cancergram identification number, available from 1978. Cancergrams are monthly current awareness publications of the Naitonal Cancer Institute with over 60 different subject related bulletins. Articles are selected by scientists. The first four characters identify the Cancergram series and the last four digits identify the publication month and year of the particular Cancergram issue. Approximately one-third of records carry one or more Cancergram Numbers which are assigned to records annually in January. The Secondary Source Identifier is the secondary supplier or source of a citation. Deviating from MEDLINE, AIDSLINE and HEALTH, only the following abbreviations without numerical codes are used in CANCERLIT: CARTH – Carcinogenesis Abstracts; CATH – Cancer Therapy Abstracts; HERN – Herner & Company; ICDB – International Cancer Research Data Bank Program.

Record composition

Abstract AB; Abstract Source AS; Author AU; Classification Code CC; CAS-Reg.No. CR; Corporate Source CS; Controlled Term CT; Document Type DT; Entry Date ED; Enzyme Code EZ; Gene Symbol GE; ITTRI/Franklin Number IF; Journal Title Code JC; Journal Title JT; Language LA; Last Revision Date LR; Number of Contract NC; Number of Document ND; Notes NO; Number of Report NR; Publication Year PY; Qualifier QF; Secondary Source Identifier SEC; Source SO; ISSN SS; Terminology TE and Title TI

The Basic Index includes the data fields Title, Abstract, Controlled Term, Gene Symbols and Terminology. All citations are indexed at least with one Document Type.

12:136. Online Japan Information Center of Science and Technology (JICST)

File name	
Alternative name(s)	Cancer Literature On-Line
Start year	
Number of records	
Update period	

12:137. Online MIC/Karolinska Institute Library and Information Center (MIC KIBIC)

File name	CANCERLIT
Alternative name(s)	Cancer Literature On-Line
Start year	1963
Number of records	680,000
Update period	Monthly

Notes

Online ordering and SDI service available.

12:138. Online National Library of Medicine

File name	Cancerlit
Alternative name(s)	Cancer Literature On-Line
Start year	
Number of records	
Update period	

12:139. Online University of Tsukuba

File name	
Alternative name(s)	Cancer Literature On-Line
Start year	
Number of records	
Update period	

Notes

Access through University of Tsukuba limited to affiliates of the University of Japan.

12:140. CD-ROM Aries Systems Corporation

File name	Cancerlit – Knowledge Finder
Format notes	Mac, IBM
Software	Knowledge Finder 2.0
Start year	1985
Number of records	650,000
Update period	Quarterly

Notes

Corresponds in part to the Cancerlit online database.

12:141. CD-ROM CD Plus

File name	CD Plus/Cancerlit
Format notes	Mac, Unix, IBM
Software	OVID 3.0
Start year	1984
Number of records	128,992
Update period	Monthly
Price/Charges	Subscription: UK£845

Notes

Covers 1984 to present on one disc. One disc. Offers the ability to limit by local journal holdings. For the experienced searcher, the software offers MeSH explodes, 'personal pre-explodes' for frequently exploded terms, SDIs and Save Searches, enhanced MeSH tree structures, and emulation of National Library of Medicine and dot-dot syntax.

Record composition

Author; Institution; Title; Personal Names as Subjects; Original Titles; Grant Numbers and Comments

This database has an index of all searchable terms together with the online *MeSh Thesaurus* which offers mapping from natural language to *MeSH* – a facility which should give significantly improved precision for the inexperienced searcher. The on-screen help provides scope notes, definitions and task descriptors.

12:142. CD-ROM   Compact Cambridge

File name	Cancerlit
Format notes	NEC, 9800, Mac, IBM
Software	SearchLITE
Start year	Most recent five years.
Number of records	190,000
Update period	Quarterly
Price/Charges	Subscription: UK£635

Notes

Contains a four year backfile, plus the current year. May be combined with PDQ – Physicians Data Query on a single disc at UK£930.

For more details of constituent databases, see:
MEDLINE

This database can also be found on:
AIDSLINE
Cancer-CD
Oncodisc

CD-GENE

Hitachi Software Engineering
National Institutes of Health
National Biomedical Research
   Foundation
European Molecular Biology Laboratory
   (EMBL)

12:145. Master record
CD-ROM   Hitachi Software Engineering

Database type	Textual, Chemical structures/DNA sequences, Bibliographic
Number of journals	
Sources	
Start year	1988
Language	English
Coverage	International
Number of records	
Update size	–
Update period	Semiannually

Description

CD-GENE is a combined software/CD system which provides a means of access to the large and rapidly growing compendium of DNA and Protein (Amino Acid) sequences in the following genetic databases: GenBank (DNA – National Institute of Health (US)); EMBL (DNA – European Molecular Biology Laboratory); PIR (Protein and Identificaton Resource) (Amino Acid – National BioMedical Research Foundation); and SWISS-PROT European Protein Database.

Sequence information can be accessed by: Author names; Keywords; Short and long directory phrases; entry or sequence name, and accession number. Also allows searches by sequence homology or relatedness, whereby up to 2,000 of the most similar sequences to a target sequence may be retrieved from the database and displayed in order of homology.

The company's literature states that CD-Gene is 'a set of compact discs that contain four major biotechnology databases together with software for similarity searches. . . . With each new release, search times increase, memory requirements increase, and database maintenance becomes more difficult . . . Together with the power of CD-ROM technology, this system provides the quickest, most efficient way of working with genetic sequence databases.' US$ 725 initial purchase, US$ 250 for updates.

For more details of constituent databases, see:
GenBank
EMBL (European Molecular Biology Laboratory)
PIR (Protein and Identificaton Resource)
SWISS-PROT

Chemical Engineering and Biotechnology Abstracts

DECHEMA Deutsche Gesellschaft für
   Chemisches Apparatewesen
Royal Society of Chemistry

12:147. Master record

Alternative name(s)	CEBA; DECHEMA; CEA; Chemical Engineering Abstracts
Database type	Bibliographic, Textual
Number of journals	1000
Sources	Journals, monographs, patents (European), conference proceedings, technical reports, press releases, dissertations, reviews, newspapers and government documents
Start year	1970
Language	English and German
Coverage	International
Number of records	300,000
Update size	6,000
Update period	Monthly
Index unit	Articles and reviews
Database aids	Current Biotechnology Abstracts Database User Aid Manual, RSC, 1989

Keywords

Analytical Chemistry; Bioagriculture; Biochemistry; Bioengineering; Biotechnology; Chemical Engineering; Chemical Equipment Manufacturing; Chemical Manufacturing; Chemical Processing; Chemical Substances; Enzymology; Food and Drink; Genetic Manipulation; Hazardous Substances; Mathematical Models; Occupational Health and Safety; Pharmaceuticals; Pollution Control

Description

During 1989 the monthly production of the Chemical Engineering Abstracts database from the Royal Society of Chemistry, UK, was merged with the DECHEMA database of Frankfurt, Germany to form this Chemical Engineering and Biotechnology Abstracts database. The combined title will be produced in English.

It contains citations, with English-language abstracts, drawn from the worldwide scientific and technical literature on biotechnology and chemical engineering.

In chemical engineering, emphasis is given to the

processing of chemicals in large or small quantities. From 1987 it also incorporates theoretical engineering abstracts. Gives full coverage of published information required by both practising chemical engineers and academics. The abstracts are written with the chemical/process engineer in mind, not chemists, and this is reflected in the content. Covers chemical reactions, mixing and separation, heating and cooling, and the transport of liquids, solids and gases. The effect of the size of the operation, the physical and other properties of the substances involved, the nature of the equipment used, corrosion and personal safety factors are also covered, as are environmental consequences.

Covers chemical processing theory and laboratory experimentation in addition to industrial practice.

Topics included are: chemical equipment manufacturing, chemical manufacturing, plant design and construction, computer-aided design (CAD), mathematical models and methods, laboratory techniques, analytical chemistry, safety engineering, hazardous materials, pollution control, environmental protection, energy and raw materials supply and conservation, chemical reaction engineering, catalysis, unit operations, process dynamics and control, measurement, instruments, materials of construction, corrosion and corrosion protection, and operating materials.

In biotechnology, it provides full coverage, with abstracts, of the technical, scientific and technocommercial literature for the industry of biotechnology. Biotechnology is defined as the development and use of biological systems and functions to realise end-products useful to mankind. Topics covered in this section include: all aspects of biotechnology such as: genetic manipulation, monoclonal antibodies, immobilized cells and enzymes, single-cell proteins and fermentation technology, in the pharmaceutical, fuel, agriculture, chemical, food and other industries.

Articles with a significant technical content are selected and documents are assigned to one of 52 sections with cross references to direct the user from one section to potentially interesting abstracts in another. Some articles are available as full text, with technical items and some book reviews also included. The scientific and technical abstracts are split into four main areas: technocommercial data, techniques, specific industrial areas and information. Technocommercial data includes business news, legal and safety issues and information on related conferences.

Techniques includes: genetic manipulation, monoclonal antibodies, enzymology, single-cell proteins and fermentation technology. Industrial areas includes pharmaceuticals, energy production, agriculture, chemical industry and food. Information includes forthcoming events, books and reviews.

The database incorporates Current Biotechnology Abstracts which is also available separately. Current Biotechnology Abstracts covers about 400 primary journals and other sources such as books and reviews are scanned: UK, USA, European and PCT patents are included. Approximately twenty per cent of the Current Biotechnology Abstracts section is patents. This section contains about 50,000 records and is updated with 400–500 records per month. All of the material published in the hard-copy version since its start-up in April 1983 is included.

Corresponds to: *Chemical Engineering Abstracts; Theoretical Chemical Engineering Abstracts; Safety, Environmental Protection and Analysis; Process and Chemical Engieering; Equipment, Corrosion and* *Corrosion Protection; Biotechnology: Apparatus, Plant and Equipment*; and *Current Biotechnology*.

Corresponds in part to *Literaturkurzberichte Chemische Technik und Biotechnologie (Dechema Chemical Engineering and Biotechnology Abstracts), and Biotechnologie, Verfahren-Anlagen-Apparate (Biotechnology, Processes-Plant-Equipment)*.

Sources include primary chemical and process engineering journals.

Bibliographic information, indexing terms and abstracts are all searchable. Users can access citations by subject, substance, or organisation name. The field Chemical Descriptors may list the names of up to fifteen chemical substances and these are searched in the same way as subject descriptors. The Patent Information field contains patent numbers, patent series, patent application (or priority) number and country, date of application (or priority).

12:148. Online   Data-Star

File name	CEAB
Alternative name(s)	CEBA; DECHEMA; CEA; Chemical Engineering Abstracts
Start year	1981
Number of records	104,036
Update period	Monthly
Database aids	Data-Star Chemical Manual, Berne, Data-Star, 1989 and Online manual (search NEWS-CEAB in NEWS)
Price/Charges	Subscription: UK£32.00
	Connect time: UK£76.00
	Online print: UK£0.75
	Offline print: UK£0.49
	SDI charge: UK£5.30

Notes

From June 1993 Data-Star have introduced an annual fee/subscription per contract (that is, not per password) of SFr 80.00 (c.UK£ 32.00) payable every June. For North American customers billed in dollars who also use DIALOG, the DIALOG fee also covers access to Data-Star. Academic customers, 'commitment' customers and customers currently billed in dollars are exempt.

12:149. Online   DIALOG

File name	File 315
Alternative name(s)	CEBA; DECHEMA; CEA; Chemical Engineering Abstracts
Start year	1971
Number of records	125,188
Update period	Monthly
Price/Charges	Connect time: US$150.00
	Online print: US$1.40
	Offline print: US$1.40
	SDI charge: US$15.00

12:150. Online   ESA-IRS

File name	File 85
Alternative name(s)	CEBA; DECHEMA; CEA; Chemical Engineering Abstracts
Start year	1970
Number of records	122,000 (October 1991)
Update period	Monthly

Notes

From 1993 ESA-IRS are charging an annual fee of 100 Accounting Units (c.UK£ 70.29) to all users. This is equivalent to the fee for full documentation and will not be charged to customers already paying for documentation.

12:151. Online   FIZ Technik

File name	DECH
Alternative name(s)	CEBA; DECHEMA; CEA; Chemical Engineering Abstracts
Start year	1976
Number of records	178,000
Update period	Monthly
Price/Charges	Connect time: DM264.00
	Online print: DM1.40 – 1.90
	Offline print: DM2.20
	SDI charge: DM18.00

12:152. Online   Hoechst

File name	
Alternative name(s)	CEBA; DECHEMA; CEA; Chemical Engineering Abstracts
Start year	1970
Number of records	122,000
Update period	Monthly

12:153. Online   ORBIT

File name	CEBA
Alternative name(s)	CEBA; DECHEMA; CEA; Chemical Engineering Abstracts
Start year	1970
Number of records	125,000+
Update period	Monthly
Database aids	Quick reference Guide (5/90) Free (single copy)

Notes

Electronic SDI service is now available within two hours on ORBIT. They can be downloaded and reformatted on a word processor. Results are retrieved in the low cost PRINTS file, $15 per connect hour.

12:154. Online   STN

File name	CEBA
Alternative name(s)	CEBA; DECHEMA; CEA; Chemical Engineering Abstracts
Start year	1975
Number of records	187,809
Update period	Monthly
Price/Charges	Connect time: DM240.00
	SDI charge: DM15.00

Notes

In English, with some abstracts in German.

12:155. Database subset

Online   CISTI, Canadian Online Enquiry Service CAN/OLE

File name	BIOTECH
Alternative name(s)	Current Biotechnology Abstracts; CBA
Start year	
Number of records	50,000
Update period	Monthly
Price/Charges	Connect time: Canadian $40.00
	Online print: Canadian $0.46 – 0.92
	Offline print: Canadian $0.26 – 0.52

Notes

CISTI accessible only in Canada. US$ 70.00 royalty per connect hour; print charges in US dollars. This is a subfile of the Chemical Engineering and Biotechnology Abstracts database.

12:156. Database subset

Online   Data-Star

File name	CUBI
Alternative name(s)	Current Biotechnology Abstracts; CBA
Start year	1983 (April)

Number of records	34,758
Update period	Monthly
Database aids	Data-Star Biomedical Manual and Online manual (search NEWS-CUBI in NEWS)
Price/Charges	Subscription: SFr80.00
	Connect time: SFr175.00
	Online print: SFr1.88
	Offline print: SFr1.36
	SDI charge: SFr13.25

Downloading is allowed

Notes

This is a subfile of the Chemical Engineering and Biotechnology Abstracts database.

From June 1993 Data-Star have introduced an annual fee/subscription per contract (that is, not per password) of SFr 80.00 (c.UK£ 32.00) payable every June. For North American customers billed in dollars who also use DIALOG, the DIALOG fee also covers access to Data-Star. Academic customers, 'commitment' customers and customers currently billed in dollars are exempt.

Record composition

Abstract AB; Accession Number and Update Code AN; Author AU; Author Affiliation IN; Chemical Descriptors ID; Company CO; Descriptors DE; Journal Coden CD; Language LG; Patent Information PA; Publication Type PT; Publisher PB; Section Code SC; Section Cross Reference; Source SO; Title TI; Update Code UP and Year YR

12:157. Database subset

Online   DIALOG

File name	File 358
Alternative name(s)	Current Biotechnology Abstracts; CBA
Start year	1983
Number of records	492,923
Update period	Monthly
Price/Charges	Connect time: US$150.00
	Online print: US$1.40
	Offline print: US$1.40
	SDI charge: US$15.00

Notes

This is a subfile of the Chemical Engineering and Biotechnology Abstracts database.

DIALINDEX Categories: AGRI, ENVIRON, FOODSCI, VETSCI.

12:158. Database subset

Online   ESA-IRS

File name	File 95
Alternative name(s)	Current Biotechnology Abstracts; CBA
Start year	1983
Number of records	43,000 (October 1991)
Update period	Monthly
Price/Charges	Subscription: UK£70.29
	Database entry fee: UK£3.49
	Online print: UK£0.56
	Offline print: UK£0.56
	SDI charge: UK£2.80

Notes

This is a subfile of the Chemical Engineering and Biotechnology Abstracts database.

From 1993 ESA-IRS are charging an annual fee of 100 Accounting Units (c.UK£ 70.29) to all users. This is equivalent to the fee for full documentation and will not be charged to customers already paying for documentation.

Record composition

Abstract /AB; Author AU; Class Code CC; Class Name CC; Coden CO; Contract Terms /CT; Corporate Source CS; Document Type DT; ISBN BN; ISSN SN; Journal Name JN; Language LA; Meeting Information MI; Native Number NN; Publisher PB; Publication Date PD; Patent Number PN; Report Number RN and Title /TI

12:159. Database subset

CD-ROM	Royal Society of Chemistry
File name	Current Biotechnology Abstracts
Alternative name(s)	Current Biotechnology Abstracts; CBA
Format notes	IBM
Start year	
Number of records	
Update period	

Notes

This is a subfile of the Chemical Engineering and Biotechnology Abstracts database.

Colleague Mail

BRS Online Service, BRS/Colleague

12:160. Master record

Alternative name(s)	MEDLINK
Database type	Directory, Textual, Computer software
Number of journals	1
Sources	Journal, Airlines, Database producers, Electronic media and Original material
Start year	
Language	English
Coverage	USA
Number of records	
Update size	—
Update period	Current six to eight months
Index unit	Classified advertisements

Keywords

Molecular Biology; HIV; Travel; Air Travel; Anaesthesia; Personal Computers; HIV; Pathology; Surgery; Gastroenterology; Intensive Care; Proctology; Dermatology; Geriatrics; Gerontology; Genetics – Human; Immunology; Health Care Administration; Neurology; Cancer; Oncology; Ophthalmology; Sickle-Cell Disease

Description

Contains a number of services for medical professionals, including classified advertisements from the *New England Journal of Medicine*, a calendar of medical events, electronic mail, gateway access to Official Airlines Guide (OAG) Electronic Edition Travel Service (see separate entry), American Airlines EASY Sabre (see separate entry) and other databases available through BT Tymnet Dialcom Service. There are also a number of bulletin boards available, operated by physician-editors: AIDS/HIV, Anesthesia Safety and Technology, Cellforum (pathology, cell biology, molecular biology), Clinical Drug Information, Colon & Rectal Surgery, Critical Care, Dermatology, Geriatrics and Gerontology, Hackers' Forum (microcomputer products and applications), Materia Eclectica, Medical Ethics, MEDLINK Help & Tips, Neurology, Oncology, Ophthalmology, Sickle-Cell Disease.

Partially equivalent to *New England Journal of Medicine* (classified advertisements).

12:161. Online   BRS, BRS/Colleague

File name	
Alternative name(s)	MEDLINK
Start year	
Number of records	
Update period	current six to eight months

For more details of constituent databases, see:
American Airlines EAASY SABRE
OAG Electronic Edition Travel Service

Current Awareness in Biological Sciences

Current Awareness in Biological Sciences

12:163. Master record

Database type	Bibliographic
Number of journals	2,500+
Sources	Journals
Start year	1983
Language	English
Coverage	International
Number of records	1,000,000+
Update size	200,000
Update period	Monthly
Index unit	Articles, Reviews and Editorials
Hosts have included	ORBIT (until 10/92)

Keywords

Cancer; Physiology; Immunology; Neuroscience

Description

Contains citations to the worldwide literature on biology. Subjects include biochemistry, cell and developmental biology, genetics and molecular biology, clinical chemistry, cancer research, immunology, endocrinology, microbiology, neurosciences, pharmacology and toxicology, physiology, ecology, and environmental and plant sciences. Includes an indication of whether articles are reviews or editorials and whether published in a language other than English.

Corresponds to *Current Awareness in Biological Sciences*. Formerly produced by Pergamon Press Ltd. Formerly available on ORBIT until Maxwell Online switched all life science files to BRS which has a much larger market for similar data.

12:164. Online   BRS

File name	CURB
Start year	1983
Number of records	1,100,000
Update period	Monthly
Price/Charges	Connect time: US$67.00/77.00
	Online print: US$0.29/0.37
	Offline print: US$0.47
	SDI charge: US$7.75

Current Contents Search Bibliographic Database

Institute for Scientific Information

12:165. Master record

Database type	Bibliographic
Number of journals	1,300
Sources	Journals
Start year	Most recent twelve months
Language	English
Coverage	International

Genetics

Number of records	1,547,676
Update size	728,000
Update period	Weekly
Index unit	Articles, reviews, letters, notes and Editorials

Keywords

Applied Science; Atmospheric Science; Clinical Medicine; Immunology; Inorganic Chemistry; Molecular Biology; Neuroscience; Organic Chemistry; Polymers; Statistics; Astrophysics; Spectroscopy; Pathology; Physics; Water Supply

Description

Contains citations to articles listed in the tables of content of leading journals in the sciences, social sciences, and arts and humanities. There are seven subsets:

Clinical medicine (CLIN): Covers allergy, anaesthesiology, biomethods, cardiology, clinical and medicinal chemistry, clinical psychiatry and psychology, dentistry, dermatology, epidemiology, family medicine, gastroenterology and hepatology, general and internal medicine, geriatrics and gerontology, hematology, infectious diseases, medical technology and laboratory medicine, neurology, oncology, ophthalmology, orthopedics, otorhinolaryngology, paediatrics, pharmacy, physical medicine and rehabilitation, radiology and nuclear medicine, reproductive systems, respiratory medicine, sports sciences, surgery, and urology.

Life sciences (LIFE): Covers anatomy, biochemistry, biophysics, cytology, endocrinology, experimental medicine, experimental biology, genetics, gerontology, hematology, histology, immunology, microbiology, molecular biology, neuroscience, parasitology, pathology, pharmaceutical chemistry, pharmacology, physiology, radiology and nuclear medicine, toxicology and virology.

Arts and humanities (ARTS).

Engineering, technology, and applied sciences (ENG).

Social and behavioural sciences (BEHA): Covers business, economics, education, geography, history, law, library and information science, management, planning and development, political science, psychiatry, psychology, public health, rehabilitation, sociology.

Agriculture, biology, and environmental sciences (AGRI): Covers agricultural chemistry, economics, engineering, agronomy, animal behaviour, animal husbandry, applied microbiology, biotechnology, botany, conservation, crop science, dairy science, ecology, entomology, environmental sciences, fishery science and technology, forestry, horticulture, marine biology, mycology, nutrition, oceanology, orinthology, pest control, soil science, taxonomy, veterinary medicine and pathology, water research and engineering, wildlife management and zoology.

Physical, chemical, and earth sciences (PHYS): Covers analytical chemistry, applied physics, astronomy, astrophysics, atmospheric sciences, chemical physics, chemistry, condensed matter, crystallography, geology and geophysics, inorganic and nuclear chemistry, mathematics, meteorology, nuclear physics, organic chemistry, paleontology, physical chemistry, physics, polymer chemistry, spectroscopy, statistics and probability.

Includes title, authors, bibliographic data, abstracts and keywords, and, when available, reprint authors' addresses.

Current Contents Search is the online version of ISI's popular Current Contents series of publications. Current Contents is a weekly service that reproduces the tables of contents from current issues of leading journals in the sciences, social sciences, and arts and humanities. All ISI databases have a linked service known as The Genuine Article which can deliver the full text of located articles by mail, facsimile transmission or courier. Orders can be placed via the host service in use, mail, facsimile transmission, telephone or telex. Diskette products have a single-keystroke order information facility. The minimum charge is US$ 11.25 within USA and Canada and US$ 12.20 elsewhere.

Leading journals in the sciences, social sciences, and arts and humanities.

Keywords supplied by the author are included. In addition, ISI adds Keywords Plus which are generated by analysis of titles of articles that appear in the list of citations.

12:166. Database subset

Online	BRS, Morning Search, BRS/Colleague
File name	LIFE
Alternative name(s)	CBIB: Life Sciences
Start year	
Number of records	
Update period	
Price/Charges	Connect time: US$85.00/95.00
	Online print: US$0.57/0.65
	Offline print: US$0.65

Notes

A special print format, CONT, allows the user to print a Table of Contents format that closely mirrors the print product.

12:167. Database subset

Online	DIMDI
File name	I583 – SCILIFE
Software	GRIPS
Start year	1983
Number of records	2,821,801
Update period	Weekly
SDI period	1 week
Database aids	User Manual SCISEARCH/SOCIAL SCISEARCH and Memocard SCISEARCH
Price/Charges	Connect time: UK£14.41–20.32 (Group I); 15.57–23.24 (Group II); 18.50–43.71 (Group III)
	Online print: UK£0.39–0.57
	Offline print: UK£0.31–0.37

Downloading is allowed

Notes

SCILIFE corresponds to the *Current Contents* edition *Life Sciences*. Approximately nine per cent of records contain abstracts. Searches are possible from January 1983.

There are preferential costs for subscribers to the printed product. Groups shown for pricing refer to: 1. Users in the Federal Republic of Germany active in the field of biosciences, with the exception of private companies. Under temporary federal grant there is a rebate for this group of users; 2. Other users who are subscribers of the equivalent printed product. These users have to inform ISI that they wish this preferential rate; 3. Other users who are not subscribers of the equivalent printed product.

Record composition

Abstract AB; Abstract Indicators AI; Author AU; Author's Keywords IT; Cluster Code CC; Cluster Term CT; Cluster Weight /W; Corporate Country CCO; Corporate Source CS; Document Type DT; Entry Date ED; Free Text FT; Journal Title JT; Keywords Plus UT; Language LA; Number of Document ND; Number of References RN; Publication Year PY; Reference RF; Referenced Journal RJ; Referenced Patent No. RP; Subject Code SC; Subject Heading SH; Source SO; Subunit SU and Title TI

The basic index includes the following data fields: Title, Controlled Term, Index Term, Uncontrolled Term and Abstract.

12:168. Database subset

Online   **DIMDI**

File name	IL89 – Current Contents/SciSearch
Software	GRIPS
Start year	Latest 12 months
Number of records	729,304
Update period	Weekly
SDI period	1 week
Database aids	User Manual SCISEARCH/Social SCISEARCH and Memocard SCISEARCH
Price/Charges	Connect time: UK£14.41–20.32 (Group I); 15.57–23.24 (Group II); 18.50–43.71 (Group III) Online print: UK£0.39–0.57 Offline print: UK£0.31–0.37

Downloading is allowed

Notes

This is a separate database on DIMDI of Current Contents/SciSearch. IL89 contains the documents of the last twelve months from Social SciSearch. It corresponds to the subject content of SciSearch, the only difference from the main file on DIMDI (IS74) is the output format. Suppliers of online documents: British Library Document Supply Centre, Boston Spa, England; Harkers Information Retrieval System, Sydney, Australia; The Information Store, San Francisco, USA; Institute for Scientific Information, Philadelphia, USA.

There are preferential costs for subscribers to the printed product. Groups shown for pricing refer to: 1. Users in the Federal Republic of Germany active in the field of biosciences, with the exception of private companies. Under temporary federal grant there is a rebate for this group of users; 2. Other users who are subscribers of the equivalent printed product. These users have to inform ISI that they wish this preferential rate; 3. Other users who are not subscribers of the equivalent printed product.

Record composition

Abstract Indicator AI; Abstract AB; Author AU; Author's Keywords IT; Cluster Code CC; Corporate Country CCO; Corporate Source CS; Document Type DT; Entry Date ED; Free Text FT; Index Term IT; Journal Title JT; Keywords Plus UT; Language LA; Number of Document ND; Number of References RN; Publication Year PY; Reference RF; Referenced Journal RJ; Referenced Patent No. RP; Source SO; Subject Code SC; Subject Heading SH; Subunit SU; Title TI and Uncontrolled Term (Keywords Plus) UT

After the SHOW-, PRINT or DLOAD- command the output of documents is displayed in the table of contents format. The basic index includes the data fields: Title, Index Term and Uncontrolled Term.

12:169. Database subset

Diskette   **Institute for Scientific Information**

File name	Current Contents on Diskette with Abstracts – Life Sciences
Format notes	IBM, NEC, Mac
Software	Proprietary Vn.3.0
Start year	
Number of records	
Update period	Weekly
Price/Charges	Subscription: US$965

Notes

Contains citations with abstracts to articles listed in the tables of contents of about 1,200 journals in the life sciences. Equivalent to the print *Current Contents/Life Sciences*; and in part to the Current Contents Search online database.

Reduced subscription for print subscribers. The latest version of the software (August 1992) allows search profiles to be run against six issues at one time; better file compression to use less hard disk space; expanded online, context sensitive help; better truncation (including left-hand) facilities; and new output options. KeyWords Plus (tm) provides users with search terms taken from an article's bibliography: in this way users should identify many more articles. KeyWords Plus (tm) also allows users to determine on inspection how closely the article pertains to their area of interest. Users are now also able to transfer multiple search terms from the dictionaries to search statements.

Record composition

ISBN; ISSN and Publisher

12:170. Database subset

Diskette   **Institute for Scientific Information**

File name	Current Contents on Diskette – Life Sciences
Format notes	IBM, NEC, Mac
Software	Proprietary Vn.3.0
Start year	
Number of records	
Update period	Weekly
Price/Charges	Subscription: US$405/575

Notes

Contains citations to articles listed in the tables of contents of about 1,200 journals in the life sciences. Data are available in two editions; one covering 1,200 journals, one 600 journals. Equivalent to the print *Current Contents/Life Sciences*; and in part to the Current Contents Search online database.

Reduced subscription for print subscribers. The latest version of the software (August 1992) allows search profiles to be run against six issues at one time; better file compression to use less hard disk space; expanded online, context sensitive help; better truncation (including left-hand) facilities; and new output options. KeyWords Plus (tm) provides users with search terms taken from an article's bibliography: in this way users should identify many more articles. KeyWords Plus (tm) also allows users to determine on inspection how closely the article pertains to their area of interest. Users are now also able to transfer multiple search terms from the dictionaries to search statements.

Record composition

ISBN; ISSN and Publisher

12:171. Database subset
Tape   Institute for Scientific
                                        Information

File name	CC Search/Life Sciences
Start year	Current
Number of records	
Update period	Weekly
Price/Charges	Subscription: US$15,000 -18,750

Notes

Contains citations to articles listed in the tables of contents of about 1,200 journals in the life sciences. Data are available in two editions; one covering 1,200 journals, one 600 journals.

Equivalent to the print *Current Contents/Life Sciences*; and in part to the Current Contents Search online database.

Reduced subscription for print subscribers. The latest version of the software (August 1992) allows search profiles to be run against six issues at one time; better file compression to use less hard disk space; expanded online, context sensitive help; better truncation (including left-hand) facilities; and new output options. KeyWords Plus (tm) provides users with search terms taken from an article's bibliography: in this way users should identify many more articles. KeyWords Plus (tm) also allows users to determine on inspection how closely the article pertains to their area of interest. Users are now also able to transfer multiple search terms from the dictionaries to search statements.

Annual lease is $15,000 (academic), $18,750 (corporate).

Record composition

ISBN; ISSN and Publisher

EMBASE
Elsevier Science Publishers

12:172. Master record

Alternative name(s)	Excerpta Medica
Database type	Bibliographic
Number of journals	4,700
Sources	Case studies, clinicians, journals, monographs, research communications, reviews, surveys and symposia
Start year	1974
Language	English
Coverage	International
Number of records	4,950,000+
Update size	350,000
Update period	Weekly
Index unit	Articles
Abstract details	Adaptations of the authors' summaries and selected on the basis of content and length by an international group of practicing medical and other qualified specialists and when necessary modified, shortened or extended to obtain the optimal information value. A group of over 2,000 biomedical specialists assists with the preparation of abstracts in particular subject areas and articles in non-Western European languages.
Thesaurus	EMTREE Thesaurus METAGS

Database aids	Guide to the Classification and Indexing System, MALIMET (available online and on microfiche), Mini-Malimet, MECLASE Drug Trade Names (DN) and EMBASE List of Journals Abstracted

Keywords

HIV; Anaesthesia; Anatomy; Anthropology; Bioengineering; Biotechnology; Cancer; Cardiology; Clinical Medicine; Clinical Neurology; Cosmetics; Drugs; Environmental Health; Environmental Pollution; Environmental Toxicology; Epilepsy; Food Additives; Food Contaminants; Forensic Medicine; Forensic Science; Gastroenterology; Gynaecology; Immunology; Industrial Medicine; Nephrology; Neuroscience; Neuromuscular Disorders; Nuclear Medicine; Obstetrics; Occupational Health and Safety; Patents; Pathology; Pharmaceuticals; Pollution; Public Health; Radiology; Toxic Substances; Waste Management

Description

EMBASE is the trademark for the English language Excerpta Medica database. Excerpta Medica was founded as a non-profit making organisation in 1946 with the goal of improving the availability and dissemination of medical knowledge through the publication of a series of abstract journals. The database contains citations, with abstracts, to the worldwide biomedical literature on human medicine and areas of biological sciences related to human medicine with an emphasis on the pharmacological effects of drugs and chemicals. The four main categories of primary literature sources are: specialist medical publications; general biomedicine publications; specialist non-medical publications and general scientific publications. Subjects covered include: anatomy; anesthesiology (including resuscitation and intensive care medicine); anthropology; pharmacology of anesthetic agents, spinal, epidural and caudal anesthesia and acupuncture (as anesthetic); autoimmunity; biochemistry; bioengineering; cancer; dangerous goods; dermatology; developmental biology; drug adverse reactions; drug dependence; drug effects; endocrinology; environmental health and pollution control (covering chemical pollution and its effect on man, animals, plants and microorganisms; measurement, treatment, prevention and control); exocrine pancreas; forensic science; gastroenterology (including diseases and disorders of: digestive systems; mouth; pharynx and more); genetics; gerontology and geriatrics; health economics; hematology; hepatobiliary system; hospital management; immunology (including immunity; hypersensitivity; histocompatibility and all aspects of the immune system); internal medicine; legal and socioeconomic aspects; mesentary; meteorological aspects; microbiology; nephrology (covering diagnosis; treatment; epidemiology; prevention; infections; glomerular and tubular disorders; blood purification; dialysis; kidney transplantation; toxic nephropathy and including important clinical abstracts with epidemiological studies and major clinical trials, with particular emphasis on hypertension and diabetes); neurosciences (especially clinical neurology and neurosurgery, epilepsy and neuromuscular disorders but also covering non-clinical articles on neurophysiology and animal models for human neuropharmacology); noise and vibration; nuclear medicine; obstetrics and gynaecology (including endocrinology and menstrual cycle, infertility, prenatal diagnosis and fetal monitoring, anti-conceptions, breast cancer diagnosis, sterilisation and psychosexual problems and neonatal care of normal children); occupational health and industrial medicine; opthalmology; otorhinolaryngology; paediatrics; pathology (including general pathology and organ pathology, pathological physiology and pathological anatomy, as well as laboratory methods and techniques used in pathology. General pathology topics range from cellular pathology, fetal and neonatal pathology, including congenital disorders, injury (both chemical and physical), inflammation and infection, immuno-pathology, collagen diseases and cancer pathology); peritoneum; pharmacology (including the effects and use of all drugs; experimental aspects of pharmacokinetics and pharmacodynamics; drug information); physiology; psychiatry and psychology (including addiction; alcoholism; sexual behaviour; suicide; mental deficiency and the clinical use or abuse of psychotropic and psychomimetic agents); public health; radiation and thermal pollution; radiology (including radiodiagnosis, radiotherapy and radiobiology, ultrasound diagnosis, thermography, adverse reactions to radiotherapy and techniques and apparatus, radiobiology of radioisotopes, aspects of radiohygiene, new labelling techniques and tracer applications); rehabilitation; surgery; toxicology (including pharmaceutical toxicology; foods, food additives, and contaminants; cosmetics, toiletries, and household products; occupational toxicology; waste material in air, soil and water; toxins and venoms; chemical teratogens, mutagens, and carcinogens; phototoxicity; regulatory toxicology; laboratory methods and techniques; and antidotes and symptomatic treatment); urology; wastewater treatment and measurement. The database is particularly strong in drug-related literature, where records include manufacturers and drug trade names and generic names. Information on veterinary medicine, nursing and dentistry is generally excluded.

Excerpta Medica is extremely current as articles are indexed within thirty days of receipt and are online very soon after that. Approximately 900 journals (the Rapid Input Processing (RIP)) are processed with priority which means that within eleven weeks of the receipt of the original document, the completely-indexed records are available. More than 100,000 records are given this priority treatment. Some hosts have companion databases giving training or details of the indexing vocabularies and thesauri.

EMBASE concentrates on journal articles although about 1,000 books per annum were indexed between 1975 and 1980. The source journals include all forty-six sections of *Excerpta Medica*, the *Drug Literature Index* and *Adverse Reactions Titles*. New titles are added and old titles deleted at a rate of about 200–300 per year. The database covers sources from 110 countries with the following geographical scope: North America 36%, Western Europe 35%, United Kingdom 14%, USSR and Eastern Europe 7%, Asia 6%, Central and South America 1%, Austalia & South Pacific 1%, Africa and Middle East 1%. Approximately 50% of the citations are from drug and pharmaceutical literature and approximately 40% of citations added to the database each year do not appear in the corresponding printed abstract journals and indexes. Approximately 65% of the citations contain abstracts of on average 200 words with a maximum of 800 words which indicate the content of the articles and are not intended to summarise the results or express opinions. This makes free-text searching of the abstracts, titles and other searchable elements of the citation valuable. This compares with approximately sixty-five per cent of the records in MEDLINE and fifty-four per cent in BIOSIS. The records of the other

leading bioscience database, SciSearch, now do contain abstracts. Approximately 75% of the articles are in the English language. Of the other leading bioscience databases, approximately eighty-eight per cent of articles on SciSearch are in English, eighty-six per cent of articles on BIOSIS and seventy-four per cent on MEDLINE. In addition approximately thirty-seven per cent of records with non-English sources contain English-language abstracts online. This compares with sixty-seven per cent on BIOSIS and twenty-six per cent on MEDLINE. SciSearch does now contain abstracts. Important publications NOT indexed in EMBASE include Meyler's *Side Effects of Drugs*, 1972–1980 published by Excerpta Medica and *Side Effects of Drugs Annual*, 1981 to the present, published by Elsevier.

A core collection of 3,500 biomedical journals supplemented by journals in the areas of agriculture, technology, economics, chemistry, environmental protection and sociology. General criteria used for selection are first that the document should be of potential relevance to medicine and secondly the information should be of lasting value for which reasons news items and comments are generally excluded.

EMBASE section headings are based on medical specialities; a total of forty-seven subfiles group together citations on topics such as anatomy, paediatrics, opthalmology, gastroenterelogy, cancer, plastic surgery, occupational health. Each subfile or section has its own hierarchical scheme. The thesaurus *MALIMET (Master List of Medical Terms)* is used which contains more than 250,000 preferred terms and 255,000 synonyms which are mapped to the preferred terms when used. It is used for indexing highly specific concepts such as names of drugs and chemicals; diseases and syndromes; anatomical and physiological aspects and diagnostic and therapeutic methods. *MALIMET* is growing at a rate of over 12,000 descriptors per annum, mainly through drug names and names of chemical compounds. The size of the complete *MALIMET* thesaurus for EMBASE (more than 250,000 preferred terms compared to 15,000 in *MeSH*) may indicate its tendency to provide a greater variety of possible terms and therefore, less consistent application in indexing. In 1993, all non-drug *MeSH* terms were included in the thesaurus mapped to *MALIMET* terms so that a search strategy can be transferred from MEDLINE.

Indexing incorporates the following rules: natural word order (acute leukemia, not leukemia acute); American spelling (tumor, not tumour), singular noun forms and not plural or adjectival forms (stomach tumor, not gastric tumors, but optic nerve, not eye nerve); the most specific term must be used. Since 1979, MALIMET terms have been weighted. Class A terms (weighted) indicate the main concepts while Class B terms (not weighted) indicate the less important concepts of a document. In addition to MALIMET broad concepts are indexed with EMCLAS and EMTAGS. EMCLAS is a poly-hierarchical decimal classification scheme of the forty-six subject subfiles which make up the sections of the printed *Excerpta Medica* containing approximately 6,500 entries. It is then further subdivided into a five level hierarchy of sub-categories. Indexing is performed by medical specialists and scientists whose specialism corresponds to the subject areas forming the major subdivisions of EMCLAS. The indexing builds up sequentially as the article is indexed by each of the sections for which it is relevant. On average each document is indexed for 3.5 different sections.

EMTAGS is a group of approximately 220 codes

which represent general concepts such as groups, gender, organ systems, experimental animals and article type. In January 1991 about 10% of the terms were changed including important descriptors such as CANCER or BENIGN NEOPLASM.

EMBASE editors also add 'uncontrolled' drug terms to augment MALIMET descriptors in selected records. EMBASE provides a hierarchical classification system (EMTREES) reflecting fifteen broad facets of biomedicine. From January 1991 a new version of EMTREE went online comprising 35,000 terms. New descriptors and changes in the hierarchy were made in the following areas: anatomy of the eye; diseases; drugs; techniques; biological phenomea and document types. Prior to 1988 Section Headings based on medical speciality areas were used instead of EMTREES to index EMBASE citations. In both classification schemes, codes are constructed to facilitate broad concept retrieval through truncation. In addition three uncontrolled vocabularies are used: Medical Secondary Text; Drug (Trade Names) and Manufacturers' Names are used. Medical Secondary Text consists of free-text words, numbers and phrases, describing concepts which are not fully covered by the controlled terms, for example quantiative information such as the number of patients or experimental animals. Drug (Trade) Names consists of trade names of drugs referred to in an original document with the main aspect of biological effects of compounds listed. Manufacturers' Names lists the names of drug manufacturers. The value of controlled indexing is important when searching for topics where a subject population has been specified.

Relatively few bioscience databases provide consistent indexing for subject populations (that is, humans or specific test animals) and related characteristics commonly requested such as age groups, gender, occupation and racial or ethnic groups. EMBASE provides extensive consistent indexing for the identification of test animals and age groups with a less consistent approach for the indexing of humans, occupational groups, racial/ethnic groups and gender. In addition, in most bioscience files a form of pharmaceutical nomenclature exists. For EMBASE the preferred search terms are generic name, classification by action/use and CAS Reigstry Number although restrictions by date, subfile and vendor may apply to the latter and vendor documentation should be consulted for guidelines. The search terms Enzyme Commission Number, investigational code, chemical name and trade name should be cross-referenced to the preferred terminology in the thesaurus. In 1993, improved CAS Registry Numbers mean that there is a single Number assigned for every substance.

12:173. Database subset

CD-ROM
SilverPlatter

File name	Excerpta Medica – Obstetrics/Gynaecology
Alternative name(s)	Excerpta Medica
Format notes	IBM, Mac
Software	SPIRS/MacSPIRS
Start year	1980
Number of records	208,000
Update period	Quarterly
Price/Charges	Subscription: UK£755 – 1,132

Notes
One of the Elsevier speciality Excerpta Medica range, this database, on CD-ROM, is a subset of EMBASE and covers human obstetrics and gynaecology. Subjects covered include endrocrinology, the men-

strual cycle, infertility, prenatal diagnosis and foetal monitoring, anticonception, breast cancer diagnosis, sterilisation, psychosexual problems and neonatal care of normal children. Relevant abstracts from other clinical and basic diciplines are also included.

Prices are: for single users UK£755, for 2–8 networked users £1,132.

This database can also be found on:
Eyenet
Cancer-CD
Medata-ROM
Logo-A Pharmaceutical Products (Discontinued)

EMBL Nucleotide Sequence Database
European Molecular Biology Laboratory (EMBL)

12:175. Master record

Alternative name(s)	European Molecular Biology Laboratory Database – EMBL
Database type	Chemical structures/DNA sequences, Factual, Bibliographic
Number of journals	
Sources	
Start year	Current Information
Language	English
Coverage	International
Number of records	44,000
Update size	—
Update period	Four times per year

Keywords
DNA Sequences; RNA Sequences; MRNA; Bacteriophages; Biotechnology; Genetics; Microbiology; Molecular Biology; Nucleotides; Viruses

Description
Nucleotide and amino acid sequences are increasingly located in separate databases such as GenBank, the European Molecular Biology Laboratory database EMBL, the Protein Identification Resource (PIR), etc. rather than being included with the original research article according to Gregory Pratt (*CD-ROM Professional* 6(3) May 1993 62–67). 'In fact, some biomedical journals require authors to submit sequences to an appropriate database before accepting a manuscript for publication. As of August 1992, over 44,000 MEDLINE references going back as far as 1971 have cross-references to sequence data in several different sequence databases.'

EMBL contains nucleotide sequences covering approximately 56 million bases, giving for each sequence its description, species, nucleotide composition, length, promoter and gene regions, topology, nucleic acid sequence and literature references. Sequences are from eukaryote, prokaryote, virus, bacteriophage genetic DNA or RNA, MRNA and functional RNA molecules.

Hibio Dnasis (CD-ROM) contains software for analysis and manipulation of sequences retrieved from this database and GenBank.

Print product: *Nucleic Acids Research* (Vol.16 no.5 1988).

12:176. Online
CISTI CAN/SND

File name	EMBL
Alternative name(s)	European Molecular Biology Laboratory Database – EMBL
Start year	Current Information

Number of records	44,000
Update period	Four times per year

12:177. Online — IntelliGenetics Inc, GenBank On-line Service

File name	EMBL Nucleotide Sequence Database
Alternative name(s)	European Molecular Biology Laboratory Database – EMBL
Start year	Current Information
Number of records	44,000
Update period	Four times per year

12:178. Online — IntelliGenetics Timesharing Service

File name	EMBL Nucleotide Sequence Database
Alternative name(s)	European Molecular Biology Laboratory Database – EMBL
Start year	Current Information
Number of records	44,000
Update period	Four times per year

12:179. Online — International Centre for Genetic Engineering and Biotechnology (ICGEB)

File name	EMBL Nucleotide Sequence Database
Alternative name(s)	European Molecular Biology Laboratory Database – EMBL
Start year	Current Information
Number of records	44,000
Update period	Four times per year

12:180. CD-ROM — IntelliGenetics Inc

File name	EMBL Nucleotide Sequence Database
Alternative name(s)	European Molecular Biology Laboratory Database – EMBL
Start year	Current Information
Number of records	44,000
Update period	Quarterly

12:181. Tape — International Centre for Genetic Engineering and Biotechnology (ICGEB)

File name	EMBL Nucleotide Sequence Database
Alternative name(s)	European Molecular Biology Laboratory Database – EMBL
Start year	Current Information
Number of records	44,000
Update period	Four times per year

This database can also be found on:
CD-GENE
PC/Gene Databanks
Genetyx
BISANCE
BISANCE CD
EMBL Sequence Database

EMBL Sequence Database
European Molecular Biology Laboratory (EMBL)

12:183. Master record
CD-ROM — European Molecular Biology Laboratory (EMBL)

Database type	Chemical structures/DNA sequences, Textual
Number of journals	
Sources	

Start year	
Language	English
Coverage	International
Number of records	–
Update size	
Update period	Quarterly
Price/Charges	Subscription: DM150 – 600

Keywords

DNA; RNA; MRNA; Bacteriophages; Biotechnology; Genetic Research; Microbiology; Nucleotides; Protein Sequences; Proteins; Viruses

Notes

Contains the European Molecular Biology Laboratory – Nucleotide Sequence Database, and SWISS-PROT Protein Sequence Database. Offers sequence data, descriptive information, ancillary databases, including abstracts.

DM 600 Commercial subscription; DM 300 Academic Subscription; DM 150 Academic (EC/EMBL Member country).

For more details of constituent databases, see:
EMBL
SWISS-PROT

Entrez: Sequences CD-ROM
National Library of Medicine
National Center for Biotechnology Information

12:185. Master record
CD-ROM — National Technical Information Service (NTIS)

Database type	Bibliographic, Factual
Number of journals	
Sources	Journals
Start year	
Language	English
Coverage	
Number of records	–
Update size	
Update period	Six times per year

Keywords

Genetic Research

Description

Nucleotide and amino acid sequences are increasingly located in separate databases such as GenBank, the European Molecular Biology Laboratory database EMBL, the Protein Identification Resource (PIR), etc. rather than being included with the original research article according to Gregory Pratt (*CD-ROM Professional* 6(3) May 1993 62–67). 'In fact, some biomedical journals require authors to submit sequences to an appropriate database before accepting a manuscript for publication. As of August 1992, over 44,000 MEDLINE references going back as far as 1971 have cross-references to sequence data in several different sequence databases.' As these databases are not generally available online, it is frequently necessary for researchers to leave the online host and move to Internet for access to the appropriate sequence database. Entrez: Sequences consists of subsets of MEDLINE, GenBank, NBRF-PIR, Swiss-Prot and the DNA Databank of Japan with pre-established links between the bibliographic records and the sequences.

Contains DNA and protein sequence information and bibliographic citations, genome mapping, molecular chemistry and other aspects of human genetics. Combining nucleotide and protein sequences and journal abstracts for papers that published them, this database eliminates the need to search separate databases. An evaluative beta test version contained the following interconnected data: 86,000 MEDLINE citations and abstracts; 35,000 GenBank nucleotide and 53,000 Protein Identification Resource protein sequences; and an NCBI translation of GenBank. The current release (Pre-release 4) contains over 44,000 MEDLINE records, 103,000 protein sequences and 77,000 nucleotide sequences.

Searching the sequence data is by way of text terms, controlled vocabularies used by the original sequence database, the Organism field, the accession numbers (again from the original databases), and the Gene Names. According to Pratt, the Organism field has no standardisation of terms (he quotes the example of fruit fly (535 records), drosophila (31) and drosophila melanogaster (1,712)) but the Gene Name field uses standardised designations although gene names are not always consistent. The name used is the one found in the Locus portion of the sequence record. His conclusion was that Entrez fills a niche that will last until disparate online systems can be linked transparently. This seems to say that Entrez has quite a long useful life.

For more details of constituent databases, see:
MEDLINE
Genbank
NBRF-PIR
Swiss-Prot
DNA Databank of Japan

Environmental Mutagens
Oak Ridge National Laboratory, Environmental Teratology Information Centre

12:187. Master record

Alternative name(s)	EMIC; Environmental Mutagen Information Center File
Database type	Bibliographic
Number of journals	
Sources	Journals
Start year	1969 (with some earlier materials)
Language	English
Coverage	International
Number of records	67,000
Update size	—
Update period	Three to four times per year

Description

Contains citations to the worldwide literature on the testing for mutagenicity and genetic toxicology of chemicals, biological agents, and selected physical agents. Covers only selected studies dealing with the mutagenicity of ionizing or ultraviolet radiation. Also includes some general references on test methods, systems, and organisms. Records also contain Chemical Abstracts Service Registry Numbers.

Only available as part of TOXLINE.

12:188. Online   BLAISE-LINK
(as a part of TOXNET)

File name	EMICBACK
Alternative name(s)	EMIC

Start year
Number of records
Update period

Notes

The backfile of Environmental Mutagens database (Environmental Mutagen Information Center Backfile), giving citations to articles published between 1950 and 1988, providing full bibliographic references, keywords, chemical names and CAS Registry numbers.

12:189. Online   CISTI MEDLARS
(as a part of TOXNET)

File name	EMICBACK
Alternative name(s)	EMIC; Environmental Mutagen Information Center File
Start year	1950
Number of records	
Update period	

Notes

The backfile of Environmental Mutagens database (Environmental Mutagen Information Center Backfile), giving citations to articles published between 1950 and 1988, providing full bibliographic references, keywords, chemical names and CAS Registry numbers.

12:190. Online   National Library of
Medicine
(as a part of TOXNET)

File name	EMICBACK
Alternative name(s)	EMIC; Environmental Mutagen Information Center File
Start year	1950
Number of records	
Update period	

Notes

The backfile of Environmental Mutagens database (Environmental Mutagen Information Center Backfile), giving citations to articles published between 1950 and 1988, providing full bibliographic references, keywords, chemical names and CAS Registry numbers.

This database can also be found on:
TOXLINE
TOXLINE Plus
PolTox I: NLM, CSA, IFIS

Environmental Teratology
Oak Ridge National Laboratory, Environmental Teratology Information Centre

12:192. Master record

Alternative name(s)	ETIC; Environmental Teratology Information Center Files
Database type	Bibliographic, Directory
Number of journals	
Sources	Journals
Start year	1975 (earliest materials from 1912)
Language	English
Coverage	International

Number of records   45,000
Update size   —
Update period   Quarterly
Index unit   Articles

Description

Produced by the Environmental Mutagens, Carcinogen and Teratogen Information Program of the ORNL, this database contains citations to the worldwide literature on teratology – the science dealing with causes, mechanisms, and manifestations of structural or functional alterations in animal development. Covers the testing and evaluation for teratogenic activity of chemical, biological, and physical agents and of dietary deficiencies in warm-blooded animals, plus developmental and reproductive teratology. Primary emphasis is on literature that covers the administration of an agent to pregnant animals and examination of offspring at or near birth for structural or functional anomalies. Records also contain Chemical Abstracts Service Registry Numbers.

12:193. Online   BLAISE-LINK
(as a part of TOXNET)

File name   ETICBACK
Alternative name(s)   ETIC
Start year
Number of records
Update period

Notes

The backfile of Environmental Teratology giving citations to articles published between 1950 and 1988, providing full bibliographic details, keywords, chemical names and CAS Registry Numbers to articles dealing with teratology and developmental/reproductive toxicology.

12:194. Online   CISTI MEDLARS
(as a part of TOXNET)

File name   ETICBACK
Alternative name(s)   ETIC
Start year
Number of records
Update period

Notes

The backfile of Environmental Teratology giving citations to articles published between 1950 and 1988, providing full bibliographic details, keywords, chemical names and CAS Registry Numbers to articles dealing with teratology and developmental/reproductive toxicology.

12:195. Online   National Library of
Medicine
(as a part of TOXNET)

File name   ETICBACK
Alternative name(s)   ETIC; Environmental Teratology
                     Information Center Files
Start year
Number of records
Update period

Notes

The backfile of Environmental Teratology giving citations to articles published between 1950 and 1988, providing full bibliographic details, keywords, chemical names and CAS Registry Numbers to articles dealing with teratology and developmental/reproductive toxicology.

This database can also be found on:
TOXLINE
TOXLINE Plus
PolTox I: NLM, CSA, IFIS
Developmental and Reproductive Toxicology – DART

GenBank
IntelliGenetics Inc
US National Institute of Health
Los Alamos National Laboratory

12:197. Master record

Alternative name(s)   Genetic Sequence Databank;
                          Genbank Nucleotide Sequence
                          Databank
Database type   Bibliographic, Textual, Chemical
                          structures/DNA sequences
Number of journals
Sources   Journals, Reports and Suppliers
Start year   1967
Language   English
Coverage   USA (primarily) and Europe
                          (primarily)
Number of records   82,000+
Update size   1,200
Update period   Monthly
Index unit   Articles, report and sequence

Keywords

DNA; RNA; MRNA; Bacteriophages; Biotechnology; Genetic Research; Genetics; Microbiology; Nucleic Acid Sequences; Nucleotides; Viruses

Description

Nucleotide and amino acid sequences are increasingly located in separate databases such as GenBank, the European Molecular Biology Laboratory database EMBL, the Protein Identification Resource (PIR), etc. rather than being included with the original research article according to Gregory Pratt (*CD-ROM Professional* 6(3) May 1993 62–67). 'In fact, some biomedical journals require authors to submit sequences to an appropriate database before accepting a manuscript for publication. As of August 1992, over 44,000 MEDLINE references going back as far as 1971 have cross-references to sequence data in several different sequence databases.'

Along with the European Molecular Biology Nucleotide Sequence Database (EMBL) and the DNA Database of Japan, GenBank is responsible for collecting, verifying and distributing nucleotide sequence data to the international scientific community. It contains over 70,000 nucleic acid sequences, together with bibliographic citations and related descriptive information. Contains more than 18,000 citations to journal articles and technical reports in genetic research, as well as descriptions of DNA and RNA sequences with fifty or more nucleotide bases.

Each record contains sixteen data items, including the sequence itself accompanied by annotations describing literature citations, bibliographic data, biological origin, sequence annotations (including significant features in each sequence), source organism, CAS Registry Numbers, CA accession numbers and starting point of sequence described.

The database contains 22 different files: release notes; directory description; a list of new and revised entries; five indexes (accession number, keyword phrase, author, citation, gene symbol); submission forms; and thirteen kinds of sequence entry (primate, rodent, other mammal, other vertebrate, invertebrate, plants including fungi and algae, eukaryotic organelles, bacteria, structural RNA, viral, phage, synthetic and chimeric sequences, unannotated).

Incoming sequences are routinely checked for vector sequence contamination.

Data are compiled by the Theoretical Biology and Biophysics Group at Los Alamos National Laboratory from several sources, including Nucleic Acids Research, Nature, Proceedings of the National Academy of Sciences (USA). IntelliGenetics Inc. has a contract with the United States National Institutes of Health GenBank System.

According to Henry and Elizabeth Urrows (*CD-ROM Librarian* 1992 7(7) p 29–35) since June 1991, satellite copies of the Los Alamos GenBank file have run at IntelliGenetics Inc, University of Texas (Austin), National Center for Biotechnology Information (NLM, Bethesda), Applied Mathematics Group (Wellington, New Zealand), Sydney University, Lawrence National Laboratory (Berkeley, California), Walter and Eliza Hall Institute (Melbourne) and Cold Spring Harbor Laboratory. These are all updated daily. However, in September 1992, GenBank moved to the National Center for Biotechnology Information (NLM, Bethesda).

To access through Bionet, users must be qualified principal investigators employed by a non-profit organisation. GenBank's software clearing house supplies a list of some 31 software suppliers and their products linked to the databanks they support. Includes program functions and capabilities; hardware requirements; price; author name, address, and telephone number; and, when available, citations to articles describing or evaluating the software. Hibio Dnasis (CD-ROM) contains software for analysis and manipulation of sequences retrieved from this database and EMBL.

GenBank does not test for compatibility.

12:198. Online   Bionet

File name	
Alternative name(s)	Genetic Sequence Databank; Genbank Nucleotide Sequence Databank
Start year	1967
Number of records	70,000+
Update period	Monthly

Notes

To access through Bionet, users must be qualified principal investigators employed by a non-profit organisation.

Online access is provided giving interactive use of FASTA similarity search program and TFASTA protein sequence comparison with nucleic acid files. It is also possible to use a software suite consisting of molecular biology, sequence entering and editing, DNA gel fragment assembly, protein and nucleic acid sequence analyses, similarity and pattern recognition searching, restricted mapping, and cloning simulation softwares.

12:199. Online   CISTI CAN/SND

File name	GenBank
Alternative name(s)	Genetic Sequence Databank; Genbank Nucleotide Sequence Databank
Start year	

Number of records	
Update period	Quarterly

12:200. Online   IntelliGenetics Inc, GenBank On-line Service

File name	GenBank
Alternative name(s)	Genetic Sequence Databank; Genbank Nucleotide Sequence Databank
Start year	1967
Number of records	70,000+
Update period	Monthly

Notes

IntelliGenetics Inc. has a contract with the United States National Institutes of Health GenBank System. Online access is provided giving interactive use of FASTA similarity search program and TFASTA protein sequence comparison with nucleic acid files. It is also possible to use a software suite consisting of molecular biology, sequence entering and editing, DNA gel fragment assembly, protein and nucleic acid sequence analyses, similarity and pattern recognition searching, restricted mapping, and cloning simulation softwares.

12:201. Online   International Centre for Genetic Engineering and Biotechnology (ICGEB)

File name	GenBank
Alternative name(s)	Genetic Sequence Databank; Genbank Nucleotide Sequence Databank
Start year	1967
Number of records	82,000+
Update period	Monthly

12:202. Online   STN

File name	Genbank
Alternative name(s)	Genetic Sequence Databank; Genbank Nucleotide Sequence Databank
Start year	1982
Number of records	82,495
Update period	Weekly
Price/Charges	Connect time: DM25.00
	Online print: DM7.73
	Offline print: DM7.97
	SDI charge: DM10.20

Notes

Online access is provided giving interactive use of FASTA similarity search program and TFASTA protein sequence comparison with nucleic acid files. It is also possible to use a software suite consisting of molecular biology, sequence entering and editing, DNA gel fragment assembly, protein and nucleic acid sequence analyses, similarity and pattern recognition searching, restricted mapping, and cloning simulation softwares.

12:203. CD-ROM   IntelliGenetics Inc

File name	GenBank Nucleotide Sequence Database
Alternative name(s)	Genetic Sequence Databank; Genbank Nucleotide Sequence Databank
Format notes	IBM, Mac
Start year	
Number of records	
Update period	Quarterly
Price/Charges	Subscription: US$100 – 125

Notes

A new format has been developed especially for the CD-ROM version of the GenBank database. Developed in collaboration with with the EMBL Data Library and the NBRF Protein Identification Resource, it includes several new indices and is designed to compensate for the slower access times of CD-ROM. It contains the full GenBank file, and each CD-ROM distribution includes the GenBank database in three different formats – as the ASCII 'flat file', found on tape releases, the floppy disk format, and a new format developed for CD-ROM.

12:204. CD-ROM — US Government Printing Office National Library of Medicine

File name	NCBI-GenBank
Alternative name(s)	Genetic Sequence Databank; Genbank Nucleotide Sequence Databank
Format notes	IBM, Mac
Start year	
Number of records	
Update period	Six times a year
Price/Charges	Subscription: UK£70

Notes

A National Library of Medicine National Center for Biotechnology Information product. Provides DNA sequence data and concerns genetic coding. This is produced in the ASCII flat file format developed for CD-ROM.

12:205. Diskette — IntelliGenetics Inc

File name	GenBank
Alternative name(s)	Genetic Sequence Databank; Genbank Nucleotide Sequence Databank
Format notes	IBM, Mac
Start year	1967
Number of records	27,000
Update period	Twice a year (March and September)
Price/Charges	Subscription: US$175

Notes

Contains citations to journal articles and technical reports in genetic research, in addition to descriptions of DNA and RNA sequences with fifty or more nucleotide bases. Includes over 22,000 reported sequences, totalling over 26 million bases.

Binary file supplied. Corresponds to the GenBank online database. Data are compiled by the Theoretical Biology and Biophysics Group at Los Alamos National Laboratory from several sources, including Nucleic Acids Research, Nature, Proceedings of the National Academy of Sciences (USA).

12:206. Tape — International Centre for Genetic Engineering and Biotechnology (ICGEB)

File name	GenBank
Alternative name(s)	Genetic Sequence Databank; Genbank Nucleotide Sequence Databank
Format notes	6250, bpi
Software	Flat ASCII file supplied.
Start year	1967
Number of records	82,000+
Update period	Quarterly

This database can also be found on:
CD-GENE

Lasergene CD-ROM
Entrez: Sequences CD-ROM
Genetyx
NCBI-Sequences (ASN.1)

Genek, feherjek es peptidek adatait elemzö programcsomag
Orszagos Sugarbiologiai es

12:208. Master record

Database type	Bibliographic, Factual
Number of journals	
Sources	
Start year	
Language	English
Coverage	
Number of records	
Update size	—
Update period	

Description

In-house DNA database, factographic.

12:209. Online — Orszagos Sugarbiologiai es

File name	BIOANAL
Start year	
Number of records	
Update period	

GeneSeq
Derwent Publications Ltd

12:210. Master record

Database type	Patents, Factual, Chemical structures/DNA sequences
Number of journals	
Sources	Patents and Patents (US)
Start year	1989, with some earlier coverage
Language	English
Coverage	International
Number of records	
Update size	—
Update period	Every two weeks

Keywords

Biotechnology; DNA; Molecular Biology; RNA; Patents; Proteins

Description

Descriptions of nucleic acid and protein sequences from patents and patent applications. Included are nucleotide sequences greater than nine bases, all protein sequences greater than three amino acids and probes of any length. Information includes type of molecule (for example, DNA, RNA, protein), molecule length, accession number, description of the sequence, genus and species of the source organism, table of sequence-specific features, patent number and publication date, patent priority details, assignee, inventors, patent title and patent sequence. Nucleotide sequences are in IUPAC format; protein sequences are in one-letter format. Sources include patents published in Europe, Japan and the USA.

12:211. Online — IntelliGenetics Inc, GenBank On-line Service

File name	
Start year	1989, with some earlier coverage

Number of records
Update period — Every two weeks

12:212. Tape — IntelliGenetics Inc

File name — GeneSeq
Start year — 1981
Number of records
Update period — Every two weeks

Notes

Derwent database of gene and protein sequence information from patents. Initially offering 1989 data relating to 4,500 sequences, it will be updated on a current basis every quarter of 1990. A backfile to at least 1981 should also be completed by end of 1990. Charges are $1.50 per sequence which gives complete ownership of the information.

Genetic Technology News
Technical Insights Inc

12:213. Master record

Database type — Textual, Directory
Number of journals — 1
Sources — Newsletters and Patents
Start year — 1982 Mead Data Central; 1988 Data-Star and DIALOG
Language — English
Coverage — USA (primarily) and International (some)
Number of records
Update size — —
Update period — Daily

Keywords

Genetic Engineering; Patents; Pharmaceutical Industry

Description

Contains full text of *Genetic Technology News*, a monthly newsletter focussing on commercial applications in the chemical, energy, food, and pharmaceutical industries of products resulting from genetic engineering. Includes market forecasts, business news from leading biotechnology firms, announcements of investment opportunities, reports on research activities at universities and research institutions, and reports of new products. Also provides information on recently granted biotechnology patents, including number, title, assignee, and issue date. Many items include names, addresses, and telephone numbers of people who may be contacted for further information.

Produced and supplied to Mead Data Central by Technical Insights Inc; supplied to Data-Star and DIALOG by Predicasts.

12:214. Online — CompuServe Information Service

File name — IQUEST File 2541
Start year — Current year
Number of records
Update period — Monthly
Price/Charges — Subscription: US$8.95 per month
Database entry fee: US$9/search; some databases carry a surcharge ($2–75)
Online print: US$10 references free; then $9 per ten; abstracts $3 each

Downloading is allowed

Notes

Accessed via IQUEST or IQMEDICAL, this database is offered by a NewsNet gateway. IQUEST can either search across all databases, a database of the user's choice or selected multiple databases.

12:215. Online — Mead Data Central (as a NEXIS database)

File name — GENTEC – NEXIS
Alternative name(s) — NEXIS – GENTEC
Start year — 1982
Number of records
Update period — Monthly, as new data are released
Price/Charges — Subscription: US$1,000 – 3,000 (Depending on needs)
Connect time: US$49.00 (Telecomms + connect time)
Database entry fee: US$6.00
Online print: US$0.04 per line

Notes

Libraries: HEALTH and PATENT.

A subscription charge which covers all transactional charges, connect time, telecommunications and the small administration charge can take the place of the individual charges. Subscriptions are negotiated with customers and vary according to the number of menus (thus, files) that are to be used – typically a minimum subscription would be about US$ 1,000. All charges include training and a 24-hour help line.

This database can also be found on:
PTS Newsletter Database
NEXIS

Genetic Toxicity
US Environmental Protection Agency (EPA), Office of Pesticides and Toxic Substances

12:217. Master record

Database type — Factual
Number of journals
Sources — Journals and Monographs
Start year — 1970
Language — English
Coverage — International
Number of records — 2,618
Update size — —
Update period — Periodically

Keywords

DNA; Toxic Substances

Description

Contains mutagenicity information (for example, chromosome aberration, DNA repair) on 2,618 chemicals (for example, dyes) that were tested against 38 biological systems (for example, the Ames test). Data are extracted from published literature.

12:218. Online — Chemical Information Systems Inc (CIS)

File name
Start year — 1970
Number of records — 2,618
Update period — Periodically

Notes

Annual subscription fee of $300 to CIS required. Chemical Information Systems is a subsidiary of Fein-Marquart Associates.

Genetyx
Software Developments

12:219. Master record

CD-ROM	Software Developments
Database type	Chemical structures/DNA sequences, Textual, Image
Number of journals	
Sources	
Start year	
Language	Japanese
Coverage	
Number of records	
Update size	—
Update period	Three times per year

Keywords

DNA; Biotechnology; Nucleic Acid Sequences; Protein Sequences

Description

Notes

Gene information: Contains the GenBank Nucleotide Sequence Database, the PIR Protein sequence database (NBRF), and the EMBL Nucleotide Sequence Database.

For more details of constituent databases, see:
GenBank
PIR
EMBL

GENTEC
Gesellschaft für Biotechnologische Forschung mbH

12:221. Master record

Alternative name(s)	Informationssystem und Datenbank Gentechnologie
Database type	Bibliographic
Number of journals	
Sources	Journals, Reviews, Books, Conference reports, Patent reports, Expert opinion, Standards, Laws/regulations and Government documents
Start year	1984
Language	German (keywords, descriptors and some abstracts) and English (some abstracts)
Coverage	
Number of records	6,949
Update size	3,500
Update period	Monthly

Keywords

Genetic Engineering

Description

GENTEC is a German-language bibliographic database on gene technology and comprises information from all over the world with an emphasis on Europe and the Federal Republic of Germany. In addition to scientific aspects the database also covers 'public opinion' on questions of gene technology and in addition to scientific publications the database also contains references to published opinions of organisations and political groups.

All of the records contain abstracts.

All subject related fields are freetext searchable. The GENTEC documents are indexed with descriptors taken from a German language alphabetic key word list. It is anticipated that a specific hierarchically structured Thesaurus will be available in the near future.

12:222. Online   DIMDI

File name	GT84
Alternative name(s)	Informationssystem und Datenbank Gentechnologie
Start year	1984
Number of records	6,949
Update period	Monthly
Price/Charges	Connect time: UK£22.48–25.31 Online print: UK£0.58–0.76 Offline print: UK£0.51–0.58 SDI charge: UK£None

Downloading is allowed

Notes

Suppliers of online documents: British Library Document Supply Centre, Boston Spa, England; Harkers Information Retrieval System, Sydney, Australia. The unit record contains author(s), title and other data as well as keywords and abstracts (100%). Key words are in German only.

This database can also be found on:
PolTox I: NLM, CSA, IFIS

Health and Safety Science Abstracts
Cambridge Scientific Abstracts
University of Southern California
Institute of Safety and Systems Management

12:224. Master record

Database type	Bibliographic, Factual
Number of journals	
Sources	Monographs, Journals, Reports, Government documents, Conference proceedings, Patents and Dissertations
Start year	1981
Language	English
Coverage	International
Number of records	78,000
Update size	—
Update period	Quarterly

Keywords

Safety; Occupational Health and Safety

Description

Contains citations to the worldwide literature on safety science and hazard control, with an emphasis on the identification, evaluation, and elimination or control of hazards. Covers industrial and occupational safety, transportation safety, aviation and aerospace safety, environmental and ecological safety, and medical safety. Within these areas the database covers liability information and phenomena which directly or indirectly threaten humanity, the environment or the technology upon which they depend, Including such topics as environmental pollution and waste disposal, fire, radiation, pesticides, natural disasters, toxicology, genetics, epidemics, drugs, injuries, diseases, and criminal acts (for example, arson).

Corresponds to *Health and Safety Science Abstracts*.

12:225. Online — ORBIT

File name	SSAB – Safety Science Abstracts
Start year	1981
Number of records	61,000
Update period	Quarterly
Database aids	Quick Reference Guide (5/90) Free (single copy) and Database Manual (1990) $15.50

12:226. Online — STN

File name	HEALSAFE
Start year	1981
Number of records	78,072
Update period	Quarterly
Price/Charges	Connect time: DM186.00
	Online print: DM1.02
	Offline print: DM1.19
	SDI charge: DM15.20

12:227. Tape — Cambridge Scientific Abstracts

File name	Health and Safety Science Abstracts on Magnetic Tape
Format notes	9-track, unlabelled, 1600 bpi, EBCDIC
Start year	1981
Number of records	78,072
Update period	Quarterly
Price/Charges	Subscription: US$Current year 4,250; single-year archival file 2,100

Notes

Corresponds to the Health and Safety Science Abstracts online database.

This database can also be found on:
PolTox I: NLM, CSA, IFIS
Cambridge Scientific Abstracts Engineering
Hard Sciences (ESA-IRS)

Hibio CD-Strains
Hitachi Software Engineering

12:229. Master record

Database type	Computer software
Number of journals	
Sources	
Start year	
Language	English
Coverage	
Number of records	
Update size	–
Update period	Annually

Keywords

Genetic Research

Notes

Additional culture collections will be added at updates.

12:230. CD-ROM — Hitachi Software Engineering

File name	Hibio CD-Strains
Format notes	IBM
Start year	
Number of records	
Update period	Annually
Price/Charges	Subscription: US$700

Hibio DNASIS
Hitachi Software Engineering

12:231. Master record

Database type	Computer software
Number of journals	
Sources	
Start year	
Language	English
Coverage	
Number of records	
Update size	–
Update period	Annually

Keywords

Genetic Research; Proteins

Description

A collection of software to manipulate and analyse DNA sequences retrieved from the GenBank and EMBL databases. DNA sequences can be added from the keyboard or via a digitiser-equiped autoradiograph while data read to a speech synthesizer can be verified for the accuracy of sequences. DNASIS permits comparison of two sequences, cloning simulations and the conversion of a sequence to its complement. Primary structure analysis includes location of restricted enzyme sites or G/C-rich regions and prediction of possible protein-coding regions. Restricted map construction automatically makes linear or circular maps from gel data.

See also Hibio PROSIS

12:232. CD-ROM — Hitachi Software Engineering

File name	Hibio DNASIS
Format notes	IBM
Start year	
Number of records	
Update period	Annually
Price/Charges	Subscription: US$1,700

This database can also be found on:
MacDNASIS Pro

Hibio PROSIS
Hitachi Software Engineering

12:234. Master record

Database type	Computer software, Factual
Number of journals	
Sources	

Start year
Language   English
Coverage
Number of records
Update size   –
Update period   Annually

Keywords
Genetic Research; Proteins

Description
Offers analytical and manipulative capacities for sequences retrieved from the NBRF-PIR and SWISS-PROT databases. Eight subfunctions include reverse-translation of an amino acid to DNA sequence, analysis for hydro-phobicity, construction of dot matrix plots for maximum homology, sequence secondary structure prediction, construction of a helical wheel, and prediction of the isoelectric point of a protein.

See also Hibio DNASIS

12:235. CD-ROM   Hitachi Software Engineering

File name   Hibio PROSIS
Format notes   IBM
Start year
Number of records
Update period   Annually
Price/Charges   Subscription: US$1,400

This database can also be found on:
MacDNASIS Pro

Human Genome Data Base
William H Welch Medical Library, Johns Hopkins University

12:237. Master record
Alternative name(s)   GDB
Database type   Bibliographic, Factual
Number of journals
Sources   Email, Journals and Databases
Start year
Language   English
Coverage   International
Number of records
Update size   –
Update period

Keywords
DNA; RNA; Bacteriophages; Biotechnology; Chromosomal Research; Genetics; Microbiology; Nucleotides; Viruses

Description
Repository of information to support the specialised on-going research of genetic scientists on chromosomal research. Items are peer-reviewed.

Effectively an electronic publishing activity for a closed user group.

12:238. Online   William H Welch Medical Library, Johns Hopkins University

File name   Human Genome Data Base
Alternative name(s) GDB
Start year

Number of records
Update period

Invittox
Invittox

12:239. Master record
Database type   Factual, Textual
Number of journals
Sources   institutions
Start year   1990
Language
Coverage
Number of records
Update size   –
Update period

Keywords
In Vitro Methods

Description
Provides in-depth technical information on the toxicology and toxicity of in vitro methods. Scientists who are developing such methods are asked to donate information on their techniques. These are used to produce guidelines which will enable others to carry out a given procedure without reference to further sources. Emphasis on methodology. Will also monitor the use of the guidelines in order to obtain feedback to add to the database. The development and evaluation of systems can be followed. Database should contribute to the standardization of in vitro methods. Service is expected to be free.

12:240. CD-ROM   Invittox
File name   Invittox
Start year   1990
Number of records
Update period

Lasergene System 190
National Biomedical Research Foundation

12:241. Master record
CD-ROM   DNAStar
Database type   Textual, Chemical structures/DNA sequences, Bibliographic, Computer software
Number of journals
Sources
Start year   1965
Language   English
Coverage   International
Number of records
Update size   –
Update period   Quarterly

Keywords
Genetic Research; Biotechnology; Proteins

Description

Contains information retrieved from several molecular biology databases plus related software for DNA and protein analysis:

GenBank; NBRF-PIR from the National Biomedical Research Foundation; and several other databases.

GenBank: contains more than 27,000 citations to journal articles and technical reports in genetic research, as well as descriptions of DNA and RNA sequences with fifty or more nucleotide bases.
PIR Protein Sequence Database: contains descriptions of over 6,700 partial and whole protein sequences representing over 1.7 million amino acids that were isolated or inferred from the gene sequences.

Priced according to combination of databases required.

For more details of constituent databases, see:
GenBank
PIR Protein Sequence Database

Lasergene System 2000

National Biomedical Research Foundation

12:243. Master record

CD-ROM   **DNAStar**

Database type	Textual, Chemical structures/DNA sequences, Bibliographic, Computer software
Number of journals	
Sources	Journals and Technical reports
Start year	1965
Language	English
Coverage	International
Number of records	
Update size	—
Update period	Quarterly
Index unit	Articles

Keywords

Biotechnology

Description

Contains molecular biology information and biotechnical data plus related softwarefor DNA and protein analysis taken from the following databases:

GenBank; NBRF-PIR from the National Biomedical Research Foundation; Vector-Bank; and several other databases.

GenBank: contains more than 27,000 citations to journal articles and technical reports in genetic research, as well as descriptions of DNA and RNA sequences with fifty or more nucleotide bases.

PIR Protein Sequence Database: contains descriptions of over 6,700 partial and whole protein sequences representing over 1.7 million amino acids that were isolated or inferred from the gene sequences.

Vector-Bank: contains the nucleotide acid sequences of 136 frequently used cloning vectors.

Priced according to combination of databases

required – not all above-listed are included in lowest-priced product.

For more details of constituent databases, see:
GenBank
Vector-Bank
PIR Protein Sequence Database

Life Sciences Collection

Cambridge Scientific Abstracts

12:245. Master record

Alternative name(s)	LSC; CSA Life Sciences Collection
Database type	Bibliographic
Number of journals	5,000
Sources	Journals, books, serial monographs, conference proceedings, patents (US), patents (UK), patents (Japanese) and reports
Start year	1978
Language	English
Coverage	International
Number of records	1,500,000
Update size	
Update period	Monthly

Keywords

Acute Poisoning; Aging; Algology; Amino-Acids; Anatomy; Antibiotics; Aquaculture; Bacteriology; Behavioural Ecology; Bioengineering; Biological Membranes; Biotechnology; Bone Disease; Calcium Metabolism; Chemoreception; Chronic Poisoning; Clinical Medicine; Clinical Toxicology; DNA; Drugs; Ecology; Ecosystems; Endocrinology; Entomology – Agricultural; Entomology – Applied; Entomology – Human; Entomology – Veterinary; Environmental Biology; Ethology; Genetic Engineering; Hazardous Substances; HIV; Histology; Human Ecology; Immune Disorders; Immunology; Infectious Diseases; Marine Biotechnology; Microbiology; Molecular Biology; Molecular Neurobiology; Mycology; Neurology; Neuropharmacology; Neurophysiology – Animal; Neuroscience; Nucleic Acids; Nutrition; Oncology; Occupational Health and Safety; Osteoporosis; Osteomalacia; Pathology; Peptides; Pharmaceuticals; Pheromones; Physiology; Pollution; Proteins; Protozoology; Psychophysics; Public Health; Radiation; Rhinology; RNA; Sleep; Smoking; Substance Abuse; Taste Perception; Viral Genetics

Description

Life Sciences Collection contains abstracts of information in the fields of (and corresponding to abstract journals from CSA): animal behaviour; biochemistry-amino-acid, peptide and protein; biochemistry – nucleic acids; biochemistry-biological membranes; biotechnology research (from 1984 to date); calcified tissue; chemoreception; ecology; endocrinology; entomology; genetics; human genomes; basic research and clinical applications; immunology, marine biotechnology, microbiology- algology, mycology and protozoology;microbiology-bacteriology;microbiology-industrial and applied microbiology; oncology-oncogenes and growth factors; neurosciences (from 1983 to date); toxicology; virology and AIDS. AIDS is covered in depth. The worldwide coverage is of journal articles, books, conference proceedings, report literature, patents, theses and dissertations.

Corresponds to the series of abstracting journals published by CSA: *Animal Behavior Abstracts; Biochemistry Abstracts-Amino-acid, Peptide & Protein; Biochemistry Abstracts-Biological Membranes; Biochemistry Abstracts-Nucleic Acids; Calcified Tissue Abstracts; Biotechnology Research Abstracts* (from 1984 to date); *Chemoreception Abstracts; Ecology Abstracts; Endocrinology Abstracts; Entomology Abstracts; Genetics Abstracts; Human Genome Abstracts; Basic Research and Clinical Applications; Immunology Abstracts; Marine Biotechnology Abstracts; Microbiology Abstracts-Algology, Mycology & Protozoology; Microbiology Abstracts-Bacteriology; Microbiology Abstracts-Industrial & Applied Microbiology; Neurosciences Abstracts* (from 1983 to date); *Oncogenes and Growth Factors Abstracts; Toxicology Abstracts; Virology and AIDS Abstracts.* Most recently added were *Marine Biotechnology Abstracts* and *Oncogenes and Growth Factors Abstracts.* Also includes *Oncology Abstracts* and *Feeding, Weight and Obesity Abstracts* for the period they were published.

12:246. Online — BIOSIS Life Science Network

File name	Life Sciences Collection
Start year	1978
Number of records	1,500,000
Update period	Monthly
Price/Charges	Connect time: US$9.00
	Online print: US$6.00 per 10; 2.25
	per abstract; 3.50 per full text article

Also available via the Internet by telnetting to LSN.COM.

Notes

On Life Science Network users can search this database or they can scan a group of subject-related databases. There is a charge of $2.00 per scan of subject-related databases. To search one database and display up to ten citations costs $6.00. Most charges are for information retrieved. There are no charges if there are no results and no charge to transfer results to a printer or diskette. Articles may also be ordered via an online document delivery request. A telecommunications software package is also available, costing $12.95, providing an automatic connection to Life Science Network for heavy users of the service, with capability to transfer to print or disk and customised colour options.

12:247. Online — DIALOG

File name	File 76
Start year	1978
Number of records	1,392,381
Update period	Monthly
Price/Charges	Connect time: US$90.00
	Online print: US$0.75
	Offline print: US$0.75
	SDI charge: US$9.50

12:248. Online — STN

File name	LIFESCI
Start year	1978
Number of records	1,500,000
Update period	Monthly

12:249. CD-ROM — Compact Cambridge

File name	Life Sciences Collection
Alternative name(s)	LSC; CSA Life Sciences Collection
Format notes	NEC, 9800, IBM
Start year	1982
Number of records	
Update period	Quarterly
Price	UK£1,165 – 2,985 (Initial with backfiles)
	Subscription: UK£985

Notes

Contains eighteen subject orientated subfiles in the life and biosciences field, covering some 5,000 core journals, books, serial monographs etc. Over 98,000 abstracts are added each year. Subscribers to CSA's life sciences print journals receive a £500 credit towards the first year's subscription to LSC CD-ROM 1982–present or 1985–present.

12:250. Tape — Cambridge Scientific Abstracts

File name	Life Sciences Collection on Magnetic Tape
Alternative name(s)	LSC; CSA Life Sciences Collection
Format notes	9-track, unlabelled, 1600 bpi, EBCDIC.
Start year	1982
Number of records	
Update period	Monthly
Price/Charges	Subscription: US$13,950

Notes

The series of abstracting journals published by CSA are available on this tape as a collection. They are also available separately as tape subsets of the Life Sciences Collection, the online database to which this tape corresponds.

Price for the current year tape is $13,950; single-year archival file is $7,100.

12:251. Database subset

Tape — Cambridge Scientific Abstracts

File name	Cambridge Biochemistry Abstracts Series on Magnetic Tape
Format notes	9-track, unlabelled, 1600 bpi, EBCDIC.
Start year	1978
Number of records	
Update period	Monthly

Notes

A subset of the Life Sciences Collection. Contains three database of information on biochemistry.

Biological Membranes contains citations, with abstracts, to the worldwide literature on cell membrane structure and function in all biological systems. Includes membrane components, physical properties, receptors, model and reconstituted systems, methodology, ultrastructure, transport and related phenomena, regulation of membrane function, immunological response, cell interaction, membrane- bound enzymes, isolation and characterization of membranes, and bioenergetics. Corresponds to the *Cambridge Biochemistry Abstracts Series, Part 1: Biological Membranes*, and in part to the Life Sciences Collection online database.

Nucleic Acids contains citations, with abstracts, to the worldwide literature on nucleic acids and molecular biology. Covers RNA,including biosynthesis, virus and phage infections, effect of hormones, and role as messenger; DNA, including effects of radiation, antibiotics and other agents, biosynthesis, virus and phage infections, gene regulation, cloning and mutagenesis; and enzymes, including RNases, DNases, polymerases, phosphorylases and DNA unwinding enzymes. Also covers enhancers, transcription factors, splicing pathways, cloning vectors, sequencing strategies, and polymerase chain reaction. Corresponds to Cambridge *Biochemistry Abstracts*

Series, Part 2: Nucleic Acids, and in part to the Life Science Collection online database.

Amino-Acids, Peptides & Proteins contains citations, with abstracts, to the worldwide literature on amino acids, peptides and proteins. Covers isolation and purification techniques, structural analysis, solution studies, biological and chemical modification of peptides and proteins, X-Ray crystallography and electron microscopy, peptide synthesis, enzyme assays, mechanisms of enzyme action, including enzyme kinetics, peptide and protein toxins, enzyme inhibitors and activators, peptide and protein analogs, and evolutionary aspects. Corresponds to Cambridge Biochemistry Abstracts Series Part 3: Amino-Acids, Peptides & Proteins, and in part to the Life Sciences Collection online database.

Contact Cambridge Scientific Abstracts for pricing information.

12:252. Database subset

Tape   **Cambridge Scientific Abstracts**

File name	Cambridge Microbiology Abstracts Series on Magnetic Tape
Format notes	9-track, unlabelled, 1600 bpi, EBCDIC.
Start year	1978
Number of records	
Update period	Monthly

Notes

A subset of the Life Sciences Collection. Contains three databases of information on microbiology.

Industrial & Applied Microbiology contains citations, with abstracts, to the worldwide literature on practical applications of microbiology. Covers pharmaceutical, food and beverage, agricultural and environmental applications, and methodology and research. Includes antibiotics and antimicrobial agents; vaccines and serum production; food contamination, ripening and fermentation processes; soil microbiology; plant diseases caused by microorganisms; composting; hydrocarbons; methane production; pollution; and isolation, identification and characterization of microorganisms. Also incudes registered US patents. Corresponds to Cambridge Microbiology Abstracts, Section A; Industrial & Applied Microbiology, and in part to the Life Sciences Collection online database.

Bacteriology contains citations, with abstracts, to the worldwide literature on bacteriology. Covers immunology, taxonomy, methods, cell properties, genetics, antibiotics and antimicrobials, toxins, medical, veterinary and invertebrate bacteriology, plant diseases, and ecological aspects. Corresponds to Cambridge Microbiology Abstracts, Section B: Bacteriology, and in part to the Life Sciences Collection online database.

Algology, Mycology & Protozoology contains citations, with abstracts, to the worldwide literature on algae, fungi, protozoa and lichens. Includes reproduction, growth, life cycles, biochemistry, genetics, and infection and immunity in humans, other animals and plants. Covers taxonomy, structure and function, ecology and distribution, effects of physical and chemical factors, methodology, media and culture, nutrition, mycotoxins, parasitism and diseases, viruses and bacteria, soil microbiolgy and mycorrhiza, spoilage and biodegradation, and pollution. Corresponds to Cambridge Microbiology Abstracts, Section C:

Algology, Mycology & Protozoology, and in part to the Life Sciences Collection online database. Pricing information may be obtained from Cambridge Scientific Abstracts.

12:253. Database subset

Tape   **Cambridge Scientific Abstracts**

File name	Biotechnology Research Abstracts on Magnetic Tape
Format notes	9-track, unlabelled, 1600 bpi, EBCDIC.
Start year	1984
Number of records	
Update period	Every two months

Notes

A subset of the Life Sciences Collection. Contains citations, with abstracts, to the worldwide literature on biotechnology, including medical, chemical, agricultural, pharmaceutical, environment and energy applications. Covers genetic engineering, cloning vectors, site-directed mutagenesis, gene manipulation, transfer and expression, biotechnology products and relevant US patents. Corresponds to Biotechnology Research Abstracts and in part to the Life Science Collection online database.

It is necessary to contact Cambridge Scientific Abstracts for pricing information.

12:254. Database subset

Tape   **Cambridge Scientific Abstracts**

File name	Genetics Abstracts on Magnetic Tape
Format notes	9-track, unlabelled, 1600 bpi, EBCDIC.
Start year	1968
Number of records	
Update period	Monthly

Notes

A subset of the Life Sciences Collection. Contains citations, with abstracts, to the worldwide literature on genetics. Covers molecular, viral, bacterial, fungal, algal, plant, human, animal and medical genetics, DNA, RNA, protein synthesis, ribosomes, nuclear proteins, chromatin, enzymes and gene regulation. Corresponds to Genetic Abstracts and in part to the Life Sciences Collection online database. Contact CSA for pricing information.

12:255. Database subset

Tape   **Cambridge Scientific Abstracts**

File name	Oncogenes and Growth Factors Abstracts on Magnetic Tape
Format notes	9-track, unlabelled, 1600 bpi, EBCDIC.
Start year	1989
Number of records	
Update period	Quarterly

Notes

A subset of the Life Sciences Collection. Contains citations, with abstracts, to the worldwide literature on cancer research and the molecular basis of malignant transformations. Covers growth factors, receptors, suppressor genes, anti-oncogenes, cellular proto-oncogenes, oncogenes in DNA and RNA tumour viruses, cell cycle control, immortalization and cellular senescence. Corresponds to *Oncogenes and Growth Factor Abstracts* and in part to the Life Sciences Collection online database. Contact Cambridge Scientific Abstracts for pricing information.

12:256. Database subset

Tape	Cambridge Scientific Abstracts
File name	Virology and AIDS Abstracts on Magnetic Tape
Format notes	9-track, unlabelled, 1600 bpi, EBCDIC.
Start year	1978
Number of records	
Update period	Monthly

Notes

A subset of the Life Sciences Collection. Contains citations, with abstracts, to the worldwide literature on human, animal and plant virology, and on Acquired Immune Deficiency Syndrome (AIDS). Covers replication cycles, oncology, viral genetics, interferon, hepatitis B virus vaccination, immunological, clinical and epidemiological aspects of AIDS, patterns of AIDS, AIDS-related diseases and investigational drugs. Corresponds to *Virology and AIDS Abstracts* and in part to the Life Sciences Collection and in part to the Life Science online database. Contact Cambridge Scientific Abstracts for pricing information.

This database can also be found on:
Cambridge Scientific Abstracts Life Sciences
Human Nutrition on CD-ROM

MacDNASIS Pro
Hitachi Software Engineering

12:258. Master record

CD-ROM	Hitachi Software Engineering
Database type	Computer software
Number of journals	
Sources	
Start year	
Language	English
Coverage	
Number of records	
Update size	—
Update period	Annually

Keywords

Genetic Research; Bioengineering

Notes

This product appears to be a combination of the two IBM-based products, Hibio PROSIS and Hibio DNASIS.

The former offers analytical and manipulative capacities for sequences retrieved from the NBRF-PIR and SWISS-PROT databases. Eight subfunctions include reverse-translation of an amino acid to DNA sequence, analysis for hydro-phobicity, construction of dot matrix plots for maximum homology, sequence secondary structure prediction, construction of a helical wheel, and prediction of the isoelectric point of a protein. Hibio DNASIS is a collection of software to manipulate and analyse DNA sequences such as those in GenBank and EMBL. DNA sequences can be added from the keyboard or via a digitiser-equiped autoradiograph while data read to a speech synthesizer can be verified for the accuracy of sequences.

DNASIS permits comparison of sequences, cloning simulations and the conversion of a sequence to its complement. Primary structure analysis includes location of restricted enzyme sites or G/C-rich regions and prediction of possible protein-coding regions. Restricted map construction automatically makes linear or circular maps from gel data.

See also Hibio PROSIS and Hibio DNASIS.

For more details of constituent databases, see:
Hibio DNASIS
Hibio PROSIS

Medical and Psychological Previews
BRS Information Technologies

12:260. Master record

Database type	Bibliographic
Number of journals	240
Sources	Journals
Start year	
Language	English
Coverage	
Number of records	19,500
Update size	7,000
Update period	
Hosts have included	BRS (until 30.9.92.)

Description

Gave bibliographic citations from 240 core medical journals prior to their appearance in MEDLINE. Covered: clinical medicine, psychology, psychiatry, nursing, hospital administration. Included editorials, notes and letters. Covered last four months. BRS discontinued this database at the end of September 1992.

Medical Science Research Database
Medical Science Research
Elsevier Science Publishers

12:261. Master record

Alternative name	IRCS Medical Science Database (former name)
Database type	Textual
Number of journals	
Sources	
Start year	1982
Language	English
Coverage	
Number of records	57,000
Update size	600
Update period	Bimonthly
Hosts have included	Data-Star and DIMDI

Keywords

Physiology; Pathology; Anatomy

Description

The Medical Science Research database consists of the full text, including tables, or peer-reviewed research articles published in *Medical Science Research* (incorporating IRCS Medical Science journals). Articles are approximately 1,000 words long and are concise but complete accounts of research with full methodological and result information. Coverage includes all areas of clinical and biomedical science, with major coverage in the following areas: alimentary system, anatomy and human biology, biochemistry, biomedical technology, cardiovascular system, cell and membrane biology, clinical medicine, clinical pharmacology and therapeutics, connective tissue, skin and bone, dentistry and oral biology, developmental biology and medicine, drug metabolism and toxicology, endocrine system, environmental biology and medicine, experimental animals, the eye, haematology, immunology and allergy, metabolism and nutrition, microbiology, parasitology and infectious diseases, nervous system, pathology, physiology, psychology and psychiatry, reproduction, obstetrics and gynaecology, social and occupational medicine, surgery and transplantation, techniques and methods.

This database appears to be no longer available.

Molecular Structures in Biology

Brookhaven National Laboratory,
   Protein Data Bank
Oxford Electronic Publishing

12:262. Master record

CD-ROM	Oxford Electronic Publishing
Database type	Bibliographic, Chemical structures/DNA sequences, Textual, Image
Number of journals	
Sources	
Start year	1991
Language	English
Coverage	
Number of records	500+
Update size	—
Update period	Annually

Description

Contains the January 1990 release Brookhaven Protein Data Bank with over 500 molecular structures; a picture bank of specially generated colour images – at least three images for each structure and also, where applicable, the depositor's preferred view; Specialist papers – texts on the structure and function of proteins and nucleic acids and on the methods of structure determination by leading international experts in the field. Programs to generate interactive graphics; Static colour images from the data and searching facilities. Structures can be rotated in three-dimensions; particular sub-units or strings of residues can be viewed, while simultaneously searching data about them or comparing images in adjacent windows.

Academic version available for £750

For more details of constituent databases, see:
Brookhaven Protein Data Bank

MTA-SOTE Genek, feherjek es peptidek adatait szolgaltato adatbazis

MTA – SOTE Egyesitett Kutatasi

12:263. Master record

Database type	
Number of journals	
Sources	
Start year	
Language	English
Coverage	
Number of records	
Update size	
Update period	

Keywords
DNA

Description
DNA mapping database.

12:264. Online   MTA – SOTE Egyesitett Kutatasi

File name	BIOSEQ
Start year	
Number of records	
Update period	

Nature of Genes, The

MedMedia

12:265. Master record

Database type	Courseware, Multimedia
Number of journals	
Sources	
Start year	
Language	English
Coverage	
Number of records	
Update size	—
Update period	

Keywords
Genetics; Molecular Biology

Description

A tutorial to teach the basics of molecular biology and genetics. Includes text, voice, realtime animation and clinical imagery and users are able to 'experience the excitement of building a double helix and splicing a gene'.

Designed for undergraduate medical students.

12:266. CD-ROM   MedMedia

File name	Nature of Genes, The
Format notes	Mac, IBM
Start year	
Number of records	
Update period	
Price	UK£1,300

NBRF-PIR Nucleic Acid Sequence Database

National Biomedical Research
   Foundation, Protein Identification
   Resource (NBRF/PIR)

12:267. Master record

Alternative name(s)	Nucleic Acid Sequence Database
Database type	Chemical structures/DNA sequences
Number of journals	
Sources	Books, Journals, Letters and Research communications
Start year	1972
Language	English
Coverage	International
Number of records	4,000
Update size	—
Update period	Irregularly

Keywords
DNA; RNA; Nucleic Acids; Proteins

Description

Descriptions of about 4,000 genetic sequences in approximately 8 million bases. Covers nucleic acid sequences for proteins and some regulatory and promoter sequences. Descriptions include function of the sequence, features of biological interest and source (RNA or DNA).

Corresponds in part to Nucleic Acid Sequence Database, with additional data available online.

12:268. Online   CISTI CAN/SND

File name	NBRF
Alternative name(s)	Nucleic Acid Sequence Database
Start year	1972
Number of records	4,000
Update period	Irregularly

12:269. Online   IntelliGenetics Inc, GenBank On-line Service

File name	
Alternative name(s)	Nucleic Acid Sequence Database
Start year	1972
Number of records	4,000
Update period	Irregularly

12:270. Online   National Biomedical Research Foundation, Protein Identification Resource (NBRF/PIR)

File name	
Alternative name(s)	Nucleic Acid Sequence Database
Start year	1972
Number of records	4,000
Update period	Irregularly

NBRF-PIR Protein Sequence Database

National Biomedical Research Foundation, Protein Identification Resource (NBRF/PIR)

12:271. Master record

Alternative name(s)	PIR Protein Sequence Database; Protein and Identification Resource Database; Protein Sequence Database; PIR
Database type	Chemical structures/DNA sequences, Bibliographic, Textual
Number of journals	
Sources	Journals, Books, Letters, Private communications and Research communications
Start year	1965
Language	English
Coverage	International
Number of records	26,700
Update size	—
Update period	Quarterly

Keywords

Amino Acids; Genetic Research; Genetics; Proteins; Protein Sequences

Description

Nucleotide and amino acid sequences are increasingly located in separate databases such as GenBank, the European Molecular Biology Laboratory database EMBL, the Protein Identification Resource (PIR), etc. rather than being included with the original research article according to Gregory Pratt (*CD-ROM Professional* 6(3) May 1993 62–67). 'In fact, some biomedical journals require authors to submit sequences to an appropriate database before accepting a manuscript for publication. As of August 1992, over 44,000 MEDLINE references going back as far as 1971 have cross-references to sequence data in several different sequence databases.'

Produced by the National BioMedical Research Foundation, NBRF-PIR Protein Sequence Database is one of the major biotechnology genetic sequence databases. Descriptions of over 26,700 partial and whole protein sequences representing more than 7.6 million amino acids that were isolated or inferred from the gene sequences. Descriptions include the function of the protein, taxonomy, sequence features of biological interest, how the sequence was experimentally determined, unambiguously determined residues within the sequence and citations to relevant literature.

Corresponds in part to NBRF *Atlas of Protein Sequence and Structure*, with more current information online. Hibio PROSIS (CD-ROM) contains software for analysis and manipulation of sequences retrieved from this database and SWISS-PROT.

12:272. Online   Bionet

File name	
Alternative name(s)	PIR; Protein and Identification Resource Database; Protein Sequence Database
Start year	1965
Number of records	
Update period	Quarterly

Notes

To access through Bionet, users must be qualified principal investigators employed by a non-profit organisation.

12:273. Online   IntelliGenetics Inc, GenBank On-line Service

File name	Protein Identification Resources
Alternative name(s)	PIR; Protein and Identification Resource Database; Protein Sequence Database
Start year	1965
Number of records	
Update period	Quarterly

12:274. Online   International Centre for Genetic Engineering and Biotechnology (ICGEB)

File name	Protein Identification Resources
Alternative name(s)	PIR; Protein and Identification Resource Database; Protein Sequence Database
Start year	1965
Number of records	
Update period	Quarterly

12:275. Online   National Biomedical Research Foundation, Protein Identification Resource (NBRF/PIR)

File name	Protein Identification Resources
Alternative name(s)	Protein and Identification Resource Database; Protein Sequence Database; PIR
Start year	1965
Number of records	26,700
Update period	Quarterly

12:276. Tape

International Centre for Genetic Engineering and Biotechnology (ICGEB)

File name	Protein Identification Resources
Alternative name(s)	PIR; Protein and Identification Resource Database; Protein Sequence Database
Format notes	UNIX
Software	IG Suite
Start year	1965
Number of records	
Update period	Quarterly

This database can also be found on:
CD-GENE
Lasergene CD-ROM
Entrez: Sequences CD-ROM
Genetyx
NCBI-Sequences (ASN.1)

NCBI-Sequences (ASN.1)
National Library of Medicine National Center Biotechnology Information

12:278. Master record
CD-ROM

US Government Printing Office (GPO)

Database type	Chemical structures/DNA sequences, Computer software
Number of journals	
Sources	
Start year	
Language	
Coverage	
Number of records	
Update size	
Update period	Six time a year

Keywords
DNA; Biotechnology; Nucleic Acid Sequences; Protein Sequences

Description
A National Library of Medicine product. Concerns genetic coding. An integrated database of DNA and protein sequence information. Uses HHS-created software.

For more details of constituent databases, see:
GenBank
NBRF-PIR

NFormation
Neurofibromatosis Institute Inc, The

12:280. Master record

Database type	Bibliographic, Textual, Encyclopedia, Dictionary, Directory
Number of journals	
Sources	Monograph, Journals, Clinicians, Associations, Groups and Original material
Start year	Varies with file
Language	English
Coverage	International

Number of records	Varies with file
Update size	—
Update period	Varies with file

Keywords
Neurofibromatosis; Neurological Diseases

Description
Contains eight separate files and services on the genetic disease, neurofibromatosis (NF).

Bibliography contains citations, with abstracts and annotations, to the international biomedical literature on NF, updated monthly.

NF References contains citations to the international literature on NF since 1960.

Textbook contains the full text (excluding figures) of *Neurofibomatosis: Phenotype, Natural History and Pathogenesis* (1986).

Journal gives the tables of contents and selected abstracts from the journal *Neurofibromatosis* since 1988, updated quarterly.

Clinical Research, updated periodically, contains clinical data on over 1,000 people with, or at risk risk from, NF, giving name and affiliation of the clinical investigator and the following data on patients: sex, race, socioeconomic status, dates of birth (and death where applicable), diagnosis and data on about ninety possible symptoms (pulmonary fibrosis, hyperpigmentation, diffuse craniofacial neurofibromas, etc) and their current severity. Physicians can add information on their own patients.

NFassist is an expert system which provides technical and diagnostic assistance to physicians and researchers, including a dictionary of NF-related terms and an encyclopaedia of related facts and concepts.

News and Comments contains a listing of professional and self-help group meetings, research opportunities and fundraising events, updated monthly.

Resource Identification contains a periodically updated directory of funding sources, health care programmes, clinical and basic research programmes and self-help groups, arranged geographically.

Partially corresponds to *Neurofibromatosis: Phenotype, Natural History and Pathogenesis* (1986).

12:281. Online

Neurofibromatosis Institute Inc, The

File name	NFormation
Start year	Varies with file
Number of records	Varies with file
Update period	Varies with file

Notes
No charges for this database.

Obstetrics and Gynaecology
Elsevier Science Publishers
CMC ReSearch

12:282. Master record

Database type	Factual, Textual, Image
Number of journals	1
Sources	Journal
Start year	1985
Language	English
Coverage	

Number of records
Update size   –
Update period   Annually

Keywords
Gynaecology; Obstetrics

Description
Full text of five years of the Elsevier journal with tables and images. Includes: Medical and surgical treatment of female conditions; Obstetric management; Clinical evaluation of drugs and instruments; etc. Covers 1985 – 1990

12:283. CD-ROM   CMC ReSearch
File name   Obstetrics and Gynaecology on
                    Disc 1985–1990
Format notes   IBM
Software   DiscPassage
Start year   1985
Number of records
Update period   Annually
Price   UK£265

This database can also be found on:
Comprehensive Core Medical Library

PASCAL
Centre National de la Recherche Scientifique, Institut de l'Information Scientifique et Technique, Science Humaines et Sociales (CNRS/INIST)

12:285. Master record
Alternative name(s)   Programme Applique a la Selection
                      et a la Compilation Automatique de
                      la Litterature
Database type   Bibliographic
Number of journals   8,500
Sources   Books, conference proceedings,
                      dissertations, journals, maps,
                      monographs, patents
                      (biotechnology), reports, technical
                      reports and theses
Start year   1973
Language   English (titles and keywords),
                      French and Spanish (keywords)
Coverage   International
Number of records   9 million
Update size   500,000
Update period   Monthly
Index unit   Articles
Thesaurus   Biomedical Thesaurus in 3 volumes
Database aids   PASCAL User Manual, PASCAL
                      Classification Scheme and PASCAL
                      Dictionary in 3 Volumes (French,
                      English, Spanish): Exact Sciences,
                      Technology, Medicine

Keywords
Bioagriculture; Biomedicine; Biotechnology; Cell Biology; Civil Engineering; Construction; Demography; Electrical Engineering; Epidemiology; Ergonomics; Immunology; Metallurgy; Microbiology; Mineralogy; Nutrition; Parasitology; Patents; Physics; Pollution; Public Health; Travel Medicine; Tropical Medicine

Description
PASCAL is a multidisciplinary and multilingual bibliographic database covering the core of scientific, technical and medical literature worldwide. Subjects covered include: Life sciences – biology, tropical

medicine, biomedical engineering, biochemistry, biotechnology, pharmacology, microbiology, ophthalmology, dermatology, anaesthesia, human diseases, animal biology, reproduction, genetics, zoology, plant biology, agronomics, agricultural science, psychology; Earth sciences – mineralogy, mining economics, cristallography, stratigraphy, hydrology, paleontology; Physical sciences physics, information science, computer science, astronomy, electrical engineering, electronics, atoms and molecules, general, physical, analytical, inorganic and organic chemistry; Engineering sciences – energy, metallurgy, pollution, mechanical industries, construction, welding and brazing, civil engineering, building and public works, transportation.

In addition there are specialised subfiles in the following areas: information science, documentation, energy, metallurgy, civil engineering, earth sciences, biotechnology, zoology of invertebrates, agriculture and tropical medicine.

On ESA-IRS, DIALOG and QUESTEL searches can be limited to one of the two subfiles PASCAL: Biotechnologies and PASCAL: Medécine Tropicale dating from 1982 on ESA-IRS and QUESTEL, but on DIALOG from 1986. Each subfile holds over 40,000 records.

Biotechnologies contains citations, with abstracts to the international biotechnology literature, covering biochemistry, cell biology, microbiology and applications of cultured microorganisms and cells in agriculture, energy, food processing, medicine, metallurgy and pollution control. Some patents are included in this area. Corresponds to *PASCAL THEMA 215: biotechnologies*.

Medécine Tropicale provides citations, with abstracts, to the international literature of tropical medicine, covering human and animal parasites and diseases, the biology and control of vectors, intermediate hosts and reservoirs, ergonomics, nutrition, physical and social demography, public health and medical issues relating to travellers. Corresponds to *PASCAL THEMA 235: Médecine Tropicale*.

These subfiles are available as part of PASCAL on DIALOG, QUESTEL and ESA-IRS.

PASCAL is the online version of the print publication *Bibliographie Internationale* (1984 onwards) and corresponds to the publication *Bulletin Signaletique* (1973–1983). The titles in the PASCAL file are in their original languages and are translated into French and/or English. Approximately fifty per cent of records have abstracts which are in French or English (from 1982 the titles and keywords are also given in English). Journal articles account for approximately ninety-three per cent of the file. 8,500 journals are regularly scanned. Source materials are published in various languages: English 63%, French 12%, Russian 10%, German 8% and other languages 7%.

The controlled terms are in French and also in English for records since 1982 and in Spanish for records since 1977. German controlled terms are also provided in the area of metallurgy.

12:286. Online   CompuServe Information
                                            Service
File name   IQUEST File 1284
Alternative name(s)   Programme Applique a la Selection
                      et a la Compilation Automatique de
                      la Litterature
Start year   1973
Number of records   9 million
Update period   Monthly

| Price/Charges | Subscription: US$8.95 per month
Database entry fee: US$9/search;
some databases carry a surcharge
($2–75)
Online print: US$10 references free;
then $9 per ten; abstracts $3 each |

Downloading is allowed

Notes

Accessed via IQUEST or IQMEDICAL, this database is offered by a Questel gateway. IQUEST can either search across all databases, a database of the user's choice or selected multiple databases.

12:287. Online   DIALOG

File name	File 144
Alternative name(s)	Programme Applique a la Selection et a la Compilation Automatique de la Litterature
Start year	1973
Number of records	3,866,245
Update period	Monthly
Price/Charges	Connect time: US$60.00
Online print: US$0.50
Offline print: US$0.50
SDI charge: US$12.00

Notes

DIALINDEX Categories: AGRI, BIOCHEM, BIOSCI, BIOTECH, CHEMLIT, EECOMP, ENERGY, ENERGYP, GEOLOGY, GEOLOGYP, GEOPHYS, MATERIAL, MEDICINE, METALS, PHYSICS, SCITECHB.

12:288. Online   ESA-IRS

File name	File 14
Alternative name(s)	Programme Applique a la Selection et a la Compilation Automatique de la Litterature
Start year	1973
Number of records	8,263,000 (October 1991)
Update period	Monthly
Price/Charges	Subscription: UK£70.29
Database entry fee: UK£3.51
Online print: UK£0.07 – 0.56
Offline print: UK£0.50
SDI charge: UK£3.51

Notes

QUESTALERT and QUESTORDER are both available on this file. The LIMIT ALL command can be used to limit all subsequent sets. This can be cancelled by entering a new LALL or a BEGIN command.

From 1993 ESA-IRS are charging an annual fee of 100 Accounting Units (c.UK£ 70.29) to all users. This is equivalent to the fee for full documentation and will not be charged to customers already paying for documentation.

Record composition

Abstract /AB; Author AU; Classification Code CC; Classification Number CN; CODEN CO; Controlled Terms (Descriptors) /CT; Controlled Terms in English /KE; Controlled Terms in French /KF; Controlled Terms in Spanish or German /KO; Corporate Source CS; Country/Place of Publication CY; Document Type DT; Domain (Subfile) DO; Generic Controlled Terms (Broader Terms) /CT*; Geographical Coordinates GC; International Patent Classification PC; ISBN BN; ISSN SN; Journal Name JN; Language LA; Language of Summary LS; Location of Document LC; Major Controlled Terms /CT* or /MAJ; Map Type CA; Meeting Date MD; Meeting Location ML; Meeting Title MT; Native Number NN; Report Number RN; Patent Application Number PA; Patent Holder (Corporate)

PH; Patent Number PN; Patent Priority PP; Publication Year PY; Publisher PB; Report Number RN; Single Controlled Terms /ST; Source SO; Titles (English) /ET; Titles (French) /FT; Titles (other) /OT and Titles (all) /TI

The titles are in their original language and are translated into French and/or English. The Controlled Terms are in French and also in English for records since 1982, and Spanish for records since 1984. German controlled terms are also provided in the area of metallurgy. Abstracts are in French or English (English especially from 1990 onwards). The EXPAND command can be used to display the PASCAL thesaurus. The basic index includes the following data fields: Abstract, Controlled Terms in any language, Controlled Terms in English, Controlled Terms in French, Controlled Terms in Spanish or German, Generic Controlled Terms, Single Controlled Terms, Titles (English), Titles (French), Titles (Other). The Classification Name is the principal hierarchical category corresponding to the classification code of the record. Some fields are searchable in both French and English. The data field Source may include: monographic source, collective source or title of collection. The prefix 'SO=' corresponds to the information displayed immediately after the title. It does not correspond to the field labelled 'Source Information' in the displayed record. To search for journal names the prefix 'JN=' should be used. Role indicators which are used with substances to identify the role they play in a chemical reaction or process are placed after the name of the substance with the symbol | as separator in file 205 and the symbol ! as separator in file 204. Role indicators have been used in chemistry-and physics-related records since 1979 and in metallurgy related reocrds since 1980. They are as follows: ENT: Primary material, FIN: End product, ACT: Active product, SUB: Substrate, solvent, etc, ANA: Analytically determined compound, SEC: Secondary material.

12:289. Online   ESA-IRS

File name	File 204
Alternative name(s)	Programme Applique a la Selection et a la Compilation Automatique de la Litterature
Start year	1973 – 1983
Number of records	4,900,000
Update period	Closed File
Price/Charges	Subscription: UK£70.29
Database entry fee: UK£3.51
Online print: UK£0.07 – 0.56
Offline print: UK£0.50
SDI charge: UK£3.51

Downloading is allowed
Thesaurus is online

Notes

QUESTALERT and QUESTORDER are both available on this file. The LIMIT ALL command can be used to limit all subsequent sets. This can be cancelled by entering a new LALL or a BEGIN command.

From 1993 ESA-IRS are charging an annual fee of 100 Accounting Units (c.UK£ 70.29) to all users. This is equivalent to the fee for full documentation and will not be charged to customers already paying for documentation.

Record composition

Abstract /AB; Author AU; Classification Code CC; Controlled Terms (Descriptors) /CT; Corporate Source CS; Country/Place of Publication CY; Document Type DT; ISBN BN; ISSN SN; Journal Name JN; Language LA; Major Controlled Terms /CT* or /MAJ; Map Type CA; Native Number NN; Report

Number RN; Single Controlled Terms /ST; Titles (English) /ET; Titles (French) /FT; Titles (other) /0T and Titles (all) /TI

The EXPAND command can be used to display the PASCAL thesaurus. The basic index includes the following data fields: Abstract, Controlled Terms (Descriptors), Major Controlled Terms, Single Controlled Terms, Titles (English), Titles (French), Titles (other), Titles (all). Examples of documents types in file 204 include: Journal Article (Code TP), Patent (TB), Conference (TC), Book (TL), Map (TM), Miscellaneous (TS), Monography (LM), Thesis (TT), Report (TR). Role indicators which are used with substances to identify the role they play in a chemical reaction or process are placed after the name of the substance with the symbol | as separator in file 205 and the symbol ! as separator in file 204. Role indicators have been used in chemistry-and physics-related records since 1979 and in metallurgy related reocrds since 1980. They are as follows: ENT: Primary material, FIN: End product, ACT: Active product, SUB: Substrate, solvent, etc, ANA: Analytically determined compound, SEC: Secondary material.

12:290. Online   ESA-IRS

File name	File 205
Alternative name(s)	Programme Applique a la Selection et a la Compilation Automatique de la Litterature
Start year	1984
Number of records	
Update period	Monthly
Price/Charges	Subscription: UK£70.29
	Database entry fee: UK£3.51
	Online print: UK£0.07 – 0.56
	Offline print: UK£0.50
	SDI charge: UK£3.51

Downloading is allowed
Thesaurus is online

Notes

QUESTALERT and QUESTORDER are both available on this file. The LIMIT ALL command can be used to limit all subsequent sets. This can be cancelled by entering a new LALL or a BEGIN command.

From 1993 ESA-IRS are charging an annual fee of 100 Accounting Units (c.UK£ 70.29) to all users. This is equivalent to the fee for full documentation and will not be charged to customers already paying for documentation.

Record composition

Abstract /AB; Author AU; Classification Code CC; Classification Number CN; CODEN CO; Controlled Terms (Descriptors) in any language /CT; Controlled Terms in English /KE; Controlled Terms in French /KF; Controlled Terms in Spanish or German /KO; Corporate Source CS; Country of Publication CY; Document Type DT; Domain (Subfile) DO; Generic Controlled Terms (Broader Terms) /CT*; Geographical Coordinates GC; International Patent Classification PC; ISBN BN; ISSN SN; Journal Name JN; Language LA; Language of Summary LS; Location of Document LC; Map Type CA; Meeting Date MD; Meeting Location ML; Meeting Title MT; Native Number NN; Patent Application Number PA; Patent Holder (Corporate) PH; Patent Number PN; Patent Priority PP; Publication Year PY; Publisher PB; Report Number RN; Single Controlled Terms /ST; Source SO and Titles /TI

The basic index includes the following data fields: Abstract, Controlled Terms in any language, Controlled Terms in English, Controlled Terms in French, Controlled Terms in Spanish or German,

Generic Controlled Terms, Single Controlled Terms, Titles. The Classification Name is the principal hierarchical category corresponding to the classification code of the record. Some fields are searchable in both French and English. The data field Source may include: monographic source, collective source or title of collection. The prefix 'SO=' corresponds to the information displayed immediately after the title. It does not correspond to the field labelled 'Source Information' in the displayed record. To search for journal names the prefix 'JN=' should be used. Role indicators which are used with substances to identify the role they play in a chemical reaction or process are placed after the name of the substance with the symbol | as separator in file 205 and the symbol ! as separator in file 204. Role indicators have been used in chemistry-and physics-related records since 1979 and in metallurgy related reocrds since 1980. They are as follows: ENT: Primary material, FIN: End product, ACT: Active product, SUB: Substrate, solvent, etc, ANA: Analytically determined compound, SEC: Secondary material.

12:291. Online   Questel

File name	PASC73
Alternative name(s)	Programme Applique a la Selection et a la Compilation Automatique de la Litterature
Start year	1973
Number of records	9 million
Update period	

12:292. CD-ROM   Centre National de la Recherche Scientifique, Institut de l'Information Scientifique et Technique, Science Humaines et Sociales (CNRS/INIST)

File name	PASCAL CD-ROM
Alternative name(s)	Programme Applique a la Selection et a la Compilation Automatique de la Litterature; CD-ROM PASCAL
Format notes	IBM
Software	GTI
Start year	1987
Number of records	450,000
Update period	Quarterly
Price/Charges	Subscription: FFr15,000 – 17,790

Notes

Each disc corresponds to one year update of the PASCAL database, that is, approximately 500,000 records. An annual subscription with quarterly updates. Costs 15,000 FFr for current year (1990, 1 disc); 7,500 Ffr for each backfile disc (1987, 1988, 1989, 1 disc each). The full collection with the current year subscription costs 35,000 – 41,150 FFr. Can be used in a LAN network provided the network conforms to the standards required for the MSCDEX extension. Several commercial packages exist to make it possible to operate PASCAL CD-ROM in a suitable network environment.

12:293. Tape   Centre National de la Recherche Scientifique, Institut de l'Information Scientifique et Technique, Science Humaines et Sociales (CNRS/INIST)

File name	PASCAL
Alternative name(s)	Programme Applique a la Selection et a la Compilation Automatique de la Litterature
Format notes	9-track 1,600 or 6,250 BPI magnetic tapes, EBCDIC character set, with or without IBM-OS label
Start year	1987

Number of records	500,000
Update period	Annually
Price/Charges	

Notes

Each tape corresponds to one year update of the PASCAL database ie. approximately 500,000 records.

12:294. Videotex   Minitel

File name	PASCAL 362936011
Alternative name(s)	Programme Applique a la Selection et a la Compilation Automatique de la Litterature
Start year	
Number of records	
Update period	

12:295. Database subset

Online   ESA-IRS

File name	File 37 – Training Pascal
Alternative name(s)	Programme Applique a la Selection et a la Compilation Automatique de la Litterature
Start year	1984–1985
Number of records	48,325(October 1991)
Update period	Not updated
Price/Charges	Connect time: UK£6.99 per hour
Downloading is allowed	
Thesaurus is online	

Notes

Training database (subfile of PASCAL main file, File 14). Neither QUESTALERT nor QUESTORDER are available. Services such as offline prints are also not available.

Record composition

Abstract /AB; Author AU; Classification Code CC; Classification Name CN; CODEN CO; Controlled terms in any language /CT; Controlled terms in English /KE; Controlled terms in French /KF; Controlled terms in Spanish or German /KO; Corporate Source CS; Country of Publication CY; Document Type DT; Domain DO; Generic controlled terms (broader terms) /CT*; Geographical Coordinates GC; ISBN BN; ISSN SN; Journal Name JN; Language LA; Language of Summary LS; Location of Document LC; Map Type CA; Meeting Title MT; Meeting Date MD; Meeting Location ML; Native Number NN; Patent Application Number PA; Patent Holder (Corporate) PH; Patent Number PN; Patent Priority PP; Publication Year PY; Publisher PB; Report Number RN; Single Controlled Terms /ST; Source SO and Titles /TI

The EXPAND command can be used to display the PASCAL thesaurus. The basic index includes the following data fields: Abstract, Controlled terms in any language, Controlled terms in English, Controlled terms in French, Controlled terms in Spanish or German, Generic controlled terms (broader terms), Single controlled terms, Titles. The classification name is the principal hierarchical category corresponding to the classification code of the record. Some fields are searchable in both French and English. Pascal can be divided into a number of subfiles (domains), a list of which can be obtained by entering the command E DO =. Source (SO=) may include: monographic source, collective source, or title of collection. The 'SO=' field is placed between title and author in the displayed record. To search for journal names the prefix 'JN=' should be used. Role indicators which are used with substances to identify the role they play in a chemical reaction or process are placed after the name of the substance with the symbol | as separator in file 205 and the symbol ! as separator in file 204. Role indicators have been used in chemistry-and physics-related records since 1979 and in metallurgy related reocrds since 1980. They are as follows: ENT: Primary material, FIN: End product, ACT: Active product, SUB: Substrate, solvent, etc, ANA: Analytically determined compound, SEC: Secondary material. The LIMIT ALL command can be used to limit all subsequent sets. The limitation can be cancelled by entering a new LALL or a BEGIN command.

This database can also be found on:
Metropolitan
Medata-ROM

PC/Gene Databanks
IntelliGenetics Inc

12:297. Master record

CD-ROM   IntelliGenetics Inc

Database type	Chemical structures/DNA sequences, Numeric
Number of journals	
Sources	Databases
Start year	
Language	
Coverage	International
Number of records	
Update size	—
Update period	Twice a year

Keywords

Genetic Research; Nucleotides; Protein Sequences

Description

Contains EMBL, the nucleotide sequence databank from the European Molecular Biology Laboratory; and SWISS-PROT, a protein sequence databank maintained at the University of Geneva. Includes the catalogues, ASCII bulk sequence files and documentation for both databanks, in addition to a listing of type 2 restriction enzymes and a database of eukaryotic promoters.

For more details of constituent databases, see:
EMBL
SWISS-PROT

Protein Data Bank (Brookhaven)
Brookhaven National Laboratory,
   Protein Data Bank

12:299. Master record

Alternative name(s)	Brookhaven Protein Data Bank; PDB
Database type	Chemical structures/DNA sequences, Textual, Bibliographic
Number of journals	
Sources	

Start year   1990 (July)
Language   English and German
Coverage   International
Number of records   554
Update size   —
Update period

Keywords
Proteins

Description
Nucleotide and amino acid sequences are increasingly located in separate databases such as GenBank, the European Molecular Biology Laboratory database EMBL, the Protein Identification Resource (PIR), etc. rather than being included with the original research article according to Gregory Pratt (*CD-ROM Professional* 6(3) May 1993 62–67). 'In fact, some biomedical journals require authors to submit sequences to an appropriate database before accepting a manuscript for publication. As of August 1992, over 44,000 MEDLINE references going back as far as 1971 have cross-references to sequence data in several different sequence databases.'

Contains the July 1990 release Brookhaven Protein Databank with 554 molecular structures. Includes the atomic coordinate entries, source codes and bibliographic records. Contains structures of proteins, enzymes and polynucleic acids.

12:300. Online   CISTI CAN/SND
File name   CRYSTPRO
Alternative name(s)   Brookhaven Protein Data Bank;
     PDB
Start year
Number of records
Update period

12:301. CD-ROM   Springer-Verlag
File name   Protein Data Bank (Brookhaven)
Alternative name(s)   Brookhaven Protein Data Bank;
     PDB
Format notes   IBM, Mac, Unix
Software   MOBY 1.5
Start year   1990 (July)
Number of records   554
Update period
Price   DM998

Notes
Software may be supplied independently and charged extra. MOBY can display structures wit up to 2,000 centres (or atoms), and its tools for probing into and modifying these structures help in analysis. Academic version available for DM498.

ISBN: 3–540–14101–4 (or 3–540–14102–2 for academic discount)

12:302. Tape   Brookhaven National Laboratory
File name   Protein Data Bank (Brookhaven)
Alternative name(s)   Brookhaven Protein Data Bank;
     PDB
Start year   1990 (July)
Number of records   554
Update period

12:303. Tape   Springer-Verlag
File name   DATAPRTP
Alternative name(s)   Brookhaven Protein Data Bank;
     PDB
Format notes   IBM
Start year   1990 (July)

Number of records   554
Update period

12:304. Tape   Springer-Verlag
File name   DATAPRFI
Alternative name(s)   Brookhaven Protein Data Bank;
     PDB
Format notes   IBM
Start year   1990 (July)
Number of records   554
Update period

This database can also be found on:
Protein Science
Molecular Structures in Biology

Protein Science
Information providers: Lightbinders

12:306. Master record
CD-ROM   Lightbinders
Database type   Chemical structures/DNA
     sequences, Textual, Image,
     Factual, Computer software
Number of journals
Sources   Journals and Monograph
Start year
Language   English
Coverage   International
Number of records
Update size   —
Update period   Annually

Description

Notes
Contains the full text and images of Protein Science volume 1, 1992 plus the Brookhaven Protein Data Bank, Kinemage 3-D protein modeling software and more.

ISSN 0961–8368

For more details of constituent databases, see:
Brookhaven Protein Data Bank

Protein
Institut obchej Genetiki

12:308. Master record
Database type   Bibliographic
Number of journals
Sources
Start year   1985
Language   English
Coverage
Number of records
Update size   —
Update period

Keywords
Biotechnology

Description
Bibliographic information in genetics and biotechnology.

12:309. Diskette   Institut obchej Genetiki
File name
Start year   1985

Number of records
Update period

PTS Newsletter Database
Predicasts International Inc

12:310. Master record

Alternative name(s)	Predicasts Newsletter Database
Database type	Textual
Number of journals	
Sources	
Start year	1988
Language	German and English
Coverage	International
Number of records	722,656
Update size	63,000
Update period	Daily
Database aids	PTS Users Manual, Cleveland, Ohio, Predicasts % x EIIA.iwr74p5.BQuint article.ukolug newsletter3(5)p11 PTS Newsletter Source Guide
Hosts have included	CORIS (Thomson Financial Network) (Until 1/92)

Keywords

Acid Rain; Advertising; Air Pollution; Alcohol Abuse; Antiviral Drugs; Asbestos; Asbestosis; Automation and Control; Beauty Care; Beauty Care; Beverages; Biotechnology; Biotechnology Industries; Brewing; Cancer; Ceramics; Chemical Industry; Chromatography; Composites; Computer Data Security; Computer Ergonomics; Company Profiles; Consumer Products; Cosmetics; Data Security; Defence Waste Disposal; Diagnosis; Diagnostic Equipment; Diagnostic Products; Drug Abuse; Drug Treatment; Drugs; Education – Cancer; Electrodialysis; Employee Benefits; Environmental Policy; Ergonomics; Explosion; Filtration; Fire; Food and Drink; Food Additives; Food Processing; Food Technology; Genetic Engineering; Greenhouse Effect; Hazardous Chemicals; Hazardous Substances; Hazardous Substances Transport; Hazardous Waste; Health and Safety; Health Care; Health Care Management; Health Care Products; Health Insurance; Health Services; HIV; Household Products; Hygiene Products; Information Services; Information Systems; Legal Liability; Legislation; Liability Insurance; Manufacturing; Marketing; Market Reports; Materials Industry; Medicare; Medical Equipment; Medical Textiles; Medical Waste Management; Membrane Technology; Metals; Nuclear Waste; Occupational Health and Safety; Packaging; Patents; Personal Hygiene; Pesticides; Pets; Pharmaceutical Industry; Pharmaceutical Products; Pharmaceuticals; Pollution; Polymers; Product Catalogues; Product Liability; Prosthetics; Public Health; Radiation; Research and Development; Separation Technology; Smoking; Standards; Textiles; Waste Management; Water Pollution; Water Purification

Description

Produced by Predicasts, PTS Newsletter is a multi-industry database providing concise information on company activities, new technologies, emerging industry trends, government regulations and international trade opportunities. It consists of the full text of over 500 business and industry newsletters cover-ing almost fifty different industries and subject areas. It is international in scope, covering all major economic and political regions of the world, including Eastern and Western Europe, the USA, the Pacific Rim, Latin America, Asia and the Middle East. Facts, figures and analyses are provided on the following industrial and geographical areas: advanced materials, biotechnology, broadcasting and publishing, computers and electronics, chemicals, defense and aerospace, energy, environment, financial services and markets, instrumentation, international trade, general technology, Japan, Middle East, manufacturing, medical and health, materials packaging, research and development, telecommunications and transportation.

Newsletters include *Multinational Service* which covers decisions and policies affecting corporations operating worldwide; and *Europe Report* which offers broad coverage of EC activities relating to economic and monetary affairs, the internal market and legislation and regulations relating to business. Both Newsletters are published by the Europe Information Service of Cooper's & Lybrand Europe. Middle East coverage includes the *Israel High-Tech Report*; *The Middle East News Network*; and *The Middle East Consultants' Newsletter*.

12.311. Online   Data-Star

File name	PTBN
Alternative name(s)	Predicasts Newsletter Database
Start year	January 1988
Number of records	533,000
Update period	Weekly
Database aids	Data-Star Business Manual, Berne and Online manual (search for NEWS-PTBN in NEWS)
Price/Charges	Subscription: UK£32.00
	Connect time: UK£80.40
	Online print: UK£0.28 – 0.55
	Offline print: UK£0.26 – 1.00
	SDI charge: UK£4.00

Also available on FIZ Technik via a gateway from Data-Star

Notes

From June 1993 Data-Star have introduced an annual fee/subscription per contract (that is, not per password) of SFr 80.00 (c. UK£ 32.00) payable every June. For North American customers billed in dollars who also use DIALOG, the DIALOG fee also covers access to Data-Star. Academic customers, 'commitment' customers and customers currently billed in dollars are exempt.

12.312. Online   DIALOG

File name	PTSNL
Alternative name(s)	Predicasts Newsletter Database
Start year	1989
Number of records	722,656
Price/Charges	Connect time: US$126.00
	Online print: US$0.90

Notes

PTSNL is a menu-access version of the PTS Newsletter Database. PTSNL provides users with the unique capability to easily retrieve the latest issue (or any available issue) of a newsletter, display a Table of Contents listing articles contained in a selected issue, and print the full text of newsletter articles selected by title. To search newsletters for information on specific subjects, use File 636 (the main PTS file), which utilizes the full range of DIALOG search commands.

12.313. Online   DIALOG

File name	File 636
Alternative name(s)	Predicasts Newsletter Database
Start year	1989
Number of records	722,656
Update period	Daily
Price/Charges	Connect time: US$126.00
	Online print: US$0.90
	Offline print: US$0.90
	SDI charge: US$1.00 (daily) – 3.00
	(weekly)

Notes

This is the main file of PTS on DIALOG. There is also a menu access version – PTSNL, which enables the user to retrieve the latest issue of a newsletter, print the full text of newspaper articles etc. It does not have the full range of DIALOG search commands.

12.314. Online   Dow Jones News/ Retrieval

File name	
Alternative name(s)	Predicasts Newsletter Database
Start year	
Number of records	
Update period	Weekly

12.315. Online   FIZ Technik (gateway)

File name	PTBN
Alternative name(s)	Predicasts Newsletter Database
Start year	1988 (January)
Number of records	Volume 1: 159,000
Update period	Weekly
Price/Charges	Connect time: SFr201.00
	Online print: SFr0.61–1.22
	Offline print: SFr0.24 – 1.83
	SDI charge: SFr10.00

Available via a gateway to Data-Star

For more details of constituent databases, see:
AIDS Weekly
Air/Water Pollution Report
Alliance Alert – Medical Health
Antiviral Agents Bulletin
Applied Genetics News
Asbestos Control Report
BBI Newsletter
Biomedical Materials
Biomedical Polymers
Cancer Weekly
Cosmetic Insiders' Report
Diagnostics Business-Matters
Environment Week
European Cosmetic Markets
FDA Medical Bulletin
Food Chemical News
Genetic Technology News
Hazmat Transport News
Health Business
Health Daily
Industrial Health and Hazards Update
International Product Alert
Japan Report: Medical Technology
Japan Science Scan
Managed Care Law Outlook
Managed Care Outlook
Managed Care Report
Medical Bulletin
Medical Scan
Medical Waste News
Medical Textiles
Membrane and Separation Technology News
National Report on Computers and Health
Nuclear Waste News
Occupational Health and Safety Letter
OTC Market Report: Update USA
OTC News and Market Report
Pesticide and Toxic Chemical News

Pharmaceutical Business News
Product Alert
PRODUCTSCAN
Report on Defense Plant Wastes
Soviet Bio/Medical Report
Toxic Materials News
Worldwide Biotech

SAGE
CSIRO Australis

12:316. Master record

Alternative name(s)	Science and Geography Education
Database type	Bibliographic
Number of journals	19+
Sources	Journals
Start year	1989, with some citations from 1986
Language	English
Coverage	Australia, South Pacific and Asian-Pacific
Number of records	2,200
Update size	1,500
Update period	Twice per year
Index unit	Articles

Keywords

Atmospheric Science; Anthropology; Archaeology; Biology; Botany; Construction; Ecology; History; Management; Microbiology; Natural Resources; Nutrition; Philosophy; Physics; Recreation; Zoology

Description

Covers a broad range of topics in the science, geography and anthropology fields with particular emphasis on the Australian and Asian-Pacific regions. Contains citations, with abstracts, to popular general science and geography journals. Topics include agriculture, anthropology, archaeology, astronomy, atmospheric sciences, biology, botany, chemistry, construction, ecology, education, engineering, environment, genetics, geography, geology, health, history, management, mathematics, microbiology, natural resources, nutrition, philosophy, physics, recreation, sociology and zoology.

Contains references to selected Australian science and geography journals. Coverage: starts 1986 for some titles, otherwise 1989.

Selected Australian journals.

12:317. Online   CSIRO Australis

File name	
Alternative name(s)	Science and Geography Education
Start year	1989, with some citations from 1986
Number of records	2,200
Update period	Twice per year

12:318. CD-ROM   INFORMIT (RMIT-INFORMIT)

File name	
Alternative name(s)	Science and Geography Education
Format notes	IBM
Software	Superfield
Start year	1989, with some citations from 1986

Number of records	2,200
Update period	Twice per year
Price/Charges	Subscription: US$100

Notes

Equivalent to SAGE on AUSTRALIS online.

SWISS-PROT

European Molecular Biology Laboratory (EMBL)

12:319. Master record

Database type	Computer software, Factual
Number of journals	
Sources	
Start year	Current
Language	English
Coverage	International
Number of records	10,000 sequences
Update size	—
Update period	Quarterly

Keywords

Biotechnology; Protein Sequences; Proteins

Description

Nucleotide and amino acid sequences are increasingly located in separate databases such as GenBank, the European Molecular Biology Laboratory database EMBL, the Protein Identification Resource (PIR), etc. rather than being included with the original research article according to Gregory Pratt (*CD-ROM Professional* 6(3) May 1993 62–67). 'In fact, some biomedical journals require authors to submit sequences to an appropriate database before accepting a manuscript for publication. As of August 1992, over 44,000 MEDLINE references going back as far as 1971 have cross-references to sequence data in several different sequence databases.'

SWISS-PROT is a protein sequence databank maintained at the University of Geneva, organized at the International Centre for Genetic Engineering and Biotechnology. Contains descriptions of more than 10,000 nucleic acid and protein sequences. Covers composition, function, length, promoter and gene regions, species, taxonomy, title, topology and literature references. Sources include EMBL Nucleotide Sequence Data Library and PIR Protein Sequence Database.

Hibio PROSIS (CD-ROM) contains software for analysis and manipulation of sequences retrieved from this database and PIR.

12:320. Online   CISTI CAN/SND

File name	SWISS-PROT
Start year	Current
Number of records	10,000 sequences
Update period	Quarterly

12:321. Online   European Molecular Biology Laboratory (EMBL)

File name	SWISS-PROT
Start year	Current
Number of records	10,000 sequences
Update period	Quarterly

12:322. Online   IntelliGenetics Inc, GenBank On-line Service

File name	SWISS-PROT
Start year	Current

Number of records	10,000 sequences
Update period	Quarterly

12:323. Online   International Centre for Genetic Engineering and Biotechnology (ICGEB)

File name	SWISS-PROT
Start year	Current
Number of records	10,000 sequences
Update period	Quarterly

12:324. Tape   International Centre for Genetic Engineering and Biotechnology (ICGEB)

File name	SWISS-PROT
Start year	Current
Number of records	10,000 sequences
Update period	Quarterly

This database can also be found on:
EMBL Sequence Database
PC/Gene Databanks
CD-GENE

Telegenline

RR Bowker Company EIC/Intelligence

12:325. Master record

Database type	Bibliographic
Number of journals	7,000
Sources	Books, conference proceedings, government reports (US), journals, monographs, research reports and symposia
Start year	1973
Language	English
Coverage	International
Number of records	25,200
Update size	—
Update period	Closed File
Database aids	EIC/Intelligence Telegenline Search Aid and Telegenline User's Manual
Hosts have included	DIMDI (Until 1.1.92)

Keywords

Genetic Engineering

Description

Telegenline contains information on the entire field of genetic engineering and biotechnology. Subjects covered include: industrial microbiology; fermentation technologies; genetics relating to plants, animals, humans, bacteria, viruses, plasma and computers; gene therapy: research techniques; applications in energy and mining; food processing; chemistry; pharmaceuticals and medicine; agriculture applications; biohazards; pollution control; public health and occupational safety; social impact; military applications; education; finance; international issues, research founding, ethics and values.

The database corresponds to the printed *Telegen Reporter*. Abstracts have been available since March 1983 and are now contained in approximately 85% of documents.

Indexing in TELEGENLINE consists of two stages. First all TELEGENLINE documents are assigned to one of the twenty-one sections of the *Telegen Reports* (the print equivalent of TELEGENLINE) as follows: 01 Business & Economics; 02 Social Impacts and Constraints; 03 Patent and Legal Issues; 04 Policy and Regulatory Issues; 05 General; 06 International;

07 Industrial Microbiology; 08 Chemical Applications; 09 Energy and Mining Applications; 10 Biohazards and Environmental Applications; 11 Food Processing and Production Applications; 12 Crop Applications; 13 Livestock Applications; 14 Pharmaceutical and Medical Applications; 15 Research on Human Genes; 16 Research on Animal Genes; 17 Research on Plant Genes; 18 Research on Yeast and Fungus Genes; 19 Research on Bacterial Genes; 20 Research on Viral Genes; 21 General Research. Secondly the documents are indexed by Key Terms taken from an alphabetical, non-structured list containing approximately 2,000 terms. The Key Terms are indexed on three levels: Level 1 – primary descriptors; Level 2 – secondary descriptors and Level 3 – tertiary descriptors. The Key Terms are searchable directly as well as through Freetext, the data fields section headings and secton codes can only be searched directly and the data fields Title and Abstracts are only searchable through freetext.

12:326. Online   ESA-IRS

File name	File 49
Start year	1976–1990
Number of records	25,477(October 1991)
Update period	No longer updated
Price/Charges	Subscription: UK£70.29
	Database entry fee: UK£3.49
	Online print: UK£0.63
	Offline print: UK£0.60
	SDI charge: UK£3.49

Downloading is allowed
Thesaurus is online

Notes

From 1993 ESA-IRS are charging an annual fee of 100 Accounting Units (c.UK£ 70.29) to all users. This is equivalent to the fee for full documentation and will not be charged to customers already paying for documentation.

Record composition

Abstract /AB; Author AU; Class Code Name CC; Classification Code CC; Controlled Terms /CT; Corporate Source CS; Document Type DT; Major Controlled Terms /CT or /MAJ; Source Data SO and Title /TI

TOXALL

National Library of Medicine

12:327. Master record

Alternative name(s)	Toxicology Information Online
Database type	Bibliographic
Number of journals	
Sources	Government documents (US), journals, monographs, research projects, Patents, Conference proceedings, Research communications and Symposia
Start year	1940, partly
Language	English
Coverage	International
Number of records	2,500,000
Update size	120,000
Update period	Monthly

Keywords

Aneuploidy; Accident Prevention; Biological Hazards; Chemical Substances; Chromosome Abnormalities; Drugs; Environmental Health; Epidemiology; Ergonomics; Hazardous Substances; Hazardous Waste; Health Physics; Industrial Materials; Industrial Processes; Metabolism; Occupational Health and Safety; Occupational Psychology; Pathology; Pesticides; Pollution; Safety Education; Standards; Vocational Training; Waste Management; Water Treatment

Description

TOXALL/TOXLINE (Toxicology Information Online) is the National Library of Medicine's extensive collection of online bibliographic information covering the toxicological effects of drugs, pesticides and other chemicals. The database contains references to published material and research in progress in areas such as adverse drug reactions, carcinogenesis, mutagenesis, teratogenesis, environmental pollution and food contamination, toxicology, pharmacology, analytical chemistry and occupational safety. Most of the citations include, in addition to the bibliographic information, abstracts and/or indexing term and/or indexing terms and/or CAS Registry numbers.

TOXALL is composed of several database segments of toxicological interest (from CA, BIOSIS Previews and MEDLINE) and of total contents of specialised toxicological data collections. As the data in the different subunits is provided by different producers, there is a relatively great number of duplicates in the database. In addition the structure of the records also varies, for example some include abstracts and some use *MeSH* Indexing, others do not.

The subfiles are, with starting date of coverage being the publication year shown:

ANEUPL (Aneuploidy file of the Environmental Mutagen Information Center) pre 1950 to the present;
Chemical-Biological Activities – CA (Chemical Abstracts);
CISDOC (International Labour Office) (ILO) Abstracts 1981 to the present;
CRISP (Toxicology Research Projects (RPROJ) 1988 to the present;
EMIC (Environmental Mutagen Information Center File of the Oak Ridge National Laboratory (ORNL) 1950 to the present;
EPIDEM (Epidemiology Information System File of the FDA) 1940 to the present;
ETIC (Environmental Teratology Information Center File of ORNL) 1950 to the present;
Federal Research in Progress (FEDRIP) 1982;
HAPAB (Health Aspects of Pesticides Abstract Bulletin of the Environmental Protection Agency (EPA) (see PESTAB));
HAYES (Hayes File on Pesticides);
HMTC (Abstract Bulletin of the US Army's Hazardous Materials Technical Center) 1982 to the present;
International Pharmaceutical Abstracts (IPA) 1969 to the present;
HEEP – see Toxicological Aspects of Environmental Health;
NIOSH (References of the National Institute for Occupational Safety and Health Technical Information Center (NIOSHTIC) database) 1984 to the present;
NTIS (Toxicology Document and Data Depository (TD3) of the National Technical Information Service (NTIS) 1979 to the present;
PESTAB (Pesticides Abstracts of the EPA (Formerly HAPAB) 1968–1981;
PPBIB (Poisonous Plants Bibliography) pre-1976;
RPROJ (Research Projects Directory);
Toxicological Aspects of Environmental Health (BIO-

SIS) (formerly BIOSIS/HEEP, Health Effects of Environmental Pollutants) 1970 to the present;
TMIC (Toxic Materials Information Center File);
TOXBIB (Toxicity Bibliography from the MEDLINE file) 1965 to the present;
TSCATS (Toxic Substances Control Act Test Submissions File of the EPA) (all relevant submissions).

References in TOXLINE are from producers that do not require royalty charges; references on toxicology from producers that do require royalty charges are placed in TOXLIT.

The database contains approximately 20,000 citations from between 1940 and 1965, 640,000 from 1965 to 1976, EMIC since 1960 and ETIC since 1965. About 45% of the records added per year are from the TOXBIB subfile, which is derived from MEDLINE. Approximately eighty-two per cent of documents contain abstracts. Some hosts only carry TOXLINE. TOXLIT comprises IPA (International Pharmaceutical Abstracts), CA (Chemical Abstracts) and Toxicological Aspects of Environmental Health (BIOSIS) (formerly BIOSIS/HEEP).

The datafield Controlled Terms contains vocabulary from all of the subunits. The datafields CAS Registry Number, Chemical Abstracts Classification Codes and ILO Classification Codes can only be searched directly. The datafield Controlled Terms can be searched directly as well as through freetext and the data fields Title and Abstract can only be searched through freetext. The following points are recommended for drugs and chemicals: always use Registry numbers when available; for a broad concept search use as many synonyms as possible in title, keywords and abstract; for TOXBIB only use controlled terms from *MeSH*.

12:328. Online DIMDI

File name	TX65 – TOXALL
Start year	1940, partly
Number of records	3,466,353
Update period	Monthly
SDI period	1 month
Price/Charges	Connect time: UK£35.99–39.78
	Online print: UK£0.52–0.70
	Offline print: UK£0.48–0.55

Downloading is allowed

Notes

As TOXALL is composed of several database segments of toxicological interest (from Chemical Abstracts Service, MEDLINE, BIOSIS Previews) and total contents of specialised toxicological data collections, single citations may occur more than once. DIMDI recommends using CHEMLINE for the retrieval of synonyms and CAS Registry Numbers of chemical substances before starting a TOXALL search. It also advises that a search for chemical substances should not be restricted to the CAS Registry Number field because several TOXALL subunits do not contain this field. The TOXALL subunits are pooled to create the subfiles TOXLINE and TOXLIT which can be accessed separately by using their poolkeys. TOXLIT contains the subunits CA, BIOSIS/HEEP (up to July 1985: HEEP) and IPA. TOXLINE contains the other subunits ANEUPL, DART, EMIC, ETIC, FEDRIP, HAYES, HMTC, ILO, NIOSH, PESTAB/HAPAB, PPBIB, RPROJ, TD3, TMIC, TOXBIB, TSCATS. Documents total over 3 million since 1965 (about 20,000 citations from 1940 to 1965, 640,000 from 1965 to 1976, EMIC since 1960, ETIC since 1950).

Suppliers of online documents: British Library Document Supply Centre, Boston Spa, England; Harkers Information Retrieval System, Sydney, Australia; Instituto de Informacion y Documentacion en Ciencia y Tecnologica, Madrid, Spain; State Central Scientific Medical Library Supplier Center, Moscow, USSR. 82% of records contain abstracts. Searches are available from January 1965.

Record composition

Abstract AB; Author AU; BIOSIS Section Heading BISH; Chemical Abstracts Section Code CASC; Chemical Abstracts Section Heading CASH; CAS Reg. No CR; Corporate Source CS; Controlled Term CT; Country CY; Document Date DT; Date Received REC; Entry Month EM; Free Text FT; Gene Symbol GE; International Labour Office Classification Code ILCC; International Labour Organisation Section Heading ILSC; International Pharmaceutical Abstracts Section Code IPSC; International Pharmaceutical Association Section Heading IPSH; ISSN SS; Journal Code JC; Journal Title JT; Language LA; Machine Date MD; Number of Document ND; Number of Supporting Agency NS; Number of Unit Record (DIMDI) NU; Order Number OD; Preprocessed Search PPS; Price PR; Publication Year PY; Qualifier AF; Secondary Source SEC; Source SO; Subunit SU; Supporting Agency SA; Title TI; Toxic Substances Control Act Section Code TSCC; Type of Award TA and ZIP Code ZP

CALL TOXDUP provides the user with a means to define its own hitlist of subunits from TOXALL and its subfiles TOXLINE and TOXLIT and thereby identify duplicate records.

12:329. Database subset

Online BLAISE-LINK

File name	TOXLINE
Start year	
Number of records	
Update period	

12:330. Database subset

Online BLAISE-LINK

File name	TOXLIT
Start year	
Number of records	
Update period	

12:331. Database subset

Online BRS

File name	TOXL
Start year	1965
Number of records	
Update period	Monthly
Price/Charges	Connect time: US$26.00/36.00
	Online print: US$0.07/0.15

Notes

Records from the IPA and BIOSIS subfiles are excluded from this database.

12:332. Database subset

Online BRS

File name	XTOL
Start year	1965
Number of records	
Update period	Monthly
Price/Charges	Connect time: US$26.00/36.00
	Online print: US$0.07/0.15

Notes

This is a subfile of BRS's TOXL database and contains documents from all TOXLINE subfiles except the MEDLINE-derived subfile TOXBIB. It contains approximately thirty per cent of the documents in TOXLINE covering the pharmacological, biomedical, physiological and toxicological effects of drugs and other chemicals. Data from proprietary sources is excluded.

12:333. Database subset

Online	CompuServe Information Service
File name	IQUEST File 2576 – TOXLINE
Start year	1965
Number of records	
Update period	Monthly
Price/Charges	Subscription: US$8.95 per month
	Database entry fee: US$9/search; some databases carry a surcharge ($2–75)
	Online print: US$10 references free; then $9 per ten; abstracts $3 each

Downloading is allowed

Notes

Coverage dates vary depending on subfile. Accessed via IQUEST or IQMEDICAL, this database is offered by a DIALOG gateway. IQUEST can either search across all databases, a database of the user's choice or selected multiple databases.

12:334. Database subset

Online	Data-Star
File name	TOXX (TOXLINE)
Start year	Current month
Number of records	1,152,262
Update period	Monthly
Database aids	Data-Star Biomedical Manual and Online Guide (search NEWS-TOXL in NEWS)
Price/Charges	Connect time: SFr78.00
	Online print: SFr0.21–0.24
	Offline print: SFr6.80
	SDI charge: SFr0.24

Notes

The current month file does not include references from Toxicology Research Projects (CRISP); Epidemiology Information System File of the FDA (EPIDEM); the Federal Research in Progress Database (FEDRIP); the Abstracts Bulletin of the US Army's Hazardous Materials Technical Centre (HMTC); or the Toxic Substances Control Act Test Submissions File of the EPA (TSCATS). For TOXBIB use also Medical Subject Headings Annotated Alphabetic List (MeSH) and Tree Structrures (TREE) published annually.

From June 1993 Data-Star have introduced an annual fee/subscription per contract (that is, not per password) of SFr 80.00 (c.UK£ 32.00) payable every June. For North American customers billed in dollars who also use DIALOG, the DIALOG fee also covers access to Data-Star. Academic customers, 'commitment' customers and customers currently billed in dollars are exempt.

Record composition

Abstract AB; Accession number and secondary source ID or by code for faster retrieval AN; Author(s) AU; Availability, Order-ID-number, Prices AV; Award type AW; CAS Registry number(s) RN; Classification code CC; Comment CM; Corporate name CA; Entry month EM; Gene symbol GS; Institution, address IN; Keywords KW; Journal coden CD; Language of original LG; MESH-Descriptors in TOXBIB DE; Publication type PT; Source and ISSN-number in TOXBIBSO; Supporting agency SA; Title TI and Year of publication YR

12:335. Database subset

Online	Data-Star
File name	TOXL (TOXLINE)
Start year	1981 to date
Number of records	1,152,262
Update period	Monthly
Database aids	Data-Star Biomedical Manual and Online guide (search NEWS-TOXL in NEWS)
Price/Charges	Subscription: SFr80.00
	Connect time: SFr78.00
	Online print: SFr0.21–0.24
	Offline print: SFr6.80
	SDI charge: SFr0.24

Notes

For TOXBIB users should also consult Medical Subject Headings Annotated Alphabet List (MeSH) and Tree Structures (TREE) published annually.

From June 1993 Data-Star have introduced an annual fee/subscription per contract (that is, not per password) of SFr 80.00 (c.UK£ 32.00) payable every June. For North American customers billed in dollars who also use DIALOG, the DIALOG fee also covers access to Data-Star. Academic customers, 'commitment' customers and customers currently billed in dollars are exempt.

Record composition

Abstract AB; Accession number and secondary source ID or by code for faster retrieval AN; Author(s) AU; Availability, Order-ID-number, Prices AV; Award type AW; CAS Registry number(s) RN; Classification code CC; Comment CM; Corporate name CA; Entry month EM; Gene symbol GS; Institution, address IN; Keywords KW; Journal coden CD; Language of original LG; MESH-Descriptors in TOXBIB DE; Publication type PT; Source and ISSN-number in TOXBIBSO; Supporting agency SA; Title TI and Year of publication YR

12:336. Database subset

Online	Data-Star
File name	TO80 (TOXLINE)
Start year	Pre 1965–1980
Number of records	
Update period	Monthly
Database aids	Data-Star Biomedical Manual and Online guide (search NEWS-TOXL in NEWS)
Price/Charges	Subscription: SFr80.00
	Connect time: SFr78.00
	Online print: SFr0.21–0.24
	Offline print: SFr6.80
	SDI charge: SFr0.24

Notes

The Health Aspects of Pesticides Abstracts Bulletin of the Environmental Protection Agency (HAPAB) is only available in the two files which extend back further than 1965 – TO80 and TOZZ – that is before it was renamed Pesticides Abstracts.

This file does not include references from Toxicology Research Projects (CRISP); Epidemiology

Information System File of the FDA (EPIDEM); the Federal Research in Progress Database (FEDRIP); the Abstracts Bulletin of the US Army's Hazardous Materials Technical Centre (HMTC); or the Toxic Substances Control Act Test Submissions File of the EPA (TSCATS). For TOXBIB users should also consult Medical Subject Headings Annotated Alphabet List (MeSH) and Tree Structures (TREE) published annually.

From June 1993 Data-Star have introduced an annual fee/subscription per contract (that is, not per password) of SFr 80.00 (c.UK£ 32.00) payable every June. For North American customers billed in dollars who also use DIALOG, the DIALOG fee also covers access to Data-Star. Academic customers, 'commitment' customers and customers currently billed in dollars are exempt.

Record composition

Abstract AB; Accession number and secondary source ID or by code for faster retrieval AN; Author(s) AU; Availability, Order-ID-number, Prices AV; Award type AW; CAS Registry number(s) RN; Classification code CC; Comment CM; Corporate name CA; Entry month EM; Gene symbol GS; Institution, address IN; Keywords KW; Journal coden CD; Language of original LG; MESH-Descriptors in TOXBIB DE; Publication type PT; Source and ISSN-number in TOXBIBSO; Supporting agency SA; Title TI and Year of publication YR

12:337. Database subset

Online   **Data-Star**

File name	TOZZ (TOXLINE)
Start year	Pre 1965
Number of records	1,152,262
Update period	Monthly
Database aids	Data-Star Biomedical Manual and Online guide (search NEWS-TOXL in NEWS)
Price/Charges	Subscription: UK£32.00
	Connect time: UK£31.20
	Online print: UK£0.00 – 0.71
	Offline print: UK£0.08 – 0.10
	SDI charge: UK£2.72

Notes

Data-Star recommends the following search tactics in relation to drugs and chemicals: always use Registry numbers when available; for a broad concept search use as many synonyms as possible in title, keyword and abstract, for multi-word names use ADJ or WITH and for TOXBIB only use specific DE-searching using online MeSH and Tree. The Health Aspects of Pesticides Abstracts Bulletin of the Environmental Protection Agency (HAPAB) is only available in the two files which extend back further than 1965 – TO80 and TOZZ – that is before it was renamed Pesticides Abstracts. For TOXBIB users should also consult Medical Subject Headings Annotated Alphabet List (MeSH) and Tree Structures (TREE) published annually.

From June 1993 Data-Star have introduced an annual fee/subscription per contract (that is, not per password) of SFr 80.00 (c.UK£ 32.00) payable every June. For North American customers billed in dollars who also use DIALOG, the DIALOG fee also covers access to Data-Star. Academic customers, 'commitment' customers and customers currently billed in dollars are exempt.

Record composition

Abstract AB; Accession number and secondary source ID or by code for faster retrieval AN; Author(s) AU; Availability, Order-ID-number, Prices AV; Award type AW; CAS Registry number(s) RN; Classification code CC; Comment CM; Corporate name CA; Entry month EM; Gene symbol GS; Institution, address IN; Keywords KW; Journal coden CD; Language of original LG; MESH-Descriptors in TOXBIB DE; Publication type PT; Source and ISSN-number in TOXBIBSO; Supporting agency SA; Title TI and Year of publication YR

12:338. Database subset

Online   **Data-Star**

File name	TRTO – Training file (TOXLINE)
Start year	
Number of records	
Update period	Monthly
Price/Charges	Connect time: UK£Free
	Online print: UK£Free

Notes

Data-Star recommends the following search tactics in relation to drugs and chemicals: always use Registry numbers when available; for a broad concept search use as many synonyms as possible in title, keyword and abstract, for multi-word names use ADJ or WITH and for TOXBIB only use specific DE-searching For TOXBIB users should also consult Medical Subject Headings Annotated Alphabet List (MeSH) and Tree Structures (TREE) published annually.

Record composition

Abstract AB; Accession number and secondary source ID or by code for faster retrieval AN; Author(s) AU; Availability, Order-ID-number, Prices AV; Award type AW; CAS Registry number(s) RN; Classification code CC; Comment CM; Corporate name CA; Entry month EM; Gene symbol GS; Institution, address IN; Keywords KW; Journal coden CD; Language of original LG; MESH-Descriptors in TOXBIB DE; Publication type PT; Source and ISSN-number in TOXBIBSO; Supporting agency SA; Title TI and Year of publication YR

12:339. Database subset

Online   **DIALOG**

File name	File 156
Start year	
Number of records	1,647,025
Update period	Monthly
Price/Charges	Connect time: US$66.00
	Online print: US$0.25
	Offline print: US$0.25
	SDI charge: US$7.50

Notes

Coverage dates vary depending on subfile.

12:340. Database subset

Online   **DIMDI**

File name	TX165 – TOXLINE
Start year	1940, partly
Number of records	1,196,643
Update period	Monthly
SDI period	1 month

Price/Charges   Connect time: UK£05.20–08.99
                 Online print: UK£0.16–0.34
                 Offline print: UK£0.09–0.15
Downloading is allowed

Notes

TOXLINE is a TOXALL-subfile containing the following subunits ANEUPL, EMIC, EPIDEM, ETIC, FEDRIP, HAYES, HMTC, ILO, NIOSH, PESTAB/HAPAB, PPBIB, RPROJ, TD3, TMIC, TOXBIB, TSCATS. Public Health Services (USA)-supported research from FEDRIP is not included in TOXLINE because that information is already available in the RPROJ subunit.

Suppliers of online documents: British Library Document Supply Centre, Boston Spa, England; Harkers Information Retrieval System, Sydney, Australia; Instituto de Informacion y Documentacion en Ciencia y Tecnologica, Madrid, Spain; State Central Scientific Medical Library Supplier Center, Moscow, USSR. 82% of records have abstracts.

Record composition

Abstract AB; Author AU; BIOSIS Section Heading BISH; Chemical Abstracts Section Code CASC; Chemical Abstracts Section Heading CASH; CAS Reg. No CR; Corporate SOurce CS; Controlled Term CT; Country CY; Date Project Begins DB; Date Project Ends DE; Date Received REC; Document Date DT; Entry Month EM; Free Text FT; Gene Symbol GE; International Labour Office Section Code ILSC; International Labour Organisation Section Heading ILSC; International Pharmaceutical Abstracts Section Code IPSC; International Pharmaceutical Association Section Heading IPSH; ISSN SS; Journal Code JC; Journal Title JT; Language LA; Machine Date MD; Number of Document ND; Number of Supporting Agency NS; Number of Unit Record (DIMDI) NU; Order Number OD; Preprocessed Search PPS; Price PR; Publication Year PY; Qualifier AF; Secondary Source SEC; Source SO; Subunit SU; Supporting Agency SA; Title TI; Toxic Substances Control Act Section Code TSCC; Type of Awared TA and ZIP Code ZP

12:341. Database subset

Online   DIMDI

File name   T265 – TOXLIT
Start year   1965
Number of records   2,269,710
Update period   Monthly
SDI period   1 month
Database aids   Online User Manual/TOXALL
Price/Charges   Connect time: UK£33.36–37.15
                 Online print: UK£0.53–0.71
                 Offline print: UK£0.50–0.56
Downloading is allowed

Notes

TOXLIT is a TOXALL-subfile containing the following subunits BIOSIS/HEEP, CA and IPA. From Chemical Abstracts the following segments are taken: CBAC Chemical/Biological Activities, plus other parts of CA referring to toxicology, pharmacology and biochemistry.

Suppliers of online documents: British Library Document Supply Centre, Boston Spa, England; Harkers Information Retrieval System, Sydney, Australia; Instituto de Informacion y Documentacion en Ciencia y Tecnologica, Madrid, Spain; State Central Scientific Medical Library Supplier Center, Moscow, USSR. Searches are possible from January 1965. 82% of records have abstracts.

Record composition

Abstract AB; Author AU; BIOSIS Section Heading BISH; Chemical Abstracts Section Code CASC; Chemical Abstracts Section Heading CASH; CAS Reg.No CR; Controlled Term CT; Corporate Source CS; Country CY; Date Received REC; Document Date DT; Entry Month EM; Free Text FT; International Labour Office Section Code ILSC; International Labour Office Section Heading ILSH; International Pharmaceutical Abstracts Section Code IPSC; International Pharmaceutical Association Section Heading IPSH; ISSN SS; Journal Code JC; Journal Title JT; Language LA; Machine Date MD; Number of Document ND; Number of Supporting Agency NS; Number of Unit Record (DIMDI) NU; Order Number OD; Preprocessed Search PPS; Price PR; Publication Year PY; Qualifier AF; Source SO; Subunit SU; Supporting Agency SA; Title TI; Toxic Substances Control Act Section Code TSCC; Type of Awared TA and ZIP Code ZP

12:342. Database subset

Online   Japan Information Center of Science and Technology (JICST)

File name   TOXLINE
Alternative name(s) Toxicology Information Online
Start year
Number of records
Update period

12:343. Database subset

Online   Japan Information Center of Science and Technology (JICST)

File name   TOXLIT
Alternative name(s) Toxicology Information Online
Start year
Number of records
Update period

12:344. Database subset

Online   National Library of Medicine

File name   TOXLINE
Start year   Varies by file
Number of records
Update period   Monthly

12:345. Database subset

Online   National Library of Medicine

File name   TOXLIT
Start year   1965
Number of records
Update period   Monthly

12:346. Database subset

Tape   National Library of Medicine

File name   TOXLINE
Format notes   IBM
Start year   Varies by file
Number of records
Update period   Monthly

Notes

Corresponds to the TOXLINE online database. Contact NLM for pricing information.

12:347. Database subset

Tape   **National Library of Medicine**

File name	TOXLIT
Format notes	IBM
Start year	1965
Number of records	
Update period	Monthly

Notes

Corresponds to the TOXLIT online database. Contact NLM for pricing information.

For more details of constituent databases, see:
TOXLIT
TOXLINE

This database can also be found on:
PolTox I: NLM, CSA, IFIS
Toxline on SilverPlatter
Toxline Plus

Toxline on SilverPlatter

National Library of Medicine
National Chemicals Inspectorate of
Sweden

12:348. Master record

CD-ROM   **SilverPlatter**

Database type	Bibliographic
Number of journals	
Sources	Journals
Start year	1966
Language	English
Coverage	International
Number of records	1 million
Update size	50,000
Update period	Quarterly

Keywords

Aneuploidy; Chromosome Abnormalities; Drugs; Occupational Health and Safety; Pesticides; Pollution; Water Treatment

Description

Toxline on SilverPlatter provides a collection of toxicological information, the majority supplied by the National Library of Medicine, but also from fifteen other separate sources. Toxline contains references to published material and research in progress in the areas of adverse material and research in progress in the areas of adverse drug reaction, air pollution, carcinogenesis via chemicals, drug toxicity, food contamination, occupational hazards, pesticides and herbicides, toxicological analysis, water treatment and more. Subjects covered include: basic and applied research in all areas of the life, physical, social, behavioural, and engineering sciences. The database contains three sections:

(1) TOXLINE which includes the public domain records in the NLM file from 1981 to the present. Information is taken from eleven sources including CAS, MEDLINE and BIOSIS.

(2) RISKLINE – A secondary bibliographic database from the National Chemicals Inspectorate in Sweden, who provide selected and evaluated material on risk assessment; and

(3) FEDRIP, containing research supported by the US Public Health Service and featuring toxicology-

related reports submitted to the National Technical Information Service.

One reviewer thought that while this product covered many of the same topics as the PolTox series, it is not as specific in its focus and does not draw on the same sources although there is some overlap.

Almost all of Toxline's citations include abstracts, indexing terms and CAS Registry Numbers.

Subscription costs are: regular subscriptions (1966+) £900 for single users and £1,1350 for 2–8 networked users; regular subscriptions (1981+) £685 for single users and £1,028 for 2–8 networked users.

For more details of constituent databases, see:
TOXLINE
RISKLINE
FEDRIP

Toxline Plus

National Library of Medicine
American Society of Hospital
  Pharmacists
BIOSIS
Chemical Abstracts Service
National Chemicals Inspectorate of
  Sweden

12:350. Master record

CD-ROM   **SilverPlatter**

Database type	Bibliographic
Number of journals	
Sources	
Start year	1985
Language	English
Coverage	International
Number of records	1.2 million
Update size	170,000
Update period	Quarterly

Keywords

Aneuploidy; Chromosome Abnormalities; Drugs; Occupational Health and Safety; Pesticides; Pollution; Water Treatment

Description

Toxline Plus combines:

TOXLINE database (National Library of Medicine database of published material and research in progress relating to drug/chemical effects);
RISKLINE a secondary database from Sweden;
TOXLIT from the Chemical Abstracts Service (CAS) and
toxicology related data from BIOSIS and the American Society of Hospital Pharmacists (ASHP) (IPA).

Toxline Plus' initial one million records include approximately 70,000 from CAS; 37,000 from BIOSIS; 12,000 from ASHP; and 50,000 from NLM and provide references with abstracts to literature in all areas of toxicology: chemicals; pharmaceuticals; pesticides; environmental pollutants; mutagens; and teratology. CAS provide interactions of chemical substances with biological systems; BIOSIS provide industrial medicine, occupational health, pollution and waste disposal; ASHP provide adverse drug reactions, toxicity, and drug evaluations; and NLM provide poisoning, adverse or environmental effects of chemicals, hazardous materials management, and health and safety. One reviewer thought that while this product covered many of the same topics as the PolTox series, it is not as specific in its focus and does not draw on the same sources although there is some overlap.

There are five discs with discounts for academic institutions, and costs are: regular subscription for single users £2,500 and £5,000 for 2–8 networked users; for academic institutions cost is £1,875 for single users, £3,750 for 2–8 networked users.

For more details of constituent databases, see:
Toxline
RISKLINE
TOXLIT
BIOSIS
IPA

TOXLINE
National Library of Medicine

12:352. Master record

Database type	Bibliographic, Factual
Number of journals	17,400
Sources	Journals
Start year	1945
Language	English
Coverage	International
Number of records	660,000
Update size	—
Update period	Monthly

Keywords

Aneuploidy; Chromosome Abnormalities; Drugs; Occupational Health and Safety; Pesticides; Pollution; Water Treatment

Description

TOXLINE is a part of TOXALL with references from producers that do not require royalty charges; references on toxicology from producers that do require royalty charges are placed in TOXLIT. The database contains approximately 20,000 citations from between 1940 and 1965, 640,000 from 1965 to 1976, EMIC since 1960 and ETIC since 1965. Approximately eighty-two per cent of documents contain abstracts. Some hosts only carry TOXLINE.

For more details of constituent databases, see:
Aneuploidy
CISDOC
Environmental Mutagens – EMIC
Environmental Teratology – ETIC
Epidemiology Information System – EPIDEM
Federal Research in Progress – FEDRIP
Hayes File on Pesticides – HAYES
Hazardous Materials Technical Center – HMTC
International Pharmaceutical Abstracts – IPA
NIOSHTIC, subset
Pesticides Abstracts – PESTAB (post-1965)
Pesticides Abstracts – HAPAB (pre-1965)
Poisonous Plants Bibliography – PPBIB
Toxic Substances Control Act Test Submissions – TSCATS
MEDLINE, subset – Toxicity Bibliography – TOXBIB
Toxicological Aspects of Environmental Health – BIOSIS (formerly HEEP) (DIALOG)
Toxicology/Epidemiology Research Projects – RPROJ – CRISP
Toxicology Document and Data Depository – NTIS, subset
Toxic Materials Information Center File – TMIC

This database can also be found on:
TOXALL
PolTox I: NLM, CSA, IFIS
Toxline on SilverPlatter
Toxline Plus

TOXLIT
National Library of Medicine

12:355. Master record

Database type	Bibliographic
Number of journals	
Sources	
Start year	
Language	
Coverage	
Number of records	
Update size	—
Update period	

Keywords

Aneuploidy; Chromosome Abnormalities; Drugs; Occupational Health and Safety; Pesticides; Pollution; Water Treatment

Description

TOXLIT is a part of TOXALL with references from producers that require royalty charges; references on toxicology from producers that do not require royalty charges are placed in TOXLINE. The database contains approximately 20,000 citations from between 1940 and 1965, 640,000 from 1965 to 1976, EMIC since 1960 and ETIC since 1965. Approximately eighty- two per cent of documents contain abstracts. Some hosts only carry TOXLINE.

For more details of constituent databases, see:
Chemical Abstracts – CA
Biological Abstracts – BIOSIS
International Pharmaceutical Abstracts – IPA

This database can also be found on:
TOXALL
PolTox I: NLM, CSA, IFIS
Toxline on SilverPlatter
Toxline Plus

X-RAY
Brookhaven National Laboratory, Protein Data Bank DNAStar

12:358. Master record

Database type	Chemical structures/DNA sequences
Number of journals	
Sources	
Start year	
Language	English
Coverage	
Number of records	
Update size	—
Update period	Quarterly

Keywords

DNA; RNA; Radiography

Description

Contains 600 crystallographic structures of proteins, RNAs, polynucleotides and polysaccharides in 3-D. Includes backbone, sidechains and secondary structures of each molecule. Molecules can be rotated to view any angle.

12:359. CD-ROM   DNAStar

File name	X-RAY
Format notes	IBM
Software	X-Ray
Start year	
Number of records	
Update period	Quarterly
Price	US$1,500
	Subscription: US$275

Zoological Record
BIOSIS
Zoological Society of London

12:360. Master record

Alternative name(s)	Zoological Record Online; ZR Online; ZRO
Database type	Bibliographic
Number of journals Sources	6,500
Start year	1978
Language	English
Coverage	International
Number of records	1,300,000
Update size	80,000
Update period	Monthly
Database aids	Zoological Record Search Guide and Zoological Record Serial Sources
Hosts have included	BRS (Until 10/92)

Keywords

Parasitology; Zoology

Description

Exhaustive coverage of worldwide literature covering all aspects of zoology with emphasis on nomenclature changes, systematics and taxonomy. The database is indexed in 27 sections devoted to various animal Phyla and Classes, including protozoa, nematoda, pisces, reptilia, aves and mammalia. Topics include behaviour, biochemistry, development, ecology, evolution, morphology, genetics, feeding and nutrition, parasitology, reproduction, physiology and zoogeography. The database contains references published in *The Zoological Record* from Volume 115 (1978) to the present day. Citations include basic bibliographical information plus systematic classification of up to six levels for the biological organisms cited.

Maxwell Online dropped the service due to low usage and the producer confirms that other services get more attention. BRS users still have access to BIOSIS database.

The *Zoological Record Search Guide* includes the controlled indexing vocabulary for Volume 128; a separate section lists taxonomic classifications in hierarchical order as well as hierarchical subject, geographical and palaeontological vocabularies.

12:361. Online   BIOSIS Life Science Network

File name	Zoological Record Online
Alternative name(s)	ZR Online; ZRO
Start year	1978
Number of records	1,300,000
Update period	Monthly
SDI period	1 month
Price/Charges	Connect time: US$9.00
	Online print: US$6.00 per 10; 2.25 per abstract; 3.50 per full text article
	SDI charge: US$8.00

Also available via the Internet by telnetting to LSN.COM.

Notes

On Life Science Network users can search this database or they can scan a group of subject-related databases. There is a charge of $2.00 per scan of subject-related databases. To search one database and display up to ten citations costs $6.00. Most charges are for information retrieved. There are no charges if there are no results and no charge to transfer results to a printer or diskette. Articles may also be ordered via an online document delivery request. A telecommunications software package is also available, costing $12.95, providing an automatic connection to Life Science Network for heavy users of the service, with capability to transfer to print or disk and customised colour options.

Record composition

Accession Number AN; Zoological Record Volume Number JA; Title TI; Author AU; Source SO; Language LA; Descriptors DE; Taxonomic Categories TX and Taxa Notes TN

12:362. Online   DIALOG

File name	File 185
Alternative name(s)	ZR Online; ZRO
Start year	1978
Number of records	1,308,826
Update period	Monthly
Price/Charges	Connect time: US$78.00
	Online print: US$0.85
	Offline print: US$0.85
	SDI charge: US$8.00

12:363. Tape   BIOSIS

File name	Zoological Record Online
Alternative name(s)	ZR Online; ZRO
Start year	1978
Number of records	1,300,000
Update period	Monthly

Notes

Corresponds to the online Zoological Record Online database. Contact BIOSIS for pricing information.

Record composition

Accession Number AN; Zoological Record Volume Number JA; Title TI; Author AU; Source SO; Language LA; Descriptors DE; Taxonomic Categories TX and Taxa Notes TN

ETHICS

AMA/NET Social and Economic Aspects of Medicine
American Medical Association

13:1. Master record

Database type	Bibliographic
Number of journals	700
Sources	Journals, Newspapers, Monographs, Legal papers and Reports
Start year	1981
Language	English
Coverage	
Number of records	
Update size	—
Update period	Monthly
Index unit	Articles

Keywords
Public Health; Sociology; Medical Insurance; Practice Management

Description
Contains citations to articles on the non-clinical aspects of health care, including economics, education, ethics, international relations, legislation, political science, psychology, public health, medical practices, and sociology. Includes such topics as cost containment, insurance reimbursement, medical staff relations, and practice management. Covers legislative reports, monographs, newspapers and over 700 journals.

13:2. Online   AMA/NET

File name	
Start year	1981
Number of records	
Update period	Monthly

Notes
Initiation fee of $30 for AMA members or $50 for non-members to AMA/NET required.

Bioethicsline
Kennedy Institute of Ethics, Georgetown University
National Library of Medicine

13:3. Master record

Database type	Bibliographic
Number of journals	2,000
Sources	A-V material, Grey literature, Journals, Laws/regulations, Legal papers, Newspapers and Monographs
Start year	1973
Language	English
Coverage	International, English-speaking countries especially USA (primarily) and International
Number of records	35,000
Update size	2,400
Update period	Every two months
Index unit	Articles (selected) and Book chapters
Abstract details	Database producer
Thesaurus	Bioethics Thesaurus – devised by Kennedy Institute of Ethics, new editions annually; Medical Subject Headings (MeSH)

Keywords
Philosophy; Abortion; HIV; Euthanasia; Genetic Intervention

Description
Bioethicsline is a cross-disciplinary database containing references to documents which deal with ethical, legal and public policy issues of medicine, health care and biomedical research. It contains citations to the literature on abortion; AIDS; euthanasia; genetic intervention; human and animal experimentation; medical confidentiality; new reproductive technologies; surrogate motherhood; organ tissue donation and transplantation; patients' rights; in-vitro fertilization; professional ethics; resource allocation in health care; torture. Covers literature of many disciplines including religion, law, behavioural science and philosophy.

Corresponds to the annual *Bibliography of Bioethics*. About fifty of the ninety journals covered are also indexed in MEDLINE. Abstracts have been added to about twenty per cent of records from fifteen Core Journals since 1982 and from court decisions since 1984. Contains information mainly from English speaking countries, especially the USA. Relevant citations from Catline, Popline and MEDLINE are transferred to Bioethicsline; the overlap between Bioethicsline and MEDLINE is approximately fifty per cent. Unlike NLM databases, multiword source names are not abbreviated. Relevant articles have been drawn from 65 indexes, more than seventy journals and newspapers, four online databases and selected other tools. Journals represent sixty-eight per cent of all citations; monographs and book chapters nineteen per cent; newspapers seven per cent; court decisions five per cent and unpublished documents/audiovisual material two per cent.

The Kennedy Institute of Ethics developed its own thesaurus with approximately 600 descriptors; about eighty per cent of which are identical to *MeSH* descriptors. Documents are indexed with both vocabularies. Following the application of Index Terms, *MeSH* descriptors (CT) are added automatically so that there is a double indexing using the two vocabularies. No MeSH Supplemental Chemical Records, Gene Symbols or Qualifiers are used. From December 1982, one of thirteen section codes have been added to each record as a coarse classification. The section codes are: BE – Bioethics and professional ethics; BR – Biomedical and behavioral research; CL – Clinical approach; DE – Death, euthanasia and the prolongation of life; GR – Genetics, reproduction and abortion; HP – Health care and health care policy; LE – Legal approach; MH – Mental health therapies and behavior control; PH – Philosophical approach; PO – Popular approach; PP – Professional patient relationship; RE – Religious approach; and XX – Miscellaneous.

13:4. Online BLAISE-LINK

File name	BIOETHICS
Start year	1973
Number of records	
Update period	Quarterly

13:5. Online CISTI MEDLARS

File name	Bioethicsline
Start year	1973
Number of records	35,000
Update period	Twice per month

13:6. Online Data-Star

File name	ETHI
Start year	1973
Number of records	34,000
Update period	Every two months
Database aids	Biomedical Manual and Online Guide (search NEWS-ETHI in NEWS)

Downloading is allowed
Thesaurus is online

Notes

The command 'AB=AB' will locate documents which contain abstracts. Publication types (JOURNAL.PT.) are: Analytic; Audiovisual-material; Bill; Court-decision; Journal-article; Law; Monograph; Newspaper-article; and Unpublished-document. Index month (IM>9210) can be used to locate documents added recently.

From June 1993 Data-Star have introduced an annual fee/subscription per contract (that is, not per password) of SFr 80.00 (c.UK£ 32.00) payable every June. For North American customers billed in dollars who also use DIALOG, the DIALOG fee also covers access to Data-Star. Academic customers, 'commitment' customers and customers currently billed in dollars are exempt.

Record composition

Accession Number AN; Author AU; Title TI; Source SO; Language LG; Publication Type PT; Descriptors (MeSH) DE; Keywords (Bioethics Thesaurus) KW; Subject Captions SC; Abstract AB; Publication Year YR; Index Month IM; Corporate Name CN and General Notes NT

Keywords (.KW.) are controlled vocabulary terms taken from the Bioethics Thesaurus: multiword terms are double posted and searchable hyphenated or as a word fragment, thus STERILIZATION.KW. and INVOLUNTARY- STERILIZATION.KW. will both work. MeSH descriptors (.DE.) are also double posted: EUTHANASIA.DE. retrieves both EUTHANASIA and EUTHANASIA as a MeSH fragment of EUTHANASIA-PASSIVE. The command '.MESH term' will display the thesaurus terms.

13:7. Online DIMDI

File name	BE73
Software	GRIPS
Start year	1973
Number of records	34,300
Update period	Every two months
SDI period	Bimonthly
Database aids	Memocard

Price/Charges

	Connect time: UK£5.84–10.58
	Online print: UK£0.17–0.35
	Offline print: UK£0.09–0.15

Downloading is allowed
Thesaurus is online

Notes

The overlap between Bioethicsline and MEDLINE is approximately fifty per cent, however, citations originating in MEDLINE are not marked as in Aidsline, Health or Cancerlit. Document supply is from the British Library Document Supply Centre, Boston Spa, England; Harkers Information Retrieval System, Sydney, Australia; Intituto de Informacion y Documentacion en Ciencia y Tecnologia, Madrid, Spain and Zentralbibliotehk der Medizin, Köln, Germany.

Record composition

Abstract AB; Abstract Source AS (Display only); Author AU; Book Title BTI; Classification Code CC; Corporate Source CS; Controlled Term CT; Document Type DT; Entry Date ED (Find only); Entry Month EM (Display only); Freetext (Basic Index) FT; Index Term IT; Journal Title JT; Language LA; Number of Document ND; Notes NO (Display only); Publication Place PL; Publisher PU (Display only); Publication Year PY; Number of References RN (Display only); ISBN SB; Section Code SC; Series Title SE; Source SO (Display only); ISSN SS; Title TI and Uncontrolled Terms UT

Bioethics Thesaurus descriptors are hierarchically arranged to three levels in the printed version of the thesaurus only. Index terms covering the main aspect of the document are weighted in the same way as MeSH terms (shown by '*' in the record). Uncontrolled Terms contain uncontrolled nouns, personal/corporate names, geographics, etc that previously were part of the datafield Index Terms (IT). With the retrospective introduction of Uncontrolled Terms, the Index Terms at Dimdi now only contain the approximately 600 descriptors of the *Bioethics Thesaurus* and other descriptors, proposed for a later integration into the Bioethics Thesaurus. Uncontrolled Terms are, like Index Terms, directly and freetext searchable.

13:8. Online National Library of Medicine

File name	Bioethicsline
Start year	
Number of records	
Update period	

13:9. Online Questel

File name	BIOETHICS
Start year	1973
Number of records	33,000
Update period	

13:10. CD-ROM SilverPlatter

File name	Bioethicsline
Format notes	IBM
Software	SPIRS
Start year	1973
Number of records	35,000
Update period	Every two months
Price/Charges	

Downloading is allowed

13:11. Videotex Minitel
Questel
INSERM

File name	BIOETHICS 36290036
Start year	1973

Number of records   33,000
Update period
Database aids   User Guide

Notes

Accessible via Minitel at either direct dial (kiosk) or subscription rates. Menu-guided searching in either French or English allow five choices of access: French keywords, English keywords, English title or abstract terms, author or journal name. Citations can be displayed or printed with or without abstracts and offline prints as well as photocopies of the original article may be ordered. Direct dial access requires no subscription and no password and charging is for connect time only with a maximum of fifteen citations sent free of charge. Subscription charging requires a password and an identity code and has three charging parameters: connection time, citations displayed and citations sent by post.

This database can also be found on:
AIDSLINE

For more details of constituent databases, see:
MEDLINE
Popline
CATLINE

Canreg
University of Western Ontario, Social Science Computing Laboratory (SSCL), Information Services

13:14. Master record

Alternative name(s)   Canadian Register of Research and Researchers in the Social Sciences
Database type   Biographical, Bibliographic
Number of journals
Sources   Databases
Start year   Current information
Language   English and French
Coverage   Canada
Number of records   5,786
Update size   —
Update period   Quarterly

Description

Contains selected professional information on memebers of the social sciences communities in Canada from the governmental, academic and industrial sectors.

Covers researchers in the traditional social sciences (for example, economics, political science, education), and in such related fields as social work, management science, library science, and biomedical ethics. Each record provides biographical information, including position, organization, discipline, areas of specialisation, language skills, and current lines of research; up to six bibliographic references to the researcher's most important publications; and information on current research projects, including title and description of project, time period covered, unpublished status reports, and principal investigator and associates.

Source of data is the Canadian Register of Research and Researchers in the Social Sciences database, maintained by the Social Science Computing Laboratory and covering over 8,900 researchers, 8,100 research projects, and 27,800 publications. CISTI accessible only in Canada. CAN/DOC not available with this database.

13:15. Online   CISTI, Canadian Online Enquiry Service CAN/OLE

File name
Alternative name(s)   Canadian Register of Research and Researchers in the Social Sciences
Start year   Current information
Number of records   5,786
Update period   Quarterly
Price/Charges   Connect time: Canadian $40.00
Online print: Canadian $0.10
Offline print: Canadian $0.10

Notes

CISTI accessible only in Canada. Can $ 10.00 royalty per connect hour.

Clinical Orthopaedics and Related Research
JB Lippincott Company

13:16. Master record

Database type   Textual, Factual
Number of journals
Sources   Newsletter
Start year   1983
Language   English
Coverage   International
Number of records
Update size   —
Update period

Keywords

Orthopaedics

Description

Contains the full text of the newsletter of the same name, a publication which chronicles current research developments and clinical topics relevant to the orthopaedic practice. Also contains information addressing scientific, educational, ethical and humanistic issues.

13:17. Online   Mead Data Central (as a NEXIS database)

File name   CLOP – NEXIS
Alternative name(s)   NEXIS – Clinical Orthopaedics and Related Research
Start year   1983
Number of records
Update period
Price/Charges   Subscription: US$1,000 – 3,000 (Depending on needs)
Connect time: US$49.00 (Telecomms + connect time)
Database entry fee: US$24.00 (Search charge)
Online print: US$0.04 per line

Notes

Library: GENMED; Group files: ARCJNL.

A subscription charge which covers all transactional charges, connect time, telecommunications and the small administration charge can take the place of the individual charges. Subscriptions are negotiated with customers and vary according to the number of menus (thus, files) that are to be used – typically a minimum subscription would be about US$ 1,000. All charges include training and a 24-hour help line.

Record composition

Publication; Cite; Date; Section; Length; Title; Source; Author; Abstract (SUM-ABS); Text; Additional supply information (SUPP-INFO); Bibliographic Citations List (BIBLIO-REF); Graphic; Correction; Correction-Date; Discussion and Editor-Note

This database can also be found on:
NEXIS

Clinical Pediatrics
JB Lippincott Company

13:19. Master record

Alternative name(s)	NEXIS – Clinical Pediatrics
Database type	Textual, Factual
Number of journals	
Sources	Newsletter
Start year	1983
Language	English
Coverage	International
Number of records	
Update size	–
Update period	

Keywords

Paediatrics

Description

Clinical Pediatrics is a publication which chronicles current research development and clinical topics relevant to the practice of pediatric medicine. *Clinical Pediatrics* also contains information addressing scientific, educational, ethical and humanistic issues. Sections which are frequently included in this newsletter include: adolescent medicine, allergy, ambulatory care, ambulatory pediatrics, anesthesia, antibiotic management, audiology, behavioral pediatrics, cardiology, child abuse, child development, clinical experiences and notes, counseling, dentistry, dermatology, developmental pediatrics, dysmorphology, emergency care, emergency medicine, endocrinology, epidemiology, ethics, gastroenterology, genetics, handicapped children, hematology, infant feeding, infectious diseases, metabolism, neonatology, neurology, oncology, opthalmology, orthopedics, otalaryngology, pharmacology, physical diagnosis, psychiatry, psychosocial medicine, public health, radiology, rehabilitation, and social pediatrics.

13:20. Online — Mead Data Central (as a NEXIS database)

File name	CLP – NEXIS
Alternative name(s)	NEXIS – Clinical Pediatrics
Start year	1983
Number of records	
Update period	
Price/Charges	Subscription: US$1,000 – 3,000 (Depending on needs) Connect time: US$49.00 (Telecomms + connect time) Database entry fee: US$24.00 (Search charge) Online print: US$0.04 per line

Notes

In GENMED library; ARCJNL group file.

A subscription charge which covers all transactional charges, connect time, telecommunications and the small administration charge can take the place of the individual charges. Subscriptions are negotiated with customers and vary according to the number of menus (thus, files) that are to be used – typically a minimum subscription would be about US$ 1,000. All charges include training and a 24-hour help line.

Record composition

Publication; Cite; Date; Section; Length; Title; Source; Author; Abstract (SUM-ABS); Text; Additional supply information (SUPP-INFO); Bibliographic Citations List (BIBLIO-REF); Graphic; Correction; Correction-Date; Discussion and Editor-Note

This database can also be found on:
NEXIS
Comprehensive Core Medical Library – CCML
IQUEST File 1189 (CompuServe)

Colleague Mail
BRS Online Service, BRS/Colleague

13:22. Master record

Alternative name(s)	MEDLINK
Database type	Directory, Textual, Computer software
Number of journals	1
Sources	Journal, Airlines, Database producers, Electronic media and Original material
Start year	
Language	English
Coverage	USA
Number of records	
Update size	–
Update period	Current six to eight months
Index unit	Classified advertisements

Keywords

Molecular Biology; HIV; Travel; Air Travel; Anaesthesia; Personal Computers; HIV; Pathology; Surgery; Gastroenterology; Intensive Care; Proctology; Dermatology; Geriatrics; Gerontology; Genetics – Human; Immunology; Health Care Administration; Neurology; Cancer; Oncology; Ophthalmology; Sickle-Cell Disease

Description

Contains a number of services for medical professionals, including classified advertisements from the *New England Journal of Medicine*, a calendar of medical events, electronic mail, gateway access to Official Airlines Guide (OAG) Electronic Edition Travel Service (see separate entry), American Airlines EASY Sabre (see separate entry) and other databases available through BT Tymnet Dialcom Service. There are also a number of bulletin boards available, operated by physician-editors: AIDS/HIV, Anesthesia Safety and Technology, Cellforum (pathology, cell biology, molecular biology), Clinical Drug Information, Colon & Rectal Surgery, Critical Care, Dermatology, Geriatrics and Gerontology, Hackers' Forum (microcomputer products and applications), Materia Eclectica, Medical Ethics, MEDLINK Help & Tips, Neurology, Oncology, Ophthalmology, Sickle-Cell Disease.

Partially equivalent to *New England Journal of Medicine* (classified advertisements).

13:23. Online — BRS, BRS/Colleague

File name	
Alternative name(s)	MEDLINK
Start year	

Number of records
Update period   current six to eight months

For more details of constituent databases, see:
American Airlines EAASY SABRE
OAG Electronic Edition Travel Service

EMBASE
Elsevier Science Publishers

13:25. Master record

Alternative name(s)	Excerpta Medica
Database type	Bibliographic
Number of journals	4,700
Sources	Case studies, clinicians, journals, monographs, research communications, reviews, surveys and symposia
Start year	1974
Language	English
Coverage	International
Number of records	4,950,000+
Update size	350,000
Update period	Weekly
Index unit	Articles
Abstract details	Adaptations of the authors' summaries and selected on the basis of content and length by an international group of practicing medical and other qualified specialists and when necessary modified, shortened or extended to obtain the optimum information value. A group of over 2,000 biomedical specialists assist with the preparation of abstracts in particular subject areas and articles in non-Western European languages
Thesaurus	EMTREE Thesaurus METAGS
Database aids	Guide to the Classification and Indexing System, MALIMET (available online and on microfiche), Mini-Malimet, MECLASE Drug Trade Names (DN) and EMBASE List of Journals Abstracted

Keywords

HIV; Anaesthesia; Anatomy; Anthropology; Bioengineering; Biotechnology; Cancer; Cardiology; Clinical Medicine; Clinical Neurology; Cosmetics; Drugs; Environmental Health; Environmental Pollution; Environmental Toxicology; Epilepsy; Food Additives; Food Contaminants; Forensic Medicine; Forensic Science; Gastroenterology; Gynaecology; Immunology; Industrial Medicine; Nephrology; Neuroscience; Neuromuscular Disorders; Nuclear Medicine; Obstetrics; Occupational Health and Safety; Patents; Pathology; Pharmaceuticals; Pollution; Public Health; Radiology; Toxic Substances; Waste Management

Description

EMBASE is the trademark for the English language Excerpta Medica database. Excerpta Medica was founded as a non-profit making organisation in 1946 with the goal of improving the availability and dissemination of medical knowledge through the publication of a series of abstract journals. The database contains citations, with abstracts, to the worldwide biomedical literature on human medicine and areas of biological sciences related to human medicine with an emphasis on the pharmacological effects of drugs and chemicals. The four main categories of primary literature sources are: specialist medical publications; general biomedicine publications; specialist non-medical publications and general scientific publications. Subjects covered include: anatomy; anesthesiology (including resuscitation and intensive care medicine); anthropology; pharmacology of anesthetic agents, spinal, epidural and caudal anesthesia and acupuncture (as anesthetic); autoimmunity; biochemistry; bioengineering; cancer; dangerous goods; dermatology; developmental biology; drug adverse reactions; drug dependence; drug effects; endocrinology; environmental health and pollution control (covering chemical pollution and its effect on man, animals, plants and microorganisms; measurement, treatment, prevention and control); exocrine pancreas; forensic science; gastroenterology (including diseases and disorders of: digestive systems; mouth; pharynx and more); genetics; gerontology and geriatrics; health economics; hematology; hepatobiliary system; hospital management; immunology (including immunity; hypersensitivity; histocompatibility and all aspects of the immune system); internal medicine; legal and socioeconomic aspects; mesentary; meteorological aspects; microbiology; nephrology (covering diagnosis; treatment; epidemiology; prevention; infections; glomerular and tubular disorders; blood purification; dialysis; kidney transplantation; toxic nephropathy and including important clinical abstracts with epidemiological studies and major clinical trials, with particular emphasis on hypertension and diabetes); neurosciences (especially clinical neurology and neurosurgery, epilepsy and neuromuscular disorders but also covering non-clinical articles on neurophysiology and animal models for human neuropharmacology); noise and vibration; nuclear medicine; obstetrics and gynaecology (including endocrinology and menstrual cycle, infertility, prenatal diagnosis and fetal monitoring, anticonceptions, breast cancer diagnosis, sterilisation and psychosexual problems and neonatal care of normal children); occupational health and industrial medicine; opthalmology; otorhinolaryngology; paediatrics; pathology (including general pathology and organ pathology, pathological physiology and pathological anatomy, as well as laboratory methods and techniques used in pathology. General pathology topics range from cellular pathology, fetal and neonatal pathology, including congenital disorders, injury (both chemical and physical), inflammation and infection, immuno-pathology, collagen diseases and cancer pathology); peritoneum; pharmacology (including the effects and use of all drugs; experimental aspects of pharmacokinetics and pharmacodynamics; drug information); physiology; psychiatry and psychology (including addiction; alcoholism; sexual behaviour; suicide; mental deficiency and the clinical use or abuse of psychotropic and psychomimetic agents); public health; radiation and thermal pollution; radiology (including radiodiagnosis, radiotherapy and radiobiology, ultrasound diagnosis, thermography, adverse reactions to radiotherapy and techniques and apparatus, radiobiology of radioisotopes, aspects of radiohygiene, new labelling techniques and tracer applications); rehabilitation; surgery; toxicology (including pharmaceutical toxicology; foods, food additives, and contaminants; cosmetics, toiletries, and household products; occupational toxicology; waste material in air, soil and water; toxins and venoms; chemical teratogens, mutagens, and carcinogens; phototoxicity; regulatory toxicology; laboratory methods and techniques; and antidotes and symptomatic treatment; urology; wastewater treatment and measurement. The database is particularly strong in drug-related literature, where records include manufacturers and drug trade names and generic names. Information on veterinary medicine, nursing and dentistry is generally excluded.

Excerpta Medica is extremely current as articles are indexed within thirty days of receipt and are online very soon after that. Approximately 900 journals (the Rapid Input Processing (RIP)) are processed with priority which means that within eleven weeks of the receipt of the original document, the completely-indexed records are available. More than 100,000 records are given this priority treatment. Some hosts have companion databases giving training or details of the indexing vocabularies and thesauri.

EMBASE concentrates on journal articles although about 1,000 books per annum were indexed between 1975 and 1980. The source journals include all forty-six sections of *Excerpta Medica*, the *Drug Literature Index* and *Adverse Reactions Titles*. New titles are added and old titles deleted at a rate of about 200–300 per year. The database covers sources from 110 countries with the following geographical scope: North America 36%, Western Europe 35%, United Kingdom 14%, USSR and Eastern Europe 7%, Asia 6%, Central and South America 1%, Austalia & South Pacific 1%, Africa and Middle East 1%. Approximately 50% of the citations are from drug and pharmaceutical literature and approximately 40% of citations added to the database each year do not appear in the corresponding printed abstract journals and indexes. Approximately 65% of the citations contain abstracts of on average 200 words with a maximum of 800 words which indicate the content of the articles and are not intended to summarise the results or express opinions. This makes free-text searching of the abstracts, titles and other searchable elements of the citation valuable. This compares with approximately sixty-five per cent of the records in MEDLINE and fifty-four per cent in BIOSIS. The records of the other leading bioscience database, SciSearch, now do contain abstracts. Approximately 75% of the articles are in the English language. Of the other leading bioscience databases, approximately eighty-eight per cent of articles on SciSearch are in English, eighty-six per cent of articles on BIOSIS and seventy-four per cent on MEDLINE. In addition approximately thirty-seven per cent of records with non-English sources contain English-language abstracts online. This compares with sixty-seven per cent on BIOSIS and twenty-six per cent on MEDLINE. SciSearch does now contain abstracts. Important publications NOT indexed in EMBASE include Meyler's *Side Effects of Drugs*, 1972–1980 published by Excerpta Medica and *Side Effects of Drugs Annual*, 1981 to the present, published by Elsevier.

A core collection of 3,500 biomedical journals supplemented by journals in the areas of agriculture, technology, economics, chemistry, environmental protection and sociology. General criteria used for selection are first that the document should be of potential relevance to medicine and secondly the information should be of lasting value for which reasons news items and comments are generally excluded.

EMBASE section headings are based on medical specialities; a total of forty-seven subfiles group together citations on topics such as anatomy, paediatrics, opthalmology, gastroenterology, cancer, plastic surgery, occupational health. Each subfile or section has its own hierarchical scheme. The thesaurus *MALIMET (Master List of Medical Terms)* is used which contains more than 250,000 preferred terms and 255,000 synonyms which are mapped to the pre-

ferred terms when used. It is used for indexing highly specific concepts such as names of drugs and chemicals; diseases and syndromes; anatomical and physiological aspects and diagnostic and therapeutic methods. *MALIMET* is growing at a rate of over 12,000 descriptors per annum, mainly through drug names and names of chemical compounds. The size of the complete *MALIMET* thesaurus for EMBASE (more than 250,000 preferred terms compared to 15,000 in MeSH) may indicate its tendency to provide a greater variety of possible terms and therefore, less consistent application in indexing. In 1993, all non-drug *MeSH* terms were included in the thesaurus mapped to *MALIMET* terms so that a search strategy can be transferred from MEDLINE.

Indexing incorporates the following rules: natural word order (acute leukemia, not leukemia acute); American spelling (tumor, not tumour); singular noun forms and not plural or adjectival forms (stomach tumor, not gastric tumors, but optic nerve, not eye nerve); the most specific term must be used. Since 1979, *MALIMET* terms have been weighted. Class A terms (weighted) indicate the main concepts while Class B terms (not weighted) indicate the less important concepts of a document. In addition to *MALIMET* broad concepts are indexed with EMCLAS and EMTAGS. EMCLAS is a poly- hierarchical decimal classification scheme of the forty-six subject subfiles which make up the sections of the printed *Excerpta Medica* containing approximately 6,500 entries. It is then further subdivided into a five level hierarchy of sub-categories. Indexing is performed by medical specialists and scientists whose specialism corresponds to the subject areas forming the major subdivisions of EMCLAS. The indexing builds up sequentially as the article is indexed by each of the sections for which it is relevant. On average each document is indexed for 3.5 different sections.

EMTAGS is a group of approximately 220 codes which represent general concepts such as groups, gender, organ systems, experimental animals and article type. In January 1991 about 10% of the terms were changed including important descriptors such as CANCER or BENIGN NEOPLASM.

EMBASE editors also add 'uncontrolled' drug terms to augment MALIMET descriptors in selected records. EMBASE provides a hierarchical classification system (EMTREES) reflecting fifteen broad facets of biomedicine. From January 1991 a new version of EMTREE went online comprising 35,000 terms. New descriptors and changes in the hierarchy were made in the following areas: anatomy of the eye; diseases; drugs; techniques; biological phenomea and document types. Prior to 1988 Section Headings based on medical speciality areas were used instead of EMTREES to index EMBASE citations. In both classification schemes, codes are constructed to facilitate broad concept retrieval through truncation. In addition three uncontrolled vocabularies are used: Medical Secondary Text; Drug (Trade Names) and Manufacturers' Names are used. Medical Secondary Text consists of free-text words, numbers and phrases, describing concepts which are not fully covered by the controlled terms, for example quantiative information such as the number of patients or experimental animals. Drug (Trade) Names consists of trade names of drugs referred to in an original document with the main aspect of biological effects of compounds listed. Manufacturers' Names lists the names of drug manufacturers. The value of controlled indexing is important when searching for topics where a subject population has been specified.

Relatively few bioscience databases provide consistent indexing for subject populations (that is, humans or specific test animals) and related characteristics commonly requested such as age groups, gender, occupation and racial or ethnic groups. EMBASE provides extensive consistent indexing for the identification of test animals and age groups with a less consistent approach for the indexing of humans, occupational groups, racial/ethnic groups and gender. In addition, in most bioscience files a form of pharmaceutical nomenclature exists. For EMBASE the preferred search terms are generic name, classification by action/use and CAS Reigstry Number although restrictions by date, subfile and vendor may apply to the latter and vendor documentation should be consulted for guidelines. The search terms Enzyme Commission Number, investigational code, chemical name and trade name should be cross-referenced to the preferred terminology in the thesaurus. In 1993, improved CAS Registry Numbers mean that there is a single Number assigned for every substance.

13:26. Database subset
CD-ROM   **SilverPlatter**

File name	Excerpta Medica – Obstetrics/Gynaecology
Alternative name(s)	Excerpta Medica
Format notes	IBM, Mac
Software	SPIRS/MacSPIRS
Start year	1980
Number of records	208,000
Update period	Quarterly
Price/Charges	Subscription: UK£755 – 1,132

Notes
One of the Elsevier speciality Excerpta Medica range, this database, on CD-ROM, is a subset of EMBASE and covers human obstetrics and gynaecology. Subjects covered include endrocrinology, the menstrual cycle, infertility, prenatal diagnosis and foetal monitoring, anticonception, breast cancer diagnosis, sterilisation, psychosexual problems and neonatal care of normal children. Relevant abstracts from other clinical and basic disciplines are also included.

Prices are: for single users UK£755, for 2–8 networked users £1,132.

This database can also be found on:
Eyenet
Cancer-CD
Medata-ROM
Logo-A Pharmaceutical Products (Discontinued)

Expert and the Law
National Forensic Center

13:28. Master record

Database type	Textual
Number of journals	1
Sources	Newsletters
Start year	1981 (December 7)
Language	English
Coverage	USA (primarily) and International (some)
Number of records	
Update size	—
Update period	Within 2 weeks after receipt of new materials

Keywords
Forensic Science

Description
Contains full text of *The Expert and the Law*, a newsletter covering the application of scientific, medical, and technical knowledge to litigation. Includes news about the use of consultants by attorneys and feature articles on the effective use of experts and consultants (for example, ethical considerations when expert witnesses incur out-of-pocket expenses).

13:29. Online   **Mead Data Central**
                             (as a NEXIS database)

File name	EXPTLW – NEXIS
Alternative name(s)	NEXIS – Expert and the law
Start year	1981 (December 7)
Number of records	
Update period	Within 2 weeks after receipt of new materials
Price/Charges	Subscription: US$1,000 – 3,000 (Depending on needs) Connect time: US$49.00 (Telecomms + connect time) Database entry fee: US$6.00 Online print: US$0.04 per line

Notes
Libraries: GENFED, HEALTH, LEGNEW, MEDMAL AND PRLIAB; Group files: ALLLEG, NWLTRS, CURRNT, ARCHIV, OMNI and LGLNEW.

A subscription charge which covers all transactional charges, connect time, telecommunications and the small administration charge can take the place of the individual charges. Subscriptions are negotiated with customers and vary according to the number of menus (thus, files) that are to be used – typically a minimum subscription would be about US$ 1,000. All charges include training and a 24-hour help line.

Record composition
Body (BODY); Byline (BYLINE); Correction; Correction Date; date; Graphic; Headline; Headline and Lead (HLEAD); Lead; Length; Publication and Section

This database can also be found on:
NEXIS

Francis
Centre National de la Recherche Scientifique, Institut de l'Information Scientifique et Technique, Science Humaines et Sociales (CNRS/INIST)

13:31. Master record

Database type	Bibliographic, Textual
Number of journals	7,500
Sources	Journals, Books, Reports, Dissertations, Conference proceedings and Research communications
Start year	1972
Language	French (keywords), English (keywords), Spanish (keywords) and Others
Coverage	France (primarily), Europe and International
Number of records	1,500,000+
Update size	80,000
Update period	Quarterly; Files 603 and 616 twice a year
Index unit	Articles

Keywords

Anthropology; Applied Linguistics; Chemical Substances; Computers and Law; Demography; Descriptive Linguistics; Environmental Health; Epidemiology; Ergonomics; Ethnolinguistics; Forensic Science; Health Care Management; Health Economics; History of Education; History of Medicine; History of Science; History of Technology; Human Ecology; Information Technology; Language Biology; Language Pathology; Linguistics; Mathematical Linguistics; Medical Education; Occupational Psychology; Occupational Medicine; Pharmaceutical Industry; Philosophy; Philosophy of Education; Psycholinguistics; Public Health; Semiotics; Social Medicine; Social Psychology; Social Services; Sociolinguistics; Sociology of Education; Vocational Training; Testing Methods

Description

Francis is a collection of twenty multidisciplinary bibliographic databases. It contains news and information, covering the core literature in: humanities, social sciences, economic sciences, computer processing, legal sciences, energy economics, health and medicine. There is especially good coverage of European and French research, with exhaustive coverage of fields where research is most active or which correspond to French national priorities. Most of the references also contain an analysis. The records include keywords for searching. Over 9,000 periodicals, books, reports, dissertations, etc. are indexed.

Databases included are:

Art and Archaeology (Near East, Asia, America) (File 526);

International Bibliography of Administrative Science (File 528);

Ethnology (File 529);

History of Science and Technology (Histoire des Sciences et des Techniques (File 522) containing citations, half with abstracts, to literature on the history of science and technology, including the exact sciences, earth sciences, life sciences, medicine and pharmacology. Corresponds to *Bulletin Signaletique Sciences Humaines: Section Histoire des Sciences et des Techniques* (522). There are 74,600 records dating from 1972, with 4,000 additions quarterly;

History of Literature and Literary Sciences (File 523);

History of Religion and Religious Sciences (File 527);

Information Technology and the Law (File 603);

Philosophy (File 519);

Prehistory and Protohistory (File 525);

Index of Art and Archaeology; Educational Sciences (Sciences de l'Education) (File 520) Contains citations, about half with abstracts, to the worldwide literature on education. Covers history and philosophy of education; education and psychology; sociology of education; planning and economics; educational research; teaching methods; testing and guidance; school life; vocational training; and adult education and employment. Corresponds to the *Bulletin Signaletique Sciences Humaines; Section Sciences de l'Education* (520). Records, approximately 40,000, date from 1979 and are updated quarterly with 4,000 additions each quarter;

Linguistic Sciences (Sciences du Langue) (File 524) contains citations, with some abstracts, to the international journal literature on linguistics, including language biology and pathology, psycholinguistics, sociolinguistics, ethnolinguistics, historical linguistics, descriptive studies, linguistics and mathematics, semiotics and communications, discursive semiotics and applied linguistics. Corresponds to *Bulletin Signaletique Sciences Humaines: Section Sciences du Langue* (524). There are 62,500 records on the file, dating from 1972, updated quarterly with 3,200 additions;

Sociology (Sociologie) (File 521) contains citations, most with abstracts, to the worldwide periodical and other literature in the field of sociology. Covers social psychology; social organization and structure; social problems; human ecology; demography; rural and urban sociology; economic and political sociology; sociology of knowledge, religion, education, art, communication, leisure, organizations, health, law, and work; and social work. The 68,000 records date from 1972, with 4,000 additions quarterly. Corresponds to the *Bulletin Signaletique Sciences Humaines: Section Sociologie* (521).

DOGE (Management) (File 616);

ECODOC (General Economics) (File 617);

Energy Economics (File 731);

Employment and Training (File 600);

RESHUS (Health-related Humanities) (Reseau documentaire en Sciences Humaines de la Santé) (File 610). A sectorial database on health economy, epidemiology, health and development, health organisation, health socio-economic aspects, medical ethic. Contains citations, with abstracts, to selected French literature from 1978 in the fields of health sciences: economics, sociology, legislation, geography, epidemiology, history, research and teaching, demography; human aspects of health: childbirth, death and illness, health developments, risk factors in failing health, ethics, health and society; health intervention systems: health organizations and politics; status, prevention and care unit management and structure, expenses and financing; and evaluation of health performances. There are 16,000 records updated quarterly with 1,300 additions per quarter. 84.5% of the documents indexed are French, 15% English and 0.5% are in other languages. 81% of references are journal articles, the other 19% coming from books, dissertations, proceedings and so on. All documents are fully analysed. Corresponds to the quarterly bulletin *RESHUS* and File 610 of *Bulletin Signaletique Sciences Humaines: Section Reseau Documentaire en Sciences Humaines de la Santé*.

Latin America (File 533);

International Geographical Bibliography (File 531); and two new releases,

Cognisciences (File 90) and

Spécial Préhistoire (File 47).

An index to author and source is cumulated annually. 7,500 periodical titles are covered, comprising 90% of the references, plus research reports, proceedings, and French dissertations.

Some of the databases can be purchased as combinations – File 521 (Sociology) and 529 (Ethnology) can be purchased as File 946; File G22 is a combination of File 525 (Prehistory and Special Prehistory (new release). Bibliographic publications are produced quarterly as hard copy, corresponding to the subject areas covered in the Francis database, Computer Science and the Law being published only twice a year.

There is very good coverage of French periodicals.

Francis has one lexicon (alphabetical list of subject terms used to index the information found in the database) per subject field. There are thesauri for the

Energy Economics, Administrative Science, Geography and RESHUS databases. There are trilingual keywords English-French-Spanish or English-French-German in some files, and a bilingual English-French classification scheme.

13:32. Online   Européenne de Données

File name	Francis
Start year	1972
Number of records	1,500,000+
Update period	Quarterly; Files 603 and 616 twice a year
Database aids	Francis User Manual (French) for Européenne de Données users

13:33. Online   Questel

File name	Francis
Start year	1972
Number of records	1,500,000+
Update period	Quarterly; Files 603 and 616 twice a year
Database aids	Francis User Manual (French or English) for Questel users

13:34. CD-ROM   Centre National de la Recherche Scientifique, Institut de l'Information Scientifique et Technique, Science Humaines et Sociales (CNRS/INIST)

File name	Francis
Format notes	IBM
Software	GTI
Start year	1984
Number of records	500,000
Update period	Annually
Price/Charges	Subscription: FFr4,000 – 17,500

Notes

The first CD-ROM produced covers the years 1984–90. Additional discs will be produced each year – 6,000 FFr for current year (1991, 1 disc); 17,500 French francs for retrospective disc 1984–1990.

13:35. Tape   Centre National de la Recherche Scientifique, Institut de l'Information Scientifique et Technique, Science Humaines et Sociales (CNRS/INIST)

File name	Francis
Format notes	9-track 1,600 or 6,250 BPI magnetic tapes, EBCDIC character, set, with or without IBM-OS label
Start year	1972
Number of records	1,500,000+
Update period	Quarterly; Files 603 and 616 twice a year

13:36. Videotex   Centre National de la Recherche Scientifique, Institut de l'Information Scientifique et Technique, Science Humaines et Sociales (CNRS/INIST)

File name	Francis
Start year	1972
Number of records	1,500,000+
Update period	Quarterly; Files 603 and 616 twice a year

13:37. Videotex   Minitel

File name	Francis (36293601)
Start year	1972

Number of records	1,500,000+
Update period	Quarterly; Files 603 and 616 twice a year

Notes

Available directly via Minitel by dialling 36.29.36.01

13:38. Database subset

Online   Européenne de Données

File name	RESH
Alternative name(s)	Reseau documentaire en Sciences Humaines de la Santé; RESHUS
Start year	1978
Number of records	16,000
Update period	Quarterly

Notes

A subfile of the multidisciplinary Francis database, *RESHUS* is a sectorial database on health economy, epidemiology, health and development, health organisation, health socio-economic aspects, medical ethic. Contains citations, with abstracts, to selected French literature from 1978 in the fields of health sciences: economics, sociology, legislation, geography, epidemiology, history, research and teaching, demography; human aspects of health: childbirth, death and illness, health developments, risk factors in failing health, ethics, health and society; health intervention systems: health organizations and politics; status, prevention and care unit management and structure, expenses and financing; and evaluation of health performances. There are 16,000 records updated quarterly with 1,300 additions per quarter. 84.5% of the documents indexed are French, 15% English and 0.5% are in other languages. 81% of references are journal articles, the other 19% coming from books, dissertations, proceedings and so on. All documents are fully analysed. Corresponds to the quarterly bulletin *RESHUS* and File 610 of *Bulletin Signaletique Sciences Humaines: Section Reseau Documentaire en Sciences Humaines de la Santé.*

13:39. Database subset

Online   Questel

File name	Francis: RESHUS
Alternative name(s)	Reseau documentaire en Sciences Humaines de la Santé; RESHUS
Start year	1978
Number of records	16,000
Update period	Quarterly

Notes

A subfile of the multidisciplinary Francis database, RESHUS is a sectorial database on health economy, epidemiology, health and development, health organisation, health socio-economic aspects, medical ethic. Contains citations, with abstracts, to selected French literature from 1978 in the fields of health sciences: economics, sociology, legislation, geography, epidemiology, history, research and teaching, demography; human aspects of health: childbirth, death and illness, health developments, risk factors in failing health, ethics, health and society; health intervention systems: health organizations and politics; status, prevention and care unit management and structure, expenses and financing; and evaluation of health performances. There are 16,000 records updated quarterly with 1,300 additions per quarter. 84.5% of the documents indexed are French, 15% English and 0.5% are in other languages. 81% of references are journal articles, the other 19% coming from books, dissertations, proceedings and so on. All documents are fully analysed. Corresponds to the quarterly bulletin *RESHUS* and File 610 of *Bulletin Signaletique Sciences Humaines: Section Reseau Documentaire en Sciences Humaines de la Santé.*

There is a thesaurus for this database.

Health Periodicals Database
Information Access Company (IAC)

13:40. Master record

Database type	Bibliographic, Textual
Number of journals	260
Sources	
Start year	Health specific articles: Index only 1987 to date/full-text 1989 to date; Health articles from general publications: Index only 1976 to date
Language	English
Coverage	International
Number of records	260,000+
Update size	39,000
Update period	Weekly
Abstract details	Either author abstracts or an abstract produced by IAC.
Database aids	Access to Access, Foster City, California, Information Access Company and The Subject Guide to IAC Databases, Foster city, California, IAC

Keywords

HIV; Consumer Protection; Drug Abuse; Mental Health; Nutrition; Occupational Health and Safety; Public Health; Sports Medicine

Description

Health Periodicals provides current and comprehensive information on a wide range of health, fitness, nutrition and specialised medical topics. It offers a mix of record types – some records in the database will contain only indexing, some indexing and author abstracts (from January 1988) and others full-text and consumer summaries (from October 1988). Subjects covered include: pre-natal care, gerontology, dieting, drug abuse, AIDS, biotechnology, cardiovascular disease, environment, medical ethics, health care costs, mental health, public health, occupational health and safety, paramedical professions, sports medicine, substance abuse, toxicology and others. The database provides a valuable resource for corporate, medical, and legal librarians, human resource professionals and product analysts. It is designed to meet the needs also of non-medical professionals. It is the only online health database that features consumer summaries for the layperson.

Articles are collected from 150 important medical journals and over 110 core health, fitness, and nutrition publications. Selected articles dealing with health topics are sourced from over 3,000 other publications indexed by IAC since 1976. Some of the database entries include author abstracts; some include summaries aimed specifically at the consumer lay-person, condensing, simplifying and explaining complex medical research terms and results. The full text of a range of 110 selected journals has been included from 1989 only.

A controlled vocabulary is used, a full list of which is available from the producer. Indexing terms are taken from Library of Congress Subject Headings, the National Library of Medicine Subject Headings (*MeSH*), Mosby's *Medical and Nursing Dictionary*,

and terms created by Information Access where no suitable term exists. The special features data field indicates inclusion of photographs, illustrations in the original article and includes the text accompanying a caption. A full list of special features is available from the producer.

13:41. Online   BRS

File name	HEAL
Start year	1987 citations; 1989 full text
Number of records	213,000
Update period	Weekly
Price/Charges	Connect time: US$80.00/90.00
	Online print: US$0.92/1.00
	Offline print: US$2.00
	SDI charge: US$3.50

13:42. Online   CompuServe Information Service

File name	IQUEST File 2847
Start year	1976, some, with most citations from 1987; 1989 full text
Number of records	34,000
Update period	Weekly
Price/Charges	Subscription: US$8.95 per month Database entry fee: US$9/search; some databases carry a surcharge ($2–75) Online print: US$10 references free; then $9 per ten; abstracts $3 each

Downloading is allowed

Notes

On CompuServe, contains more than 34,000 articles, including more than 26,000 in full text.

Accessed via IQUEST or IQMEDICAL, this database is offered by a DIALOG gateway. IQUEST can either search across all databases, a database of the user's choice or selected multiple databases.

13:43. Online   Data-Star

File name	HLTH
Start year	Health specific articles: Index only 1987 to date/full-text 1989 to date; Health articles from general publications: Index only 1976 to date/full-text 1983 to date.
Number of records	187,000
Update period	Weekly
Database aids	Data-Star Biomedical Manual and Data-Star Online Manual (search NEWS-HLTH in NEWS)
Price/Charges	Subscription: SFr80.00 Connect time: SFr147.00 Online print: SFr0.56 Offline print: SFr0.64 SDI charge: SFr6.80

Notes

From June 1993 Data-Star have introduced an annual fee/subscription per contract (that is, not per password) of SFr 80.00 (c.UK£ 32.00) payable every June. For North American customers billed in dollars who also use DIALOG, the DIALOG fee also covers access to Data-Star. Academic customers, 'commitment' customers and customers currently billed in dollars are exempt.

Record composition

Abstract AB; Article Type AT; Author AU; Availability AV; Accession Number and Update Code AN; Case Law CS; Column Inches CI; Company Name CO; Copyright CP; Date of Publication DT; Descriptor(s) DE; Full-text FT; Geographic Code and Name CN; Lead paragraph LP; Length LE; Personal Name PE;

Product Name TN; Source SO; Special Features and Letter Grade SF; Statute/Jurisdiction LW; Text TX; Title TI; Update Code UP; US SIC Code CC; Year YR; Year/Month YM and Year/Month/Day DT

13:44. Online   DIALOG

File name	File 149
Start year	January 1988
Number of records	264,870
Update period	Weekly
Price/Charges	Connect time: US$90.00
	Online print: US$0.90 – 1.20
	Offline print: US$0.90 – 1.20
	SDI charge: US$3.50

Notes

The DIALOG file contains records from January 1988, when the author abstracts were added to the database by IAC. DIALINDEX Categories: CONSUMER, MEDICINE, NUTRIT, PRODINFO. Daily updates to indexing and displayable abstracts, summaries and full text are available in Newsearch database, File 211 on DIALOG. DIALOG Alert Service available weekly. Available on DIALOG menus.

13:45. Database subset
Tape   Information Access
                                Company (IAC)

File name	Health Index
Format notes	IBM
Start year	1987
Number of records	125,000+
Update period	Monthly
Price/Charges	Subscription: US$9,000

Notes

A subset of Health Periodicals Database containing the citations only (not the full text of articles) from the contents of the Health Periodicals Database. It is a comprehensive index to over 150 journals, magazines, newspapers, newsletters in health, fitness, medicine, nutrition, and other related consumer health topics. Prices are: annual subscription to current and previous year, $9,00; archival files, $2,500 per year of data.

This database can also be found on:
Health Reference Center

Health Reference Center
Information Access Company (IAC)

13:46. Master record
CD-ROM   Information Access
                                Company (IAC)

Alternative name(s)	Health Index Plus (former name)
Database type	Factual, Bibliographic, Textual, Dictionary, Courseware
Number of journals	
Sources	
Start year	1987
Language	English
Coverage	International
Number of records	
Update size	–
Update period	Monthly

Keywords

HIV; Consumer Protection; Occupational Health and Safety; Nutrition; Sports Medicine

Description

Claimed by Information Access Company to be a 'complete consumer health library in one integrated system, including periodicals, pamphlets and reference books.' Contains the Health Periodicals Database which comprises:

a comprehensive index to over 150 core medical journals, plus 110 core magazines, newspapers and newsletters in health, fitness, medicine, nutrition, and other related consumer health topics;

indexes to selected health related articles from over 3,000 other magazines and newspapers, ranging from business to academic journals, popular magazines and newsletters;

the full text of articles from 106 professional medical journals. Articles are indexed from January 1987, and full text from January 1989 to the present.

In addition to the Health Periodicals Database, the disc also includes: the full text of leading medical and drug reference books including *Physicians and Surgeons Complete Home Medical Guide, People's Book of Medical Tests* and *USP DI Volume II Advice for the Patient*; a medical dictionary (Mosby's *Medical and Nursing Dictionary*); the full text of 500 medical pamphlets by health organisations such as Muscular Dystrophy Association, Juvenile Diabetes Foundation and the National Cancer Institute; and a proprietary tutorial database of background information on 300 diseases and medical conditions.

The system permits the viewing and printing of the full text of medical definitions, pamphlets, periodical articles and abstracts of articles. US$ 12,000 subscription including hardware rental.

For more details of constituent databases, see:
Health Periodicals Database
USP DI Volume 2: Advice for the Patient

Legal Resource Index
Information Access Company (IAC)

13:47. Master record

Database type	Bibliographic
Number of journals	750+
Sources	Journals, Monographs, Newspapers and Government publications
Start year	1980
Language	English
Coverage	International
Number of records	474,507
Update size	42,000
Update period	Monthly (daily into Newsearch)
Index unit	Reviews and articles
Database aids	Subject guide to IAC databases, Access to Access and IAC 1992 Source Guide

Keywords

Environmental Hazards; Taxation; Occupational Health and Safety

Description

Legal Resource Index provides cover-to-cover indexing of over 800 key law and legal-related journals, seven law newspapers, legal monographs, abstracts of legal reviews and journal articles on US law. Indexes articles, news, case notes, commentaries, book reviews, letters to the editor, president's pages, columns, obituaries, transcripts, biographical pieces and editorials providing access to valuable secondary information for the legal profession and others. The most comprehensive index to English-language articles that contain information on non-U.S. jurisdiction legal topics, as well as U.S. legal issues, providing the legal profession with access to developing legal trends, extensive background information on all areas of law and historical analysis of cases. Canada, Europe, Australia and Asia are also represented. For general researchers, the database is a useful source of material on the legal aspects of environmental hazards, taxation, ethics, mergers and acquisitions, human rights and environmental laws and case and statute names, and for tracking rulings that affect the workplace and employees.

Corresponds to *Legal Resource Index* on microform, and the law journal portion corresponds to *Current Law Index*. Records are added daily to the database Newsearch and are transferred to this database monthly. Sources include all major law reviews, seven legal newspapers, speciality publications, and bar association journals as well as law-related articles from over a thousand other business and general interest periodicals. The subject guide to IAC databases, Access to Access, and IAC 1992 Source Guide are all available from the producer.

Major law journals and newspapers, legal material in general, and selected coverage of relevant law materials periodicals and newspapers from the databases Magazine Index, National Newspaper Index and Trade and Industry Index. Law related articles from 1,000 additional U.S. publications are also indexed.

13:48. Online — BRS, Morning Search, BRS/Colleague

File name	LAWS
Start year	1980
Number of records	
Update period	Monthly (daily into Newsearch)
Price/Charges	Connect time: US$102.00/112.00
	Online print: US$0.17/0.25
	Offline print: US$0.38
	SDI charge: US$10.00

13:49. Online — Data-Star

File name	LAWS
Start year	1980
Number of records	
Update period	Monthly
Database aids	Data-Star Guide to LAWS

Notes

From June 1993 Data-Star have introduced an annual fee/subscription per contract (that is, not per password) of SFr 80.00 (c.UK£ 32.00) payable every June. For North American customers billed in dollars who also use DIALOG, the DIALOG fee also covers access to Data-Star. Academic customers, 'commitment' customers and customers currently billed in dollars are exempt.

Record composition

Accession Number and Update Code AN; Title TI; Author AU; Source SO; Publication Date DT; Special Features SF; Article Type AT; Names Person PE; Jurisdiction and Geographic Code CN; Case Name and Citation CS; Statute LW; US SIC Code and Subject Category CC; Company CO; Product Name TN; Descriptors DE; Article Type AT; Column Inches

CI; Publication Month YM; Publication Year YR; Update Date UD; Update Month UP and Abstract AB Type DOCZ to retrieve total number of records currently in the database. Only a small percentage of the records in the file have abstracts; to ensure only those with abstracts are retrieved add the 'AND AB=AB' to the search statement.

13:50. Online — DIALOG, Knowledge Index

File name	File 150
Start year	1980
Number of records	474,507
Update period	Monthly
Price/Charges	Subscription: US$120.00
	Online print: US$0.35
	Offline print: US$0.35
	SDI charge: US$9.95

Notes

This database is also available to home users during evenings and weekends at a reduced rate on the Knowledge Index service of DIALOG – file name in this case is Legal Resource Index and searches are made with simplified commands or menus. Relevant law articles from Magazine Index (File 47), National Newspaper Index (File 111) and Trade and Industry Index (File 148) are also included.

13:51. Online — Mead Data Central (as a NEXIS database)

File name	LGLIND – NEXIS
Alternative name(s)	NEXIS – Legal Resource Index
Start year	1980
Number of records	
Update period	Monthly
Price/Charges	Subscription: US$1,000 – 3,000
	(Depending on needs)
	Connect time: US$49.00
	(Telecomms + connect time)
	Database entry fee: US$16.00
	(Search charge)
	Online print: US$0.04 per line

Notes

Libraries: LAWREV and LEXREF.

A subscription charge which covers all transactional charges, connect time, telecommunications and the small administration charge can take the place of the individual charges. Subscriptions are negotiated with customers and vary according to the number of menus (thus, files) that are to be used – typically a minimum subscription would be about US$ 1,000. All charges include training and a 24-hour help line.

13:52. Online — West Publishing Company (as part of WESTLAW)

File name	
Start year	1980
Number of records	
Update period	Monthly

Notes

Subscription to West Publishing Company required.

13:53. CD-ROM — Information Access Company (IAC)

File name	Legaltrac
Format notes	IBM
Software	InfoTrac EF
Start year	1980

Number of records 325,000
Update period Monthly
Price/Charges Subscription: UK£5,000

Notes

Corresponds to the online and microform Legal *Resource Index*. The law journal part corresponds to *Current Law Index*. Software has PowerTrac option for experienced users. Subscription fee includes all hardware, software, maintainance, customer service and monthly updates.

Differential prices for subscribers to other Information Access Company CD-ROM products.

13:54. Tape — Information Access Company (IAC)

File name Legal Resource Index
Start year 1980
Number of records 325,000
Update period Monthly

Notes

Annual subscription to current and previous year, $8000; archival files, $2500 per year of data. Corresponds to Legal Resource Index online and microform. The law journal part corresponds to *Current Law Index*.

This database can also be found on:
NEXIS

Medical Malpractice Lawsuit Filings

Medical Malpractice Verdicts, Settlements & Experts

13:56. Master record

Alternative name(s) MEDMAL; WESTLAW Medical
 Malpractice Lawsuit Filings
Database type Textual
Number of journals
Sources
Start year 1986
Language English
Coverage USA
Number of records 33,000
Update size 6,000
Update period Six times per year

Keywords

Medical Malpractice

Description

Summaries of malpractice suits in US District Courts and 51 state courts, giving the state in which the complaint was filed, medical speciality concerned and a description of the complaint. Includes plaintiff's allegations only. Complete texts of complaints can be ordered from Medical Malpractice Verdicts, Settlements & Experts.

13:57. Online — West Publishing Company (as part of WESTLAW)

File name
Alternative name(s) MEDMAL; WESTLAW Medical
 Malpractice Lawsuit Filings
Start year 1986

Number of records 33,000
Update period Six times per year

Notes

Subscription to West Publishing Company required.

Obstetrics & Gynecology – Personal MEDLINE

National Library of Medicine

13:58. Master record

CD-ROM — **Macmillan New Media**

Database type Bibliographic
Number of journals
Sources
Start year Most recent five years
Language
Coverage
Number of records 230,000
Update size –
Update period Annually

Keywords

Gynaecology

Description

Notes

References and abstracts on obstetric and gynaecological-related clinical and patient management issues. Covers: anatomy, diagnostic procedures and techniques, chemicals and drugs, including hormones, hormone antagonists and other related topics. A subset of MEDLINE, plus all abstracts from major obstetrics and gynaecology journals. As of December 1992, no longer available.

For more details of constituent databases, see:
MEDLINE

Obstetrics and Gynaecology

Elsevier Science Publishers
CMC ReSearch

13:60. Master record

Database type Factual, Textual, Image
Number of journals 1
Sources Journal
Start year 1985
Language English
Coverage
Number of records
Update size –
Update period Annually

Keywords

Gynaecology; Obstetrics

Description

Full text of five years of the Elsevier journal with tables and images. Includes: Medical and surgical treatment of female conditions; Obstetric management; Clinical evaluation of drugs and instruments; etc. Covers 1985 – 1990

13:61. CD-ROM   CMC ReSearch

File name	Obstetrics and Gynaecology on Disc 1985–1990
Format notes	IBM
Software	DiscPassage
Start year	1985
Number of records	
Update period	Annually
Price	UK£265

This database can also be found on:
Comprehensive Core Medical Library

Popline
Johns Hopkins University School of Public Health

13:63. Master record

Alternative name(s)	Population Information Online
Database type	Bibliographic
Number of journals	
Sources	Journals, monographs, Technical reports, conference proceedings, theses, newspapers, laws, manuals, Court decisions, grey literature and international agencies
Start year	1970, with earliest material from 1827
Language	English
Coverage	International
Number of records	200,000
Update size	—
Update period	Monthly

Keywords

HIV; Demography; Family Planning; Population

Description

Citations and abstracts to the worldwide literature on population, fertility, family planning and related health care, law and policy issues. Areas covered include AIDS in developing countries; breastfeeding; censuses; child immunization; contraceptive methods; demography; effects of overpopulation on ecology; family planning programs; family planning technology; health care instruction; health care training materials; infant and maternal mortality; law/policy on reproduction; maternal and child health; methods used to regulate fertility; migration trends; overpopulation; policies on migration; population dynamics; population and natural resources; practices to ensure child survival; primary health care; reproductive performance; research in human fertility; safe motherhood; sexually transmitted diseases; and vital statistics. Comprehensive coverage from 1970, selective coverage of earlier materials. The database is maintained by the Population Information Program at the Johns Hopkins University, with assistance from Population Index, Princetown University, funded primarily by the US Agency for International Development.

13:64. Online   BLAISE-LINK

File name	Popline
Alternative name(s)	Population Information Online
Start year	1970, with earliest material from 1827
Number of records	200,000
Update period	Monthly

Notes

Ninety per cent of references have an English abstract.

13:65. Online   CISTI MEDLARS

File name	Popline
Alternative name(s)	Population Information Online
Start year	1970, with earliest material from 1827
Number of records	200,000
Update period	Monthly

13:66. Online   National Library of Medicine

File name	Popline
Alternative name(s)	Population Information Online
Start year	1970, with earliest material from 1827
Number of records	200,000
Update period	Monthly

13:67. CD-ROM   National Information Services Corporation (NISC)

File name	Popline
Alternative name(s)	Population Information Online
Format notes	IBM
Software	ROMWright
Start year	1827
Number of records	200,000
Update period	Semiannually
Price/Charges	Subscription: US$695

Notes

The software offers both novice and expert search modes with context sensitive help. Field indexes may be browsed. The full text of most documents is available from the University at a charge of US$5.00 per document plus 10 cents per page.

13:68. CD-ROM   SilverPlatter

File name	Popline
Alternative name(s)	Population Information Online
Format notes	Mac, IBM
Software	SPIRS/MacSPIRS
Start year	1970; some records back to 1827
Number of records	189,000
Update period	Twice a year
Price/Charges	Subscription: UK£545 – 818

Notes

Regular subscriptiopn cost is £545 for single users, £818 for 2–8 networked users.

This database can also be found on:
Bioethicsline
Aidsline

Spriline
Planning and Rationalization Institute for the Health and Social Services
Spri Bibliotek och utredningsbanken Stiftelsen Stockholms läna Äldrecentrum

13:70. Master record

Alternative name(s)	Spri Library and Research Report Bank
Database type	Bibliographic, Textual
Number of journals	350
Sources	Journals, Research reports and Grey literature
Start year	1988
Language	Swedish (primarily) and English
Coverage	International

Number of records	16,000
Update size	3,000
Update period	Irregular

Keywords

Health Care Planning

Description

Concerns the area of health and medical care, with the exception of medical literature of a purely scientific character. Spri stands for Sjukvardens och socialvardens planerings-och rationaliseringsinstitut. Spriline consists of two parts: the library collections and journal articles from about 350 journals which are mainly Swedish; Spri's Research Report Bank (Spri's utredningsbank), that is, unpublished research reports from the health care sector in Sweden and in other Scandinavian countries.

The Spri Library and Research Bank offers a complete document delivery service. Other products – Spri litteraturtjänst, Nytt fran Spris utredninngsbank, Utredninsgbankens jkatalog, Fou-primavard.

Terms in Swedish from an inhouse thesaurus. Retrieval from all fields of the reference.

13:71. Online — MIC/Karolinska Institute Library and Information Center (MIC KIBIC)

File name	Spriline
Alternative name(s)	Spri Library and Research Report Bank
Start year	1988
Number of records	16,000
Update period	Irregular

Notes

Online ordering available.

Telegenline

RR Bowker Company
EIC/Intelligence

13:72. Master record

Database type	Bibliographic
Number of journals	7,000
Sources	Books, conference proceedings, government reports (US), journals, monographs, research reports and symposia
Start year	1973
Language	English
Coverage	International
Number of records	25,200
Update size	–
Update period	Closed File
Database aids	EIC/Intelligence Telegenline Search Aid and Telegenline User's Manual
Hosts have included	DIMDI (Until 1.1.92)

Keywords

Genetic Engineering

Description

Telegenline contains information on the entire field of genetic engineering and biotechnology. Subjects covered include: industrial microbiology; fermentation technologies; genetics relating to plants, animals, humans, bacteria, viruses, plasma and computers; gene therapy: research techniques; applications in energy and mining; food processing; chemistry; pharmaceuticals and medicine; agriculture applications; biohazards; pollution control; public health and occupational safety; social impact; military applications; education; finance; international issues, research founding, ethics and values.

The database corresponds to the printed *Telegen Reporter*. Abstracts have been available since March 1983 and are now contained in approximately 85% of documents.

Indexing in TELEGENLINE consists of two stages. First all TELEGENLINE documents are assigned to one of the twenty-one sections of the *Telegen Reports* (the print equivalent of TELEGENLINE) as follows: 01 Business & Economics; 02 Social Impacts and Constraints; 03 Patent and Legal Issues; 04 Policy and Regulatory Issues; 05 General; 06 International; 07 Industrial Microbiology; 08 Chemical Applications; 09 Energy and Mining Applications; 10 Biohazards and Environmental Applications; 11 Food Processing and Production Applications; 12 Crop Applications; 13 Livestock Applications; 14 Pharmaceutical and Medical Applications; 15 Research on Human Genes; 16 Research on Animal Genes; 17 Research on Plant Genes; 18 Research on Yeast and Fungus Genes; 19 Research on Bacterial Genes; 20 Research on Viral Genes; 21 General Research. Secondly the documents are indexed by Key Terms taken from an alphabetical, non-structured list containing approximately 2,000 terms. The Key Terms are indexed on three levels: Level 1 – primary descriptors; Level 2 – secondary descriptors and Level 3 – tertiary descriptors. The Key Terms are searchable directly as well as through Freetext, the data fields section headings and secton codes can only be searched directly and the data fields Title and Abstracts are only searchable through freetext.

13:73. Online — ESA-IRS

File name	File 49
Start year	1976–1990
Number of records	25,477(October 1991)
Update period	No longer updated
Price/Charges	Subscription: UK£70.29
	Database entry fee: UK£3.49
	Online print: UK£0.63
	Offline print: UK£0.60
	SDI charge: UK£3.49

Downloading is allowed
Thesaurus is online

Notes

From 1993 ESA-IRS are charging an annual fee of 100 Accounting Units (c.UK£ 70.29) to all users. This is equivalent to the fee for full documentation and will not be charged to customers already paying for documentation.

Record composition

Abstract /AB; Author AU; Class Code Name CC; Classification Code CC; Controlled Terms /CT; Corporate Source CS; Document Type DT; Major Controlled Terms /CT or /MAJ; Source Data SO and Title /TI

WESTLAW Medical Malpractice Topical Highlights Data Base

West Publishing Company

13:74. Master record

Database type	Textual
Number of journals	
Sources	Newspapers, Law reports, Laws/regulations and Courts
Start year	Current three months
Language	English
Coverage	USA

Ethics

WESTLAW MEDICAL MALPRACTICE TOPICAL HIGHLIGHTS DATA BASE

Number of records
Update size   —
Update period   Daily

Keywords
Medical Malpractice

Description
Contains summaries of significant recent state and federal cases in medical malpractice. Also provides summaries of relevant statutes, federal administrative materials and news items.

13:75. Online   West Publishing Company
(as part of WESTLAW)

File name
Start year   Current three months
Number of records
Update period   Daily

Notes
Subscription to West Publishing Company required.

DRUGS AND PHARMACY

21CFR Online
Diogenes

14:1. Master record

Database type	Textual
Number of journals	
Sources	Laws/regulations
Start year	Current information
Language	English
Coverage	USA
Number of records	7,000
Update size	–
Update period	Monthly
Database aids	21CFR Online Users Guide 1991, Rockville, DIOGENES

Description
Contains the full text of Title 21 of the Code of Federal Regulations (CFR) – official regulations from two US government departments: the Food and Drug Administration (FDA), concerned with administering food and drugs; and the Drug Enforcement Agency (DEA), involved in drug enforcement. Covers drugs, food, cosmetics, medical devices and veterinary products.

Title 21 is divided into two chapters:

Chapter I: Food and Drug Administration (Department of Health and Human services) –
Subchapter A: General, covering general regulations, hearings, patent term restoration and colour additives.

Subchapter B: Food for Human Consumption, covering food labelling, quality standards, infant formula, general and specific food standards, food additives and seafood inspection.
Subchapter C: Drugs, General, covering drug labelling and advertising, Good Manufacturing Practices, controlled drugs and manufacturer registration.
Subchapter D: Drugs for Human Use, covering approval applications, and requirements for specific drug and antibiotic categories.
Subchapter E: Animal Drugs, Feeds, and Related Products, covering animal food labelling and packaging, and new animal drug and antibiotic approval applications.
Subchapter F: Biologics, covering licensing, standards and Good Manufacturing Practices for biological products.
Subchapter G: Cosmetics, covering labelling, establishment registration and experience reporting for cosmetics.
Subchapter H: Medical Devices, covering labelling, manufacturer registration, device classes, adverse experience reporting and premarket approvals for medical devices.
Subchapter I: Reserved.
Subchapter J: Radiological Health, covering general requirements, records and reports and performance standards for radiological health products.
Subchapter K: Reserved.
Subchapter L: Regulations Under certain Other Acts Administered by the Food and Drug Administration,

covering Federal Import Milk Act, Tea Importation Act, Federal Caustic Poison Act, communicable diseases, interstate conveyance sanitation.
Chapter II: Drug Enforcement Administration (Department of Justice) – covering manufacturer registration, labelling, prescriptions, schedules and import/export of controlled substances.

14:2. Online · BRS

File name	CF21
Start year	
Number of records	
Update period	
Price/Charges	Connect time: US$89.00/99.00
	Online print: US$0.91/0.99
	Offline print: US$0.99

14:3. Online · Data-Star

File name	CF21
Start year	Current information
Number of records	7,000
Update period	Monthly
Database aids	Data-Star Business and Biomedical Manuals, Berne, Data-Star and Online guide (search NEWS-CF21 in NEWS)
Price/Charges	Subscription: UK£32.00
	Connect time: UK£60.00
	Online print: UK£0.60
	Offline print: UK£0.90
	SDI charge: UK£5.12

Notes
From June 1993 Data-Star have introduced an annual fee/subscription per contract (that is, not per password) of SFr 80.00 (c.UK£ 32.00) payable every June. For North American customers billed in dollars who also use DIALOG, the DIALOG fee also covers access to Data-Star. Academic customers, 'commitment' customers and customers currently billed in dollars are exempt.

This database can also be found on:
FDA on CD-ROM

A-V Online
Access Innovations Inc
National Information Center for Educational Media – NICEM

14:5. Master record

Alternative name(s)	NICEM (former name); LC Audio-Visual catalogue database; AV Online
Database type	Bibliographic, Directory
Number of journals	
Sources	A-V material
Start year	1964; with selective earlier coverge
Language	English, French (titles), Spanish (titles), German (titles) and Others (titles)
Coverage	International (excluding South Africa)
Number of records	336,000
Update size	14,000 – 20,000
Update period	Varies

Keywords

Drug Abuse; Human Resources Development Programmes; Occupational Health and Safety; Office Management; Religion; Smoking; Sport; Vocational Training

Description

Formerly named NICEM, A-V Online provides comprehensive coverage with citations and abstracts, to non-print educational materials for all educational levels, from pre-school to professional or graduate programmes, and is intended for use in education and professional training. It is a comprehensive index of the Library of Congress audiovisual catalogue and 6,500 producers and distributors. Contains a wealth of information on documentaries, instructional, informational and recreational programmes. Covers the following media: 16mm films, 35mm filmstrips, overhead transparencies, audio tapes, video tapes, phonograph records, slide sets, slide/tape, overhead transparencies and 8mm motion picture cartridges. The file now also has more than 10,000 non-English-language titles, including French, English, Spanish, German and other languages.

Some records date back as far as 1900. Subjects include academic, industrial, corporate and professional training, health, safety, sport, religion and more.

A subfile, Training Media Database, contains citations, with abstracts, to audiovisual materials for use in workplace training and human resources development programmes. Covers career development, management principles, supervision techniques, job satisfaction and motivation, leadership, smoking and drugs, industrial safety and law. Also includes selected vocational areas such as office procedures, computers, engineering and foreign languages.

Corresponds to NICEM Audiocassette Finder and Film and Video Finder, LC audiovisual catalogue, and HRIN Training Media Database.

14:6. Online   DIALOG

File name	File 46
Alternative name(s)	NICEM (former name); LC Audio-Visual catalogue database; AV Online
Start year	1964; with selective earlier coverage
Number of records	336,613
Update period	Quarterly
Price/Charges	Subscription: US$72.00 Online print: US$0.15 Offline print: US$0.20

14:7. CD-ROM   SilverPlatter

File name	AV Online
Alternative name(s)	NICEM (former name); LC Audio-Visual catalogue database; AV Online
Format notes	Mac, IBM
Software	SPIRS/MacSPIRS
Start year	1964; with selective earlier coverage
Number of records	380,000
Update period	Annually
Price	UK£865 – 1,295 Subscription: UK£575 – 863

Notes

Pricing: for a single user the regular subscription is £575, for 2–8 networked users £863. A one-time purchase costs £865 for a single user, £1,295 for 2–8 networked users.

14:8. Database subset

Online	Executive Telecom System International, Human Resource Information Network (ETSI/HRIN)
File name	Training Media Database
Alternative name(s)	NICEM (former name); LC Audio-Visual catalogue database; AV Online
Start year	Current information
Number of records	136,000
Update period	Twice per year

Notes

Citations, with abstracts, to audiovisual materials for use in workplace training and human resources development programmes. Covers career development, management principles, supervision techniques, job satisfaction and motivation, leadership, smoking and drugs, industrial safety and law. Also includes selected vocational areas such as office procedures, computers, engineering and foreign languages. This is a subset of the A-V Online database (formerly NICEM).

ABDA-Pharma

Ärzneibüro Bundesvereinigung Deutscher Apothekerverbaende (ABDA)

14:9. Master record

Alternative name(s)	ABDA-Datenbank
Database type	Directory, Textual
Number of journals	
Sources	Journals, Monographs, Pharmacopoeias, Suppliers and Handbooks
Start year	Current information
Language	German
Coverage	Germany (Western) and International
Number of records	278,050
Update size	—
Update period	Monthly
Index unit	Drug
Downloading is allowed	

Keywords

Drugs; Pharmaceuticals; Pharmaceutical Industry

Description

A database from ABDA consisting of subfiles of information on drug preparations, interactions and pharmaceutical substances. The subfiles are:

Substances with data of the Pharmazeutische Stoffliste (Pharmaceutical Substances List) of ABDA, offering information on 19,000 drug ingredients and adjuvants, including chemical elements and compounds, plant and animal products and microorganisms;

Drugs contains data on German and non-German commercial drugs and information in the German Drug catalogues, about 23,500 German and 77,000 non-German drugs. For all drugs includes trade names, active ingredients, dosage forms; for German drugs only, also includes administration and dosage, composition, indications, contraindications, side effects, interactions, producers, shelf life and storage, date of initial marketing and delivery regulations.

Corresponds to Mikropharm 3, Indikationsverzeichnis: other subfiles are:

Central file, containing data on approximately 70,00 drugs available in Germany;

Manufacturers file containing names and addresses of about 2,000 manufacturers in Germany and 7,500 outside the country;

Interactions file containing monographs from the worldwide journal and monographic literature on about 450 drug-food, drug-alcohol and drug-drug interactions, covering pharmacological effect, clinical significance, clinical observations, mechanism, recommendations and interaction management. Corresponds to Mikropharm 1, Ärzneimittel-interaktionen.

14:10. Online   CompuServe Information Service

File name	
Alternative name(s)	ABDA-Datenbank
Start year	Current
Number of records	278,050
Update period	Monthly
Price/Charges	Subscription: US$8.95 per month
Downloading is allowed	

14:11. Database subset
Online   DIMDI

File name	AD00 – ABDA-Pharma-Ärzneistoffe
Alternative name(s)	ABDA-Datenbank
Start year	Current information
Number of records	19,119
Update period	Monthly
Price/Charges	Connect time: UK£Group 1: 3.88–8.62; Group II: 15.80–20.55 Online print: UK£0.16–0.34 Offline print: UK£0.13–0.20

Notes

This is a subfile of ABDA-Pharma on DIMDI, of which the Substance file corresponds to Pharmazeutische Stoffliste (List of Pharmaceutical Substances), containing information on approximately 19,000 drug ingredients and adjuvants. Stoffdaten file ingredients include chemical elements and compounds and their naturally occurring mixtures and solutions, plants and plant components (processed and unprocessed), animal bodies (dead or alive) and components of the bodies and metabolites of man or animal (processed or unprocessed), microorganisms and viruses and their components or metabolites. Provides nomenclature from the International Non-Proprietary Names and the International Union of Pure and Applied Chemistry nomenclature, Chemical Abstracts Service Registry Numbers, Arzneimittel-Stoff Katalog numbers, synonyms, molecular formulas and weight, basicity, refractive index, solubility, boiling point, melting point, specific rotation, physiochemical properties, substance classifications, plus data for medical use: drug delivery regulations in Germany, maximum dosage that can be prescribed, indications and dosage. Formerly loaded together with DIMDI file ABDA-Pharma-Interaktionen, which is now file AI00 since DIMDI reloaded the ABDA database. The other subfile available on DIMDI ABDA-Pharma is AE00 ABDA-Pharma- Fertigarzneimittel. Other changes are planned by DIMDI so that searching for ingredients or interactions will be possible directly. Pricing for online users is in two user group categories : Group I, pharmacists in public pharmacies and hospital pharmacies within the Federal Republic of Germany; Group II, other users.

The file is arranged by chemical record. Unit records contain chemical substance identification (group: IDEN), for example, name of ingredient with synonyms, CAS Registry Number, molecular formula, classification of the substance and references to related drugs; chemical and physical properties (group: CHEM), for example, molecular weight, basicity, refractive index, solubility, boiling point, melting point and specific rotation; data for medical use (group: PHAR) (PHARMACOLOGY)), for example, dosage, maximum dose, indication and maximal prescription amount. As with the other factual files on DIMDI searching for chemical substances can be done using the descriptor-identifiers TE(Terminology), CR(CAS Registry Number, resp. FT(Freetext). With SHOW F=CONTENTS the user receives lists of the available fields without data for the individual ingredients. WithSHOW F=ALL, SHOW F=STD, SHOW F=fieldname for example, SHOW D=DOST (dosierung Stoff) the data in the individual fields is shown.

14:12. Database subset
Online   DIMDI

File name	AE00 – ABDA-Pharma-Fertigarzneimittel
Alternative name(s)	ABDA-Datenbank
Software	GRIPS
Start year	Current information
Number of records	111,474
Update period	Monthly
Price/Charges	Connect time: UK£Group 1: 3.88–8.62; Group II: 15.80–20.55 Online print: UK£0.16–0.34 Offline print: UK£0.13–0.20
Downloading is allowed	

Notes

This is a subfile of ABDA-Pharma on DIMDI. ABDA-Pharma-Fertigarzneimittel contains data on German and non-German commercial drugs and information in the German Drug catalogues, plus national drug catalogues of other countries: Mikropharm 2 (general drug information), and Mikropharm 3 (Indications, Indikationsverzeichnis). The data includes approximately 99% of the German drugs, 6,500 of which have detailed information, 22,500 German drugs with basic information, plus a file of 72,000 non-German drugs with basic information. For all drugs, includes trade name, active ingredients, dosage forms; for German drugs only, also includes administration and dosage, composition, indications, contraindications, information of the 'Pharmazeutische Stoffliste' (substance information) for the ingredients, side effects, interactions, producers, shelf life and storage, date of initial marketing and delivery regulations. Subunit titles include: Central file (Zentraldaten) of drugs available in Germany; Manufactures/producers (Hersteller) which lists names and addresses of about 2,000 manufacturers in Germany; plus two auxiliary subunits – Application forms and dosage forms (Darreichungsformen) and Indications (Indikationen), which is Mikropharm 3, together providing vocabulary for drug application forms and drug indications. Corresponds to the catalogue Micropharm 3, Indikationsverzeichnis and to the Novitaetenkartei. The data of Mikropharm 1 (drug interactions) and of the Phaemazeutisch Stoffliste are integrated in the individual drug records. After the reload of the ABDA-Pharma database in 1992 the commercial drugs resp. products of the 'Große Spezialitäten Taxe' have been removed from the DIMDI file because they contain only limited information. To simplify searching for interactions and pharmaceutical substances, there are two other sub-files on DIMDI, AD00 ABDA-Pharma-Ärzneistoffe and AI00 ABDA-Pharma-Interaktionen. Pricing for online users is in two user group categories : Group I, pharmacists in public pharmacies and hospital pharmacies within the Federal Republic of Germany; Group II, other users.

Menu driven user guidance is available in German and English. After DIMDI's reload of ABDA-Pharma data on interactions are available as in the past with the SHOW-formats SHOW F=INT, SHOW F=STD, SHOW F=INTALL, SHOW F=ALL. The output of lists of interacting partners (SHOW F=INTPL) which contain the interacting commercial drugs ingredients is no longer possible. Data on ingredients are obtained as before, with SHOW F=STO, SHOW F=ALL or SHOW F=fieldnme. All fields belonging to an interaction monograph (as INTND) (number of document INT), INTG (group of interaction), INTSTO (interacting substance), BED (significance), INTYP (type of interaction), EFF (effect), MEC (mechanism of action), MAS (special directives), KOM (comment) and LIT (literature) references are now exclusively searchable in ABDA-Pharma-Interaktionen with which this file was formerly loaded. Other changes are planned by DIMDI so that seaching for ingredients or interactions will be possible directly.

14:13. Database subset
Online   DIMDI

File name	AI00 – ABDA-Pharma-Interaktionen
Alternative name(s)	ABDA-Datenbank
Start year	Current information
Number of records	438 monographs
Update period	4–5 times a year
Price/Charges	Connect time: UK£Group 1: 3.88–8.62; Group II: 15.80–20.55 Online print: UK£0.16–0.34 Offline print: UK£0.13–0.20
Downloading is allowed	

Notes

A subfile on DIMDI of the ABDA-Pharma database. ABDA-Pharma- Interaktionen, built and maintained by ABDA and the Association of Pharmacists of Switzerland contains 438 monographs compiled from the worldwide journal and monographic literature on drug-food, drug-alcohol and drug-drug reactions. The records include short information on the two interacting substance groups, significance of interaction, type of interaction and a short description of the effect, textfields for effect, mechanism of action, special directives and comments, a complete list of interacting partners (ingredients, commercial drugs) which are listed in two separated groups. Covers pharmacological effect, clinical significance, clinical observations, recommendations and interaction management of 8,500 different drugs. Corresponds to Mikropharm 1, Ärnzneimittelinteraktionen. There are two other subfiles available on DIMDI since they reloaded the database, AD00 ABDA-Pharma-Ärzneistoffe and AE00 ABDA-Pharma-Fertigarzneimittel. Other changes are planned by DIMDI so that seaching for ingredients or interactions will be possible directly. Pricing for online users is in two user group categories : Group I, pharmacists in public pharmacies and hospital pharmacies within the Federal Republic of Germany; Group II, other users.

Search results must be interpreted with care. A search result > 0 means that a true interaction has been found only, when the searched substances, substance groups or drug preparations occur in different interaction groups. However, a result > 0 is also obtained when the searched substances, substance groups or drug preparations occur in the same interaction group. In this case the search result does not represent a true interaction. It is therefore essential to use the SHOW-command to check the kind of search result obtained. The records include short information, textfields, and a list of interacting partners. The short information contains the two interacting substance groups (INTGA, INTGB), significance of interaction (grave, less than grave, unsignificant) (BED), the type of interaction, (eg pharmacodynamic interaction) and a short description of the effect (INTYP). The textfields are: effect (EFF), mechanism of action (MEC), special directives (MAS), comment (KOM), and bibliographic references (LIT). In the list of interacting partners the ingredients and trade names are listed in two interacting roups: Terminology A and Terminology B. The interacting partners are arranged according to: interaction approved, interaction expect, interaction excluded, no assertion yet possible.

14:14. Database subset
CD-ROM   Pharma Daig & Lauer

File name	AIS – Ärzneimittel Informations System
Alternative name(s)	ABDA-Datenbank
Format notes	IBM
Start year	
Number of records	
Update period	Six times per year
Price	DM3,500

Notes

Pharmaceutical product information taken from the ABDA databases. Monthly updates cost an additional 150 DM.

14:15. Database subset
CD-ROM   Pharma Daig & Lauer

File name	ABDA Datenbank Mikropharm 1 + 2
Alternative name(s)	ABDA-Datenbank
Format notes	IBM
Software	Cobra
Start year	
Number of records	
Update period	Monthly
Price/Charges	Subscription: DM2,000

Notes

Comtains the ABDA-Pharm database, Mikropharm 1, the Interactions file and Micropharm 2, general drug information, plus the Substances file. Contains basic information for German and international (46 countries) drugs, giving producer, country, application forms and compounds. For German drugs: gives preparations, doses, indications, effects and pharmokinetics. Also includes a list of pharmaceutical substances (chemical elements and compounds, plants and plant substances, microorganisms); international nonproprietary names and other designations, formulae and physicochemical references.

14:16. Database subset
CD-ROM   Pharma Daig & Lauer

File name	ABDA Datenbank Mikropharm 2
Alternative name(s)	ABDA-Datenbank
Format notes	IBM
Software	Cobra
Start year	
Number of records	
Update period	Six times per year
Price/Charges	Subscription: DM2,500

Notes

The Central subfile of ABDA-Pharma, containing basic information on approximately 20,000 pharmaceutical products approved in Germany. Costs 2,500 DM for first disc, then 65 DM for each upgrade.

This database can also be found on:
Grosse Deutsche Spezialitätemtaxe – Lauertaxe und BADA – Datenbank

ADONIS
ADONIS BV

14:17. Master record

Database type	Bibliographic, Image
Number of journals	500
Sources	journals
Start year	1991
Language	
Coverage	International
Number of records	180,000
Update size	—
Update period	Weekly
Index unit	articles

Description

Contains scanned facsimile images of the editorial contents of more than 400 (rising to 500 in 1993) scientific journals for document delivery from local CD-ROM based workstations. Covers medicine, biotechnology, drug information, environment, food science and health care. From 1993, chemistry and related disciplines will be added.

14:18. CD-ROM ADONIS BV

File name	
Start year	1991
Number of records	
Update period	Weekly

Advanced Medical Information Services
AMS Corporation

14:19. Master record

Database type	Bibliographic, Textual, Factual
Number of journals	
Sources	Press releases, News releases, Journals and Reports
Start year	1985 (June)
Language	Japanese
Coverage	Japan
Number of records	350,000+
Update size	—
Update period	Continuously/Weekly/Monthly
Index unit	Drug and articles

Description

Contains news, literature references, and other information and electronic services for physicians, hospital administrators and public health officials in Japan.

News: Contains full text of news stories related to medicine and health care. Also includes press releases from public agencies, infectious disease surveillance alerts, adverse drug reaction reports, health care product recalls, and other news items of interest of interest to health care providers.

AMS Database: Contains approximately 190,000 citations to Japanese medical literature. Also provides information on approximately 160,000 therapeutic drugs.

News: updated continuously, throughout the day. AMS Database: citations updated weekly; drug information updated monthly. Other information services include bulletin boards, classified advertisements, electronic mail, a directory of users, and access to databases available through AMA/NET and BRS/Colleague.

14:20. Online AMS Corporation

File name	Advanced Medical Information Services
Start year	1985 (June)
Number of records	350,000+
Update period	Continuously/Weekly/Monthly

Notes

Monthly subscription required.

Ärzte Zeitung Datenbank
Ärzte Zeitung Verlagsgesellschaft mbH

14:21. Master record

Alternative name(s)	Arzte Zeitung Datenbank
Database type	Textual
Number of journals	450
Sources	Journals, newspapers, press releases, research reports and surveys
Start year	1984
Language	German
Coverage	Germany (primarily) and International (some)
Number of records	100,000
Update size	—
Update period	Weekly

Keywords

Clinical Research; Diagnosis; Therapy

Description

This database covers medical trends, management of health services and the pharmaceutical industry. The main subjects covered include: developments in current medical and clinical research, diagnosis, therapy and treatment, health-care planning and social issues, national and international health policies, health management, office management and relevant company and industry news, market data and trends in the pharmaceutical industry.

This is the online equivalent to the printed *Ärzte-Zeitung* (daily) and selected articles from *Arzneimittel Zeitung* (bi-weekly). Approximately seventy per cent of the news is devoted to West Germany and the database is also strong on developments in Eastern Europe; other countries (including Western Europe and North America) are covered to a lesser extent. Information is taken from 450 national and international newspapers and journals and from press releases of companies, government agencies, and national and international organisations. Original research and statistical surveys on specific topics is also provided from Ärzte Zeitung's editorial staff in Munich, Frankfurt, Bonn, Hamburg, Berlin and New York.

There are seven broad groups of subject categories: Forschung-und-Prazis, Gesundheitspolitik, Kultur, Medizin, Panorama, WIrtachaft-Politik and Undefined.

14:22. Online — Bertelsmann Informations Service GmbH – BIS

File name	AEZT
Alternative name(s)	Arzte Zeitung Datenbank
Start year	
Number of records	
Update period	

14:23. Online — Data-Star

File name	AEZT
Alternative name(s)	Arzte Zeitung Datenbank
Start year	1984
Number of records	100,000
Update period	Weekly
Database aids	Data-Star Business Manual and Online manual (search NEWS-AEZT in NEWS)
Price/Charges	Subscription: SFr80.00 Connect time: SFr115.00 Online print: SFr0.45 Offline print: SFr0.73 SDI charge: SFr7.80

Thesaurus is online

Notes

From June 1993 Data-Star have introduced an annual fee/subscription per contract (that is, not per password) of SFr 80.00 (c.UK£ 32.00) payable every June. For North American customers billed in dollars who also use DIALOG, the DIALOG fee also covers access to Data-Star. Academic customers, 'commitment' customers and customers currently billed in dollars are exempt.

Record composition

Accession Number and Update Code AN and Date of Publication DT

Aesculapius Project – WHO
ETI SpA
IKONA Srl
World Health Organisation

14:24. Master record

Database type	Bibliographic, Textual, Image
Number of journals	
Sources	Monographs
Start year	1986
Language	English and French
Coverage	International
Number of records	
Update size	–
Update period	Quarterly

Keywords

Immunology

Description

Contains the full text and graphics of six years (1986–1991) of the *WHO Technical Support Series, WHO Bulletin, WHO Weekly Epidemiological Record* and other selected WHO monographs.

14:25. CD-ROM — IKONA Srl

File name	Aesculapius Project – WHO
Format notes	IBM
Software	Proprietary
Start year	1986

Number of records	
Update period	Quarterly
Price/Charges	Subscription: US$6,000

AfterCare Instructions: Injury and Illness
Micromedex Inc

14:26. Master record

Alternative name(s)	Computerized Clinical Information System: AfterCare Instructions: Injury and Illness; CCIS: AfterCare Instructions: Injury and Illness; Injury and Illness: AfterCare Instructions; AfterCare Instructions
Database type	Factual, Textual, Numeric, Directory
Number of journals	
Sources	
Start year	1988
Language	English and Spanish
Coverage	International
Number of records	
Update size	–
Update period	Quarterly

Keywords

Clinical Medicine; Drugs

Description

The AfterCare database consists of two individual modules, available separately or as a combination. Injury and Illness contains instructions for injury and illness, which can be personalized for each patient, and can be accessed by more than 500 titles in 22 subject categories. The other module is USP DI Volume 2. Injury and Illness which provides printed instructions for health care professionals to give to patients who have been discharged from the emergency department or clinic or who have received medication from a pharmacy. Each instruction sheet can be located by the medical or common name of the sign, symptom or diagnosis. Brief information regarding thirty generic drugs specific to the emergency department or clinic setting is included. All instructions are researched, prepared and reviewed by members of the Micromedex editorial staff and board, comprising over 350 physicians and pharmacists. Information is available in both English and Spanish.

14:27. CD-ROM — Micromedex Inc

File name	AfterCare Instructions: Injury and Illness
Alternative name(s)	Computerized Clinical Information System: AfterCare Instructions: Injury and Illness; CCIS: AfterCare Instructions: Injury and Illness; Injury and Illness: AfterCare Instructions; AfterCare Instructions
Start year	1988
Number of records	
Update period	Quarterly

Notes

This database is available as a standalone product, as well as being a part of CCIS, Computerized Clinical Information System.

This database can also be found on:
CCIS

AfterCare Instructions: USP DI Drug Information Leaflets

Micromedex Inc
US Pharmacopeial Convention

14:29. Master record

Alternative name(s)	USP DI Volume 2: Advice for the Patient; CCIS: AfterCare Instructions: USP DI Drug Information Leaflets; Computerised Clinical Information Systems: AfterCare Instructions: USP DI Drug Information Leaflets; USP DI Drug Information Leaflets; Advice for the Patient
Database type	Bibliographic, Factual, Textual
Number of journals	
Sources	
Start year	1988
Language	English
Coverage	USA
Number of records	5,000+
Update size	–
Update period	Quarterly

Keywords

Drugs

Description

This is one module of the AfterCare Instructions Database from Micromedex (the other is AfterCare Instructions: Injury and Ilness). Published by the US Pharmacopeial Convention this database has been prepared specifically for the consumer and written in an easy-to-understand form with little technical data and terminology. It includes drug information from the US Pharmacopoeial Convention (USP) for more than 5,000 drug products which can be accessed by both generic and US or foreign trade names. Gives drug instructions for patients who have received a medication from a pharmacy, including use and pronunciation; dosage forms available; information to be considered before using the drug; proper use directions; precautions to be observed; and side effects. All drug information leaflets are reviewed and updated by the USP Committee of Revision and by 34 expert Advisory Panels. In an overview of general health CD-ROMs, Nicholas Tomaiuolo noted that the major difference between Physicians' Desk Reference and USP DI is that 'the latter is the only published reference work that uses a structured review system contributed to by experts. The PDR contains basically recapitulated drug package inserts provided by pharmaceutical manufacturers' (*CD-ROM World* 8(1) January 1993 p 38–49).

14:30. CD-ROM   Micromedex Inc

File name	USP DI Drug Information Leaflets
Alternative name(s)	USP DI Volume 2: Advice for the Patient; CCIS: AfterCare Instructions: USP DI Drug Information Leaflets; Computerised Clinical Information Systems: AfterCare Instructions: USP DI Drug Information Leaflets; USP DI Drug Information Leaflets; Advice for the Patient
Start year	1988
Number of records	5,000+
Update period	Quarterly
Price/Charges	Subscription: UK£180 – 360

Notes

This database is available as a standalone product, as well as being a part of CCIS, Computerized Clinical Information System. It can also be purchased as part of an AfterCare combo.

14:31. CD-ROM   SilverPlatter

File name	USP DI Volume 2: Advice for the Patient
Alternative name(s)	USP DI Volume 2: Advice for the Patient; CCIS: AfterCare Instructions: USP DI Drug Information Leaflets; Computerised Clinical Information Systems: AfterCare Instructions: USP DI Drug Information Leaflets; USP DI Drug Information Leaflets; Advice for the Patient
Format notes	IBM
Software	SPIRS
Start year	
Number of records	
Update period	Quarterly
Price/Charges	Subscription: US$495

Notes

This is also available on the same CD with USP DI Volume 1, Drug Information for the Health Care Professional from 1993.

This database can also be found on:
CCIS
Health Reference Center
STAT!-Ref

AIDSDRUGS

National Library of Medicine
National Institute of Allergy and Infectious Diseases (US)

14:33. Master record

Database type	Directory
Number of journals	
Sources	
Start year	Current information
Language	English
Coverage	USA
Number of records	80
Update size	–
Update period	Monthly

Keywords

HIV

Description

Gives information on the drugs being tested in the clinical trials for AIDS which are described in the AIDSTRIALS database. Contains references to more than eighty drugs being tested for use against Acquired Immune Deficiency Syndrome (AIDS), AIDS-Related Complex (ARC), and related diseases. Gives: agent name and synonyms, including trade names and generic name; Chemical Abstracts Service (CAS) Registry Number; adverse reactions and contraindications; pharmacology – synergistic, antagonistic or other interaction of the drug with other agents; physical and chemical properties; manufacturer.

Drugs are indexed by Medical subject Headings (MeSH). For details of the associated clinical trials see AIDSTRIALS.

14:34. Online   National Library of Medicine

File name	AIDSDRUGS
Start year	Current information
Number of records	80
Update period	Monthly

This database can also be found on:
AIDS Compact Library
Physician's AIDSLINE

AIDSline
National Library of Medicine

14:36. Master record

Database type	Bibliographic
Number of journals	4,000
Sources	Journals, government publications, technical reports, meeting papers, meeting abstracts, monographs, special publications, theses, A-V material, software, Databases (National Library of Medicine) and National Library of Medicine
Start year	1980
Language	English, primarily
Coverage	International
Number of records	54,000+
Update size	15,000
Update period	Three times per month
Index unit	Articles and letters
Abstract details	Taken directly from the published articles
Thesaurus	Medical Subject Headings (MeSH)

Keywords
HIV

Description

Contains citations, with some abstracts (around 60% of the records), to the worldwide literature on Acquired Immune Deficiency Syndrome (AIDS), AIDS related subjects and HIV infections. Contains information from seventy countries. Covers biomedical, epidemiological, social, behavioural, clinical and research aspects of the disease as well as health policy issues. AIDSLINE contains all AIDS-related citations from 1980 to date with 70% of the citations deriving from three different NLM-databases: MEDLINE (approximately 19,000 citations), Health Planning and Administration (approximately 1,000 citations), CANCERLIT (approximately 1,500 citations); in addition to more recent AIDS-related records from other NLM-databases – BIOETHICSLINE, CATLINE, AVLINE and POPLINE – which will provide access to abstracts of papers presented at conferences, meetings, symposia reports, research, dissertations, theses, monographs, government reports, newspaper articles and audiovisuals.

The file structure is very similar to MEDLINE, with the exception of the supplementary SSI (Secondary Source Identifier) and PT (Publication Type) paragraph. About 60% of the references have an English abstract and about 85% of references come from articles written in English. AIDSLINE offers the possibility of searching a relatively small file together with the advantage of the features of a MEDLINE-like structure including the MESH controlled vocabulary and the subheadings.

All citations are indexed with Medical Subject Headings (MeSH) and subheadings according to MEDLINE rules. The hierarchical structure of MeSH makes it possible to search for a whole group of related descriptors in one step.

14:37. Online   BIOSIS Life Science Network

File name	AIDSLINE
Start year	1980
Number of records	45,000
Update period	Three times per month
Price/Charges	Connect time: US$9.00
	Online print: US$6.00 per 10; 2.25 per abstract; 3.50 per full text article

Also available via the Internet by telnetting to LSN.COM.

Notes

On Life Science Network users can search AIDS Abstracts or AIDSLINE or they can scan a group of subject-related databases. There is a charge of $2.00 per scan of subject-related databases. To search one database and display up to ten citations costs $6.00. Most charges are for information retrieved. There are no charges if there are no results and no charge to transfer results to a printer or diskette. Articles may also be ordered via an online document delivery request. A telecommunications software package is also available, costing $12.95, providing an automatic connection to Life Science Network for heavy users of the service, with capability to transfer to print or disk and customised colour options.

14:38. Online   BLAISE-LINK

File name	AIDSLINE
Start year	1980
Number of records	
Update period	Three times a month

14:39. Online   CISTI MEDLARS

File name	AIDSLINE
Start year	1980
Number of records	39,378
Update period	Twice per monthly

14:40. Online   Data-Star

File name	ACQS
Start year	1980
Number of records	48,091
Update period	Monthly
Database aids	Data-Star Biomedical Manual and Online manual (search NEWS-ACQS in NEWS)
Price/Charges	Subscription: SFr80.00
	Connect time: SFr78.00
	Online print: SFr0.18
	Offline print: SFr0.21–0.24
	SDI charge: SFr6.80

Downloading is allowed
Thesaurus is online

Notes

From June 1993 Data-Star have introduced an annual fee/subscription per contract (that is, not per password) of SFr 80.00 (c.UK£ 32.00) payable every June. For North American customers billed in dollars who also use DIALOG, the DIALOG fee also covers access to Data-Star. Academic customers, 'commitment' customers and customers currently billed in dollars are exempt.

Record composition

Abstract AB; Accession Number AN; Author(s) AU; Author Affiliation IN; CAS Registry number or Enzyme Commission Number RN; Corporate name CN; Country of publication ZN; Descriptors (MeSH/subheadings) DE; Entry date on NLM computer ED; Gene Symbol GS; General Notes GN; Index month IM; Journal coden JC; Journal subset SB; Language of original LG; Original language title TT; Publication Type PT; Secondary source identifier SI; Source SO; Title TI and Year of publication YR

14:41. Online — Data-Star

File name	ACQX
Start year	Current month
Number of records	
Update period	Monthly
Database aids	Data-Star Biomedical Manual and Online manual (search NEWS-ACQS in NEWS)
Price/Charges	Subscription: SFr80.00
	Connect time: SFr78.00
	Online print: SFr0.18
	Offline print: SFr0.21–0.24
	SDI charge: SFr6.80

Downloading is allowed
Thesaurus is online

Notes

From June 1993 Data-Star have introduced an annual fee/subscription per contract (that is, not per password) of SFr 80.00 (c.UK£ 32.00) payable every June. For North American customers billed in dollars who also use DIALOG, the DIALOG fee also covers access to Data-Star. Academic customers, 'commitment' customers and customers currently billed in dollars are exempt.

Record composition

Abstract AB; Accession Number AN; Author(s) AU; Author Affiliation IN; CAS Registry number or Enzyme Commission Number RN; Corporate name CN; Country of publication ZN; Descriptors (MeSH/subheadings) DE; Entry date on NLM computer ED; Gene Symbol GS; General Notes GN; Index month IM; Journal coden JC; Journal subset SB; Language of original LG; Original language title TT; Publication Type PT; Secondary source identifier SI; Source SO; Title TI and Year of publication YR

14:42. Online — DIALOG

File name	File 157
Start year	1980
Number of records	54,219
Update period	Monthly
Price/Charges	Connect time: US$36.00
	Online print: US$0.12
	Offline print: US$0.12
	SDI charge: US$5.25

Notes

Dialindex categories: Medicine, RNMED.

14:43. Online — DIMDI

File name	AX80
Software	GRIPS
Start year	1980
Number of records	68,115
Update period	Monthly
SDI period	1 month
Database aids	User Manual MEDLINE; AIDSLINE; BIOETHICSLINE; CANCERCILT; HEALTH;, Memocard AIDSLINE, MeSH Annotated Alphabetic List, MeSh Tree Structures, MeSH Supplementary Chemical Records and Permutated MeSH
Price/Charges	Connect time: UK£05.84–10.58
	Online print: UK£0.17–0.35
	Offline print: UK£0.09–0.15

Downloading is allowed

Notes

Menu driven user guidance is available in German and English. Suppliers of online documents: British Library Document Supply Centre, Boston Spa, England; Bayerische Staatsbibliothek München, München, Germany; Harkers Information Retrieval System, Sydney, Australia; The Information Store, San Francisco, USA; Institute for Scientific Information, Philadelphia, USA; Koninklijke Nederlandse Akademie van Wetenschapen, Amsterdam, The Nederlands.

Record composition

Abstract AB; Abstract Source AS; Author AU; Classification Code CC; Conference Name CF; Corporate Name CNA; CAS-Reg.No CR; Corporate Source CS; Controlled Term CT; Country CY; Document Type DT; Entry Date ED; Enzyme Code EZ; Gene Symbol GE; ITTRI/Franklin Number IF; Index Medicus Date IMD; Journal TItle Code JC; Journal Priority JP; Journal TItle JT; Language LA; Last Revision Date LR; Number of Document ND; Notes NO; Numer of Report NR; Personal Name as Subject PS; Publication Year PY; Qualifier QF; Number of References RN; ISBN SB; Series Title SE; Secondary Source SEC; Source SO; ISSN-NO SS; Subunit SU; Terminology TE and Title TI

14:44. Online — National Library of Medicine

File name	AIDSline
Start year	1980
Number of records	52,000+
Update period	Three times per month

14:45. CD-ROM — Aries Systems Corporation

File name	AIDSLINE AIDS
Format notes	IBM, Mac
Software	Knowledge Finder
Start year	1980
Number of records	52,000
Update period	Quarterly
Price/Charges	Subscription: US$245

Notes

Knowledge Finder uses fuzzy logic to allow users to create natural language searches with results displayed in order of likely relevance to the query.

14:46. CD-ROM — SilverPlatter

File name	AIDSLine
Format notes	IBM, Mac
Software	SPIRS
Start year	1980
Number of records	67,000
Update period	Quarterly
Price/Charges	Subscription: UK£430 – 645

Notes

Pricing – For a single user price is UK£430, for 2–8 users networked, UK£645. This database is also available on fixed disk.

14:47. Fixed disk — SilverPlatter

File name	AIDSLine
Format notes	IBM
Software	SPIRS
Start year	1980
Number of records	67,000
Update period	Quarterly
Price/Charges	Subscription: UK£645 – 1,075

Notes

Contains the entire database on fixed disk, with updates supplied on CD-ROM. This means that up to thirty networked users can have access to a single file containing the complete database. Search speeds are up to ten times faster than CD-ROM searching.

Pricing varies according to number of users on network: 2–8 users UK£645, 9–16 users £860, 17–25 users £1,075. The fee for the hard disk is US$1,000.

14:48. Tape
National Library of Medicine

File name	AIDSline
Start year	1980
Number of records	52,000+
Update period	Twice a month

Notes

Corresponds to the AIDSline online database.

AIDSTRIALS

National Library of Medicine
National Institute of Allergy and
Infectious Diseases (US)

14:49. Master record

Database type	Textual, Directory
Number of journals	
Sources	
Start year	Current information
Language	English
Coverage	USA (primarily) and International (some)
Number of records	230
Update size	—
Update period	Every two weeks

Keywords

HIV

Description

Describes clinical trials currently under way for AIDS. Contains references to approximately 230 clinical trials of agents being evaluated for use against Acquired Immune Deficiency Syndrome (AIDS), AIDS-Related Complex (ARC), and related diseases. Covers both open and closed or completed trials. For each trial, gives: title and purpose, agent name, diseases under study, patient inclusion and exclusion criteria, trial sites, and trial status. For some trials, covers three phases: 1) tests to determine drug dosage and safety or toxicity before testing for effectiveness; 2) tests to determine side effects and tests to determine efficacy of agent, alone or in combination with other drugs, against specific diseases; 3) tests for additional use-related information. Also includes telephone contact numbers for sites or sponsors of trials.

For more information on drugs used see AIDSDRUGS.

14:50. Online
National Library of Medicine

File name	AIDSTRIALS
Start year	Current information
Number of records	230
Update period	Every two weeks

This database can also be found on:
AIDS Compact Library
Physician's AIDSLINE

Alcohol and Alcohol Problems Science Database

National Institute on Alcohol Abuse and Alcoholism (NIAAA)

14:52. Master record

Database type	Bibliographic
Number of journals	
Sources	Books, conference papers, conference proceedings, dissertations, journals, monographs and reports
Start year	1972
Language	English
Coverage	International
Number of records	75,000
Update size	—
Update period	Monthly
Index unit	Articles, conference papers, book chapters and books

Keywords

Alcohol Abuse

Description

This database consists of bibliographic citations, with abstracts of alcohol related scientific references from US and foreign sources, to the worldwide literature on alcoholism research. Subjects covered include: psychology, psychiatry, physiology, biochemistry, epidemiology, animal studies, sociology, prevention, education, treatment, safety and accidents, employment, legislation, labour and industry and public policy.

14:53. Online
BIOSIS Life Science Network

File name	AAPS
Start year	1972
Number of records	75,000
Update period	Monthly
Price/Charges	Connect time: US$9.00 Online print: US$6.00 per 10; 2.25 per abstract; 3.50 per full text article

Also available via the Internet by telnetting to LSN.COM.

Notes

On Life Science Network users can search this database or they can scan a group of subject-related databases. There is a charge of $2.00 per scan of subject-related databases. To search one database and display up to ten citations costs $6.00. Most charges are for information retrieved. There are no charges if there are no results and no charge to transfer results to a printer or diskette. Articles may also be ordered via an online document delivery request.

A telecommunications software package is also available, costing $12.95, providing an automatic connection to Life Science Network for heavy users of the service, with capability to transfer to print or disk and customised colour options.

14:54. Online
BRS

File name	ETOH
Start year	1972
Number of records	75,000
Update period	Monthly
Price/Charges	Connect time: US$44.00/54.00 Online print: US$0.46/0.54 Offline print: US$0.54

Alcohol Information for Clinicians and Educators Database

Project CORK Institute, Dartmouth Medical School

14:55. Master record

Database type	Bibliographic, Library catalogue/cataloguing aids
Number of journals	
Sources	Conference papers, government documents, journals, monographs and reports
Start year	1978
Language	English
Coverage	International
Number of records	9,000+
Update size	1,200
Update period	Quarterly
Hosts have included	BRS (until 31.12.92.)

Keywords

Alcohol Abuse; Drug Abuse

Description

This database provides an index to the collection of information about alcohol and alcoholism and other drugs in the Project Cork Resource Center which was started in 1978 to provide information services to physicians and medical educators as they worked to integrate alcohol education into the medical school curriculum. It also includes biomedical, social science and social policy literature. The scope of the collection was expanded throughout 1990 to include drugs other than alcohol. The multidisciplinary collection is used by health care providers, administrators, policy makers and educators. Materials selected for the collection include journals, books, government reports, and documents and presentations.

The database corresponds in part to *Alcohol Clinical Update*, a newsletter that contains selected material from the database.

Controlled vocabulary developed by the Project Cork Resource Center.

BRS discontinued this database at the end of 1992.

Alconarc

Centralförbundet för Alkohol- och Narkotikaupplysning

14:56. Master record

Database type	Library catalogue/cataloguing aids
Number of journals	
Sources	
Start year	1980
Language	Danish, English, Swedish and Norwegian
Coverage	International
Number of records	6,500
Update size	700
Update period	Weekly

Keywords

Drugs

Description

Alconarc is a catalogue of the collections of the CAN library. Exhaustive coverage of Swedish, Norwegian and Danish literature, selective coverage of monographs and research reports from other countries on alcohol and drugs. Alconarc is one of the files in the Drugab information system. See also Dalctraf and Nordrug.

Equivalent to *Alkohol Och Narkotika. Svensk Litteratur. ; Cans Bibliotek Och Dokumentationscentral Nyförvärvad Litteratur.*

Alconarc is indexed by *Medical Subject Headings* (*MeSH*).

14:57. Online   DAFA Data AB

File name	Alconarc
Start year	1980
Number of records	6,500
Update period	Weekly

This database can also be found on:
Drugab

Alconline

Centralforbundet for Alkohol- och Narkotikaupplysning

14:59. Master record

Database type	Bibliographic, Textual
Number of journals	
Sources	Journals and Books
Start year	Late 1970s
Language	English
Coverage	International
Number of records	8,000
Update size	—
Update period	

Keywords

Accidents; Alcohol Abuse; Drug Abuse; Safety

Description

Citations with abstracts, to literature on road safety, and alcohol and drug abuse.

14:60. Online   MIC/Karolinska Institute Library and Information Center (MIC KIBIC)

File name	Alconline
Start year	Late 1970s
Number of records	8,000
Update period	

ALERTS

Adis International Ltd

14:61. Master record

Alternative name(s)	LMS Drug Alerts Online; Adis Alerts Online
Database type	Bibliographic
Number of journals	1,900
Sources	Journals
Start year	Varies; earliest data from 1983
Language	
Coverage	International

Number of records	30,000
Update size	—
Update period	Three times per week
Database aids	Adis Drugs and Disease Thesaurus, Auckland, Adis International, 1990

Keywords

Drugs

Description

Citations, with evaluative summaries by two independent editors and a consulting clinical specialist in the area, to drug trials, focussing on drugs, disease and therapeutics. The database is based on the Adis Literature Monitoring and Evaluation Service (LMS) which is centred on thirteen major therapeutic areas.

Services available (with date of first issue online) are: *Antibacterials* (Jan 1985); *Antivirals* (Jan 1989); *Arrhythmias* (Oct 1983); *Cancer Chemotherapy* (Jan 1988); *Diabetes* (Jan 1990); *Heart Failure* (Oct 1983); *Hyperlipidaemia* (Jan 1989); *Hypertension* (Oct 1983); *Ischaemic Heart Disease* (Oct 1983); *Obstructive Airways*; *Disease* (Jan 1986); *Neuropsychotherapeutics* (Jul 1986); *Peptic Ulcer Disease* (Jan 1986); *Rheumatic Disease* (Jan 1983). The documents are highly structured and authoritative. Each summary includes information on the purpose, evaluation of trial design and reporting, summary of trial details, drugs and regimens in easy to read tables (1990 onwards), results and side effects tabulated (1990 onwards) for review at a glance, and this is enhanced by an Adis score for quality of trial design and reporting, with Adis comments on the strengths and weaknesses of the trial design.

Corresponds to Adis Literature Monitoring and Evaluation Service (LMS).

Major international medical and biomedical journals are selected for their coverage of drugs, disease and therapeutics, and include the major Japanese publications.

Adis descriptor indexing is designed to highlight key article features by allocating drug or disease tags from the following lists:

Drug Tags: abuse; antimicrobial activity; adverse reactions; drug interactions; general; overdose; pharmacodynamics; pharmacokinetics; therapeutic use; poisoning; diagnostic use; laboratory test modifications.

Disease Tags: assessment; contributory factors; diagnosis; drug-induced; epidemiology; general; management; pathogenesis; prevention; treatment; incidence. These tags are combined with descriptors in order to qualify the term. Associated descriptors and sub-descriptors can be matched by use of the WITH operator to confine searches to terms in the same sentence.

14:62. Online   Data-Star

File name	AALR
Alternative name(s)	LMS Drug Alerts Online
Start year	1983 up to approximately four weeks ago
Number of records	30,000
Update period	c.12 times per month
Database aids	Data-Star Biomedical Manual, Berne, Data-Star 1991
Price/Charges	Subscription: UK£32.00
	Connect time: UK£70.00
	Online print: UK£5.00
	Offline print: UK£5.22
	SDI charge: UK£4.72

Notes

From June 1993 Data-Star have introduced an annual fee/subscription per contract (that is, not per password) of SFr 80.00 (c.UK£ 32.00) payable every June. For North American customers billed in dollars who also use DIALOG, the DIALOG fee also covers access to Data-Star. Academic customers, 'commitment' customers and customers currently billed in dollars are exempt.

14:63. Online   Data-Star

File name	AALC
Alternative name(s)	LMS Drug Alerts Online
Start year	Current, including the AALD file, holding approx. four weeks of data
Number of records	
Update period	c.12 times per month
Database aids	Data-Star Biomedical Manual, Berne, Data-Star 1991
Price/Charges	Subscription: UK£32.00
	Connect time: UK£70.00
	Online print: UK£6.60
	Offline print: UK£6.82
	SDI charge: UK£4.72

Notes

From June 1993 Data-Star have introduced an annual fee/subscription per contract (that is, not per password) of SFr 80.00 (c.UK£ 32.00) payable every June. For North American customers billed in dollars who also use DIALOG, the DIALOG fee also covers access to Data-Star. Academic customers, 'commitment' customers and customers currently billed in dollars are exempt.

14:64. Online   Data-Star

File name	AALD
Alternative name(s)	LMS Drug Alerts Online
Start year	Current, holds the latest update data
Number of records	
Update period	Twelve times per month
Database aids	Data-Star Biomedical Manual, Berne, Data-Star 1991
Price/Charges	Subscription: UK£32.00
	Connect time: UK£70.00
	Online print: UK£6.60
	Offline print: UK£6.82
	SDI charge: UK£4.72

Notes

From June 1993 Data-Star have introduced an annual fee/subscription per contract (that is, not per password) of SFr 80.00 (c.UK£ 32.00) payable every June. For North American customers billed in dollars who also use DIALOG, the DIALOG fee also covers access to Data-Star. Academic customers, 'commitment' customers and customers currently billed in dollars are exempt.

14:65. Online   Data-Star

File name	AAZZ
Alternative name(s)	LMS Drug Alerts Online
Start year	1983 to date
Number of records	
Update period	c.12 times per month
Database aids	Data-Star Biomedical Manual, Berne, Data-Star 1991
Price/Charges	Subscription: UK£32.00
	Connect time: UK£70.00
	Online print: UK£6.60
	Offline print: UK£6.82
	SDI charge: UK£4.72

Notes

From June 1993 Data-Star have introduced an annual fee/subscription per contract (that is, not per password) of SFr 80.00 (c.UK£ 32.00) payable every June. For North American customers billed in dollars who also use DIALOG, the DIALOG fee also covers access to Data-Star. Academic customers, 'commitment' customers and customers currently billed in dollars are exempt.

14:66. CD-ROM — ADIS International Ltd

File name	Alerts (Retrospective file)
Alternative name(s)	LMS Drug Alerts Online
Format notes	IBM
Start year	
Number of records	
Update period	

Notes

Retrospective file of the ALERTS database.

Allied and Alternative Medicine

Medical Information Systems, Reference & Index Services

14:67. Master record

Alternative name(s)	AMED
Database type	Bibliographic
Number of journals	350+
Sources	Journals, monographs and newspapers
Start year	1985
Language	English
Coverage	International
Number of records	40,000
Update size	—
Update period	Monthly
Thesaurus	CATS Thesaurus, 1991 version in preparation
Database aids	List of journals indexed, 1991

Keywords

Acupuncture; Alexander Technique; Alternative Medicine; Herbal Remedies; Homeopathy; Occupational Therapy; Osteopathy; Physiotherapy; Psychotherapy; Rehabilitation

Description

This database provides coverage of the wider areas of clinical medicine – complementary or alternative medicine. Subjects covered include: acupuncture; homeopathy; hypnosis; chiropractic; osteopathy; psychotherapy; diet therapy; herbalism; holistic treatment; traditional Chinese medicine; occupational therapy; physiotherapy; rehabilitation; Ayurvedic medicine; reflexology; iridology; moxibustion; meditation; yoga; healing research; Alexander technique. The database will be of interest to those who need to know more about alternatives to conventional medicine – doctors, nurses, therapists, health care libraries, self help groups and the pharmaceutical industry.

350 biomedical journals are indexed regularly and relevant articles are taken from other journals. Few documents on AMED contain abstracts. Newspapers and books are indexed as well as journals. Only original language titles appear in the title field as there are no English translations. The Notes field indicates whether there is an English summary present in the original document. In addition both English

and American spellings should be used where appropriate, for example HOMEOPATHY OR HOMOEOPATHY.

Descriptors are based on MeSH, free text searching is also available.

14:68. Online — Data-Star

File name	AMED
Alternative name(s)	AMED
Start year	1985
Number of records	40,000
Update period	Monthly
Database aids	Data-Star Biomedical Manual and Online manual (search NEWS-AMED in NEWS)
Price/Charges	Subscription: SFr80.00
	Connect time: SFr106.40
	Online print: SFr0.58
	Offline print: SFr0.73
	SDI charge: SFr8.10

Notes

From June 1993 Data-Star have introduced an annual fee/subscription per contract (that is, not per password) of SFr 80.00 (c.UK£ 32.00) payable every June. For North American customers billed in dollars who also use DIALOG, the DIALOG fee also covers access to Data-Star. Academic customers, 'commitment' customers and customers currently billed in dollars are exempt.

Record composition

Abstract AB; Accession Number and Update Code AN; Author AU; Descriptors DE; Identifiers ID; Language LG; Major descriptors MJ; Minor descriptors MN; Notes NT; Publication Type PT; Source SO; Title TI; Update date (YYMMDD) UD; Update date (YYMM) UP and Year of Publication YR

American Bulletin of Technology Transfer

International Advancement Inc

14:69. Master record

Database type	Textual, Directory
Number of journals	1
Sources	
Start year	1988
Language	English
Coverage	International
Number of records	
Update size	—
Update period	Monthly

Keywords

Technology Transfer; Construction; Transport; Plastics; Instrumentation; Packaging; Mechanical Engineering; Mechanics; Consumer Products; Pharmaceuticals

Description

A newsletter listing descriptions of offers and requests for international joint-venture and licensing agreements, covering technologies, processes and products in construction, transportation, chemicals, consumer goods, medicine, plastics, instrumentation, packaging, mechanics and electronics. Also provides abstracts of industry and market studies, executive employment listings and a question and answer forum.

Corresponds to *American Bulletin of Technology Transfer* newsletter.

14:70. Online   International Advancement Inc

File name
Start year   1988
Number of records
Update period   Monthly

Notes

Annual subscription of $75 required.

AMNIS
Nederlandse Associatie van de Farmaceutische Industrie

14:71. Master record

Database type   Textual
Number of journals
Sources
Start year   1988
Language   Dutch
Coverage
Number of records   2,000
Update size   150
Update period   Daily

14:72. Online   Medimatica BV

File name   AMNIS
Start year   1988
Number of records   2,000
Update period   Daily

Analytical Abstracts
Royal Society of Chemistry

14:73. Master record

Database type   Bibliographic
Number of journals   2,000
Sources   Conference proceedings, journals, monographs, technical reports and standards
Start year   1978
Language   English
Coverage   International
Number of records   150,000+
Update size   15,000
Update period   Monthly
Index unit   Conference papers and articles
Abstract details   RSC – abstracts are written specifically aimed at the analytical user
Database aids   Analytical Abstracts Online User Manual UK£30 ($50), Analysis Hotline (newletter) Free and Analytical Abstracts Information Pack – Free

Keywords

Analytical Chemistry; Forensic Science; Inorganic Chemistry

Description

Analytical Abstracts is the only abstracting service devoted solely to analytical chemistry. It covers all aspects of analytical chemistry appearing world-wide including applications of analytic techniques in inorganic, organic, agricultural, pharmacy, food chemistry, agriculture, analytical methods, analytical instruments, biochemical, environmental, food and pharmaceutical chemistry. The database contains citations with, since 1984, high quality English-language abstracts enabling the user to assess the analytical relevance of the original paper. Subjects covered include: the application of various analytical techniques, including use of computers and instruments in general, inorganic, organic, biochemical, pharmaceutical, food, agricultural and environmental chemistry. Records include chemical names, trade names, Chemical Abstracts Service (CAS) Registry Numbers and analytical techniques used (for example, gas chromatography).

The data correspond to the printed *Analytical Abstracts*. Journal articles represent 98% of the file. Items are selected from over 2,000 journals world-wide, originally published in more than 20 languages. The 'core' list of journals totals more than 300 primary titles.

All Analytical Abstracts material has been indexed by the producer to facilitate the retrieval of Analytes (the chemical substances being separated, determined, identified or detected), the Matrix (the medium or type of sample in which the analyte is present) and the Concept (techniques, reagents, apparatus, or fields of study that is anything which is not an analyte or a matrix). Chemical nomenclature is based on that recommended by the International Union of Pure and Applied Chemistry; organic compounds are indexed at the parent compound, followed by substituent groups. Esters and salts of organic acids are indexed under the name of the acid constituent. Colour Index names are used for the names of dyes; enzymes are named according to the approved names of the International Union of Biochemistry; drugs according to the British Pharmacopoeia Commission and pesticides according to the British Standards Institute. CAS Registry Numbers are included for all compounds that are indexed as an ANALYTE or a MATRIX. Note that if the compound of interest is not indexed (that is, it is a solvent, interferent or reagent), or is indexed as a CONCEPT (for example, a novel reagent), CAS Registry Numbers will not help.

Abbreviations for techniques such as gas chromatography and atomic-absorption spectrophotometry are given in the form of capital letters, with no full stops (GC, AAS, etc.) However, references dating from prior to 1986 have an 'old-style' abbreviation viz 'g.c.' or 'a.a.s.' and so proximity operators must be used.

Analytical Abstracts modified its index categorisation in 1991 as a result of editorial changes in its print equivalent. The modifications are in Section and Subsection headings. Cross-reference headings have also changed in format and content. In January 1993, the producers changed to the American spelling 'Sulfur' rather than the English 'Sulphur' – the change will be implemented on all chemical names containing the term or 'sulp', 'sulph', 'sulpho', 'sulphate', etc. The only exceptions are approved drug and pesticide names. Pre-1993 data will NOT be altered.

14:74. Online   Data-Star

File name   ANAB
Start year   1978

Number of records	126,018
Update period	Monthly
Database aids	Data-Star Chemical Manual, Berne, Data-Star, 1989 and Online manual (search NEWS-ANAB in NEWS)
Price/Charges	Subscription: SFr80.00
	Connect time: SFr200.00
	Online print: SFr2.57
	Offline print: SFr1.56
	SDI charge: SFr15.51

Downloading is allowed

Notes

From June 1993 Data-Star have introduced an annual fee/subscription per contract (that is, not per password) of SFr 80.00 (c.UK£ 32.00) payable every June. For North American customers billed in dollars who also use DIALOG, the DIALOG fee also covers access to Data-Star. Academic customers, 'commitment' customers and customers currently billed in dollars are exempt.

Record composition

Abstract AB; Accession Number and Update Code AN; Author AU; Author Affiliation IN; Availability AV; Coden CD; Conference Data CT; Cross Reference XR; Descriptor superlabel for DA, DC, DM; Descriptor/s: analyte DA; Descriptor/s: concept DC; Descriptor: matrix DM; Language of Article LG; Publication Type PT; Publisher PB; Section Details SC; Source SO; Title TI; Update Code UP; Year YR and Year of Publication PY

14:75. Online — DIALOG, Knowledge Index

File name	File 305
Start year	1980
Number of records	150,000+
Update period	Monthly
Price/Charges	Connect time: US$174.00
	Online print: US$1.30
	Offline print: US$1.30
	SDI charge: US$6.50

Downloading is allowed

Notes

This database is also available to home users during evenings and weekends at a reduced rate on the Knowledge Index service of DIALOG – file name in this case is CHEM2, and searches are made with simplified commands or menus.

Record composition

Accession Number; Title; Author; Corporate Source; Journal; Coden; Publication Date; Language; Abstract; Analyte; Matrix and Section Code

DIALINDEX Categories: BIOCHEM, CHEMLIT, FOODSCI, POLLUT, RNCHEM, RNMED, SCITECHB.

14:76. Online — ORBIT

File name	ANAB
Start year	1980
Number of records	150,000+
Update period	Monthly
Database aids	Quick Reference Guide (1/89) Free (single copy) and Database Manual (1986) $7.50

Price/Charges	Connect time: US$142
	Online print: US$1.05
	Offline print: US$0.70
	SDI charge: US$8.50

Downloading is allowed

Notes

Electronic SDI service is now available within two hours on ORBIT. They can be downloaded and reformatted on a word processor. Results are retrieved in the low cost PRINTS file, $15 per connect hour.

Record composition

Accession Number AN; Title TI; Author AU; Corporate Source OS; Source SO; Language LA; CODEN JC; ISSN NU; Document Type DT; Classification Codes CC; Index Terms IT and Abstract AB

14:77. Online — STN

File name	ANABSTR
Start year	1980
Number of records	159,929
Update period	Monthly
Price/Charges	Connect time: DM220.00
	Online print: DM2.70
	Offline print: DM2.70
	SDI charge: DM18.00

Downloading is allowed

Record composition

Accession Number AN; Title TI; Author AU; Source SO; Document Type DT; Language LA; Abstract AB; Classification Codes CC and Index Terms IT

14:78. CD-ROM — SilverPlatter

File name	Analytical Abstracts
Format notes	IBM, Mac
Software	SPIRS/MacSPIRS
Start year	1980
Number of records	160,000
Update period	Quarterly
Price/Charges	Subscription: UK£885 – 2,212

Downloading is allowed

Notes

Requires a signed subscription and licence agreement. Regular subscription is UK£885 for a single user, £2,212 for 2–8 networked users. Discounts are available to print subscribers – £585 for a single user, ££1,462 for 2–8 networked users. Chuck Huber, the reviewer in *CD-ROM Professional* (5(4) p.120–121) thought the SilverPlatter implementation good, the software allowing searching by CAS Registry Number and by the substance's role as either analyte or matrix. He makes the point that with the excellence of the Royal Society's indexing in the print version, the advantages of searching the CD-ROM are reduced but, as the print index does not cumulate annually, there is an advantage to set against the high price differential.

14:79. Database subset
Online — DIALOG

File name	File 385 – ONTAP Analytical Abstracts Training File
Start year	January to June 1987
Number of records	6,041
Update period	Closed File
Price/Charges	Connect time: US$15.00

Notes

The training file for Analytical Abstracts contains records from the January to June updates to File 305, the main Analytical Abstracts file on DIALOG. Offline prints are not available in ONTAP files.

Antiviral Agents Bulletin

OMEC International Inc
Biotechnology Information Institute

14:80. Master record

Database type	Textual, Bibliographic
Number of journals	1
Sources	Newsletter
Start year	1988
Language	English
Coverage	USA (primarily) and International (some)
Number of records	
Update size	—
Update period	Monthly

Keywords

Antiviral Drugs; HIV

Description

Contains full text of *Antiviral Agents Bulletin*, a monthly newsletter on the development of natural and synthetic antiviral products. Provides news and abstracts of AIDS and antiviral drug and vaccine research and development, significant results from screening and drug development programs and patents relating to natural and synthetic products, biological and immunological agents. Covers clinical drug trials; legal and regulatory developments; corporate news, including summaries of licensing and marketing agreements; and announcements of proposals, contracts and awards. Also provides announcements of patent applications available for licensing from the US federal government, citations to antiviral and virus-related patents granted in the USA and in other countries, and selected citations to worldwide literature on antiviral drug development.

Supplied to Data-Star and DIALOG by Predicasts.

This database can be found on:
PTS Newsletter

APINMAP Database

UNESCO Asian and Pacific Information Network on Medicinal and Aromatic Plants (APINMAP)

14:84. Master record

Alternative name(s)	Asian and Pacific Information Network on Medicinal and Aromatic Plants
Database type	Bibliographic
Number of journals	
Sources	
Start year	Current
Language	English
Coverage	Asia and Pacific
Number of records	
Update size	—
Update period	Daily

Keywords

Alternative Medicine; Medicinal Plants

Description

A database of information on the medicinal and aromatic plants and spices of Asia and the Pacific region. Available to network members and to external users with restrictions. Also available as a printout.

Indexing terms are drawn from the *Medical Subject Headings* of the US National Library of Medicine (*MeSH*), *Index Kiwensis* and *PIDVOC*. The Chemical Abstracts Registry Number is also indexed.

14:85. Diskette UNESCO Asian and Pacific Information Network on Medicinal and Aromatic Plants (APINMAP)

File name	APINMAP Database
Alternative name(s)	Asian and Pacific Information Network on Medicinal and Aromatic Plants
Format notes	IBM
Software	CDS/ISIS (Mini-micro version)
Start year	Current
Number of records	
Update period	Daily

Arthur D Little/Online

Arthur D Little
Decision Resources

14:86. Master record

Database type	Bibliographic, Factual, Textual
Number of journals	
Sources	Own publications
Start year	1977
Language	English
Coverage	USA (primarily) and International (some)
Number of records	2,300
Update size	—
Update period	Bimonthly
Index unit	Books

Keywords

Applied Science; Telecommunications

Description

Arthur D. Little Online is derived from the publications of Arthur D. Little Decision Resources, plus the non-exclusive publications of Arthur D. Little Inc., its divisions and subsidiaries. Influential industry forecasts, product and market reviews, technology, corporate profiles, opinion research, product and market overviews, public opinion surveys and management commentaries are included. Industries and technologies include information processing, telecommunications, electronics, especially office automation, computers, equipment manufacturere and services; topics covered include: health care, medical equipment, chemicals including speciality chemicals, petrochemicals, packaging, diagnostic products, plastics, fibres, transport, energy, food processing, biotechnology and environmental issues. In addition to indexing and document availability information, most records contain the Table of Contents and List of Tables and Figures from the print document. Most records prior to 1989 contain the complete text of reports. From 1989 forward records contain extensive summaries of the research report.

Indexes or full text for Arthur D. Little publications, including full text of executive summaries of *Industry Outlook Reports*, *Research Letters*, *Public Opinion Index Reports*.

14:87. Online

DIALOG

File name	File 192
Start year	1977
Number of records	2,300
Update period	Bimonthly
Price/Charges	Connect time: US$114.00
	Online print: US$1.00
	Offline print: US$0.50

Arzneimittel-Interaktionen des SAV

Schweizerischer Apothekerverein

14:88. Master record

Database type	Textual, Factual
Number of journals	
Sources	
Start year	
Language	German
Coverage	Switzerland
Number of records	
Update size	–
Update period	
Hosts have included	AEK (AerzteKasse)

Keywords

Drugs; Pharmaceuticals; Surgery

Description

This is one of ten databases in the medical and pharmaceutical fields on the MediROM database. It is possible to establish logical links between the data of some of the databases.

This database can be found on:
MediROM

ASSIA

Bowker-Saur Ltd

14:92. Master record

Alternative name(s)	Applied Social Sciences Index and Abstracts
Database type	Bibliographic, Textual
Number of journals	550
Sources	Journals and Newspapers
Start year	1987
Language	English
Coverage	International
Number of records	68,000
Update size	18,000
Update period	Every two months
Index unit	Articles
Abstract details	Subject specialists
Database aids	ASSIA Thesaurus, Bowker-Saur UK£53

Keywords

HIV; Child Abuse; Child Development; Child Psychiatry; Criminology; Drug Abuse; Dyslexia; Ethnic Problems; Geriatrics; Health Services; Housing; Immigration; Industrial Relations; Legislation; Pensions; Pollution; Prison Services; Probation; Public Administration; Race Relations; Riots; Rural Studies; Social Welfare; Television; Unemployment; Urban Studies

Description

Citations, with abstracts, to the international English-language literature on applied social science. Covers the information needs of all those engaged in the caring services and the core sociology which sup-

ports these services. Aspects of law, business, national politics as well as nursing and health sciences, social studies, communication and, in particular, local government are included. It has a strong emphasis on the applied aspects of the social sciences. About 40% of ASSIA's coverage is on the United Kingdom, 45% on North America and 15% on the rest of the world. Coverage is of both theoretical and practical articles. Covers child development, industrial relations, social welfare, criminology, politics, child abuse, pollution, geriatrics, immigration, housing, child psychiatry, probation, prison services, nervous disorders, European regulations, unemployment, social effects of television, dyslexia, public administration, drug problems, AIDS, health services retirement pensions, riots, race relations, manpower, inner city problems, rural depredation and ethnic problems.

Corresponds to bi-monthly *Applied Social Sciences Index and Abstracts*. The print version of Applied Social Science Index and Abstracts has been described variously as 'one of the most useful of the many databases in the social sciences'; 'an essential resource'; and 'an excellent source of information . . . with highly developed and accurate indexing'.

Non-selective coverage of core journals; coverage of all major social sciences and related media. About 80% abstracted from cover-to-cover, 20% selectively.

Cross references, synonym references and related headings. All documents contain a short informative abstract, full bibliographic details and index terms which facilitate both general and specific subject searches. Bowker-Saur have produced a thesaurus containing around 8,259 terms which have appeared in ASSIA since its first publication. Its coverage is comprehensive, embracing social science in the widest sense.

14:93. Online

Data-Star

File name	ASSI
Alternative name(s)	Applied Social Sciences Index and Abstracts
Start year	1987
Number of records	68,000
Update period	Every two months
Database aids	Data-Star Biomedical Manual, Berne, Data-Star, 1990 and Online manual (search for NEWS-ASSI in NEWS)
Price/Charges	Subscription: UK£32.00
	Connect time: UK£45.68
	Online print: UK£0.55
	Offline print: UK£0.62
	SDI charge: UK£3.76

Notes

From June 1993 Data-Star have introduced an annual fee/subscription per contract (that is, not per password) of SFr 80.00 (c.UK£ 32.00) payable every June. For North American customers billed in dollars who also use DIALOG, the DIALOG fee also covers access to Data-Star. Academic customers, 'commitment' customers and customers currently billed in dollars are exempt.

14:94. CD-ROM

Bowker-Saur Ltd

File name	ASSIA Plus
Alternative name(s)	Applied Social Sciences Index and Abstracts
Format notes	IBM
Software	Bowker Plus
Start year	1987

Number of records	100,000
Update period	Quarterly
Price/Charges	Subscription: UK£1,150

Australasian Medical Index

National Library of Australia
Department of Community Services
and Health

14:95. Master record

Database type	Bibliographic
Number of journals	
Sources	Journals, Monographs and Conference proceedings
Start year	1980
Language	English
Coverage	Australia and New Zealand
Number of records	28,000+
Update size	8,400
Update period	Monthly

Keywords

Clinical Medicine; Drug Abuse; Aging; Health: Aborigines

Description

Contains citations, with abstracts, to the biomedical literature of Australia and New Zealand. Covers clinical practice, research, policy, health services, drug abuse, the biology of aging, and Aboriginal health.

Biomedical literature of Australia and New Zealand. Journals exclude those covered in MEDLINE.

14:96. Online   Australian MEDLINE Network

File name	Australasian Medical Index
Start year	1980
Number of records	28,000+
Update period	Monthly

Notes

Permission of the National Library of Australia required.

Badekurorte

14:97. Master record

Database type	Textual, Factual
Number of journals	
Sources	
Start year	
Language	German
Coverage	Switzerland
Number of records	
Update size	—
Update period	
Hosts have included	AEK (AerzteKasse)

Keywords

Drugs; Pharmaceuticals; Surgery

Description

This is one of ten databases in the medical and pharmaceutical fields on the MediROM database. It is possible to establish logical links between the data of some of the databases.

This database can also be found on:
MediROM

Banque d'Informations Automatisée sur les Medicaments

Banque d'Informations Automatisée sur les Medicaments

14:99. Master record

Alternative name(s)	BIAM
Database type	Factual, Bibliographic
Number of journals	
Sources	
Start year	Current information
Language	French
Coverage	France
Number of records	11,000
Update size	—
Update period	Weekly

Keywords

Drugs

Description

Information on about 8,000 proprietary drugs and 3,000 substances authorised for use in France, giving composition, toxicology, uses, actions, interactions, effects on foetuses, contraindications, dosage and administration, corresponding foreign names, and bibliographic references.

14:100. Online   Université de Paris V, CITI

File name	
Alternative name(s)	BIAM
Start year	Current information
Number of records	11,000
Update period	Weekly

BGA-Pressedienst

Bundesgesundheitsamt – BGA

14:101. Master record

Database type	Textual
Number of journals	
Sources	Press releases
Start year	1980
Language	German
Coverage	Germany
Number of records	462 documents
Update size	50 documents
Update period	As needed

Keywords

Drugs; HIV; Infectious Diseases; Pollution

Description

This is a full text database in the German language in the field of human and veterinary medicine and related fields. It corresponds to the printed press releases from the Bundesgesundheitsamt (BGA that is, Federal Health Office) of the Federal Republic of Germany. The database contains the full text of the original documents. Subject coverage includes especially: drugs (for example, express information on drugs), infectious diseases (for example, AIDS), social medicine and epidemiology, toxicology, water, soil, air pollution, environmental chemicals in food, radiation health.

14:102. Online DIMDI

File name	BP80
Start year	1980
Number of records	418 documents
Update period	As needed
Price/Charges	Connect time: UK£0.16–0.34
	Online print: UK£03.88–08.62
	Offline print: UK£0.07–0.14

Downloading is allowed

Record composition

DIMDI Number ENR; Machine Date MD; Number of Document ND; Publication Year PY; Source SO and Title TI

Since January 29, 1992 the database can be searched using DIMDI's User guidance GRIPS-Menu. Freetext searches have to be carried out. There is neither controlled nor uncontrolled vocabulary in the database. Only the user guidance is in English, search terms have to entered in German.

The press releases are continuously numbered per year by the BGA, for example, the thirty first press release in 1991 has the number 31/91. In the field ND (Number of Document) this number is transformed to the format YYnn (YY=two digits for the year, nn=serial number), thus 9131.

BIFOS

Federal Ministry for Youth, Family Affairs, Women and Health

14:103. Master record

Alternative name(s)	Betaeubungsmittelrecht-Informationssystem
Database type	Factual, Textual
Number of journals	
Sources	Law reports
Start year	1984–1987
Language	German
Coverage	Germany
Number of records	99,000
Update size	30,000
Update period	Annually

Keywords

Drug Abuse

Description

BIFOS is a non-bibliographic German Language database containing references to Federal Republic of Germany and West Berlin court decisions for cases involving the law on dangerous drugs (Beteaubungsmittelgesetz – BtMG). Records include defendant's age, sex, and nationality, charge, relevant statutes applied, sentence, and location and type of court, names of the drugs and sanctions.

For the year 1984 only approximately 50% of all decisions were stored. From 1985 onwards all annual decisions are available. The annual data can only be released after the report to parliament on drugs of the Federal Minister for Youth, Family Affairs, Women and Health has been published.

14:104. Online DIMDI

File name	BT84
Alternative name(s)	Betaeubungsmittelrecht-Informationssystem
Start year	1984
Number of records	17,162
Update period	Not updated

Price/Charges	Connect time: UK£03.88–08.62
	Online print: UK£0.16–0.34
	Offline print: UK£0.07–0.14

Downloading is allowed

Notes

For 1984 only 50% of all decisions have been stored.

14:105. Online DIMDI

File name	BT85
Alternative name(s)	Betaeubungsmittelrecht-Informationssystem
Start year	1985
Number of records	25,364
Update period	Not updated
Price/Charges	Connect time: UK£03.88–08.62
	Online print: UK£0.16–0.34
	Offline print: UK£0.07–0.14

Downloading is allowed

14:106. Online DIMDI

File name	BT86
Alternative name(s)	Betaeubungsmittelrecht-Informationssystem
Start year	1986
Number of records	26,638
Update period	Not updated
Price/Charges	Connect time: UK£03.88–08.62
	Online print: UK£0.16–0.34
	Offline print: UK£0.07–0.14

14:107. Online DIMDI

File name	BT87
Alternative name(s)	Betaeubungsmittelrecht-Informationssystem
Start year	1987
Number of records	29,856
Update period	Not updated
Price/Charges	Connect time: UK£03.88–08.62
	Online print: UK£0.16–0.34
	Offline print: UK£0.07–0.14

BioBusiness

BIOSIS

14:108. Master record

Database type	Bibliographic
Number of journals	500
Sources	Conference proceedings, journals, monographs, newsletters, research reports and patents (US)
Start year	1985
Language	English
Coverage	International
Number of records	480,000
Update size	42,000
Update period	Monthly
Database aids	BioBusiness Search Guide, Philadelphia, BIOSIS, How to search BioBusiness,Philadelphia, BIOSIS and Newsletters: BioSearch, BioScene

Keywords

Cosmetics; Fishing; Forestry; Genetic Engineering; Immunology

Description

BioBusiness is a bibliographic database which focuses specifically on the business applications of biomedical research. It contains citations, with abstracts, to the worldwide periodical literature on business applications of biological and biomedical research. Subjects covered include: agriculture and forestry, animal production, biomass conversion, crop production, diet and nutrition, fermentation, food technology, cosmetics, genetic engineering, health care, industrial microbiology, pharmaceutical products, medical technology, medical diagnostics, medical instrumentation, occupational health, pesticides, pharmaceuticals, protein production, toxicology, veterinary science, waste treatment, energy and the environment, and other industries affected by biotechnological developments. Also covers patents in such areas as immunological testing, food processes, and fishing. For each patent record, includes inventor's name and address, patent title and number, patent classes, date granted, and assignee. BioBusiness can be used to discover: the latest legislation and regulatory controls affecting implementation of biotechnology research; the impact of economic fluctuations on price and production forecasts for agricultural commodities; the financial effects of recycling programs on business; the increased use of natural ingredients in cosmetic and personal care products; the applications of bioengineering in pharmaceuticals; trends in the development and marketing of food products; etc.

A broad spectrum of life science, business and management journals are scanned. Abstracts are included for approximately 55–60% of the records.

Both controlled and uncontrolled terms are used for indexing. The concept codes used are different from the BIOSIS concept codes.

14:109. Online   BIOSIS Life Science Network

File name	
Start year	1985
Number of records	480,000
Update period	Monthly
Price/Charges	Connect time: US$9.00
	Online print: US$6.00 per 10; 2.25 per abstract; 3.50 per full text article

Downloading is allowed
Also available via the Internet by telnetting to LSN.COM.

Notes

On Life Science Network users can search this database or they can scan a group of subject-related databases. There is a charge of $2.00 per scan of subject-related databases. To search one database and display up to ten citations costs $6.00. Most charges are for information retrieved. There are no charges if there are no results and no charge to transfer results to a printer or diskette. Articles may also be ordered via an online document delivery request. A telecommunications software package is also available, costing $12.95, providing an automatic connection to Life Science Network for heavy users of the service, with capability to transfer to print or disk and customised colour options.

14:110. Online   BRS

File name	BBUS
Start year	1985
Number of records	480,000
Update period	Weekly
Price/Charges	Connect time: UK£88.00/98.00
	Online print: UK£0.46/0.54
	Offline print: UK£0.52

Downloading is allowed

14:111. Online   CISTI, Canadian Online Enquiry Service CAN/OLE

File name	
Start year	1985

Number of records 480,000
Update period Monthly
Downloading is allowed

14:112. Online   Data-Star

File name	BBUS
Start year	1985
Number of records	277,972
Update period	Weekly
Database aids	Data-Star Business Manual and Online manual (search NEWS-BBUS in NEWS)
Price/Charges	Subscription: UK£32.00
	Connect time: UK£63.60
	Online print: UK£0.41
	Offline print: UK£0.36
	SDI charge: UK£3.94

Downloading is allowed

Notes

From June 1993 Data-Star have introduced an annual fee/subscription per contract (that is, not per password) of SFr 80.00 (c.UK£ 32.00) payable every June. For North American customers billed in dollars who also use DIALOG, the DIALOG fee also covers access to Data-Star. Academic customers, 'commitment' customers and customers currently billed in dollars are exempt.

Record composition

Abstract AB; Accession Number and Update Code AN; Author AU; Author Affliation IN; Company Name CO; Concept Codes CC; Descriptors DE; Language of Article LG; Named Person(s) NA; Publication Details PU; Source SO; Title TI; Update Codes UP and Year of Publication YR

14:113. Online   DIALOG

File name	File 285
Start year	1985
Number of records	371,575
Update period	Weekly
Price/Charges	Connect time: US$126.00
	Online print: US$0.85
	Offline print: US$0.85
	SDI charge: US$10.50

Downloading is allowed

Notes

DIALINDEX Categories: AGRIBUS, BIOBUS, BIOTECH, PHARMINA.

14:114. Online   ESA-IRS

File name	File 137
Start year	1985
Number of records	372,000 (October 1991)
Update period	Weekly
Price/Charges	Subscription: UK£70.29
	Database entry fee: UK£3.49
	Online print: UK£0.74
	Offline print: UK£0.79
	SDI charge: UK£3.49

Downloading is allowed

Notes

The default supplier of original document is British Library Documentation Supply Centre.

From 1993 ESA-IRS are charging an annual fee of 100 Accounting Units (c.UK£ 70.29) to all users. This is equivalent to the fee for full documentation and will not be charged to customers already paying for documentation.

Record composition

Abstract /AB; Additional Source Information NT; Author AU; Concept Code CC; Concept Code Name CN; Corporate Source CS; ISBN BN; Journal Name JN; Language LA; Named Company NM; Named Person SP; Native Number NN; Patent Assignee PH; Patent Number PN; Publication Year PY; Subfile (1) SF; Title /TI; Uncontrolled Terms /UT and US Patent Classification PC

14:115. Online   STN

File name	BIOBUS
Start year	1985
Number of records	480,000
Update period	Weekly
Downloading is allowed	

14:116. Tape   BIOSIS

File name	
Format notes	9-track, 800, 1600 or 6250 bpi, variable length records, variable block size.
Start year	1985
Number of records	480,000
Update period	Monthly

Notes

Corresponds to the BioBusiness online database. Annual lease price is $2,350 plus additional usage charges; contact BIOSIS for archival tape prices.

BIOCAS
BIOSIS
Chemical Abstracts Service

14:117. Master record

Alternative name(s)	BIOSIS/CAS Registry Number Concordance
Database type	Directory
Number of journals	
Sources	
Start year	1969–1985
Language	English
Coverage	International
Number of records	1.2 million
Update size	–
Update period	Quarterly

Keywords

Animal Sciences; Bioengineering; Biophysics; Fishing; Immunology; Patents; Plant Sciences

Description

Contains references to citations common to both CA Search and BIOSIS Previews. Each record currently includes the BIOSIS Document Number, the equivalent CA Search Abstract Number and, for approximately 78 percent of the references, CAS Registry Numbers (see Registry Nomenclature and Structure Service). In subsequent updates, CAS Registry Numbers will be available for the remaining BIOSIS citations.

14:118. Online   STN

File name	BIOCAS
Alternative name(s)	BIOSIS/CAS Registry Number Concordance
Start year	

Number of records	
Update period	

BIOLIS
Informationzentrum für Biologie am Forschungsinstitut Senckenberg

14:119. Master record

Alternative name(s)	Biologische Literaturinformation Senckenberg
Database type	Bibliographic
Number of journals	
Sources	Periodicals and serials
Start year	1970
Language	German and English
Coverage	Germany, Switzerland and Austria
Number of records	53,3532,214
Update size	6,000
Update period	Every two months
Index unit	Articles

Keywords

Animal Sciences; Bioengineering; Biophysics; Fishing; Immunology; Patents; Plant Sciences

Description

BIOLIS is a bilingual (German/English) database in the field of biology. It is intended as a supplement to the American database BIOSIS Previews. Subjects covered include: biology; botany; zoology; ecology; environmental protection and paleontology. Each record contains details of authors, title and other bibliographic data as well as free key words and the codes and terms of the BIOSIS classification system.

Sources are publications in the Federal Republic of Germany, Switzerland or Austria which are not listed in BIOSIS Previews.

Articles from serials and periodicals which are published in the Federal Republic of Germany, Switzerland and Austria.

14:120. Online   DIMDI

File name	BS70
Alternative name(s)	Biologische Literaturinformation Senckenberg
Start year	1970
Number of records	53,353
Update period	Every two months
SDI period	2 months
Price/Charges	Connect time: UK£10.55–13.39
	Online print: UK£0.30–0.48
	Offline print: UK£0.23–0.30
Downloading is allowed	

Notes

Suppliers of online documents: British Library Document Supply Centre, Boston Spa, England; Harkers Information Retrieval System, Sydney, Australia.

The unit record contains information about author(s), title, and other bibliographic data as well as free key words and the codes and terms of the BIOSIS classification system. At present there are no abstracts. Searches are possible from January 1970. The

English biosystematic names in BIOLIS are associated to the Latin biosystematic names in BIOSIS Previews. BIOLIS is the only database into which Latin biosystematic names have been introduced.

Biosis Previews Vocabulary
BIOSIS

14:121. Master record

Database type	Factual, Directory, Thesaurus
Number of journals	
Sources	
Start year	
Language	English
Coverage	
Number of records	
Update size	–
Update period	Irregular

Keywords

Immunology; Fishing; Animal Sciences; Plant Sciences; Bioengineering; Biophysics; Patents

Description

Contains the meaning of the numeric code in natural language.

Corresponds to the *Alphabetic Directory of Concept Headings*.

14:122. Online   Data-Star

File name	BVOC
Start year	
Number of records	
Update period	
Price/Charges	Subscription: SFr80.00
	Connect time: SFr147.00
	Online print: SFr0.00
	Offline print: SFr0.83

Notes

From June 1993 Data-Star have introduced an annual fee/subscription per contract (that is, not per password) of SFr 80.00 (c.UK£ 32.00) payable every June. For North American customers billed in dollars who also use DIALOG, the DIALOG fee also covers access to Data-Star. Academic customers, 'commitment' customers and customers currently billed in dollars are exempt.

BIOSIS Previews
BIOSIS

14:123. Master record

Alternative name(s)	Biological Abstracts
Database type	Bibliographic
Number of journals	9,300
Sources	Bibliographies, conference proceedings, government documents, journals, letters, meeting abstracts, monographs, notes, patents, reviews, reports, research communications, symposia and theses
Start year	1969
Language	English
Coverage	International

Number of records	7,826,768
Update size	535,000
Update period	Weekly
Index unit	Articles, book chapters, letters, meeting abstracts, reports and reviews
Database aids	BIOSIS Previews Search Guide, BIOSCENE BIOSEARCH, BIOSIS Previews Search Guide Master Index and Discovering BIOSIS Previews: An Interactive Disk (IBM-compatible CAL software US$ 45.00)

Keywords

Animal Sciences; Bioengineering; Biophysics; Fishing; Immunology; Patents; Plant Sciences

Description

Biosis Previews, the world's largest English language indexing and abstracting service for biology and biomedicine, contains citations, with abstracts, to the worldwide literature on research in the life sciences: microbiology; plant and animal science; experimental medicine; agriculture; pharmacology; ecology; biochemistry; bioengineering; biophysics; including the basic biological disciplines of zoology, genetics, botany; related interdisciplinary fields including food science, veterinary medicine and research medicine, and associated areas of life sciences such as instrumentation.

It covers original research reports, reviews of original research, history and philosophy of biology and biomedicine, and documentation and retrieval of biological information, including references to accounts of field, laboratory, clinical, experimental and theoretical work. The database presents research findings and literature references on all living things and emphasizes their identification (taxonomy), their life processes, environments and applications. From 1986 to 1989 the database covers selective US patents in such areas as immunological testing, food processes, and fishing. For each patent record, the database includes the inventor's name and address, patent title and number, patent classes, date granted, and assignee.

The database corresponds in coverage to *Biological Abstracts (BA)* (1969+) and *Biological Abstracts/RRM (Reports, Reviews, Meetings) (BA/RRM)* (1980+) and BioResearch Index (BioI), the major publications of BIOSIS (*BA/RRM* is the successor to *BioI* beginning in 1980). Biological Abstracts includes approximately 275,000 accounts of original research yearly and *Biological Abstracts/RRM* includes 260,000 citations yearly. As to the origin or sources, approximately fifty per cent of the items in the database originate from Europe and Middle East, twenty six per cent from North America, fifteen per cent from Asia and Australia, six per cent from Central and South America and three per cent from Africa. Approximately forty-five per cent of database records relate to non-journal literature which means that of the leading bioscience databases, BIOSIS offers the most extensive coverage of this type of literature, EMBASE and MEDLINE both having ceased coverage of non-journal literature in 1980 and 1981 respectively. The references to non-journal literature do not contain abstracts but title keywords augmented by natural language descriptors provide access to scientific communications not found in many other life science databases. Approximately eighty six per cent of records contain citations to English-language sources. This compares to seventy five per cent in EMBASE, seventy four per cent in MEDLINE and eighty-eight per cent in SciSearch. In addition fifty-four per cent of records contain abstracts (from 1986 onwards). This compares with sixty- five per cent of records in MEDLINE and sixty per cent in Embase. The other leading bioscience database, SciSearch, now does contain abstracts. In BIOSIS sixty-seven per cent of records with non-English sources contain English-language abstracts online. This compares with thirty-seven per cent on EMBASE and twenty-six per cent on MEDLINE (since 1980). In the UK, the Royal Society of Chemistry operates an SDI service against the tapes of the latest two weeks of BIOSIS and Chemical Abstracts under the name of BIOSCAN. Results are mailed on diskette ready for use with most PC-based searching packages. Printed output is also available. Abstracts from July 1976 to date (from BA on Tape) are available online through BRS, Data-Star, DIALOG, DIMDI, ESA-IRS, and STN International. Abstracts from 1982 to date are available through CISTI.

Most BIOSIS PREVIEWS descriptors are natural language terms added by editors to enrich or claify information provided in titles, identifying such factors as: specific scientific or common names or organisms discussed in a source if not included in the citationtitle; virus names; organ systems or tissues used or affected; diseases discussed; geographic location, if pertinent and instrumentation, apparatus methodology. Three data elements are indexed: Keywords, Cross Codes and Biosystematic Codes. The free-text file comprises two data fields: title and added keywords or uncontrolled terms. The added keywords are a data element of indexing whereas the title is a bibliographic data element and is taken from the original publication. The following categories of keywords are added to explain or supplement the title: Descriptors describing the type of the work for example, Review, Book, Letter, Abstract; Organisms; Virus-affiliation terms; organs, tracts, tissues; geographic terms; drugs and their affiliation terms; chemical substances and their affiliation terms; enzymes; instrumentation, apparatus, methods; diseases; topics and purposes of a publication. Organisms: each organism is indexed twice – by a keyword and by a Biosystematic code. Categories of keywords used for organism-related concepts include scientific and/or colloquial names, depending on how they appear in the article; abbreviations which characterise the taxonomical classification of an organism (for example SP for species, VAR for variety); pathogenic organisms as causes of diseases and keywords characterising the sex and/or age groups for human beings and animals. Drugs and their affiliation terms: the name of a drug is taken from the publication in the form in which it is given, that is as a commercial or generic name. For each drug mentioned in the title or in the added keywords one or more drug affiliation terms are indexed. Chemical substances and their affiliation terms: for every chemical substance mentioned in the title or added to the title as a keyword, BIOSIS indexes an affiliation term if the effect of the substance is described in the article (herbicide, insecticide). Enzymes: are only indexed with their Enzyme Commission Number (EC) when the EC-number is mentioned in the article. Spelling: prior to 1985 BIOSIS used word segmentation for some biological, anatomical, chemical and enzyme terms in title and added descriptors. This segmentation was dropped from January 1985 to standardise spelling in the freetext sections. Hyphenated words: in the title and added keywords field the words which form a logical unit are linked by a hypen. This spelling is not used in the abstract. Concept Headings: there are more than 500 concept headings used to index according to broader concepts. These are hierarchically ordered with the section names in the hierarchy corresponding to the section headings in the printed issues. The Concept Headings are weighted into three categories according to the emphasis of an aspect of an article: primary level for the main aspect of an article, secondary level for important aspects and teritary level for incidental aspects.

The availability of weighted indexing is useful as it provides a method for reducing output while maintainin high precision. Biosystematic Codes are also used to denote concept terms and groups of organisms which removes the need to list individually all the items and their synonyms within a group and automatically produces a context of further, more specific queries within that category. Strategy Recommendations (See References) are also given as part of the scope notes on concept codes, providing pointers towards other areas of possibly fruitful examination. The Biosystematic Codes group organisms by accepted taxonomic rules which make it possible to search references to large taxonomic groupings. New Biosystematic Codes for bacteria, based primarily on Bergey's Manual of Systematic Bacteriology, were effective from the first update of 1992. 140 new Biosystematic Codes (BCs) for bacteria replaced the 81 codes in use up to the end of 1991. To avoid incorrect use the names of the respective BCs have been supplemented with the years of their validity, for example BS:RHODOSPIRILLACEAE (1979–91). As there was a comparable change with viruses in 1979 respective in 1981, these BCs have been supplemented in the same way, for example BS : COMOVIRUS (1979–). The group known as the blue-green algae or Cyanophyta or Cyanobacteria, indexed till the end of 1991 as algae (BS : CYANOPHYTA, BC : 13900) will now be indexed as bacteria (BS : CYANOBACTERIA (1992–), BC : 09200). Entering the new text version of Biosystematic Codes for viruses and bacteria may cause errors and the use of the numeric version of BC is therefore recommended.

According to Snow in Chapter Five of the *Manual of Online Search Strategies* (2nd Ed. Aldershot: Ashgate, 1992) the Master Index in the *Biosis Previews Search Guide* should not be regarded as an authority list or thesaurus, since it does not include all words or concepts that are searchable as indexer-added keywords in the online database. Snow also points out the value of controlled vocabulary when searching for topics where a subject population has been specified. Relatively few bioscience databases provide consistent indexing for subject populations (for example humans or specific test animals) and related characteristics commonly requested such as age groups, gender, occupation and racial or ethnic groups. BIOSIS provides consistent indexing for the identification of humans and test animals with less consistent indexing of occupational groups and racial/ethnic groups and uses a natural language approach for the identification of gender. She also notes that American spellings are used as standard. In most bioscience files a form of pharmaceutical nomenclature exists. For BIOSIS the preferred terminology consists of generic names, classification by use/action and CAS Registry Numbers although certain restrictons apply to the latter (for example date, subfile or vendor restrictions). The use of enzyme commission number, investigational code, chemical name or trade name is inconsistent and it is recommended that alternative names should be used in search strategies. In addition retrospective searching may require entry of other names used for the same substance at earlier stages in its development life cycle.

Review articles can be retrieved by adding the word 'review', restricted to title and added keywords, to a search strategy.

14:124. Online — BRS, Morning Search, BRS/Colleague

File name	BIOL
Alternative name(s)	Biological Abstracts
Start year	1976
Number of records	
Update period	Monthly
Price/Charges	Connect time: US$53.00/83.00
	Online print: US$0.44/0.52
	Offline print: US$0.52
	SDI charge: US$10.75

Notes

Users can search in BIOZ, the merged file for both the current file BIOL and the back file BIOB. Abstracts from July 1976 to date are available.

14:125. Online — BRS, Morning Search, BRS/Colleague

File name	BIOB
Alternative name(s)	Biological Abstracts
Start year	1976
Number of records	
Update period	Monthly
Price/Charges	Connect time: US$53.00/83
	Online print: US$0.44/0.52
	Offline print: US$0.52
	SDI charge: US$10.75

Notes

Users can search in BIOZ, the merged file for both the current file BIOL and the back file BIOB. Abstracts from July 1976 to date are available.

14:126. Online — BRS, Morning Search, BRS/Colleague

File name	BIOZ
Alternative name(s)	Biological Abstracts
Start year	1976
Number of records	
Update period	Monthly
Price/Charges	Connect time: US$53.00/83
	Online print: US$0.44/0.52
	Offline print: US$0.52
	SDI charge: US$10.75

Notes

Users can search in BIOZ, the merged file for both the current file BIOL and the back file BIOB. Abstracts from July 1976 to date are available.

14:127. Online — CISTI, Canadian Online Enquiry Service CAN/OLE

File name	BA69
Alternative name(s)	Biological Abstracts
Start year	1969–1984
Number of records	4,267,300
Update period	Closed File
Price/Charges	Connect time: Canadian $40.00
	Online print: Canadian $0.275 – 0.33
	Offline print: Canadian $0.275 – 0.33

Notes

Abstracts from 1982 to date are available. CISTI is accessible only in Canada.

14:128. Online — CISTI, Canadian Online Enquiry Service CAN/OLE

File name	BA85
Alternative name(s)	Biological Abstracts
Start year	1985–1991
Number of records	3,532,472
Update period	Closed File
Price/Charges	Connect time: Canadian $40.00
	Online print: Canadian $0.275 – 0.33
	Offline print: Canadian $0.275 – 0.33

Notes

Abstracts from 1982 to date are available. CISTI is accessible only in Canada.

14:129. Online — CISTI, Canadian Online Enquiry Service CAN/OLE

File name	BA92
Alternative name(s)	Biological Abstracts
Start year	1992
Number of records	185,400
Update period	48 per year
Price/Charges	Connect time: Canadian $40.00
	Online print: Canadian $0.275 – 0.33
	Offline print: Canadian $0.275 – 0.33

Notes

Abstracts from 1982 to date are available. CISTI is accessible only in Canada.

14:130. Online — CompuServe Information Service

File name	IQUEST File 1182
Alternative name(s)	Biological Abstracts
Start year	1969
Number of records	7,713,784
Update period	Twice per month
Price/Charges	Subscription: US$8.95 per month
	Database entry fee: US$9/search; some databases carry a surcharge ($2–75)
	Online print: US$10 references free; then $9 per ten; abstracts $3 each

Downloading is allowed

Notes

Accessed via IQUEST or IQMEDICAL, this database is offered by a DIALOG gateway. IQUEST can either search across all databases, a database of the user's choice or selected multiple databases.

14:131. Online — Council of Scientific Research

File name	
Alternative name(s)	Biological Abstracts
Start year	
Number of records	
Update period	

14:132. Online — Data-Star

File name	BIOL
Alternative name(s)	Biological Abstracts
Start year	1985

Number of records	6,000,000
Update period	Every two weeks
Database aids	Data-Star Biomedical Manual and Data-Star Online Manual (search for NEWS-BIOL in NEWS)
Price/Charges	Subscription: SFr80.00 Connect time: SFr147.00 Online print: SFr0.40–1.03 Offline print: SFr0.90 SDI charge: SFr4.94

Notes

Abstracts are provided for about two-thirds of the database.

From June 1993 Data-Star have introduced an annual fee/subscription per contract (that is, not per password) of SFr 80.00 (c.UK£ 32.00) payable every June. For North American customers billed in dollars who also use DIALOG, the DIALOG fee also covers access to Data-Star. Academic customers, 'commitment' customers and customers currently billed in dollars are exempt.

Record composition

Abstract AB; Accession Number or and Update Code AN; Authors AU; Author Affiliation IN; Biosystematic Codes BC; Coden CD; Concept Codes CC; Keywords KW; Language LG; Supertaxa ST; Source SO; Title TI and Year of Publication YR

14:133. Online   Data-Star

File name	BI84
Alternative name(s)	Biological Abstracts
Start year	1970–1984
Number of records	
Update period	
Database aids	Data-Star Biomedical Manual and Data-Star Online Manual (search NEWS-BIOL in NEWS)
Price/Charges	Subscription: SFr80.00 Connect time: SFr147.00 Online print: SFr0.40–1.03 Offline print: SFr0.90 SDI charge: SFr4.94

Notes

Abstracts from July 1976 are available.

From June 1993 Data-Star have introduced an annual fee/subscription per contract (that is, not per password) of SFr 80.00 (c.UK£ 32.00) payable every June. For North American customers billed in dollars who also use DIALOG, the DIALOG fee also covers access to Data-Star. Academic customers, 'commitment' customers and customers currently billed in dollars are exempt.

Record composition

Abstract AB; Accession Number or and Update Code AN; Authors AU; Author Affiliation IN; Biosystematic Codes BC; Coden CD; Concept Codes CC; Keywords KW; Language LG; Supertaxa ST; Source SO; Title TI and Year of Publication YR

14:134. Online   Data-Star

File name	BIZZ
Alternative name(s)	Biological Abstracts
Start year	1970+
Number of records	6 million
Update period	Every two weeks
Database aids	Data-Star Biomedical Manual and Data-Star Online Manual
Price/Charges	Subscription: SFr80.00 Connect time: SFr147.00 Online print: SFr0.40–1.03 Offline print: SFr0.90 SDI charge: SFr4.94

Notes

Abstracts from July 1976 to date are available. Abstracts are provided for about two-thirds of the database.

From June 1993 Data-Star have introduced an annual fee/subscription per contract (that is, not per password) of SFr 80.00 (c.UK£ 32.00) payable every June. For North American customers billed in dollars who also use DIALOG, the DIALOG fee also covers access to Data-Star. Academic customers, 'commitment' customers and customers currently billed in dollars are exempt.

Record composition

Abstract AB; Accession Number or and Update Code AN; Authors AU; Author Affiliation IN; Biosystematic Codes BC; Coden CD; Concept Codes CC; Keywords KW; Language LG; Supertaxa ST; Source SO; Title TI and Year of Publication YR

14:135. Online   DIALOG

File name	File 5
Alternative name(s)	Biological Abstracts
Start year	1969
Number of records	7,713,784 Files 5, 55
Update period	Weekly
Price/Charges	Connect time: US$90.00 Online print: US$0.75 Offline print: US$0.75 SDI charge: US$10.50 (biweekly)/14.95 (monthly)

Notes

Abstracts from July 1976 to date are available and for book synopses in BA/RRM from 1985. Most BA/RRM records do not contain abstracts; no BioResearch Index records contain abstracts. On DIALOG there are two files – File 5 covers 1969 to the present, File 55 1985 to the present.

DIALINDEX categories: AGRI, BIOCHEM, BIOSCI, BIOTECH, ENRION, FOODSCI, MARINE, MEDENG, MEDICINE, NUTRIT, PHARM, PHARMR, SAFETY, TOXICOL, VETSCI.

14:136. Online   DIALOG

File name	File 55
Alternative name(s)	Biological Abstracts
Start year	1985
Number of records	
Update period	
Price/Charges	Connect time: US$90.00 Online print: US$0.75 Offline print: US$0.75 SDI charge: US$10.50 (biweekly)/14.95 (monthly)

Notes

Abstracts from July 1976 to date are available and for book synopses in BA/RRM from 1985. Most BA/RRM records do not contain abstracts and no BioResearch Index records contain abstracts. On DIALOG there are two files – File 5 covers 1969 to the present, File 55 1985 to the present.

DIALINDEX categories: AGRI, BIOCHEM, BIOSCI, BIOTECH, ENRION, FOODSCI, MARINE, MEDENG, MEDICINE, NUTRIT, PHARM, PHARMR, SAFETY, TOXICOL, VETSCI.

14:137. Online   DIMDI

File name	BA70
Alternative name(s)	Biological Abstracts
Software	GRIPS

Start year	1970–1982
Number of records	8,033,918
Update period	Monthly
Database aids	User Manual BIOSIS Previews and Memocard Biosis Previews
Price/Charges	Connect time: UK£23.42–32.18
	Online print: UK£0.37–0.55
	Offline print: UK£0.29–0.36

Downloading is allowed
Thesaurus is online

Notes

Abstracts (52% of the records) are available from July 1976 to date. Searches are possible from January 1970. The Basic Index includes the data fields: Title, Abstract, Uncontrolled Terms. Suppliers of online documents: British Library Document Supply Centre, Boston Spa, England; Bayerishe Staatsbibliothek München, München, Germany; Harkers Information Retrieval System, Sydney, Australia; Koninklijke Nederlandse Akademie van Wetenschapen, Amsterdam, The Netherlands.

Record composition

Abstract AB; Author AU; Biosystematic Code BC; Biosystematic Code-New /NEW; Biosystematic Heading BS; Biosystematic Heading-New /NEW; Coden CD; Corporate Source CS; Entry Date ED; Free Text FT; Index Term IT; Journal Title JT; Language LA; Document Number ND; Publication Year PY; Subject Code SC; Subject Heading SH; Source SO; Title TI and Uncontrolled Terms UT

14:138. Online   DIMDI

File name	BA83
Alternative name(s)	Biological Abstracts
Software	GRIPS
Start year	1983
Number of records	4,681,303
Update period	Monthly
SDI period	1 month
Database aids	User Manual BIOSIS Previews and Memocard Biosis Previews
Price/Charges	Connect time: UK£23.42–32.18
	Online print: UK£0.37–0.55
	Offline print: UK£0.29–0.36

Downloading is allowed
Thesaurus is online

Notes

Abstracts are available from July 1976 to date. The Basic Index includes the data fields: Title, Abstract, Uncontrolled Terms. Suppliers of online documents: British Library Document Supply Centre, Boston Spa, England; Bayerishe Staatsbibliothek München, München, Germany; Harkers Information Retrieval System, Sydney, Australia; Koninklijke Nederlandse Akademie van Wetenschapen, Amsterdam, The Netherlands.

Record composition

Abstract AB; Author AU; Biosystematic Code BC; Biosystematic Code-New /NEW; Biosystematic Heading BS; Biosystematic Heading-New /NEW; Coden CD; Corporate Source CS; Entry Date ED; Free Text FT; Index Term IT; Journal Title JT; Language LA; Document Number ND; Publication Year PY; Subject Code SC; Subject Heading SH; Source SO; Title TI and Uncontrolled Terms UT

14:139. Online   ESA-IRS

File name	File 7
Alternative name(s)	Biological Abstracts
Start year	1970

Number of records	7,517,000 (October 1991)
Update period	Every two weeks

Downloading is allowed

Notes

From 1973–84 the records contain terms physically split into their components for example PHOSPHO LIPID (not PHOSPHOLIPID). From 1984 the splitting has been interrupted by the Biosis producer. Abstracts from July 1976 to date are available. BIOSIS on ESA-IRS from February 1992 includes new biosystematic codes.

From 1993 ESA-IRS are charging an annual fee of 100 Accounting Units (c.UK£ 70.29) to all users. This is equivalent to the fee for full documentation and will not be charged to customers already paying for documentation.

Record composition

Author AU; Biosystematic Codes BC; Biosystematic Code Name BN; CODEN CO; Concept Codes CC; Concept Code Name CN; Descriptors /UT; Journal Name JN and Title /TI

14:140. Online   Japan Information Center of Science and Technology (JICST)

File name	BIOSIS
Alternative name(s)	Biological Abstracts
Start year	1969
Number of records	6,800,000
Update period	
SDI period	Monthly/bi-weekly
Database aids	Thesaurus Translation List: Japanese-English 1987: English-Japanese 1987.
Price/Charges	Connect time: US$85.00
	Online print: US$0.32
	Offline print: US$0.38
	SDI charge: US$6.10

14:141. Online   OCLC EPIC; OCLC FirstSearch

File name	BIOSIS Previews
Alternative name(s)	Biological Abstracts
Start year	1976
Number of records	
Update period	

14:142. Online   STN

File name	BIOSIS Previews/RN
Alternative name(s)	Biological Abstracts
Start year	1969
Number of records	8,334,568
Update period	Weekly
Price/Charges	Connect time: DM139.00
	Online print: DM1.32
	Offline print: DM1.40
	SDI charge: DM10.70

Downloading is allowed

Notes

Abstracts from July 1976 to date are available.

CAS Registry Numbers, derived from a computer check for chemical names in the title and added keyword fields are present for citations from July 1980 onwards. There is an online thesaurus for for the Biosystematic Code Superterms (/BC) field.

14:143. Online   University of Tsukuba

File name	
Alternative name(s)	Biological Abstracts
Start year	

Number of records
Update period

Notes

Access through University of Tsukuba is limited to affiliates of the University of Japan.

14:144. Tape BIOSIS

File name	BIOSIS Previews
Alternative name(s)	Biological Abstracts
Start year	1969
Number of records	7,826,768
Update period	4 times a month
Price/Charges	Subscription: US$9,125

Notes

Two tapes correspond to Biological Abstracts and two tapes correspond to Biological Abstracts/Reports, Reviews, Meeting Literature (BA/RRM). Corresponds in coverage to Biological Abstracts (BA) and Biological Abstracts/RRM (BA/RRM) (formerly BioResearch Index), and to the BIOSIS Previews online database.

Annual licence fee is $9,125 plus additional usage charges; contact BIOSIS for archival tape prices.

14:145. Database subset
Online CISTI, Canadian Online Enquiry Service CAN/OLE

File name	ABC3
Alternative name(s)	Biological Abstracts
Start year	1989
Number of records	47,138
Update period	Closed File

Notes

Static training file for BIOSIS Previews enabling users to practice searching using free-text terms, Concept Codes, Biosystematic Codes, Super Taxonomic Codes and bibliographic information.

14:146. Database subset
Online Data-Star

File name	TRBI – Biosis Training File
Alternative name(s)	Biological Abstracts
Start year	1984
Number of records	100,000
Update period	Fortnightly
Database aids	Data-Star Biomedical Manual and Data-Star Online Manual (search for NEWS-BIOL in NEWS)
Price/Charges	Connect time: Free

Notes

Static training file for BIOSIS Previews enabling users to practice searching using free-text terms, Concept Codes, Biosystematic Codes, Super Taxonomic Codes and bibliographic information. Records are taken from 1984, 1990 and 1992 from both the Biological Abstracts and the Biological Abstracts/RRM subfiles of the database.

Record composition

Abstract AB; Accession Number or and Update Code AN; Authors AU; Author Affiliation IN; Biosystematic Codes BC; Coden CD; Concept Codes CC; Keywords KW; Language LG; Supertaxa ST; Source SO; Title TI and Year of Publication YR

14:147. Database subset
Online DIALOG

File name	File 205 – ONTAP BIOSIS Previews Training File
Alternative name(s)	Biological Abstracts

Start year	January 1986 updates to File 5, BIOSIS Previews
Number of records	43,406
Update period	Closed File
Price/Charges	Connect time: US$15.00

Notes

The training file from the January updates of File 5, the main BIOSIS Preview file on DIALOG. It includes records from both Biological Abstracts and Biological Abstracts/Reports, Reviews, Meetings. Allows for low-cost practice using the BISOIS biosystematic and concept codes for searching. Offline prints are not available in ONTAP files.

14:148. Database subset
Online ESA-IRS

File name	File 209 – Training Biosis
Alternative name(s)	Biological Abstracts
Start year	References from 1970, 1980, 1986
Number of records	40,000
Update period	Not updated

Notes

A fixed subset of the main BIOSIS database (File 7), enabling the user to practise ESA-QUEST at low cost. Services such as offline prints, automatic current awareness and document ordering are not available.

Record composition

Author AU; Biosystematic Codes BC; Biosystematic Code Name BN; CODEN CO; Concept Codes CC; Concept Code Name CN; Descriptors /UT; Journal Name JN and Title /TI

14:149. Database subset
CD-ROM SilverPlatter

File name	BA on CD
Alternative name(s)	Biological Abstracts
Format notes	Mac, IBM
Software	SPIRS v.2.0/MacSPIRS
Start year	1985
Number of records	280,000
Update period	Quarterly
Database aids	The SilverPlatter Users' Manual and Quick Reference Card
Price/Charges	Subscription: UK£1,647 – 6,762

Notes

When combined with BA/RRM on CD, BA on CD forms the equivalent of the online database BIOSIS Previews, incorporating the concept codes, biosystematic codes and super taxonomical codes used by searchers of the online database. On its own this CD-ROM version includes only Biological Abstracts whereas BIOSIS online includes Biological Abstracts and Biological Abstract/RRM (Reports, Reviews, Meetings). This version only provides initials to authors' first and middle names. According to Condic (Condic, K.S. *CD-ROM Librarian* 6(3) 1991 29–33) each year of the database will appear on a separate CD-ROM, making searching cumbersome for multiple-year access.

In early 1993, SilverPlatter prices for BA on CD were: regular subscriptions UK£5,880 for single users, £6,762 for 2–8 networked users. Prices for those who subscribe to the print or microfilm version – for single users £1,489 and £3,797 for 2–8 networked users. For subscribers to the cumulative index £1,647 for single users and £2,529. For the collection starting with the calendar year 1993 (1985–88, 1989, 1990, 1991 and 1992) prices vary, depending on the user's current subscriptions – prices on application. There are now available back files to 1985. BA on CD requires a signed subscription and licence agreement.

Record composition

Abreviated Journal Title AJ; Abstract AB; Author AU; Biosystematic Codes; Coden CO; Concept Codes CC; Corporate Source CS; Descriptors DE; Journal Anouncement JA; Language of Article LA; Language of Summary LS; Major Concept Codes MJCC; Minor Concept Codes MNCC; Publication Year PY; Source Journal SO; Super Taxa ST; Title TI and Update Code UD

Subject access is via concept codes, biosystematic codes, super taxonomic groups and descriptors. The disc contains over 600 concept codes from the BIOSIS Search Guides. Articles have from one to ten codes assigned to them which are divided into major and minor categories resembling major or minor descriptors found in other databases. Most articles also have one to twelve biosystematic codes assigned to them. Supertaxonomic groups consist of related groups of biosystematic codes which search the English names of groups of animals. Descriptors consist of natural language or controlled vocabulary terms.

14:150. Database subset

CD-ROM **SilverPlatter**

File name	BA/RRM on CD
Alternative name(s)	Biological Abstracts
Format notes	IBM, Mac
Software	SPIRS
Start year	1989
Number of records	260,000
Update period	Quarterly
Database aids	Software Manual, Database Manual and Quick Reference Cards
Price/Charges	Subscription: UK£841 – 6,762

Notes

Most records in this database do not contain abstracts as abstracts are included only in the form of book sysnopses. Equivalent to the printed Biological Abstracts/RRM (Reports, Reviews and Meetings), previously entitled BioResearch Index. Records in the database cover notes, short communications, technical reports, bibliographies and taxonomic keys. Books are also included as are abstracts from meetings. When combined with BA on CD, forms the equivalent of the online database BIOSIS Previews. According to Shirley Cousin's review (*CD-ROM Information Products: The Evaluative Guide* 1993 4(1) p.1–12), the majority of records are from Europe and the Middle East (48%) with a further 28 per cent from North America, 16 per cent from Asia and Australia, 6 per cent from South and Central America and the final 2 per cent from Africa.

Pricing, as of January 1993 is: for regular subscribers, single user UK£3,021, and for 2–8 networked users £3,903; Discounts are available for subscribers to the print or microfilm versions of BA – £1,480 for single users, £2,362 for 2–8 networked users; for cumulative index subscribers prices are £841 for single users and £1,723 for 2–8 networked users. For the collection starting with the calendar year 1993 (1985–88, 1989, 1990, 1991 and 1992) prices vary, depending on the user's current subscriptions – prices on application. BA on CD requires a signed subscription and licence agreement.

14:151. Database subset

Tape **BIOSIS**

File name	BAT – Biological Abstracts on Tape
Alternative name(s)	Biological Abstracts
Format notes	9-track, 800, 1600, or 6250 bpi, variable, length record, variable block size.
Start year	1976
Number of records	
Update period	Twice a month
Price/Charges	Subscription: US$11,000

Notes

Contains abstracts of the worldwide literature on research in the life sciences. Covers articles from over 9,000 periodicals cited in BIOSIS Previews. Corresponds to the abstracts appearing in *Biological Abstracts*, and in part to the BIOSIS Previews online database.

Annual licence fee $11,000 plus additional usage charges; contact BIOSIS for archival tape prices.

This database can also be found on:
TOXLIT
BA/RRM on CD
Foods Intelligence on CD
Toxline Plus

Biotechnology Abstracts
Derwent Publications Ltd

14:153. Master record

Database type	Bibliographic
Number of journals	1,200
Sources	Journals, Patents and Conference proceedings
Start year	1982 (June)
Language	English
Coverage	International
Number of records	110,000
Update size	15,000
Update period	Monthly

Keywords

Biochemical Engineering; Genetic Engineering; Waste Management

Description

Contains citations, with abstracts and indexing, to the worldwide journal and patent literature on biotechnology. It covers all aspects of biotechnology, including genetic engineering, biochemical engineering, fermentation, cell culture, microbiology, down-stream processing, pharmaceuticals, industrial uses of microorganisms, plant breeding, cell hybridization, and industrial waste management.

Each record in the database comprises a detailed abstract of up to 200 words together with controlled-language indexing. Literature records also include complete bibliographic information, and patent documents include patent number, patentee, and publication details. Approximately 27% of the records are patent records.

Corresponds to *Biotechnology Abstracts*.

Differential charges for subscribers and non-subscribers to *Biotechnology Abstracts*.

14:154. Online **DIALOG**

File name	File 357
Start year	1982

Number of records	123,404
Update period	Monthly
Price/Charges	Subscription: US$96.00 – 155.00
	Online print: US$0.27 – 0.70
	Offline print: US$0.49 – 0.75
	SDI charge: US$9.75

Notes

Differential pricing for subscribers and non-subscribers.

14:155. Online   ORBIT

File name	BIOT
Start year	1982 (July)
Number of records	110,000
Update period	Monthly
Database aids	Quick Reference Guide (9/88) Free (single copy)

Notes

Differential charges for subscribers and non-subscribers to Biotechnology Abstracts. Electronic SDI service is now available within two hours on ORBIT. They can be downloaded and reformatted on a word processor. Results are retrieved in the low cost PRINTS file, $15 per connect hour.

14:156. CD-ROM   SilverPlatter

File name	Biotechnology Abstracts
Format notes	IBM, Mac
Software	SPIRS/MacSPIRS
Start year	1982
Number of records	140,000
Update period	Quarterly
Price/Charges	Subscription: UK£1,000 – 2,800

Notes

Data can be displayed in individual fields: title; abstract; journal; classification; etc. There is a discount for academics – subscription cost is £1,000 for single users, £2,000 for 2–8 networked users. The regular subscription is £ 1,400 for single users, £2,800 for 2–8 networked users. Requires a signed subscription and licence agreement.

Biotechnology Newswatch
McGraw-Hill Inc

14:157. Master record

Alternative name(s)	McGraw-Hill Biotechnology Newswatch
Database type	Textual
Number of journals	1
Sources	Newsletter
Start year	1981 (May)
Language	English
Coverage	International
Number of records	
Update size	–
Update period	Twice per month

Keywords

Genetic Engineering

Description

Contains full text of *Biotechnology Newswatch*, a newsletter on bioengineering, biotechnology and the international biotechnology industry. Technical coverage includes biomass conversion, enzyme and fermentation processes, genetic engineering, monoclonal antibodies, and recombinant DNA technology. Business coverage includes emerging companies, company products and earnings, financing and new ventures. Recurring topics are updates on European and Japanes patent disclosures, biotechnology ventures of established firms in the pharmaceutical or chemical industries and biotechnology developments in the United States and key countries around the world.

14:158. Online   Mead Data Central (as a NEXIS database)

File name	BIOTEC – NEXIS
Alternative name(s)	McGraw-Hill Biotechnology Newswatch
Start year	1981 (May)
Number of records	
Update period	Twice per month
Price/Charges	Subscription: US$1,000 – 3,000 (Depending on needs)
	Connect time: US$49.00 (Telecomms + connect time)
	Database entry fee: US$6.00 (Search charge)
	Online print: US$0.04 per line

Notes

Library: NEXIS; Group files: NWLTRS, TRDTEC, CURRNT, ARCHIV and OMNI.

Sections include BIOBUSINESS which provides a brief summary of research contracts awarded to biotech companies, joint ventures of biotech firms and a brief description of the project or end product; JAPANWATCH which reports briefly on new developments in Japanese biotechnology; and PATENTSCAN which provides information on patent disclosures in the field of biotechnology from the British, European or Japanese Patent Offices, including an abstracts of the patent, file number, date, inventor's name and associated company or country.

A subscription charge which covers all transactional charges, connect time, telecommunications and the small administration charge can take the place of individual charges. Subscriptions are negotiated with customers and vary according to the number of menus (thus, files) that are to be used – typically a minimum subscription would be about US$ 1,000. All charges include training and a 24-hour help line.

Record composition

Body of text BODY; Correction CORRECTION; Correction Date CORRECTION-DATE; Date DATE; Filing Location of Story DATELINE; Headline HEADLINE; Summary HIGHLIGHT; First 50 Words LEAD; Headline and Lead HLEAD; Length LENGTH; Name of Publication PUBLICATION; Section SECTION and Series SERIES

This database can also be found on:
NEXIS

BNA Alcohol & Drugs in the Workplace: Costs, Controls, and Controversies
Bureau of National Affairs Inc

14:160. Master record

Alternative name(s)	Alcohol & Drugs in the Workplace: Costs, Controls, and Controversies
Database type	Textual
Number of journals	
Sources	Report

Start year	1986 only
Language	English
Coverage	USA
Number of records	
Update size	—
Update period	Not updated

Keywords

Alcohol Abuse; Drug Abuse

Description

Contains full text of *Alcohol & Drugs in the Workplace: Costs, Controls and Controversies*, a special report covering drug and alcohol abuse in the workplace and strategies for employer and union responses. Includes fourteen case studies and a discussion of current and proposed laws and regulations.

Corresponds to *Alcohol & Drugs in the Workplace: Costs, Controls and Controversies*.

14:161. Online   Executive Telecom System International, Human Resource Information Network (ETSI/HRIN)

File name	
Alternative name(s)	Alcohol & Drugs in the Workplace: Costs, Controls, and Controversies
Start year	1986 only
Number of records	
Update period	Not updated

Notes

Annual subscription to ETSI/HRIN required.

BNA Drug Testing: A Select Bibliography
Bureau of National Affairs Inc

14:162. Master record

Alternative name(s)	Drug Testing: A Select Bibliography
Database type	Bibliographic
Number of journals	
Sources	Journals, Newspapers, Reports and Conference reports
Start year	1985–1986 Closed File
Language	English
Coverage	USA
Number of records	
Update size	—
Update period	Not updated
Index unit	Articles

Keywords

Drug Abuse; Alcohol Abuse; Human Resources Management

Description

Contains citations to articles on employee drug testing. Sources include journals, newspapers, and BNA information services, reports, and conferences.

14:163. Online   Executive Telecom System International, Human Resource Information Network (ETSI/HRIN)

File name	DTB
Alternative name(s)	Drug Testing: A Select Bibliography
Start year	1985–1986 Closed File

Number of records	
Update period	Not updated

Notes

Annual subscription to ETSI/HRIN required.

Boirondoc
Institut Boiron

14:164. Master record

Database type	Bibliographic
Number of journals	
Sources	Journals and Theses
Start year	
Language	French
Coverage	France
Number of records	3,200
Update size	—
Update period	Every two weeks
Index unit	Articles and Theses

Keywords

Homeopathy

Description

Citations to articles and theses on homeopathy. Documents can be ordered online.

14:165. Online   SUNIST

File name	
Start year	
Number of records	3,200
Update period	Every two weeks

Cambridge Scientific Abstracts Engineering
Cambridge Scientific Abstracts

14:166. Master record

Alternative name(s)	CSAE; Hard Sciences
Database type	Bibliographic, Factual
Number of journals	
Sources	Journals, Monographs, Conference proceedings, Technical reports, Patents, Theses and Dissertations
Start year	1981
Language	English
Coverage	International
Number of records	450,000
Update size	—
Update period	Monthly

Keywords

Computer Science; Health and Safety; Mechanical Engineering; Safety; Occupational Health and Safety

Description

A superfile, comprising five subfiles, providing access to the following abstracting services:
Electronics and Communications Abstracts;
ISMEC: Mechanical Engineering Abstracts;
Computer and Information Systems Abstracts;
Solid State/Superconductivity Abstracts;
Health and Safety Science Abstracts.

It includes references selected from a wide range of worldwide literature including journals, government reports, technical reports, conference proceedings, dissertations, theses and patents. Subject coverage includes: communications, telecommunications, information and computer sciences, electronics, medicine, health and safety and mechanical engineering.

14:167. Online   BRS

File name	Cambridge Scientific Abstracts Engineering
Alternative name(s)	CSAE; Hard Sciences
Start year	
Number of records	
Update period	Monthly

14:168. Online   ESA-IRS

File name	Hard Sciences
Alternative name(s)	Cambridge Scientific Abstracts Engineering; CSAE
Start year	1981
Number of records	454,000 (October 1991)
Update period	Monthly

Notes

From 1993 ESA-IRS are charging an annual fee of 100 Accounting Units (c.UK£ 70.29) to all users. This is equivalent to the fee for full documentation and will not be charged to customers already paying for documentation.

For more details of constituent databases, see:
Electronics and Communications Abstracts
ISMEC: Mechanical Engineering Abstracts
Computer and Information Systems Abstracts
Solid State/Superconductivity Abstracts
Health and Safety Science Abstracts

Cambridge Scientific Abstracts Life Sciences
Cambridge Scientific Abstracts

14:170. Master record

Alternative name(s)	CSAL
Database type	Bibliographic
Number of journals	
Sources	Journals, Books, Conference papers, Technical reports, Patents, Theses and Dissertations
Start year	1978
Language	English
Coverage	International
Number of records	1,164,810
Update size	—
Update period	Monthly

Keywords

Acute Poisoning; Aging; Air Pollution; Algology; Amino-Acids; Anatomy; Antibiotics; Aquaculture; Atmospheric Science; Bacteriology; Behavioural Ecology; Bioengineering; Biological Membranes; Biotechnology; Bone Disease; Calcium Metabolism; Chemoreception; Chronic Poisoning; Clinical Medicine; Clinical Toxicology; DNA; Drugs; Ecology; Ecosystems; Endocrinology; Entomology – Agricultural; Entomology – Applied; Entomology – Human; Entomology – Veterinary; Environmental Biology; Ethology; Genetic Engineering; Hazardous Substances; HIV; Histology; Human Ecology; Immune Disorders; Immunology; Infectious Diseases; Land Pollution; Marine Biotechnology; Marine Engineering; Microbiology; Molecular Biology; Molecular Neurobiology; Mycology; Naval Engineering; Noise Pollution; Oceanography; Neurology; Neuropharmacology; Neurophysiology –

Animal; Neuroscience; Nucleic Acids; Nutrition; Oncology; Occupational Health and Safety; Osteoporosis; Osteomalacia; Pathology; Peptides; Pharmaceuticals; Pheromones; Physiology; Pollution; Proteins; Protozoology; Psychophysics; Public Health; Radiation; Rhinology; RNA; Sleep; Smoking; Substance Abuse; Taste Perception; Thermal Pollution; Viral Genetics; Water; Water Pollution

Description

A superfile providing access to the following abstracting services:

Life Sciences Collection;
Aquatic Sciences and Fisheries Abstracts;
Oceanic Abstracts;
Pollution Abstracts.

Covers the worldwide technical literature on medical and biological disciplines from journals, books, conference papers, technical reports, patents, theses and dissertations.

14:171. Online   BRS

File name	Cambridge Scientific Abstracts Life Sciences
Alternative name(s)	CSAL
Start year	1978
Number of records	1,164,810
Update period	Monthly

Notes

A superfile providing access to the following abstracting services: the Life Science Collection, Aquatic Sciences and Fisheries Abstracts, Oceanic Abstracts and Pollution Abstracts.

For more details of constituent databases, see:
Life Sciences Collection
Aquatic Sciences and Fisheries Abstracts
Oceanic Abstracts
Pollution Abstracts

Cancer Treatment Symposia
US Department of Health and Human Services

14:173. Master record

Database type	Textual, Factual
Number of journals	1
Sources	Newsletter
Start year	1983
Language	English
Coverage	International
Number of records	
Update size	—
Update period	
Index unit	articles

Keywords

Cancer; Drugs; Surgery

Description

The publication chronicles symposia in any of the following topical areas of investigation: surgery, radiotherapy, chemotherapy, biologic response modification, supportive care, pharmacology, cell biology and kinetics, mechanisms of drug action and medicinal chemistry. Cancer Treatment Symposia also contains information addressing scientific, educational, ethical and humanistic issues.

14:174. Online
Mead Data Central (as a NEXIS database)

File name	CTS – NEXIS
Alternative name(s)	NEXIS – Cancer Treatment Symposia
Start year	1983–1985
Number of records	
Update period	
Price/Charges	Subscription: US$1,000 – 3,000 (Depending on needs) Connect time: US$49.00 (Telecomms + connect time) Database entry fee: US$24.00 (Search charge) Online print: US$0.04 per line

Notes

Library name: GENMED; Group files: ARCJNL.

A subscription charge which covers all transactional charges, connect time, telecommunications and the small administration charge can take the place of the individual charges. Subscriptions are negotiated with customers and vary according to the number of menus (thus, files) that are to be used – typically a minimum subscription would be about US$ 1,000. All charges include training and a 24-hour help line.

Record composition

Publication; Cite; Section; Length; Title; Author; Abstract (SUM-ABS); Text; Additional information (SUPP-INFO); Reference (BIBLIO-REF); Graphic; Correction and Correction Date

This database can also be found on:
NEXIS

Cancer Weekly
CDC AIDS Weekly/NCI Cancer Weekly
Charles W. Henderson

14:176. Master record

Alternative name(s)	NCI Cancer Weekly
Database type	Textual
Number of journals	1
Sources	Newsletter
Start year	1988
Language	English
Coverage	International
Number of records	
Update size	—
Update period	Daily or weekly
Index unit	articles

Keywords

Education – Cancer; Cancer

Description

A newsletter on developments in detection, treatment and prevention of cancer. Reports news on cancer-related drugs in clinical trials, FDA approvals, cancer studies and therapy, findings from research programs at universities, government laboratories and companies, and includes summaries of articles appearing in important scientific journals dealing with cancer. It is international in scope and includes news from health-care agencies and organisations, development and testing of drugs and procedures, announcements of

research grants and educational programmes, information from the periodical literature and a calendar of events and meetings.
Full text of *Cancer Weekly*.

14:177. Online
CANCERQUEST Online

File name	
Alternative name(s)	NCI Cancer Weekly
Start year	
Number of records	
Update period	

14:178. Online
CompuServe Information Service

File name	IQUEST File 2444
Alternative name(s)	NCI Cancer Weekly
Start year	Current year
Number of records	
Update period	Weekly
Price/Charges	Subscription: US$8.95 per month Database entry fee: US$9/search; some databases carry a surcharge ($2–75) Online print: US$10 references free; then $9 per ten; abstracts $3 each

Downloading is allowed

Notes

Accessed via IQUEST or IQMEDICAL, this database is offered by a NewsNet gateway. IQUEST can either search across all databases, a database of the user's choice or selected multiple databases.

14:179. Online
NewsNet Inc

File name	
Alternative name(s)	NCI Cancer Weekly
Start year	
Number of records	
Update period	

This database can also be found on:
PTS Newsletter Database

Cancer-CD
Elsevier Science Publishers
National Library of Medicine
National Cancer Institute, US National Institutes of Health
Year Book Medical Publishers Inc

14:180. Master record
CD-ROM   **SilverPlatter**

Database type	Bibliographic
Number of journals	
Sources	
Start year	1984
Language	English
Coverage	International
Number of records	340,000
Update size	77,000
Update period	Quarterly
Database aids	Comprehensive printed documentation and Quick Reference Card

Keywords

Cancer; Drugs

Notes

In addition to the complete Cancerlit file, this database contains references to, abstracts of and commentaries on the world's literature in cancer and related subjects from the following sources: Elsevier Science

Publishers; Year Book Medical Publishers; National Cancer Institute (in conjunction with the National Library of Medicine). Duplicate citations are merged into one record, whilst preserving information that is specific to each information provider. It also includes drug/clinical data. *The Year Book of Cancer* contains articles which are the result of an annual search of the world literature on oncology conducted by a professional board of editors and advisors in whose opinion the selected articles warrant the attention of clinicians. Each Year Book record includes a concise summary of the journal article with commentaries by the editors and medical advisors. The database covers the current year together with its five preceding years. The database consists of two CD-ROM discs. Prices are for single users or for 2–8 networked users.

For more details of constituent databases, see:
Cancerlit
EMBASE
Year Book of Cancer

CCINFOdisc Series A1 – MSDS

Canadian Centre for Occupational Health and Safety (CCOHS)

14:182. Master record
CD-ROM   **Canadian Centre for Occupational Health and Safety (CCOHS)**

Alternative name(s)	MSDS
Database type	Textual, Factual, Directory, Numeric
Number of journals	
Sources	Chemical manufacturers, Chemical distributors, data sheets, Government documents, Journals, Monographs and Suppliers
Start year	Current information
Language	English and French
Coverage	Canada (primarily), International (some) and USA (some)
Number of records	
Update size	–
Update period	Quarterly

Keywords
Dangerous Chemicals; First Aid; Hazardous Substances; Occupational Health and Safety; Waste Management

Description
Contains full text of two databases, in both French and English, containing trade names, chemical information, regulatory information on pesticide products and pest management research information systems:

MSDS/FTSS includes over 72,500 Material Safety Data Sheets on chemical trade name products, as supplied by the manufacturers.

Cheminfo/Infochim, produced by the CCOHS, covers the properties, uses, occurrences, health effects and hazards of pure chemicals, natural substances, and mixtures resulting from industrial processes – for each chemical it provides name, synonyms, CAS number, molecular and structural formula, as well as information about its uses and occurrences, physical properties, appearance, reactivity, warning properties (odours, irritation), animal toxicity data; information is

gathered from journals, monographs, government documents, and from MSDS from chemical manufacturers.

Equivalent to the online databases: MSDS/FTSS; Cheminfo/Infochim. FTSS is the French-language equivalent of MSDS, Infochim is the French-language equivalent of Cheminfo, MSDS is also known as Trade Names, the French-language equivalent being Noms de Marque.

For more details of constituent databases, see:
MSDS/FTSS
Cheminfo/Infochim

CCINFOdisc Series A2 – CHEM Data

Canadian Centre for Occupational Health and Safety (CCOHS)

14:184. Master record
CD-ROM   **Canadian Centre for Occupational Health and Safety (CCOHS)**

Alternative name(s)	CHEM Data; Chemical Information
Database type	Bibliographic, Textual, Numeric, Factual, Directory, Computer software
Number of journals	
Sources	Chemical manufacturers, Databases, data sheets, Journals, Government departments, Government documents, Monographs, Producers documents, Research communications, Research reports, Suppliers, Thesaurus and Laws/regulations
Start year	Current information
Language	English and French
Coverage	Canada (primarily), USA (some) and International (some)
Number of records	
Update size	–
Update period	Quarterly

Keywords
Biological Control; Chemical Hazards; Chemicals; Chemical Toxicology; Dangerous Chemicals; Environmental Health; Hazardous Materials; First Aid; Herbicides; Mineralogy; Nickel; Occupational Health and Safety; Occupational Medicine; Pest Control; Pesticide Residues; Pesticides; Pharmaceuticals; Teratology; Transport; Weed Control

Description
Contains both full-text and bibliographic information in several files of descriptive, toxicological and transportation data for chemical substances, and educational meterials on a variety of occupational safety and health topics.

Cheminfo/Infochim (English and French), which is produced by the CCOHS, on the properties, uses, occurrences, health effects and hazards of pure chemicals, natural substances, and mixtures resulting from industrial processes – for each chemical, provides name, synonyms, CAS number, molecular and structural formula, as well as information about its uses and occurrences, physical properties, appearance, reactivity, warning properties (odours, irritation), animal toxicity data; information is gathered from journals, monographs, government documents, and from MSDS from chemical manufacturers;

RIPP/RIPA (English and French), which is Agriculture Canada's Regulatory Information on Pesticide Products.

PRIS/SILD (English and French), six of Agriculture Canada's databases on pesticide research.

TDG/Hazardous Materials, giving US and Canadian regulations on the transportation of dangerous goods.

New Jersey Hazardous Substance Fact Sheets, information sheets from the NJ Department of Health.

DSL/NDSL, LI/EDS (English and French), Environment Canada's listing of chemicals in use in Canada.

NiPERA CAB, Nickel Producer's ERA bibliographic database of nickel- related health documents.

CESARS, contains toxicological data on approximately 195 chemicals, covering their physical and chemical properties and toxicity.

OH&S Software database, the equivalent of the hard copy publication Occupational Health & Safety Software Packages, offers descriptions of commercial computer software programs. The database currently contains some 186 Canadian and US programs.

Contains full text of *Chemical Hazard Summaries*, covering chemicals in common use in Canadian workplaces, *Fiches Toxologiques* (French-language equivalent of Chemical Hazard summaries) and *New Jersey Hazardous Substance Fact Sheets*.

For more details of constituent databases, see:
Cheminfo/Infochim
RIPP/RIPA
PRIS/SILD
TDG/Hazardous Materials
New Jersey Hazardous Substance Fact Sheets
DSL/NDSL, LI/EDS
NiPERA CAB
CESARS
OH&S Software database

CCINFOdisc Series B1 – OHS CanData
Canadian Centre for Occupational Health and Safety (CCOHS)

14:186. Master record
CD-ROM	Canadian Centre for Occupational Health and Safety (CCOHS)
Alternative name(s)	CanData; OHS CanData; Canadian Occupational Health and Safety Databases
Database type	Bibliographic, Textual, Factual, Directory
Number of journals	

Sources	Accident reports, Books, Conference proceedings, Courts, Government departments, Government publications, Grey literature, Institutions, Journals, Law reports, Laws/regulations, Monographs, Periodicals, Producers catalogues, Questionnaires, Reports, Research reports, Standards, Surveys and Technical reports
Start year	Current information
Language	English, English (field labels), French, French (field labels), English, if provided by contributors and French, if provided by contributors
Coverage	Canada, Canada (primarily), International (some) and USA (some)
Number of records	
Update size	—
Update period	Quarterly
Index unit	Case reports

Keywords
Accidents; HIV; Air Pollution; Business Management; Construction; Dangerous Chemicals; Electrical Safety; Electromagnetic Radiation; Environmental Health; Farm Safety; Hazardous Materials; Industrial Noise; Information Services; Infrared Radiation; Light; Magnetic Field Radiation; Microwave Radiation; Mine Safety; Mortality; Noise Pollution; Non-Ionising Radiation; Occupational Health and Safety; Organisations; Pesticides; Pharmaceuticals; Product Catalogues; Radiation; Radiation Protection; Radio Waves; Standards; Ultraviolet Radiation

Description
Canadian occupational health and safety information, with English/French access, in directories and full-text documents. Includes:

Canadian Studies/Etudes Canadienne – directories of studies;
Resource Organisations/Organismes Ressources – organisations;
Resource People/Personnes Ressources – persons related to Canadian occupational health and safety;
Case Law/Jurisprudence – legislation related to Canadian occupational health and safety;
Standards and Directories/Normes et Répertoires – directory of Canadian standards;
Canadiana – summaries of Canadian occupational health and safety cases;
Fatality Reports – Canadian occupational fatality reports;
Mining Incidents/Accidents Minieres – reports on occupational incidents in the mining industry;
Aidscan for Health Care Workers – bibliographic databases on occupational aspects of AIDS;
Directory of Occupational Safety and Health Legislation in Canada/Répertoire de la Legislation en Matiére de Santé et Sécurité au Travail au Canada -general occupational health and safety topics;
Noise Levels/Niveaux de Bruit – specialised databases on occupational aspects of noise; and
Non-Ionizing Radiation Leveles/Niveaux de Rayonnements Non-Ionisants – non-ionising radiation.

For more details of constituent databases, see:
Canadian Studies
Etudes Canadiennes
Resource Organizations
Organismes Ressources

Resource People
Personnes Ressources
Case Law
Jurisprudence
Standards and Directories
Normes et Répertoires
Canadiana
Fatality Reports
Mining Incidents
Accidents Miniers
Aidscan for health care workers
Directory of Occupational Safety and Health Legislation in Canada
Répertoire de la Legislation en Matière de Santé et Securité au Travail au Canada
Noise Levels
Niveaux de Bruit
Non-Ionizing Radiation Levels
Niveaux de Rayonnements Non-Ionisants

CCIS
Micromedex Inc

14:188. Master record

CD-ROM	Micromedex Inc
Alternative name(s)	Computerized Clinical Information System
Database type	Bibliographic, Factual, Textual, Directory, Numeric
Number of journals	
Sources	
Start year	1974
Language	English and Spanish (some)
Coverage	International
Number of records	
Update size	—
Update period	Quarterly

Keywords

Acute Medicine; Clinical Medicine; Dangerous Chemicals; Diagnosis; Drugs; Drug Therapy; Emergency Medicine; Epidemiology; Hazardous Substances; Occupational Health and Safety; Pharmaceutical Products; Pharmaceuticals; Pharmacokinetics; Poisons; Radiography

Description

The Computerized Clinical Information System (CCIS) is a compilation of the Micromedex databases: the Poisindex, Drugdex and Emergindex databases are referred to as primary databases; all other databases are referred to as supplementary databases: Martindale, AfterCare Instructions (in two modules, Injury and Illness and USP DI Drug Information Leaflets), TOMES system (including TOMES Plus), Identidex, Dosing & Therapeutic Tools, USP DI Volume I, Reprorisk and P&T Quik.

The primary databases (Poisindex, Drugdex and Emergindex) are offered on annual subscription with a choice of – System I: any one of the primary titles, System II: any two of the primary titles, System III: all three of the primary titles. Any of the primary databases can be purchased separately for a cost plus a first year software licence fee of £280. There are optional and variable subscriptions for the supplementary databases. The price is determined by the primary system type purchased and the price is added to the cost for the primary system selected. They are also available on a standalone basis, for which a £65 licence fee per standalone product at list price applies. Prices are as follows (first price is standalone cost, price in brackets is cost when combined with a primary

system) : AfterCare Instructions: Injury/Illness £425 (£215); AfterCare Instructions: AfterCare USP DI £360 (£180); AfterCare Combo (a combination of the latter two databases) £620 (£310); Drug Interactions £230 (£115); Identidex £520 (the supplementary Identidex system is included with Poisindex free of charge); Martindale £250 (£125); P&T Quik £195 (available only as diskette); Reprorisk £455 (£230); TOMES £1,300 (£650); Know Abuse £100; Identidex and Dosing & Therapeutic Tools are included with the primary systems at no extra cost; Martindale, Reprorisk, P&T Quik (diskette version), Know Abuse, USP DI Volume 1, Identidex and AfterCare may be purchased as standalone products. Reprorisk may also be purchased as a part of TOMES Plus, but is not included in the standard subscription.

TOMES and TOMES Plus are important standalone products, they are not designated as 'primary' for the purpose of pricing to facilitate the system's concept of pricing. TOMES Plus is a separate disc and product, not part of the CCIS system. Licence fees are not charged for these two products. Additional disc pricing is available for customers wanting to add additional systems to the same physical facility – price for this additional disc is £685 plus the licence fee (which is required for each new installation). Contact Micromedex for details.

For more details of constituent databases, see:

CCIS: AfterCare Instructions: Injury and Illness
CCIS: AfterCare Instructions: Drug Information for the Health Professional: USP DI Volume 1
CCIS: AfterCare Instructions: USP DI Drug Information Leaflets – USP DI Volume 2
CCIS: Dosing & Therapeutic Tools
CCIS: Drugdex
CCIS: Emergindex
CCIS: Identidex
CCIS: Martindale: The Extra Pharmacopoeia
CCIS: P&T Quik
CCIS: Poisindex
CCIS: Reprorisk
CCIS: TOMES

CDID on Disc
Knowledge Access

14:190. Master record

Database type	Factual
Number of journals	
Sources	
Start year	
Language	
Coverage	
Number of records	250
Update size	—
Update period	

Keywords

Drugs

Description

Consumer Drug Information on 250 prescription drugs.

14:191. CD-ROM   Knowledge Access

File name	CDID on Disc
Format notes	IBM
Start year	
Number of records	250
Update period	

Chapman and Hall Chemical Database
Chapman and Hall Ltd
BRS EPI-Centre

14:192. Master record

Alternative name(s)	CHCD;Natural Products and Organic Compounds; Dictionary of Natural Products CD-ROM
Database type	Directory, Chemical structures
Number of journals	
Sources	
Start year	
Language	English
Coverage	International
Number of records	80,000
Update size	–
Update period	Twice per year

Keywords

Biochemistry; Antibiotics; Drugs

Description

Major database of natural products which have appeared in any of the Chapman and Hall Chemical Dictionaries – between 70,000 and 80,000 structures. It is said that chemists will appreciate the way in which the information is organised as compounds which are closely related chemically are grouped together in families – the substances are grouped together in some 33,000 entries. Great care has been taken with the display of text and graphics, using different type faces, subscripts and superscripts to make the screen resemble a page from a book.

Equivalent to the *Dictionary of Organic Compounds*, the *Dictionary of Antibiotics*, and the *Dictionary of Drugs*.

14:193. Online   DIALOG

File name	File 303
Alternative name(s)	Heilbron (former name)
Start year	Current
Number of records	97,976
Update period	Twice a year
Price/Charges	Connect time: US$95.00
	Online print: US$0.65 – 1.50
	Offline print: US$0.85 – 1.50

Notes

The DIALOG version does not contain chemical structures. There is information on 200,000 substances.

14:194. Tape   Questel

File name	Chapman & Hall Chemical Database
Start year	
Number of records	80,000
Update period	Twice per year

Notes

Available for use from Questel based on Darc Inhouse.

14:195. Database subset
CD-ROM   Chapman and Hall Ltd

File name	CHCD Dictionary of Natural Products
Alternative name(s)	Natural Products and Organic Compounds; Dictionary of Natural Products CD-ROM
Format notes	IBM
Software	Headfast and PsiBase
Start year	

Number of records	
Update period	Twice per year
Price	UK£2,950
	Subscription: UK£1,750

Notes

Database is a subset of the Chapman and Hall Chemical Database (CHCD) available for use with DARC INHOUSE and via Questel based on Darc Inhouse, as well as via DIALOG without chemical structures. Subsets are also available on tape. Initial payment for first year is £2,950; thereafter £1,750 per year. Substructure searching is facilitated by PsiBase software specially adapted for the application which allows users to draw substructures on screen using a mouse. Headfast and PsiBase have both been adapted to run in the Microsoft Windows graphic user interface environment, which will enable users to combine text and structure searches, making it possible to find, for example, all compounds containing a benzene ring with an attached chlorine atom, which crystallise as red needles and have a boiling point around 188°. Although only one set of 3-D coordinates is stored for each structure, special keys in the database enable a range of 'low-energy conformations' to be searched using ChemDBS-3D software. The aim is to identify molecules that meet specific 3-D criteria in some low energy formulation – for example, potential drug molecules that could bind with a receptor site of known geometry.

Record composition

CAS Registry Number; Accession number; Name; Synonyms; Structure display; Connection tables; Molecular formula; Molecular weight; Toxicity data; Botanical sources; Pharmacological activity; Physical properties and Bibliography with references to publications and patents

14:196. Database subset
CD-ROM   Chapman and Hall Ltd

File name	CHCD Dictionary of Organic Compounds
Alternative name(s)	Dictionary of Organic Compounds on CD-ROM; DOC on CD-ROM
Format notes	IBM
Software	Headfast and PsiBase
Start year	1993
Number of records	145,000 substances
Update period	Twice per year
Price/Charges	

Notes

Database is a subset of the Chapman and Hall Chemical Database (CHCD) containing chemical, structural and bibliographic data. The database can be interrogated by text or by substructure and contains all entries and data from the DOC Main Work (1982) to the latest Tenth Supplement (Published December 1992), making this the most selective and up-to-date set of data on organic compunds. There are over 145,000 organic compounds organised in over 50,000 entries. The executive editor is J Buckingham. Substructure searching is facilitated by PsiBase software specially adapted for the application which allows users to draw substructures on screen using a mouse. Headfast and PsiBase have both been adapted to run in the Microsoft Windows graphic user interface environment, which will enable users to combine text and structure searches, making it possible to find, for example, all compounds containing a benzene ring with an attached chlorine atom, which crystallise as red needles and have a boiling point around 188°. Although only one set of 3-D coordinates is stored for each structure, special keys in the database enable a range of 'low-energy conformations' to be searched using ChemDBS-3D software. The aim is to identify molecules that meet specific 3-D criteria in some low energy formulation – for example, potential drug molecules that could bind with a receptor site of known geometry.

According to Chapman & Hall, reviews of the print product have said, 'It is recommended for every library . . . as a most time-saving and convenient source of information' (*Journal of Pharmaceutical Science*) and 'Excellent value . . . an essential adjunct wherever organic compounds are used' (*Nature*).

Record composition

CAS Registry Number; Accession number; Name; Synonyms; Structure display; Connection tables; Molecular formula; Molecular weight; Toxicity data; Botanical sources; Pharmacological activity; Physical properties; Melting point; Boiling point; Freezing point; Relative density; Refractive index; Optical rotation; Solubility; Dissociation constants for acids and bases; Bibliography with references to publications and patents; Author; Publication year and Journal

14:197. Database subset

CD-ROM	Chapman and Hall Ltd
File name	CHCD Dictionary of Inorganic Compounds
Alternative name(s)	Dictionary of Inorganic Compounds on CD-ROM; DIC on CD-ROM
Format notes	IBM
Software	Headfast and PsiBase
Start year	1993
Number of records	42,000
Update period	Twice per year

Notes

Database is a subset of the Chapman and Hall Chemical Database (CHCD). Recently published as a five-volume printed work, this is a unique database of inorganic compounds with full-text retrieval and substructure searching covering the elements; fundamental inorganic compounds of simple structure; a wide range of coordinate compounds; compounds of industrial importance; and reagents, solvents and other chemicals of structural or chemical interest. The substructure searching has been specially enhanced and upgraded for inorganics and users can search by ligand, metal or a combination of the two. Invaluable to scientists from all disciplines including inorganic, organic and organometallic chemists, materials scientists, biochemists, geologists and metallurgists. Each entry contains extensive bibliographies, labelled to show their contents and allowing ready access to primary material. Substructure searching is facilitated by PsiBase software specially adapted for the application which allows users to draw substructures on screen using a mouse. Headfast and PsiBase have both been adapted to run in the Microsoft Windows graphic user interface environment, which will enable users to combine text and structure searches, making it possible to find, for example, all compounds containing a benzene ring with an attached chlorine atom, which crystallise as red needles and have a boiling point around 188°. Although only one set of 3-D coordinates is stored for each structure, special keys in the database enable a range of 'low-energy conformations' to be searched using ChemDBS-3D software. The aim is to identify molecules that meet

specific 3-D criteria in some low energy formulation – for example, potential drug molecules that could bind with a receptor site of known geometry.

The executive editor is J E Macintyre.

Record composition

CAS Registry Number; Accession number; Name; Synonyms; Structure display; Connection tables; Molecular formula; Molecular weight; Hazard data; Toxicity data; Botanical sources; Pharmacological activity; Physical properties; Melting point; Boiling point; Freezing point; Relative density; Refractive index; Optical rotation; Solubility; Dissociation constants for acids and bases; Bibliography with references to publications and patents; Author; Publication year and Journal

Full-text searching enables users to locate compounds using a search term of their choice and bibliographic references are searchable by author, year and journal.

CHEMEST
Technical Database Services Inc (TDS)

14:198. Master record

Database type	Factual
Number of journals	
Sources	Handbook
Start year	
Language	English
Coverage	
Number of records	
Update size	—
Update period	Periodically, as new data become available

Keywords

Chemical Substances; Pharmaceuticals; Pollution

Description

Contains data for estimating properties of pharmaceuticals and chemicals of environmental concern. Data are given for water solubility, soil absorption, bioconcentration factor, dissociation constant, activity coefficient, boiling point, vapour pressure, water volatization rate, melting point and Henry's Law Constant.

Partially corresponds to the *Handbook of Chemical Property Estimation Methods*.

14:199. Online

File name	
Start year	
Number of records	
Update period	Periodically, as new data become available

Chemical Business Newsbase
Royal Society of Chemistry

14:200. Master record

Database type	Bibliographic
Number of journals	500
Sources	Journals, press releases, newspapers, directories, publishers' lists, government reports, company reports and advertments
Start year	1984
Language	English
Coverage	Europe (primarily), USA and Japan

Number of records	260,000
Update size	52,000
Update period	Weekly

Keywords

Pharmaceutical Products; Cosmetics; Dyes; Paper and Packaging; Agrochemicals; Marketing; Production

Description

Chemical Business NewsBase, produced by the Royal Society of Chemistry, provides direct access to business information related to the chemicals industry. Originally developed as an information resource for the chemicals industry itself, its presentation makes it a database which can be used easily by business and investment researchers analysing chemicals companies, the sector and developments. The database concentrates on companies, products and the industry, so that precise technical knowledge of compounds and chemical structures is not required. Coverage is extensive within Europe, and embraces major events in the United States and Japan, and elsewhere as appropriate; about 70% of the sources are published in Europe. The database covers journal articles, government publications, stockbroker and market research reports, advertisements, and other significant sources. Subject coverage includes trends in supply and demand, production and the factors affecting it, quantities, prices, merger information, environmental aspects, government policies and legislation. The coverage extends into all major end-use sectors for chemicals, including pharmaceuticals, dyes, paper products, cosmetics and agrochemicals. The databases can be used in conjunction with the Royal Society of Chemistry's technical databases, Analytical Abstracts, Chemical Engineering Abstracts, Biotechnology Abstracts, and Chemical Safety NewsBase, as well as other services, for a comprehensive view of the subject. Chemical Business NewsBase provides informative abstracts, as well as bibliographic data and factual data regarding production figures, sales, etc. which also can be used for current awareness as part of an selective dissemination of information service. Much of the source material is originally in languages other than English (14% translated from French, 11% translated from German, for instance).

Although some of the information covered is also available in general business databases, the specialist nature of Chemical Business NewsBase makes it the prime source of information on the chemicals business in Europe.

Complete description furnished by business editor, Jacqueline Cropley.

14:201. Online — Data-Star

File name	CBNB
Start year	1984
Number of records	260,000
Update period	Weekly
Database aids	Data-Star Business Manual and Chemical Manual, Berne, Data-Star 1989 and Online User Guide (search NEWS-CBNB in NEWS)
Price/Charges	Subscription: UK£32.00
	Connect time: UK£111.20
	Online print: UK£1.24
	Offline print: UK£0.82
	SDI charge: UK£5.58

Notes

The identifiers (ID) include controlled vocabulary for chemicals, companies, countries and economic and business terms. Since July 1988, US SIC Codes have been added: all codes in the '28' (Chemicals and Allied Products) section are listed in the Chemical Manual.

From June 1993 Data-Star have introduced an annual fee/subscription per contract (that is, not per password) of SFr 80.00 (c.UK£ 32.00) payable every June. For North American customers billed in dollars who also use DIALOG, the DIALOG fee also covers access to Data-Star. Academic customers, 'commitment' customers and customers currently billed in dollars are exempt.

Record composition

Accession Number AN; Source SO; Publication Year YR; Title TI; Abstract AB; Subject Identifiers ID; Descriptors DE; US SIC Code CC; Publication Type PT; Language of Article LG; Authors AU; Author Affiliation IN; Journal Coden CD; CAS Registry Number RN; Reference RE; Duplicate Cross Reference XR and Update Code UP

14:202. Online — DIALOG

File name	File 319
Start year	1984 (October)
Number of records	214,771
Update period	Weekly
Price/Charges	Connect time: US$180.00
	Online print: US$2.30
	Offline print: US$2.30
	SDI charge: US$6.50

14:203. Online — Reuters (as a part of Textline)

File name	CBNB
Start year	1986
Number of records	260,000
Update period	Weekly
Delay	Updated 7 days after publication

Notes

Can be found in Reuter Textline Database F – Chemicals. Comprehensive coverage of CBNB – between 600–800 stories per week.

14:204. Online — STN

File name	CBNB
Start year	1984
Number of records	260,000
Update period	Weekly
Price/Charges	Connect time: DM320.00
	Online print: DM3.30
	Offline print: DM3.30
	SDI charge: DM18.00

Record composition

Accession Number AN; Title TI; Source SO; Document Type DT; Language LA; Abstract AB; SIC Code CC; SIC Code Terms (English) CC; SIC Code Terms (German) CCDE; SIC Code Terms (French) CCFR; Geographic Term GT; Company CO; Note NTE; Publication Type CT; Publication Type (French) CTFR and Publication Type (German) CTDE

14:205. Tape — Royal Society of Chemistry

File name	Chemical Business Newsbase
Start year	1984
Number of records	260,000
Update period	Weekly

This database can also be found on:
Textline

Chemical Engineering and Biotechnology Abstracts

DECHEMA Deutsche Gesellschaft für
Chemisches Apparatewesen
Royal Society of Chemistry

14:206. Master record

Alternative name(s)	CEBA; DECHEMA; CEA; Chemical Engineering Abstracts
Database type	Bibliographic, Textual
Number of journals	1000
Sources	Journals, monographs, patents (European), conference proceedings, technical reports, press releases, dissertations, reviews, newspapers and government documents
Start year	1970
Language	English and German
Coverage	International
Number of records	300,000
Update size	6,000
Update period	Monthly
Index unit	Articles and reviews
Database aids	Current Biotechnology Abstracts Database User Aid Manual, RSC, 1989

Keywords

Analytical Chemistry; Bioagriculture; Biochemistry; Bioengineering; Biotechnology; Chemical Engineering; Chemical Equipment Manufacturing; Chemical Manufacturing; Chemical Processing; Chemical Substances; Enzymology; Food and Drink; Genetic Manipulation; Hazardous Substances; Mathematical Models; Occupational Health and Safety; Pharmaceuticals; Pollution Control

Description

During 1989 the monthly production of the Chemical Engineering Abstracts database from the Royal Society of Chemistry, UK, was merged with the DECHEMA database of Frankfurt, Germany to form this Chemical Engineering and Biotechnology Abstracts database. The combined title is produced in English.

It contains citations, with English-language abstracts, drawn from the worldwide scientific and technical literature on biotechnology and chemical engineering.

In chemical engineering, emphasis is given to the processing of chemicals in large or small quantities. From 1987 it also incorporates theoretical engineering abstracts. Gives full coverage of published information required by both practising chemical engineers and academics. The abstracts are written with the chemical/process engineer in mind, not chemists, and this is reflected in the content. Covers chemical reactions, mixing and separation, heating and cooling, and the transport of liquids, solids and gases. The effect of the size of the operation, the physical and other properties of the substances involved, the nature of the equipment used, corrosion and personal safety factors are also covered, as are environmental consequences.

Covers chemical processing theory and laboratory experimentation in addition to industrial practice.

Topics included are: chemical equipment manufacturing, chemical manufacturing, plant design and construction, computer-aided design (CAD), mathematical models and methods, laboratory techniques, analytical chemistry, safety engineering, hazardous materials, pollution control, environmental protection, energy and raw materials supply and conservation, chemical reaction engineering, catalysis, unit operations, process dynamics and control, measurement, instruments, materials of construction, corrosion and corrosion protection, and operating materials.

In biotechnology, it provides full coverage, with abstracts, of the technical, scientific and technocommercial literature for the industry of biotechnology. Biotechnology is defined as the development and use of biological systems and functions to realise end-products useful to mankind. Topics covered in this section include: all aspects of biotechnology such as: genetic manipulation, monoclonal antibodies, immobilized cells and enzymes, single-cell proteins and fermentation technology, in the pharmaceutical, fuel, agriculture, chemical, food and other industries.

Articles with a significant technical content are selected and documents are assigned to one of 52 sections with cross references to direct the user from one section to potentially interesting abstracts in another. Some articles are available as full text, with technical items and some book reviews also included. The scientific and technical abstracts are split into four main areas: technocommercial data, techniques, specific industrial areas and information. Technocommercial data includes business news, legal and safety issues and information on related conferences.

Techniques includes: genetic manipulation, monoclonal antibodies, enzymology, single-cell proteins and fermentation technology. Industrial areas includes pharmaceuticals, energy production, agriculture, chemical industry and food. Information includes forthcoming events, books and reviews.

The database incorporates Current Biotechnology Abstracts which is also available separately. Current Biotechnology Abstracts covers about 400 primary journals and other sources such as books and reviews are scanned: UK, USA, European and PCT patents are included. Approximately twenty per cent of the Current Biotechnology Abstracts section is patents. This section contains about 50,000 records and is updated with 400–500 records per month. All of the material published in the hard-copy version since its start-up in April 1983 is included.

Corresponds to: *Chemical Engineering Abstracts; Theoretical Chemical Engineering Abstracts; Safety, Environmental Protection and Analysis; Process and Chemical Engieering; Equipment, Corrosion and Corrosion Protection; Biotechnology: Apparatus, Plant and Equipment*; and *Current Biotechnology*.

Corresponds in part to *Literaturkurzberichte Chemische Technik und Biotechnologie (Dechema Chemical Engineering and Biotechnology Abstracts), and Biotechnologie, Verfahren-Anlagen-Apparate (Biotechnology, Processes-Plant-Equipment).*

Sources include primary chemical and process engineering journals.

Bibliographic information, indexing terms and abstracts are all searchable. Users can access citations by subject, substance, or organization name. The field Chemical Descriptors may list the names of up to fifteen chemical substances and these are searched in the same way as subject descriptors. The Patent Information field contains patent numbers, patent series, patent application (or priority) number and country, date of application (or priority).

14:207. Online — Data-Star

File name	CEAB
Alternative name(s)	CEBA; DECHEMA; CEA; Chemical Engineering Abstracts
Start year	1981
Number of records	104,036
Update period	Monthly
Database aids	Data-Star Chemical Manual, Berne, Data-Star, 1989 and Online manual (search NEWS-CEAB in NEWS)
Price/Charges	Subscription: UK£32.00
	Connect time: UK£76.00
	Online print: UK£0.75
	Offline print: UK£0.49
	SDI charge: UK£5.30

Notes

From June 1993 Data-Star have introduced an annual fee/subscription per contract (that is, not per password) of SFr 80.00 (c.UK£ 32.00) payable every June. For North American customers billed in dollars who also use DIALOG, the DIALOG fee also covers access to Data-Star. Academic customers, 'commitment' customers and customers currently billed in dollars are exempt.

14:208. Online — DIALOG

File name	File 315
Alternative name(s)	CEBA; DECHEMA; CEA; Chemical Engineering Abstracts
Start year	1971
Number of records	125,188
Update period	Monthly
Price/Charges	Connect time: US$150.00
	Online print: US$1.40
	Offline print: US$1.40
	SDI charge: US$15.00

14:209. Online — ESA-IRS

File name	File 85
Alternative name(s)	CEBA; DECHEMA; CEA; Chemical Engineering Abstracts
Start year	1970
Number of records	122,000 (October 1991)
Update period	Monthly

Notes

From 1993 ESA-IRS are charging an annual fee of 100 Accounting Units (c.UK£ 70.29) to all users. This is equivalent to the fee for full documentation and will not be charged to customers already paying for documentation.

14:210. Online — FIZ Technik

File name	DECH
Alternative name(s)	CEBA; DECHEMA; CEA; Chemical Engineering Abstracts
Start year	1976
Number of records	178,000
Update period	Monthly
Price/Charges	Connect time: DM264.00
	Online print: DM1.40 – 1.90
	Offline print: DM2.20
	SDI charge: DM18.00

14:211. Online — Hoechst

File name	
Alternative name(s)	CEBA; DECHEMA; CEA; Chemical Engineering Abstracts
Start year	1970
Number of records	122,000
Update period	Monthly

14:212. Online — ORBIT

File name	CEBA
Alternative name(s)	CEBA; DECHEMA; CEA; Chemical Engineering Abstracts
Start year	1970
Number of records	125,000+
Update period	Monthly
Database aids	Quick reference Guide (5/90) Free (single copy)

Notes

Electronic SDI service is now available within two hours on ORBIT. They can be downloaded and reformatted on a word processor. Results are retrieved in the low cost PRINTS file, $15 per connect hour.

14:213. Online — STN

File name	CEBA
Alternative name(s)	CEBA; DECHEMA; CEA; Chemical Engineering Abstracts
Start year	1975
Number of records	187,809
Update period	Monthly
Price/Charges	Connect time: DM240.00
	SDI charge: DM15.00

Notes

In English, with some abstracts in German.

14:214. Database subset
Online — CISTI, Canadian Online Enquiry Service CAN/OLE

File name	BIOTECH
Alternative name(s)	Current Biotechnology Abstracts; CBA
Start year	
Number of records	50,000
Update period	Monthly
Price/Charges	Connect time: Canadian $40.00
	Online print: Canadian $0.46 – 0.92
	Offline print: Canadian $0.26 – 0.52

Notes

CISTI accessible only in Canada. This is a subfile of the Chemical Engineering and Biotechnology Abstracts database.

14:215. Database subset
Online — Data-Star

File name	CUBI
Alternative name(s)	Current Biotechnology Abstracts; CBA
Start year	1983 (April)
Number of records	34,758
Update period	Monthly
Database aids	Data-Star Biomedical Manual and Online manual (search NEWS-CUBI in NEWS)
Price/Charges	Subscription: SFr80.00
	Connect time: SFr175.00
	Online print: SFr1.88
	Offline print: SFr1.36
	SDI charge: SFr13.25
Downloading is allowed	

Notes

This is a subfile of the Chemical Engineering and Biotechnology Abstracts database.

From June 1993 Data-Star have introduced an annual fee/subscription per contract (that is, not per password) of SFr 80.00 (c.UK£ 32.00) payable every June. For North American customers billed in dollars who also use DIALOG, the DIALOG fee also covers access to Data-Star. Academic customers, 'commitment' customers and customers currently billed in dollars are exempt.

Record composition

Abstract AB; Accession Number and Update Code AN; Author AU; Author Affiliation IN; Chemical Descriptors ID; Company CO; Descriptors DE; Journal Coden CD; Language LG; Patent Information PA; Publication Type PT; Publisher PB; Section Code SC; Section Cross Reference; Source SO; Title TI; Update Code UP and Year YR

14:216. Database subset

Online   DIALOG

File name	File 358
Alternative name(s)	Current Biotechnology Abstracts; CBA
Start year	1983
Number of records	492,923
Update period	Monthly
Price/Charges	Connect time: US$150.00
	Online print: US$1.40
	Offline print: US$1.40
	SDI charge: US$15.00

Notes

This is a subfile of the Chemical Engineering and Biotechnology Abstracts database.

DIALINDEX Categories: AGRI, ENVIRON, FOODSCI, VETSCI.

14:217. Database subset

Online   ESA-IRS

File name	File 95
Alternative name(s)	Current Biotechnology Abstracts; CBA
Start year	1983
Number of records	43,000 (October 1991)
Update period	Monthly
Price/Charges	Subscription: UK£70.29
	Database entry fee: UK£3.49
	Online print: UK£0.56
	Offline print: UK£0.56
	SDI charge: UK£2.80

Notes

This is a subfile of the Chemical Engineering and Biotechnology Abstracts database.

From 1993 ESA-IRS are charging an annual fee of 100 Accounting Units (c.UK£ 70.29) to all users. This is equivalent to the fee for full documentation and will not be charged to customers already paying for documentation.

Record composition

Abstract /AB; Author AU; Class Code CC; Class Name CC; Coden CO; Contract Terms /CT; Corporate Source CS; Document Type DT; ISBN BN; ISSN SN; Journal Name JN; Language LA; Meeting Information MI; Native Number NN; Publisher PB; Publication Date PD; Patent Number PN; Report Number RN and Title /TI

14:218. Database subset

CD-ROM   Royal Society of Chemistry

File name	Current Biotechnology Abstracts
Alternative name(s)	Current Biotechnology Abstracts; CBA
Format notes	IBM
Start year	
Number of records	
Update period	

Notes

This is a subfile of the Chemical Engineering and Biotechnology Abstracts database.

Chemical Exposure

Science Applications International Corporation

14:219. Master record

Database type	Factual, Bibliographic
Number of journals	
Sources	journals and conference reports
Start year	1974 to 1987 Closed File
Language	English
Coverage	International
Number of records	25,607
Update size	–
Update period	Not updated
Index unit	articles

Keywords

Chemical Substances; Drugs; Pharmaceuticals; Toxic Substances

Description

Contains citations to the worldwide literature on over 1,800 chemicals that have been identified in human and animal biological media (for example, tissues, body fluids) and reported effects of drugs (through 1984 only), metals, pesticides, and other substances on the body. It spans the range of body-burden information that is, information related to human and animal exposure to food, air, and water contaminants and pharmaceuticals. Toxic chemicals and other substances can be traced to evaluate their effects.

Each record covers information about one chemical in a particular tissue; there may be more than one record for articles on multiple chemicals and/or multiple tissues. Each record includes bibliographic information, Chemical Abstracts Service preferred name and Registry Number, chemical properties, formulas, synonyms, tissue levels measured, analytical method used, number and sex of cases, demographic information on sources of samples, health effects, geographic location, and animal studied.

Corresponds to *Chemicals Identified in Human Biological Media* and *Chemicals Identified in Feral and Food Animals.*

14:220. Online   DIALOG

File name	File 138
Start year	1974 to 1987 Closed File
Number of records	25,607
Update period	Not updated

| Price/Charges | Subscription: US$45.00 |
| | Offline print: US$0.15 |

Chemical Industry Notes
American Chemical Society Chemical Abstracts Service

14:221. Master record

Database type	Bibliographic
Number of journals	80
Sources	Journals, Trade Magazines, Newspapers, Newsletters, Reviews, Market reports, Digests, Survey reports, Technical reports and Commercial reports
Start year	1974 (December)
Language	English
Coverage	International
Number of records	937,230
Update size	52,000
Update period	Weekly

Keywords

Agricultural Industry; Chemical Engineering; Chemical Substances; Paper and Packaging; Petroleum; Pharmaceutical Industry

Description

Contains citations, with abstracts, to the worldwide business literature and news on chemical processing in the chemical, pharmaceutical, petroleum, paper and pulp, and agriculture industries. Topics covered include production, pricing, sales, facilities, products, processes, corporate and government activities, and people. About eighty US and non-US publications are covered.

Corresponds to *Chemical Industry Notes*.

14:222. Online   Data-Star

File name	CIND
Start year	1983
Number of records	355,500+
Update period	Weekly
Database aids	Data-Star Chemical Manual, Berne, Data-Star 1989 and Online Manual (search NEWS-CIND in NEWS)
Price/Charges	Subscription: UK£32.00
	Connect time: UK£61.28
	Online print: UK£0.58
	Offline print: UK£0.61
	SDI charge: UK£4.64

Notes

From June 1993 Data-Star have introduced an annual fee/subscription per contract (that is, not per password) of SFr 80.00 (c.UK£ 32.00) payable every June. For North American customers billed in dollars who also use DIALOG, the DIALOG fee also covers access to Data-Star. Academic customers, 'commitment' customers and customers currently billed in dollars are exempt.

14:223. Online   DIALOG

File name	File 19
Start year	1974 (December)
Number of records	886,034
Update period	Weekly
Price/Charges	Connect time: US$126.00
	Online print: US$0.75
	Offline print: US$0.75
	SDI charge: US$15.25

14:224. Online   ORBIT

File name	CINF
Start year	1974
Number of records	795,000+
Update period	Weekly
Database aids	Quick Reference Guide (1/88) Free (single copy) and Database manual (1981) $7.50

Notes

Electronic SDI service is now available within two hours on ORBIT. They can be downloaded and reformatted on a word processor. Results are retrieved in the low cost PRINTS file, $15 per connect hour.

14:225. Online   STN

File name	CIN
Start year	1974
Number of records	937,230
Update period	Weekly
Price/Charges	Connect time: DM50.00
	Offline print: DM0.24
	SDI charge: DM10.30

Thesaurus is online

Notes

An online thesaurus is available for the Geographic Terms (/GT) field.

Bibliographical information, indexing terms, titles, abstracts, CAS Registry Numbers and chemical names are searchable.

Chinese Medical Plant Database
Computing Institute, Chinese Academy of Sciences

14:226. Master record

Alternative name(s)	CMP
Database type	Factual, Directory, Bibliographic
Number of journals	
Sources	Dictionaries
Start year	1989
Language	English and Chinese
Coverage	China
Number of records	27,000
Update size	—
Update period	Continuously

Keywords

Alternative Medicine; Herbal Remedies; Plant Sciences

Description

Contains both bibliographic and factual data covering Chinese native medical plants used in traditional Chinese medicine and western medicine and plants transplanted into China from abroad. Data sources are dictionaries of traditional Chinese medicines and Chinese herb books of medicinal plants. All data has been evaluated by Chinese specialists before being incorporated into the database.

Botanical data covers plant family, medicinal components, medicinal features, name, region where found, preservation instructions and curative properties.

As of 1993, the database contains details of 2,000 medicinal plants, 5,000 traditional Chinese medicines and 20,000 bibliographic references.

14:227. Online — Scientific Database System

File name	Chinese Medical Plant Database
Alternative name(s)	CMP
Start year	1989
Number of records	27,000
Update period	Continuously

Notes

Retrieval is by key word, CAS Registry Number, chemical name, chemical structures, molecular formula and molecular weight.

Record composition

Index terms; CAS Registry Number; Chemical Name; Chemical Structure; Molecular Formula and Molecular Weight

CIPSLINE PC

Prous Science Publishers

14:228. Master record

Database type	Factual
Number of journals	
Sources	
Start year	
Language	English
Coverage	
Number of records	22,000
Update size	3,000
Update period	Quarterly

Keywords

Drugs

Description

CIPSLINE is made up of eleven different databases, categorised by therapeutic class and which include chemical structures and abridged text on more than 20,000 compounds. Subject are medicinal chemistry and pharmacology. The database was developed for use with ChemBase from Molecular Design Ltd and ISIS/Base software. It also links through a reference citation to Drug Data Report database and Drugs of the Future database.

14:229. Diskette — Prous

File name	CIPSLINE
Start year	
Number of records	22,000
Update period	Quarterly
Price/Charges	Subscription: US$5,000

Clinical Protocols

National Cancer Institute, US National Institutes of Health

14:230. Master record

Alternative name(s)	Clinical Cancer Protocols; CLINPROT
Database type	Factual, Textual
Number of journals	
Sources	Clinical trial protocols
Start year	1960s
Language	English
Coverage	International
Number of records	
Update size	–
Update period	

Keywords

Cancer; Clinical Oncology; Pathology

Description

The database comprises summaries of clinical trials of anticancer drugs and treatment modalities. All records contain a detailed abstract. Gives patient entry criteria, therapy regimen and special study parameters. Includes open (active) and closed protocols. Investigators' names and addresses are given, together with the supporting agency. The data is of special interest to clinical oncologists who are actively engaged in the development and evaluation of clinical therapy methods.

The US National Cancer Institute ceased production of CLINPROT in June 1991 as the content is duplicated within Physician's Data Query (PDQ) database. On some hosts the protocol file is accessible separately.

Colleague Mail

BRS Online Service, BRS/Colleague

14:231. Master record

Alternative name(s)	MEDLINK
Database type	Directory, Textual, Computer software
Number of journals	1
Sources	Journal, Airlines, Database producers, Electronic media and Original material
Start year	
Language	English
Coverage	USA
Number of records	
Update size	–
Update period	Current six to eight months
Index unit	Classified advertisements

Keywords

Molecular Biology; HIV; Travel; Air Travel; Anaesthesia; Personal Computers; HIV; Pathology; Surgery; Gastroenterology; Intensive Care; Proctology; Dermatology; Geriatrics; Gerontology; Genetics – Human; Immunology; Health Care Administration; Neurology; Cancer; Oncology; Ophthalmology; Sickle-Cell Disease

Description

Contains a number of services for medical professionals, including classified advertisements from the *New England Journal of Medicine*, a calendar of medical events, electronic mail, gateway access to Official Airlines Guide (OAG) Electronic Edition Travel Service (see separate entry), American Airlines EASY Sabre (see separate entry) and other databases available through BT Tymnet Dialcom Service. There are also a number of bulletin boards available, operated by physician-editors: AIDS/HIV, Anesthesia Safety and Technology, Cellforum (pathology, cell biology, molecular biology), Clinical Drug Information, Colon & Rectal Surgery, Critical Care, Dermatology, Geriatrics and Gerontology, Hackers' Forum (microcomputer products and applications), Materia Eclectica, Medical Ethics, MEDLINK Help & Tips, Neurology, Oncology, Ophthalmology, Sickle-Cell Disease.

Partially equivalent to *New England Journal of Medicine* (classified advertisements).

14:232. Online — BRS, BRS/Colleague

File name	
Alternative name(s)	MEDLINK
Start year	
Number of records	
Update period	current six to eight months

For more details of constituent databases, see:
American Airlines EAASY SABRE
OAG Electronic Edition Travel Service

COMLINE: Japan News Wire
COMLINE Business Data Inc

14:233. Master record

Alternative name(s)	Japan News Wire: COMLINE; COMLINE Daily News; COMLINE Daily
Database type	Factual, Textual, Bibliographic, Directory
Number of journals	130
Sources	Companies, Press releases, Newspapers and Trade journals
Start year	Data-Star: 1986; SIS: 1989; NewsNet: 1990
Language	English
Coverage	Japan (primarily)
Number of records	75,000
Update size	15,000
Update period	Daily

Keywords

Bioreactors; Biotechnology; Cancer; Computer Technology; HIV; Medical Equipment; Physics; Telecommunications

Description

The database provides detailed English language summaries, abstracted from over 130 Japanese publications, plus exclusive interviews and research giving information on commercially important Japanese product and technology news covering corporate, industrial, financial, economic affairs as well as information on high-techology developments and research and development. Extensive interviews are conducted by qualified writers and researchers to uncover information that is often exclusive to the Comline database. Data is re-confirmed by fact-checkers, while American and English editors ensure proper, standard and understandable use of English. The activities of Japanese companies in Europe, the US and elsewhere, are also covered. Japan News Wire is the only English language daily business and technical news service from Japan. Subject areas covered include: electronics, biotechnology, medical technology, chemicals and materials, industrial automation, physics, computers, telecommunications, transportation, agriculture, environment, economy, defence and construction. The database does not include political or socio-economic issues.

The database contains original material collected and indexed by COMLINE.

Sourced from major Japanese financial and industrial newspapers and trade journals – all Japanese publications.

14:234. Online — FT Profile

File name	COMLINE Daily
Alternative name(s)	COMLINE: Japan News Wire; COMLINE Daily News
Start year	1991 (January)

Number of records	
Update period	Daily
Price/Charges	Connect time: UK£2.40
	Online print: UK£0.04 – 0.10 per line
	Offline print: UK£0.01 per line

Notes

A Japanese business information source which combines the Daily News Service (Industrial Monitor) with the Tokyo Financial Wire and 100 Japanese language publications.

Registration fee required, including free documentation and training. Usage charges for access consist of two elements: a connect rate for time online, and a display rate (applies only to lines of file text). There is no charge for blank lines, system messages, menus or help information.

14:235. Online — NewsNet Inc

File name	
Alternative name(s)	Japan News Wire: COMLINE; COMLINE Daily News
Start year	1990
Number of records	
Update period	Daily
Database aids	Comline Data Descriptor Table

Notes

This is the daily update version of Japan News Wire database.

14:236. CD-ROM — SilverPlatter

File name	COMLINE
Alternative name(s)	Japan News Wire: COMLINE; COMLINE Daily News; COMLINE
Format notes	IBM
Software	SPIRS
Start year	1986
Number of records	75,000
Update period	6 times per year
Price/Charges	Subscription: UK£719 – 1,150

Notes

Annual subscription price for first time subscribers is reduced to UK £719 for single users, £1,150 for networked users. Subscribers may retain previous disc on update.

14:237. Database subset
Online — NewsNet Inc

File name	COMLINE Daily News: Biotechnology and Medical Technology
Alternative name(s)	Japan News Wire: COMLINE; COMLINE Daily News; COMLINE
Start year	1990
Number of records	
Update period	Daily

Notes

A subset of the Japan News Wire: Comline database, giving summaries of biotechnology industry news and information from Japanese publications. Covers new pharmaceuticals, medical equipment, agricultural science developments, industrial applications of bioreactors and research on anti-cancer and anti-AIDS agents. Gives citations to sources and some contact numbers for further information.

Monthly subscription required, with differential charges to subscribers and non-subscribers to Comline Japan Daily.

Compact Library – AIDS
Medical Publishing Group
San Francisco General Hospital
National Library of Medicine
Bureau of Hygiene and Tropical
   Diseases
Massachusetts Medical Society,
   Medical Publishing Group

14:239. Master record

CD-ROM	Macmillan New Media
Alternative name(s)	Compact Library: AIDS; AIDS CD-ROM
Database type	Textual, Bibliographic, Factual, Directory
Number of journals	11
Sources	Journals, conference proceedings, monographs and A-V material
Start year	1983
Language	English
Coverage	International
Number of records	100,000 refs; 10,000 full-text
Update size	–
Update period	Quarterly

Keywords
HIV

Description
Contains full-text articles, citations, critical abstracts, from various sources, together with annotations from the AIDS Subset of MEDLINE. It includes the AIDS Knowledge Base from San Francisco General Hospital/UCSF (produced by the Massachusetts Medical Society), with new updates on Varicella-Zoster Virus, transmission of HIV in blood products, HIV-associated non-Hodgkin's Lymphoma, new CDC statistics, etc. The Full Text of Articles database contains the complete text of more than 10,000 journal articles selected from *AIDS* (Jan 1989-March 1991); *Annals of Internal Medicine* (August 1984 – April 1991); *British Medical Journal* (21 May 1983 – 23 March 1991); *Journal of Infectious Diseases* (February 1984 – February 1991); Lancet (7 May 1983 – 20 April 1991); *MMWR* (7 June 1985 – 21 September 1991); *Nature* (31 October 1985 – 28 September 1991); *New England Journal of Medicine* (6 January 1983 – 3 May 1991 plus selected articles prior to 1983); *Science* (2 April 1986 – 12 April 1991) and, unique to this disc, the complete text of two leading AIDS newsletters: *AIDS Clinical Care* (June 1989-) and *AIDS Newsletter* (November 1987-).

Also included are the AIDS database from the Bureau of Hygiene and Tropical Diseases (more than 15,000 abstracts); the AIDS subset of MEDLINE with more than 45,000 citations and abstracts from 3,200 medical journals worldwide; AIDSLINE with a total of nearly 60,000 citations drawn from from MEDLINE (about 30,000), CancerLit, CatLine, and Health Planning and Administration databases plus abstracts from the 5th and 6th International Conference on AIDS; and AIDSTRIALS and AIDSDRUGS, which contain information from the National Institute of Allergy and Infectious Diseases and the NLM describing 321 clinical trials currently in progress and the 101 drugs being tested in the trials. For each drug, the generic, trade and standard chemical name, the physical and chemical properties, pharmacological data and adverse effects, uses, contradictions and manufacturer's information are given. The AIDS Knowledge Base is an electronic textbook divided into twelve chapters covering AIDS/HIV topics from epidemiology to therapy; chapters are constantly revised.

Dudee Chiang, writing in *CD-ROM Professional* (1992 5(6) p112–116) feels that the major strength of Compact Library: AIDS, apart from its ease of use, is the scope and range of material included – physicians and researchers should find it informative and useful, while it would also be a good educational source for students and lay people. Its major disadvantage is the overlap between AIDSLINE and MEDLINE with no simple way to eliminate duplicates.

Aimed at the AIDS specialist.

Notes
Subscriptions: Quarterly updates for institutions is UK£510; quarterly updates for individuals is UK£370. The May 1993 *CD-ROM World* reported that US prices have been significantly lowered (by $200) to US$ 495.00 for individuals and US$ 695.00 for institutions.

For more details of constituent databases, see:
AIDS Knowledge Base
AIDS (BHTD)
MEDLINE
AIDSLINE
AIDSTRIALS
AIDSDRUGS

Conference Fast Track
Derwent Publications Inc

14:240. Master record

Database type	Bibliographic, Factual, Directory
Number of journals	
Sources	
Start year	1993
Language	English
Coverage	International
Number of records	
Update size	–
Update period	

Keywords
Drugs

Description
Supplies the latest information on new drugs gleaned from conference reports.

Initially supplied as a printed bulletin.

14:241. Diskette   Derwent Publications Inc

File name	Conference Fast Track
Format notes	IBM
Start year	1993
Number of records	
Update period	

Consult Scientific American Medicine
Scientific American Inc

14:242. Master record

CD-ROM	Scientific American Inc
Alternative name(s)	Scientific American Medicine/Consult
Database type	Textual, Image, Factual
Number of journals	1
Sources	Journal

Start year	
Language	English
Coverage	USA
Number of records	
Update size	—
Update period	Quarterly
Price/Charges	Subscription: UK£280 – 995

Keywords

Cardiovascular Medicine; Dermatology; Endocrinology; Gastroenterology; Haematology; Immunology; Infectious Diseases; Interdisciplinary Medicine; Internal Medicine; Metabolism; Nephrology; Neurology; Oncology; Respiratory Medicine; Rheumatology

Description

Contains the full text, including graphics, of the looseleaf textbook and each update/issue of *Scientific American Medicine*. Covers current developments in all areas of internal medicine including chapters on diagnosis, treatment, drug dosage and laboratory values. It holds more than 2,300 pages of text, charts, tables and many full colour and black and white illustrations, plus photographs. Each article includes references. Also includes the complete library of Discotest Interactive Patient Management Problems, initially 45 cases, two to be added at each update, available for CME credits. Contains timely clinical information on diagnosis, treatment, drug dosage, lab values etc.

Corresponds to print and online versions of *Scientific American Medicine*.

Price: £420 for institutions; £280 for individuals. Network licence: £995 for up to 15 workstations.

Requires VGA monitor.

For more details of constituent databases, see:
Scientific American Medicine

Consumer Drug Information
American Society of Hospital Pharmacists

14:244. Master record

Alternative name(s)	CDIF
Database type	Textual
Number of journals	1
Sources	Journal and Monographs
Start year	Current information
Language	English
Coverage	USA
Number of records	1,940
Update size	—
Update period	3 times a year
Hosts have included	BRS, BRS After Dark, BRS/Colleague (until 10/92)

Keywords

Drug Therapy; Drugs

Description

Contains full text of *Consumer Drug Digest*, covering most drugs prescribed in the USA. Provides in-depth descriptions of each of more than 260 drug entities, which make up over 80% of all prescription drugs, and a number of important non-prescription drugs. It is a database for the consumer. There is information on how they work, possible side effects and how to manage them, precautions, instructions on dosage and use, including the foods and activities that are permitted during medication and what to do if a dosage is missed, and advice on storage. Includes monographs on nearly 300 of the top drugs marketed in the US (representing 95% of the brand names prescribed in the US).

This popular version of drug information offers all the information consumers need to work with their physicians to ensure effective drug therapy. According to Barbara Quint in her article, The 'Dead' Database: Where do databases go when they leave online? (*Database* October 1992 15–31), BRS dropped the file because ASHP wanted a complete file reload and redesign to implement major changes and improvements and Maxwell Online (now InfoPro Technologies) found the cost too high. It is suggested that BRS searchers might try the 'larger and more technical' companion file, Drug Information Fulltext.

The database is written for the general public.

14:245. Online   DIALOG, Knowledge Index

File name	File 271
Alternative name(s)	CDIF
Start year	Current information
Number of records	1,940
Update period	3 times a year with annual reloads
Price/Charges	Connect time: US$45.00
	Online print: US$0.20
	Offline print: US$0.30

Notes

The number of records represents 260 drugs.

Record composition

Monograph Title MT; Name NA; Synonyms SY; Section Heading SH; Text TX; Descriptors DE; Accession Number AN; Pronunciation PN; Section PC; Uses US (Display only); Undesired Effects UE (Display only); Storage ST (Display only); Product Information PI (Display only); Precautions PC (Display only) and Dosage DO (Display only)

Corporate Technology Database
Corporate Technology Information Services

14:246. Master record

Database type	Directory
Number of journals	
Sources	Direct contacts
Start year	Current information
Language	English
Coverage	USA
Number of records	35,000
Update size	—
Update period	Quarterly
Database aids	CorpTech Technology Classification System Manual $45, CorpTech TCS Manual (with 1 year of updates) $95 and CorpTech Products Listing Free

Keywords

Chemical Industry; Defence; Manufacturing; Marketing; Medical Technology; Pharmaceuticals; Telecommunications

Description

The database is a directory of public and private American corporations and operating units of large corporations in all areas of high technology design, development, manufacture, production and marketing. It is a comprehensive source of company information on over 35,000 US manufacturers for market analysis, sales prospecting, mergersd and acquisitions, recruiting and new business developing. Ninety per cent of the listed companies are private or operating units of larger corporations. The products include factory automation, biotechnology, chemicals, computer hardware, the defence industrires, energy and environment, advanced materials, medical technology, pharmaceuticals, photonics, computer software, subassemblies and components, test and measurement, telecommunications and transport, robotics and artificial intelligence. The descriptive information includes company and alternate name, address and contact numbers icluding fax, names and titles of executive officers, annual sales, export activities, number of employees, rate of growth, ownership (for example, public, private, foreign parent), subsidiaries and divisions, year founded, company description, 4-digit Standard Industrial Classification (SIC) codes, and product lists classified by the producer's proprietary high-technology classification system.

Print equivalent is *Corporate Technology Directory, Regional Sales Guide to High-Tech Companies; Fast 5,000 Company Locator*. Information is obtained direct from company sources by telephone interviews followed by written verification. The database contains entirely original data collected and indexed by CorpTech.

14:247. Online — Data-Star

File name	CTCO
Start year	Current information
Number of records	35,000
Update period	Quarterly
Database aids	Data-Star Business Manual, Berne and Online manual (search NEWS-CTCO in NEWS)
Price/Charges	Subscription: SFr80.00
	Connect time: SFr123.33
	Online print: SFr2.40
	Offline print: SFr2.88

Notes

From June 1993 Data-Star have introduced an annual fee/subscription per contract (that is, not per password) of SFr 80.00 (c.UK£ 32.00) payable every June. For North American customers billed in dollars who also use DIALOG, the DIALOG fee also covers access to Data-Star. Academic customers, 'commitment' customers and customers currently billed in dollars are exempt.

14:248. Online — ORBIT

File name	CORP
Start year	Current information
Number of records	35,000
Update period	Quarterly
Database aids	Quick Reference Guide (6/89) Free (single copy) and Database Manual (1990) $15
Price/Charges	Subscription: US$7,500

14:249. CD-ROM — Corporate Technology Information Services

File name	CorpTech
Start year	Current information

Number of records	35,000
Update period	Quarterly
Price/Charges	Subscription: US$7,500

Cosmetic Insiders' Report

Edgell Communications Inc.
Biotechnology Information Institute

14:250. Master record

Database type	Textual, Bibliographic
Number of journals	1
Sources	
Start year	1990
Language	English
Coverage	
Number of records	
Update size	–
Update period	Monthly

Keywords

Beauty Care; Cosmetics

Description

Contains the full text of *Cosmetic Insiders' Report*. Covers news and insider views on the beauty care industry, comprising cosmetics, toiletries and fragrances with an editorial focus on companies, marketing, advertising, regulatory issues and consumer buying trends.

This database can be found on:
PTS Newsletter

Criminal Justice Periodical Index

University Microfilms International

14:252. Master record

Database type	Bibliographic
Number of journals	120
Sources	Journals and Newsletters
Start year	1975
Language	English
Coverage	Canada, UK and USA
Number of records	182,778
Update size	12,000
Update period	Monthly
Index unit	articles

Keywords

Forensic Science; Child Abuse; Computer Crime; Drug Abuse

Description

The Criminal Justice Periodical Index database provides cover-to-cover indexing of over 100 journals, newsletters, and law reporters. Contains citations to articles in magazines, journals, newsletters, and law reporting publications on the administration of justice and law enforcement. Subjects covered include abortion, arrest (police methods), child abuse, the justice system, penology, commercial crime, computer crime, court reform, crime prevention, drug abuse, due process of law, evidence, family law, fingerprinting, forensic science, jail administration, judges, juvenile offenders, legal aid, narcotics trafficking, negligence, environmental and industrial crime, political and social crime, organized crime, parole officers prisons, recidivism, security forces, victimless crimes, violence, and more.

Corresponds to *Criminal Justice Periodical Index*.

14:253. Online · DIALOG

File name	File 171
Start year	1975
Number of records	182,778
Update period	Monthly
Price/Charges	Subscription: US$66.00
	Online print: US$0.25
	Offline print: US$0.25
	SDI charge: US$7.95

CSIC
Consejo Superior de Investigaciones Científicas de España (CSIC)
La Ley

14:254. Master record
CD-ROM · Micronet

Database type	Bibliographic, Library catalogue/cataloguing aids
Number of journals	2,300
Sources	Journals and books
Start year	
Language	Spanish
Coverage	Spain (primarily) and International (some)
Number of records	625,000
Update size	—
Update period	Three times per year
Index unit	Articles, journals and Books

Keywords

Agronomy; Astrophysics; Earth Sciences; Logic; Physics; Technology; Urban Studies

Description

Contains the databases of ICYT, ISOC and CEDIB, plus CIRBIC. Bibliographic references to articles in specialised Spanish scientific and technical journals.

Also contains a complete listing of all the books and journals held by CSIC libraries. Made up of four databases: social sciences and humanities (ISOC); medicine (CEDIB); science and technology (ICYT); and libraries' holdings (CIRBIC). The CIRBIC database is prepared by PRIBIC.

Equivalent to the ICYT, ISOC, CEDIB and CIRBIC online databases. CSIC is a state body made up of 100 research and scientific institutes throughout Spain.

For more details of constituent databases, see:
ICYT
ISOC
CEDIB
CIRBIC

Current Awareness in Biological Sciences
Current Awareness in Biological Sciences

14:256. Master record

Database type	Bibliographic
Number of journals	2,500+
Sources	Journals

Start year	1983
Language	English
Coverage	International
Number of records	1,000,000+
Update size	200,000
Update period	Monthly
Index unit	Articles, Reviews and Editorials
Hosts have included	ORBIT (until 10/92)

Keywords

Cancer; Physiology; Immunology; Neuroscience

Description

Contains citations to the worldwide literature on biology. Subjects include biochemistry, cell and developmental biology, genetics and molecular biology, clinical chemistry, cancer research, immunology, endocrinology, microbiology, neurosciences, pharmacology and toxicology, physiology, ecology, and environmental and plant sciences. Includes an indication of whether articles are reviews or editorials and whether published in a language other than English.

Corresponds to *Current Awareness in Biological Sciences*. Formerly produced by Pergamon Press Ltd. Formerly available on ORBIT until Maxwell Online switched all life science files to BRS which has a much larger market for similar data.

14:257. Online · BRS

File name	CURB
Start year	1983
Number of records	1,100,000
Update period	Monthly
Price/Charges	Connect time: US$67.00/77.00
	Online print: US$0.29/0.37
	Offline print: US$0.47
	SDI charge: US$7.75

Current Contents Search Bibliographic Database
Institute for Scientific Information

14:258. Master record

Database type	Bibliographic
Number of journals	1,300
Sources	Journals
Start year	Most recent twelve months
Language	English
Coverage	International
Number of records	1,547,676
Update size	728,000
Update period	Weekly
Index unit	Articles, reviews, letters, notes and Editorials

Keywords

Applied Science; Atmospheric Science; Clinical Medicine; Immunology; Inorganic Chemistry; Molecular Biology; Neuroscience; Organic Chemistry; Polymers; Statistics; Astrophysics; Spectroscopy; Pathology; Physics; Water Supply

Description

Contains citations to articles listed in the tables of content of leading journals in the sciences, social sciences, and arts and humanities. There are seven subsets:

Clinical medicine (CLIN): Covers a broad range of disciplines including: allergy, anaesthesiology, biomethods, cardiology, clinical and medicinal chemistry, clinical psychiatry and psychology, dentistry, dermatology, epidemiology, family medicine, gastroenterology and hepatology, general and internal medicine, geriatrics and gerantology, hematology, infectious diseases, medical technology and laboratory medicine, neurology, oncology, ophthalmology, orthopedics, otorhinolaryngology, paediatrics, pharmacy, physical medicine and rehabilitation, radiology and nuclear medicine, reproductive systems, respiratory medicine, sports sciences, surgery, and urology.

Life sciences (LIFE): Covers anatomy, biochemistry, biophysics, cytology, endocrinology, experimental medicine, experimental biology, genetics, gerontology, hematology, histology, immunology, microbiology, molecular biology, neuroscience, parasitology, pathology, pharmaceutical chemistry, pharmacology, physiology, radiology and nuclear medicine, toxicology and virology.

Arts and humanities (ARTS)

Engineering, technology, and applied sciences (ENG)

Social and behavioural sciences (BEHA): Covers: business, economics, education, geography, history, law, library and information science, management, planning and development, political science, psychiatry, psychology, public health, rehabilitation, sociology.

Agriculture, biology, and environmental sciences (AGRI): Covers agricultural chemistry, economics, engineering, agronomy, animal behaviour, animal husbandry, applied microbiology, biotechnology, botany, conservation, crop science, dairy science, ecology, entomology, environmental sciences, fishery science and technology, forestry, horticulture, marine biology, mycology, nutrition, oceanology, orinthology, pest control, soil science, taxonomy, veterinary medicine and pathology, water research and engineering, wildlife management and zoology.

Physical, chemical, and earth sciences (PHYS): Covers analytical chemistry, applied physics, astronomy, astrophysics, atmospheric sciences, chemical physics, chemistry, condensed matter, crystallography, geology and geophysics, inorganic and nuclear chemistry, mathematics, meteorology, nuclear physics, organic chemistry, paleontology, physical chemistry, physics, polymer chemistry, spectroscopy, statistics and probability.

Includes title, authors, bibliographic data, abstracts and keywords, and, when available, reprint authors' addresses.

Current Contents Search is the online version of ISI's popular Current Contents series of publications. Current Contents is a weekly service that reproduces the tables of contents from current issues of leading journals in the sciences, social sciences, and arts and humanities. All ISI databases have a linked service known as The Genuine Article which can deliver the full text of located articles by mail, facsimile transmission or courier. Orders can be placed via the host service in use, mail, facsimile transmission, telephone or telex. Diskette products have a single-keystroke order information facility. The minimum charge is US$ 11.25 within USA and Canada and US$ 12.20 elsewhere.

Leading journals in the sciences, social sciences, and arts and humanities.

Keywords supplied by the author are included. In addition, ISI adds Keywords Plus which are generated by analysis of titles of articles that appear in the list of citations.

14:259. Database subset

Online **BRS, Morning Search, BRS/Colleague**

File name	CLIN
Alternative name(s)	CBIB: Clinical Medicine
Start year	
Number of records	
Update period	
Price/Charges	Connect time: US$85.00/95.00
	Online print: US$0.57/0.65
	Offline print: US$0.65

Notes

A special print format, CONT, allows the user to print a Table of Contents format that closely mirrors the print product.

14:260. Database subset

Online **BRS, Morning Search, BRS/Colleague**

File name	LIFE
Alternative name(s)	CBIB: Life Sciences
Start year	
Number of records	
Update period	
Price/Charges	Connect time: US$85.00/95.00
	Online print: US$0.57/0.65
	Offline print: US$0.65

Notes

A special print format, CONT, allows the user to print a Table of Contents format that closely mirrors the print product.

14:261. Database subset

Online **DIMDI**

File name	I383 – SCICLIN
Software	GRIPS
Start year	1983
Number of records	1,569,589
Update period	Weekly
SDI period	1 week
Database aids	User Manual SCISEARCH/SOCIAL SCISEARCH and Memocard SCISEARCH
Price/Charges	Connect time: UK£14.41–20.32 (Group I); 15.57–23.24 (Group II); 18.50–43.71 (Group III)
	Online print: UK£0.39–0.57
	Offline print: UK£0.31–0.37

Downloading is allowed

Notes

SCICLIN corresponds to the Current Contents edition Clinical Practice. Approximately eight per cent of records contain abstracts. Searches are possible from January 1983.

There are preferential costs for subscribers to the printed product. Groups shown for pricing refer to: 1. Users in the Federal Republic of Germany active in the field of biosciences, with the exception of private companies. Under temporary federal grant there is a rebate for this group of users; 2. Other users who are subscribers of the equivalent printed product. These users have to inform ISI that they wish this preferential rate; 3. Other users who are not subscribers of the equivalent printed product.

Record composition

Abstract AB; Abstract Indicators AI; Author AU; Author's Keywords IT; Cluster Code CC; Cluster Term CT; Cluster Weight /W; Corporate Country CCO; Corporate Source CS; Document Type DT; Entry Date ED; Free Text FT; Journal Title JT; Keywords Plus UT;

Language LA; Number of Document ND; Number of References RN; Publication Year PY; Reference RF; Referenced Journal RJ; Referenced Patent No. RP; Subject Code SC; Subject Heading SH; Source SO; Subunit SU and Title TI

The basic index includes the following data fields: Title, Controlled Term, Index Term, Uncontrolled Term and Abstract.

14:262. Database subset
Online   DIMDI

File name	I583 – SCILIFE
Software	GRIPS
Start year	1983
Number of records	2,821,801
Update period	Weekly
SDI period	1 week
Database aids	User Manual SCISEARCH/SOCIAL SCISEARCH and Memocard SCISEARCH
Price/Charges	Connect time: UK£14.41–20.32 (Group I); 15.57–23.24 (Group II); 18.50–43.71 (Group III) Online print: UK£0.39–0.57 Offline print: UK£0.31–0.37

Downloading is allowed

Notes

SCILIFE corresponds to the Current Contents edition Life Sciences. Approximately nine per cent of records contain abstracts. Searches are possible from January 1983.

There are preferential costs for subscribers to the printed product. Groups shown for pricing refer to: 1. Users in the Federal Republic of Germany active in the field of biosciences, with the exception of private companies. Under temporary federal grant there is a rebate for this group of users; 2. Other users who are subscribers of the equivalent printed product. These users have to inform ISI that they wish this preferential rate; 3. Other users who are not subscribers of the equivalent printed product.

Record composition

Abstract AB; Abstract Indicators AI; Author AU; Author's Keywords IT; Cluster Code CC; Cluster Term CT; Cluster Weight /W; Corporate Country CCO; Corporate Source CS; Document Type DT; Entry Date ED; Free Text FT; Journal Title JT; Keywords Plus UT; Language LA; Number of Document ND; Number of References RN; Publication Year PY; Reference RF; Referenced Journal RJ; Referenced Patent No. RP; Subject Code SC; Subject Heading SH; Source SO; Subunit SU and Title TI

The basic index includes the following data fields: Title, Controlled Term, Index Term, Uncontrolled Term and Abstract.

14:263. Database subset
Online   DIMDI

File name	IL89 – Current Contents/SciSearch
Software	GRIPS
Start year	Latest 12 months
Number of records	729,304
Update period	Weekly
SDI period	1 week
Database aids	User Manual SCISEARCH/Social SCISEARCH and Memocard SCISEARCH
Price/Charges	Connect time: UK£14.41–20.32 (Group I); 15.57–23.24 (Group II); 18.50–43.71 (Group III) Online print: UK£0.39–0.57 Offline print: UK£0.31–0.37

Downloading is allowed

Notes

This is a separate database on DIMDI of Current Contents/ SciSearch. IL89 contains the documents of the last 12 months from Social SciSearch. It corresponds to the subject content of SciSearch, the only difference from the main file on DIMDI (IS74) is the output format. Suppliers of online documents: British Library Document Supply Centre, Boston Spa, England; Harkers Information Retrieval System, Sydney, Australia; The Information Store, San Francisco, USA; Institute for Scientific Information, Philadelphia, USA.

There are preferential costs for subscribers to the printed product. Groups shown for pricing refer to: 1. Users in the Federal Republic of Germany active in the field of biosciences, with the exception of private companies. Under temporary federal grant there is a rebate for this group of users; 2. Other users who are subscribers of the equivalent printed product. These users have to inform ISI that they wish this preferential rate; 3. Other users who are not subscribers of the equivalent printed product.

Record composition

Abstract Indicator AI; Abstract AB; Author AU; Author's Keywords IT; Cluster Code CC; Corporate Country CCO; Corporate Source CS; Document Type DT; Entry Date ED; Free Text FT; Index Term IT; Journal Title JT; Keywords Plus UT; Language LA; Number of Document ND; Number of References RN; Publication Year PY; Reference RF; Referenced Journal RJ; Referenced Patent No. RP; Source SO; Subject Code SC; Subject Heading SH; Subunit SU; Title TI and Uncontrolled Term (Keywords Plus) UT

After the SHOW-, PRINT or DLOAD- command the output of documents is displayed in the table of contents format. The basic index includes the data fields: Title, Index Term and Uncontrolled Term.

14:264. Database subset
Diskette   Institute for Scientific Information

File name	Current Contents on Diskette with Abstracts – Life Sciences
Format notes	IBM, NEC, Mac
Software	Proprietary Vn.3.0
Start year	
Number of records	
Update period	Weekly
Price/Charges	Subscription: US$965

Notes

Contains citations with abstracts to articles listed in the tables of contents of about 1,200 journals in the life sciences. Equivalent to the print Current Contents/Life Sciences; and in part to the Current Contents Search online database.

Reduced subscription for print subscribers. The latest version of the software (August 1992) allows search profiles to be run against six issues at one time; better file compression to use less hard disk space; expanded online, context sensitive help; better truncation (including left-hand) facilities; and new output options. KeyWords Plus (tm) provides users with search terms taken from an article's bibliography: in this way users should identify many more articles. KeyWords Plus (tm) also allows users to determine on inspection how closely the article pertains to their area of interest. Users are now also able to transfer multiple search terms from the dictionaries to search statements.

Record composition

ISBN; ISSN and Publisher

14:265. Database subset
Diskette   **Institute for Scientific Information**

File name	Current Contents on Diskette with Abstracts – Clinical Medicine
Format notes	IBM, NEC, Mac
Software	Proprietary Vn.3.0
Start year	
Number of records	
Update period	Weekly
Price/Charges	Subscription: US$750

Notes

Contains citations with abstracts to articles listed in the tables of contents of journals and book series in clinical medicine.

Equivalent in part to the Current Contents Search online database.

Reduced subscription for print subscribers. The latest version of the software (August 1992) allows search profiles to be run against six issues at one time; better file compression to use less hard disk space; expanded online, context sensitive help; better truncation (including left-hand) facilities; and new output options. KeyWords Plus (tm) provides users with search terms taken from an article's bibliography: in this way users should identify many more articles. KeyWords Plus (tm) also allows users to determine on inspection how closely the article pertains to their area of interest. Users are now also able to transfer multiple search terms from the dictionaries to search statements.

Record composition

ISBN; ISSN; Publisher; Author keywords; Key Words Plus; Bibliographic details and Abstracts

14:266. Database subset
Diskette   **Institute for Scientific Information**

File name	Current Contents on Diskette – Life Sciences
Format notes	IBM, NEC, Mac
Software	Proprietary Vn.3.0
Start year	
Number of records	
Update period	Weekly
Price/Charges	Subscription: US$405/575

Notes

Contains citations to articles listed in the tables of contents of about 1,200 journals in the life sciences. Data are available in two editions; one covering 1,200 journals, one 600 journals. Equivalent to the print *Current Contents/Life Sciences*; and in part to the Current Contents Search online database.

Reduced subscription for print subscribers. The latest version of the software (August 1992) allows search profiles to be run against six issues at one time; better file compression to use less hard disk space; expanded online, context sensitive help; better truncation (including left-hand) facilities; and new output options. KeyWords Plus (tm) provides users with

search terms taken from an article's bibliography: in this way users should identify many more articles. KeyWords Plus (tm) also allows users to determine on inspection how closely the article pertains to their area of interest. Users are now also able to transfer multiple search terms from the dictionaries to search statements.

Record composition

ISBN; ISSN and Publisher

14:267. Database subset
Diskette   **Institute for Scientific Information**

File name	Current Contents on Diskette – Clinical Medicine
Format notes	IBM, NEC, Mac
Software	Proprietary Vn.3.0
Start year	
Number of records	
Update period	Weekly
Price/Charges	Subscription: US$427

Notes

Contains citations to articles listed in the tables of contents of journals and book series in clinical medicine. Equivalent in part to the Current Contents Search online database.

Reduced subscription for print subscribers. The latest version of the software (August 1992) allows search profiles to be run against six issues at one time; better file compression to use less hard disk space; expanded online, context sensitive help; better truncation (including left-hand) facilities; and new output options. KeyWords Plus (tm) provides users with search terms taken from an article's bibliography: in this way users should identify many more articles. KeyWords Plus (tm) also allows users to determine on inspection how closely the article pertains to their area of interest. Users are now also able to transfer multiple search terms from the dictionaries to search statements.

Record composition

ISBN; ISSN; Publisher; Author keywords; Key Words Plus and Bibliographic details

14:268. Database subset
Tape   **Institute for Scientific Information**

File name	CC Search/Life Sciences
Start year	Current
Number of records	
Update period	Weekly
Price/Charges	Subscription: US$15,000 -18,750

Notes

Contains citations to articles listed in the tables of contents of about 1,200 journals in the life sciences. Data are available in two editions; one covering 1,200 journals, one 600 journals.

Equivalent to the print *Current Contents/Life Sciences*; and in part to the Current Contents Search online database. Covers a broad range of disciplines including: biochemistry, biomedical research, biophysics, chemistry, cytology/histology, endocrinology, experimental medicine, genetics, hematology, immunology, microbiology, molecular biology, neurosciences, oncology, pathology, pharmacology/pharmaceutics, physiology and toxicology.

Reduced subscription for print subscribers. The latest

version of the software (August 1992) allows search profiles to be run against six issues at one time; better file compression to use less hard disk space; expanded online, context sensitive help; better truncation (including left-hand) facilities; and new output options. KeyWords Plus (tm) provides users with search terms taken from an article's bibliography: in this way users should identify many more articles. KeyWords Plus (tm) also allows users to determine on inspection how closely the article pertains to their area of interest. Users are now also able to transfer multiple search terms from the dictionaries to search statements.

Annual lease is $15,000 (academic), $18,750 (corporate).

Record composition

ISBN; ISSN and Publisher

14:269. Database subset
Tape   Institute for Scientific
Information

File name	CC Search/Clinical Medicine
Start year	Current
Number of records	
Update period	Weekly
Price/Charges	Subscription: US$15,000 – 18,750

Notes

Contains citations to articles listed in the tables of contents of journals and book series in clinical medicine. Equivalent in part to the Current Contents Search online database.

Reduced subscription for print subscribers. The latest version of the software (August 1992) allows search profiles to be run against six issues at one time; better file compression to use less hard disk space; expanded online, context sensitive help; better truncation (including left-hand) facilities; and new output options. KeyWords Plus (tm) provides users with search terms taken from an article's bibliography: in this way users should identify many more articles. KeyWords Plus (tm) also allows users to determine on inspection how closely the article pertains to their area of interest. Users are now also able to transfer multiple search terms from the dictionaries to search statements.

Annual lease is $15,000 (academic), $18,750 (corporate).

Record composition

ISBN; ISSN; Publisher; Author keywords; Key Words Plus and Bibliographic Details

Current Drugs Group Files
Current Drugs Ltd

14:270. Master record

Database type	Bibliographic, Factual
Number of journals	
Sources	
Start year	
Language	English
Coverage	International
Number of records	
Update size	–
Update period	Weekly

Keywords

Drugs; Biotechnology; Immunology; Therapeutic Medicine; DNA; Molecular Biology

Description

Covers five areas of drug research and development: Serotonin, Neurodegenerative Disorders, RAS Agents, Potassium Channel Activators, and Anti-atherosclerotic Agents.

14:271. Tape   Current Drugs Ltd

File name
Start year
Number of records
Update period

Current Patents Evaluation
Current Drugs Ltd

14:272. Master record

Alternative name(s)	CPEV
Database type	Patents, Bibliographic
Number of journals	3
Sources	Journals
Start year	1990
Language	English
Coverage	International
Number of records	
Update size	–
Update period	Monthly
Index unit	Patents
Database aids	International Patent Classification
Hosts have included	Data-Star (until 12/92)

Keywords

Patents – Pharmaceutical; Cardiovascular Diseases; Chemotherapy; Haematology; Neurological Diseases; Alzheimer's Disease; Parkinson's Disease; Stroke; Cancer; Pain; Epilepsy; Hormone Disorders; Metabolic Disorders; Migraine; Gastroenterology; Allergy

Description

A patent database of 'informed summary' and bibliographic data for agrochemical and pharmaceutical patents in selected therapeutic areas. Citations, with abstracts and evaluations, to pharmaceutical patents and patent applications for antimicrobials (antivirals, antiparasitics, antibacterials and antifungals), cardiovascular patents (including chemotherapy and blood products), central nervous system patents (including antidepressants, antipsychotics, analgesics, antiepileptics, antimigraines and treatments for Alzheimer's Disease, Parkinson's Disease and stroke) and anticancer, anti-inflammatory, anti-allergic, gastrointestinal, hormonal and metabolic disease therapies, plus immunology. Patent documents come from Great Britain, the United States and the European Patent Office, included also are PCT applications, with coverage of the various therapeutic categories, beginning at various times since 1989. Each entry includes publication date, assignee and inventor names, International Patent Classification and therapeutic classification. Summaries and evaluations are written by professionals in patent information and the relevant research areas. The evaluations are written in English and commentaries made in the context of latest research findings. Approximately 35–40 patents are selected each month from patents appearing in the Therapeutic Patent Fast Alert Database. The focus of these services is to inform the scientific community of advances in drug development, rather than to provide access to patents as legal documents or prior art. The emphasis is on the pharmaceutical utility disclosed in the patent and focuses on the specific compounds exemplified in the patent; although the abstract identifies the novel features of the claims in a general sense there is no attempt to define the generic scope of the claims. There is an extensive evaluation of the claimed invention in the EV field. It takes into account the pharmacological data provided in the patent specification and compares the invention with products currently available and under clinical development in the same therapeutic category. Much of the material in the evaluation is taken from sources outside the patent under discussion and is based on the subjective opinion of the expert author. These critical evaluations are later printed in the monthly *Current Opinion in Therapeutic Patents*, which forms the basis of this database.

Corresponds to *Current Antimicrobial Patents*, *Current Cardiovascular Patents* and *Current CNS Patents*, plus *Current Opinion in Therapeutic Patents*. Data-Star says the database is 'no longer being maintained and updated by the producers'.

14:273. Online ORBIT

File name	CPEV
Start year	1990 to date
Number of records	30 – 40 patents
Update period	Monthly
Database aids	Quick Reference Guide (9/91) Free (single copy)

Notes

Approximately 30–40 patents are selected each month from patents appearing in the Therapeutic Patent Fast Alert database. Discounts are available online to subscribers to the printed Current Patents' bulletins in two or more therapeutic areas. Electronic SDI service is now available within two hours on ORBIT. They can be downloaded and reformatted on a word processor. Results are retrieved in the low cost PRINTS file, $15 per connect hour.

Record composition

Accession Number AN; Title TI; Patent Number PN; Designated States DS; Priority Country and Number PR; Patent Assignee PA; Inventors IN; Priotity Data Field PY; Priority Date PY; Filing Date FD; Publication Date PD; Abstract AB; Evaluation EV; Annotated Title Field AT; Key References KR; Section Codes SC and Descriptors DE

The descriptor terms are not based upon a controlled thesaurus. A maximum of six IPC codes are listed, each searchable at the sub-class, group and sub-group level.

Dalctraf

Dalctraf HB

14:274. Master record

Database type	Bibliographic
Number of journals	
Sources	
Start year	1980
Language	English
Coverage	International
Number of records	3,000
Update size	450
Update period	Monthly

Keywords

Alcohol Abuse; Drug Abuse; Road Safety

Description

Dalctraf registers international literature in the biomedical and social sciences related to the incidence and effects of alcohol and drugs on traffic safety. It is one of the files in the DRUGAB information system. See also Alconarc and Nordrug.

14:275. Online DAFA Data AB

File name	Dalctraf
Start year	1980
Number of records	3,000
Update period	Monthly

This database can also be found on:
Drugab

DataStat

National Data Corporation, Health Care Data Services Division

14:277. Master record

Database type	Directory, Factual
Number of journals	
Sources	Pharmacopoeias and Suppliers
Start year	
Language	English
Coverage	USA (primarily)
Number of records	
Update size	—
Update period	Weekly
Index unit	Drug

Keywords

Drug Therapy; Drugs; Pharmaceutical Industry; Pharmaceutical Products

Description

Contains descriptions of drug interactions at the ingredient level for individual drugs and therapeutic classes of drugs. Each interaction is classified according to its level of seriousness to the patient. Also includes drug packaging and pricing data.

Sources of data include manufacturers' catalogues and standard pharmaceutical reference works.

14:278. Online National Data Corporation, Health Care Data Services Division

File name	
Start year	
Number of records	
Update period	Weekly

Notes

Monthly subscription fee required.

De Haen Drug Data

Paul de Haen International Inc

14:279. Master record

Database type	Bibliographic, Factual
Number of journals	1,200+
Sources	Journals, Newsletters and Conference proceedings
Start year	1980
Language	English
Coverage	International

Number of records   94,879
Update size   15,000
Update period   Every two months
Index unit   Drug

Keywords

Drug Therapy; Drugs; Pharmaceutical Products

Description

The database includes four subfiles, each covering a different aspect of drug information, which can be searched individually or simultaneously. Contains specially prepared reports on drugs that summarise information from the worldwide biomedical literature, over 1,200 journals and more than twenty other respected secondary references and numerous abstracts and summaries of papers presented at international meetings. Topics covered include: adverse drug reactions, clinical studies, drug efficacy, drug interactions, drug toxicity, investigational drugs, marketed drugs, pharmaceutical chemistry and more. Each report provides generic and trade name of drug, manufacturer, country of manufacture, usage status (for example, investigational), type (for example, efficacy), description, purpose, and results and conclusions of study.

Drugs in Prospect (DIP). Covers newly synthesized compounds exhibiting pharmacological activity.
Drugs in Research (DIR). Covers investigational drugs involved in pre- clinical and clinical studies.
Drugs in Use (DIU). Covers commercially available and investigational drugs used in clinical studies.
ADRID (Adverse Drug Reactions & Interactions Database). Covers adverse reactions and interactions of commercially available and investigational drugs.

14:280. Online   DIALOG

File name   File 267
Start year   1980
Number of records   94,879
Update period   Every two months
Price/Charges   Subscription: US$66.00
     Connect time: US$66.00
     Online print: US$0.25
     Offline print: US$0.30

Derwent Drug File
Derwent Publications Ltd

14:281. Master record

Alternative name(s)   Ringdoc (Previous name);
     Pharmaceutical Literature
     Documentation (Previous name);
     Derwent Ringdoc
Database type   Bibliographic
Number of journals   1,000
Sources   Journals and conference
     proceedings
Start year   1964
Language   English
Coverage   International
Number of records   1.2m
Update size   50,000
Update period   Monthly

Keywords

Biochemistry; Drugs; Endocrinology; Nutrition;
Pharmaceuticals; Side Effects

Description

This database was originally called Pharmaceutical Literature Documention from 1964 until 1983, when Derwent Publications took over the production, redesigned and reformatted the database and named it Ringdoc, then recently renamed it Derwent Drug File. Derwent have reorganised their collection of drug databases, resulting in three new names: Derwent Drug Registry (formerly Standard Drug File); Derwent Drug File (formerly Ringdoc); and, with the launch of a CD-ROM in Spring 1993, the World Drug Index (formerly the Standard Drug File with Graphics). These databases provide access to information important to the pharmaceutical industry. Coverage includes information on the chemistry, biochemistry, pharmacology, therapeutic effects, and toxicology of drugs. This includes the preparation and testing of potential drugs, analysis, pharmacokinetics, and isolation from natural sources.

Derwent Drug File is a bibliographic database. Detailed abstracts from articles in over 800 key worldwide journals are included, covering all aspects of drugs. Includes: chemistry, synthesis, pharmacology, toxicology, and clinical applications.

The non-bibliographic parts of the files (chemical structures only) are in a separate database called Derwent Drug Registry (formerly named Standard Drug File). Searches should be conducted in Derwent Drug Registry for chemical structures of standard drugs and then transferred to the sister Derwent Unified Drug File for bibliographic information.

Corresponds to *RINGDOC Abstract Journal* weekly. Derwent report that the Derwent Drug File and Derwent Drug Register will shortly be available online on STN as well as on DIALOG and ORBIT.

Indepth keywording; fragmentation coding.

14:282. Online   DIALOG

File name   File 912
Alternative name(s)   Ringdoc (former name);
     Pharmaceutical Literature
     Documentation (former name);
     Derwent Ringdoc Unified Database
     File
Start year   1983
Number of records
Update period   Monthly

Notes

This is the current unified Ringdoc database file on DIALOG, dating from January 1983 when Derwent redesigned and reformatted the database. Online access to RINGDOC is restricted to subscribers to RINGDOC Abstracts Journal. DIALOG's collection of three files that make up their Derwent Ringdoc, totalling 1.2 million records are: File 911 (an authoritative file on drugs, once the Standard Drug File, now called Derwent Drug Registry, DDR, a sister database); File 912 (current unified file from 1983 updated on a monthly basis, adding approximately 4,000 records per month); and File 913 (the historical file dating from 1964-1982), containing over 800,000 records.

14:283. Online   DIALOG

File name   File 913
Alternative name(s)   Ringdoc (former name);
     Pharmaceutical Literature
     Documentation (former name);
     Derwent Ringdoc Codeless
     Scanning File
Start year   1964 – 1982

Number of records   800,000
Update period   Not updated

Notes

This is the Ringdoc historical database on DIALOG, containing over 800,000 records from 1964–1982, before Derwent managed the database. Online access to RINGDOC is restricted to subscribers to RINGDOC Abstracts Journal. DIALOG's collection of three files that make up their Derwent Ringdoc, totalling 1.2 million records are: File 911 (an authoritative file on drugs, once the Standard Drug File, now called Derwent Drug Registry, DDR, a sister database); File 912 (current unified file from 1983 updated on a monthly basis, adding approximately 4,000 records per month); and File 913 (the historical file dating from 1964- 1982), containing over 800,000 records.

14:284. Online   ORBIT

File name   RGBK
Alternative name(s) Ringdoc (former name);
                     Pharmaceutical Literature
                     Documentation (former name);
                     Derwent Ringdoc
Start year   1976–1982
Number of records
Update period   Not updated

Notes

This is a backfile of Ringdoc on ORBIT, containing records from 1976-1982. There is another backfile, RING, on ORBIT, for the years 1964–1975. The unified database name is UDBR on ORBIT, dating from January 1983, when Derwent took over production of the database. Online access is restricted to RINGDOC print subscribers. Electronic SDI service is now available within two hours on ORBIT. They can be downloaded and reformatted on a word processor. Results are retrieved in the low cost PRINTS file, $15 per connect hour.

14:285. Online   ORBIT

File name   RING
Alternative name(s) Ringdoc (former name);
                     Pharmaceutical Literature
                     Documentation (former name);
                     Derwent Ringdoc
Start year   1964–1975
Number of records
Update period   Not updated

Notes

This is a backfile of Rindoc on ORBIT, containing records from 1964-1975. There is another backfile called RGBK containing records from 1976- 1982. The unified database name is UDBR on ORBIT, dating from January 1983, when Derwent took over production of the database. Online access to RINGDOC is restricted to subscribers to RINGDOC Abstracts Journal.

Electronic SDI service is now available within 2 hours on ORBIT. They can be downloaded and reformatted on a word processor. Results are retrieved in the low cost PRINTS file, $15 per connect hour.

14:286. Online   ORBIT

File name   UDBR
Alternative name(s) Ringdoc (former name);
                     Pharmaceutical Literature
                     Documentation (former name);
                     Derwent Ringdoc
Start year   1983
Number of records   1.2m
Update period   Monthly

Notes

This is the unified database on ORBIT, dating from January 1983 when Derwent took over production. There are two backfiles also – RING; 1964-1975, and RGBK; 1976–1982. Online access to RINGDOC is restricted to subscribers to RINGDOC Abstracts Journal. Electronic SDI service is now available within two hours on ORBIT. They can be downloaded and reformatted on a word processor. Results are retrieved in the low cost PRINTS file, $15 per connect hour.

14:287. CD-ROM   SilverPlatter

File name   Ringdoc
Alternative name(s) Ringdoc (former name);
                     Pharmaceutical Literature
                     Documentation (former name);
                     Derwent Ringdoc
Format notes   IBM
Software   WINSPIRS
Start year   1983
Number of records   450,000
Update period   Quarterly

Notes

The database was formerly called Ringdoc. Complete abstracts as in the print (but not online) versions are included. The CD-ROM will include only the unified database, which covers January 1983 to the present. Also includes the graphical data, which is excluded from the online version.

Three discs each containing three years. Only available to subscribers of print version of the Derwent service. The software provides fully displayable images with scroll and zoom facility and rapid access to data.

14:288. Tape   Derwent Publications Ltd

File name   Derwent Drug File
Alternative name(s) Ringdoc (former name);
                     Pharmaceutical Literature
                     Documentation (former name);
                     Derwent Ringdoc
Start year   1964
Number of records   1.2m
Update period   Monthly

Derwent Drug Registry
Derwent Publications Ltd

14:289. Master record

Alternative name(s) DDR; Standard Drug File (Previous
                     name); SDF (Previous name)
Database type   Factual, Chemical structures
Number of journals   1,000
Sources   journals, patents and conference
                     proceedings
Start year   1983
Language   English
Coverage   International
Number of records   37,800
Update size   —
Update period   Irregular

Keywords

Drugs

Description

This database was formerly called the Standard Drug File. Derwent have reorganised their collection of drug databases, resulting in three new names: Derwent Drug Registry (formerly Standard Drug File); Derwent

Drug File (formerly Ringdoc); and, with the launch of a CD-ROM in Spring 1993, the World Drug Index (formerly the Standard Drug File with Graphics, part of this database).

These databases provide access to information important to the pharmaceutical industry. Coverage includes information on the chemistry, biochemistry, pharmacology, therapeutic effects, and toxicology of drugs. Derwent Drug Registry is a database listing of pharmaceutical compounds. For each compound listed the following information is provided: Name, standard registry name, pharmacological classification of standard activities, substructure keywords, chemical Ring codes, and other codes. The 37,800 drugs in the file at the time of writing are represented by 10,000 official names, 19,000 drug code numbers, and 106,000 trade names or synonyms. Some 4,700 of the drugs have medical fields included – five fields of information have been extracted from official compendia: Indications, Contra-Indications; Interactions; Precautions; and Adverse Effects. The Mechanism of Action and the Pharmaceuticalogical Activity of the drug are also shown. DDR allows users to ask questions such as 'How many benzimidazoles are drugs?'; 'Which of these have antihistamine-H1 activity?' and 'Are any of these marketed in Spain, and if so, by whom and under what names?'

Derwent Drug Registry is a companion dictionary database to the sister bibliographic Derwent Drug File database. Derwent report that the Derwent Drug File and Derwent Drug Register will shortly be available online on STN as well as on DIALOG and ORBIT.

To be included in the file, a drug must have appeared in the Derwent Drug File more than once; searches should be conducted in DDR for standard drugs and then transferred to the Derwent Unified Drug File.

14:290. Online   DIALOG

File name	File 911
Alternative name(s)	DDRR; Standard Drug File (Previous name); SDF (Previous name)
Start year	1983
Number of records	37,800
Update period	Irregular

Notes

An authoritative file providing detailed information on each drug, its biological activity and chemical substructures, keywords and codes. Online access to RINGDOC is restricted to subscribers to *RINGDOC Abstracts Journal*. A companion to the bibliographic Derwent Unified Drug File (previously Ringdoc) database, File 912 on DIALOG. Searches should be conducted in Derwent Drug Registry for chemical structures of standard drugs and then transferred to the sister Derwent Drug File for bibliographic information.

14:291. Online   ORBIT

File name	DDRR
Alternative name(s)	DDRR; Standard Drug File (Previous name); SDF (Previous name)
Start year	1983
Number of records	37,800
Update period	Irregular

Notes

Previously called the Standard Drug File, this is an authoritative file providing detailed information on each drug, its biological activity and chemical substructures, keywords and codes. A companion to the

bibliographic Derwent Drug File (formerly Ringdoc Database). Searches should be conducted in Derwent Drug Registry for chemical structures of standard drugs and then transferred to the sister Derwent Unified Drug File (UDBR on ORBIT) for bibliographic information. Access is limited to subscribers of the print publication RINGDOC.

14:292. Tape   Derwent Publications Ltd

File name	Derwent Drug Registry
Alternative name(s)	DDRR; Standard Drug File (Previous name); SDF (Previous name)
Start year	1983
Number of records	37,800
Update period	Irregular

Notes

A companion to the bibliographic Derwent Unified Drug File (previously Ringdoc) database. Searches should be conducted in Derwent Drug Registry for chemical structures of standard drugs and then transferred to the sister Derwent Drug File for bibliographic information.

DHSS-MEDTEH
UK Departments of Health and Social Security Library

14:293. Master record

Alternative name(s)	Medical Toxicology and Environmental Health
Database type	Bibliographic, Textual
Number of journals	2,000
Sources	Administrative circulars, books, conference proceedings, government documents, government publications, journals, pamphlets, official publications and reports
Start year	1888
Language	English
Coverage	International
Number of records	26,600
Update size	—
Update period	Weekly
Index unit	Articles
Thesaurus	DHSS-Data Thesaurus, Dept of Health, London, 1985

Keywords

Air Pollution; Cancer; Cosmetics; Food Additives; Food Contaminants; Laboratory Practice; Mutation; Noise Pollution; Nutrition; Pesticides; Radiation Biology; Smoking; Veterinary Medicines; Water Pollution

Description

DHSS-MEDTECH offers specialised information covering medical toxicology and environmental health, using the resources of the Department of Health library in London. It includes more strictly scientific and medical information than the wider ranging DHSS-DAT database. It contains citations with abstracts to literature on environmental, chemical, toxicological, food and nutrition issues, and includes more strictly scientific and medical information in these subject areas than the wider ranging DHSS-DATA database. Subjects covered include: government and regulatory authorities, carcinogenicity and mutagenicity, chemicals in food (such as contaminants, preservatives and additives); consumer products; industrial chemicals; pesticides, radiation, air, water and noise pollution; radiation biology; veterinary medicines; laboratory practices; cosmetics; toxicology and the health consequences of smoking. An important feature of the database is the inclusion of full details, including sources of supply, of DOH publications.

Materials from 1888 to 1983 have recently been added to the database. Abstracts are available for documents added to the database from 1984.

The data field Note contains information such as: Bibliography, annual, named individuals and additional publication details. DHMT covers a variety of multi-word sources, not all of which are hyphenated, for example details of monographs, reports etc. These should be searched in freetext using adjacency operators to link terms and qualified by the use of .SO.

14:294. Online   Data-Star

File name	DHMT
Alternative name(s)	Medical Toxicology and Environmental Health
Start year	1888
Number of records	26,600
Update period	Weekly
Database aids	Data-Star Biomedical Manual and Online manual (search NEWS-DHMT in NEWS)
Price/Charges	Subscription: SFr80.00
	Connect time: SFr127.20
	Online print: SFr0.39
	Offline print: SFr0.80
	SDI charge: SFr6.80

Notes

To search DHSS-DATA and DHSS-MEDTEH simultaneously use the DHZZ-Superlabel.

From June 1993 Data-Star have introduced an annual fee/subscription per contract (that is, not per password) of SFr 80.00 (c.UK£ 32.00) payable every June. For North American customers billed in dollars who also use DIALOG, the DIALOG fee also covers access to Data-Star. Academic customers, 'commitment' customers and customers currently billed in dollars are exempt.

Record composition

Accession Number and Update Code AN; Author(s) AU; Corporate Author(s) CA; Descriptor(s) DE; Language LG; Notes NT; Publication Type PT; Publication Year PY; Publication Year (archive) YA; Source SO; Title TI and Update Code UP

DIAGNOSIS (Datenbank)
Georg Thieme Verlag

14:295. Master record

Database type	Bibliographic, Factual, Textual
Number of journals	
Sources	Clinicians, direct contacts, journals and monographs
Start year	1985
Language	German
Coverage	
Number of records	2,061
Update size	—
Update period	Varies

Keywords

Drugs; Drug Therapy; Gynaecology; Internal Medicine; Medical Diagnosis; Rheumatology; Urology

Description

The Diagnosis database contains medical case reports and structured portions from medical textbooks providing descriptions of about 2,000 diseases, leading from signs and symptoms to suggestions of possible diagnoses. It aims to offer suggestions for diagnoses and therapy together with citations to relevant literature based on signs and given symptoms and is intended to be used as a diagnostic aid for physicians. Assistance is provided by the presentation of plausible explanations for clinical data entered by the user. It is emphasised that the doctor himself is responsible for any decision concerning diagnoses or treatment which may be based on the database.

The primary emphasis of the database is on internal medicine, but its coverage also includes diseases in urology, gynaecology, and rheumatology.

The database is based on case notes by Georg Thieme Verlag, Stuttgart and Elsevier Excerpta Medica, London. Small sections out of textbooks complete the content.

Medical textbooks, journals and personal communication with physicians.

Indexing is through the use of Controlled Terms.

14:296. Online   DIMDI

File name	DI85
Start year	1985
Number of records	2,061
Update period	Irregular
SDI period	1 week
Price/Charges	Connect time: UK£07.85–12.60
	Online print: UK£0.56–0.74
	Offline print: UK£0.47–0.54

Downloading is allowed

Notes

For the DIAGNOSIS database a self-explaining menu-guided dialog in German and English has been developed which can be used on all BTX- or page-mode terminals.

Record composition

GRIPS; Author AU; Befunde (Findings) BF; Controlled Terms CT; Corporate Source CS; Diagnosis DG; Differential Diagnosis DD; Document Origin HERK; Freetext fields FT; Number of Document ND; Pathologische Refunde (Pathological Findings) PB; Resuemee und Verlauf (Summary and Further Progress) VE; Symptome (Symptoms) SP; Therapie (Therapy) TH and Title TI

The unit record contains bibliographic information about title, author(s), signs and symptoms, diagnoses, differential diagnoses, in the case notes mostly suggestions for therapy and controlled terms. There are several synonyms for every Controlled Term which are all searchable but only the preferred terms can be seen in the records.

This database can also be found on:
MediROM
DIAGNOSIS, Vergiftungen, Radiolab

DIAGNOSIS, Vergiftungen, Radiolab
Georg Thieme Verlag

14:297. Master record
CD-ROM   **Medisoft GmbH**

Database type	
Number of journals	
Sources	

Start year
Language   German
Coverage
Number of records
Update size   —
Update period   Annually

Keywords

Drugs; Drug Therapy; Gynaecology; Internal Medicine; Medical Diagnosis; Pharmaceuticals; Rheumatology; Surgery; Urology

Description

This database enables the user to enter signs and symptoms and the program will then find the corresponding diseases. Full text descriptions of the diseases are available.

For more details of constituent databases, see:
DIAGNOSIS
Vergiftungen
Radiolab

Diagnostics Business-Matters

Fortia Marketing Consultants Ltd

14:298. Master record

Database type   Textual
Number of journals   1
Sources   Newsletters
Start year   1988
Language   English
Coverage   International
Number of records
Update size   —
Update period   Daily
Index unit   articles

Keywords

Company Profiles; Diagnostic Products; Marketing; Research and Development

Description

A monthly newsletter on companies that develop and market medical diagnostic products. Provides busines intelligence on the companies involved, along with information on the latest trends and events in research, development, markets, product introduction, joint ventures and merger and acquisition activity. Also features company profile articles. On DIALOG, CORIS and Data-Star this newsletter is part of the PTS Newsletter Database.

Full text of the monthly *Diagnostics Business-Matters* newsletter.

This database can also be found on:
PTS Newsletter Database

Dictionnaire Vidal

Bureau van Dijk
OVP – Editions du Vidal

14:300. Master record

Alternative name(s)   Vidal 1992; CD-ROM Vidal
Database type   Directory, Textual
Number of journals
Sources   Book

Start year
Language   French
Coverage   France
Number of records   9,000
Update size   —
Update period   Annually
Index unit   drug

Keywords

Drugs; Pharmaceuticals; Surgery

Description

The *Dictionnaire Vidal*: the reference book in France for physicians and pharmacists. It contains fully detailed prescribing information on more than 9,000 pharmaceuticals, plus information on drug interaction and side effects. Features include automatic interaction checking and split screen comparisons. Covers 31st May 1990 to 31st May 1991.

Equivalent to the *Dictionnaire Vidal* or Vidal Directory, the drug reference book of France.

Free-text searching on every word. Can be searched by product name, active ingredient, therapeutic category, company name, or word.

14:301. CD-ROM   OVP – Editions du Vidal

File name   CD-ROM Vidal
Alternative name(s)   Vidal 1992; CD-ROM Vidal
Format notes   IBM
Software   Proprietary
Start year
Number of records   9,000
Update period   Annually
Price/Charges   Subscription: US$710

Notes

Extra subscription options include: 'Rote Liste' (Bundesverband der Pharazeutischen Industrie eV) in German (US$155); 'Physician's Desk Reference' (Medical Economics Company) in English (US$710); 'Index Nominum' (Société Suisse de Pharmacie) in English (US$460); 'Breviaire Des Medicaments' (Documed) in French and German (US$460).

This database can also be found on:
MediROM
PharmaROM

Diogenes

Diogenes
FOI Services
Washington Business Information Inc

14:303. Master record

Database type   Bibliographic, Textual
Number of journals
Sources   Grey literature, laws/regulations, letters, newsletters, press releases, reports and speeches
Start year   Varies by source, earliest data from 1938
Language   English
Coverage   USA

Number of records   320,000+
Update size   –
Update period   Weekly

Keywords
Pharmaceutical Products; Drugs

Description
DIOGENES contains citations to unpublished US Food and Drug Administration (FDA) regulatory documents covering pharmaceuticals and over-the-counter drugs and medical devices (for example, sunlamps and pacemakers). It is made up of three major types of information:

(1) Unpublished Food and Drug Administration (FDA) documents acquired under the Freedom of Information Act. These documents include: Advisory Committee Minutes, Drug and Device Approval information, Regulatory Letters, Establishment Inspections Reports, Industry/FDA correspondence, and many others. Many of the more timely or substantive documents are included full-text online.
(2) Newsletters published by Washington Business Information Inc. and FDA. These include: *Washington Drug Letter, The GMP Letter, Washington Health Costs Letter, The Food & Drug Letter, Devices & Diagnostics Letter, The Drug Bulletin* and *The Radiological Health Bulletin* which are all online full-text.
(3) Other FDA documentation full-text online includes: Federal Register Notice summaries, complete listings of FDA-approved drugs and devices, Enforcement Reports, Medical Device Report incident summaries, press releases and talk papers.

The following publications are included in the database: (FT denotes full text; coverage and update schedule is given): *Advisory Committees* (ADV) – *Advisory Committee Minutes* (selected; as available); *Advisory Committee Manuscripts* (selected; as available). *Medical Devices* (DEV) – *FDA Premarket Approval List (PMAs)* (all, 1976+; quarterly); *FDA 510(k) List* (all, 1976+; quarterly); *Device Approvals* from *FDA Drug & Device Product Approvals* (all, 1984+; monthly); *Medical Device Reports (MDRs)* (FT; all, 1985+; quarterly); FDA Medical Devices Bulletin (FT; all, 1986+; irregularly, as published); FDA Radiological Health Bulletin (FT; all, 1986+; irregularly, as published); *Device Documentation (510(k) Notices)* (selected; as available); Device Documentation (PMA Summaries) (selected; as available). *Drug (DRG)* – FDA New Drug Application List (all, 1938+; quarterly); *Drug Approvals from FDA Drug & Device Product Approvals* (all, 1984+; monthly); *FDA Drug Bulletin* (FT; all, 1985+; irregularly, as published); *FOI Services Drug Documentation* (SBOAs, Reviews, etc.) (selected; as available). *Establishment Inspection Report* (EIR) – Establishment Inspection Reports (selected; as available). *Federal Register* (FED) – Federal Register Notice Summaries (FT; all, 1985+; weekly). *Guidelines* (GLS) – Guidelines (selected; as available). Letters, Meetings & Telecons (LTR & MTG) – Correspondence (selected; as available). Newsletter (NEW) – Newsletters (FT; all, 1981+; weekly). Press Releases & Talk Papers (PRL & TLP) – Press Releases (FT; all, 1984+; as available) and Talk Papers (FT; all, 1984+; as available). Speech (SPE) – Speeches (selected; as available). *Regulatory Action* (REG) – FDA Enforcement Report (FT; all, 1984+; weekly); *Warning (Regulatory) Letters* (FT; all, 1984+; weekly); *Recall Documentation* (selected; as available).

14:304. Online   BRS
File name	DIOG
Start year	Varies by source, earliest data from 1938
Number of records	320,000+
Update period	Weekly
Price/Charges	Connect time: US$104.00/114.00
	Online print: US$1.96/2.04
	Offline print: US$2.08
	SDI charge: US$6.50

14:305. Online   CompuServe Information Service
File name	IQUEST File 1945
Start year	Varies by source, earliest data from 1938
Number of records	
Update period	Weekly
Price/Charges	Subscription: US$8.95 per month
	Database entry fee: US$9/search; some databases carry a surcharge ($2–75)
	Online print: US$10 references free; then $9 per ten; abstracts $3 each

Downloading is allowed

Notes
Accessed via IQUEST, this database is offered by a BRS gateway. IQUEST can either search across all databases, a database of the user's choice or selected multiple databases.

14:306. Online   Data-Star
File name	DIOG
Start year	Unpublished documents 1976+; Newsletters 1981+; Drug approval listings 1938+;
Number of records	320,000+
Update period	Weekly
Database aids	Data-Star Biomedical Manual and Online Manual (search NEWS-DIOG in NEWS)
Price/Charges	Subscription: SFr80.00
	Connect time: SFr195.00
	Online print: SFr2.38
	Offline print: SFrNot applicable
	SDI charge: SFrNot applicable

Notes
From June 1993 Data-Star have introduced an annual fee/subscription per contract (that is, not per password) of SFr 80.00 (c.UK£ 32.00) payable every June. For North American customers billed in dollars who also use DIALOG, the DIALOG fee also covers access to Data-Star. Academic customers, 'commitment' customers and customers currently billed in dollars are exempt.

Record composition
Accession Number and Update Code; Advisory Committee/Speaker AU; Company Name CO; Descriptors DE; Drug/device number or FDA number NU; Generic/Trade/name/s PH; Occurence Paragraph OC; Publication Type PT; Source SO; Text TX; Title TI; Year YR; Year/month YM; Year/date YD; Year of publication or occurrence YR and Update Code UP

14:307. Online   DIALOG
File name	File 158
Start year	1976
Number of records	1,196,482
Update period	Weekly

Price/Charges
Connect time: US$129.00
Online print: US$2.25
Offline print: US$4.95
SDI charge: US$3.50

Notes

DIALINDEX Categories: BIOTECH, CHEMBUS, MEDENG, PHARMINA, PHARM, PHARMR, REGS.

Dosing & Therapeutic Tools
Micromedex Inc

14:308. Master record

Alternative name(s)
Computerized Clinical Information System: Dosing & Therapeutic Tools; CCIS: Dosing & Therapeutic Tools

Database type
Bibliographic, Factual, Textual, Directory, Numeric

Number of journals
Sources
Start year   1985
Language   English
Coverage   International
Number of records
Update size   —
Update period   Quarterly

Keywords

Clinical Medicine; Diagnosis; Drug Therapy; Drugs; Pharmaceuticals

Description

Contains a library of resources related to medical dosages and therapeutic tools.

Diagnostic and Therapeutic Pearls contains brief charts or tables of significant medical, pharmaceutical or toxicological information not readily available separately. Covers medical terms and jargon, abbreviations and statistics.

Differential Diagnostic Lists contains lists of possible causes (for example, disease, drug, toxic agent) of clinical signs or symptoms, or laboratory findings that enable health care officials to narrow the possible causes of a specific finding.

EKG Rhythm Strips contains EKG rhythm strips that represent one-lead electrocardiogram of various cardiac rhythms and their descriptions. EKG rhythm strips are used as a teaching tool for medical personnel to recognise irregularities in heartbeats. Users can compare any two EKG strips in the database.

Nomograms contains nomograms (charts and graphs) that show correlation of potential clinical outcome with plasma or serum drug levels in an overdose situation. Users can compare serum drug level obtained at a known time after ingestion with the nomogram to predict ther potential for development of toxicity. Nomograms are available for acetaminophen, ibuprofen and salicylates.

Drug Dosing contains software that can be used to calculate the dosage and administration of medication for a specific patient. Users can calculate adult or paediatric dosages for emergency drugs and for selected other drugs (Dobutamine, Dopamine, Ethanoi, Epinephrine, Lidocaine, N-Acetylcysteine, Nitroglycerin, Nitroprusside and Norephinephrine).

Calculators contains software that can be used to perform these calculations: alveolar-arterial oxygen gradient, anion gap, body weight and surface area, creatinine clearance, alcohols/ethylene glycol blodod level and SIU.

This database can be found on:
CCIS

DRI Health Care Cost Forecasting
Data Resources Inc (DRI)

14:310. Master record

Database type   Statistical
Number of journals
Sources   Databases
Start year   4-year forecasts, with historical series from 1976
Language
Coverage   USA
Number of records   100
Update size   —
Update period   Quarterly

Keywords

Health Care Costs; Medical Equipment; Pharmaceuticals

Description

Contains quarterly forecast indexes of United States health care costs. Covers labour, food, utilities, medical equipment, supplies, pharmaceuticals, physician services, and capital. Also provides forecasts of the 'market basket' indexes developed by the United States Health Care Financing Administration (HCFA) for hospitals, nursing homes, and home health-care agencies. Some series are available at a regional level.

Sources include DRI data banks and models, and the Health Care Financing Administration.

14:311. Online   Data Resources Inc (DRI)

File name
Start year   4-year forecasts, with historical series from 1976
Number of records   100
Update period   Quarterly

Notes

Subscription to DRI required.

Drug and Cosmetic Industry
Advanstar Communications

14:312. Master record

Database type   Textual, Factual
Number of journals   1
Sources   Journal
Start year   1989
Language   English
Coverage   International
Number of records
Update size   —
Update period   Monthly
Index unit   Articles and Reviews

Keywords

Beauty Care; Cosmetics; Marketing; Drugs; Packaging

Description

Written for executives and managers in the drug and cosmetic industry, this trade magazine covers the production, packaging, marketing, industry news and events for both manufacturers and distributors of drugs and cosmetics.

The editorial criteria for inclusion on the database are set by IAC and state all feature articles, DCI People and Compounders Corner will be included along with substantial editorial and industry related articles that are half a page or more in length plus book reviews of more than 200 words. Specifically excluded are international news, Washington Letter, articles without separate headlines and news in packaging.

14:313. Online   Mead Data Central (as a NEXIS database)

File name	DRGCOS – NEXIS
Start year	1989
Number of records	
Update period	Monthly
Price/Charges	Subscription: US$1,000 – 3,000 (Depending on needs) Connect time: US$49.00 (Telecomms + connect time) Database entry fee: US$6.00 (Search charge) Online print: US$0.04 per line

Notes

Libraries: CONSUM and NEXIS; Group files: ALLCON, COSM, RETAIL, MAGS, TRDTEC, CURRNT, ARCHIV, OMNI and ASAP.

On NEXIS, this publication is available as a part of ASAP Publications.

A subscription charge which covers all transactional charges, connect time, telecommunications and the small administration charge can take the place of the individual charges. Subscriptions are negotiated with customers and vary according to the number of menus (thus, files) that are to be used – typically a minimum subscription would be about US$ 1,000. All charges include training and a 24-hour help line.

Record composition

Publication PUBLICATION; Subject SUBJECT; Date DATE; Section SECTION; Terms TERMS; Type TYPE; Body BODY; Byline BYLINE; Company COMPANY; Geographic GEOGRAPHIC; Graphic GRAPHIC; Headline HEADLINE; Headline and Lead HLEAD; Lead LEAD; Length LENGTH; Name NAME and Product Name PRODUCT-NAME

This database can also be found on:
NEXIS

Drug Data Report
Prous Science Publishers

14:315. Master record

Database type	Chemical structures/DNA sequences
Number of journals	
Sources	
Start year	1989
Language	English
Coverage	

Number of records	45,000
Update size	10,000
Update period	Quarterly

Keywords

Drugs

Description

A comprehensive database containing chemical structures and textual information, including chemical name, biological action, generic names, trademarks and company codes, source, CAS Registry Number, patent numbers, titles, authors, and other bibliographic references, on more than 40,000 bioactive compounds appearing in Drug Data Report since 1989. Information is obtained from a very wide range of sources including patents from 10 different patent offices and through screening of 1,500 medical and science journals combined with proceedings and information from company communications. There is a backfile of records 1989 -1991.

Corresponds to the print *Drug Data Report*.

14:316. CD-ROM   Prous

File name	Drug Data Report
Format notes	IBM
Start year	1989
Number of records	45,000
Update period	Quarterly
Price	US$5,000

Notes

Drug Data Report on CD-ROM has been entirely prepared by Prous, not only in the compilation process but also in the development of the software used to access the data. Prous has developed a technique where, by treating chemical structures as a text language, text and images can be merged in the database. In this way, access time has been dramatically improved and the storage requirements have been reduced to allow records for the 45,000 presently held compounds to be stored on the CD-ROM.

14:317. Tape   Prous

File name	Drug Data Report
Format notes	IBM
Start year	
Number of records	43,000
Update period	Twice a year

Notes

Developed in conjunction with Molecular Design Ltd this is the magnetic tape version of the database in MDDR MACCS-II database format. It is available in both two-dimensional and three-dimensional versions.

Drug Information Fulltext
American Society of Hospital Pharmacists

14:318. Master record

Alternative name(s)	DIF
Database type	Textual, Directory, Bibliographic
Number of journals	
Sources	Journals, monographs and suppliers
Start year	Current information
Language	English
Coverage	USA

Number of records	50,000
Update size	–
Update period	Three times per year
Index unit	Articles and drug

Keywords

Chemical Substances

Description

Drug Information Fulltext contains the full text of about 1,400 monographs covering about 50,000 commercially available and experimental drugs in the United States, including selected investigational drugs and intravenous infusion solutions. Drug Information Fulltext is completely unbiased – the editors and reviewers have no connection or financial interest with the drugs discussed. Subjects covered include: uses, interactions, toxicity, cautions, concentration, pharmacology, pharmacokinetics, dosage, administration, chemistry, stability, adverse reactions, pharmacology, pharmakinetics and preparation information. information on unlabeled uses of drugs and the availability of investigational drugs is also included. The file also includes Chemical Abstracts Service Registry Numbers, trade names, manufacturers, and references to journal articles. A typical discussion of a drug incorporates information from more than a hundred references, while some incorporate as many as a thousand.

The file is recognised by the US government as a source of drug information for determining reimbursement of outpatient presecriptions under Medicaid.

The database corresponds to the printed *American Hospital Formulary Service Drug Information* which contains information on 1,000 drugs available commercially in the US and the *Handbook on Injectable Drugs* which covers 217 commercially available and 57 investigational drugs in use in the US, plus enhancements. References are available only online.

14:319. Online   BRS

File name	DIFT
Start year	
Number of records	
Update period	Three times per annum with annual reload
Price/Charges	Connect time: US$45.00/55.00 Online print: US$1.67/1.75 Offline print: US$0.42

Record composition

Access Number .AN.; Monograph Title .TI.; Generic Name .GN.; Trade Name .TN.; Manufacturer .TN.; Abbreviated Name .DI.; Synonyms .SY.; Investigational Name .DI.; Chemical Name .DI.; Molecular Formula .DI.; CAS Registry Number .RN.; AHFS Classification Name .TC.; AHFS Classification Number .TC.; Section Heading .SH.; Subsection Heading .SH.; Text .TX.; Text Primary .AB.; Text (Additional) .AT.; Tables .TA; Table Heading .TH.; References .CR.; Descriptor .DE.; Descriptor Code .DE. and Subfile .SO.

14:320. Online   Chemical Information Systems Inc (CIS)

File name	File 103
Start year	
Number of records	
Update period	

Notes

Annual subscription fee of $300 to CIS required.

Record composition

Access Number MN; Monograph Title MT; Generic Name MAT; Trade Name TM; Manufacturer TM; Abbreviated Name DDP; Synonyms SYN; Investigational Name IN; Chemical Name SYN; Molecular Formula MF; CAS Registry Number CAS; AHFS Classification Name AD; AHFS Classification Number AF; Section Heading US; Subsection Heading PK; Text; Text Primary; Text (Additional); Tables TA; Table Heading CP; References; Descriptor DE; Descriptor Code DE and Subfile BK

14:321. Online   CompuServe Information Service

File name	IQUEST File 1063
Start year	Current
Number of records	1,274
Update period	Quarterly
Price/Charges	Subscription: US$8.95 per month Database entry fee: US$9/search; some databases carry a surcharge ($2–75) Online print: US$10 references free; then $9 per ten; abstracts $3 each
Downloading is allowed	

Notes

Accessed via IQUEST, this database is offered by a DIALOG gateway. IQUEST can either search across all databases, a database of the user's choice or selected multiple databases.

Record composition

Access Number; Monograph Title MT; Generic Name GN; Trade Name TN; Manufacturer MN; Abbreviated Name TN; Synonyms SY; Investigational Name IN; Chemical Name CN; Molecular Formula MF; CAS Registry Number RN; AHFS Classification Name SH; AHFS Classification Number AH; Section Heading US; Subsection Heading SH; Text TX; Text Primary TX; Text (Additional) TX; Tables TA; Table Heading TX; References RF; Descriptor DE; Descriptor Code DC and Subfile SF

14:322. Online   DIALOG, Knowledge Index

File name	File 229
Start year	Current
Number of records	1,274
Update period	Quarterly
Price/Charges	Connect time: US$60.00 Online print: US$2.50 Offline print: US$2.50

Notes

This database is also available to home users during evenings and weekends at a reduced rate on the Knowledge Index service of DIALOG – file name in this case is MEDI8, and searches are made with simplified commands or menus.

Record composition

Access Number; Monograph Title MT; Generic Name GN; Trade Name TN; Manufacturer MN; Abbreviated Name TN; Synonyms SY; Investigational Name IN; Chemical Name CN; Molecular Formula MF; CAS Registry Number RN; AHFS Classification Name SH; AHFS Classification Number AH; Section Heading US; Subsection Heading SH; Text TX; Text Primary TX; Text (Additional) TX; Tables TA; Table Heading

TX; References RF; Descriptor DE; Descriptor Code DC and Subfile SF

DIALINDEX Categories: DRUGDIR, PHARM, PHARMR, RNMED, TOXICOL, TRADENMS.

14:323. Online
Mead Data Central (as a NEXIS database)

File name	DIF – NEXIS
Alternative name(s)	NEXIS – Drug Information Fulltext
Start year	
Number of records	
Update period	
Price/Charges	Subscription: US$1,000 – 3,000 (Depending on needs) Connect time: US$49.00 (Telecomms + connect time) Database entry fee: US$24.00 (Search charge) Online print: US$0.04 per line

Notes
Library GENMED.

This is a group file which includes both the American Hospital Formulary Service (AHFS) and Handbook on Injectable Drugs (HID) files.

A subscription charge which covers all transactional charges, connect time, telecommunications and the small administration charge can take the place of the individual charges. Subscriptions are negotiated with customers and vary according to the number of menus (thus, files) that are to be used – typically a minimum subscription would be about US$ 1,000. All charges include training and a 24-hour help line.

Record composition
Acute Toxicity ACUTE-TOX; AHFS Classification Descriptor AD; Additional Compatibility Data AD-COMPAT; Administration ADMINISTRATION; Classification Text AD-TEXT; AHFS Classification Number AF; Text Information ALL-TEXT; Abbreviated Name AR; Cautions CAUTIONS; Chemical Name CHEM-NAME; Chemical Stability CHEM-STABIL; Toxic Effects CHRONIC-TOX; AHFS Class Numbers CLASS; Chemical Name CN; Dosage Administration DOSAGE-ADMIN; Drug Interactions DRUG-INTER-ACT; Formula MF; General Information GENERAL-INFO; Interpretation INTERPRETATION; Compatibility COMPATIBILITY; Dosage DOSAGE; Investigative Drug Number INVEST-ID; Laboratory Test Interferences LAB-TEST-INTERF; Monograph Title MT; Drug Name NAME; CAS Registry Number RN; Additional Information OTHER-INFO; Pharmokinetics PHARMOKINETICS; Pharmacology PHARMACOLOGY; Products PRODUCTS; Primary Text PR-TEXT; Stability STABILITY; Synonyms SY; Tables TABLES and Drug Trade Name TM

14:324. Database subset
Online
Mead Data Central (as a NEXIS database)

File name	AHFS – NEXIS (American Hospital Formulary Service)
Start year	Current
Number of records	
Update period	Quarterly
Price/Charges	Subscription: US$1,000 – 3,000 (Depending on needs) Connect time: US$49.00 (Telecomms + connect time) Database entry fee: US$24.00 (Search charge) Online print: US$0.04 per line

Notes
Library: GENMED; Group file: DIF.

The AHFS file contains the full text of the most recent edition of the *American Hospital Formulary Service Drug Information*, a collection of drug monographs kept current by quarterly supplements and a complete revision of the master volume annually. The publication's purpose is to provide a comprehensive and authoritative source of evaluative drug information. The file is recommended or required standard reference for drug information by entities such as the US Public Health Service, the National Association of Board of Pharmacy, the Standard for Medicare and third-party health-care insurance providers. AHFS Drug Information contains a monograph on most drugs available in the United States. Each monograph text online is divided into two portions: primary text and additional text. The Primary Text contains basic information about the drug while the Additional Text provides in-depth discussion about various aspects of the drug.

A subscription charge which covers all transactional charges, connect time, telecommunications and the small administration charge can take the place of the individual charges. Subscriptions are negotiated with customers and vary according to the number of menus (thus, files) that are to be used – typically a minimum subscription would be about US$ 1,000. All charges include training and a 24-hour help line.

Record composition
Acute Toxicity ACUTE-TOX; AHFS Classification Descriptor AD; Classification Text AD-TEXT; AHFS Classification Number AF; Text Information ALL-TEXT; Abbreviated Name AR; Cautions CAUTIONS; Chemical Name CHEM-NAME; Chemical Stability CHEM-STABIL; Toxic Effects CHRONIC-TOX; AHFS Class Numbers CLASS; Chemical Name CN; Dosage Administration DOSAGE-ADMIN; Drug Interactions DRUG-INTER-ACT; Formula MF; General Information GENERAL-INFO; Interpretation INTERPRETATION; Investigative Drug Number INVEST-ID; Laboratory Test Interferences LAB-TEST-INTERF; Drug Name NAME; CAS Registry Number RN; Additional Information OTHER-INFO; Pharmokinetics PHARMOKINETICS; Pharmacology PHARMACOLOGY; Primary Text PR-TEXT; Synonyms SY; Tables TABLES and Drug Trade Name TM

The file can be searched using special Concept Codes/Descriptors or American Hospital Formulary Service Therapeutic classification Number/Descriptors. The Concept Codes are organised by a three-digit numeric code and a descriptor name; each sentence, or group of sentences, discussing the same concept has been indexed and assigned a code. Using these concept codes when searching provides more comprehensive results. Each tag (which appears in brackets within the text) represents a particular idea or concept. The drug monographs are also classified according to the AHFS Pharmacologic-Therapeutic Classification system which allows searches to be easily restricted to certain types of drugs.

14:325. Database subset
Online
Mead Data Central (as a NEXIS database)

File name	HID – NEXIS (Handbook on Injectable Drugs)
Start year	Current

Number of records	300
Update period	Quarterly
Price/Charges	Subscription: US$1,000 – 3,000
	(Depending on needs)
	Connect time: US$49.00
	(Telecomms + connect time)
	Database entry fee: US$24.00
	(Search charge)
	Online print: US$0.04 per line

Notes

Library: GENMED; Group file: DIF.

The Handbook of Injectable Drugs contains the full text of the most recent edition of the handbook produced by the American Society of Hospital Pharmacists' Special Projects Division. Its aim is to organise and summarise in a concise, standardised format the results of primary research on parenteral drug stability and compatibility. HIS covers 240 drugs as well as 58 investigational drugs.

A subscription charge which covers all transactional charges, connect time, telecommunications and the small administration charge can take the place of the individual charges. Subscriptions are negotiated with customers and vary according to the number of menus (thus, files) that are to be used – typically a minimum subscription would be about US$ 1,000. All charges include training and a 24-hour help line.

Record composition

AHFS Classification Descriptor AD; Additional Compatibility Data AD-COMPAT; Administration ADMINISTRATION; AHFS Classification Number AF; Chemical Name CHEM-NAME; AHFS Class Numbers CLASS; Compatibility COMPATIBILITY; Dosage DOSAGE; Generic Drug Name GN; Investigative Drug Number INVEST-ID; Monograph Title MT; Drug Name NAME; CAS Registry Number RN; Additional Information OTHER-INFO; Products PRODUCTS; Primary Text PR-TEXT; References REFERENCES; Stability STABILITY; Synonyms SY; Tables TA and Drug Trade Name TM

The file can be searched using special Concept Codes/Descriptors or American Hospital Formulary Service Therapeutic classification Number/ Descriptors. The Concept Codes are organised by a three-digit numeric code and a descriptor name; each sentence, or group of sentences, discussing the same concept has been indexed and assigned a code. Using these concept codes when searching provides more comprehensive results. Each tag (which appears in brackets within the text) represents a particular idea or concept. The drug monographs are also classified according to the AHFS Pharmacologic-Therapeutic Classification system which allows searches to be easily restricted to certain types of drugs.

This database can also be found on:
NEXIS
Drug Information Source CD

Drug Information Source CD
American Society of Hospital Pharmacists

14:327. Master record

CD-ROM	Compact Cambridge
Database type	Factual, Directory, Textual, Bibliographic
Number of journals	700 journals; 1,400 monographs.
Sources	Journals and Monographs

Start year	Monographs: current; citations: 1970.
Language	
Coverage	USA
Number of records	150,000 citations; 50,000 drugs.
Update size	—
Update period	Quarterly
Index unit	Drug and articles

Keywords
Drugs

Description

Contains three American Society of Hospital Pharmacists databases:

American Hospital Formulary Service Drug Information, which provides full-text information, from 1,400 monographs, on drug action, dosage, toxicity, interactions, side effects, cautions, interactions, adverse effects, chemistry, stability, pharmacology, pharmokinetics, and so on, relating to nearly 50,000 trade names, synonyms, and generic names. It covers practically every drug available in the USA. It also includes recommendations from leading health authorities such as the American Heart Association, National Institute of Health and the US Public Health Association.

International Pharmaceutical Abstracts, containing over 250,000 citations and abstracts on drug related subjects from over 800 international journals covering pharmaceutical literature since 1970; and

Handbook on Injectable Drugs, a directory of about 270 commercially available and investigational drugs, giving stability and compatibility information. The Handbook is said to be 'the most trusted reference' on commercial drugs used in admixtures and includes coverage of investigational drugs and infusion solutions.

Corresponds to the print: *Handbook on Injectable Drugs; International Pharmaceutical Abstracts; and American Hospital Formulary Service Drug Information*; and to the online databases: Drug Information Full Text; and International Pharmaceutical Abstracts.

Notes

One or all of the databases can be searched simultaneously in both command or menu mode. US$ 2,750 initial purchase, US$ 1,500 for renewal.

For more details of constituent databases, see:
Drug Information Fulltext
International Pharmaceutical Abstracts

Drug License Opportunities
IMS AG, International Services Division

14:329. Master record

Database type	Directory, Textual
Number of journals	
Sources	Patents
Start year	1977
Language	English
Coverage	International
Number of records	
Update size	—
Update period	Weekly

Keywords

Pharmaceutical Products; Pharmaceuticals; Therapeutic Drugs; Patents; Drugs

Description

One of the four files in the IMSworld Online Service Database, Drug License Opportunities contains information on therapeutic drugs under development or available for licensing worldwide. For each drug, the record includes phase of development, names (chemical, labcode, generic and brand), therapeutic class, pharmacological actions and indications, clinical details, formulations, patent, trademark, regulatory approval status, expected launch date, licensing availability and contact information for companies associated with the product.

Corresponds to *Drug License Opportunities*.

14:330. Online   IMS AG, International Services Division

File name	
Start year	1977
Number of records	
Update period	Weekly

Drug News & Perspectives
Prous Science Publishers

14:331. Master record

Database type	Textual
Number of journals	
Sources	
Start year	
Language	English
Coverage	
Number of records	
Update size	–
Update period	

Keywords

Drugs

14:332. CD-ROM   Prous

File name	Drug News & Perspectives
Format notes	IBM
Start year	
Number of records	
Update period	
Price/Charges	

Drug Patents International
IMSWorld Publications Ltd

14:333. Master record

Database type	Patents
Number of journals	
Sources	Patents
Start year	1987
Language	English
Coverage	International
Number of records	13,000
Update size	240 compounds
Update period	Monthly
Index unit	Patents

Keywords

Patents; Drugs; Pharmaceutical Products

Description

Provides evaluated product patent coverage for more than 750 drug molecules in drug patents, either marketed or in active R & D. Each entry comprises one patent in one country and includes drug name, synonyms, trade names, therapeutic class, compound name, CAS Registry Number, description, patent number, assignee, priority numbers and dates, publication date, patent country and estimated patent expiration dates. There is emphasis on the marketing aspects of the industry rather than the scientific aspects of other databases such as Current Patents. It has been designed to provide pharmaceutical executives with information about the patents that cover marketed single-entity drugs. Data is derived from searches of other databases to identify patents claiming a drug, the patent specification is 'evaluated' to determine the scope of its claims, and equivalent patents are found by consulting INPADOC and/or Derwent's patent family databases. The expiration date of the patent, with information about the availability of patent term extensions, is calculated for each patent, and the data is published in the printed Patents International. The data from the 1987–1989 publications were made available online in early 1991, with additional information to be added through monthly updates. The currency of database updates has nothing to do with the currency of the patents added to the file. Newly added records will cover additional drugs, and most drugs have already been patented by the time they are eligible for coverage by this database. It does not puropt to provide the entire patent status of the drug; comments on additional patent families are provided only as Notes and Comments in the record for the original patent on the drug. It does not provide the entire answer for most questions, but since most drugs are eventually covered by numerous patents on pharmaceutical compsitions and processes, it does have the information deemed most important by senior managers. Links generic drug names, laboratory codes and trade names to evaluated product patent families.

Corresponds to *Patents International*. Corresponds to one of the files available in IMSworld Online Service Database.

Although a record in this database relates to a patent, the title of the record is the generic name of the compound the patent covers provided in several official versions. The patent PN number can be searched in Derwent format or as the publication number independent of the ISO country code. For countries that grant patents after unexamined publication, both numbers are provided, but dates may not be provided for unexamined publications. The patent country can be searched by name or ISO code. Application dates are searchable, but the application serial number is not provided. Priority numbers and dates are provided, with the priority number searchable in Derwent format or as the serial number recorded from the patent. The name of the assignee and its country of residence can be searched, and the corporate producer of the marketed drug is indexed. It should be noted that the database producer does not identify producers other than the original marketer of the drug except when a licence agreement is noted in the Country Comments field or when patents belonging to other companies are discussed in the Notes field. Technical information about the patent is sparse. The type of patent claim, for example, product, process or product-by-procss, is reported. The CAS registry number of the compound is provided along with synonyms for its generic name , trade names, descriptors for the drug's activity, and IMSworld's therapeutic class codes. There is no title, abstract or claim text. The expected expiration date is given in the field. For most patents this data has been estimated, but some extended terms are noted. The availability of patent term extensions or imposition of licences of right is indicated where the patent law provides for them. IMSworld does not promise that the expiry date reflects the actual status of the patent. The expiry field is accessible online only to hardcopy subscribers, and thus others must obtain this information from other sources.

14:334. Online   IMSWorld Publications Ltd

File name   Drug Patents International
Start year   1987
Number of records   13,000
Update period   Monthly

Notes

Access to patent expiration data is restricted to subscribers to Patents International.

14:335. Online   ORBIT

File name   DPIN
Start year   Current
Number of records   13,000
Update period   Monthly
Database aids   Quick reference Guide (2/91) Free (single copy)

Notes

Access to patent expiration data is restricted to subscribers to Patents International. Electronic SDI service is now available within two hours on ORBIT. They can be downloaded and reformatted on a word processor. Results are retrieved in the low cost PRINTS file, $15 per connect hour.

Record composition

Accession Number – AN; Compound Name – NA; Patent Number – PN; Patent Country – PC; Priority Number and Date – PR; Patentee – PA; Country of Patentee Residence – AR; Corporate Producer – CP; Country Comments – CM; Notes – NO; Patent Claim Type – PT; CAS Registry Number – RN; Synonym for Generic Name – SY; Trade Names – TN; Descriptor for Drug Activity – DE; IMSworld Therapeutic Class Code – TC and Expected Exxpiration Date – EX

This database can also be found on:
IMSWorld Online Service

Drug Topics
Medical Economics Company Inc

14:337. Master record

Database type   Textual, Factual
Number of journals   1
Sources   Journal
Start year   1983
Language   English
Coverage   International
Number of records
Update size   –
Update period   Twice per week
Index unit   Articles

Keywords

Drugs; Health Care Products; Marketing

Description

Drug Topics is a trade magazine written for pharmacy professionals and retail, hospital and nursing home pharmacists. It contains articles that focus on health products, health care trends and the health care industry's marketing and legislative activity. Special feature articles cover drug research and developments, updates on disease detection testing and drug programmes.

14:338. Online   CompuServe Information Service

File name   IQUEST File 7134
Start year   1983
Number of records
Update period   Twice per week
Price/Charges   Subscription: US$8.95 per month
Database entry fee: US$9/search; some databases carry a surcharge ($2–75)
Online print: US$10 references free; then $9 per ten; abstracts $3 each
Downloading is allowed

Notes

Accessed via IQUEST, this database is offered by a DIALOG gateway; DIALOG mount the file as a part of the Trade and Industry ASAP database. IQUEST can either search across all databases, a database of the user's choice or selected multiple databases.

14:339. Online   Mead Data Central (as a NEXIS database)

File name   DRUGTP – NEXIS
Start year   1983
Number of records
Update period   Twice per week
Price/Charges   Subscription: US$1,000 – 3,000 (Depending on needs)
Connect time: US$49.00 (Telecomms + connect time)
Database entry fee: US$6.00 (Search charge)
Online print: US$0.04 per line

Notes

Libraries: CONSUM and NEXIS; Group files: ALLCON, COSM, MAGS, TRDTEC, CURRNT, ARCHIV, OMNI and ASAP.

On NEXIS, this publication is available as a part of ASAP Publications.

A subscription charge which covers all transactional charges, connect time, telecommunications and the small administration charge can take the place of the individual charges. Subscriptions are negotiated with customers and vary according to the number of menus (thus, files) that are to be used – typically a minimum subscription would be about US$ 1,000. All charges include training and a 24-hour help line.

Record composition

Publication PUBLICATION; Subject SUBJECT; Date DATE; Section SECTION; Terms TERMS; Type TYPE; Body BODY; Byline BYLINE; Company COMPANY; Geographic GEOGRAPHIC; Graphic GRAPHIC; Headline HEADLINE; Headline and Lead HLEAD; Lead LEAD; Length LENGTH; Name NAME and Product Name PRODUCT-NAME

This database can also be found on:
NEXIS

Drugab
Dalctraf HB
Swedish Council for Information on Alcohol and Other Drugs

14:341. Master record

Database type   Bibliographic
Number of journals
Sources   Journals

Start year	1980
Language	Original language, English keywords and English
Coverage	International
Number of records	13,500
Update size	–
Update period	Quarterly

Keywords

Drug Abuse; Alcohol Abuse

Description

Contains citations, with abstracts, to the Scandinavian and worldwide literature on alcohol and drug abuse. Covers diagnosis, education, epidemiology, legal and social aspects, medical complications, pharmacology, pharmacotherapy, prevention and control, psychotherapy, public policy, and rehabilitation. Items are grouped into three files.

Alconarc. Contains citations to all documents held by the Swedish Council for Information on Alcohol and Other Drugs library, indexed by *Medical Subject Headings (MeSH)*. Produced by the Swedish Council on Alcohol and Other Drugs.

Dalctraf. Contains citations, with abstracts, to the worldwide literature in the biomedical and social sciences on the incidence and impact of alcohol and drug use on road safety. Produced by Dalctraf.

Nordrug. Contains citations, with abstracts, to Scandinavian and selected worldwide scientific literature on alcohol and drug abuse. Produced by the Swedish Council on Alcohol and Other Drugs.

Scandinavian and worldwide literature.

14:342. Online — Swedish Council for Information on Alcohol and Other Drugs

File name	Drugab
Start year	1980
Number of records	13,500
Update period	Quarterly

For more details of constituent databases, see:
Nordrug
Alconarc
Dalctraf

Drugdex
Micromedex Inc

14:344. Master record

Alternative name(s)	Computerized Clinical Information System: Drugdex; CCIS: Drugdex
Database type	Factual, Textual, Directory
Number of journals	
Sources	Monographs
Start year	1974
Language	English
Coverage	USA (primarily) and International (some)
Number of records	61,000
Update size	–
Update period	Quarterly

Keywords

Drugs

Description

An unbiased and referenced drug information system containing three databases.

Drug Evaluations contains about 775 monographs, each on a particular drug. Each monograph covers one drug and includes summaries and reviews of the drug and drug use in the clinical setting, as well as information on dosage, pharmokinetics, cautions, clinical applications, drug-food interactions and disease states. Covers Federal Drug Administration approved, non-US and investigational drugs, plus OTC preparations. Also includes an adverse drug reactions index and a product trade name index

Drug Consults – contains over 5,300 patient-based consultations, case histories and documents from drug information centres and clinical pharmacological services worldwide. Includes pharmaceutical and clinical data on disease states, use of drugs and drug-related problems.

Drugdex Index – contains 55,000 listings by generic drug name, brand names and disease states, with secondary access through such topics as interactions, adverse side effects and clinical applications.

The data is indexed by: US and foreign brand/trade names; generic names; disease states; dosage; pharmokinetics; cautions; interactions; and clinical applications.

14:345. Tape — Micromedex Inc

File name	Drugdex
Alternative name(s)	Computerized Clinical Information System: Drugdex; CCIS: Drugdex
Software	Proprietary
Start year	1973
Number of records	61,000
Update period	Quarterly

Notes

Annual subscription to CCIS required. Martindale: the Extra Pharmacopoeia on CCIS and Identidex are available to subscribers of this database for an additional fee.

14:346. Database subset
Online — Mead Data Central (as a NEXIS database)

File name	EVAL – NEXIS
Alternative name(s)	Computerized Clinical Information System: Drugdex; CCIS: Drugdex
Start year	1974
Number of records	61,000
Update period	Quarterly
Price/Charges	Subscription: US$1,000 – 3,000 (Depending on needs) Connect time: US$49.00 (Telecomms + connect time) Database entry fee: US$24.00 (Search charge) Online print: US$0.04 per line

Notes

Library: GENMED; Group files: DRUGDX, MEDEX.

On NEXIS, Drugdex is divided into two files: Drug Evaluation Monographs (EVAL) and Drug Consults (CONSLT). The EVAL file contains the full text of the Drug Evaluation Monographs which are unbiased reviews providing specific information relevant to the clinical use of drugs and covering FDA-approved, investigational drugs, over-the-counter and non-US preparations. Professionals in clinical pharmacy, medicine and pharmacology who are actively involved clinical practice, teaching and research update the information every ninety days. Each evaluation contains discussion on dosage, adverse reactions, comparative efficacy and clinical applications. References and clinical studies from the world's medical literature are also included. Each evaluation contains a list of specific segments for that particular document. This list may be viewed by pressing the SEGMNTS key (.se command) and selecting OUTLINE.

A subscription charge which covers all transactional charges, connect time, telecommunications and the small administration charge can take the place of the individual charges. Subscriptions are negotiated with customers and vary according to the number of menus (thus, files) that are to be used – typically a minimum subscription would be about US\$ 1,000. All charges include training and a 24-hour help line.

Record composition

Drug Classification CLASS; Overview OVERVIEW; Dosage Information DOSE; Dosage Forms FORM; Storage STOR; Adult Dosage ADOSE; Pediatric Dose PDOSE; Pharmokinetics PKINET; Onset and Duration ONSET; Drug Concentration Levels CONC; Absorption, Distribution, Metabolism, Ecretion ADME; Cautions CAUT; Contraindications CONTR; Precautions PREC; Adverse Reactions ADR; Teratogenicity/Effects in Pregnancy TERAT; Drug Interactions INTERACT; Clinical Applications APPL; Monitoring Parameters MONIT; Patient Instructions INSTR; Place in Therapy THER; Therapeutic Indications INDIC; Comparative Efficacy EFFIC; Manufacturer Information MFR; Title of the Document NAME and References REFS

14:347. Database subset

Online	Mead Data Central (as a NEXIS database)
File name	CONSLT – NEXIS
Alternative name(s)	Computerized Clinical Information System: Drugdex; CCIS: Drugdex
Start year	1974
Number of records	61,000
Update period	Quarterly
Price/Charges	Subscription: US\$1,000 – 3,000 (Depending on needs) Connect time: US\$49.00 (Telecomms + connect time) Database entry fee: US\$24.00 (Search charge) Online print: US\$0.04 per line

Notes

Library: GENMED; Group files: DRUGDX, MEDEX.

On NEXIS, Drugdex is divided into two files: Drug Evaluation Monographs (EVAL) and Drug Consults (CONSLT). The CONSLT file contains the full text of Drugdex Drug Consults which are patient-related reference consultations answering specific questions regarding disease states, use of drugs and drug-related problems. The case histories and documents are gathered from major drug information centres and clinical pharmacology services throughout the world. In contrast to Drug Evaluations, Consults are individualised responses to a specific problem regarding the use of drugs, and providing more detailed information about the problem.

Each document consists of a single consultation article and accompanying index terms. Although there are occasional references to a drug by its trade name, most drug consults refer to a drug only by its generic name. Each consultation follows a specific format for ease of use and thoroughness and includes patient data, response, conclusion and references.

A subscription charge which covers all transactional charges, connect time, telecommunications and the

small administration charge can take the place of the individual charges. Subscriptions are negotiated with customers and vary according to the number of menus (thus, files) that are to be used – typically a minimum subscription would be about US\$ 1,000. All charges include training and a 24-hour help line.

Record composition

Title TITLE; Body of consult TEXT; Summary of Findings CONCLUSION and References REFS

This database can also be found on:
CCIS
NEXIS

Druginfo and Alcohol Use and Abuse

University of Minnesota, College of Pharmacy, Drug Information Services

14:349. Master record

Database type	Bibliographic
Number of journals	
Sources	Monographs, Journals, Conference proceedings, Handbooks and Grey literature
Start year	Druginfo: 1968; Alcohol Use and Abuse: 1968–1978
Language	English
Coverage	International
Number of records	
Update size	–
Update period	Quarterly
Index unit	Conference papers, articles, Book chapters and Guides

Keywords

Adolescents; Alcohol Abuse; Drug Abuse; Gerontology; Psychological Tests; Sociology

Description

Contains two files on alcohol and drug use/abuse that may be searched together or separately.

Druginfo. Contains citations, with abstracts, to monographs, journals, conference papers, instructional guides, and other materials that deal with the educational, sociological, medical, and psychological aspects of alcohol and drug use/abuse. As from 1980 this file also covers research and problems of alcohol use/abuse.

Alcohol Use/Abuse. Contains citations to journal articles, reprints, unpublished papers, and chapters from books relating to research into chemical dependency, including evaluations of treatments, family therapy, use of the Minnesota Multiphasic Personality Inventory and selected material dealing with the alcohol problems of adolescents and the elderly. File ends in 1978.

As from 1980, the Druginfo file also covers research and problems of alcohol use and abuse. On BRS there are three interrelated databases: DRSC covers the educational, sociological and psychological aspects of alcohol and drug use and abuse; HAZE includes material on treatment evaluation, chemical dependence, family therapy, the MMPI, and alcoholism among various populations; DRUG represents a combination of these two databases.

14:350. Online — BIOSIS Life Science Network

File name	
Start year	Druginfo: 1968; Alcohol Use and Abuse: 1968–1978
Number of records	
Update period	Four times per year
Price/Charges	Connect time: US$9.00
	Online print: US$6.00 per 10; 2.25 per abstract; 3.50 per full text article

Also available via the Internet by telnetting to LSN.COM.

Notes

On Life Science Network users can search this database or they can scan a group of subject-related databases. There is a charge of $2.00 per scan of subject-related databases. To search one database and display up to ten citations costs $6.00. Most charges are for information retrieved. There are no charges if there are no results and no charge to transfer results to a printer or diskette. Articles may also be ordered via an online document delivery request. A telecommunications software package is also available, costing $12.95, providing an automatic connection to Life Science Network for heavy users of the service, with capability to transfer to print or disk and customised colour options.

14:351. Online — BRS

File name	DRSC
Start year	Druginfo: 1968; Alcohol Use and Abuse: 1968–1978
Number of records	
Update period	Four times per year
Price/Charges	Connect time: US$53.00/63.00
	Online print: US$0.52/0.60
	Offline print: US$0.71

Notes

On BRS there are three interrelated databases: DRSC covers the educational, sociological and psychological aspects of alcohol and drug use and abuse. DRUG is a combination of DRSC and HAZE.

14:352. Online — BRS

File name	HAZE
Start year	
Number of records	
Update period	

Notes

On BRS there are three interrelated databases: HAZE includes material on treatment evaluation, chemical dependence, family therapy, the MMPI, and alcoholism among various populations. DRUG is a combination of DRSC and HAZE.

14:353. Online — BRS

File name	DRUG
Start year	
Number of records	
Update period	

Notes

On BRS there are three interrelated databases: DRSC covers the educational, sociological and psychological aspects of alcohol and drug use and abuse. DRUG is a combination of DRSC and HAZE.

14:354. Online — CompuServe Information Service

File name	IQUEST File 1206
Start year	1968
Number of records	
Update period	Quarterly
Price/Charges	Subscription: US$8.95 per month
	Database entry fee: US$9/search; some databases carry a surcharge ($2–75)
	Online print: US$10 references free; then $9 per ten; abstracts $3 each

Downloading is allowed

Notes

Accessed via IQUEST, this database is offered by a BRS gateway. IQUEST can either search across all databases, a database of the user's choice or selected multiple databases.

Drugline
Läkemedelsinformationscentralen, Huddinge sjukhus

14:355. Master record

Database type	Factual, Textual
Number of journals	
Sources	Request forms
Start year	1982
Language	Swedish, English (some) and English (indexing)
Coverage	International
Number of records	3,500
Update size	400
Update period	Quarterly
Index unit	Drug

Keywords

Clinical Pharmacology; Drugs; Drug Therapy

Description

A problem-oriented drug information data bank. The information is based on questions received and answers prepared by clinical pharmacologists and pharmacists at the Drug Information Center (DIC), a subunit of the Institution for Clinical Pharmacology, Karolinska Institute at Huddinge Hospital, Sweden. Clinical pharmacologists and pharmacists help by reviewing information from the medical literature and databases not readily available to community physicians. Clinical questions are personally answered by referenced reviews after a literature search. Most requests deal with adverse drug reactions, including safety of drug treatment during pregnancy or breast feeding. There are also questions concerning choice of drug, pharmacokinetics and drug interactions. Drugline was created in cooperation with the Medical Information Centre (MIC). The records include all data and text from the rquest forms, except names of requester and patient.

Previously produced by MIC/Karolinska Institute Library and Information Center.

Topics are indexed by *Medical Subject Headings (MeSH)*

14:356. Online — MIC/Karolinska Institute Library and Information Center (MIC KIBIC)

File name	DRUGLINE
Start year	1982

Number of records   3,500
Update period   Quarterly

Notes
Special conditions for use apply.

DrugNews
Adis International Ltd
Adis Press Ltd

14:357. Master record

Alternative name(s)	Adis DrugNews
Database type	Bibliographic, Textual
Number of journals	1,900
Sources	Journals, Press releases, Company reports, News reports, Market launches and Conferences
Start year	1983
Language	English
Coverage	International
Number of records	45,000
Update size	—
Update period	Daily
Thesaurus	Adis Drugs and Diseases Thesaurus
Database aids	Adis Drugs and Diseases Thesaurus, Auckland, Adis 1990

Keywords
Drugs; Drug Therapy; Biotechnology

Description
Adis DrugNews is the world's first daily updated clinical news service, to provide current information on the most significant clinical and therapeutic drug research, including product news, significant side effects or adverse reactions, competitor information, product launches and meeting reports. There are citations with evaluative summaries and highly current analyses of the literature on drugs, drug therapy, product introductions,biotechnology and adverse drug experience. The database contains the full text of the weekly publications *Inpharma and Reactions*, fortnightly *BioInpharma*, and unpublished news. Inpharma focuses on significant new findings in clinical pharmacology and therapeutics, highlighting new promotional directions, drug licensing opportunities and research developments. It also reports on the biotechnological advances in these areas. *BioInpharma* reports on the biotechnological advances in these areas. Reactions gives details of all adverse drug experiencess, overdose, abuse and dependence reports published in the international medical literature. 'First reports' and 'serious' drug reactions are highlighted to assist in regulatory and other reporting requirements. Evaluative summaries written by Adis' own scientific editors are included for most documents. Covers clinical pharmacology, therapeutics and biotechnology. Entries include drug generic and trade names, manufacturer, purpose and design of study and results.

Corresponds to *Inpharma and Reactions*. Over 1.800 major international medical and biomedical are routinely scanned, and concise, substantive summaries are prepared from those papers of clinical, marketing and strategic significance to the international pharmaceutical industry. Over 100 of the sources come from Japan alone. In addition, product news from press releases, company annual reports, market launches, conferences and other sources are included. US English is used up to the end of 1989, UK English is used from 1990 onwards. For a comprehensive search covering both periods it is recommended to use both.

Adis descriptor indexing is designed to highlight key article features by allocating drug or disease tags from the following lists (1) Drug Tags: abuse; antimicrobial activity; adverse reactions; drug interactions; general; overdose; pharmacodynamics; pharmacokinetics; therapeutic use; poisoning; diagnostic use; laboratory test modifications and (2) Disease Tags: assessment; contributory factors; diagnosis; drug-induced; epidemiology; general; management; pathogenesis; prevention; treatment; incidence. These tags are combined with descriptors in order to qualify the term. Adverse reaction tracking: all adverse reaction reports are flagged with ADR. Generic drugs names (INN/Adis preferred terms) are used. Trade names are only used in the text of Product Introductions and when specified in the original or press releases and summaries/citations.

14:358. Online   BRS

File name	ADNR
Alternative name(s)	Adis DrugNews
Start year	
Number of records	
Update period	Daily
Price/Charges	Connect time: US$104.00/114.00
	Online print: US$0.45/0.53
	Offline print: US$0.63

Notes
Drug tags and Disease tags are combined with descriptors in order to qualify the term. Adverse reaction tracking: all adverse reaction reports are flagged with ADR, in the HL field on BRS. First reports: FIRST ADJ REPORTS.HL.; Serious ADRs (FDA criteria): SERIOUS.HL.; and Product launches: LAUNCH ADJ RECORD:HL.

14:359. Online   BRS

File name	ADND
Alternative name(s)	Adis DrugNews
Start year	Current
Number of records	
Update period	Daily
Price/Charges	Connect time: US$104.00/114.00
	Online print: US$1.42/1.50
	Offline print: US$1.60

Notes
Drug tags and Disease tags are combined with descriptors in order to qualify the term. Adverse reaction tracking: all adverse reaction reports are flagged with ADR, in the HL field on BRS. First reports: FIRST ADJ REPORTS.HL.; Serious ADRs (FDA criteria): SERIOUS.HL.; and Product launches: LAUNCH ADJ RECORD:HL.

14:360. Online   BRS

File name	ADNC
Alternative name(s)	Adis DrugNews
Start year	Current
Number of records	
Update period	Daily
Price/Charges	Connect time: US$104.00/114.00
	Online print: US$1.42/1.50
	Offline print: US$1.60

Notes

Drug tags and Disease tags are combined with descriptors in order to qualify the term. Adverse reaction tracking: all adverse reaction reports are flagged with ADR, in the HL field on BRS. First reports: FIRST ADJ REPORTS.HL.; Serious ADRs (FDA criteria): SERIOUS.HL.; and Product launches: LAUNCH ADJ RECORD:HL.

14:361. Online   BRS

File name	ADZZ
Alternative name(s)	Adis DrugNews
Start year	1983
Number of records	45,000
Update period	Daily
Price/Charges	Connect time: US$104.00/114.00
	Online print: US$1.42/1.50
	Offline print: US$1.60

Notes

Drug tags and Disease tags are combined with descriptors in order to qualify the term. Adverse reaction tracking: all adverse reaction reports are flagged with ADR, in the HL field on BRS. First reports: FIRST ADJ REPORTS.HL.; Serious ADRs (FDA criteria): SERIOUS.HL.; and Product launches: LAUNCH ADJ RECORD:HL.

14:362. Online   CompuServe Information Service

File name	IQUEST File 2759
Alternative name(s)	Adis DrugNews
Start year	1983
Number of records	
Update period	Daily
Price/Charges	Subscription: US$8.95 per month
	Database entry fee: US$9/search; some databases carry a surcharge ($2–75)
	Online print: US$10 references free; then $9 per ten; abstracts $3 each

Downloading is allowed

Notes

Accessed via IQUEST, this database is offered by a Data-Star gateway. IQUEST can either search across all databases, a database of the user's choice or selected multiple databases.

Record composition

Accession Number and Update Code AN; Cited References CR; Date DA; Date of Entry; Descriptors DE; Month of Entry YM; Number of cited references NU; Occurrence OC; Source SO; Text TX; Title TI; Update Code and Year of Entry YR

14:363. Online   Data-Star

File name	ADNR
Alternative name(s)	Adis DrugNews
Start year	1983 – date less current month
Number of records	40,000+
Update period	Daily
Database aids	Data-Star Biomedical Manual, Berne, Data-star, 1990
Price/Charges	Subscription: SFr80.00
	Connect time: SFr175.00
	Online print: SFr2.28
	Offline print: SFr2.45
	SDI charge: SFr11.80

Notes

From June 1993 Data-Star have introduced an annual fee/subscription per contract (that is, not per password) of SFr 80.00 (c.UK£ 32.00) payable every June. For North American customers billed in dollars who also use DIALOG, the DIALOG fee also covers access to Data-Star. Academic customers, 'commitment' customers and customers currently billed in dollars are exempt.

Record composition

Accession Number and Update Code AN; Cited References CR; Date DA; Date of Entry; Descriptors DE; Month of Entry YM; Number of cited references NU; Occurrence OC; Source SO; Text TX; Title TI; Update Code and Year of Entry YR

Drug tags and Disease tags are combined with descriptors in order to qualify the term. Adverse reaction tracking: all adverse reaction reports are flagged with ADR, in the TI field on Data-Star. First reports: FIRST ADJ REPORTS.TI.; Serious ADRs (FDA criteria): SERIOUS.TI.; Product launches: LAUNCH ADJ RECORD:TI.

14:364. Online   Data-Star

File name	ADND
Alternative name(s)	Adis DrugNews
Start year	Daily news
Number of records	
Update period	Daily
Database aids	Data-Star Biomedical Manual, Berne, Data-star, 1990
Price/Charges	Subscription: SFr80.00
	Connect time: SFr175.00
	Online print: SFr2.28
	Offline print: SFr2.45
	SDI charge: SFr11.80

Notes

From June 1993 Data-Star have introduced an annual fee/subscription per contract (that is, not per password) of SFr 80.00 (c.UK£ 32.00) payable every June. For North American customers billed in dollars who also use DIALOG, the DIALOG fee also covers access to Data-Star. Academic customers, 'commitment' customers and customers currently billed in dollars are exempt.

Record composition

Accession Number and Update Code AN; Cited References CR; Date DA; Date of Entry; Descriptors DE; Month of Entry YM; Number of cited references NU; Occurrence OC; Source SO; Text TX; Title TI; Update Code and Year of Entry YR

Drug tags and Disease tags are combined with descriptors in order to qualify the term. Adverse reaction tracking: all adverse reaction reports are flagged with ADR, in the TI field on Data-Star. First reports: FIRST ADJ REPORTS.TI.; Serious ADRs (FDA criteria): SERIOUS.TI.; Product launches: LAUNCH ADJ RECORD:TI.

14:365. Online   Data-Star

File name	ADNC (Current news incl. ADND)
Alternative name(s)	Adis DrugNews
Start year	Current, including the ADND file, holding up to four weeks of data
Number of records	
Update period	Daily
Database aids	Data-Star Biomedical Manual, Berne, Data-star, 1990
Price/Charges	Subscription: SFr80.00
	Connect time: SFr175.00
	Online print: SFr2.28
	Offline print: SFr2.45
	SDI charge: SFr11.80

Notes

From June 1993 Data-Star have introduced an annual fee/subscription per contract (that is, not per password) of SFr 80.00 (c.UK£ 32.00) payable every June. For North American customers billed in dollars who also use DIALOG, the DIALOG fee also covers access to Data-Star. Academic customers, 'commitment' customers and customers currently billed in dollars are exempt.

Record composition

Accession Number and Update Code AN; Cited References CR; Date DA; Date of Entry; Descriptors DE; Month of Entry YM; Number of cited references NU; Occurrence OC; Source SO; Text TX; Title TI; Update Code and Year of Entry YR

Drug tags and Disease tags are combined with descriptors in order to qualify the term. Adverse reaction tracking: all adverse reaction reports are flagged with ADR, in the TI field on Data-Star. First reports: FIRST ADJ REPORTS.TI.; Serious ADRs (FDA criteria): SERIOUS.TI.; Product launches: LAUNCH ADJ RECORD:TI.

14:366. Online   Data-Star

File name	ADZZ
Alternative name(s)	Adis DrugNews
Start year	1983 to date
Number of records	40,000
Update period	Daily
Database aids	Data-Star Biomedical Manual, Berne, Data-star, 1990
Price/Charges	Subscription: SFr80.00
	Connect time: SFr175.00
	Online print: SFr2.28
	Offline print: SFr2.45
	SDI charge: SFr11.80

Notes

From June 1993 Data-Star have introduced an annual fee/subscription per contract (that is, not per password) of SFr 80.00 (c.UK£ 32.00) payable every June. For North American customers billed in dollars who also use DIALOG, the DIALOG fee also covers access to Data-Star. Academic customers, 'commitment' customers and customers currently billed in dollars are exempt.

Record composition

Accession Number and Update Code AN; Cited References CR; Date DA; Date of Entry; Descriptors DE; Month of Entry YM; Number of cited references NU; Occurrence OC; Source SO; Text TX; Title TI; Update Code and Year of Entry YR

Drug tags and Disease tags are combined with descriptors in order to qualify the term. Adverse reaction tracking: all adverse reaction reports are flagged with ADR, in the TI field on Data-Star. First reports: FIRST ADJ REPORTS.TI.; Serious ADRs (FDA criteria): SERIOUS.TI.; Product launches: LAUNCH ADJ RECORD:TI;

Drugs in Japan, 1991, 'Ethical Drugs' (Nihon Iyakuhin Shu)
Yakugyo Jiho Co Ltd
Japan Pharmaceutical Information Centre

14:367. Master record

Alternative name(s)	Ethical Drugs; Nihon Iyakuhin Shu
Database type	Directory, Textual
Number of journals	
Sources	
Start year	
Language	Japanese
Coverage	Japan
Number of records	
Update size	—
Update period	Annually

Keywords

Drugs; Pharmaceuticals

Description

A drug information sourcebook, covering all drugs listed on the *Japanese Drug Tariff*.

Equivalent to print *Nihon Iyakuhin Shu*.

14:368. CD-ROM   Yakugyo Jiho Co Ltd

File name	Drugs in Japan, 1991, 'Ethical Drugs' (Nihon Iyakuhin Shu)
Alternative name(s)	Ethical Drugs; Nihon Iyakuhin Shu
Format notes	NEC
Start year	
Number of records	
Update period	Annually

Drugs of the Future
Prous Science Publishers

14:369. Master record

Database type	Chemical structures/DNA sequences
Number of journals	
Sources	
Start year	
Language	English
Coverage	
Number of records	
Update size	—
Update period	

Keywords

Drugs

Description

This is a database covering medicinal chemistry and paharmacology.

14:370. CD-ROM   Prous

File name	Drugs of the Future
Format notes	IBM
Start year	
Number of records	
Update period	
Price/Charges	

Drugs of Today
Prous Science Publishers

14:371. Master record

Database type	Chemical structures/DNA sequences
Number of journals	
Sources	
Start year	
Language	English
Coverage	
Number of records	
Update size	–
Update period	

Keywords

Drugs

Description

A medicinal chemistry/pharmacology database.

14:372. CD-ROM   Prous

File name	Drugs of Today
Format notes	IBM
Start year	
Number of records	
Update period	
Price/Charges	

DSI
Dansk Sygehus Institut

14:373. Master record

Alternative name(s)	Dansk Sygehus Institut
Database type	Bibliographic
Number of journals	
Sources	Books, Reports and Journals
Start year	1977
Language	Danish
Coverage	
Number of records	18,000
Update size	–
Update period	Daily
Index unit	Articles

Description

DSI contains references to literature on hospitals, nursing and health services. Disciplines covered are: Medicine, nursing, pharmacology, economics, management, building, technology, law, sociology etc. Document types indexed are: books, reports, serials and articles.

14:374. Online   DSI

File name	DSI
Alternative name(s)	Dansk Sygehus Institut
Start year	1977
Number of records	18,000
Update period	Daily

East European Chemical Monitor
Business International Corporation

14:375. Master record

Alternative name(s)	EECM
Database type	Bibliographic, Textual
Number of journals	
Sources	News bureaux, Newspapers, Journals, Trade press, Correspondents and Statistical reports
Start year	1984
Language	English
Coverage	Yugoslavia and Soviet-bloc
Number of records	12,000
Update size	3,000
Update period	Monthly

Keywords

Agrochemicals; Chemical Industry; Chemical Substances; Cosmetics; Petrochemicals; Pharmaceutical Industry; Plastics; Rubber Technology; Surface Coatings

Description

Contains citations, with abstracts, and some full-text translations of Eastern European periodical literature on the pharmaceutical and chemical industries. Includes company information, market information, new capacity, details on new products in the chemical industry sector for East-Europe.

It is arranged in six groups and a general section:

General – this section contains all items which refer to trends or output in the chemical industry as a whole. It also contains material which spans several categories at once.

Basics and General – contains material on organics, inorganics, base chemicals, reagents and chemical auxiliaries, including tanning agents, dyes, paints, photographic chemicals and so on.

Agrochemicals – covers material on oil, gas and coal processing, together with material on petrochemicals and downstream products.

Plastics and Rubber – items on plastics, synthetic resins, synthetic rubber and products manufactured from plastics and rubber.

Chemical Fibre – contains material on chemical and synthetic fibres and filaments, both on their production and use in the textile industry.

Pharmaceuticals – items on the production of medicines, cosmetics, soaps and detergents as well as occasional items on biotechnology and animal food products.

Petrochemicals – contains material on oil, gas and coal processing, together with material on basic petrochemicals and downstream products.

Data are collected from the East European popular, commercial and trade press in Russian, Serbo-Croat, Slovenian, Hungarian, Czech, Slovak, Polish, German, Bulgarian and Romanian. Primary sources are eighty-five cyrillic-language (as above) news sources, including newspapers such as *Pravda, Izvestiya, Ekonomicheskaya Gazeta* from the Soviet Union; *Maly Rocznik Statystyczny* from Poland; *Plaste und Kautschuk* from the Democratic Republic of

Germany; *Rude Pravo* from Czechoslovakia) and news agencies (for example, TASS, from the Soviet Union; Tanjug, from Yugoslavia; PAP, from Poland; CTK, from Czechoslovakia). Approximately 100 sources are scanned, of which 80% are newspapers, 8% periodials, 8% statistical sources and 4% material received from correspondents (source: TV, radio, interviews, etc.) Corresponds to *East European Monitor: The Chemical Industry, a Monthly Report on Chemicals and Related Industries in Eastern Europe.*

Cyrillic-language news sources.

14:376. Online   Data-Star

File name	EECM
Alternative name(s)	EECM
Start year	1984
Number of records	12,000
Update period	Monthly
Database aids	Data-Star Chemical Manual, Berne, Data-Star, 1989 and Online Manual (search NEWS-EECM in NEWS)
Price/Charges	Subscription: UK£32.00
	Connect time: UK£88.40
	Online print: UK£0.44
	Offline print: UK£0.54

Notes

From June 1993 Data-Star have introduced an annual fee/subscription per contract (that is, not per password) of SFr 80.00 (c.UK£ 32.00) payable every June. For North American customers billed in dollars who also use DIALOG, the DIALOG fee also covers access to Data-Star. Academic customers, 'commitment' customers and customers currently billed in dollars are exempt.

Easy Vet
IMS America Ltd, Hospital/Laboratory/Veterinary Database Division

14:377. Master record

Database type	Statistical, Textual
Number of journals	
Sources	Journal
Start year	1982
Language	English
Coverage	USA
Number of records	21,000
Update size	—
Update period	Quarterly

Keywords

Animal Health Care Products; Drugs; Pharmaceutical Industry; Pharmaceutical Products; Veterinary Science

Description

Contains time series on sales of animal health-care products. Includes pharmaceuticals, biologicals, and diagnostic aids purchased for therapy, diagnosis, and health maintenance. Provides estimated total national sales and breakdowns of sales by veterinarians, drug stores, livestock supply stores, farming cooperatives,

poultry owners, feed lots, feed mills, and feed manufacturers.

Corresponds to *US Pharmaceutical Market: Animal and Poultry.*

14:378. Online   IMS America Ltd

File name	
Start year	1982
Number of records	21,000
Update period	Quarterly

Notes

Subscription to *US Pharmaceutical Market: Animal and Poultry* required.

Electronic Library of Medicine
Little, Brown and Company

14:379. Master record

Database type	Factual
Number of journals	
Sources	Books
Start year	
Language	
Coverage	
Number of records	
Update size	—
Update period	Quarterly

Keywords

Drugs; Pharmaceuticals

Description

Contains diagnostic and therapeutic information for some thirteen medical disciplines. Also includes volume one of the *US Pharmacopoetal Drug Information.*

14:380. CD-ROM   Little, Brown and Company

File name	Electronic Library of Medicine
Format notes	IBM
Software	Proprietary
Start year	
Number of records	
Update period	Quarterly

EMBASE
Elsevier Science Publishers

14:381. Master record

Alternative name(s)	Excerpta Medica
Database type	Bibliographic
Number of journals	4,700
Sources	Case studies, clinicians, journals, monographs, research communications, reviews, surveys and symposia
Start year	1974
Language	English
Coverage	International

Number of records	4,950,000+
Update size	350,000
Update period	Weekly
Index unit	Articles
Abstract details	Adaptations of the authors' summaries and selected on the basis of content and length by an international group of practicing medical and other qualified specialists and when necessary modified, shortened or extended to obtain the optimal information value. A group of over 2,000 biomedical specialists assists with the preparation of abstracts in particular subject areas and articles in non-Western European languages
Thesaurus	EMTREE Thesaurus METAGS
Database aids	Guide to the Classification and Indexing System, MALIMET (available online and on microfiche), Mini-Malimet, MECLASE Drug Trade Names (DN) and EMBASE List of Journals Abstracted

Keywords

HIV; Anaesthesia; Anatomy; Anthropology; Bioengineering; Biotechnology; Cancer; Cardiology; Clinical Medicine; Clinical Neurology; Cosmetics; Drugs; Environmental Health; Environmental Pollution; Environmental Toxicology; Epilepsy; Food Additives; Food Contaminants; Forensic Medicine; Forensic Science; Gastroenterology; Gynaecology; Immunology; Industrial Medicine; Nephrology; Neuroscience; Neuromuscular Disorders; Nuclear Medicine; Obstetrics; Occupational Health and Safety; Patents; Pathology; Pharmaceuticals; Pollution; Public Health; Radiology; Toxic Substances; Waste Management

Description

EMBASE is the trademark for the English language Excerpta Medica database. Excerpta Medica was founded as a non-profit making organisation in 1946 with the goal of improving the availability and dissemination of medical knowledge through the publication of a series of abstract journals. The database contains citations, with abstracts, to the worldwide biomedical literature on human medicine and areas of biological sciences related to human medicine with an emphasis on the pharmacological effects of drugs and chemicals. The four main categories of primary literature sources are: specialist medical publications; general biomedicine publications; specialist non-medical publications and general scientific publications. Subjects covered include: anatomy; anesthesiology (including resuscitation and intensive care medicine); anthropology; pharmacology of anesthetic agents, spinal, epidural and caudal anesthesia and acupuncture (as anesthetic); autoimmunity; biochemistry; bioengineering; cancer; dangerous goods; dermatology; developmental biology; drug adverse reactions; drug dependence; drug effects; endocrinology; environmental health and pollution control (covering chemical pollution and its effect on man, animals, plants and microorganisms; measurement, treatment, prevention and control); exocrine pancreas; forensic science; gastroenterology (including diseases and disorders of: digestive systems; mouth; pharynx and more); genetics; gerontology and geriatrics; health economics; hematology; hepatobiliary system; hospital management; immunology (including immunity; hypersensitivity; histocompatibility and all aspects of the immune system); internal medicine; legal and socioeconomic aspects; mesentary; meteorological aspects; microbiology; nephrology (covering diagnosis; treatment; epidemiology; prevention; infections; glomerular and tubular disorders; blood purification; dialysis; kidney transplantation; toxic nephropathy and including important clinical abstracts with epidemiological studies and major clinical trials, with particular emphasis on hypertension and diabetes); neurosciences (especially clinical neurology and neurosurgery, epilepsy and neuromuscular disorders but also covering non-clinical articles on neurophysiology and animal models for human neuropharmacology); noise and vibration; nuclear medicine; obstetrics and gynaecology (including endocrinology and menstrual cycle, infertility, prenatal diagnosis and fetal monitoring, anti-conceptions, breast cancer diagnosis, sterilisation and psychosexual problems and neonatal care of normal children); occupational health and industrial medicine; opthalmology; otorhinolaryngology; paediatrics; pathology (including general pathology and organ pathology, pathological physiology and pathological anatomy, as well as laboratory methods and techniques used in pathology. General pathology topics range from cellular pathology, fetal and neonatal pathology, including congenital disorders, injury (both chemical and physical), inflammation and infection, immuno-pathology, collagen diseases and cancer pathology); peritoneum; pharmacology (including the effects and use of all drugs; experimental aspects of pharmacokinetics and pharmacodynamics; drug information); physiology; psychiatry and psychology (including addiction; alcoholism; sexual behaviour; suicide; mental deficiency and the clinical use or abuse of psychotropic and psychomimetic agents); public health; radiation and thermal pollution; radiology (including radiodiagnosis, radiotherapy and radiobiology, ultrasound diagnosis, thermography, adverse reactions to radiotherapy and techniques and apparatus, radiobiology of radioisotopes, aspects of radiohygiene, new labelling techniques and tracer applications); rehabilitation; surgery; toxicology (including pharmaceutical toxicology; foods, food additives, and contaminants; cosmetics, toiletries, and household products; occupational toxicology; waste material in air, soil and water; toxins and venoms; chemical teratogens, mutagens, and carcinogens; phototoxicity; regulatory toxicology; laboratory methods and techniques; and antidotes and symptomatic treatment); urology; wastewater treatment and measurement. The database is particularly strong in drug-related literature, where records include manufacturers and drug trade names and generic names. Information on veterinary medicine, nursing and dentistry is generally excluded.

Excerpta Medica is extremely current as articles are indexed within thirty days of receipt and are online very soon after that. Approximately 900 journals (the Rapid Input Processing (RIP)) are processed with priority which means that within eleven weeks of the receipt of the original document, the completely-indexed records are available. More than 100,000 records are given this priority treatment. Some hosts have companion databases giving training or details of the indexing vocabularies and thesauri.

EMBASE concentrates on journal articles although about 1,000 books per annum were indexed between 1975 and 1980. The source journals include all forty-six sections of *Excerpta Medica*, the *Drug Literature Index* and *Adverse Reactions Titles*. New titles are added and old titles deleted at a rate of about 200–300 per year. The database covers sources from 110 countries with the following geographical scope: North

America 36%, Western Europe 35%, United Kingdom 14%, USSR and Eastern Europe 7%, Asia 6%, Central and South America 1%, Austalia & South Pacific 1%, Africa and Middle East 1%. Approximately 50% of the citations are from drug and pharmaceutical literature and approximately 40% of citations added to the database each year do not appear in the corresponding printed abstract journals and indexes. Approximately 65% of the citations contain abstracts of on average 200 words with a maximum of 800 words which indicate the content of the articles and are not intended to summarise the results or express opinions. This makes free-text searching of the abstracts, titles and other searchable elements of the citation valuable. This compares with approximately sixty-five per cent of the records in MEDLINE and fifty-four per cent in BIOSIS. The records of the other leading bioscience database, SciSearch, now do contain abstracts. Approximately 75% of the articles are in the English language. Of the other leading bioscience databases, approximately eighty-eight per cent of articles on SciSearch are in English, eighty-six per cent of articles on BIOSIS and seventy-four per cent on MEDLINE. In addition approximately thirty-seven per cent of records with non-English sources contain English-language abstracts online. This compares with sixty-seven per cent on BIOSIS and twenty-six per cent on MEDLINE. SciSearch does now contain abstracts. Important publications NOT indexed in EMBASE include *Meyler's Side Effects of Drugs*, 1972–1980 published by Excerpta Medica and *Side Effects of Drugs Annual*, 1981 to the present, published by Elsevier.

A core collection of 3,500 biomedical journals supplemented by journals in the areas of agriculture, technology, economics, chemistry, environmental protection and sociology. General criteria used for selection are first that the document should be of potential relevance to medicine and secondly the information should be of lasting value for which reasons news items and comments are generally excluded.

EMBASE section headings are based on medical specialities; a total of forty-seven subfiles group together citations on topics such as anatomy, paediatrics, opthalmology, gastroenterelogy, cancer, plastic surgery, occupational health. Each subfile or section has its own hierarchical scheme. The thesaurus *MALIMET (Master List of Medical Terms)* is used which contains more than 250,000 preferred terms and 255,000 synonyms which are mapped to the preferred terms when used. It is used for indexing highly specific concepts such as names of drugs and chemicals; diseases and syndromes; anatomical and physiological aspects and diagnostic and therapeutic methods. *MALIMET* is growing at a rate of over 12,000 descriptors per annum, mainly through drug names and names of chemical compounds. The size of the complete *MALIMET* thesaurus for EMBASE (more than 250,000 preferred terms compared to 15,000 in MeSH) may indicate its tendency to provide a greater variety of possible terms and therefore, less consistent application in indexing. In 1993, all non-drug *MeSH* terms were included in the thesaurus mapped to *MALIMET* terms so that a search strategy can be transferred from MEDLINE.

Indexing incorporates the following rules: natural word order (acute leukemia, not leukemia acute); American spelling (tumor, not tumour), singular noun forms and not plural or adjectival forms (stomach tumor, not gastric tumors, but optic nerve, not eye nerve); the most specific term must be used. Since 1979,

MALIMET terms have been weighted. Class A terms (weighted) indicate the main concepts while Class B terms (not weighted) indicate the less important concepts of a document. In addition to *MALIMET* broad concepts are indexed with EMCLAS and EMTAGS. EMCLAS is a poly-hierarchical decimal classification scheme of the forty-six subject subfiles which make up the sections of the printed Excerpta Medica containing approximately 6,500 entries. It is then further subdivided into a five level hierarchy of sub-categories. Indexing is performed by medical specialists and scientists whose specialism corresponds to the subject areas forming the major subdivisions of EMCLAS. The indexing builds up sequentially as the article is indexed by each of the sections for which it is relevant. On average each document is indexed for 3.5 different sections.

EMTAGS is a group of approximately 220 codes which represent general concepts such as groups, gender, organ systems, experimental animals and article type. In January 1991 about 10% of the terms were changed including important descriptors such as CANCER or BENIGN NEOPLASM.

EMBASE editors also add 'uncontrolled' drug terms to augment MALIMET descriptors in selected records. EMBASE provides a hierarchical classification system (EMTREES) reflecting fifteen broad facets of biomedicine. From January 1991 a new version of EMTREE went online comprising 35,000 terms. New descriptors and changes in the hierarchy were made in the following areas: anatomy of the eye; diseases; drugs; techniques; biological phenomea and document types. Prior to 1988 Section Headings based on medical speciality areas were used instead of EMTREES to index EMBASE citations. In both classification schemes, codes are constructed to facilitate broad concept retrieval through truncation. In addition three uncontrolled vocabularies are used: Medical Secondary Text; Drug (Trade Names) and Manufacturers' Names are used. Medical Secondary Text consists of free-text words, numbers and phrases, describing concepts which are not fully covered by the controlled terms, for example quantiative information such as the number of patients or experimental animals. Drug (Trade) Names consists of trade names of drugs referred to in an original document with the main aspect of biological effects of compounds listed. Manufacturers' Names lists the names of drug manufacturers. The value of controlled indexing is important when searching for topics where a subject population has been specified.

Relatively few bioscience databases provide consistent indexing for subject populations (that is, humans or specific test animals) and related characteristics commonly requested such as age groups, gender, occupation and racial or ethnic groups. EMBASE provides extensive consistent indexing for the identification of test animals and age groups with a less consistent approach for the indexing of humans, occupational groups, racial/ethnic groups and gender. In addition, in most bioscience files a form of pharmaceutical nomenclature exists. For EMBASE the preferred search terms are generic name, classification by action/use and CAS Reigstry Number although restrictions by date, subfile and vendor may apply to the latter and vendor documentation should be consulted for guidelines. The search terms Enzyme Commission Number, investigational code, chemical name and trade name should be cross-referenced to the preferred terminology in the thesaurus. In 1993, improved CAS Registry Numbers mean that there is a single Number assigned for every substance.

14:382. Database subset
Online   AMA/NET

File name	AMA/NET Empires
Alternative name(s)	Excerpta Medica
Start year	1984
Number of records	
Update period	Weekly

Notes

AMA/NET Empires contains citations, with some abstracts, to articles in key clinical journals. Articles are coded by medical specialty. Citations include full bibliographic information, subject indexing, drug terminology and drug manufacturers. The source of the database is EMBASE. A subscription fee of $30 for members or $50 for non-members of AMA/NET required.

14:383. Database subset
Online   BRS, BRS/Colleague

File name	EMDR
Alternative name(s)	Excerpta Medica
Start year	1974
Number of records	700,000
Update period	Weekly
Price/Charges	Connect time: US$62.00/90.00
	Online print: US$0.60/0.68
	Offline print: US$0.68

Notes

This database is a subset of EMBASE. EMBASE Drug Information contains citations, with abstracts, to the worldwide literature on therapeutic drugs. It covers development, applications, interactions, adverse effects, and toxicity and includes manufacturers, drug trade and generic names. BRS is the only host to provide full journal titles.

Record composition

EMTREE Term .DE.; Explosion term; Explosion code; Descriptor .DE.; Single-word term .SJ,SN.; Link Subheading AE; EMTAG Code .ii.; EMCLAS 37 .CC.; EMCLAS Section Heading .MC.; CAS Registry Number .RN.; Title .TI.; Title (Non-English) .TT.; Abstract .AB.; Manufacturer's Name .MF.; Trade Name .TN.; Author .AU.; Author Address .IN.; Author Country .IN.; Journal Abbreviation .SO.; Coden .CD.; ISSN .CD.; Country of Publication .CP.; Year of Publication .YR.; Language .LG.; Summary Language .LS.; EMBASE Accession Number .AN. and Update Year and Week .UP.

Hedges or limit capability is available to limit to human and/or full text in CCML.

14:384. Database subset
Online   DIMDI

File name	E274 – EMDRUGS
Alternative name(s)	Excerpta Medica
Software	GRIPS
Start year	1974
Number of records	1,583,665
Update period	Weekly
SDI period	1 week
Database aids	User Manual EMBASE and Memocard EMBASE
Price/Charges	Connect time: UK£11.66–23.56
	Online print: UK£0.41–0.59
	Offline print: UK£0.34–0.41
Thesaurus is online	

Notes

This is a subfile of EMBASE. EMDRUGS contains citations to the worldwide literature on drugs. It corresponds to the 'Pharmacology', 'Drug Literature Index', and 'Adverse Reactions Titles' sections of Excerpta Medica, and to citations from those sections contained in EMBASE. Approximately 58% of the records contain abstracts. The corresponding file E283 contains records covering the period 1983 to date. Searches are possible from January 1974. The EMBASE subfiles have different groupings for costing – EMDRUGS is in Group 2.

Record composition

Abstract AB; Abstract Language AL; ADONIS Number ANR; Author AU; Classification Code CC; Conference CF; Coden CO; CAS-Reg No CR; Corporate Source CS; Controlled Terms CT; Qualifier /QF; Weighting /W1; Country CY; Drug Trade Name DN; Document Name DT; EMCLAS Code EC; Entry Date ED; Editor EDR; EMCLAS Term ET; EMTAGS-Code IC; EMTAGS-Term IT; CY/JT JC; Journal Title JT; Language LA; Manufacturer's Name MN; Number of Document ND; Publisher PU; Publication Year PY; Qualifier QF; ISBN-NO SB; Source SO; ISSN-NO and Title TI

Hedges or limit capabilities are provided to limit to (pps=) human; adverse drug reactions; AIDS; animals, birds; animals, cold-blooded; animals, vertebrate; cancer; developing countries; and ecotoxicity. The basic Index includes the data fields: Abstract, Controlled Term, Drug Trade Name, EMTAGS-Term, Manufacturer's Name, Title. EMDRUGS is defined as subfile to EMBASE with: FIND EC DOWN (30;37;38).

14:385. Database subset
Online   DIMDI

File name	E283 – EMDRUGS
Alternative name(s)	Excerpta Medica
Software	GRIPS
Start year	1983
Number of records	810,882
Update period	Weekly
SDI period	1 week
Database aids	User Manual EMBASE and Memocard EMBASE
Price/Charges	Connect time: UK£11.66–23.56
	Online print: UK£0.41–0.59
	Offline print: UK£0.34–0.41
Downloading is allowed	
Thesaurus is online	

Notes

This is a subfile of EMBASE. EMDRUGS contains citations to the worldwide literature on drugs. It corresponds to the 'Pharmacology', 'Drug Literature Index', and 'Adverse Reactions Titles' sections of Excerpta Medica, and to citations from those sections contained in EMBASE. Approximately 61% of the records contain abstracts. The corresponding file E274 contains records covering the period 1974 to date. The EMBASE subfiles have different groupings for costing – EMDRUGS is in Group 2.

Record composition

Abstract AB; Abstract Language AL; ADONIS Number ANR; Author AU; Classification Code CC; Conference CF; Coden CO; CAS-Reg No CR; Corporate Source CS; Controlled Terms CT; Qualifier /QF; Weighting /W1; Country CY; Drug Trade Name DN; Document

Name DT; EMCLAS Code EC; Entry Date ED; Editor EDR; EMCLAS Term ET; EMTAGS-Code IC; EMTAGS-Term IT; CY/JT JC; Journal Title JT; Language LA; Manufacturer's Name MN; Number of Document ND; Publisher PU; Publication Year PY; Qualifier QF; ISBN-NO SB; Source SO; ISSN-NO and Title TI

Hedges or limit capabilities are provided to limit to (pps=) human; adverse drug reactions; AIDS; animals, birds; animals, cold-blooded; animals, vertebrate; cancer; developing countries; and ecotoxicity. The basic Index includes the data fields: Abstract, Controlled Term, Drug Trade Name, EMTAGS-Term, Manufacturer's Name, Title. EMDRUGS is defined as subfile to EMBASE with: FIND EC DOWN (30;37;38).

14:386. Database subset
Online
DIMDI

File name	E474 – EMTOX
Alternative name(s)	Excerpta Medica
Software	GRIPS
Start year	1974
Number of records	402,514
Update period	Weekly
SDI period	1 week
Database aids	User Manual EMBASE and Memocard EMBASE
Price/Charges	Connect time: UK£08.06- 16.35
	Online print: UK£0.41–0.59
	Offline print: UK£0.34–0.41
Downloading is allowed	
Thesaurus is online	

Notes

This is a subfile of EMBASE. EMTOX contains citations to the worldwide literature on drug toxicity and environmental toxicology (until 1992 containing pharmacology). It corresponds to the 'Toxicology' and 'Pharmacology and Toxicology' sections of Excerpta Medica and to the citations from those sections contained in EMBASE. Approximately 58% of the records contain abstracts. The corresponding file E483 contains records covering the period 1983 to date. Searches are possible from January 1974. The EMBASE subfiles have different groupings for costing – EMTOX is in Group 1, with EMFORENSIC, EMCANCER and EMHEALTH.

Record composition

Abstract AB; Abstract Language AL; ADONIS Number ANR; Author AU; Classification Code CC; Conference CF; Coden CO; CAS-Reg No CR; Corporate Source CS; Controlled Terms CT; Qualifier /QF; Weighting /W1; Country CY; Drug Trade Name DN; Document Name DT; EMCLAS Code EC; Entry Date ED; Editor EDR; EMCLAS Term ET; EMTAGS-Code IC; EMTAGS-Term IT; CY/JT JC; Journal Title JT; Language LA; Manufacturer's Name MN; Number of Document ND; Publisher PU; Publication Year PY; Qualifier QF; ISBN-NO SB; Source SO; ISSN-NO and Title TI

The basic Index includes the data fields: Abstract, Controlled Term, Drug Trade Name, EMTAGS-Term, Manufacturer's Name, Title. Hedges or limit capabilities are provided to limit to (pps=) human; adverse drug reactions; AIDS; animals, birds; animals, cold-blooded; animals, vertebrate; cancer; developing countries; and ecotoxicity. EMTOX is defined as subfile to EMBASE with: FIND EC DOWN 52 or (EC DOWN 30 AND ED < 83).

14:387. Database subset
Online
DIMDI

File name	E483 – EMTOX
Alternative name(s)	Excerpta Medica
Software	GRIPS
Start year	1983
Number of records	138,139
Update period	Weekly
SDI period	1 week
Database aids	User Manual EMBASE and Memocard EMBASE
Price/Charges	Connect time: UK£08.06- 16.35
	Online print: UK£0.41–0.59
	Offline print: UK£0.34–0.41
Downloading is allowed	
Thesaurus is online	

Notes

This is a subfile of EMBASE. EMTOX contains citations to the worldwide literature on drug toxicity and environmental toxicology. It corresponds to the 'Toxicology' and 'Pharmacology and Toxicology' sections of Excerpta Medica and to the citations from those sections contained in EMBASE. Approximately 61% of the records contain abstracts. The corresponding file E474 contains records covering the period 1974 to date. The EMBASE subfiles have different groupings for costing – EMTOX is in Group 1, with EMFORENSIC, EMCANCER and EMHEALTH.

Record composition

Abstract AB; Abstract Language AL; ADONIS Number ANR; Author AU; Classification Code CC; Conference CF; Coden CO; CAS-Reg No CR; Corporate Source CS; Controlled Terms CT; Qualifier /QF; Weighting /W1; Country CY; Drug Trade Name DN; Document Name DT; EMCLAS Code EC; Entry Date ED; Editor EDR; EMCLAS Term ET; EMTAGS-Code IC; EMTAGS-Term IT; CY/JT JC; Journal Title JT; Language LA; Manufacturer's Name MN; Number of Document ND; Publisher PU; Publication Year PY; Qualifier QF; ISBN-NO SB; Source SO; ISSN-NO and Title TI

The basic Index includes the data fields: Abstract, Controlled Term, Drug Trade Name, EMTAGS-Term, Manufacturer's Name, Title. Hedges or limit capabilities are provided to limit to (pps=) human; adverse drug reactions; AIDS; animals, birds; animals, cold-blooded; animals, vertebrate; cancer; developing countries; and ecotoxicity. EMTOX is defined as subfile to EMBASE with: FIND EC DOWN 52 or (EC DOWN 30 AND ED < 83).

14:388. Database subset
CD-ROM
CD Plus

File name	Excerpta Medica Drugs and Pharmacology
Alternative name(s)	Excerpta Medica
Format notes	IBM, Mac, Unix
Software	OVID 3.0
Start year	1980
Number of records	1,300,000
Update period	Quarterly
Price/Charges	

Notes

This CD-ROM database, a six-disc subset of EMBASE, contains citations and abstracts covering drugs and pharmacology literature, including: the effects and use of all drugs and potential drugs, clinical and experimental aspects of pharmacokinetics and pharmacodynamics. It also covers extensively the side effects of and adverse reactions to drugs. Relevant abstracts from other clinical and basic disciplines are also included.

14:389. Database subset

CD-ROM **Compact Cambridge**

File name	PolTox II: Excerpta Medica
Alternative name(s)	Excerpta Medica
Format notes	IBM, NEC, 9800
Software	Proprietary
Start year	1981
Number of records	260,000
Update period	Quarterly
Price/Charges	Subscription: UK£635

Notes

This CD-ROM database contains a subset of EMBASE giving citations and abstracts to the worldwide literature on scientific, industrial and social concerns on toxic items and environmental health. Subjects covered include environmental pollution and toxicology. Pollution-related topics include chemical pollution and its effect on man, animals, plants and micro-organisms; environmental impact of chemical pollution, including measurement, treatment, prevention and control; radiation and thermal pollution; noise and vibration; dangerous goods; wastewater treatment and measurement; meteorological aspects of pollution; and legal and socioeconomic aspects of pollution. Toxicology coverage includes pharmaceutical toxicology; foods, food additives and contaminants; cosmetics, toiletries and household products; occupational toxicology; waste materials in air, soil and water; toxins and venoms; chemical teratogens, mutagens and carcinogens; phototoxicity, toxic mechanisms; predictive toxicology; regulatory toxicology; laboratory methods and techniques; and antidotes and symptomatic treatment. The database, together with PolTox I, seeks to provide the beginnings of a CD-ROM library on environmental pollution and toxic substances. One reviewer especially liked the bringing together of material from so many different sources but pointed out there are drawbacks in the different indexing for the various source databases and in the frustration of having to switch between discs.

See also PolTox I and PolTox III. Special discount is available for combined purchase of all three volumes.

14:390. Database subset

CD-ROM **Compact Cambridge**

File name	Excerpta Medica – Drugs and Pharmacology (1980 to date)
Alternative name(s)	Excerpta Medica
Format notes	IBM
Software	CORE
Start year	1980
Number of records	1,300,000
Update period	Quarterly
Price/Charges	Subscription: US$3,495

Notes

This database, consisting of four CD-ROM discs, is a subset of EMBASE and contains citations and abstracts covering drugs and pharmacology literature. It includes the effects and use of all drugs and potential drugs, clinical and experimental aspects of pharmacokinetics and pharmacodynamics. It also covers extensively the side effects of and adverse reactions to drugs. Relevant abstracts from other clinical and basic disciplines are also included.

14:391. Database subset

CD-ROM **Compact Cambridge**

File name	Excerpta Medica – Drugs and Pharmacology (1989 to date)
Alternative name(s)	Excerpta Medica
Format notes	IBM
Software	CORE
Start year	1989
Number of records	
Update period	Quarterly
Price/Charges	Subscription: US$1,495

Notes

This database, consisting of two CD-ROM discs, is a subset of EMBASE and contains citations and abstracts covering drugs and pharmacology literature. It includes the effects and use of all drugs and potential drugs, clinical and experimental aspects of pharmacokinetics and pharmacodynamics. It also covers extensively the side effects of and adverse reactions to drugs. Relevant abstracts from other clinical and basic disciplines are also included.

14:392. Database subset

CD-ROM **SilverPlatter**

File name	Excerpta Medica – Drugs and Pharmacology (1980 to date)
Alternative name(s)	Excerpta Medica
Format notes	Mac, IBM
Software	SPIRS/MacSPIRS
Start year	1980
Number of records	1,382,000
Update period	Quarterly
Price/Charges	Subscription: UK£2,295 – 3,443

Notes

One of the Elsevier speciality Excerpta Medica range, this database, comprising five CD-ROM discs, is a subset of EMBASE and contains citations and abstracts covering drugs and pharmacology literature. It includes the effects and use of all drugs and potential drugs, clinical and experimental aspects of pharmacokinetics and pharmacodynamics. It also covers extensively the side effects of and adverse reactions to drugs. Relevant abstracts from other clinical and basic disciplines are also included. It is available from 1980 to the present; 1989 to the present (two CD-ROMs) is also available.

Prices for discs covering 1980 to present are: UK£2,295 for single users, £3,443 for 2–8 networked users; 1989 to present, for single users UK£755, for 2–8 networked users £1,132.

14:393. Database subset

CD-ROM **SilverPlatter**

File name	Excerpta Medica – Pathology
Alternative name(s)	Excerpta Medica
Format notes	IBM, Mac
Software	SPIRS/MacSPIRS
Start year	1980
Number of records	266,000
Update period	Quarterly
Price/Charges	Subscription: UK£755 – 1,132

Notes

One of the Elsevier speciality Excerpta Medica range, this CD-ROM database is a subset of EMBASE covering pathology. Subjects covered include general pathology and organ pathology, pathophysiology, pathological anatomy and laboratory methods and techniques used in pathology. General pathology topics range from cellular pathology, foetal and neonatal pathology including congenital disorders, injury (both chemical and physical), inflammation and infection, immunopathology, collagen diseases and cancer pathology. Relevant abstracts from other clinical and basic disciplines are also included.

Prices are: for single users UK£755, for 2–8 networked users £1,132.

14:394. Database subset

CD-ROM	SilverPlatter
File name	Excerpta Medica – Psychiatry
Alternative name(s)	Excerpta Medica
Format notes	IBM, Mac
Software	SPIRS/MacSPIRS
Start year	1980
Number of records	253,000
Update period	Quarterly
Price/Charges	Subscription: UK£755 – 1,132

Notes

One of the Elsevier speciality Excerpta Medica range, this CD-ROM database is a subset of EMBASE and covers all aspects of medical psychology and psychiatry. Subjects covered include addiction, alcoholism, sexual behaviour and suicide. Mental deficiency and the clinical use or abuse of psychotropic and psychomimetic agents are also included. Normal psychology, experimental psychology and neurophysiology of the mental processes are not included unless there is some relevance to a psychiatric disorder. Relevant abstracts from other clinical and basic disciplines are also included.

Prices are: for single users UK£755, for 2–8 networked users £1,132.

14:395. Database subset

CD-ROM	SilverPlatter
File name	Excerpta Medica – Radiology and Nuclear Medicine
Alternative name(s)	Excerpta Medica
Format notes	IBM, Mac
Software	SPIRS/MacSPIRS
Start year	1980
Number of records	356,000
Update period	Quarterly
Price/Charges	Subscription: UK£755 – 1,132

Notes

One of the Elsevier speciality Excerpta Medica range, this CD-ROM database is a subset of EMBASE and covers information on radiology and nuclear medicine. Radiology subjects covered include radiodiagnosis, radiotherapy and radiobiology, ultrasound diagnosis, thermography, adverse reactions to radiotherapy and techniques and apparatus. Nuclear medicine subjects covered include diagnostic and therapeutic applications of radioisotopes in biomedicine, the radiobiology of radioisotopes, aspects of radiohygiene, new labelling techniques and tracer applications. Relevant abstracts from other clinical and basic disciplines are also included.

Prices are: for single users UK£755, for 2–8 networked users £1,132.

14:396. Database subset

CD-ROM	SilverPlatter
File name	Excerpta Medica – Drugs and Pharmacology (1989 to date)
Alternative name(s)	Excerpta Medica
Format notes	Mac, IBM
Software	SPIRS/MacSPIRS
Start year	1989

Number of records	
Update period	Quarterly
Price/Charges	Subscription: UK£755 – 1,132

Notes

One of the Elsevier speciality Excerpta Medica range, this database, consisting of two CD-ROM discs, is a subset of EMBASE and contains citations and abstracts covering drugs and pharmacology literature. It includes the effects and use of all drugs and potential drugs, clinical and experimental aspects of pharmacokinetics and pharmacodynamics. It also covers extensively the side effects of and adverse reactions to drugs. Relevant abstracts from other clinical and basic disciplines are also included. It is available from 1980 to the present or 1989 to the present (two CD-ROMs) is also available. Prices for discs covering 1980 to present are: UK£2,295 for single users, £3,443 for 2–8 networked users; 1989 to present, for single users UK£755, for 2–8 networked users £1,132.

This database can also be found on:
Eyenet
Cancer-CD
Medata-ROM
Logo-A Pharmaceutical Products (Discontinued)

Emergindex
Micromedex Inc

14:398. Master record

Alternative name(s)	Computerized Clinical Information System: Emergindex; CCIS: Emergindex
Database type	Bibliographic, Factual, Textual, Directory
Number of journals	50
Sources	
Start year	
Language	English
Coverage	USA and International
Number of records	
Update size	—
Update period	Quarterly
Thesaurus	MeSH-based

Keywords

Acute Medicine; Diagnosis; Emergency Medicine; Epidemiology; Pharmaceuticals; Radiography

Description

A clinical support tool for the diagnosis and treatment of diseases and trauma seen in acute care settings. A referenced clinical information system that presents pertinent data for the practice of acute care medicine. It is designed to help those who deal with acute medical/surgical disease and traumatic injuries to more quickly and efficiently diagnose and treat the multitude of problems encountered daily. The system comprises three files of information on emergency, traumatic injury and acute care medicine, diagnosis and treatment.

Clinical Reviews contains over 285 reviews of emergency and acute care treatment protocols. Covers clinical presentation, including etiology and epidemiology, laboratory and radiographic studies, diagnostic aids, differential diagnoses, non-pharmacologic and pharmacologic therapeutics and disposition.

Clinical Abstracts contains about 17,000 citations, with abstracts, to about fifty journals on emergency and critical care medicine worldwide. Includes clinical and experimental studies on nearly 300 diseases and injuries. Each record includes study problem or purpose, study type, population data, study design, methodology, results, conclusions, and references.

Prehospital Care Protocols contains over thirty protocols for emergency medical service (EMS) personnel for diagnosis and treatment of the injured or ill patient in the prehospital environment. Each protocol includes presentation, stabilisation, base contact, special concerns and references.

A primary product of the Computerized Clinical Information System from Micromedex. The primary databases are offered on annual subscription with a choice of – System I: any one of the primary titles, System II: any two of the primary titles, System III: all three of the primary titles. Any of the primary databases can be purchased separately. Any combination of these systems attracts a first year software licence fee of £280.

Users can search by subjects in a 40,000 term medical thesaurus based on the National Library of Medicine Medical Subject Headings (MeSH).

14:399. Tape   Micromedex Inc

File name	Emergindex
Alternative name(s)	Computerized Clinical Information System: Emergindex; CCIS: Emergindex
Start year	1973
Number of records	
Update period	Quarterly

Notes

Annual subscription to CCIS required. AfterCare Instructions, also on CCIS, is available to subcribers of this database for an additional fee.

14:400. Database subset

Online   Mead Data Central (as a NEXIS database)

File name	ABSTR – NEXIS
Start year	1980
Number of records	285 in Clinical Reviews; 17,000 in Clinical Abstracts
Update period	Quarterly
Price/Charges	Subscription: US$1,000 – 3,000 (Depending on needs) Connect time: US$49.00 (Telecomms + connect time) Database entry fee: US$24.00 (Search charge) Online print: US$0.04 per line

Notes

Library: GENMED; Group files: EMERDX and MEDEX.

On NEXIS, Emergindex is divided into two files: Clinical Abstracts (ABSTR) and Clinical Reviews (DISEAS). ABSTR is designed as authoritative information to assist in the diagnosis and treatment of acute diseases and injuries. The clinical abstracts are an ongoing cumulative review of the world's medical literature specifically related to emergency and critical care medicine. When the file is selected, an introductory note about searching the file and a list of topics is automatically displayed.

A subscription charge which covers all transactional charges, connect time, telecommunications and the small administration charge can take the place of the individual charges. Subscriptions are negotiated with customers and vary according to the number of menus (thus, files) that are to be used – typically a minimum subscription would be about US$ 1,000. All charges include training and a 24-hour help line.

Record composition

Copyright Information PUBLICATION; Citation SOURCE; Descriptive Phrase TOPIC; Statement of Purpose/Problem PURPOSE; Population (Study Subjects) POPULATION; Number in Study TOTAL; Number of Males in Study MALE; Number of Females in Study FEMALE; Methodology METHODOLOGY; Results RESULTS; Descriptive Terms TERMS; Study Design DESIGN and Study Definition STUDY-TYPE Each abstract is indexed by key terms for easy reference to any topic relevant to acute care medicine.

14:401. Database subset

Online   Mead Data Central (as a NEXIS database)

File name	DISEAS – NEXIS
Start year	1980
Number of records	285 in Clinical Reviews; 17,000 in Clinical Abstracts
Update period	Quarterly
Price/Charges	Subscription: US$1,000 – 3,000 (Depending on needs) Connect time: US$49.00 (Telecomms + connect time) Database entry fee: US$24.00 (Search charge) Online print: US$0.04 per line

Notes

Library: GENMED; Group files: EMERDX and MEDEX.

On NEXIS, Emergindex is divided into two files: Clinical Abstracts (ABSTR) and Clinical Reviews (DISEAS). DISEAS is an information system which includes reviews of acute medical/surgical diseases and traumatic injuries. The reviews are written primarily by physicians who are involved in the practice, research and teaching of emergency and critical medicine. The system includes a comprehensive dictionary of over 40,000 index terms and synonyms based on the National Library of Medicine's subject headings (MeSH) and special headings devised by a panel of emergency and critical care physicians.

A document in DISEAS consists of a single Clinical Review and accompanying index terms. Most of the documents are several screens long.

A subscription charge which covers all transactional charges, connect time, telecommunications and the small administration charge can take the place of the individual charges. Subscriptions are negotiated with customers and vary according to the number of menus (thus, files) that are to be used – typically a minimum subscription would be about US$ 1,000. All charges include training and a 24-hour help line.

Record composition

Topic TOPIC; Summary Information SUMM; Critical Focus CRIT; Clinical Presentation CLNP; Diagnosis DGNS; Differential Diagnosis DDGN; Clinical Information CLPR; Clinical Information Introduction INTRO; Clinical Information Associated Conditions ASSOC; Clinical Information Vital Signs VITS; Clinical Information Dermatologic Presentation; Clinical Information HEENT Presentation HENT; Clinical Information Neck Presentation NECK; Clinical Information Respiratory Presentation RESP; Clinical

Information Cardiovascular Presentation CARD; Clinical Information Gastrointestinal Presentation GAST; Clinical Information Genitourinary Presentation GENT; Clinical Information Musculoskeletal Presentation MUSC; Clinical Information Neurologic Presentation NEUR; Clinical Information Endocrine Presentation ENDO; Clinical Information Infectious Presentation INFT; Clinical Information Hematologic Presentation HEMP; Clinical Information Psychiatric Presntation PSYCH; Clinical Information Miscellaneous Presentation MSYMP; Clinical Information Complications COMP; Laboratory Studies LAB; Laboratory Studies General Discussion LAB-DCSSN; Laboratory Studies Hematologic Data HEME; Laboratory Studies Electrolytes ELEC; Laboratory Studies Chemical Survey CHEM; Laboratory Studies Urinalysis URNL; Laboratory Studies Arterial Blood Gases ABGS; Laboratory Studies Bacteriology BACT; Laboratory Studies Serology SEROL; Laboratory Studies Electrocardiogram EKG; Laboratory Studies Miscellaneous MISC; Radiographic Studies XRAY; Radiographic Studies Plain Films FILM; Radiographic Studies Contrast Studies CONT; Radiographic Studies Nuclear Scans NUCL; Radiographic Studies CT Scans CT; Radiographic Studies Ultrasound SONO; Radiographic Studies Magnetic Resonance Imaging MRI; Diagnostic Aids DIAG; Diagnostic Aids Invasive Procedures INVS; Diagnostic Aids Noninvasive Procedures NINV; Differential Diagnosis DIFF; Differential Diagnosis General Discussion DIFF-DCSSN; Differential Diagnosis Trauma TRMA; Differential Diagnosis Infectious INFC; Differential Diagnosis Inflammatory INFL; Differential Diagnosis Metabolic META; Differential Diagnosis Vascular VASC; Differential Diagnosis Neoplastic NEOP; Differential Diagnosis Toxicologic TOXC; Differential Diagnosis Physical Agents PHYS; Differential Diagnosis Miscellaneous MDGN; Treatment TRMT; Treatment Management Overview MGMT; Treatment Therapy, Non-Pharmacologic THNP; Treatment Therapy, Pharmacologic THPH; Criteria DISP; Admission Criteria ADMIT; Home Criteria HOME; Consult Criteria CONS; Transfer Criteria TRNS and References REFS

Synonyms for Clinical Review document titles are built into the TOPIC segment to retrieve valuable equivalents for document titles which are acronyms or variations of disease names (for example, CARDIO-VASCULAR will retrieve several documents, each covering a specific symptom or type of cardiovascular disease). The standard form of author's name in the REFS segment is LAST NAME-COMMA-SPACE-INITIAL(s). Depending on the information available from the publisher, there may be one initial or two initials without spaces between them.

This database can also be found on:
CCIS
NEXIS

Environmental Bibliography
Environmental Studies Institute, Internat Academy, Santa Barbara

14:403. Master record

Alternative name(s)	EPB; Environmental Periodicals Bibliography
Database type	Bibliographic
Number of journals	450
Sources	Journals

Start year	1973
Language	English
Coverage	International
Number of records	450,000
Update size	24,000
Update period	Every two months

Keywords
Drug Abuse; Urban and Regional Planning; Public Health; Waste Management; Pollution; Water Pollution; Air Pollution; Noise Pollution; Soil Pollution; Drugs

Description
Contains citations to literature on the environment, covering the fields of general human ecology, atmospheric studies, energy, land resources, water resources, nutrition and health, and air quality. Human ecology covers federal, state and local government planning; laws programs, policies and regulations; recycling and management of world wastes; environmental pollution – both ecological and biological issues; environmental education and information; and transportation studies. Energy issues covered include: fossil fuels and synthesis; nuclear power generation; chemical, fission and fusion energy; solar, geothermal, wind, and wave and tide energy; hydroelectrical and pumped storage energy; and the handling and disposal of radioactive material. Water resources cover fertiliser and phosphate eutrophication; detergents, sewage and waste; treatment systems and processes; agricultural effluents; and thermal, oil and chemical pollution. Air quality includes air quality control; emissions and detection; thermal air pollution; climatic change; meteorology; and atmospheric chemistry. Land resources information includes material on animal habitat; wilderness preservation; hunting and fishing; soil erosion and conservation; mining and land reclamation; and agriculture and forestry. Nutrition and health covers drug use and abuse; food poisoning and contamination; population planning and control; public health; and toxicological studies.

Corresponds to the printed *Environmental Periodicals Bibliography*.

14:404. Online   DIALOG

File name	File 68
Alternative name(s)	EPB; Environmental Periodicals Bibliography
Start year	1973
Number of records	426,075
Update period	Twice a month
Price/Charges	Connect time: US$60.00 Offline print: US$0.15

14:405. CD-ROM   National Information Services Corporation (NISC)

File name	Environmental Periodicals Bibliography
Alternative name(s)	EPB; Environmental Periodicals Bibliography
Format notes	IBM
Software	CD-Answer
Start year	1972
Number of records	442,000
Update period	Six times per year

Notes
One reviewer thought that while this product covered many of the same topics as the PolTox series, it is not as specific in its focus and does not draw on the same sources although there is some overlap.

14:406. CD-ROM National Information Services Corporation (NISC)

File name	Environmental Periodicals Bibliography – junior
Alternative name(s)	EPBjr
Format notes	IBM
Start year	1987
Number of records	100,000
Update period	Every two months
Price/Charges	Subscription: US$895

Notes

A sub-set of the world's most extensive collection of bibliographic records on environmental issues covering the most recent five years of the literature.

Especialidades Consumidas por la Seguridad Social

Ministerio de Sanidad y Consumo de España, Dirección General de Farmacia y Productos Sanitarios, Servicio de Gestión del Banco de Datos de Medicamentos

14:407. Master record

Database type	Statistical
Number of journals	
Sources	Government documents (Spanish)
Start year	1980
Language	Spanish
Coverage	Spain
Number of records	21,000
Update size	—
Update period	Annually
Index unit	Drug

Keywords

Drug Consumption; Pharmaceutical Products

Description

Contains consumption data on drugs distributed under authority of the Social Security system of Spain. Includes quantities (that is, units sold) and prices. Data are aggregated by province.

14:408. Online Ministerio de Sanidad y Consumo de España, Dirección General de Farmacia y Productos Sanitarios, Servicio de Gestión del Banco de Datos de Medicamentos

File name	
Start year	1980
Number of records	21,000
Update period	Annually

Especialidades de Exportacion

Ministerio de Sanidad y Consumo de España, Dirección General de Farmacia y Productos Sanitarios, Servicio de Gestión del Banco de Datos de Medicamentos

14:409. Master record

Database type	Textual, Factual
Number of journals	
Sources	
Start year	1962
Language	Spanish
Coverage	Spain
Number of records	3,700
Update size	—
Update period	Periodically, as new data become available

Keywords

Pharmaceuticals

Description

Descriptions of Spanish pharmaceutical products authorised for export. Records include trade name, manufacturer, form, active and excipient ingredients, indications and dosage and administration.

14:410. Online Ministerio de Sanidad y Consumo de España, Dirección General de Farmacia y Productos Sanitarios, Servicio de Gestión del Banco de Datos de Medicamentos

File name	
Start year	1962
Number of records	3,700
Update period	Periodically, as new data become available

Especialidades Farmaceuticas de España

Consejo General de Colegios Oficiales de Farmaceuticos de España

14:411. Master record

Alternative name(s)	Especialidades Farmaceuticas de Espana
Database type	Directory
Number of journals	
Sources	Government documents, Journals, Reports and Suppliers
Start year	1972
Language	Spanish
Coverage	Spain
Number of records	22,000
Update size	—
Update period	Varies

Keywords

Drug Therapy; Drugs; Pharmaceutical Industry

Description

Contains data on drugs marketed in Spain, including repealed and discontinued drugs. Provides trade name, manufacturer code, therapeutic category as defined in Grupos Terapeuticos (see), dosage forms and prices, posological data, cautions, pharmacological actions, indications, contraindications, interactions, and side effects.

Sources include the pharmaceuticals register of the Ministerio de Sanidad y Consumo, international scientific literature, and technical documentation from pharmaceutical manufacturers.

14:412. Online

Consejo General de Colegios Oficiales de Farmaceuticos de España

File name	
Alternative name(s)	Especialidades Farmaceuticas de España
Start year	1972
Number of records	22,000
Update period	Varies

Especialidades Farmaceuticas en Tramite de Registro

Ministerio de Sanidad y Consumo de España, Dirección General de Farmacia y Productos Sanitarios, Servicio de Gestión del Banco de Datos de Medicamentos

14:413. Master record

Alternative name(s)	Pharmaceutical Specialities in the Process of Authorization Marketing
Database type	Factual
Number of journals	
Sources	
Start year	Current information
Language	Spanish
Coverage	Spain
Number of records	4,500
Update size	1,200
Update period	Daily

Keywords

Drugs; Pharmaceuticals

Description

Data on drugs awaiting registration for use in Spain. Records include name, definition, active and excipient ingredients, usgae and benefits, dosage and administration, manufacturer and price, evaluation reports and current status in the process of registration.

14:414. Online

Ministerio de Sanidad y Consumo de España, Dirección General de Farmacia y Productos Sanitarios, Servicio de Gestión del Banco de Datos de Medicamentos

File name	
Alternative name(s)	Pharmaceutical Specialities in the Process of Authorization Marketing
Start year	Current information
Number of records	4,500
Update period	Daily

Especialidades Farmaceuticas Españolas

Ministerio de Sanidad y Consumo de España, Dirección General de Farmacia y Productos Sanitarios, Servicio de Gestión del Banco de Datos de Medicamentos

14:415. Master record

Alternative name(s)	Especialidades Farmaceuticas Espanolas
Database type	Directory
Number of journals	
Sources	Suppliers
Start year	1979
Language	Spanish
Coverage	Spain
Number of records	12,000
Update size	—
Update period	Varies
Index unit	Drug

Keywords

Drugs; Pharmaceutical Industry

Description

Contains descriptions of drugs registered for use in Spain. Includes trade name, form and size, definition, active and excipient ingredients, usage and benefits, dosage and administration, manufacturer, and price.

14:416. Online

Ministerio de Sanidad y Consumo de España, Dirección General de Farmacia y Productos Sanitarios, Servicio de Gestión del Banco de Datos de Medicamentos

File name	
Alternative name(s)	Especialidades Farmaceuticas Espanolas
Start year	1979
Number of records	12,000
Update period	Varies

European Chemical News

European Chemical News
Reed Business Publishing Ltd

14:417. Master record

Database type	Textual
Number of journals	1
Sources	Newspapers
Start year	1984 (April)
Language	English
Coverage	International
Number of records	28,962
Update size	5,200
Update period	Weekly; CNEX updated every Friday before next issue

Keywords

Agrochemicals; Chemical Substances; Fertilizers; Fibres; Marketing; Patents; Petrochemicals; Pharmaceuticals; Pharmaceutical Industry; Plastics; Rubber Technology

Description

Contains full text of *European Chemical News*, a newspaper on market, technical, and corporated developments in the chemical and related industries. It focuses on every aspect from manufacturing through distribution, trading and engineering to market analysis and planning. Covers petrochemicals, plastics, rubber, specialty chemicals, pharmaceuticals, synthetic fibres, fertilizers, agrochemicals, and chemical applications of biotechnology. Provides weekly summaries and commentary on contract and spot prices for bulk petrochemicals; business news, including mergers and acquisitions, new plant investments, and corporate financial information; and articles on such issues as trade legislation and environmental regulations. In line with the regular sections appearing in the magazine, articles in the text include: Newsdesk – news items, often exclusive, on major business developments affecting the chemicals industry; Market Trends – weekly update and commentary on contract and spot price movements for bulk petrochemicals; Market Report – what's happening in the marketplace, product analysis, plant start-ups, trade legislation issues such as dumping, as well as shipping and distribution news; Technology – new developments in process and environmental technologies, agricultural biotechnology and patents; Company News – a weekly round up of interim and year-end financial results, combined with informed commentary on performance; New Projects – hot news on new plant, investment and existing plant expansion worldwide; Pharm Report – important news on the pharmaceutical industry, including new products, biotechnology, patents and litigation; Environment Monitor – fortnightly round up of environmental news, legislation and regulation, and other environmental isssues of concern to the chemical industry; People – who's moving where in the chemical industry.

The database also features articles from ECN's monthly monitors on plastics, shipping and the environment, as well as its in-depth special reports which appear most weeks.

Corresponds to European Chemical News.

14:418. Online   Data-Star

File name	CNEW
Start year	1984 (April) (excluding latest issue)
Number of records	28,962
Update period	Weekly
Database aids	Data-Star Chemical Manual, Berne, Dta-Star and Online Manual (search NEWS-CNEW in NEWS)
Price/Charges	Subscription: UK£32.00
	Connect time: UK£92.48
	Online print: UK£0.47
	Offline print: UK£0.66

Notes

CNEW also features articles from ECN's monthly monitors on plastics, shipping and the environment, as well as its in-depth special reports which appear most weeks.

From June 1993 Data-Star have introduced an annual fee/subscription per contract (that is, not per password) of SFr 80.00 (c.UK£ 32.00) payable every June. For North American customers billed in dollars who also use DIALOG, the DIALOG fee also covers access to Data-Star. Academic customers, 'commitment' customers and customers currently billed in dollars are exempt.

14:419. Online   Data-Star

File name	CNEX
Start year	1984 (April)

Number of records	
Update period	Weekly (every Friday before the following Monday's issue is published)
Database aids	Data-Star Chemical Manual, Berne, Dta-Star and Online Manual (search NEWS-CNEW in NEWS)
Price/Charges	Subscription: UK£32.00
	Connect time: UK£92.48
	Online print: UK£1.19
	Offline print: UK£1.51
	SDI charge: UK£2.72

Notes

From June 1993 Data-Star have introduced an annual fee/subscription per contract (that is, not per password) of SFr 80.00 (c.UK£ 32.00) payable every June. For North American customers billed in dollars who also use DIALOG, the DIALOG fee also covers access to Data-Star. Academic customers, 'commitment' customers and customers currently billed in dollars are exempt.

14:420. CD-ROM   Reed Information Services Ltd

File name	European Chemical News
Format notes	IBM
Start year	Current year
Number of records	28,962
Update period	Quarterly
Price/Charges	Subscription: UK£900

Notes

Initial subscription is inclusive of a six-month backfile. Publicity says 'additional material may be ordered from Asia-Pacific Chemicals, Performance Chemicals and Chemscope. At the same time relevant news from these journals is being used to update the Kompass file'.

European Cosmetic Markets
Nicholas Hall & Company

14:421. Master record

Database type	Textual
Number of journals	1
Sources	Reports
Start year	1989
Language	English
Coverage	Europe
Number of records	
Update size	—
Update period	Monthly

Keywords

Beauty Care; Company Profiles; Cosmetics; Marketing; Personal Hygiene; Research and Development

Description

Reports on what's happening of importance in the major European markets for beauty care and personal hygiene products. Includes special reports on the market for classes of products, company profiles, reviews of key industry seminars and conferences, new product introductions, company news and summaries of industry research studies.

Full text of the monthly *European Cosmetic Markets Report*.

This database can be found on:
PTS Newsletter Database

European Pharmaceutical Market Research Association Database
Resource Group, The

14:423. Master record

Alternative name(s)	EPhMRA
Database type	Bibliographic
Number of journals	150
Sources	Journals, Conference reports, Books and Surveys
Start year	1988, with some earlier materials
Language	English
Coverage	Europe, USA and International (some items)
Number of records	2,500
Update size	—
Update period	Weekly
Database aids	Thesaurus available from producer

Keywords

Pharmaceutical Industry; Health Care; Market Research

Description

EPHM contains market research information from journals and pharmaceutical multi-client and syndicated studies. There are citations, with abstracts, to the worldwide literature on market reesearch in the pharmaceutical and health care industries. Includes author, title, source, publication date, type, language, country of origin and abstract. Abstracts are provided for articles and studies from around the world on all aspects of market research in the industry. Each document contains full bibliographical details and precise descriptors to facilitate effective retrieval. About 50% of the information is on Europe, 35% on USA and 15% on the rest of the world. Sources include over 600 market research companies.

14:424. Online   Data-Star

File name	EPHM
Alternative name(s)	EPhMRA
Start year	1988, with some earlier materials
Number of records	2,500
Update period	Weekly
Price/Charges	Subscription: UK£32.00
	Connect time: UK£61.28
	Online print: UK£2.20
	Offline print: UK£2.31
	SDI charge: UK£0.94

Notes

Discounted prices are available to both clients and members. From June 1993 Data-Star have introduced an annual fee/subscription per contract (that is, not per password) of SFr 80.00 (c.UK£ 32.00) payable every June. For North American customers billed in

dollars who also use DIALOG, the DIALOG fee also covers access to Data-Star. Academic customers, 'commitment' customers and customers currently billed in dollars are exempt.

Eyenet
American Society of Contemporary Ophthalmology (ASCO)

14:425. Master record

Database type	Bibliographic, Directory, Textual
Number of journals	
Sources	Journals, Suppliers and Monographs
Start year	Current information; Literature Search, 1983
Language	English
Coverage	International
Number of records	
Update size	—
Update period	Varies by file
Index unit	Articles, Book reviews, Editorials, Letters to the editor, Classified advertisements, News items, Product announcements, Calendar, Drug and products

Keywords

Eye Disorders; Ophthalmic Instruments; Ophthalmology; Pharmaceuticals

Description

Contains five files of information for opthalmologists and physicians on eye disorders and their treatment.

Electronic Eye Journal Monthly. Contains full text of selected articles, book reviews, editorials, letters to the editor, and classified advertisements to be published in *Annals of Ophthalmology, Glaucoma*, and *Journal of Ocular Therapy and Surgery*. Also contains news bulletins, product announcements and warnings, and a calendar of conferences and meetings. Updated monthly; bulletins and product news updated daily.

Eye Disorders. Contains information on disorders of the eye (for example, of the eyelid, cornea, optic nerve) and preferred and alternate treatments.

Pharmaceuticals. Provides information on drugs by brand name. Includes manufacturer, form of application (for example, ointment), and concentration.

Instruments. Provides descriptions of about 3,000 instruments, lenses, and other equipment used in the practice of ophthalmology. Descriptions include manufacturer and price.

Literature Search. Provides citations from Excerpta Medica to the worldwide literature in the field of opthalmology (see EMBASE). Updated weekly.

Database no longer maintained.

For more information on constituent databases, see:
EMBASE.

14:426. Online General Electric Information Services Company

File name	Eyenet
Start year	Current information; Literature Search, 1983
Number of records	
Update period	Varies by file

Notes
Access limited to ophthalmologists, physicians, and the ophthalmic industry; monthly maintenance fee to ASCO required. Database no longer maintained.

Fachinformation

14:427. Master record

Database type	Factual
Number of journals	
Sources	
Start year	
Language	German
Coverage	Germany
Number of records	
Update size	–
Update period	

Keywords
Drugs

Description
One of the databases on Lauer Mobi-med 3 plus CD-ROM.

This database can be found on:
Lauer Mobi-med 3 plus

Family Doctor, The
CMC ReSearch

14:429. Master record

Database type	Textual, Image, Directory, Factual
Number of journals	
Sources	
Start year	1991
Language	English
Coverage	
Number of records	1,500 questions; 1,600 drugs.
Update size	–
Update period	Varies

Keywords
Anatomy; Drugs; Home Health Care

Description
Written and edited by Dr Allen H Bruckheim – a US nationally-recognised physician and medical expert, this is a medical guide for do-it-yourself diagnosis and advice consisting of colour illustrations and text covering common diseases, symptoms, medical procedures, and human anatomy. It brings together a substantial amount of medical information written in plain English for lay users. Includes a wide-ranging question-and-answer section-over a thousand commonly asked questions covering subjects as diverse as ultrasound scans and why limbs swell in aeroplanes. Health update booklets provide answers in further detail on selected subjects, inlcuding the heart, ageing, arthritis, diabetes, colon cancer and cholesterol control.

Also includes details of support groups, photographs to help identify medications and data on a large number of drugs commonly prescribed for everyday ailments: the comprehensive *Consumer Guide to Prescription Drugs* – the equivalent of a 992-page book providing detailed information on over 1,600 brand name products, including: brand names, type of drug, ingredients, dosage forms, storage, uses, treatment, side effects, interactions and warnings, common abbreviations and over two hundred images to assist in drug identification.

Dr Bruckheim was awarded the Vincent Downing Award by the metropolitan New York Chapter of the American Medical Writers Association for this product in 1992. Previous winners have been the originator of the *Merck Manual* and the author of the *Complete Guide to Prescription and Nonprescription Drugs*.

Full-text word searching, browsing, or table of contents.

14:430. CD-ROM CMC ReSearch

File name	Family Doctor, The
Format notes	IBM, Mac
Software	DiscPassage
Start year	1991
Number of records	1,500 questions; 1,600 drugs
Update period	Varies
Price	UK£80

14:431. CD-ROM 8cm CMC ReSearch

File name	Portable Family Doctor, The
Format notes	Sony, Data, Discman
Start year	1991
Number of records	1,500 questions; 1,600 drugs.
Update period	Varies
Price	US$49.95

Family Resources
National Council on Family Relations

14:432. Master record

Database type	Bibliographic, Directory, Organisational/Biographical
Number of journals	1,200+
Sources	Journals, Reports, Research communications, Project descriptions, Monographs, Conference proceedings, Dissertations, Government documents, A-V material, Newsletters, Films, Filmstrips and Databases
Start year	1970, with some earlier data; journals, 1973
Language	English
Coverage	International
Number of records	121,563
Update size	–
Update period	Monthly
Index unit	Articles and Professional

Keywords
Alcohol Abuse; Child Abuse; Drug Abuse; Family; Counselling; Therapy

Description
Provides more than 120,000 citations to journal and non-journal psychosocial literature and references to other resources (for example, family study centres, community resource centres) on marriage and the

family. Subjects covered include trends and changes in marriage and family; organisations and services to families; family relationships and dynamics; mate selection; marriage and divorce; issues related to reproduction; sexual attitudes and behaviour; families with special problems (for example, violence, drug abuse, child abuse, learning disabilities, alcoholism); family counselling and education; minority groups; and aids for theory and research.

Inventory of Marriage and Family Literature (MFL). Contains citations to family-related articles in over 1,000 journals. Corresponds to the printed index of the same name.

Human Resources Bank. Contains biographical summaries and references to over 1,000 professionals who can be contacted by the general public. Includes psychologists, sociologists, researchers, family life educators, and marriage and family therapists.

Idea Bank. Contains references to work in progress, work planned, and new ideas. Abstracts are submitted by individuals in family-related programmes, research, service agencies, and educational institutions.

From 1970 to 1990 audiovisuals, newsletters, government publications, instructional materials, dissertations, human resource publications and other miscellaneous sources of information were indexed. Currently, only citations to journals are being added to the database.

14:433. Online   BRS

File name	NCFR
Start year	1970, with some earlier data; journals, 1973
Number of records	121,563
Update period	Monthly
Price/Charges	Connect time: US$50.00/60.00
	Online print: US$0.97/1.05
	Offline print: US$1.10

14:434. Online   DIALOG

File name	File 291
Start year	1970+ journals; 1970–1990 other media
Number of records	129,709
Update period	6 times per year
Price/Charges	Subscription: US$66.00
	Online print: US$0.35
	Offline print: US$0.40
	SDI charge: US$10.00

14:435. Online   Executive Telecom System International, Human Resource Information Network (ETSI/HRIN)

File name	
Start year	1970, with some earlier data; journals, 1973
Number of records	121,563
Update period	Monthly

Notes

Annual subscription to Executive Telecom System Inc, The Human Resource Information Network.

14:436. CD-ROM   National Council on Family Relations

File name	Family Resources on Disc (FROD)
Start year	1970
Number of records	
Update period	

Notes

Contains citations and abstracts from over 1,200 journals, books, dissertations, films, and videos: Includes organizations, names, addresses, and telephone numbers of experts in the family field. Cover marriage and family life, etc. Covers 1970 – 1989.

Farmadisco
CD Systems
OEMF

14:437. Master record

Alternative name(s)	Informatore, L' Farmaceutico; Info-Farmadisco
Database type	Textual, Directory, Bibliographic, Factual
Number of journals	
Sources	Databases
Start year	1970
Language	Italian
Coverage	Italy
Number of records	
Update size	—
Update period	Semiannually

Keywords

Drugs; Pharmaceutical Products

Description

Pharmaceutical data on all medicinal products, with active ingredients and their anatomic, therapeutic, and chemical classification. Also includes cosmetic, dietary, and veterinary products; and names and addresses of manufacturers of drugs and borderline products. Contains:

Useful telephone numbers;

List of ASS.INDE members;

Medicinal products only available on non-repeatable prescriptions;

Summary table of mandatory drugs to be stocked by pharmacies;

Alphabetical list of the pharmaceutical substances monographs with the relative type of confection;

Adverse reaction to drugs – Definition and Codes – WHO/OMS list;

Medicinal herbs, listed with the necessary instructions for preparing magistral galenic preparations;

Laboratories (full addresses, deposits and representatives, and relative level of production, plus a list of Italian wholesalers); and

Index Magnus, with over 60,000 references.

In addition, one section has medicinal products subdivided by ATC in order of active element. A description of the type of confection is given for each medicinal product and its SSN Therapeutical Manual (A-B-C) category and producing company is also given. Users can move from any of the archives to others, for example, from a substance card to all specialities in Informatore Farmaceutico containing that substance, or to all the firms producing that same substance.

Contains the contents of the two volumes of the print edition. Equivalent to the online L'Informatore Farmaceutico.

14:438. CD-ROM   OEMF

File name	Farmadisco
Alternative name(s)	Informatore, L' Farmaceutico; Info-Farmadisco
Format notes	IBM
Software	CD-Hyper

Start year   1970
Number of records
Update period   Semiannually
Price/Charges   Subscription: US$1,089

Fascinating World of CD-ROM

Springer-Verlag

14:439. Master record

Database type	Factual, Image, Bibliographic
Number of journals	
Sources	
Start year	
Language	
Coverage	
Number of records	
Update size	—
Update period	

Keywords

CD-ROM; Hazardous Substances

Description

Example uses: Dangerous Goods, Machine parts, Maths & Maps databanks

14:440. CD-ROM   Springer-Verlag

File name	Fascinating World of CD-ROM
Format notes	IBM
Start year	
Number of records	
Update period	

FDA Electronic Bulletin Board

Food and Drug Administration

14:441. Master record

Database type	Bibliographic, Textual, Directory
Number of journals	
Sources	Speeches, Reports, Press releases, Journals, Trade journals, Newsletters and Laws/regulations
Start year	Current month
Language	English
Coverage	USA
Number of records	
Update size	—
Update period	Daily
Index unit	Articles, Drug and products

Description

Contains full text of reports, press releases, articles, speeches, and other items issued by the FDA. Includes the weekly enforcement report of FDA-regulated products under recall; citations to articles and full text of selected articles from the monthly *FDA Consumer* magazine; the monthly list of drug and device product approvals; citations to FDA Federal Register announcements; newsletters of interest to physicians and other health professionals; prepared speeches delivered by the FDA Commissioner and Deputy Commissioner; prepared statements delivered by FDA officials at congressional oversight meetings; and a schedule of upcoming FDA-sponsored meetings and conferences.

14:442. Online   Dialcom Inc

File name	FedNews
Start year	Current month

Number of records
Update period   Daily

FDA Medical Bulletin

Food and Drug Administration

14:443. Master record

Alternative name(s)	FDA Drug Bulletin
Database type	Textual
Number of journals	1
Sources	Newsletters
Start year	1988
Language	English
Coverage	USA
Number of records	
Update size	—
Update period	Quarterly

Keywords

Drugs; Food Additives; Pharmaceuticals

Description

Contains full text of *FDA Medical Bulletin* (formerly *FDA Drug Bulletin*), a quarterly newsletter providing information of importance to physicians, medical research and other health professionals related to new drugs, clinical drug testing, approvals of new drugs by the United States Food and Drug Administration (FDA), and information on food additives and processes used in food preparation and packaging.

Corresponds to the quarterly *FDA Medical Bulletin*. Supplied by Predicasts to DIALOG and Data-Star.

This database can be found on:
PTS Newsletter

FDA on CD-ROM

FD Inc
US Food and Drug Administration

14:445. Master record

Database type	Textual, Factual
Number of journals	
Sources	Laws/regulations, law reports, speeches, press releases, reports, manuals and government documents (US)
Start year	1938
Language	English
Coverage	USA
Number of records	
Update size	—
Update period	Monthly

Keywords

Cosmetics; Drugs; Health Care

Description

Full text of the law relating to US food and drug administration. Federal Statutes, regulations, FDA Manuals and Judicial Decisions on CD-ROM including over twenty Federal Statutes, 9 CFR and 21 CFR updated since last publication, Judicial Decisions from 1938 to 1991, and the Food and Drug Administration's staff manual guides, regulatory procedures manual, compliance policy guide, compliance program guidance manual, inspection operations manual and import alerts relating to foods, drugs, cosmetics and medical devices. Also monthly updates of FDA talk papers, press releases, speeches, congrssional testimony of FDA officials, enforcement reports, new and proposed statutes and regulations and FDA- related Federal Register notices, Congressional record entries and changes in FDA guides and manuals.

14:446. CD-ROM   FD Inc

File name	FDA on CD-ROM
Format notes	IBM
Start year	1938
Number of records	
Update period	Monthly
Price/Charges	Subscription: US$2,300

This database can also be found on:
21CFR Online

FDC Reports
FDC Reports Inc

14:448. Master record

Database type	Textual
Number of journals	3
Sources	Conference reports, courts, direct contacts, government documents (US), journals, laws/regulations, ministry reports, newsletters, press releases, reports and trade journals
Start year	1984
Language	English
Coverage	USA (primarily) and International (some)
Number of records	22,767
Update size	—
Update period	Weekly
Index unit	Articles and trademarks

Keywords

Applied Science; Beauty Care; Biomedical Research; Cosmetics; Dermatology; Drugs; Health Care Management; Marketing; Perfumes; Pharmaceuticals; Skin Care

Description

FDC Reports contains the full text of five related paramedical newsletters: Prescription and OTC Pharmaceuticals (*The Pink Sheet*), Medical Devices, Diagnostics and Instrumentation Reports (*The Gray Sheet*), and Toiletries, Fragrances and Skin Care (*The Rose Sheet*), health policy and biomedical research (*The Blue Sheet*) and pharmaceuticals (*The Green Sheet*).

Together the newsletters provide up-to-date information about companies, product development, marketing, packaging, scientific news, personnel, retailing and advertising, trade association news, United States Food and Drug Administration regulatory activities, and corporate news, including financial operations, mergers and acquisitions, marketing and licensing agreements, legal news and market share of importance to the worldwide health care industry. *The Pink Sheet* focuses on the pharmaceutical industry and includes over-the-counter drugs as well as prescription products. New products are profiled through all phases of the approval process, from early investigational stages through marketing. Personnel changes, marketing/licensing agreements, and mergers/acquisitions are covered regularly. Activities of major trade associations and regulatory bodies such as the Food and Drug Administration are reported. *The Gray Sheet* provides varied and detailed information pertinent to the costmetics industry, including toiletries, fragrances and skin care. Coverage includes marketing information, new product introduc-

tions, line extensions, promotions and advertising activities at retail. A Trademark Review is also provided which is a compilation of cosmetics-related product trademarks registered and filed for opposition with the US Patent and Trademark Office. *The Rose Sheet* also includes descriptions of cosmetics trademarks registered and filed for opposition with the United States Patent and Trademark Office. The database contains six types of records: full-text journal articles, FDA Recalls & Court Actions, Weekly Trademark Review records, Medical Device Approvals, New Drug Approvals and Abbreviated New Drug Approvals. *The Blue Sheet* deals with news and information concerning health policy and biomedical research topics including government funding and legal issues. *The Green Sheet* is particularly valuable in tracking the latest developments in drug sales and marketing.

Sources for all newsletters include new product announcements, market research reports, press releases, sales and earnings reports, United States Securities and Exchange Commission filings, government and trade association reports, reports from conferences, meetings, and conventions, and interviews with industry leaders. News coverage is focused primarily on US and multi- national activities and accounts for approximately eighty five per cent of the database. Approximately ten per cent is focused on Europe and five per cent on Japan and other countries.

The accession numbers field contains volume number, publication code, issue number and article number. The source field contains five options: pink-sheet, gray-sheet, green-sheet, blue-sheet and rose-sheet.

14:449. Online   BRS

File name	FDCR
Start year	1984
Number of records	22,767
Update period	Weekly
Price/Charges	Connect time: US$110.00/120.00
	Online print: US$0.92/1.00
	Offline print: US$1.00
	SDI charge: US$10.00

Notes

Contains the entire text of the following FDC Report publications: *The Pink Sheet*, *The Gray Sheet* and *The Rose Sheet*.

14:450. Online   Data-Star

File name	FDCR
Start year	January 1988
Number of records	620+ documents
Update period	Weekly
Database aids	Data-Star Business Manual and Data-Star Online Manual (search for NEWS-FDCR in NEWS)
Price/Charges	Subscription: SFr80.00
	Connect time: SFr187.00
	Online print: SFr1.64
	Offline print: SFr1.89
	SDI charge: SFr10.00
Downloading is allowed	

Notes

From June 1993 Data-Star have introduced an annual fee/subscription per contract (that is, not per password) of SFr 80.00 (c.UK£ 32.00) payable every June. For North American customers billed in dollars who also use DIALOG, the DIALOG fee also covers access to Data-Star. Academic customers, 'commitment' customers and customers currently billed in dollars are exempt.

Record composition

Accession Number and Update Code AN; Date of Publication DT; Month of Publication YM; Occurence Table OC; Source SO; Text of article TX; Title TI; Update Code UP and Year of Publication YR

14:451. Online   DIALOG

File name	File 187
Start year	1987
Number of records	31,232
Update period	Weekly
Price/Charges	Connect time: US$120.00
	Online print: US$1.20
	Offline print: US$1.50
	SDI charge: US$3.95

Notes

DIALINDEX Categories: BIOBUS, PHARMINA, REGS.

14:452. Online   Mead Data Central
                            (as a NEXIS database)

File name	FDC – NEXIS
Alternative name(s)	NEXIS – FDC Reports
Start year	1984
Number of records	
Update period	Weekly
Price/Charges	Subscription: US$1,000 – 3,000
	(Depending on needs)
	Connect time: US$49.00
	(Telecomms + connect time)
	Database entry fee: US$24.00
	(Search charge)
	Online print: US$0.04 per line

Notes

Library: GENMED. FDC is the Group File containing all five reports: Blue, Gray, Green, Pink and Rose.

A subscription charge which covers all transactional charges, connect time, telecommunications and the small administration charge can take the place of the individual charges. Subscriptions are negotiated with customers and vary according to the number of menus (thus, files) that are to be used – typically a minimum subscription would be about US$ 1,000. All charges include training and a 24-hour help line.

14:453. Database subset

Online   Mead Data Central
                     (as a NEXIS database)

File name	GREEN – NEXIS
Alternative name(s)	NEXIS – FDC Reports
Start year	1984
Number of records	
Update period	Weekly
Price/Charges	Subscription: US$1,000 – 3,000
	(Depending on needs)
	Connect time: US$49.00
	(Telecomms + connect time)
	Database entry fee: US$24.00
	(Search charge)
	Online print: US$0.04 per line

Notes

Library: GENMED; Group File: FDC.

The full text of the weekly newsletter, *The Green Sheet*, reporting news about pharmaceuticals to professionals in the industry. Although *The Green Sheet* is considered a valuable reference for most professionals seeking information regarding practice of pharmacy and related issues in pharmacology, it is particularly valuable for tracking the latest develop-

ments in drug sales and marketing, new products, government actions and official pronouncements for pharmacy professional organisations.

A subscription charge which covers all transactional charges, connect time, telecommunications and the small administration charge can take the place of the individual charges. Subscriptions are negotiated with customers and vary according to the number of menus (thus, files) that are to be used – typically a minimum subscription would be about US$ 1,000. All charges include training and a 24-hour help line.

Record composition

Publication; Cite; Date; Length; Title; Text; Graphic; Correction; Correction Date and Editor's Note

14:454. Database subset

Online   Mead Data Central
                     (as a NEXIS database)

File name	PINK – NEXIS
Alternative name(s)	NEXIS – FDC Reports
Start year	1984
Number of records	
Update period	Weekly
Price/Charges	Subscription: US$1,000 – 3,000
	(Depending on needs)
	Connect time: US$49.00
	(Telecomms + connect time)
	Database entry fee: US$24.00
	(Search charge)
	Online print: US$0.04 per line

Notes

Library: GENMED; Group File: FDC.

The full text of the weekly newsletter, *The Pink Sheet*, dealing with prescription and over-the-counter pharmaceutical industries and reporting on items of national and international interest. Topics include new products, product research, marketing and advertising campaigns, government regulations and oversight, legal issues, and corporate and industry performances.

A subscription charge which covers all transactional charges, connect time, telecommunications and the small administration charge can take the place of the individual charges. Subscriptions are negotiated with customers and vary according to the number of menus (thus, files) that are to be used – typically a minimum subscription would be about US$ 1,000. All charges include training and a 24-hour help line.

Record composition

Publication; Cite; Date; Section; Length; Title; Text; Correction; Correction Date; Discussion and Editor's Note

14:455. Database subset

Online   Mead Data Central
                     (as a NEXIS database)

File name	ROSE – NEXIS
Alternative name(s)	NEXIS – FDC Reports
Start year	1984
Number of records	
Update period	Weekly
Price/Charges	Subscription: US$1,000 – 3,000
	(Depending on needs)
	Connect time: US$49.00
	(Telecomms + connect time)
	Database entry fee: US$24.00
	(Search charge)
	Online print: US$0.04 per line

Notes

Library: GENMED; Group File: FDC.

The full text of the weekly newsletter, *The Rose Sheet*, covering the toiletry, fragrance and skin care industry and reporting items of national and international interest. Topics include news of new products, product research, government regulations, legal issues, marketing and advertising and corporate and industry performance.

A subscription charge which covers all transactional charges, connect time, telecommunications and the small administration charge can take the place of the individual charges. Subscriptions are negotiated with customers and vary according to the number of menus (thus, files) that are to be used – typically a minimum subscription would be about US$ 1,000. All charges include training and a 24-hour help line.

Record composition

Publication; Cite; Date; Section; Length; Title; Text; Correction; Correction Date; Discussion and Editor's Note

This database can also be found on:
NEXIS
Pharmaceutical News Index

Fine Chemicals Database

Chemron Inc

14:457. Master record

Database type	Directory
Number of journals	
Sources	
Start year	Current information
Language	English
Coverage	USA, Canada, Europe and International (some)
Number of records	207,580
Update size	—
Update period	Twice per year reloads

Keywords

Chemical Substances; Perfumes; Pharmaceuticals; Product Catalogues

Description

Gives current product and supplier information for about 207,000 chemical substances available from over fifty manufacturers and distributors in North America and Europe. Concentrates on sources for laboratory, speciality and unusual chemicals and reagents used in scientific research and new product development, and normally produced in small quantities for applications such as pharmaceuticals, biological products, perfumes and photography. Information includes common, chemical and trade names, synonyms, systematic nomenclature, CAS Registry number, molecular formula and catalogue number. Supplier information includes company name, address and contact numbers.

14:458. Online   DIALOG

File name	File 360
Start year	Current information
Number of records	207,580
Update period	Two times per year reloads

Price/Charges	Connect time: US$90.00
	Online print: US$0.70
	Offline print: US$0.70

Fish and Fisheries Worldwide

National Information Services Corporation (NISC)

14:459. Master record
CD-ROM   National Information Services Corporation (NISC)

Database type	Bibliographic, Directory, Addresses/Telephone directory
Number of journals	
Sources	Journals, monographs, pamphlets, conference proceedings, reports, government publications, theses and grey literature
Start year	1971
Language	English
Coverage	International
Number of records	135,000
Update size	—
Update period	Twice per year
Index unit	Articles

Keywords

Ichthyology; Toxicology; Oceanography

Description

Citations of the world's literature on fisheries and fish-related topics. Drawn from several leading sources, including:

Fisheries Review from the US Fish and Wildlife Service (76,000 entries from 1971 onwards);

FISHLIT database from the JLB Smith Institute of Ichthyology, Rhodes University (30,000 records drawn from over 1,000 relevant journals – 1985 to present);

Fish Health News Abstracts (1978–1985, equivalent to the publication produced by the US Fish and Wildlife Service) fish health references up to 1985 when they were first included in the Fisheries Review database; and

Aquaculture which covers marine, freshwater and brackish organisms (over 10,000 citations from 1970 to 1984). Covers such topics in Aquaculture as: fish culture and propagation; fish farming; hatcheries and propogation; aquarium fish; warmwater culture; growing requirements culture techniques and equipment; management of aquaria; farm ponds; small impoundments; dams; cage culture and marine ranching; intensive and extensive culture; and regulations and legislation. Ecology and the Environment covers marine, brackish, estuarine and freshwater environments; habitats; aquatic communities and fish assemblages; limnology and oceanography; species interactions and food webs; natural history; mathematical models; biogeography; and freshwater and marine fish. Physiology topics include biology and physiology; biochemistry; histochemistry; age and growth; nutrition; and reproduction. Fisheries subject areas cover fishery regulations and legislation; management topics; fishery stations; surveys, marking; tagging and returns, data analysis; stock assessment and identification; fishing gear and techniques; management techniques and equipment; and mathematical modelling. Fish diseases are covered: parasitic, viral and bacterial diseases; nutritional and physiological diseases; fungal and protozoan diseases; diagnostic procedures; pathology; fish health studies; immunization; drug clearance; and disease treatment and control measures. Experimental research coverage includes research technologies and equipment; cell and tissue culture; genetics and behaviour; genetic engineering; genetics variation studies; electrophoretic studies; mathematical modelling; biochemistry; and hybridisation. Academic ichthyology covers taxonomy, phylogeny and evolution; morphological studies; meristics and morphometrics; and electron microscopy and histology. Also covered are distribution (biogeography; movement, seasonal and depth distributions; geographic distribution; and migration), economic aspects (aquatic plants and their control; fisheries management) and pollution studies (pesticides and industrial pollution; toxicology and bioassays). There is also a directory with the latest addresses of fish scientists with over 5,000 publishing ichthyologists and fishery scientists.

Notes

For related CD-ROMs see 'Fisheries Review/Wildlife Review' and 'Wildlife Worldwide'. The combination of these four databases means that gaps which may exist in one database have been greatly reduced or eliminated by the other files. Searches can be performed on all databases simultaneously, individually or in user-designated groups. Extensive keyword indexing as well as taxonomic and geographic identifiers mean that searches can be performed by species or by geographic areas from broad, regional basis to a narrow, specific locality.

For more details of constituent databases, see:
Fisheries Review/Wildlife Review
FISHLIT
Fish Health News Abstracts
Aquaculture

Forensic Science Database
Home Office Forensic Science Service – HOFSS

14:461. Master record

Database type	Bibliographic
Number of journals	300
Sources	Conference proceedings, government documents, grey literature, journals, monographs and reports
Start year	1976, with some earlier materials
Language	English
Coverage	International
Number of records	35,000
Update size	—
Update period	Nine times per year
Thesaurus	Thesaurus of Forensic Science, 3rd ed., Aldermaston, HOFSS
Database aids	FORS Users Guide, Aldermaston, HOFSS

Keywords

Biotechnology; Drugs; Forensic Science; Pathology

Description

Forensic Science Database contains citations, with abstracts, to the worldwide literature on forensic sciences. The database is multidisciplinary and covers literature relevant to the examination of evidential materials, analytical methods and the presentation and interpretation of findings. Subjects covered include: drugs and toxicology, forensic biology, forensic chemistry, documents and firearms examination, safety and management aspects of running a Forensic Science Service, pathology, case law, information management and use of computers and the management of forensic science laboratories and programmes. The database also covers techniques and problems which are also encountered in many analytical laboratories, especially areas of toxicology and body fluid identification. The database is a valuable infomation tool for forensic scientists and other professionals involved in crime investigation and the provision of expert testimony to the Courts.

Sources include about 300 journals and over 1,500 books, periodicals, conference proceedings, technical reports, government documents, and grey literature together with a series of abstracting and bibliographic services.

14:462. Online — CompuServe Information Service

File name	IQUEST File 2657
Start year	1977
Number of records	35,000
Update period	Monthly
Price/Charges	Subscription: US$8.95 per month Database entry fee: US$9/search; some databases carry a surcharge ($2–75) Online print: US$10 references free; then $9 per ten; abstracts $3 each

Downloading is allowed

Notes

Accessed via IQUEST or IQMEDICAL, this database is offered by a Data-Star gateway. IQUEST can either search across all databases, a database of the user's choice or selected multiple databases.

Record composition

Abstract AB; Accession Number and Update Code AN; Author AU; Author Affiliation IN; Availability of Original Article AV; Descriptors DE; Language of article LG; Source SO; Title TI; Update Code and Year of Publication YR

The data field, Title, deals with conference proceedings by listing the title of the paper, the collective title of the proceedings and the name, location and date of the conference.

14:463. Online — Data-Star

File name	FORS
Start year	1976, with some earlier materials
Number of records	35,000
Update period	Nine times per year
Database aids	Data-Star Biomedical Manual, Berne, Data-Star, 1989 and Online manual (search NEWS-FORS in NEWS)
Price/Charges	Subscription: SFr80.00 Connect time: SFr101.20 Online print: SFr0.42 Offline print: SFr0.65

Downloading is allowed

Notes

From June 1993 Data-Star have introduced an annual fee/subscription per contract (that is, not per password) of SFr 80.00 (c.UK£ 32.00) payable every June. For North American customers billed in dollars who

also use DIALOG, the DIALOG fee also covers access to Data-Star. Academic customers, 'commitment' customers and customers currently billed in dollars are exempt.

Record composition

Abstract AB; Accession Number and Update Code AN; Author AU; Author Affiliation IN; Availability of Original Article AV; Descriptors DE; Language of article LG; Source SO; Title TI; Update Code and Year of Publication YR

The data field title deals with conference proceedings by listing the title of the paper, the collective title of the proceedings and the name, location and date of the conference.

Francis

Centre National de la Recherche Scientifique, Institut de l'Information Scientifique et Technique, Science Humaines et Sociales (CNRS/INIST)

14:464. Master record

Database type	Bibliographic, Textual
Number of journals	7,500
Sources	Journals, Books, Reports, Dissertations, Conference proceedings and Research communications
Start year	1972
Language	French (keywords), English (keywords), Spanish (keywords) and Others
Coverage	France (primarily), Europe and International
Number of records	1,500,000+
Update size	80,000
Update period	Quarterly; Files 603 and 616 twice a year
Index unit	Articles

Keywords

Anthropology; Applied Linguistics; Chemical Substances; Computers and Law; Demography; Descriptive Linguistics; Environmental Health; Epidemiology; Ergonomics; Ethnolinguistics; Forensic Science; Health Care Management; Health Economics; History of Education; History of Medicine; History of Science; History of Technology; Human Ecology; Information Technology; Language Biology; Language Pathology; Linguistics; Mathematical Linguistics; Medical Education; Occupational Psychology; Occupational Medicine; Pharmaceutical Industry; Philosophy; Philosophy of Education; Psycholinguistics; Public Health; Semiotics; Social Medicine; Social Psychology; Social Services; Sociolinguistics; Sociology of Education; Vocational Training; Testing Methods

Description

Francis is a collection of twenty multidisciplinary bibliographic databases. It contains news and information, covering the core literature in: humanities, social sciences, economic sciences, computer processing, legal sciences, energy economics, health and medicine. There is especially good coverage of European and French research, with exhaustive coverage of fields where research is most active or which correspond to French national priorities. Most of the references also contain an analysis. The records

include keywords for searching. Over 9,000 periodicals, books, reports, dissertations, etc. are indexed.

Databases included are:

Art and Archaeology (Near East, Asia, America) (File 526);

International Bibliography of Administrative Science (File 528);

Ethnology (File 529);

History of Science and Technology (Histoire des Sciences et des Techniques (File 522) containing citations, half with abstracts, to literature on the history of science and technology, including the exact sciences, earth sciences, life sciences, medicine and pharmacology. Corresponds to *Bulletin Signaletique Sciences Humaines: Section Histoire des Sciences et des Techniques* (522). There are 74,600 records dating from 1972, with 4,000 additions quarterly;

History of Literature and Literary Sciences (File 523);

History of Religion and Religious Sciences (File 527);

Information Technology and the Law (File 603); Philosophy (File 519);

Prehistory and Protohistory (File 525);

Index of Art and Archaeology; Educational Sciences (Sciences de l'Education) (File 520) Contains citations, about half with abstracts, to the worldwide literature on education. Covers history and philosophy of education; education and psychology; sociology of education; planning and economics; educational research; teaching methods; testing and guidance; school life; vocational training; and adult education and employment. Corresponds to the *Bulletin Signaletique Sciences Humaines; Section Sciences de l'Education* (520). Records, approximately 40,000, date from 1979 and are updated quarterly with 4,000 additions each quarter;

Linguistic Sciences (Sciences du Langue) (File 524) contains citations, with some abstracts, to the international journal literature on linguistics, including language biology and pathology, psycholinguistics, sociolinguistics, ethnolinguistics, historical linguistics, descriptive studies, linguistics and mathematics, semiotics and communications, discursive semiotics and applied linguistics. Corresponds to *Bulletin Signaletique Sciences Humaines: Section Sciences du Langue* (524). There are 62,500 records on the file, dating from 1972, updated quarterly with 3,200 additions;

Sociology (Sociologie) (File 521) contains citations, most with abstracts, to the worldwide periodical and other literature in the field of sociology. Covers social psychology; social organization and structure; social problems; human ecology; demography; rural and urban sociology; economic and political sociology; sociology of knowledge, religion, education, art, communication, leisure, organizations, health, law, and work; and social work. The 68,000 records date from 1972, with 4,000 additions quarterly. Corresponds to the *Bulletin Signaletique Sciences Humaines: Section Sociologie* (521).

DOGE (Management) (File 616);

ECODOC (General Economics) (File 617);

Energy Economics (File 731);

Employment and Training (File 600);

RESHUS (Health-related Humanities) (Reseau documentaire en Sciences Humaines de la Santé) (File 610). A sectorial database on health economy, epidemiology, health and development, health organisation, health socio-economic aspects, medical ethic. Contains citations, with abstracts, to selected French literature from 1978 in the fields of health sciences: economics, sociology, legislation, geography, epidemiology, history, research and teaching, demography; human aspects of health: childbirth, death and illness, health developments, risk factors in failing health, ethics, health and society; health intervention systems: health organizations and politics; status, prevention and care unit management and structure, expenses and financing; and evaluation of health performances. There are 16,000 records updated quarterly with 1,300 additions per quarter. 84.5% of the documents indexed are French, 15% English and 0.5% are in other languages. 81% of references are journal articles, the other 19% coming from books, dissertations, proceedings and so on. All documents are fully analysed. Corresponds to the quarterly bulletin *RESHUS* and File 610 of *Bulletin Signaletique Sciences Humaines: Section Reseau Documentaire en Sciences Humaines de la Santé*.

Latin America (File 533);

International Geographical Bibliography (File 531); and two new releases,

Cognisciences (File 90) and

Spécial Préhistoire (File 47).

An index to author and source is cumulated annually. 7,500 periodical titles are covered, comprising 90% of the references, plus research reports, proceedings, and French dissertations.

Some of the databases can be purchased as combinations – File 521 (Sociology) and 529 (Ethnology) can be purchased as File 946; File G22 is a combination of File 525 (Prehistory and Special Prehistory (new release). Bibliographic publications are produced quarterly as hard copy, corresponding to the subject areas covered in the Francis database, Computer Science and the Law being published only twice a year.

There is very good coverage of French periodicals.

Francis has one lexicon (alphabetical list of subject terms used to index the information found in the database) per subject field. There are thesauri for the Energy Economics, Administrative Science, Geography and RESHUS databases. There are trilingual keywords English-French-Spanish or English-French-German in some files, and a bilingual English-French classification scheme.

14:465. Online   Européenne de Données

File name	Francis
Start year	1972
Number of records	1,500,000+
Update period	Quarterly; Files 603 and 616 twice a year
Database aids	Francis User Manual (French) for Européenne de Données users

14:466. Online   Questel

File name	Francis
Start year	1972
Number of records	1,500,000+
Update period	Quarterly; Files 603 and 616 twice a year
Database aids	Francis User Manual (French or English) for Questel users

14:467. CD-ROM   Centre National de la Recherche Scientifique, Institut de l'Information Scientifique et Technique, Science Humaines et Sociales (CNRS/INIST)

File name	Francis
Format notes	IBM
Software	GTI

Start year	1984
Number of records	500,000
Update period	Annually
Price/Charges	Subscription: FFr4,000 – 17,500

Notes

The first CD-ROM produced covers the years 1984–90. Additional discs will be produced each year – 6,000 FFr for current year (1991, 1 disc); 17,500 French francs for retrospective disc 1984–1990.

14:468. Tape   Centre National de la Recherche Scientifique, Institut de l'Information Scientifique et Technique, Science Humaines et Sociales (CNRS/INIST)

File name	Francis
Format notes	9-track, 1,600 or 6,250 BPI magnetic tapes, EBCDIC character set, with or without IBM-OS label
Start year	1972
Number of records	1,500,000+
Update period	Quarterly; Files 603 and 616 twice a year

14:469. Videotex   Centre National de la Recherche Scientifique, Institut de l'Information Scientifique et Technique, Science Humaines et Sociales (CNRS/INIST)

File name	Francis
Start year	1972
Number of records	1,500,000+
Update period	Quarterly; Files 603 and 616 twice a year

14:470. Videotex   Minitel

File name	Francis (36293601)
Start year	1972
Number of records	1,500,000+
Update period	Quarterly; Files 603 and 616 twice a year

Notes

Available directly via Minitel by dialling 36.29.36.01

14:471. Database subset
Online   Européenne de Données

File name	RESH
Alternative name(s)	Reseau documentaire en Sciences Humaines de la Santé; RESHUS
Start year	1978
Number of records	16,000
Update period	Quarterly

Notes

A subfile of the multidisciplinary Francis database, RESHUS is a sectorial database on health economy, epidemiology, health and development, health organisation, health socio-economic aspects, medical ethic. Contains citations, with abstracts, to selected French literature from 1978 in the fields of health sciences: economics, sociology, legislation, geography, epidemiology, history, research and teaching, demography; human aspects of health: childbirth, death and illness, health developments, risk factors in failing health, ethics, health and society; health intervention systems: health organizations and politics; status, prevention and care unit management and structure, expenses and financing; and evaluation of health performances. There are 16,000 records updated quarterly with 1,300 additions per quarter. 84.5% of the documents indexed are French, 15% English and 0.5% are in other languages. 81% of references are journal articles, the other 19% coming from books, dissertations, proceedings and so on. All documents are fully analysed. Corresponds to the quarterly bulletin *RESHUS* and File 610 of *Bulletin Signaletique Sciences Humaines: Section Reseau Documentaire en Sciences Humaines de la Santé.*

14:472. Database subset

Online   Questel

File name	Francis: RESHUS
Alternative name(s)	Reseau documentaire en Sciences Humaines de la Santé; RESHUS
Start year	1978
Number of records	16,000
Update period	Quarterly

Notes

A subfile of the multidisciplinary Francis database, RESHUS is a sectorial database on health economy, epidemiology, health and development, health organisation, health socio-economic aspects, medical ethic. Contains citations, with abstracts, to selected French literature from 1978 in the fields of health sciences: economics, sociology, legislation, geography, epidemiology, history, research and teaching, demography; human aspects of health: childbirth, death and illness, health developments, risk factors in failing health, ethics, health and society; health intervention systems: health organizations and politics; status, prevention and care unit management and structure, expenses and financing; and evaluation of health performances. There are 16,000 records updated quarterly with 1,300 additions per quarter. 84.5% of the documents indexed are French, 15% English and 0.5% are in other languages. 81% of references are journal articles, the other 19% coming from books, dissertations, proceedings and so on. All documents are fully analysed. Corresponds to the quarterly bulletin *RESHUS* and File 610 of *Bulletin Signaletique Sciences Humaines: Section Reseau Documentaire en Sciences Humaines de la Santé.*

There is a thesaurus for this database.

Frost & Sullivan Market Research Reports Summaries
Frost & Sullivan Inc

14:473. Master record

Alternative name(s)	F & S Market Research Reports Summaries
Database type	Bibliographic
Number of journals	
Sources	Research reports
Start year	Current 2–3 years
Language	English
Coverage	International
Number of records	409 documents
Update size	—
Update period	Monthly

Keywords

Chemical Substances; Defence; Electronics; Data Processing; Transport; Food and Drink; Manufacturing; Marketing; Machinery; Instrumentation; Pharmaceuticals; Drugs

Description

Contains citations, with detailed abstracts, to Frost & Sullivan market research reports. Reports provide analyses and forecasts of market size and share by product and company. Industries analysed include chemicals, communications, consumer products, data processing, defense, electronics, food, health, instrumentation, machinery and transportation. Includes forecasts by country for a five year period plus appraisal of technological developments and applications. Reports are written by consultants who are experts within their field.

The database contains only references to the full published Frost and Sullivan Market Research reports. Original reports may be obtained from Frost and Sullivan; each document records the report number and price information for the original report.

14:474. Online   Data-Star

File name	FSFS
Alternative name(s)	F & S Market Research Reports Summaries
Start year	Current 2–3 years
Number of records	409 documents
Update period	Monthly
Database aids	Data-Star Business Manual, Berne, Data-Star and Online manual (search NEWS-FSFS in NEWS)
Price/Charges	Subscription: UK£32.00 Connect time: UK£40.00 Online print: UK£0.30 Offline print: UK£0.20

Notes

From June 1993 Data-Star have introduced an annual fee/subscription per contract (that is, not per password) of SFr 80.00 (c.UK£ 32.00) payable every June. For North American customers billed in dollars who also use DIALOG, the DIALOG fee also covers access to Data-Star. Academic customers, 'commitment' customers and customers currently billed in dollars are exempt.

General Practitioner
Haymarket Marketing Publications Ltd

14:475. Master record

Database type	Textual
Number of journals	3
Sources	journals and newspapers
Start year	January 1987
Language	English
Coverage	International
Number of records	22,174
Update size	—
Update period	Varies with publication

Keywords

Clinical Medicine; General Practice; Primary Health Care

Description

General Practitioner contains the full text of three publications of interest to general practitioners and others involved in primary health care, nursing, or administration.

(1) *GP-General Practitioner* is the best-read newspaper for Britain's family doctors. It includes news coverage of medico-political matters, medical scientific developments and financial affairs and is seen as

a principal source of clinical, business and general news for GPs. GP-General Practitioner on GPGP is updated weekly.

(2) Mims Magazine is the leading fortnightly journal for GPs and concentrates on issues relating to pharmaceutical developments, prescription trends, therapeutics and detection and analysis of side effects. It contains news items about new products together with indications and side-effects by outside experts including GPS. The journal is currently looking at the many issues concerned with prescribing under the GP contract and in particular is performing a systematic anaysis of the cost-effectiveness of drugs in major therapeutic areas. Mims Magazine on GPGP is updated every fortnight.

(3) Medeconomics is a journal covering the business, management, finance and organisational aspects of general practice within the British National Health Service. Subjects relate to the business efficiency of GPs practices and cover: taxation, pensions, control of practice expenses, accounting in the practice, computers, personal finance, surgery premises and the implications for the GP of major changes in government legislation. Medeconomics on GPGP is updated on a monthly basis.

14:476. Online   Data-Star

File name	GPGP
Start year	1987
Number of records	22,174
Update period	Varies with publication
Database aids	Data-Star Biomedical Manual and Data-Star Online Manual (search NEWS-GPGP in NEWS)
Price/Charges	Subscription: SFr80.00
	Connect time: SFr101.20
	Online print: SFr0.77
	Offline print: SFr1.58
	SDI charge: SFrNot applicable

Downloading is allowed

Notes

The special features paragraph lists additional pictorial and graphical information available in the original article but not reproduced online. The following special features are available: Charts, Figures, Illustrations, Photographs, Drawings, Graphs, Maps, Tables.

From June 1993 Data-Star have introduced an annual fee/subscription per contract (that is, not per password) of SFr 80.00 (c.UK£ 32.00) payable every June. For North American customers billed in dollars who also use DIALOG, the DIALOG fee also covers access to Data-Star. Academic customers, 'commitment' customers and customers currently billed in dollars are exempt.

Record composition

Accession Number and Update Code AN; Author(s) AU; Length of Document LE; Publication Date YD; Publication Month YM; Publication Year YR; Source SO; Special Feature(s) SF; Text TE; Title TI and Update Code UP

Genetic Technology News
Technical Insights Inc

14:477. Master record

Database type	Textual, Directory
Number of journals	1
Sources	Newsletters and Patents

Start year	1982 Mead Data Central; 1988 Data-Star and DIALOG
Language	English
Coverage	USA (primarily) and International (some)
Number of records	
Update size	–
Update period	Daily

Keywords

Genetic Engineering; Patents; Pharmaceutical Industry

Description

Contains full text of Genetic Technology News, a monthly newsletter focussing on commercial applications in the chemical, energy, food, and pharmaceutical industries of products resulting from genetic engineering. Includes market forecasts, business news from leading biotechnology firms, announcements of investment opportunities, reports on research activities at universities and research institutions, and reports of new products. Also provides information on recently granted biotechnology patents, including number, title, assignee, and issue date. Many items include names, addresses, and telephone numbers of people who may be contacted for further information.

Produced and supplied to Mead Data Central by Technical Insights Inc; supplied to Data-Star and DIALOG by Predicasts.

14:478. Online   CompuServe Information Service

File name	IQUEST File 2541
Start year	Current year
Number of records	
Update period	Monthly
Price/Charges	Subscription: US$8.95 per month
	Database entry fee: US$9/search; some databases carry a surcharge ($2–75)
	Online print: US$10 references free; then $9 per ten; abstracts $3 each

Downloading is allowed

Notes

Accessed via IQUEST or IQMEDICAL, this database is offered by a NewsNet gateway. IQUEST can either search across all databases, a database of the user's choice or selected multiple databases.

14:479. Online   Mead Data Central (as a NEXIS database)

File name	GENTEC – NEXIS
Alternative name(s)	NEXIS – GENTEC
Start year	1982
Number of records	
Update period	Monthly, as new data are released
Price/Charges	Subscription: US$1,000 – 3,000 (Depending on needs)
	Connect time: US$49.00 (Telecomms + connect time)
	Database entry fee: US$6.00
	Online print: US$0.04 per line

Notes

Libraries: HEALTH and PATENT.

A subscription charge which covers all transactional charges, connect time, telecommunications and the small administration charge can take the place of the individual charges. Subscriptions are negotiated with customers and vary according to the number of menus (thus, files) that are to be used – typically a minimum subscription would be about US$ 1,000. All charges include training and a 24-hour help line.

This database can also be found on:
PTS Newsletter Database
NEXIS

Grosse Deutsche Spezialitätentaxe – Lauertaxe und ABDA – Datenbank
Ärzneibüro Bundesvereinigung Deutscher Apothekerverbaende (ABDA)

14:480. Master record
CD-ROM   **Pharm-Daig & Lauer**

Database type	Textual, Numeric
Number of journals	
Sources	
Start year	
Language	German
Coverage	Germany
Number of records	
Update size	–
Update period	Quarterly

Keywords

Drugs; Pharmaceuticals; Pharmaceutical Industry

Description

Grosse Deutsche Spezialitäten Taxe combines information from the ABDA database and Lauer Taxe, two databases containing information on drugs and chemicals in the pharmaceutical industry. Gives prices, dates of expiry, details of contents and manufacturers.

For more details of constituent databases, see:
Abda-Pharma
Lauer Taxe

Grupos Terapeuticos
Consejo General de Colegios Oficiales de Farmaceuticos de España

14:481. Master record

Database type	Factual
Number of journals	
Sources	Government documents
Start year	Current information
Language	Spanish
Coverage	Spain
Number of records	
Update size	–
Update period	Periodically
Index unit	Drug

Keywords

Drugs; Pharmaceuticals

Description

Contains data on 423 therapeutic categories of drugs available in Spain. Provides trade name, number of dosage forms available, shelf life, conditions of dispensation (for example, prescription required), and method of administration.

Source is the pharmaceuticals register of the Ministerio de Sanidad y Consumo.

14:482. Online   Consejo General de Colegios Oficiales de Farmaceuticos de España

File name	Grupos Terapeuticos
Start year	Current information
Number of records	
Update period	Periodically

Health and Fitness Forum
CompuServe Information Service

14:484. Master record

Database type	Textual, Factual
Number of journals	
Sources	
Start year	
Language	English
Coverage	International
Number of records	
Update size	–
Update period	Daily

Keywords

Alternative Medicine; Elderly; Environmental Hazards; Family Medicine; Health Care; Mental Health; Nutrition; Substance Abuse

Description

A bulletin board providing members with general health-related information and support groups. Included are discussions of exercise, nutrition, fitness, mental health, emotional and family health, the elderly, food, substance abuse, environmental hazards and alternative health care. In the alternative health care section, regular summaries of published research and new developments on nutritional therapy and herbal remedies can be found.

14:485. Online   CompuServe Information Service

File name	GOODHEALTH
Start year	
Number of records	
Update period	Daily
Price/Charges	Subscription: US$8.95 per month
Downloading is allowed	

Health and Safety Science Abstracts
Cambridge Scientific Abstracts
University of Southern California Institute of Safety and Systems Management

14:486. Master record

Database type	Bibliographic, Factual
Number of journals	
Sources	Monographs, Journals, Reports, Government documents, Conference proceedings, Patents and Dissertations
Start year	1981
Language	English
Coverage	International

Number of records   78,000
Update size   –
Update period   Quarterly

Keywords
Safety; Occupational Health and Safety

Description
Contains citations to the worldwide literature on safety science and hazard control, with an emphasis on the identification, evaluation, and elimination or control of hazards. Covers industrial and occupational safety, transportation safety, aviation and aerospace safety, environmental and ecological safety, and medical safety. Within these areas the database covers liability information and phenomena which directly or indirectly threaten humanity, the environment or the technology upon which they depend, Including such topics as environmental pollution and waste disposal, fire, radiation, pesticides, natural disasters, toxicology, genetics, epidemics, drugs, injuries, diseases, and criminal acts (for example, arson).

Corresponds to *Health and Safety Science Abstracts.*

14:487. Online   ORBIT
File name   SSAB
Start year   1981
Number of records   61,000
Update period   Quarterly
Database aids   Quick Reference Guide (5/90) Free (single copy) and Database Manual (1990) $15.50

14:488. Online   STN
File name   HEALSAFE
Start year   1981
Number of records   78,072
Update period   Quarterly
Price/Charges   Connect time: DM186.00
                        Online print: DM1.02
                        Offline print: DM1.19
                        SDI charge: DM15.20

14:489. Tape   Cambridge Scientific Abstracts
File name   Health and Safety Science Abstracts on Magnetic Tape
Format notes   9-track, unlabelled, 1600 bpi, EBCDIC
Start year   1981
Number of records   78,072
Update period   Quarterly
Price/Charges   Subscription: US$Current year 4,250; single-year archival file 2,100

Notes
Corresponds to the *Health and Safety Science Abstracts* online database.

This database can also be found on:
PolTox I: NLM, CSA, IFIS
Cambridge Scientific Abstracts Engineering
ESA-IRS File 25 – Hard Sciences

Health Business
Faulkner & Gray Inc.

14:491. Master record
Database type   Textual
Number of journals   1
Sources
Start year
Language   English
Coverage   USA

Number of records
Update size   –
Update period   DIALOG, as new data are added to the next daily update of PTS; Data-Star, as new data are added to the next weekly update of PTS

Keywords
Health Care; Pharmaceutical Industry

Description
Tracks important news events and trends in the health care industry dealing with health care provider organizations, pharmaceutical and insurance companies covering business, financial, legal and regulatory developments.

Corresponds to the weekly *Health Business* publication. Supplied by Predicasts to DIALOG and Data-Star.

This database can be found on:
PTS Newsletter

Health Industry Research Reports
JA Micropublishing Inc

14:493. Master record
Database type   Bibliographic
Number of journals
Sources   Reports and Research communications
Start year   1982
Language   English
Coverage   International
Number of records   6,000
Update size   –
Update period   Quarterly

Description
Contains citations, with abstracts, to research reports issued by about seventy security and investment firms on the health industry and individual industry firms. Covers hospital management, pharmaceuticals, medical hardware, life insurance, hospitals, and health care. Citations include title, author, publisher, date, and for companies, geographic location and product listings. Each abstract contains a description of the type of statistical data to be found in the original article.

Users can order full text of documents online.

14:494. Online   BRS, Morning Search, BRS/Colleague
File name   HIRR
Start year   1982
Number of records   6,000
Update period   Quarterly

Health Legislation
World Health Organisation – Health and Biomedical Information Programme. Health Legislation Unit

14:495. Master record
Database type   Bibliographic, Textual
Number of journals
Sources   Government documents and Monographs
Start year   1919
Language
Coverage   International

Number of records   40,000
Update size   –
Update period   Daily

Keywords

Health Care Law; Occupational Hygiene; Pharmaceuticals; Tobacco; Smoking; Nutrition; Environmental Health; HIV

Description

A bibliographic and textual database of information on all aspects of health legislation worldwide. Subjects include AIDS, environmental legislation, health, human nutrition, occupational hygiene, pharmaceuticals and tobacco.

Available to UN system organisations; also to external users. Printed products: *International Digest of Health Legislation* (English and French editions).

14:496. Diskette   World Health Organisation – HLE

File name   Health Legislation
Start year   1919
Number of records   40,000
Update period   Daily

Health News Daily

FDC Reports Inc

14:497. Master record

Alternative name(s)   Health Daily (formerly)
Database type   Textual
Number of journals   1
Sources   Government committee meetings, Government reports, Meeting papers, Newsletters, Press releases, Press conferences, Trade association meetings and Direct contacts
Start year   1988
Language   English
Coverage   USA
Number of records   4,400+
Update size   –
Update period   Daily

Keywords

Cosmetics; Pharmaceuticals

Description

Health News Daily Online contains the full text of *Health News Daily*, a daily newsletter on health care delivery. Subjects covered include: policy and legislation, insurance, funding, manufacturing and new technology, medical breakthroughs and treatments, pharmaceuticals and pharmacy, medical devices and diagnostics, biomedical research, cosmetics, health policy, provider payment policies and cost-containment. Using the FDC reports' staff of thirty reporters and editors, each issue provides up-to-date information about companies, products, markets, personnel, regulatory and legislative activities, financial performances and scientific and legal developments. Regular departments include: Product News, People, Litigation, Legislative News, Industry News, Research, Regulatory News, Financings, Reimbursement and Public Health. 'Washington This Week' lists scheduled congressional hearings, agency meetings and industry conferences in the DC area. 'Calendar' presents notices of forthcoming meetings, conferences and seminars around the USA. 'Legislative Roundup' tracks recently introduced bills, committee activities and congressional votes on health care legislation.

Corresponds to the FDC daily publication *Health News Daily*. Formerly produced by Warren Publishing, Inc. Primary news sources include: press conferences, government committee and panel meetings, briefings to financial analysts, company annual meetings, trade association annual meetings and conventions, activities of scientific and standards-setting groups, legislative and regulatory testimony in Congress, professional organizations and direct interviews with industry newsmakers. In addition, the following secondary sources are utilized: new product announcements, market research reports, press releases, consultant studies, wire services, sales and earnings reports, Securities and Exchange Commission (SEC) filings, and government reports.

14:498. Online   BRS

File name   HNDY
Alternative name(s)   Health Daily (formerly)
Start year   1988
Number of records   4,400+
Update period   Daily
Price/Charges   Connect time: US$120.00/130.00
Online print: US$1.92/2.00
Offline print: US$2.10

14:499. Online   Data-Star

File name   HNDO
Alternative name(s)   Health Daily (formerly)
Start year   March 1989
Number of records   4,400
Update period   Daily
Database aids   Data-Star Business Manual and Data-Star Online Manual (search for NEWS-FDCR or NEWS-HNDO in NEWS)
Price/Charges   Subscription: SFr80.00
Connect time: SFr212.60
Online print: SFr3.25
Offline print: SFr3.42
SDI charge: SFr10.00
Downloading is allowed

Notes

This file contains the latest day's update plus the archive from March 1989.

From June 1993 Data-Star have introduced an annual fee/subscription per contract (that is, not per password) of SFr 80.00 (c.UK£ 32.00) payable every June. For North American customers billed in dollars who also use DIALOG, the DIALOG fee also covers access to Data-Star. Academic customers, 'commitment' customers and customers currently billed in dollars are exempt.

Record composition

Accession Number AN; Date of Publication DT; Month of Publication YM; Occurence table OC; Source SO; Text of article (in full) TX; Title TI; Update Code UP and Year of Publication YR

14:500. Online   Data-Star

File name   HNDD
Alternative name(s)   Health Daily (formerly)
Start year   Current – latest day's update

Number of records	
Update period	Daily
Database aids	Data-Star Business Manual and Data-Star Online Manual (search for NEWS-FDCR or NEWS-HNDO in NEWS)
Price/Charges	Subscription: SFr80.00 Connect time: SFr212.60 Online print: SFr3.25 Offline print: SFr3.42 SDI charge: SFr10.00
Downloading is allowed	

Notes

From June 1993 Data-Star have introduced an annual fee/subscription per contract (that is, not per password) of SFr 80.00 (c.UK£ 32.00) payable every June. For North American customers billed in dollars who also use DIALOG, the DIALOG fee also covers access to Data-Star. Academic customers, 'commitment' customers and customers currently billed in dollars are exempt.

Record composition

Accession Number AN; Date of Publication DT; Month of Publication YM; Occurence table OC; Source SO; Text of article (in full) TX; Title TI; Update Code UP and Year of Publication YR

14:501. Online   NewsNet Inc

File name	Health News Daily
Alternative name(s)	Health Daily (formerly)
Start year	1988
Number of records	
Update period	

Notes

Monthly subscription to NewsNet required; differential charges for subscribers and non-subscribers to Health News Daily.

This database can also be found on:
PTS Newletter

Health Periodicals Database
Information Access Company (IAC)

14:503. Master record

Database type	Bibliographic, Textual
Number of journals Sources	260
Start year	Health specific articles: Index only 1987 to date/full-text 1989 to date; Health articles from general publications: Index only 1976 to date
Language	English
Coverage	International
Number of records	260,000+
Update size	39,000
Update period	Weekly
Abstract details	Either author abstracts or an abstract produced by IAC.
Database aids	Access to Access, Foster City, California, Information Access Company and The Subject Guide to IAC Databases, Foster city, California, IAC

Keywords

HIV; Consumer Protection; Drug Abuse; Mental Health; Nutrition; Occupational Health and Safety; Public Health; Sports Medicine

Description

Health Periodicals provides current and comprehensive information on a wide range of health, fitness, nutrition and specialised medical topics. It offers a mix of record types – some records in the database will contain only indexing, some indexing and author abstracts (from January 1988) and others full-text and consumer summaries (from October 1988). Subjects covered include: pre-natal care, gerontology, dieting, drug abuse, AIDS, biotechnology, cardiovascular disease, environment, medical ethics, health care costs, mental health, public health, occupational health and safety, paramedical professions, sports medicine, substance abuse, toxicology and others. The database provides a valuable resource for corporate, medical, and legal librarians, human resource professionals and product analysts. It is designed to meet the needs also of non-medical professionals. It is the only online health database that features consumer summaries for the layperson.

Articles are collected from 150 important medical journals and over 110 core health, fitness, and nutrition publications. Selected articles dealing with health topics are sourced from over 3,000 other publications indexed by IAC since 1976. Some of the database entries include author abstracts; some include summaries aimed specifically at the consumer lay- person, condensing, simplifying and explaining complex medical research terms and results. The full text of a range of 110 selected journals has been included from 1989 only.

A controlled vocabulary is used, a full list of which is available from the producer. Indexing terms are taken from *Library of Congress Subject Headings*, the National Library of Medicine Subject Headings (*MeSH*), *Mosby's Medical and Nursing Dictionary*, and terms created by Information Access where no suitable term exists. The special features data field indicates inclusion of photographs, illustrations in the original article and includes the text accompanying a caption. A full list of special features is available from the producer.

14:504. Online   BRS

File name	HEAL
Start year	1987 citations; 1989 full text
Number of records	213,000
Update period	Weekly
Price/Charges	Connect time: US$80.00/90.00 Online print: US$0.92/1.00 Offline print: US$2.00 SDI charge: US$3.50

14:505. Online   CompuServe Information Service

File name	IQUEST File 2847
Start year	1976, some, with most citations from 1987; 1989 full text
Number of records	34,000
Update period	Weekly
Price/Charges	Subscription: US$8.95 per month Database entry fee: US$9/search; some databases carry a surcharge ($2–75) Online print: US$10 references free; then $9 per ten; abstracts $3 each
Downloading is allowed	

Notes

On CompuServe, contains more than 34,000 articles, including more than 26,000 in full text.

Accessed via IQUEST or IQMEDICAL, this database is offered by a DIALOG gateway. IQUEST can either search across all databases, a database of the user's choice or selected multiple databases.

14:506. Online   Data-Star

File name	HLTH
Start year	Health specific articles: Index only 1987 to date/full-text 1989 to date; Health articles from general publications: Index only 1976 to date/full-text 1983 to date.
Number of records	187,000
Update period	Weekly
Database aids	Data-Star Biomedical Manual and Data-Star Online Manual (search NEWS-HLTH in NEWS)
Price/Charges	Subscription: SFr80.00 Connect time: SFr147.00 Online print: SFr0.56 Offline print: SFr0.64 SDI charge: SFr6.80

Notes

From June 1993 Data-Star have introduced an annual fee/subscription per contract (that is, not per password) of SFr 80.00 (c.UK£ 32.00) payable every June. For North American customers billed in dollars who also use DIALOG, the DIALOG fee also covers access to Data-Star. Academic customers, 'commitment' customers and customers currently billed in dollars are exempt.

Record composition

Abstract AB; Article Type AT; Author AU; Availability AV; Accession Number and Update Code AN; Case Law CS; Column Inches CI; Company Name CO; Copyright CP; Date of Publication DT; Descriptor(s) DE; Full-text FT; Geographic Code and Name CN; Lead paragraph LP; Length LE; Personal Name PE; Product Name TN; Source SO; Special Features and Letter Grade SF; Statute/Jurisdiction LW; Text TX; Title TI; Update Code UP; US SIC Code CC; Year YR; Year/Month YM and Year/Month/Day DT

14:507. Online   DIALOG

File name	File 149
Start year	January 1988
Number of records	264,870
Update period	Weekly
Price/Charges	Connect time: US$90.00 Online print: US$0.90 – 1.20 Offline print: US$0.90 – 1.20 SDI charge: US$3.50

Notes

The DIALOG file contains records from January 1988, when the author abstracts were added to the database by IAC. DIALINDEX Categories: CONSUMER, MEDICINE, NUTRIT, PRODINFO. Daily updates to indexing and displayable abstracts, summaries and full text are available in Newsearch database, File 211 on DIALOG. DIALOG Alert Service available weekly. Available on DIALOG menus.

14:508. Database subset
Tape   Information Access Company (IAC)

File name	Health Index
Format notes	IBM
Start year	1987

Number of records	125,000+
Update period	Monthly
Price/Charges	Subscription: US$9,000

Notes

A subset of Health Periodicals Database containing the citations only (not the full text of articles) from the contents of the Health Periodicals Database. It is a comprehensive index to over 150 journals, magazines, newspapers, newsletters in health, fitness, medicine, nutrition, and other related consumer health topics. Prices are: annual subscription to current and previous year, $9,000; archival files, $2,500 per year of data.

This database can also be found on:
Health Reference Center

Health Source
EBSCO

14:510. Master record

Alternative name(s)	Source Line: Health Source CD-ROM; Health and Consumer Source
Database type	Textual
Number of journals	160
Sources	Journals
Start year	
Language	English
Coverage	International
Number of records	
Update size	—
Update period	Three times a year/Six times a year
Index unit	Articles

Keywords

Diet; Drugs; Nutrition

Description

A consumer health reference product that provides abstracts and indexing for 160 journals in the fields of consumer products, diet and nutrition, exercise, drugs and alcohol plus medical self care. Contains searchable full-text articles for approximately fifteen of the journals.

EBSCO report the disc was released in August 1992. Also available on one disc updated six times a year.

14:511. CD-ROM   EBSCO

File name	Health Source CD-ROM
Alternative name(s)	Source Line: Health Source CD-ROM; Health and Consumer Source
Format notes	IBM
Start year	
Number of records	
Update period	Three times a year/Six times a year
Price/Charges	Subscription: US$495 – 570

Notes

Cost for the alternative (six times a year update) disc is $995 inside US and Canada, $1095 outside US and Canada.

Healthcom Medical Information Service
Robert L Walter Communications

14:512. Master record

Database type	Textual, Bibliographic, Directory
Number of journals	
Sources	Journals and Groups

Start year	Current information
Language	English
Coverage	USA
Number of records	
Update size	—
Update period	Continuously; tutorials, monthly

Keywords

HIV; Drug Abuse; Alcohol Abuse; Women's Studies

Description

Contains health care information and advice for consumers. Covers diet and nutrition, mental health, sexuality, traditional and alternative therapies, alcohol and drug abuse, family health care, women's health issues, and dental care. Provides a forum for exchanges between health care professionals and users, as well as interactive tutorials on subjects of current interest (for example, Acquired Immune Deficiency Syndrome (AIDS)). Each tutorial is accompanied by references to selected materials from popular and professional journals. Also contains full text of Health Resources Directory, providing descriptions of United States health organizations and self-help groups.

14:513. Online CompuServe Information Service

File name	
Start year	Current information
Number of records	
Update period	Continuously; tutorials, monthly
Price/Charges	Subscription: US$8.95 per month
Downloading is allowed	

Healthnet
HealthNet Ltd

14:514. Master record

Database type	Textual, Factual
Number of journals	
Sources	
Start year	Current information
Language	English
Coverage	USA
Number of records	
Update size	—
Update period	Monthly

Keywords

HIV; Cancer

Description

Contains health care information for consumers. Covers symptoms and diseases, drugs, medical tests and procedures, first aid, nutrition, sexuality, exercise, sports medicine, preventive medicine, and environmental health. Also includes topical articles (for example, effects of caffeine consumption, updates on Acquired Immune Deficiency Syndrome (AIDS), lung cancer, near sightedness), a self-administered health quiz, and a question and answer forum.

14:515. Online CompuServe Information Service

File name	HNT
Start year	Current information
Number of records	
Update period	Monthly
Price/Charges	Subscription: US$8.95 per month
Downloading is allowed	

14:516. Online General Videotex Corporation, Delphi

File name	
Start year	Current information
Number of records	
Update period	Monthly

Herbalist CD-ROM
Hopkins Technology

14:517. Master record

Database type	Textual, Factual
Number of journals	
Sources	
Start year	
Language	English
Coverage	
Number of records	180
Update size	—
Update period	

Keywords

Alternative Medicine; Herbal Remedies

Description

The Herbalist CD-ROM covers the use of herbal medicines within a holistic perspective and includes information on basic principles of herbalism, human systems, herbal actions and their activity, and Materia Medica covering over 180 herbs. Medical and scientific citations and illustrations are included. The text is written by David L Hoffmann.

14:518. CD-ROM Hopkins Technology

File name	
Format notes	IBM
Start year	
Number of records	180
Update period	
Price	US$99.95

Notes

It is possible to search by herb, ailment, body area or generic topic. Software runs under DOS or Windows.

Human Sexuality Databank and Forums
Clinical Communications Inc

14:519. Master record

Database type	Textual
Number of journals	
Sources	Periodicals, Interviews and Discussions
Start year	Current information
Language	English
Coverage	USA
Number of records	
Update size	—
Update period	Every one or two weeks

Keywords

Social Medicine; Pathology; Sexuality; HIV; Homosexuality; Reproduction; Contraception; Sexually Transmitted Diseases; Urology; Gynaecology; Endocrinology; Sexual Dysfunction

Description

Contains information and advice on all aspects of human sexuality, including contraception, relationships, sexual dysfunction, homosexuality, sexually transmitted diseases, urology, gynaecology, psychiatry, pharmacology and endocrinology. Includes articles, interview and discussion transcripts, interactive programs and answers to commonly asked questions. Users can submit comments and questions online via two fora; experts answer topics on a variety of topics.

14:520. Online — CompuServe Information Service

File name	HUMAN
Start year	Current information
Number of records	
Update period	Every one or two weeks
Price/Charges	Subscription: US$8.95 per month
Downloading is allowed	

ICYT

Consejo Superior de Investigaciones Científicas de España (CSIC)

14:521. Master record

Alternative name(s)	Indice Español de Ciencia y Tecnología
Database type	Bibliographic
Number of journals	365
Sources	
Start year	1979
Language	Spanish
Coverage	Spain
Number of records	56,500
Update size	–
Update period	Twice per year

Keywords

Agronomy; Astrophysics; Earth Sciences; Logic; Physics; Technology

Description

Bibliographic referential database containing citations to Spanish literature and research articles in the scientific and technical field extracted from 365 Spanish periodicals. Covers the following areas: agriculture, astronomy and astrophysics, life sciences, earth sciences and space, physics, mathematics, logic, pharmacology, chemistry and technology.

Corresponds to *Indice Español de Ciencia y Technología*.

Material published in Spain.

14:522. Online — Consejo Superior de Investigaciones Científicas de España (CSIC)

File name	ICYT
Start year	1979
Number of records	56,500
Update period	Twice per year

14:523. Online — Ministerio de Educación y Ciencia de España (MEC), Centro de Proceso de Datos

File name	
Start year	1979
Number of records	56,500
Update period	Twice per year

14:524. Online — Ministerio de Cultura de España, Secretaria General Técnica

File name	
Start year	1979
Number of records	56,500
Update period	Twice per year

This database can also be found on:
CSIC

Identidex

Micromedex Inc

14:526. Master record

Alternative name(s)	Computerized Clinical Information System: Identidex; CCIS: Identidex
Database type	Factual, Textual, Directory
Number of journals	
Sources	
Start year	1985
Language	English (primarily)
Coverage	USA
Number of records	
Update size	–
Update period	Quarterly

Keywords

Drugs

Description

Contains two databases providing identification of prescription, over the counter (OTC), trademarked and generic drugs in tablet or capsule form, primarily by the manufacturer's imprint code with secondary characteristics, such as colour and shape, as descriptors. Descriptions of manufacturer's logos assist in differentiating among similar logos. Manufacturer's telephone numbers are also included.

Slang listing – a file containing over 4700 contemporary slang terms for abusive substances. Includes ethnic and non-English terms, and, when available, place of origin and literature references.

Tablet & Capsule Identification – contains identification information on over 40,000 pharmaceuticals including prescription and over the counter, trademarked and generic drugs, 'look-alike' stimulants and street drugs, in tablet and capsule form. Users can search by manufacurer imprint code. Information on each drug includes physical description (for example, size, colour, shape, logo description), ingredient information, historical data (date of imprint code change or discontinuation)

14:527. CD-ROM — Micromedex Inc

File name	Identidex
Alternative name(s)	Computerized Clinical Information System: Identidex; CCIS: Identidex
Start year	1985
Number of records	
Update period	Quarterly

Notes

This database is available as a standalone product, as well as being a part of CCIS, Computerized Clinical Information System.

14:528. Tape — Micromedex Inc

File name	Identidex
Alternative name(s)	Computerized Clinical Information System: Identidex; CCIS: Identidex
Software	Proprietary

Start year	1973
Number of records	
Update period	Quarterly

Notes

Annual subscription to CCIS required. This database is also available on CD-ROM as a standalone product, and as part of the CCIS, Computerized Clinical Information System.

This database can also be found on:
CCIS

IDIS Drug File
Iowa Drug Information Service

14:530. Master record

Database type	Bibliographic
Number of journals	160
Sources	Journals
Start year	1966
Language	English
Coverage	International
Number of records	300,000
Update size	—
Update period	Monthly
Index unit	Articles
Database aids	Drug and disease cross-reference lists with the IDIS controlled vocabulary terms are available from the producer

Keywords

Drug Therapy; Pathology

Description

IDIS Drug File presents an online index to the IDIS drug literature microfilm file, which contains some 240,000 articles, relating to drugs and drug therapy in humans published since 1965 in over 160 biomedical journals. Subjects covered include age group of study population, study design, treatment efficacy, dosage administration technique, pharmacokinetics, pharmaceutics, incompatibilities, drug interactions, toxicology and side effects. Animal studies are not included. Each record contains title, author(s), bibliographic details.

Articles are taken from over 140 of the top English language medical and pharmaceutical journals.

Documents are extensively indexed with terms for drugs, diseases and type of information. The corresponding microfilm number is also given, directing users to the microfilmed journal article, which is available from the producer as IDIS Drug Literature Microfilm File. There may be multiple index documents for the same journal article to reflect a group of concepts presented within the article. Drug and disease cross-reference lists with the IDIS controlled vocabulary terms are available from the producer.

Drug indexing terms are adapted from the United States Adapted Names; Disease indexing terms are adapted from the International Classification of Diseases, 9th Revision, Clinical Modification.

14:531. Online   BRS

File name	IDIS
Start year	1966
Number of records	300,000
Update period	Monthly

Price/Charges	Connect time: US$42.00/52.00
	Online print: US$0.27/0.35
	Offline print: US$0.45
	SDI charge: US$6.95
Downloading is allowed	

14:532. Online   Data-Star

File name	IOWA
Start year	1966
Number of records	336,000
Update period	Monthly
Database aids	Data-Star Biomedical Manual, Berne, Data-Star, 1988 and Online Manual (search in NEWS for NEWS-IOWA)
Price/Charges	Subscription: SFr80.00
	Connect time: SFr87.80
	Online print: SFr0.63
	Offline print: SFr0.79
	SDI charge: SFr8.40
Downloading is allowed	

Notes

From June 1993 Data-Star have introduced an annual fee/subscription per contract (that is, not per password) of SFr 80.00 (c.UK£ 32.00) payable every June. For North American customers billed in dollars who also use DIALOG, the DIALOG fee also covers access to Data-Star. Academic customers, 'commitment' customers and customers currently billed in dollars are exempt.

Record composition

Accession Number and Update Code AN; Author(s) AU; Descriptors DE; Microfilm Number MF; Publication Type PT; Source SO; Title TI; Update Code UP and Year of Publication YR

IMS Marketletter
IMSWorld Publications Ltd

14:533. Master record

Alternative name(s)	Marketletter
Database type	Textual
Number of journals	1
Sources	Interviews, Journals, Press releases and Conferences
Start year	1985
Language	English
Coverage	International
Number of records	
Update size	—
Update period	Daily
Index unit	Articles

Keywords

Health Care; Legislation; Marketing; Pharmaceutical Industry; Stock Market

Description

The full text of IMSworld publication *Marketletter*, a weekly newsletter covering up-to-date news and information on all aspects of the pharmaceuticals and health care industries worldwide. On Data-Star prepublication material appears in the daily (IMLD) and current (IMLC) files within one day of writing. *Marketletter* focuses on current news and information about the following aspects of the pharmaceutical and health care industry: Company news, including financial reports, marketing development trends and strategies, corporate developments, detailed company profiles, legal influences, research and devlopment trends, multinational deals, in-depth stock market analysis, mergers and acquisitions, sales performance and personnel appointments. Product news includes drug submissions, approvals and rejections, licensing arrangements, clinical trial developments and results, product developments and new product introductions. Current news (USA, European and world news) includes conference reports, regulatory developments and reviews of new and proposed market legislation and regulations.

14:534. Online — CompuServe Information Service

File name	IQUEST File 2844
Alternative name(s)	Marketletter
Start year	1985
Number of records	
Update period	Weekly
Price/Charges	Subscription: US$8.95 per month
	Database entry fee: US$9/search; some databases carry a surcharge ($2–75)
	Online print: US$10 references free; then $9 per ten; abstracts $3 each

Downloading is allowed

Notes

Accessed via IQUEST, this database is offered by a Data-Star gateway. IQUEST can either search across all databases, a database of the user's choice or selected multiple databases.

14:535. Online — Data-Star

File name	IMLA
Alternative name(s)	Marketletter
Start year	1985
Number of records	
Update period	Daily
Price/Charges	Subscription: UK£32.00
	Connect time: UK£87.60
	Online print: UK£0.51
	Offline print: UK£0.69

Notes

IMLA is the archive database for IMS Marketletter, containing all records from the start date (1985) to prior to four weeks ago.

From June 1993 Data-Star have introduced an annual fee/subscription per contract (that is, not per password) of SFr 80.00 (c.UK£ 32.00) payable every June. For North American customers billed in dollars who also use DIALOG, the DIALOG fee also covers access to Data-Star. Academic customers, 'commitment' customers and customers currently billed in dollars are exempt.

14:536. Online — Data-Star

File name	IMLC
Alternative name(s)	Marketletter
Start year	Current (latest four weeks of data)
Number of records	
Update period	Daily
Price/Charges	Subscription: UK£32.00
	Connect time: UK£87.60
	Online print: UK£1.82
	Offline print: UK£1.94
	SDI charge: UK£4.32

Notes

IMLC contains all the current news from the IMS Marketletter database, including IMLD (the latest four weeks of data), and pre-publication material, which appears within one day of writing.

From June 1993 Data-Star have introduced an annual

fee/subscription per contract (that is, not per password) of SFr 80.00 (c.UK£ 32.00) payable every June. For North American customers billed in dollars who also use DIALOG, the DIALOG fee also covers access to Data-Star. Academic customers, 'commitment' customers and customers currently billed in dollars are exempt.

14:537. Online — Data-Star

File name	IMLD
Alternative name(s)	Marketletter
Start year	Current
Number of records	
Update period	Daily
Price/Charges	Subscription: UK£32.00
	Connect time: UK£87.60
	Online print: UK£1.82
	Offline print: UK£1.94
	SDI charge: UK£4.32

Notes

IMLD contains the daily news from the IMS Marketletter database, pre-publication material which appears within one day of writing.

From June 1993 Data-Star have introduced an annual fee/subscription per contract (that is, not per password) of SFr 80.00 (c.UK£ 32.00) payable every June. For North American customers billed in dollars who also use DIALOG, the DIALOG fee also covers access to Data-Star. Academic customers, 'commitment' customers and customers currently billed in dollars are exempt.

14:538. Online — Data-Star

File name	IMZZ
Alternative name(s)	Marketletter
Start year	1985
Number of records	
Update period	Daily
Price/Charges	Subscription: UK£32.00
	Connect time: UK£87.60
	Online print: UK£1.82
	Offline print: UK£1.94
	SDI charge: UK£4.32

Notes

IMZZ contains the full text of the IMSworld Marketletter, from 1985 to date.

From June 1993 Data-Star have introduced an annual fee/subscription per contract (that is, not per password) of SFr 80.00 (c.UK£ 32.00) payable every June. For North American customers billed in dollars who also use DIALOG, the DIALOG fee also covers access to Data-Star. Academic customers, 'commitment' customers and customers currently billed in dollars are exempt.

Imspact
IMS America Ltd, Hospital/Laboratory/Veterinary Database Division

14:539. Master record

Database type	Numeric, Textual
Number of journals	7
Sources	Trade journals
Start year	Current six years
Language	English
Coverage	USA

Number of records
Update size   —
Update period   Weekly

Keywords

Marketing; Advertising; Pharmaceutical Industry;
Drugs

Description

Gives reports of seven audits performed by IMS
America of the pharmaceuticals industry. Provides
monthly sale data, including hospital and chemist
(drugstore) purchases by company, product class and
individual product (at the package level); medical
data, including NDTI information on the usage of
drugs (by product, form and strength) per diagnosis;
prescription data, including new prescriptions written
and new and repeat (refill) prescriptions dispensed;
and promotional data, including number of units and
dollars spent on mail and journal advertising. Also
gives data on the number of kilogrammes sold of
pharmaceutically active chemicals. Product characteristics covered include formula, price, date of introduction, chemical family, medical usage, application form
and corporate structure of the manufacturer.

Full texts of *Pharmaceutical Markets, Drugstores*;
*Pharmaceutical Markets, Hospitals; National Disease
& Therapeutic Index (NDTI)*; *National Prescription
Audit*; *National Journal Audit*; *National Mail Audit*; and
National Detailing Audit.

14:540. Online   IMS America Ltd

File name
Start year   Current six years
Number of records
Update period   Weekly

Notes

Subscription to the printed audits required.

IMSWorld New Product Launch Letter

IMSWorld Publications Ltd

14:541. Master record

Alternative name(s)   New Product Launch Letter; New
                       Product Card Index (former name)
Database type   Directory, Factual
Number of journals
Sources   Newsletters and technical reports
Start year   1977
Language   English and European languages
                       (some paragraphs)
Coverage   International
Number of records   23,000
Update size   4,800
Update period   Monthly
Database aids   EPhMRA Classification Codes, free
                       from IMSWorld Publications Ltd

Keywords

Pharmaceutical Products

Description

This database is a source of new pharmaceutical
product launch information worldwide. The launching
of new ethical pharmaceuticals in 47 countries is
monitored for inclusion in the database, which contains details of ethical pharmaceutical products

launched since the beginning of 1987. Each record
contains the following details: brand name, local marketing company and its international parent company,
launch date, country of launch, launch price, active
ingredients, formulation and strength, retail sales price
at launch, therapeutic class and code, indications and
presentation (pack information). Biotechnology and
new chemical entity launches can be identified.

The database is equivalent to the Compendium section of *New Product Launch Letter* published monthly
by IMSWorld

Therapeutic class codes used are derived from the
EPhMRA classification system. Product names are
those under which drugs are marketed in the country
of launch. Broader retrieval will result from a search by
drug-name qualified to composition. Launches in
other countries may be made by local subsidiaries of
larger multinationals it is therefore recommended that
the corporate name field is searched to check as to
'who owns whom' among the manufacturers. The language of text field refers to the language of indications
and pack information in the country of launch. English
is used for many countries worldwide and Spanish for
most of Central and South America as well as Spain.
Biotechnology classification can be used either as a
search term or as a limit option to enable products to
be found or excluded from a search. The launch indicator field is displayed only for first world launches.

14:542. Online   Data-Star

File name   IPLL
Alternative name(s)   New Product Launch Letter; New
                       Product Card Index (former name)
Start year   1977
Number of records   23,000
Update period   Monthly
Database aids   Data-Star Business Manual and
                       Data-Star Online Guide (search
                       NEWS-IPLL in NEWS)

Downloading is allowed
Thesaurus is online

Notes

From June 1993 Data-Star have introduced an annual
fee/subscription per contract (that is, not per password) of SFr 80.00 (c.UK£ 32.00) payable every June.
For North American customers billed in dollars who
also use DIALOG, the DIALOG fee also covers
access to Data-Star. Academic customers, 'commitment' customers and customers currently billed in
dollars are exempt.

Record composition

Accession Number and Update Code AN; Biotech
classification BC; Composition CP; Corporate Name
CO; Country of Launch CN; Entry Date ED;
Indications IN; Language of Text LG; Launch Date DT;
Manufacturer MF; Number of Components IG; Pack
Information PI; Product Name PN; Therapeutic Class
TC; Update Code (YYMMDD) UD; Update Code
(YYMM) UP and Year of Launch YR

14:543. CD-ROM   IMSWorld Publications Ltd

File name   Drug Launches
Alternative name(s)   New Product Launch Letter; New
                       Product Card Index (former name)
Format notes   IBM
Start year   1977

Number of records	23,000
Update period	Monthly
Price/Charges	Subscription: UK£2,400

Notes

For non-profit organisations the subscription cost is £1,000, updated quarterly.

This database can also be found on:
IMSWorld Online Service

IMSWorld Online Service
IMS AG, International Services Division

14:545. Master record

Database type	Directory, Textual
Number of journals	
Sources	
Start year	DLO: 1977; DPI: 1987; NPLL: 1977; PM: Current information
Language	English
Coverage	International
Number of records	DPI: 13,000; PM: 230,000
Update size	—
Update period	DLO: Weekly; DPI: Monthly; NPLL: Monthly; PM: Annually or twice per year, depending on country

Keywords

Pharmaceutical Products; Pharmaceuticals; Therapeutic Drugs; Marketing; Patents; Drugs

Description

Contains four files.

Drug License Opportunities contains information on therapeutic drugs under development or available for licensing worldwide, from 1977 to date. For each drug, the record includes phase of development, names (chemical, labcode, generic and brand), therapeutic class, pharmacological actions and indications, clinical details, formulations, patent, trademark, regulatory approval status, expected launch date, licensing availability and contact information for companies associated with the product. Corresponds to *Drug License Opportunities*.

Drug Patents International contains information on over 800 drug molecules covering more than 13,000 drug patents. Each record includes drug name, synonyms, trade names, therapeutic class, compound name, CAS Registry number, description, patent information (patent number, assignee, priority numbers and dates, publication date, country, and for subscribers to the printed version, estimated expiry dates).

New Product Launch Letter contains the full text of *New Product Launch Letter* (previous title: *New Product Card Index*), covering pharmaceutical introductions in 48 countries from 1977 to date. Records give compound and brand names, indication, ingredients, country and date of launch, marketing company, formulation, packaging and price.

Product Monographs contains standardised profiles for about 230,000 pharmaceutical products marketed in 44 countries, giving international product name, brand name, packaging size and description, ingredients, formulation and strength, price, marketing company

14:546. Online
IMS AG, International Services Division

File name	
Start year	DLO: 1977; DPI: 1987; NPLL: 1977; PM: Current information
Number of records	DPI: 13,000; PM: 230,000
Update period	DLO: Weekly; DPI: Monthly; NPLL: Monthly; PM: Annually or twice per year, depending on country

For more details of constituent databases, see:
IMSWorld New Product Launch Letter
Drug Patents International

IMSWorld Product Monographs
IMSWorld Publications Ltd

14:549. Master record

Alternative name(s)	Product Monographs
Database type	Directory, Factual
Number of journals	
Sources	
Start year	1993
Language	English
Coverage	International
Number of records	350,000
Update size	—
Update period	Monthly (May to December)
Index unit	Drugs
Database aids	EPhMRA Anatomical Therapeutic Classification Codes and IMS Dose Form Codes

Description

IMS Product Monographs contains comprehensive details on launched pharmaceuticals. Each monograph details brand name, composition, country, therapeutic class and country of launch together with date and marketing company for that country. For each brand retail and hospital prices (at ex-manufacturer prices) are given for each pack presentation or formulation.

The producers suggest that the database can answer such questions as:

– What is the price and pack availability for Capoten in the USA?
– What injectable formulations of ranitidine are available?
– What cardiovascular drugs were launched in 1990?
– How many drugs has a competitor company launched in the last year?
– In how many countries has aciclovir been launched?

The pricing data is exclusive to the pharmaceutical industry; while the database is available to all business sectors, product pricing is not included outside of the pharamceutical industry for reasons of confidentiality. For market research intelligence on the pharmaceutical industry the IMS Product Monographs files provide invaluable competitor information on marketed drugs worldwide. For this reason the database is split between two files on Data-Star.

The database contains unique data collected and audited by IMSWorld Publications from more than fifty countries throughout the world.

14:550. Online
Data-Star

File name	IPOP
Alternative name(s)	Product Monographs
Start year	1993

Number of records	350,000
Update period	Monthly (May to December)
Price/Charges	Connect time: US$158.00
	Online print: US$1.45
	Offline print: US$1.80

Notes

IPOP does not contain product pricing; in all other aspects it is an identical file to IPPP. IPPP is available to the pharmaceutical industry only – users should contact IMS for more details.

The product information includes: ingredients, launch date, the number of active ingredients, the formulation, the dose form code, the therapeutic class code and the availability.

Record composition

Accession Number AN; Occurences OC; Trade Name TN/TP; First Launch Date DT; Country CN; Company CO; Parent Company PA; Composition CP; Source and Publication Date SO; Product Information PI; Therapeutic Class Code CC; Ingredients IN; Availability AV (AV=R Retail/AV=H Hospital); Entry Date ED; Update UD and Update Month UP

14:551. Online   Data-Star

File name	IPPP
Alternative name(s)	Product Monographs
Start year	1993
Number of records	350,000
Update period	Monthly (May to December)
Price/Charges	Connect time: US$158.00
	Online print: US$1.65
	Offline print: US$1.99

Notes

IPPP contains product pricing; in all other aspects IPOP is an identical file. IPPP is available to the pharmaceutical industry only – users should contact IMS for more details.

The product information includes: ingredients, launch date, the number of active ingredients, the formulation, the dose form code, the therapeutic class code and the availability.

Record composition

Accession Number AN; Occurences OC; Trade Name TN/TP; First Launch Date DT; Country CN; Company CO; Parent Company PA; Composition CP; Source and Publication Date SO; Product Information PI; Therapeutic Class Code CC; Ingredients IN; Availability AV (AV=R Retail/AV=H Hospital); Entry Date ED; Update UD and Update Month UP

IMSWorld's Pharmaceutical Company Profiles
IMSWorld Publications Ltd

14:552. Master record

Alternative name(s)	Pharmaceutical Company Profiles
Database type	Factual, Textual
Number of journals	
Sources	Annual reports, Analyst reports, News wire services and Trade press
Start year	1991
Language	English
Coverage	International

Number of records	110
Update size	–
Update period	Monthly
Index unit	Companies

Keywords

Drugs; Pharmaceuticals

Description

In depth profiles of 110 pharmaceutical companies around the world, reporting on and reviewing each company's activity in finance, research and development, product portfolio, historical development and major events. Its strategic and competitive analysis of the worldwide pharmaceutical industry includes interviews with key company executives wherever possible, gathering inside information unobtainable elsewhere.

The views of independent financial analysts are include in many reports, to add breadth of viewpoint. Coverage in IPCP includes a wide range of companies – both large and small, private and public, national and multinational within the international arena.

Data are collected from the following principal sources: IMS own in- house information from IMS services; interviews with executives within the profiled companies, independent analysts, press conferences; investor meetings. Pharmaceutical subsidiaries will be available on IPDR.

14:553. Online   Data-Star

File name	IPCP
Alternative name(s)	Pharmaceutical Company Profiles
Start year	1991
Number of records	110 reports
Update period	Monthly
Database aids	Data-Star Guide to IPCP in Data-Star Business Manual and Online manual (search NEWS-IPCP in NEWS)

Notes

From June 1993 Data-Star have introduced an annual fee/subscription per contract (that is, not per password) of SFr 80.00 (c.UK£ 32.00) payable every June. For North American customers billed in dollars who also use DIALOG, the DIALOG fee also covers access to Data-Star. Academic customers, 'commitment' customers and customers currently billed in dollars are exempt.

Index Nominum
Société Suisse de Pharmacie

14:554. Master record

Database type	
Number of journals	
Sources	
Start year	
Language	English
Coverage	Switzerland
Number of records	
Update size	–
Update period	
Index unit	Drug

Keywords

Drugs; Pharmaceuticals; Surgery

Description

One of the databases contained on the CD-ROMs MediROM and PharmaROM in the medical and health care fields, produced for Swiss physicians and pharmacists. Also included as an option with the CD-ROM Vidal.

This database can also be found on:
MediROM
CD-ROM Vidal
PharmaROM

Industry Data Sources
Information Access Company (IAC)

14:556. Master record

Alternative name(s)	Harfax; Harfax Industry Data Sources
Database type	Bibliographic, Textual
Number of journals	
Sources	Reports, Trade journals, Databases, Monographs, Dissertations and Conference reports
Start year	1979 to 1990
Language	English
Coverage	International
Number of records	133,686
Update size	–
Update period	Closed File
Hosts have included	Data-Star (HARF) (until 12/90) DIALOG (File 189) (until 10/92) BRS (HARF) (until 12/90)

Keywords

Drugs; Pharmaceutical Industry; Pharmaceuticals

Description

Major bibliographic index of sources for financial and marketing data in 65 major industries worldwide, including market research, investment banking studies, forecasts, etc. More than 100,000 primary and secondary sources, including market research reports, investment banking studies, special issues of trade journals, economic forecast and numeric databases. It covers industries and sectors such as advertising, agriculture, broadcasting, chemicals, commercial banking, construction, drugs, pharmaceuticals. Each record includes a short abstract of the item, plus full information for ordering from the publisher (that is, contact person, address, telephone number). Detailed classification scheme and indexing.

Also known as Harfax, IAC discontinued the file in December 1990 according to The 'Dead' Database: Where do databases go when they leave online? (*Database* October 1992 15–31) after many years of poor updates; BRS and Data-Star dropped the file but DIALOG continues to carry it until late 1992. Barbara Quint recommends searchers to try FIND/SVP Information Catalog (NewsNet: GB51E) or the Cambridge Information Group's Findex (DIALOG File 196); full-text market reports can be found on Investext, or – for a more European focus – on ICC Key Note Market Analyses (Data-Star, DIALOG, Mead and MAID) while directory information is available in the Gale Database of Publications and Broadcast Media (DIALOG File 469).

Entries are indexed in several ways, including SIC codes, data descriptors and country designations.

14:557. Online — Society of Petroleum Engineers (SPE), Petro-Link

File name	
Alternative name(s)	Harfax; Harfax Industry Data Sources
Start year	1979 to 1990
Number of records	133,686
Update period	Closed File

Infomat
Infomat Ltd
Predicasts Europe

14:559. Master record

Alternative name(s)	Infomat International Business News; Infomat International Business
Database type	Bibliographic, Textual
Number of journals	560
Sources	Newspapers, Trade journals and Reports
Start year	1991 (January)
Language	English
Coverage	International (some) and Europe (primarily)
Number of records	914,467
Update size	234,000
Update period	Daily

Keywords

Automotive Industry; Biotechnology; Food and Drink; Construction; Civil Engineering; Pharmaceutical Industry; Information Technology

Description

Infomat International Business, a wholly-owned subsidiary of Predicasts, extracts and provides concise summaries of news stories and press cuttings services from around 600 business and trade newspapers and journals, translated into English from ten languages, from 22 countries in Europe and the world. Covers marketing, advertising, competitors' activities, sales leads, new products and services, technology, legislation, mergers and acquisitions, business trends, economic forecasts, new technologies, key appointments, company news: results, mergers and acquisitions, business trends. Abstracts included in the database are selected to meet the specific information requests of Infomat's client companies in the key companies monitored – sectors such as: advanced engineering, food, beverages, leisure, transport, automotive industry, construction/civil engineering, science, technology, biotechnology, electronics, communications, engineering, chemicals, energy, forest products, media/marketing, oil/gas/chemicals, packaging/paper/printing/publishing, financial services, health care, pharmaceuticals, communications, information technology. Comprehensive attempt to provide abstracts of relevant foreign-language material in English.

Sources include such varied titles as *Computerwoche* (West Germany), *Dinero* (Spain) *Food and Drug Packaging* (USA), *Marketing Week* (UK), *Moniteur du Commerce International* (France) *Singapore Business Times*, and *Il Sole 24 Ore* (Italy).

14:560. Online — Data-Star

File name	EBUS
Alternative name(s)	Infomat International Business News; Infomat International Business
Start year	1984 (April)

Number of records — 514,000
Update period — Weekly
Price/Charges — Subscription: UK£32.00
Connect time: UK£56.40
Online print: UK£0.58
Offline print: UK£0.54
SDI charge: UK£3.92

Notes

Also available on FIZ Technik via a gateway. From June 1993 Data-Star have introduced an annual fee-/subscription per contract (that is, not per password) of SFr 80.00 (c.UK£ 32.00) payable every June. For North American customers billed in dollars who also use DIALOG, the DIALOG fee also covers access to Data-Star. Academic customers, 'commitment' customers and customers currently billed in dollars are exempt.

14:561. Online   DIALOG

File name — File 583
Alternative name(s) — Infomat International Business News; Infomat International Business
Start year — 1984 (April)
Number of records — 914,467
Update period — Weekly
Price/Charges — Connect time: US$108.00
Online print: US$0.90
Offline print: US$0.90
SDI charge: US$4.95

14:562. Online   ESA-IRS

File name — File 156
Alternative name(s) — Infomat International Business News; Infomat International Business
Start year — 1984
Number of records — 830,000 (October 1991)
Update period — Weekly

Notes

From 1993 ESA-IRS are charging an annual fee of 100 Accounting Units (c.UK£ 70.29) to all users. This is equivalent to the fee for full documentation and will not be charged to customers already paying for documentation.

14:563. Online   FIZ Technik

File name — EBUS
Alternative name(s) — Infomat International Business News; Infomat International Business
Start year — 1986
Number of records — 852,000
Update period — Weekly
Price/Charges — Connect time: SFr141.00
Online print: SFr1.46
Offline print: SFr1.35
SDI charge: SFr9.80

Available via a gateway to Data-Star, accessible with the user codes of FIZ Technik. For usage and invoicing the fees and subscription conditions of Data-Star with respect to the database producer are valid

14:564. Online   FT Profile

File name — INF
Alternative name(s) — Infomat International Business News; Infomat International Business
Start year — 1991 (January)
Number of records — 914,467
Update period — Daily

Price/Charges — Connect time: UK£2.40
Online print: UK£0.04 – 0.10 per line
Offline print: UK£0.01 per line

Notes

Registration fee required, including free documentation and training. Usage charges for access consist of two elements: a connect rate for time online, and a display rate (applies only to lines of file text). There is no charge for blank lines, system messages, menus or help information.

14:565. Database subset
Online   Data-Star

File name — TREB – Infomat International Business Training File
Alternative name(s) — Infomat International Business News; Infomat International Business
Start year —
Number of records —
Update period — Closed File
Price/Charges — Connect time: Free

Notes

This is the free training file for EBUS on Data-Star, the Infomat International Business database.

Information Catalog, The
FIND/SVP

14:566. Master record

Database type — Bibliographic
Number of journals —
Sources — Publishers, Database producers, Own publications, Reports and Investment firms
Start year — Current information
Language — English
Coverage — USA
Number of records —
Update size — —
Update period — Annually

Keywords

Alcoholic Beverages; Transport; Industry Forecasts; Company Profiles; Health Care; Retailing; Telecommunications; Tobacco; Beverages; Food and Drink; High Technology; Natural Resources; Marketing; Packaging; Media; Publishing; Biotechnology; Business Planning; Business Strategy; Chemical Industry; Plastics; Office Products; Manufacturing; Consumer Products; Construction; Defence

Description

Contains citations, with abstracts, to business reports, studies, surveys and reference books covering 38 industries, including biotechnology, business planning and strategy, chemicals and plastics, computers and office products, construction, consumer and personal products, defence, electronics, environment and natural resources, finance and economics, food and beverages, high technology and manufacturing, markets and packaging, media and publishing, medical and health care, pharmaceuticals, retailing, telecommunications, tobacco and alcohol and transportation.

Typical reports give information on new products, market size and share, industry forecasts, competitor profiles and technological advances.

Corresponds to *The Information Catalog*.

14:567. Online NewsNet Inc

File name	
Start year	Current information
Number of records	
Update period	Annually

Notes

Monthly subscription to NewsNet required.

Interacciones con Analisis Clinicos

Consejo General de Colegios Oficiales de Farmaceuticos de España

14:568. Master record

Database type	Factual, Textual
Number of journals	
Sources	Databases, Journals and Monographs
Start year	Current Information
Language	Spanish
Coverage	Spain
Number of records	200
Update size	—
Update period	Periodically, as new data become available

Keywords

Drugs; Haematology; Pharmaceuticals; Urology

Description

Descriptions of the effects of about 200 drugs or their active ingredients on chemicals in the human body, as determined by blood and urine tests for such substances as bilirubin, calcium, cholesterol, corticosteroids, glucose, lactic acid, magnesium, potassium, prolactin, proteins, triglycerides, urea and uric acid.

14:569. Online Consejo General de Colegios Oficiales de Farmaceuticos de España

File name	
Start year	Current Information
Number of records	200
Update period	Periodically, as new data become available

Interacciones entre Medicamentos

Consejo General de Colegios Oficiales de Farmaceuticos de España

14:570. Master record

Database type	Bibliographic, Textual
Number of journals	
Sources	Databases, Journals and Monographs
Start year	1978
Language	Spanish
Coverage	Spain

Number of records	7,000
Update size	—
Update period	Periodically, as new data become available

Keywords

Drugs

Description

Descriptions of interactions between pairs of drugs or active ingredients available in Spain, giving names of drugs, mechanism of interaction, clinical effects and frequency of appearance, means of halting or preventing interaction, summaries of relevant published clinical studies and bibliography.

14:571. Online Consejo General de Colegios Oficiales de Farmaceuticos de España

File name	
Start year	1978
Number of records	7,000
Update period	Periodically, as new data become available

Interactions de la Société Suisse de Pharmacie

Société Suisse de Pharmacie

14:572. Master record

Database type	
Number of journals	
Sources	
Start year	
Language	French
Coverage	Switzerland
Number of records	
Update size	—
Update period	
Index unit	Drug

Keywords

Drugs; Pharmaceuticals; Surgery

Description

One of the databases on both PharmaROM and MediROM.

This database can be found on:
MediROM
PharmaROM

Interactions of the Medical Letter

14:574. Master record

Alternative name(s)	Medical Letter's Interactions
Database type	
Number of journals	
Sources	
Start year	
Language	English
Coverage	Switzerland
Number of records	
Update size	—
Update period	

Keywords

Drugs; Pharmaceuticals; Surgery

Description

This database in the medical and pharmaceutical field forms part of the MediROM and PharmaROM CD-ROMs, originally intended for Swiss pharmacists.

This database can be found on:
MediROM
PharmaROM

Interactive Drug Interactions

Medi-Span Development Corporation
Micromedex Inc

14:576. Master record

Alternative name(s)	Computerized Clinical Information System: Interactive Drug Interactions; Drug Interactions; CCIS: Interactive Drug Interactions
Database type	Factual, Textual, Directory
Number of journals	
Sources	
Start year	
Language	English
Coverage	International
Number of records	
Update size	–
Update period	Quarterly

Keywords

Drugs; Drug Therapy

Description

Drug therapy screening system from Medi-Span. This package allows a clinician to check for interacting drug ingredients, their effects and clinical significance. Drug-drug interactions, drug-food interactions and previous adverse reactions can all be reviewed for individual drugs or any combination of drugs, as in the case of several medications being prescribed for a specific patient.

This database can be found on:
CCIS

International Drug Library

Abt Books
US Information Agency

14:578. Master record

Alternative name(s)	IDL
Database type	Factual, Textual, Statistical, Image
Number of journals	
Sources	
Start year	
Language	English and Spanish
Coverage	International
Number of records	
Update size	–
Update period	Annually

Keywords

Crime; Drugs

Description

Contains information on the worldwide illegal drug industry and United States policy. Covers: current situation by type of drug and by geography, US Policy on illegal drugs, US public opinion on illegal drugs, glossary. Also covers: US market, US measures, demand reduction, supply reduction, legislation, alternative economic development, drug chain production, processing, export import and trafficking, finance, sales, distribution, consumption data, effects of illegal drugs, economic effects, political effects, public safety effects, national and international security effects, social impacts, health impacts, results of international and national drug control efforts, internationl cooperation.

14:579. CD-ROM   Abt Books

File name	International Drug Library
Alternative name(s)	IDL
Format notes	IBM
Software	KAware 2
Start year	
Number of records	
Update period	Annually
Price/Charges	

International Nonproprietary Names for Pharmaceutical Substances

World Health Organisation – Division of Drug Management and Policies

14:580. Master record

Alternative name(s)	INN for Pharmaceutical Substances Data Base
Database type	Textual, Directory
Number of journals	
Sources	
Start year	1976–1989
Language	English, French, Latin, Russian and Spanish
Coverage	International
Number of records	8,383
Update size	–
Update period	Annually

Keywords

Pharmaceuticals

Description

A full text and referral database of data and terminology with listings of pharmaceuticals substances. The 8,000 plus records refer to 5,675 international nonproprietary names.

Available to UN system organisations; external users; data provided free of charge on tape provided on request. Printed product: *International Nonproprietary names (INN) for Pharmaceutical Substances (Cumulative List No.7)*. Available also as a printout.

14:581. Tape   World Health Organisation – Division of Drug Management and Policies

File name	International Nonproprietary Names for Pharmaceutical Substances
Alternative name(s)	INN for Pharmaceutical Substances Data Base
Format notes	IBM
Software	Mark IV
Start year	1976–1989
Number of records	8,383
Update period	Annually

International Pharmaceutical Abstracts

American Society of Hospital Pharmacists

14:582. Master record

Alternative name(s)	IPA
Database type	Bibliographic
Number of journals	600+
Sources	Journals, Editorials, Letters, Reviews and Notes
Start year	1970
Language	English
Coverage	International
Number of records	182,535
Update size	17,000
Update period	Monthly
Thesaurus	Thesaurus of Subject Terms & Cross References to International Pharmaceutical Abstracts (6th Ed.)
Database aids	IPA Users Guide (3rd Ed.) and Drug Trade Name cross reference list

Keywords

Drugs; Pharmacy Practice

Description

IPA contains citations and abstracts from medical and health journals giving comprehensive coverage of the worldwide pharmaceutical literature. Subjects covered include: pharmaceutical technology; institutional pharmacy practice; adverse drug reactions; toxicity; investigational drugs; drug evaluations; drug interactions; biopharmaceutics; pharmaceutics; drug stability; pharmacology; preliminary drug testing; drug research; pharmaceutical chemistry; drug analysis; drug metabolism and body distribution; microbiology; pharmacognosy; methodology; environmental toxicity; legislation, laws and regulations; history, sociology, economics; ethics; pharmaceutical education and information processing and literature. Coverage was expanded in early 1985 to include state pharmacy journals that deal with state regulations, salaries, guidelines, human resources studies, laws and related topics. A unique feature of abstracts reporting clinical studies is the inclusion of the study design, number of patients, dosage, dosage forms and dosage schedule. Problems concerning over 10,000 drugs are referred to. In addition IPA identifies articles which qualify for continuing education credit for pharmacists. The IPA database is used by professionals in every area of health care, medical librarians and pharmaceutical and cosmetic industry researchers.

The database includes abstracts from all United States state pharmacy journals and ASHP's Annual and Midyear Clinical Meetings. Abstracts are also included for all foreign literature records. The database corresponds to the printed *International Pharmaceutical Abstracts*.

Launched at the start of 1993, a new drug classification system is designed to give one-number coverage to each group of therapeutic drugs; the system will eventually be applied to all drugs dating back to 1970. IPA is also part of the TOXLIT file. Some hosts apparently hold the database separately as well as on TOXLIT. DIALOG alone reports that IPA is part of their TOXLINE, not TOXLIT file, as well as a file on its own.

14:583. Online BIS

File name	IPA
Alternative name(s)	IPA
Start year	
Number of records	
Update period	

14:584. Online BRS

File name	IPAB
Alternative name(s)	IPA
Start year	
Number of records	
Update period	Monthly
Price/Charges	Connect time: US$65.00/75.00
	Online print: US$0.42/0.50
	Offline print: US$0.60
	SDI charge: US$8.00

14:585. Online CompuServe Information Service

File name	IQUEST File 1252
Alternative name(s)	IPA
Start year	1970
Number of records	
Update period	Monthly
Price/Charges	Subscription: US$8.95 per month
	Database entry fee: US$9/search; some databases carry a surcharge ($2–75)
	Online print: US$10 references free; then $9 per ten; abstracts $3 each

Downloading is allowed

Notes

Accessed via IQUEST, this database is offered by a PRS gateway. IQUEST can either search across all databases, a database of the user's choice or selected multiple databases.

14:586. Online Data-Star

File name	IPAB
Alternative name(s)	IPA
Start year	1970
Number of records	182,535
Update period	Monthly
Database aids	Data-Star Business Manual and Online manual (search NEWS-IPAB in NEWS)
Price/Charges	Subscription: SFr80.00
	Connect time: SFr123.00
	Online print: SFr0.88
	Offline print: SFr0.84
	SDI charge: SFr11.60

Downloading is allowed
Thesaurus is online

Notes

From June 1993 Data-Star have introduced an annual fee/subscription per contract (that is, not per password) of SFr 80.00 (c.UK£ 32.00) payable every June. For North American customers billed in dollars who also use DIALOG, the DIALOG fee also covers access to Data-Star. Academic customers, 'commitment' customers and customers currently billed in dollars are exempt.

Record composition

Abstract AB; Accession Number and Update Code AN; Author(s) AU; CAS Registry Number RN; Descriptors DE; Human H; Institution IN; Language LG; Notes NT; Section Code SC; Source SO; Title TI; Trade Name TN; Update Code UP and Year of IPA Publication YR

14:587. Online DIALOG, Knowledge Index

File name	File 74
Alternative name(s)	IPA
Start year	1970
Number of records	182,802
Update period	Monthly

Price/Charges	Connect time: US$90.00
	Online print: US$0.80
	Offline print: US$0.80
	SDI charge: US$9.95

Notes

This database is also available to home users during evenings and weekends at a reduced rate on the Knowledge Index service of DIALOG – file name in this case is IPA, and searches are made with simplified commands or menus.

DIALINDEX Categories: MEDICINE, PHARM, PHARMINA, PHARMR, REGS, RNMED, TOXICOL.

14:588. Online   DIMDI

File name	IA70
Alternative name(s)	IPA
Start year	
Number of records	203,233
Update period	Monthly
SDI period	1 month
Price/Charges	Connect time: UK£18.50–23.24
	Online print: UK£0.33–0.51
	Offline print: UK£0.28–0.35
Downloading is allowed	

Notes

IPA is a separate database and at the same time a subunit of TOXALL and TOXLIT on DIMDI. Searches are possible from January 1970.

14:589. Online   ESA-IRS

File name	File 102
Alternative name(s)	IPA
Start year	1970
Number of records	194,400 (October 1991)
Update period	Monthly
Price/Charges	Subscription: UK£70.29
	Database entry fee: UK£3.51
	Online print: UK£0.07 – 0.49
	Offline print: UK£0.46
	SDI charge: UK£2.80
Downloading is allowed	
Thesaurus is online	

Notes

From 1993 ESA-IRS are charging an annual fee of 100 Accounting Units (c.UK£ 70.29) to all users. This is equivalent to the fee for full documentation and will not be charged to customers already paying for documentation.

Record composition

Abstract /AB; Author Name AU; CAS Registry No RN; Controlled Terms /CT; Corporate Source CS; Coden CO; Document Type DT; File Update UP; Journal Name JN; Language LA; Publication Year PY; Section Headings CC; Summary Language LS; Title /TI; Trade Name /TN and Uncontrolled Terms /UT

The basic index includes Title, Trade Name, Controlled Terms, Uncontrolled Terms, Abstracts.

14:590. Online   University of Tsukuba

File name	IPA
Alternative name(s)	IPA
Start year	
Number of records	
Update period	

14:591. CD-ROM   Compact Cambridge

File name	International Pharmaceutical
	Abstracts
Format notes	NEC, 9800, IBM
Software	Proprietary

Start year	1970
Number of records	200,000
Update period	Quarterly
Price	UK£1,105
	Subscription: UK£635

Notes

Annual subscription is from 1970-present. Subscription renewal cost is £635. Discount for ASHP members.

14:592. CD-ROM   SilverPlatter

File name	International Pharmaceutical
	Abstracts
Format notes	Mac, IBM
Software	SPIRS/MacSPIRS
Start year	1970
Number of records	202,000
Update period	Quarterly
Database aids	Database Guide and Quick
	Reference Card
Price/Charges	Subscription: UK£1,155 – 1,733

Notes

Regular subscription is UK£1,155 for single users, £1,733 for 2–8 networked users.

Record composition

Title TI; Author AU; Address of Author AD; Abstract AB; Publication Year PY; Source SO; Country of Publication; Document Number DN; References RF; Descriptors DE; Drug Names DR; Human HU; CODEN CO; Combination Indicator; Note; CAS Registry Number RN; Classification Code CC; Language LA and Accession Number AN

Drugs are indexed by trade name as well as generic name.

This database can also be found on:
Drug Information Source CD
Toxline Plus
TOXLIT
TOXALL
TOXLINE

International Product Alert
Marketing Intelligence Service Ltd

14:594. Master record

Database type	Textual
Number of journals	1
Sources	Newsletter
Start year	1988
Language	English
Coverage	Europe, USA, Canada, Central America, South America, Japan and Australia
Number of records	8,000
Update size	—
Update period	Twice per month

Keywords

Beauty Care; Beverages; Cosmetics; Food and Drink; Health Care Products; Household Products; Packaging; Pets

Description

Descriptions of about 8,000 packaged foods and beverages, household products, pet supplies, and health and beauty aids each year. Products are selected from those introduced in Europe, Latin America, Japan and Australia as being of commercial potential in North America. Information includes product description, key ingredients, retail price, packaging and manufacturer's name and location.

Corresponds to *International Product Alert* semi-monthly newsletter. On CORIS, DIALOG and Data-Star this newsletter is made available as part of the PTS Newsletter database, supplied by Predicasts.

This database can be found on:
PTS Newsletter Database

Price/Charges	Connect time: UK£03.88–08.62
	Online print: UK£0.16–0.34
	Offline print: UK£0.07–0.14
	SDI charge: UK£None
Downloading is allowed	

Notes
DIMDI's aim is to extend the number of institutions supplying data for INTOX to create an instrument for representative evaluations on cases of poisoning in Germany.

INTOX
Technische Universitët München, Toxikologishe Abteilung DIMDI

14:596. Master record

Alternative name(s)	Datenbank über Vergiftungsfälle; Database on Poisoning
Database type	Factual
Number of journals	
Sources	Case studies
Start year	1975
Language	German
Coverage	Germany
Number of records	259,638
Update size	20,000
Update period	Monthly

Keywords
Clinical Toxicology; Drugs; Poisons; Forensic Science

Description
INTOX is a non-bibliographic database containing data on individual cases of poisoning from German poison control centres and clinical-toxicological departments of hospitals. Subjects covered include: epidemiology of poisoning; clinical toxicology; forensic medicine and drug dependence. Records of poison control centres and institutes of forensic medicine in the Federal Republic of Germany are evaluated. Information on individual cases of poisoning given includes the name of the poison, the year of poisoning, the age group of the patient, the degree of severity, etiology, poisoning symptoms, therapy, outcome and analytical data. In addition almost all records contain data on toxicological analytics which is the determination of poisons and their metabolites in body fluids and tissues.

None of the records contain abstracts. Institutions supplying INTOX data include: Toxikologishe Abteilung (Giftnotruf), Klinikum rechts der Isar, Technical University, Munich, Giftinformations-zentrale, Land Baden-Württemberg, Universitäts-Kinderklinik, Mathildenstr.1, Freiburg, the Department of Clinical Toxicology of the Municipal Hospital Friedrichshain, Berlin and the Reanimation Centre of the Rudolf Virchow Medical School, Charlottenburg, Berlin.

14:597. Online   DIMDI

File name	GI00
Alternative name(s)	Datenbank über Vergiftungsfälle; Database on Poisoning
Start year	1975
Number of records	259,638
Update period	Monthly

Investext
Thomson Financial Networks Inc

14:598. Master record

Database type	Textual, Bibliographic
Number of journals	
Sources	Reports
Start year	1982
Language	English
Coverage	USA, Canada, European Community and Japan
Number of records	320,000
Update size	125,000 pages per year
Update period	Weekly
Hosts have included	CORIS (Thomson Financial Network) (Until 1/92)

Keywords
Aerospace; Automotive Industry; Banking Industry; Broadcasting; Chemical Industry; Computer Industry; Insurance Industry; Metals Industry; Pharmaceutical Industry; Social Policy; Telecommunications; Transport; Utilities Industry

Description
The world's largest database of full-text, company, industry research, geographical and topical reports produced by professional research analysts at almost 200 top international brokers and investment bankers in major investment banking and financial research firms in the United States, Australia, Canada, Europe and Japan. This is the largest, long-running database covering investment research information. It provides hard-to-find information on companies and industries – information that is not available from any other source, according to Sharon Ladner in her review of the product (*CD-ROM Professional* 5(4) p. 77–83). Information includes all tabular data plus indexing and abstracts.

Gives historical analyses of firms, together with short and long-term forecasts of sales, financial information, prospects, earnings, research and development expenditures, market share, production and distribution, consumer spending etc. Industries covered include aerospace, automotive, banking, broadcasting, computers, insurance, metals, pharmaceuticals, telecommunications, utilities.

Company information covers sales, stock prices, balance sheets, financial results, cash flow, capital expenditure. Includes material on 21,000 companies internationally, and 53 industry groups, covering high tech industries, chemical and medical areas as well as consumer goods and trade. Investext can be used for a wide range of business intelligence activities, including competitive analysis, market research, evaluation of companies for acquisition, corporate planning, sales planning, etc. Each analyst report has on average eight pages. Information covered is originally produced as investment advice for the clients of the investment houses and financial advisers. It is placed on the database after a delay, and recommendations should no longer be considered as investment recommendations. The information remains useful for analytical purposes. Covers 53 industries with good coverage of smaller, regional companies. Most of the recent growth in the Investext database comes by including reports from foreign and regional brokerage firms – as of September 1991, Investext listed 198 contributors to its database – more than half from outside the United States and 35 from outside of New York City.

The archive covers the current twelve months of supplied material. During 1992, the Europe Information Service of Cooper's & Lybrand Europe added their bulletins on the EC to the service. Each bulletin provides detailed coverage of debates, projects and agreements relating to the EC through the bi-weekly European Report and a series of monthly and bi-monthly titles looking at specific areas such as transport, energy and social policy.

US sources for Investext reports written by professional analysts within such investment houses as: Bear Stearns & Co.; J.C. Bradford & Co.; Alex. Brown & Sons Inc.; Butcher & Singer Inc.; Cable Howse & Ragen; Craig- Hallum Inc.; Dain Bosworth Inc.; Dean Witter Reynolds Inc.; Dillon Read & Company Inc.; Donaldson, Lufkin & Jenrette Securities Corp.; Drexel Burnham Lambert Inc.; Eberstadt Fleming Inc.; First Boston Corp.; Fitch Investors Service Inc.; Fox-Pitt, Kelton; Hibbard Brown & Company; E.F. Hutton & Company Inc.; Interstate Securities Corp.; Janney Montgomery Scott inc.; Kidder Peabody and Co. Inc.; C.J. Lawrence, Morgan Grenfell Inc.; Mabon, Nugent & Company; Market Guide Inc.; Merrill Lynch, Pierce, Fenner & Smith Inc.; Morgan Stanley & Co. Inc; Moseley Securities Corporation; The New York Society of Security Analysts; Nomura Securities international Inc.; Oppenheimer & Co. Inc.; Paine webber Inc.; Pershing; Piper, Jaffray & Hopwood Inc.; Prudential-Bache Securities; Rauscher Pierce Refsnes Inc.; Salomon Brothers inc.; Sanyo Securities America Inc.; Stephens Inc.; Tucker, Anthony and R.L.Day Inc.; and Van Kasper & Company.

Other sources of financial research in major industrial countries worldwide include: Algemene Bank Nederland N.V.; Banca Commerciale Italiana; Citicorp Scrimgour Vickers; DAFSA; DEGAB; Kredietbank N.V.; Phillips and Drew Ltd. (Member UBS group); Richardson Greenshields of Canada Limited; Roach Tilley Grice Inc.; Sutro & Company; McLeod Young Weir Limited; Union Bank of Switzerland; Barclays de Zoete Wedd and Yamaichi Research Institute of Securities and Economics Inc.

Complete presentation-style, laser-printed reports corresponding to the individual analyses are available from Investext.

Significant research reports from major investment research institutions willing to make their material publicly available once it has outlived its utility for investment purposes.

14:599. Online   BRS, BRS/Colleague

File name	
Start year	1982

Number of records	320,000
Update period	Weekly

Notes

On this host Investext includes the Market Guide Data Base

14:600. Online   CompuServe Information Service

File name	
Start year	1982
Number of records	200,000
Update period	Weekly
Price/Charges	Subscription: US$8.95 per month
Downloading is allowed	

Notes

Apparently Market Guide Data Base is not included in Investext on this host.

14:601. Online   Data-Star

File name	INVE
Start year	January 1987
Number of records	263,000
Update period	Weekly (Daily in 1992)
Database aids	Data-Star Smart Search Guide to Investext, Investext Product Terms Plus Directory: available free from Data-Star,, Data-Star Business Manual, Berne, Data-Star, and Online guide (search NEWS-INVE in NEWS)
Price/Charges	Subscription: UK£32.00
	Connect time: UK£76.00
	Online print: UK£0.53 – 3.52
	Offline print: UK£0.56 – 3.81

Also available on FIZ Technik via a gateway from Data-Star

Notes

From June 1993 Data-Star have introduced an annual fee/subscription per contract (that is, not per password) of SFr 80.00 (c.UK£ 32.00) payable every June. For North American customers billed in dollars who also use DIALOG, the DIALOG fee also covers access to Data-Star. Academic customers, 'commitment' customers and customers currently billed in dollars are exempt.

On this host Investext includes the Market Guide Data Base

14:602. Online   Data-Star

File name	IV86
Start year	1982 to 1986
Number of records	137,800
Update period	Weekly (Daily in 1992)
Database aids	Data-Star Smart Search Guide to Investext, Investext Product Terms Plus Directory: available free from Data-Star,, Data-Star Business Manual, Berne, Data-Star, and Online guide (search NEWS-INVE in NEWS)
Price/Charges	Subscription: UK£32.00
	Connect time: UK£76.00
	Online print: UK£0.53 – 3.52
	Offline print: UK£0.56 – 3.81

Also available on FIZ Technik via a gateway from Data-Star

Notes

On this host Investext includes the Market Guide Data Base.

From June 1993 Data-Star have introduced an annual fee/subscription per contract (that is, not per password) of SFr 80.00 (c.UK£ 32.00) payable every June.

For North American customers billed in dollars who also use DIALOG, the DIALOG fee also covers access to Data-Star. Academic customers, 'commitment' customers and customers currently billed in dollars are exempt.

14:603. Online   Data-Star

File name	IVZZ
Start year	July 1982
Number of records	401,000
Update period	Weekly (Daily in 1992)
Database aids	Data-Star Smart Search Guide to Investext, Investext Product Terms Plus Directory: available free from Data-Star,, Data-Star Business Manual, Berne, Data-Star, and Online guide (search NEWS-INVE in NEWS)
Price/Charges	Subscription: UK£32.00
	Connect time: UK£76.00
	Online print: UK£0.53 – 3.81
	Offline print: UK£0.56 – 3.81

Also available on FIZ Technik via a gateway from Data-Star.

Notes

On this host Investext includes the Market Guide Data Base. From June 1993 Data-Star have introduced an annual fee/subscription per contract (that is, not per password) of SFr 80.00 (c.UK£ 32.00) payable every June. For North American customers billed in dollars who also use DIALOG, the DIALOG fee also covers access to Data-Star. Academic customers, 'commitment' customers and customers currently billed in dollars are exempt.

14:604. Online   DIALOG

File name	File 545
Start year	1982 (July)
Number of records	1,742,965 representing 283,096 reports
Update period	Weekly
Price/Charges	Connect time: US$96.00
	Online print: US$5.50
	Offline print: US$5.50
	SDI charge: US$4.00

Notes

There may be differences between search results on the CD-ROM and on the DIALOG online file: one review (*CD-ROM Professional* 5(4) p. 77–83) reported that 'during the 12-month review period, InfoTrac Investext did not include reports published by Market Guide, a financial research firm which specializes in smaller publicly owned companies. More recent InfoTrac CD-ROM discs do include Market Guide Reports.' while the DIALOG file does. Because names of subsidiaries of public companies are not included in the Subject Index, searches for information on subsidiaries result in 'no hits' even though the data on these corporate forms is often included in the investment reports.

14:605. Online   Dow Jones

File name	
Start year	1982
Number of records	320,000
Update period	Weekly

Notes

Annual fee of $12 to Dow Jones required On this host Investext includes the Market Guide Data Base.

14:606. Online   FIZ Technik (gateway)

File name	INVE
Start year	1987

Number of records	263,000
Update period	Weekly (Daily in 1992)
Database aids	Data-Star Smart Search Guide to Investext, Investext Product Terms Plus Directory: available free from Data-Star,, Data-Star Business Manual, Berne, Data-Star, and Online guide (search NEWS-INVE in NEWS)
Price/Charges	Connect time: SFr190.00
	Online print: SFr1.33 – 8.80 (per paragraph)
	Offline print: SFr1.41 – 9.52 (per paragraph)

Available via Data-Star on a gateway

Notes

On this host Investext includes the Market Guide Data Base

14:607. Online   FIZ Technik (gateway)

File name	IV89
Start year	1982 to 1989
Number of records	137,800
Update period	Weekly (Daily in 1992)
Database aids	Data-Star Smart Search Guide to Investext, Investext Product Terms Plus Directory: available free from Data-Star,, Data-Star Business Manual, Berne, Data-Star, and Online guide (search NEWS-INVE in NEWS)
Price/Charges	Connect time: SFr190.00
	Online print: SFr1.33 – 8.80 (per paragraph)
	Offline print: SFr1.41 – 9.52 (per paragraph)

Available via Data-Star on a gateway

Notes

On this host Investext includes the Market Guide Data Base.

14:608. Online   FIZ Technik (gateway)

File name	IVZZ
Start year	1987
Number of records	401,000
Update period	Weekly (Daily in 1992)
Database aids	Data-Star Smart Search Guide to Investext, Investext Product Terms Plus Directory: available free from Data-Star, Data-Star Business Manual, Berne, Data-Star and Online guide (search NEWS-INVE in NEWS)
Price/Charges	Connect time: SFr190.00
	Online print: SFr1.33 – 8.80 (per paragraph)
	Offline print: SFr1.41 – 9.52 (per paragraph)

Available via Data-Star on a gateway

Notes

On this host Investext includes the Market Guide Data Base

14:609. Online   FT Profile

File name	INV
Start year	Current information only
Number of records	
Update period	
Delay	Reports are generally available online on FT Profile within four to six weeks of publication.
Price/Charges	Connect time: UK£2.40
	Online print: UK£0.04 – 0.10 per line
	Offline print: UK£0.01 per line

Notes

Registration fee required, including free documentation and training. Usage charges for access consist of two elements: a connect rate for time online, and a display rate (applies only to lines of file text). There is no charge for blank lines, system messages, menus or help information.

14:610. Online   Mead Data Central (as a NEXIS database)

File name	INTL
Start year	1982
Number of records	200,000
Update period	Daily
Delay	Varies but usually within thirty days of printed source.

Notes

Libraries: COMPNY and INVEST which have all Investext reports; other libraries have selected reports (for example, transportation industry reports in TRAN). Also: ASIAPC, MDEAFR, NSAMER and WORLD.

Investext sources are listed (with their addresses) in the documentation; individual file names can be used for each source (given in parenthesis with coverage start date):

A.G. Edwards and Sons (AGE 10/88); ABN AMRO Bank NV Advest Inc. (ADV 5/84); Alex Brown and Sons Inc. (AB 1/84); Altman Brenner & Wasserman Inc. (ABW 6/90); Argus Research Corporation (ARG 12/90); B. Metzler Seel (BMS 5/91); Bain Securities Inc. (BSI 10/90); Baird, Patrick & Co. Inc. (BDP 6/90); Balis & Zorn Inc. (BZG 10/88); Banca Commerciale Italiana Piazza (BCI 6/83); Bank in Liechtenstein (BIL 2.91); Barclays de Zoete Wedd Securities Ltd. (BZW 2/90); Bateman Eichler, Hill Richards Inc. (BEH 4/90); Bayerische Vereinsbank AG (BVB 7/91); BDMI Limited (BDM 8/90); Bear Stearns & Co. (BDS 4/83); Beeson Gregory Ltd. (BSG 7/91); Bell Lawrie White & Co (BLL 4/89); Boettcher & Company (BOE 5/89); Booz- Allen & Hamilton (BAH 2/89); B.W.D. Rensburg Ltd. (BWD 1/90); C.J. Lawrence Inc (CJL 1/83); CCF Elysees Bourse (CCF 1/90); Charterhouse Tilney (CHT 11/89); Coburn & Meredith Inc. (CMI 4/90); Coopers & Lybrand Europe (CLE 5/90); County NatWest Securities Asia Ltd (CNA 7/90); County NatWest Securities Japan Ltd. (CNJ 2/91); Craig-Hallum Inc. (CH 4/88); Credit-Lyonnais Securities (Japan) (CLJ 5/91); Credit Suisse First Boston Ltd. (CSF 7/90); Crowell, Weedon & Co. (CRW 12/90); DAFSA (DAF 2/82); Dain Bosworth Inc. (DB 1/83); Daiwa Institute of Research Europe Ltd. (DIR 4/92); Daiwa Securities Co., Ltd. (DAI 10/90); Dean Witter Reynolds Inc. (DW 3/88) Decision Resources Inc. (ADL 2/87); DEGAB (DGB 3/82); Deloitte & Touche Europe Services (DRT 4/91); Dillon Read & Company Inc. (DR 11/88); Donaldson, Lufkin & Jenrette Securities Corp. (DLJ 3/83); Duff & Phelps Inc. (DNP 12/90); Fahnestock/B.C. Christopher (FHN 6/91); First Boston Corp. (FB 7/86); Fitch Investors Service Inc. (FIT 9/84); Fox-Pitt, Kelton (FOX 7/84); FT Analysis Corporation (PLC 3/90); George K. Baum & Co. (GKB 9/90); Gerard Klauer Mattison (GKM 9/90); H.C. Wainwright & Co. (HCW 8/90); Hambrecht & Quist Inc. (HMQ 6/90); Hanifen Imhoff Inc. (HAN 8/91); Henderson Crosthwaite Inst. Brokers Ltd. (HCR 3/90); Henry Cooke, Lumsden (HCL 11/89); Hibbard Brown & Company (HBC 10/88); Hoare Govett Investment Research Ltd. (HGV 1/90); Interstate/ Johnson Lane (INT 5/83); J.C. Bradford & Co. (JCB

11/83); James Capel & Co. Ltd. (JCC 2/90); Janney Montgomery Scott Inc. (JMS 8/88); Jesup, Josephthal & Co. (JSJ 9/90); Johnson Rice & Co. (JR 1/89); Johnston, Lemon & Co. (JL 5/89); Kankaku Securities Co. (KKS 3/91); Kemper Securities Group (KSG 3/91); Kenneth, Jerome & Co. (KJR 9/90); Kidder Peabody and Co. Inc. (KP 1/83); Kredietbank NV (KB 9/83); Ladenburg, Thalman (LDB 9/90); Loewen, Ondaatje, McCutcheon & Co. (LOM 1/91); Mabon Securities Corp. (MNC 10/86); MacDonald, Grippo & Riely (MGR 12/90); Matheson Securities Ltd. (MTH 8/91); McDonald & Company Securities Inc. (MCD 11/89); McIntosh & Company Ltd. (MIH 7/90); Merrill Lynch Capital Markets (MER 9/88); Morgan Stanley & Co. (MRG 6/86); New York Society of Security Analysts (NYSSA 1/84); Oppenheim Finanzanalyse GmbH (OFA 9/90); Oppenheimer & Co. (OPP 12/84); Paine Webber Inc. (PNW 4/85); Panmure Gordon & Co. (PMG 8/89); Paribas Capital Markets (PAR 2/91); Pasfin Sevizi Finanzzziari (PSF 7/90); Pauli & Company Inc. (PLI 1/91); Pershing Division (PER 8/83); Peterbroeck, Van Campenhout & CIE (PCM 8/90); Piper, Jaffray & Hopwood Inc. (PJH 4/83); PNC Institutional Investment Service (PNB 11/88); Prudential-Bache Securities (PB 9/83); Raffensperger, Hughes (RPH 12/89); Rauscher Pierce Refsnes Inc. (RPR 11/83); Research Capital Corporation (RCC 7/91); Riada & Co. (RDA 4/91); Richardson Greenshields (RG 9/83); Robert W. Baird & Co. (RWB 5/90); Rothschild Inc. (RTH 7/91); Rowan Dartington & Co. (RDT 9/90); S.G. Warburg Securities (SGW 6/91); Salomon Brothers Inc. (SB 8/88); Sanford C. Bernstein (SCB 3/89); Sanwa McCarthy Limited (SMC 6/91); SBCI Hong Kong Limited (SBC 6/91); Schroder Securities (Japan) Ltd. (SHJ 4/91); Scotia McLeod Inc. (MYW 2/83); Scott & Stringfellow Investment Corporation (SCT 9/89); Securities Data Company (SDC 1/90); Shearson Lehman Brothers Holdings Inc. (SLH 2/88); Sheppards (SHE 1/90); Smith Barney, Harris Upham & Co. (SBH 6/82); Smith New Court Far East Limited (SFE 12/89); Smith New Court Securities plc (SNC 6/91); SNL Securities (SNL 6/91); Societé General Strauss Turnbull (STN 9/90); Stephens Inc. (SI 5/87); Sun Hung Kai Research (SHK 6/90); Sutro & Company Inc. (STR 6/88); Svenska Handelsbanken (SVK 10/90); The Chicago Corporation (CHC 10/90); The Principal/Eppler, Guerin & Turner, Inc. (EGT 1/90); The Robinson-Humphrey Company Inc. (RHC 10/89); The Stuart-James Co. (STJ 6/90); Thomas James Associates (TJA 2/89); Thomson BankWatch (KBW 1/89); Tucker, Anthony and R.L.Day Inc. (TAD 10/85); UBS Phillips & Drew Global Research Group (PDI 5/84); UBS Phillips & Drew International Ltd. (UPJ 5/91); Union Bank of Switzerland (UBS 9/82); Van Kasper & Company (VNK 1/84); Vereins- und Westbank AG (VWB 10/89); W.I. Carr (Far East) Ltd. (WIC 4/90); Wedbush Morgan Securities Inc. (WDM 9/89); Wertheim Schroder & Co. (WRS 2/89); Wheat First Securities (BUS 6/83); William Blair & Co. (WBC 3/90); Wise Speke Ltd. (WSD 4/91); and Yamaichi Research Institute (YAM 10/82).

Apparently Market Guide Data Base is not included in Investext on this host. The index segments include the following: Company Index lists all companies that are identified at the page level of the report with page references; Subject Index contains subject terms assigned to specific pages, again with page numbers; Product Index contains a list of products reported with references; SIC Index contains the four-digit codes that relate to products reported; and the Associated Industry Index contains a list of industries that are associated with the SIC Codes.

Format FULL2 displays complete report including index segments and FULL3 displays the full report except for the Table of Contents and index segments.

A subscription charge which covers all transactional charges, connect time, telecommunications and the small administration charge can take the place of the individual charges. Subscriptions are negotiated with customers and vary according to the number of menus (thus, files) that are to be used – typically a minimum subscription would be about US$ 1,000. All charges include training and a 24-hour help line.

Record composition

Source SOURCE; Date DATE; Company CO; Ticker Symbols TS; Hierarchical Geographic Company Location GEOCO/GEOREG/GEOSRC; Name NAME; Title TITLE; Type TYPE; Length LENGTH; Analyst ANALYST; Report Number REPORT-NO; Industry INDUSTRY; Abstract ABSTRACT; Contents CONTENTS; Company Index COMPANY-INDEX; Subject Index SUBJECT-INDEX; Product Index PRODUCT-INDEX; SIC Index SIC-INDEX; Associated Industry Index ASSOC-IND-INDEX; Text TEXT; Tables TABLES and Body BODY

14:611. Online NewsNet Inc

File name	
Start year	1982 (July)
Number of records	234,000
Update period	Weekly (Daily in 1992)

Notes

Monthly subscription to NewsNet required On this host Investext includes the Market Guide Data Base

14:612. Online SOURCE, The

File name	
Start year	1982
Number of records	234,000
Update period	Weekly

Notes

Monthly minimum of $10 to THE SOURCE required On this host Investext includes the Market Guide Data Base

14:613. CD-ROM Information Access Company (IAC)

File name	Investext on InfoTrac
Format notes	IBM
Software	Proprietary InfoTrac
Start year	1984
Number of records	289,400
Update period	Monthly
Price/Charges	Subscription: US$7,000

Notes

There may be differences between search results on the CD-ROM and on the DIALOG online file: one review (*CD-ROM Professional* 5(4)p.77–83) reported that 'during the 12-month review period, InfoTrac Investext did not include reports published by Market Guide, a financial research firm which specializes in smaller publicly owned companies More recent InfoTrac CD-ROM discs do include Market Guide Reports . . .'. Because names of subsidiaries of public companies are not included in the Subject Index, searches for information on subsidiaries result in 'no hits' even though the data on these corporate forms is often included in the investment reports. Sharyn Ladner, in the above-mentioned review, states that InfoTrac Investext is both simple to use and more

cost-effective than online searching on DIALOG for its intended users. The search software is not intended for – and indeed the product is not available to – corporate analysts, but even so it does have some shortcomings (for instance, searching lacks precision and reports can only be printed in full) which might upset some its intended users. Despite this, she has no reservations in recommending the product to academic and public libraries as excellent.

It provides hard-to-find information on companies and industries – information that is not available from any other source.

Subscription includes 386 IBM PC workstation. (Without workstation: $6,000). Due to IAC contractual arrangements with Thomson, this disc is only sold to academic and public libraries.

14:614. Database subset

Online Data-Star

File name	TRST – Investext Training File
Start year	
Number of records	
Update period	Closed file
Price/Charges	Connect time: UK£Free

14:615. Database subset

Online DIALOG

File name	File 277 – ONTAP Investext Training File
Start year	Selected record from 1988 and 1991
Number of records	50,000
Update period	Closed File
Price/Charges	Connect time: US$15.00

Notes

The low-cost training file contains selected records from File 545, the main Investxt file on DIALOG. Offline prints are not available in ONTAP files.

Investigational Drugs Data-Base

Current Drugs Ltd

14:617. Master record

Alternative name(s)	IDdb
Database type	Factual, Textual
Number of journals	
Sources	Patents, Journals, Reports, News releases and News bureaux
Start year	1993
Language	English
Coverage	International
Number of records	
Update size	—
Update period	Weekly
Index unit	Drug

Keywords

Drugs

Description

An Oracle-based application which provides evaluated information on the research and development programmes of the international pharmaceutical industry. A fully-integrated competitor-monitoring service covering pharmaceutical research and development in patents, scientific journals, scientific meetings, analysis reports and news services. The company's managing director, describes the database, modelled on the Current Drugs Group Files, as 'an entirely new method of electronically presenting and integrating patent information on drugs in development, including primary literature, with expert evaluation'. All information is evaluated and analysed by a board of internationally recognised experts, providing an informative guide to the wealth of data in the database. Section editors, experts in their own field, comment on the information published on each clinical drug. For any investigational drug there is: a complete bibliography of published information; published data classified under standard headings: chemistry, biology (in vitro, in vivo, drug metabolism/pharmacokinetics, toxicology), pharmaceutics, clinical, and sales potential; standard structure information (chemical structure, CAS Registry Number, INN, synonyms, etc); a scientific review of the bibliography; and a 'current opinion' – editorial comment in context. For each company, there is also an analysis of its Discovery Research Programme, based on the latest patent information and early information on possible lead compounds. It is always stated whether the information has yet been made public – that is, the user knows that Current Drugs has performed a full literature search for the information and updated that search every week.

For licensing executives, there is a country-by-country analysis of licensing opportunities within any therapeutic area and company profile information helps to build a complete picture of a potential partner's strengths and weaknesses.

Corresponds to the monthly journal *Current Opinion in Investigational Drugs*.

14:618. Diskette — Current Drugs Ltd

File name	Investigational Drugs Data-Base
Alternative name(s)	IDdb
Format notes	IBM, Mac
Software	Oracle Card; ISIS/Base
Start year	1993
Number of records	
Update period	Weekly

Notes

Oracle Card and ISIS/Base front-ends provide user-friendly access to the data. The Oracle Card front end provides a guided search and browsing environment with an initial menu which allows the user to obtain summary information from the database from five different perspectives: Executive Review; Latest Reports; Licensing Analysis; Clinical Compounds; and Discovery Research. Each option takes the user to a guided search card which builds a query based on tailored question-and-answer approach. Lists of appropriate search terms are provided whenever necessary (for instance, company names, therapeutic classes). Structure-searchable patent records are stored on the TDdb (Therapeutic Patent Fast Alert database) which can be linked to patent records analysed in IDdb. With this option, the company offers free structure records for lead compounds covered in IDdb. Version 6 or 7 of Oracle RDBMS is required.

Japan Report: Biotechnology

Business Information & Solutions Ltd,
Japan Report Division
Newmedia International Japan

14:619. Master record

Database type	Textual
Number of journals	1
Sources	Newsletter
Start year	1988
Language	English
Coverage	Japan
Number of records	
Update size	–
Update period	Daily

Keywords

Biotechnology; Brewing; Food Processing

Description

A monthly newsletter on events occurring in the Japanese biotechnology industry, covering research, developments and applications in agriculture, brewing, food processing and pharmaceuticals.

Corresponds to *Japan Report: Biotechnology* monthly newsletter. Data-Star and DIALOG are supplied with PTS Newsletter Database by Predicast.

This database can be found on:
PTS Newsletter Database

Japan Report: Medical Technology

Business Information & Solutions Ltd,
Japan Report Division
Newmedia International Japan

14:621. Master record

Database type	Textual
Number of journals	1
Sources	Newsletter
Start year	1988
Language	English
Coverage	Japan
Number of records	
Update size	–
Update period	Monthly

Keywords

Diagnostic Equipment; Prosthetics

Description

The full text of a newsletter on Japanese medical technology and the production of medical diagnostic equipment and materials, therapeutic substances and prosthetics. Covers new developments and activities in Japan dealing with medical diagnostic reagents, instrumentation and artificial products, production and processes.

Corresponds to *Japan Report: Medical Technology* monthly newsletter. On DIALOG and Data-Star this newsletter is made available as part of the PTS Newsletter Database.

This database can be found on:
PTS Newsletter Database

Japanese Government and Public Research in Progress

Japan Information Center of Science and Technology (JICST)

14:623. Master record

Database type	Bibliographic, Factual
Number of journals	
Sources	Questionnaires
Start year	1990
Language	English
Coverage	Japan

Number of records	20,000
Update size	–
Update period	Annually
Index unit	Questionnaire

Keywords
Physics; Building; Applied Science

Description
Japanese Government and Public Research in Progress is a databank which contains information on current and completed research projects in all fields of science and technology carried out by government research establishments in Japan. The entries are in English, and include abstracts. Subject fields: agriculture, applied thermodynamics, biosciences, building, chemical industry, construction engineering, electrical engineering, environment, food science and engineering, fundamental chemistry, information technology, management, mechanical engineering, medicine, metallurgy and the extractive industries, nuclear technology, outer space and earth sciences, pharmacology, physics and system control engineering, thermal engineering and applied thermodynamics, transportation and traffic engineering.

14:624. Online   STN

File name	JGRIP
Start year	1990
Number of records	20,000
Update period	Annually
Price/Charges	Connect time: US$83.00
	Online print: US$0.31
	Offline print: US$0.44
	SDI charge: Not applicable

JIGSAW
ISIS Ltd

14:625. Master record

Database type	Factual
Number of journals	
Sources	
Start year	1980
Language	English
Coverage	
Number of records	
Update size	–
Update period	Monthly

Description
The database contains responses from a panel of 400 doctors to prescriptions written by General Practitioners for chronic diseases and the numeric relationship between sales representation of the pharmaceutical companies selling those products.

14:626. Online   ISIS Ltd

File name	JIGSAW
Start year	1980
Number of records	
Update period	Monthly

KINETIDEX System
Micromedex Inc

14:627. Master record

Database type	Factual, Textual
Number of journals	
Sources	

Start year	
Language	English
Coverage	
Number of records	
Update size	–
Update period	
Index unit	Drug

Keywords
Drugs

Description
A therapeutic drug monitoring system for clinicians, designed to optimise drug therapy and provide drug utilisation evaluations for patients.

14:628. CD-ROM   Micromedex Inc

File name	KINETIDEX System
Format notes	IBM
Start year	
Number of records	
Update period	

Kirk-Othmer Encyclopedia of Chemical Technology
John Wiley and Sons Inc

14:629. Master record

Database type	Textual, Encyclopedia, Bibliographic
Number of journals	
Sources	Encyclopedia
Start year	Current
Language	English
Coverage	International
Number of records	1,140
Update size	–
Update period	Irregular
Index unit	Articles

Keywords
Fuels; Drugs; Cosmetics

Description
This is the online version of the printed *Kirk-Othmer Encyclopedia of Chemical Technology*. The 25 volume *Kirk-Othmer Encyclopedia of Chemical Technology* (3rd edition) has long been recognised as the standard reference work in the field of chemical science and technology. Articles are provided on chemistry technology in the areas of energy, health, safety, and new materials: agricultural chemicals; chemical engineering; coatings and inks; composite materials; drugs, cosmetics and biomaterials; dyes, pigments and brighteners; ecology and industrial hygiene; energy conversion and technology; fats and waxes; fermentation and enzyme technology; fibres, textiles and leather; food and animal nutrition; fossil fuels and derivatives; glass, ceramics and cement; industrial organic and inorganic chemicals; metals, metallurgy and metal alloys; plastics and elastomers; semiconductors and electronic materials; surfactants, detergents and emulsion technology; water supply, purification and reuse; and wood, paper, and industrial carbohydrates. The database also contains articles relevant to the manufacture and distribution of chemicals in these areas: computers, instrumentation and control; information retrieval; market research and project planning; patents and trademarks; process development and design; product development and technical service; purchasing, materials allocation and supply; research and operations management and

transportation of chemical products. Scientists, engineers, researchers, teachers and students have access to authoritative information covering a wide range of subject disciplines. Kirk-Othmer also provides information on specific chemicals by CAS Registry Number, including uses, physical and chemical properties, preparation, specific chemical reactions and industrial processes.

Equivalent to the *Encyclopedia of Chemical Technology*, 1977 to date with selected older materials. All 1,200 full text articles from the 25 volume set are included together with supplements, indexing, abstracts, tables and bibliographic citations.

14:630. Online BRS

File name	KIRK
Start year	Current
Number of records	1,140
Update period	Irregular
Price/Charges	Connect time: US$73.00/83.00
	Online print: US$0.29/0.37
	Offline print: US$0.55

Downloading is allowed

14:631. Online CompuServe Information Service

File name	IQUEST File 1256
Start year	Current
Number of records	1,140
Update period	Irregular
Price/Charges	Subscription: US$8.95 per month
	Database entry fee: US$9/search; some databases carry a surcharge ($2–75)
	Online print: US$10 references free; then $9 per ten; abstracts $3 each

Downloading is allowed

Notes

Accessed via IQUEST, this database is offered by a Data-Star gateway. IQUEST can either search across all databases, a database of the user's choice or selected multiple databases.

Record composition

Abstract AB; Accession number and update code AN; Author AU; Author affiliation IN; Cited references CR; Descriptors DE; Figure titles FT; General references GR; List of tables TC; Occurrences OC; Source SO; Tables TA; Text TX; Title TI and Update code UP

14:632. Online Data-Star

File name	KIRK
Start year	Current
Number of records	1,140
Update period	Irregular
Database aids	Data-Star Chemical Manual, Berne, Data-Star, 1989 and Data-Star Online Manual (search NEWS-KIRK in NEWS)
Price/Charges	Subscription: SFr80.00
	Connect time: SFr163.00
	Online print: SFr0.24
	Offline print: SFrNot applicable
	SDI charge: SFrNot applicable

Notes

From June 1993 Data-Star have introduced an annual fee/subscription per contract (that is, not per password) of SFr 80.00 (c.UK£ 32.00) payable every June. For North American customers billed in dollars who also use DIALOG, the DIALOG fee also covers access to Data-Star. Academic customers, 'commitment' customers and customers currently billed in dollars are exempt.

Record composition

Abstract AB; Accession number and update code AN; Author AU; Author affiliation IN; Cited references CR; Descriptors DE; Figure titles FT; General references GR; List of tables TC; Occurrences OC; Source SO; Tables TA; Text TX; Title TI and Update code UP

The SAME or AND operators should not be used in this database to combine terms as a specified word might appear at the beginning of an article and another at the end. The data field Occurrence (OC) should be used with the PRINT command to locate search terms by displaying the relevant text section numbers where the terms occur. For example to find which section deals with animal pests enter ANIMAL ADJ PEST$1.TX followed by .P OC/1. The data field Author (AU) lists all contributing authors. The Cited references field (CR) contains references to books, journal articles etc which are cited within the body of KIRK articles. The Descriptors field (DE) contains keyword descriptive phrases, chemical names or expressions and CAS Registry numbers. The Figure titles field (FT) contains the titles of figures which enable the user to locate valuable figures, tables and graphs. The Source (SO) is always Kirk-Othmer. The edition, volume number and page numbers are searchable. The List of tables (TC) field lists the titles of the tables contained in the document. The Title (TI) field contains the title of the Kirk-Othmer article. Brief subheadings may be merged with the lead title to create informative titles for the document. As the database is updated irregularly it is better to search for the information regardless of date, thereby disregarding the Update code (UP).

14:633. Online DIALOG

File name	File 302
Start year	3rd edition of the Kirk-Othmer Encyclopedia of Chemical Techology
Number of records	33,293 records representing 1,200 chapters
Update period	Irregular
Price/Charges	Connect time: US$85.00
	Online print: US$0.25
	Offline print: US$0.55

Notes

DIALINDEX Categories: CHEMENG, CHEMLIT, RNCHEM, SCITECHB.

14:634. CD-ROM DIALOG OnDisc

File name	Kirk-Othmer Encyclopedia of Chemical Technology
Format notes	Mac, IBM
Software	DIALOG OnDisc Manager
Start year	
Number of records	
Update period	Not updated
Price	UK£3,000
	Subscription: UK£1,000

Notes

Four types of record allow flexibility in searching: a summary record of each chapter; text records for each subject heading; individual records for each table; and bibliography records for groups of citations from each chapter.

14:635. CD-ROM John Wiley and Sons Inc

File name	Kirk-Othmer Encyclopedia of Chemical Technology, 3rd Edition
Format notes	IBM
Software	FindIt
Start year	

Number of records
Update period
Price/Charges   Subscription: US$1,500

Notes

The complete text of the entire nine million word encyclopedia is available and searchable including tables, cited and general references and tables, and abstracts from text. All tables are fully searchable and displayable.

14:636. Database subset

Online   **DIALOG**

File name   File 386 – ONTAP Kirk-Othmer
                       Online Training File
Start year   12 chapters
Number of records   452
Update period   Closed File
Price/Charges   Connect time: US$15.00

Notes

The low-cost training file contains twelve chapters of Kirk-Othmer Online, File 302 on DIALOG. The twelve chapters include: Ammonia; Beer; Ceramics as Electric Materials; Chocolate and Cocoa; Cosmetics; Food Additives; Insect Control Technology; Mixing and Blending; Plant Safety; Semiconductors, Theory and Applications; Solar Energy; and Vaccine Technology. Offline prints are not available in ONTAP files.

KOMBI-ROM
ID/Farma BV

14:637. Master record

Database type   Textual, Image, Directory
Number of journals
Sources
Start year
Language   Dutch and English
Coverage   Netherlands
Number of records
Update size   –
Update period   Monthly

Keywords

Drugs

Description

Contains drug information, including prices, of the Pharmacists Association four wholesale organisations in the Netherlands. Also provides details on additional sources of software and courseware.

14:638. CD-ROM   **ID/Farma BV**

File name   KOMBI-ROM
Format notes   IBM
Software   HiCare
Start year
Number of records
Update period   Monthly
Price/Charges   Subscription: DFl1,200

Kosmet
International Federation of the Societies of Cosmetics Chemists (IFSCC)

14:639. Master record

Database type   Bibliographic
Number of journals
Sources

Start year   1968
Language   German and English
Coverage   International
Number of records   4,000
Update size   1,200
Update period

Keywords

Dermatology; Physics; Applied Science

Description

Contains citations, with some abstracts, on cosmetic and perfume science and technology, specifically dealing with raw materials, manufacture, analysis, control and use. KOSMET covers articles from periodicals, congresses and seminars on all matters related to cosmetics and perfumes, in particular the scientific, technical and biomedical areas. It covers different aspects of product development, the knowledge of healthy skin and its adnexa (hair, nails, teeth, glands), the trading of perfumes and cosmetics, the research and development of raw materials, active ingredients, formulations, manufacture, analysis, safety, physico-chemical properties, biological properties, stability, packaging and clinical studies.

14:640. Online   **Data-Star**

File name   KOSM
Start year   January 1985 periodicals and
                       meetings; 1968 for IFSCC
                       Congresses
Number of records   6,152
Update period   Monthly
Database aids   Data-Star Biomedical Manual,
                       Berne, Data-Star 1989 and Online
                       Manual (search NEWS-KOSM in
                       NEWS)
Price/Charges   Subscription: UK£32.00
                       Connect time: UK£51.60
                       Online print: UK£0.50
                       Offline print: UK£0.60
                       SDI charge: UK£4.32

Notes

From June 1993 Data-Star have introduced an annual fee/subscription per contract (that is, not per password) of SFr 80.00 (c.UK£ 32.00) payable every June. For North American customers billed in dollars who also use DIALOG, the DIALOG fee also covers access to Data-Star. Academic customers, 'commitment' customers and customers currently billed in dollars are exempt.

Laboratorios Farmaceuticos Españoles
Consejo General de Colegios Oficiales de Farmaceuticos de España

14:641. Master record

Database type   Directory
Number of journals
Sources   Government publication and
                       Pharmacopoeias
Start year   1972
Language   Spanish
Coverage   Spain
Number of records
Update size   –
Update period   Periodically, as new data become
                       available

Keywords

Drugs; Pharmaceutical Industry; Product Catalogues

Description

Gives data on drugs produced by about 550 Spanish pharmaceutical manufacturers since 1972, including firms which have ceased trading. Provides drug trade name, therapeutic category (as defined in the Grupos Therapeuticos database), number of dosage forms available, shelf life, conditions of dispensation, for example, whether a prescription is required, and the method of administration.

Source is the pharmaceutial register of the Ministerio de Sanidad y Consumo.

14:642. Online   Consejo General de Colegios Oficiales de Farmaceuticos de España

File name	
Start year	1972
Number of records	
Update period	Periodically, as new data become available

Lauer Mobi-med 3 plus
Pharma Daig & Lauer
Information providers: Pharma Daig & Lauer

14:643. Master record
CD-ROM   **Pharma Daig & Lauer**

Database type	Directory, Textual
Number of journals	
Sources	
Start year	
Language	German
Coverage	Germany
Number of records	
Update size	–
Update period	Quarterly
Index unit	Drug

Keywords
Drugs; Pharmaceuticals

Description
Contains the following drug databases: Lauer-Taxe, Rote Liste, Fachinformation.

For more details of constituent databases, see:
Lauer-Taxe
Rote Liste
Fachinformation

Lauer-Taxe
Pharma Daig & Lauer

14:645. Master record

Database type	Factual, Directory
Number of journals	
Sources	
Start year	
Language	German
Coverage	Germany
Number of records	120,000
Update size	–
Update period	Weekly
Index unit	Drug

Keywords
Drugs; Pharmaceuticals

Description

Contains information on 120,000 medicines: dosage, effects, side effects, interaction, prices, dates of expiration, information on contents and manufacturers, etc.

14:646. CD-ROM   Pharma Daig & Lauer

File name	Lauer-Taxe
Format notes	IBM
Software	Cobra
Start year	
Number of records	120,000
Update period	Weekly

This database can also be found on:
Lauer Mobi-med 3 plus

Life Sciences Collection
Cambridge Scientific Abstracts

14:648. Master record

Alternative name(s)	LSC; CSA Life Sciences Collection
Database type	Bibliographic
Number of journals	5,000
Sources	Journals, books, serial monographs, conference proceedings, patents (US), patents (UK), patents (Japanese) and reports
Start year	1978
Language	English
Coverage	International
Number of records	1,500,000
Update size	Monthly
Update period	Monthly

Keywords
Acute Poisoning; Aging; Algology; Amino-Acids; Anatomy; Antibiotics; Aquaculture; Bacteriology; Behavioural Ecology; Bioengineering; Biological Membranes; Biotechnology; Bone Disease; Calcium Metabolism; Chemoreception; Chronic Poisoning; Clinical Medicine; Clinical Toxicology; DNA; Drugs; Ecology; Ecosystems; Endocrinology; Entomology – Agricultural; Entomology – Applied; Entomology – Human; Entomology – Veterinary; Environmental Biology; Ethology; Genetic Engineering; Hazardous Substances; HIV; Histology; Human Ecology; Immune Disorders; Immunology; Infectious Diseases; Marine Biotechnology; Microbiology; Molecular Biology; Molecular Neurobiology; Mycology; Neurology; Neuropharmacology; Neurophysiology – Animal; Neuroscience; Nucleic Acids; Nutrition; Oncology; Occupational Health and Safety; Osteoporosis; Osteomalacia; Pathology; Peptides; Pharmaceuticals; Pheromones; Physiology; Pollution; Proteins; Protozoology; Psychophysics; Public Health; Radiation; Rhinology; RNA; Sleep; Smoking; Substance Abuse; Taste Perception; Viral Genetics

Description
Life Sciences Collection contains abstracts of information in the fields of (and corresponding to abstract journals from CSA): animal behaviour; biochemistry-amino-acid, peptide and protein; biochemistry – nucleic acids; biochemistry-biological membranes; biotechnology research (from 1984 to date); calcified tissue; chemoreception; ecology; endocrinology; entomology; genetics; human genomes; basic research and clinical applications; immunology, marine biotechnology, microbiology- algology, mycology and protozoology; microbiology-bacteriology; microbiology-industrial & applied microbiology; oncology-oncogenes and growth factors; neurosciences (from

1983 to date); toxicology; virology and AIDS. AIDS is covered in depth. The worldwide coverage is of journal articles, books, conference proceedings, report literature, patents, theses and dissertations.

Corresponds to the series of abstracting journals published by CSA: *Animal Behavior Abstracts; Biochemistry Abstracts-Amino-acid, Peptide & Protein; Biochemistry Abstracts-Biological Membranes; Biochemistry Abstracts-Nucleic Acids; Calcified Tissue Abstracts; Biotechnology Research Abstracts* (from 1984 to date); *Chemoreception Abstracts; Ecology Abstracts; Endocrinology Abstracts; Entomology Abstracts; Genetics Abstracts; Human Genome Abstracts; Basic Research and Clinical Applications; Immunology Abstracts; Marine Biotechnology Abstracts; Microbiology Abstracts-Algology, Mycology & Protozoology; Microbiology Abstracts-Bacteriology; Microbiology Abstracts-Industrial & Applied Microbiology; Neurosciences Abstracts* (from 1983 to date); *Oncogenes and Growth Factors Abstracts; Toxicology Abstracts; Virology and AIDS Abstracts.* Most recently added were *Marine Biotechnology Abstracts* and *Oncogenes and Growth Factors Abstracts.* Also includes *Oncology Abstracts* and Feeding, Weight and Obesity Abstracts for the period they were published.

14:649. Online — BIOSIS Life Science Network

File name	Life Sciences Collection
Start year	1978
Number of records	1,500,000
Update period	Monthly
Price/Charges	Connect time: US$9.00
	Online print: US$6.00 per 10; 2.25 per abstract; 3.50 per full text article

Also available via the Internet by telnetting to LSN.COM.

Notes

On Life Science Network users can search this database or they can scan a group of subject-related databases. There is a charge of $2.00 per scan of subject-related databases. To search one database and display up to ten citations costs $6.00. Most charges are for information retrieved. There are no charges if there are no results and no charge to transfer results to a printer or diskette. Articles may also be ordered via an online document delivery request. A telecommunications software package is also available, costing $12.95, providing an automatic connection to Life Science Network for heavy users of the service, with capability to transfer to print or disk and customised colour options.

14:650. Online — DIALOG

File name	File 76
Start year	1978
Number of records	1,392,381
Update period	Monthly
Price/Charges	Connect time: US$90.00
	Online print: US$0.75
	Offline print: US$0.75
	SDI charge: US$9.50

14:651. Online — STN

File name	LIFESCI
Start year	1978
Number of records	1,500,000
Update period	Monthly

14:652. CD-ROM — Compact Cambridge

File name	Life Sciences Collection
Alternative name(s)	LSC; CSA Life Sciences Collection
Format notes	NEC, 9800, IBM

Start year	1982
Number of records	
Update period	Quarterly
Price	UK£1,165 – 2,985 (Initial with backfiles)
	Subscription: UK£985

Notes

Contains eighteen subject orientated subfiles in the life and biosciences field, covering some 5,000 core journals, books, serial monographs etc. Over 98,000 abstracts are added each year. Subscribers to CSA's life sciences print journals receive a £500 credit towards the first year's subscription to LSC CD-ROM 1982-present or 1985-present.

14:653. Tape — Cambridge Scientific Abstracts

File name	Life Sciences Collection on Magnetic Tape
Alternative name(s)	LSC; CSA Life Sciences Collection
Format notes	9-track,, unlabelled,, 1600, bpi,, EBCDIC.
Start year	1982
Number of records	
Update period	Monthly
Price/Charges	Subscription: US$13,950

Notes

The series of abstracting journals published by CSA are available on this tape as a collection. They are also available separately as tape subsets of the Life Sciences Collection, the online database to which this tape corresponds.

Price for the current year tape is $13,950; single-year archival file is $7,100.

14:654. Database subset

Online — Cambridge Scientific Abstracts

File name	Toxicology Abstracts
Start year	1974
Number of records	14,000
Update period	Monthly

Notes

A subset of the Life Sciences Collection online database. Corresponds to *Toxicology Abstracts.* Contains citations to the worldwide literature on toxicology. Covers clinical toxicology, including acute or chronic poisoning from drugs, medicines and chemicals; toxic risks in the workplace; and environmental toxicology. Sources include about 2,500 journals.

14:655. Database subset

Tape — Cambridge Scientific Abstracts

File name	Toxicology Abstracts on Magnetic Tape
Format notes	9-track, unlabelled, 1600 bpi, EBCDIC.
Start year	1978
Number of records	
Update period	Monthly

Notes

A subset of the Life Sciences Collection. Contains citations to the international literature on toxicology, covering clinical toxicology (including acute and chronic poisoning from drugs, medicines and chemicals), toxic risks in the workplace and environmental toxicology. Includes social poisons and substance abuse;

natural toxins; legislation and recommended standards; studies of industrial and agricultural chemicals; household products, pharmaceuticals and other substances; effects of alcohol and smoking; radiation and radioactive materials; and toxicology methodology and analytical procedures. Corresponds to *Toxicology Abstracts* and in part to the Life Sciences Collection online database. Contact Cambridge Scientific Abstracts for pricing information.

14:656. Database subset

Tape	Cambridge Scientific Abstracts
File name	Biotechnology Research Abstracts on Magnetic Tape
Format notes	9-track, unlabelled, 1600 bpi, EBCDIC.
Start year	1984
Number of records	
Update period	Every two months

Notes
A subset of the Life Sciences Collection. Contains citations, with abstracts, to the worldwide literature on biotechnology, including medical, chemical, agricultural, pharmaceutical, environment and energy applications. Covers genetic engineering, cloning vectors, site-directed mutagenesis, gene manipulation, transfer and expression, biotechnology products and relevant US patents. Corresponds to *Biotechnology Research Abstracts* and in part to the Life Science Collection online database.

It is necessary to contact Cambridge Scientific Abstracts for pricing information.

14:657. Database subset

Tape	Cambridge Scientific Abstracts
File name	Industrial and Applied Microbiology on Magnetic Tape
Format notes	9-track, unlabelled, 1600, bpi, EBCDIC
Start year	1978
Number of records	
Update period	Monthly

Notes
A subset of the Life Sciences Collection. Contains three databases of information on microbiology.

Industrial and Applied Microbiology contains citations, with abstracts, to the worldwide literature on practical applications of microbiology. Covers pharmaceutical, food and beverage, agricultural and environmental applications, and methodology and research. Includes antibiotics and antimicrobial agents; vaccines and serum production; food contamination, ripening and fermentation processes; soil microbiology; plant diseases caused by microorganisms; composting; hydrocarbons; methane production; pollution; and isolation, identification and characterization of microorganisms. Also incudes registered US patents. Corresponds to *Cambridge Microbiology Abstracts, Section A: Industrial and Applied Microbiology*, and in part to the Life Sciences Collection online database.

Bacteriology contains citations, with abstracts, to the worldwide literature on bacteriology. Covers immunology, taxonomy, methods, cell properties, genetics, antibiotics and antimicrobials, toxins, medical, veterinary and invertebrate bacteriology, plant dis-

eases, and ecological aspects. Corresponds to *Cambridge Microbiology Abstracts, Section B: Bacteriology*, and in part to the Life Sciences Collection online database. Algology, Mycology & Protozoology contains citations, with abstracts, to the worldwide literature on algae, fungi, protozoa and lichens. Includes reproduction, growth, life cycles, biochemistry, genetics, and infection and immunity in humans, other animals and plants. Covers taxonomy, structure and function, ecology and distribution, effects of physical and chemical factors, methodology, media and culture, nutrition, mycotoxins, parasitism and diseases, viruses and bacteria, soil microbiolgy and mycorrhiza, spoilage and biodegradation, and pollution. Corresponds to *Cambridge Microbiology Abstracts, Section C: Algology, Mycology and Protozoology*, and in part to the Life Sciences Collection online database. Pricing information may be obtained from Cambridge Scientific Abstracts.

14:658. Database subset

Tape	Cambridge Scientific Abstracts
File name	Entomology Abstracts on Magnetic Tape
Format notes	9-track, unlabelled, 1600, bpi, EBCDIC
Start year	1982
Number of records	
Update period	Monthly

Notes
A subset of the Life Sciences Collection. Contains citations, with abstracts, to the worldwide literature on insects, arachnids, myriapods, onychophorans and terrestrial isopods. Covers geographic distribution, nomenclature, new species, techniques and methodology, morphology of all life cycle stages, physiology, anatomy, histology, biochemistry, toxicology and resistance, ecology, behaviour, and medical, veterinary, agricultural and applied entomology. Corresponds to *Entomology Abstracts* and in part to the Life Sciences Collection online database. Contact Cambridge Scientific Abstracts for pricing information.

14:659. Database subset

Tape	Cambridge Scientific Abstracts
File name	Animal Behavior Abstracts on Magnetic Tape
Format notes	9-track, unlabelled, 1600 bpi, EBCDIC
Start year	1978
Number of records	
Update period	Quarterly

Notes
A subset of the Life Sciences Collection. Contains citations, with abstracts, to the worldwide literature on ethology, the study of animal behaviour. Covers neurophysiology, behavioural ecology, biochemical, anatomical and neurophysiological correlates, sleep, brain stimulation, drug studies, hormones, habituation, reinforcement, avoidance, discrimination, complex learning, memory, theoretical models, communication, aggression, social spacing and dominance in animals.

Corresponds to *Animal Behavior Abstracts* and in part to the Life Sciences Collection online database. Contact Cambridge Scientific Abstracts for pricing information.

14:660. Database subset

Tape   Cambridge Scientific
                                    Abstracts

File name	Virology and AIDS Abstracts on Magnetic Tape
Format notes	9-track, unlabelled, 1600, bpi, EBCDIC
Start year	1978
Number of records	
Update period	Monthly

Notes

A subset of the Life Sciences Collection. Contains citations, with abstracts, to the worldwide literature on human, animal and plant virology, and on Acquired Immune Deficiency Syndrome (AIDS). Covers replication cycles, oncology, viral genetics, interferon, hepatitis B virus vaccination, immunological, clinical and epidemiological aspects of AIDS, patterns of AIDS, AIDS-related diseases and investigational drugs. Corresponds to *Virology and AIDS Abstracts* and in part to the Life Sciences Collection and in part to the Life Science online database. Contact Cambridge Scientific Abstracts for pricing information.

This database can also be found on:
Cambridge Scientific Abstracts Life Sciences
Human Nutrition on CD-ROM

Literature Analysis System on Road Safety

Australia Department of Transport and Communications, Transport Group Library

14:662. Master record

Alternative name(s)	LASORS
Database type	Bibliographic
Number of journals	
Sources	Journals, Books, Reports, Conference proceedings and A-V material
Start year	1970
Language	English
Coverage	Australia
Number of records	10,000
Update size	—
Update period	Six times per year

Keywords

Road Safety; Driver Licensing; Driver Training; Alcohol Abuse; Driver Behaviour; Drug Abuse; Road Construction; Urban Planning; Road Accidents; Health and Safety

Description

Gives citations to the international literature on road safety relevant to Australia, including driver licensing and improvement; road safety training, education and publicity; legislation, enforcement and sanctions; impact of alcohol and other drugs; road user behaviour; pedestrians; safety aspects of traffic control, town planning and road design; bicycle, motorcycle and motor vehicle safety; accident research and statistics; medical, psychological, sociological and policy aspects of safety and general literature of interest to road safety researchers.

14:663. Online   Ferntree Computer
                           Corporation Ltd, AUSINET

File name	
Alternative name(s)	LASORS
Start year	1970
Number of records	10,000
Update period	Six times per year

Notes

Monthly minimum to Ferntree required; fees vary depending on service selected.

This database can also be found on:
Engineering and Applied Science

Lithium Consultation

University of Wisconsin-Madison, Department of Psychiatry, Lithium Information Center

14:665. Master record

Database type	Textual, Computer software
Number of journals	
Sources	
Start year	Current information
Language	English
Coverage	International
Number of records	
Update size	—
Update period	Periodically, as new data become available

Keywords

Biochemistry; Lithium – Pharmacology; Patient Management

Description

Contains information to help physicians select patients suitable for treatment with lithium and to help in patient management. Patient data are input and information is retrieved on the patient's suitability for treatment, expected responsiveness, possible contraindications, procedures for initiating lithium therapy, managing side-effects and alternative treatments.

14:666. Online   University of
                           Wisconsin-Madison,
                           Department of Psychiatry,
                           Lithium Information Center

File name	
Start year	Current information
Number of records	
Update period	Periodically, as new data become available

Lithium Index

University of Wisconsin-Madison, Department of Psychiatry, Lithium Information Center

14:667. Master record

Database type	Bibliographic, Textual (reviews)
Number of journals	
Sources	
Start year	Current information
Language	English
Coverage	International

Number of records	125
Update size	–
Update period	Periodically, as new data become available

Keywords

Biochemistry; Clinical Medicine; Lithium – Clinical Uses

Description

Contains analyses of the international literature on medical uses of lithium, including interactions with other drugs, side effects, medical conditions and treatment guidelines. Summaries can be retrieved by clinical topics (pregnancy, teratogenesis, neurological side effects, kidney damage, sexual function, fertility, cardiovascular system, cutaneous side effects, etc).

14:668. Online
University of Wisconsin-Madison, Department of Psychiatry, Lithium Information Center

File name	
Start year	Current information
Number of records	125
Update period	Periodically, as new data become available

Lithium Library

University of Wisconsin-Madison, Department of Psychiatry, Lithium Information Center

14:669. Master record

Database type	Bibliographic
Number of journals	
Sources	Databases, Bibliographies, Indexes, Books, Journals, Government publications and Meeting abstracts
Start year	1800s
Language	English
Coverage	International
Number of records	15,000
Update size	1,000
Update period	Periodically

Keywords

Biochemistry; Biology; Lithium

Description

Citations to the international literature on medical and biological uses of lithium. Records give title, subject headings, author, source and date.

14:670. Online
University of Wisconsin-Madison, Department of Psychiatry, Lithium Information Center

File name	
Start year	1800s
Number of records	15,000
Update period	Periodically

Logo-A Pharmaceutical Products

Adviseur Informatisering en Organisatie

14:671. Master record

Database type	Factual
Number of journals	
Sources	

Start year	1988
Language	English
Coverage	
Number of records	–
Update size	–
Update period	Quarterly

Keywords

Drugs; Pharmaceuticals

Notes

This database contained medical/pharmaceutical information including EMBASE and SEDBASE. It was available to pharmacists only, but is no longer available.

For more details of constituent databases, see:
EMBASE
SEDBASE

MarkIntel Master

Investext

14:673. Master record

Database type	Factual, Textual
Number of journals	
Sources	Reports
Start year	1988
Language	English
Coverage	International
Number of records	2,155
Update size	–
Update period	

Keywords

Chemical Industry; Computer Industry; Construction; Gas Industry; Market Reports; Oil Industry; Pharmaceutical Industry

Description

Market studies prepared for clients by five consulting firms, including Kline & Co, Forrester Research and Decision Resources. The reports provide extensive primary research, detailed market share information and hard-to-find provate company data. The major industry areas covered are chemical, construction, pharmaceuticals, oil and gas, and computers. Companies and industries in the United States, Europe and Asia are included.

The company reports run to about five pages and discuss products, market share, financial data, and customer and company official interviews. Industry reports range from ten to thirty pages and examine technologies, trends, new markets and projections.

Database is embargoed by the consultant firms for several weeks to several months.

14:674. Online
I/PLUS Direct (Investext)

File name	
Start year	1988
Number of records	2,155
Update period	

MarkIntel

Investext

14:675. Master record

Database type	Factual, Textual
Number of journals	
Sources	Reports

Start year 1990
Language English
Coverage International
Number of records 1,000
Update size –
Update period

Keywords

Chemical Industry; Market Reports; Medical Supply Industry; Pharmaceutical Industry; Textiles

Description

Full-text database of Frost & Sullivan research reports in fourteen categories including chemicals, pharmaceuticals, medical supply and textiles. Industry reports cover new products, market share, business environment and trends. Company reports include a profile of the company, brief history, larketing strategies and a five-year projection.

Database is embargoed by the consultant firms for several weeks to several months.

14:676. Online   I/PLUS Direct (Investext)

File name
Start year 1990
Number of records 1,000
Update period

Martindale
Royal Pharmaceutical Society of Great Britain

14:677. Master record

Alternative name(s) CCIS: Martindale: The Extra Pharmacopoeia; Martindale – The Extra Pharmacopoeia on CCIS
Database type Bibliographic, Factual, Textual
Number of journals
Sources Government reports, journals, laws/regulations, official publications and WHO publications
Start year Current
Language English
Coverage International
Number of records 60,000
Update size –
Update period Annually
Index unit Articles
Thesaurus Martindale Online: Drug Information Thesaurus. London: Pharmaceutical Society of Great Britain, 2nd ed., 1990
Database aids Martindale Online help-desk (9 am. to 5pm. UK time) Tel. +44 1 582 8455 and Martindale Online User's Guide (Data-Star), London, Pharmaceutical Society of Great Britain, 1985

Keywords

Clinical Medicine; Hazardous Substances; Drugs; Drug Therapy; Pharmacokinetics

Description

Martindale is a full text database based on the textbook, *Martindale, The Extra Pharmacopoeia* published by the Royal Pharmaceutical Society of Great Britain. It offers an extensive resource of evaluated information on drugs and medicines in clinical and therapeutic use throughout the world, and on investigational drugs, compounds liable to abuse and ancillary substances including diagnostic agents,

pharmaceutical adjuvants and toxic substances. The database contains information on more than 25,000 compounds that are used in the many thousands of preparations also included. The compounds cover most drugs and medicines used to treat diseases as well as many investigational drugs. It also covers ancilliary substances such as asbestos. The database supplies information on groups of compounds as well as on individual substances and is supported by selected abstracts.

The information available for each compound will usually include: nomenclature (synonyms, generic names, chemical names), CAS Registry numbers, physical and pharmaceutical properties such as appearance, pharmacopoeial status, units adverse effects and their treatment, precautions, standards, contra-indications and interactions, pharmacokinetics, actions, uses, dosage and administration, proprietary names and preparations.

The database corresponds to the printed *Martindale: The Extra Pharmacopoeia* (30th edition). It is updated annually over a five-year cycle, so that at the end of the cycle the whole database has been reassessed. Conditions for use note that all the information provided through Martindale Online and is copyright of the Royal Pharmaceutical Society of Great Britain. Payment for information obtained through Martindale Online includes the right to store the information in memory and to print and display it for private use only. Martindale Online has been prepared assuming that the user has the necessary training to interpret the information it provides.

Martindale Online developed a hierarchical thesaurus of more than 9,600 descriptors to facilitate searching on classes of drugs (a feature omitted from printed editions). The database can be searched by: old English terms or their modern synonyms; international trade name; generic name; chemical name; disease state.

14:678. Online   Data-Star

File name MART
Start year Current
Number of records 46,000
Update period Annually on a 5 year cycle
Database aids Data-Star Biomedical Manual and Data-Star Online Manual (search NEWS-MART in NEWS)
Price/Charges Subscription: SFr80.00
Connect time: SFr107.00
Online print: SFr1.19
Offline print: SFr0.92
Downloading is allowed

Notes

From June 1993 Data-Star have introduced an annual fee/subscription per contract (that is, not per password) of SFr 80.00 (c.UK£ 32.00) payable every June. For North American customers billed in dollars who also use DIALOG, the DIALOG fee also covers access to Data-Star. Academic customers, 'commitment' customers and customers currently billed in dollars are exempt.

Record composition

Abstract AB; Accession Number AN; Author(s) AU; CAS Registry Number RN; Cross reference(s) XR; Descriptors DE; Document Length LE; Document Type RF; Entry Date ED; Headings HE; Molecular formula and Molecula Weight MO; Notes and Warnings NT; Pharmacopoeia(s) PC; Preparations

PR; Preparation Licence Holder and Number PL; Publication Year PY; Radiopharmaceutical Data RP; Source(s) SO; Synonym(s) SY; Text TX; Title TI; Update Code UP and Warning WA

14:679. Online   DIALOG

File name	File 141
Start year	Current edition
Number of records	43,393 describing 25,000 preparations or compunds
Update period	Annually
Price/Charges	Connect time: US$63.00
	Online print: US$0.50
	Offline print: US$0.50

Notes

DIALINDEX Categories: DRUGDIR, PHARM, PHARMR, RNMED, TOXICOL, TRADENMS.

14:680. CD-ROM   Micromedex Inc

File name	Martindale – The Extra Pharmacopoeia on CCIS
Alternative name(s)	CCIS: Martindale: The Extra Pharmacopoeia; Martindale – The Extra Pharmacopoeia on CCIS
Format notes	IBM
Software	Proprietary
Start year	Current
Number of records	60,000
Update period	Quarterly

Notes

This database is available as a standalone product, as well as being a part of CCIS, Computerized Clinical Information System. The 30th edition of Martindale is now available both in print and on this CD-ROM.

14:681. Tape   Micromedex Inc

File name	Martindale – The Extra Pharmacopeia on CCIS
Alternative name(s)	CCIS: Martindale: The Extra Pharmacopoeia; Martindale – The Extra Pharmacopoeia on CCIS
Software	Proprietary
Start year	1987
Number of records	
Update period	Quarterly

Notes

Annual subsription to CCIS required. This database is also available as a standalone CD product, as well as being a part of CCIS, Computerized Clinical Information System.

This database can also be found on:
CCIS

Medical Bulletin
US Food and Drug Administration

14:683. Master record

Database type	Textual
Number of journals	1
Sources	Newsletter and Government departments
Start year	1988
Language	English
Coverage	USA
Number of records	
Update size	—
Update period	Quarterly

Keywords

Drugs; Food Additives

Description

A newsletter, updated quarterly, covering clinical drug testing, approvals of new drugs and medical devices by the US FDA, and information on food additives and food preparation processes.

Corresponds to Medical Bulletin quarterly newsletter. On DIALOG and Data-Star, this newsletter is available as part of the PTS Newsletter Database.

This database can be found on:
PTS Newsletter Database

Medical Scan
Market Intelligence Research Company (MIRC)

14:685. Master record

Alternative name(s)	Medical Market Scan
Database type	Textual
Number of journals	
Sources	Newsletter
Start year	1988
Language	English
Coverage	USA (primarily) and International (some)
Number of records	
Update size	—
Update period	Monthly

Keywords

Health Care; Medical Equipment; Pharmaceutical Industry

Description

Contains the full text of Medical Scan, a monthly newsletter on the medical electronics and pharmaceutical industries. Covers market analyses, legal and regulatory developments and business news. Focuses on developing medical technology and treatments and the emerging markets in medical equipment and health care. Provides in-depth analysis of trends in the medical industry and the competitive environment for medical products, equipment and health services.

Corresponds to the monthly Medical Scan newsletter. The newsletter on DIALOG and Data-Star is available on PTS Newsletter Database, supplied by Predicasts.

This database can be found on:
PTS Newsletter Database

Medical Science Research Database
Medical Science Research
Elsevier Science Publishers

14:686. Master record

Database type	Textual
Number of journals	
Sources	
Start year	1982
Language	English
Coverage	

Number of records	57,000
Update size	600
Update period	Bimonthly

Keywords

Physiology; Pathology; Anatomy

Description

The Medical Science Research database (formerly IRCS Medical Science database) consists of the full text, including tables, or peer-reviewed research articles published in *Medical Science Research* (incorporating IRCS Medical Science journals). Articles are approximately 1,000 words long and are concise but complete accounts of research with full methodological and result information. Coverage includes all areas of clinical and biomedical science, with major coverage in the following areas: alimentary system, anatomy and human biology, biochemistry, biomedical technology, cardiovascular system, cell and membrane biology, clinical medicine, clinical pharmacology and therapeutics, connective tissue, skin and bone, dentistry and oral biology, developmental biology and medicine, drug metabolism and toxicology, endocrine system, environmental biology and medicine, experimental animals, the eye, haematology, immunology and allergy, metabolism and nutrition, microbiology, parasitology and infectious diseases, nervous system, pathology, physiology, psychology and psychiatry, reproduction, obstetrics and gynaecology, social and occupational medicine, surgery and transplantation, techniques and methods.

This database appears to be no longer available.

Medicamentos en el Embarazo
Consejo General de Colegios de Farmaceuticos de España

14:687. Master record

Database type	Bibliographic, Textual
Number of journals	
Sources	Journals, Pharmacopoeias and Databases
Start year	Articles: current information; Bibliographies: 1980
Language	Spanish
Coverage	Spain
Number of records	390
Update size	—
Update period	Periodically, as new data become available

Keywords

Drugs; Obstetrics; Pharmaceuticals

Description

Complete texts of articles, with bibliographies, on the risks associated with about 390 drugs available in Spain for pregnant women. Includes description, mechanism and frequency of adverse reactions on mother and foetus, relevant research results and recommendations on usage.

14:688. Online
Consejo General de Colegios Oficiales de Farmaceuticos de España

File name	
Start year	Articles: current information; Bibliographies: 1980
Number of records	390
Update period	Periodically, as new data become available

Medicamentos en Enfermedades Crónicas
Consejo General de Colegios Oficiales de Farmaceuticos de España

14:689. Master record

Database type	Textual
Number of journals	
Sources	Journals, Pharmacopoeias and Databases
Start year	Current information
Language	Spanish
Coverage	Spain
Number of records	1,700
Update size	—
Update period	Periodically, as new data become available

Keywords

Allergy; Angina; Asthma; Cardiovascular Diseases; Chronic Diseases; Depression; Diabetes; Drugs; Epilepsy; Glaucoma; Hepatic Disease; Hypertension; Renal Disease; Ulcers

Description

Complete texts of articles on risks associated with over 1,700 drugs or active ingredients available in Spain for patients with chronic diseases such as penicillin or salicilate allergy, angina, asthma, depression, diabetes, epilepsy, glaucoma, hypertension, peptic ulcers or insufficient function of the heart, liver or kidneys. Covers general actions of each drug, possible side effects on patients with chronic conditions, contraindications and precautions.

14:690. Online
Consejo General de Colegios Oficiales de Farmaceuticos de España

File name	
Start year	Current information
Number of records	1,700
Update period	Periodically, as new data become available

Medicinal Herbs
ArmNIINTI

14:691. Master record

Database type	Bibliographic
Number of journals	
Sources	
Start year	1989
Language	English
Coverage	
Number of records	1,000
Update size	—
Update period	

Keywords

Alternative Medicine; Homeopathy

Description

Bibliographic source on medicinal herbs and homeopathy.

14:692. Diskette
ArmNIINTI

File name	
Start year	1989

Number of records   1,000
Update period

Medicorom
Inter CD

14:693. Master record

Database type	Encyclopedia, Directory, Dictionary, Factual
Number of journals	
Sources	Books
Start year	
Language	French
Coverage	France
Number of records	
Update size	–
Update period	Twice a year
Index unit	Drugs, doctors, hospitals, clinics and trade shows

Description
Contains: a drug dictionary with 3,400 entries; drug interactions; professional encyclopedia; directory of doctors in France; directories of hospitals and clinics; diary of medical trade shows; six-language medical glossary, and other encyclopaedic and directory information of use to the medical community.

14:694. CD-ROM   Inter CD

File name	Medicorom
Format notes	IBM
Start year	
Number of records	
Update period	Semiannually
Price/Charges	Subscription: FFr14,600

MediROM

Société Suisse de Pharmacie
Bureau van Dijk
Médecine et Hygiéne
OVP – Editions du Vidal
Schweizerischer Apothekerverein
Telmed
Georg Thieme Verlag

14:695. Master record
CD-ROM   AEK (AerzteKasse)

Database type	Textual, Factual
Number of journals	
Sources	
Start year	
Language	English, German and French
Coverage	Switzerland
Number of records	
Update size	–
Update period	Semiannually

Keywords
Drugs; Drug Therapy; Gynaecology; Internal Medicine; Medical Diagnosis; Pharmaceuticals; Rheumatology; Surgery; Travel; Urology

Description
This CD-ROM uses records from ten databases in the medical and pharmaceutical fields including: Index Nominum; Arzneimittel-Interaktionen des SAV; Medical Letter's Interactions; Dictionnaire Vidal;

Phytotherapie; Diagnosis; Vergiftungen; Reisemedizin; Badekurorte. It is possible to establish logical links between the data of some of the databases.

This disc is intended primarily for Swiss physicians.

For more details of constituent databases, see:
Index Nominum
Arzneimittel-Interaktionen des SAV
Medical Letter's Interactions
Dictionnaire Vidal
Phytotherapie
Diagnosis
Vergiftungen
Reisemedizin
Badekurorte

Membrane & Separation Technology News
Business Communications Company (BCC)

14:697. Master record

Database type	Textual
Number of journals	1
Sources	Newsletter
Start year	1989
Language	English
Coverage	USA
Number of records	
Update size	–
Update period	Monthly

Keywords
Biotechnology; Chromatography; Electrodialysis; Filtration; Membrane Technology; Pollution; Separation Technology; Water Purification

Description
A monthly newsletter on the filtration and separation technology industry, covering research developments and patents in microfiltration, reverse osmosis, ultrafiltration, cross filtration, gas separation, electrodialysis and specialty chromatography, and an array of other separation opportunities and potential commercial applications in pharmaceuticals, biotechnology, beverages, electronics, pollution control and water purification. Includes a calendar of events. On DIALOG and Data-Star, available as part of the PTS Newsletter Database.

Corresponds to *Membrane & Separation Technology News* monthly newsletter.

14:698. Online   NewsNet Inc

File name	
Start year	1989
Number of records	
Update period	

This database can also be found on:
PTS Newsletter Database

Merck Index, The
Merck and Company Inc

14:700. Master record

Database type	Textual, Directory
Number of journals	
Sources	pharmacopoeias

Drugs and Pharmacy

MPHARM

Start year	1889
Language	English
Coverage	International
Number of records	30,000
Update size	–
Update period	Twice a year reloads

Keywords

Drugs

Description

This is the online version of *The Merck Index* encyclopaedia (10th edition 1983), consisting of 10,000 monographs describing 30,000 chemical products, biopharmaceutical products, agricultural products, preparations, properties, uses and the therapeutic/toxicological effects of substances. It provides patent information, chemical, generic and trivial names, nomenclatures, trademarks and their owners, preparations, molecular formulae and weights for title substances and derivatives, physical properties, CAS Registry number, principal pharmacological actions and toxicity information. It also includes monographs that have been written or revised *since* publication of this tenth edition. The monographs which describe the synthesis and properties of chemical compounds refer the reader to patents as the source of much of the information in the database.

This file is the online equivalent to the printed *Merck Index* an internationally recognised one-volume encyclopedia of chemicals, drugs and biologicals.

14:701. Online   BRS

File name	MRCK
Start year	
Number of records	
Update period	
Price/Charges	Connect time: US$35.00/45.00
	Online print: US$0.15/0.23
	Offline print: US$0.43

14:702. Online   Chemical Information Systems Inc (CIS)

File name	Merck Index
Start year	
Number of records	
Update period	

Notes

Annual subscription fee of US$300 required.

14:703. Online   CompuServe Information Service

File name	IQUEST File 1951
Start year	1900
Number of records	
Update period	Twice per year
Price/Charges	Subscription: US$8.95 per month
	Database entry fee: US$9/search; some databases carry a surcharge ($2–75)
	Online print: US$10 references free; then $9 per ten; abstracts $3 each

Downloading is allowed

Notes

Accessed via IQUEST, this database is offered by a BRS gateway. IQUEST can either search across all databases, a database of the user's choice or selected multiple databases.

14:704. Online   DIALOG

File name	File 304
Start year	1889

Number of records	10,160
Update period	Twice a year reloads
Price/Charges	Connect time: US$50.00
	Online print: US$0.20
	Offline print: US$0.40

Notes

This database is also available to home users during evenings and weekends at a reduced rate on the Knowledge Index service of DIALOG – file name in this case is CHEM4, and searches are made with simplified commands or menus.

DIALINDEX Categories: CHEMILIT, CHEMPROP, CHEMSUBS, DRUGDIR, RNMED, TRADENMS.

14:705. Online   Questel

File name	MERCK
Start year	
Number of records	
Update period	

MPHARM

Institut National de la Propriété Industrielle (INPI)

14:706. Master record

Alternative name(s)	Markush Pharmsearch
Database type	Factual
Number of journals	
Sources	Patents (US) and Patents (European)
Start year	1987
Language	English and French
Coverage	France, USA and Europe
Number of records	70,578
Update size	–
Update period	Twice a month

Keywords

Pharmaceutical Products; Patents

Description

This database complements the Pharmsearch database covering US, European and French pharmaceutical patents. Contains graphic representations of generic (Markush) and defined structures used in patents for new therapeutically active compounds with novel preparation processes or activities, and active ingredients of new drug compositions. Structures are grouped under 21 concepts, called 'superatoms', which specify a particular attribute. Users can transfer search results to Pharmsearch to facilitate retrieval of complete patent information. The databases are linked by compound number. Structure records are searchable and displayable. Patents are added to the database within six to ten weeks of publication date (fourteen weeks for US Patents). Records are sourced from all US, European and French patents covering pharmaceutical, chemical and biological topics. Included in the 70,000 plus structures are over 8,000 peptides. Both databases also cover the older French BSM (Brevets Speciaux de Medicaments) system which ran from 1961–1971. The training file for this, is iPAT.

Coverage of European and US patents since 1978 and French patents since 1961 will be added.

14:707. Online   Questel

File name	MPHARM
Alternative name(s)	Markush Pharmsearch

Start year	1987
Number of records	500
Update period	Twice a month

14:708. Database subset

Online   Questel

File name	IPAT
Alternative name(s)	Markush Pharmsearch
Start year	1987
Number of records	500
Update period	Twice a month

Notes

The training file for the MPHARM database.

MSI Market Research Reports

Marketing Strategies for Industry (UK) Ltd

14:709. Master record

Alternative name(s)	MSI Databriefs; Market Research Reports from MSI
Database type	Textual, Factual
Number of journals	
Sources	Reports and Statistical tables
Start year	1987 (February)
Language	English
Coverage	UK (primarily) and Europe (some)
Number of records	
Update size	70
Update period	Varies

Keywords

Marketing; Pharmaceuticals

Description

Variety of marketing reports, mainly for the UK, with some European coverage. Reports analyse a specific market and industry and provide a concise review, a summary of trends and informed predictions for over ninety UK markets, industries and busines sectors. The reports are written and researched by consultants of the authoritative Marketing Strategies for Industry (UK) Ltd. and each report uses both primary and secondary sources of information and is supported by statistical tables. Covers market size and segmentation, industry sector, distributions, advertising, trade, company profiles, brand shares, production analysis, sales, prospects. Sectors include banking and services, building, decorating, do-it-yourself, chemists' goods, pharmaceuticals, drinks, food, engineering, garden, horticulture, agriculture, household goods, leisure goods, office equipment, packaging, printing, retailing, distribution, textiles, footwear, miscellaneous.

14:710. Online   FT Profile

File name	MSR
Alternative name(s)	MSI Databriefs; Market Research Reports from MSI
Start year	1987 (February)
Number of records	
Update period	As MSI databriefs are published
Price/Charges	Connect time: UK£2.40
	Online print: UK£0.04 – 0.10 per line
	Offline print: UK£0.01 per line

Notes

Information is online between two to three weeks of publication. Registration fee required, including free documentation and training. Usage charges for access consist of two elements: a connect rate for time online, and a display rate (applies only to lines of file text). There is no charge for blank lines, system messages, menus or help information.

This database can also be found on:
FT Profile

National Epilepsy Library Database

Epilepsy Foundation of America

14:712. Master record

Database type	Bibliographic
Number of journals	
Sources	Journals, Symposia, Books and Reports
Start year	1982
Language	English
Coverage	International
Number of records	
Update size	—
Update period	Quarterly
Index unit	Book chapters
Thesaurus	NEL Thesaurus

Keywords

Epilepsy; Neurology; Paediatrics; Internal Medicine; Vocational Rehabilitation

Description

A database from the Epilepsy Foundation of America, covering the clinical and psychosocial aspects of epilepsy. Journal articles, symposia, book chapters and reports are included. Specific subject areas are epileptology, neurology, psychiatry, pharmacology, paediatrics, internal medicine and vocational rehabilitation.

14:713. Online   BRS

File name	EPIL
Start year	1982
Number of records	
Update period	Quarterly
Database aids	Aidpage (8/91) Free (single copy)
Price/Charges	Connect time: US$25.00/35.00
	Online print: US$0.12/0.20
	Offline print: US$0.25

National Report on Substance Abuse, The

Bureau of National Affairs Inc

14:714. Master record

Alternative name(s)	BNA National Report on Substance Abuse
Database type	Textual
Number of journals	1
Sources	Newsletter and Companies
Start year	1987
Language	English
Coverage	USA
Number of records	
Update size	—
Update period	Every two weeks

Keywords

Alcohol Abuse; Drug Abuse; Occupational Health and Safety; Employee Benefits; Substance Abuse

Description

A newsletter on corporate policies towards substance abuse in the workplace, including drug testing and privacy rights, types of tests and accuracy assessments, employer liability issues and employee assistance programmes.

Corresponds to *The National Report on Substance Abuse* newsletter.

14:715. Online   Executive Telecom System International, Human Resource Information Network (ETSI/HRIN)

File name	
Alternative name(s)	BNA National Report on Substance Abuse
Start year	1987
Number of records	
Update period	Every two weeks

Notes

Annual subscription to ETSI/HRIN required.

National Survey of Worksite Health Promotion Activities

US Department of Health and Human Services, Office of Disease Prevention and Health Promotion

14:716. Master record

Database type	Textual
Number of journals	
Sources	Government departments and Surveys
Start year	1987
Language	English
Coverage	USA
Number of records	
Update size	—
Update period	Not updated

Keywords

Diet; Occupational Health and Safety; Smoking; Physical Fitness; Hypertension; Stress; Nutrition

Description

Information on employer-sponsored activities to improve employee health. Covers programme characteristics (for example, location, eligibility, funding, employee involvement) in health risk assessment, smoking control, high blood pressure control, stress management, exercise and physical fitness, weight control and nutrition.

14:717. Online   Executive Telecom System International, Human Resource Information Network (ETSI/HRIN)

File name	
Start year	1987
Number of records	
Update period	Not updated

Notes

Annual subscription to ETSI/HRIN required.

Natural Products Alert

University of Illinois at Chicago, College of Pharmacy, Program for Collaborative Research in the Pharmaceutical Sciences (PCRPS)

14:718. Master record

Alternative name(s)	NAPRALERT
Database type	Bibliographic, Textual, Factual
Number of journals	200
Sources	Books, Journals, Databases, Pharmacopoeias and Indexes
Start year	1975, with some earlier material
Language	English
Coverage	International
Number of records	140,000
Update size	91,000
Update period	Monthly

Keywords

Ethnomedicine; Zoology; Marine Biology; Botany; Microbiology; Phytochemistry

Description

Citations to articles and books on the chemical constituents and pharmacology of plant, microbial and animal (primarily marine) extracts. The database has records on over 40,000 organisms and 100,000 compounds. Also contains data on the chemistry and pharmacology of secondary metabolites reported present in or isolated from natural sources. In addition to customised reports, ethnomedical, pharmacological and phytochemical profiles are available for specified plants, animals, microbes, extracts of a given species and secondary constituents. Ethnomedical profiles for plants include synonymous names (Latin binomials), common names and ethnomedical uses. Pharmacological profiles for extracts include Latin name, family name, organism part, country where grown or collected, type of pharmacologic test, type of extract tested, route of administration, test species and sex, dosage and qualitative results (for example, active, weak active, strong active, equivocal, inactive). Phytochemistry profiles for secondary constitutents include name and major chemical class of the constituent, percentage yield of the constituent and country or region where the plant was collected. All profiles include relevant literature citations.

14:719. Online   STN

File name	NAPRALERT
Alternative name(s)	NAPARALERT
Start year	1975, with some earlier material
Number of records	140,000
Update period	Monthly
Price/Charges	Connect time: DM85.00 SDI charge: DM33.90

14:720. Online   University of Illinois at Chicago, College of Pharmacy, Program for Collaborative Research in the Pharmaceutical Sciences (PCRPS)

File name	
Alternative name(s)	NAPRALERT
Start year	1975, with some earlier material
Number of records	140,000
Update period	Monthly

Notes

Annual subscription required.

NIJ Drugs and Crime CD-ROM Library – US National Institute of Justice
Abt Books
National Institute of Justice (US)

14:721. Master record

Alternative name(s)	Drugs and Crime CD-ROM Library – US National Institute of Justice
Database type	Factual, Textual, Statistical, Image
Number of journals	
Sources	Journals, Books, Reports, Data sets and Laws/regulations
Start year	1970
Language	English
Coverage	USA, Europe, Australasia, Asia and Latin America
Number of records	
Update size	–
Update period	Annually
Index unit	Articles and images

Keywords
Criminology; Drugs; Drug Therapy

Description
A comprehensive collection of books, reports, articles, data sets, abstracts, graphics and images related to drugs and crime, including several of the most important scholarly works on drugs, crime and law enforcement, providing historical and international perspectives. Also includes research results, with statistics and case histories, from various government and private sector studies.

Subjects covered: health care (drug treatment and rehabilitation); law and legislation (fifty state drug laws, federal acts); social sciences (criminology, economics, psychology, sociology and anthropology of illegal drugs and crime); banking (money laundering laws and law enforcement); crime and criminal law; drug information (all kinds).Includes: 40,000 pages of text; 1,000 images from books and articles. Covers 1970 – 1989. Information is provided by the NCJRS (National Criminal Justice Reference Service).

14:722. CD-ROM US National Institute of Justice

File name	Drugs and Crime CD-ROM Library – US National Institute of Justice
Alternative name(s)	Drugs and Crime CD-ROM Library – US National Institute of Justice
Format notes	IBM
Software	KAware
Start year	1970
Number of records	
Update period	Annually
Price/Charges	Subscription: US$195

NMD'S Tablettidentifikasjonsdatabase
Arbeids- og administrasjons-
departementet Dagens Nöringsliv
Norsk Medisinaldepot

14:723. Master record

Alternative name(s)	TABID
Database type	Factual, Textual
Number of journals	
Sources	
Start year	1987
Language	Norwegian and English
Coverage	
Number of records	1,200
Update size	–
Update period	

Keywords
Pharmaceutical Products

Description
Database for identification of unknown tablets and capsules. Description of known products. Listings available on demand.

14:724. Online AET

File name	Tabid Eregin
Start year	1987
Number of records	1,200
Update period	

14:725. Online LOVDATA

File name	LOVDATA
Start year	1987
Number of records	1,200
Update period	

14:726. Online Norsk Medisinaldepot (NMD)

File name	Tabid (NMD)
Start year	1987
Number of records	1,200
Update period	
Price/Charges	Subscription: Norwegian krone500.00 (connection fee) Connect time: Free

Notes
Open to pharmacies and hospitals. Other users may be admitted. Applications to the Norwegian Medicinal Depot.

Nordrug
Centralförbundet för Alkohol- och Narkotikaupplysning

14:727. Master record

Database type	Bibliographic
Number of journals	
Sources	
Start year	1980
Language	English and Swedish (Keywords)
Coverage	International
Number of records	6,100
Update size	700
Update period	Monthly

Keywords
Drug Abuse; Alcohol Abuse

Description
Contains citations, with abstracts, to scientific literature on alcohol and drug abuse. Exhaustive coverage of Nordic literature, selective coverage of literature from other countries. Nordrug is one of the files in the Drugab information system. See also Alconarc and Dalctraf.

Drug abuse and research on treatment of alcohol and drug dependence.

14:728. Online   DAFA Data AB

File name	Nordrug
Start year	1980
Number of records	6,100
Update period	Monthly

Obstetrics & Gynecology – Personal MEDLINE
National Library of Medicine

14:730. Master record

CD-ROM   **Macmillan New Media**

Database type	Bibliographic
Number of journals	
Sources	
Start year	Most recent five years.
Language	
Coverage	
Number of records	230,000
Update size	–
Update period	Annually

Keywords

Gynaecology

Description

References and abstracts on obstetric and gynaecological-related clinical and patient management issues. Covers: anatomy, diagnostic procedures and techniques, chemicals and drugs, including hormones, hormone antagonists and other related topics. A subset of MEDLINE, plus all abstracts from major obstetrics and gynecology journals. As of December 1992, no longer available.

For more details of constituent databases, see:
MEDLINE

Obstetrics and Gynaecology
Elsevier Science Publishers
CMC ReSearch

14:732. Master record

Database type	Factual, Textual, Image
Number of journals	1
Sources	Journal
Start year	1985
Language	English
Coverage	
Number of records	
Update size	–
Update period	Annually

Keywords

Gynaecology; Obstetrics

Description

Full text of five years of the Elsevier journal with tables and images. Includes: Medical and surgical treatment of female conditions; Obstetric management; Clinical evaluation of drugs and instruments; etc. Covers 1985 – 1990

14:733. CD-ROM   CMC ReSearch

File name	Obstetrics and Gynaecology on Disc 1985–1990
Format notes	IBM
Software	DiscPassage

Start year	1985
Number of records	
Update period	Annually
Price	UK£265

This database can also be found on:
Comprehensive Core Medical Library

Occupational Health & Safety Letter
Business Publishers Inc

14:735. Master record

Database type	Textual
Number of journals	1
Sources	Newsletter
Start year	1990
Language	English
Coverage	USA
Number of records	
Update size	–
Update period	Twice per month

Keywords

Air Pollution; Alcohol Abuse; Computer Ergonomics; Drug Abuse; Ergonomics; Hazardous Chemicals; HIV; Legal Liability; Occupational Health and Safety; Radiation; Smoking

Description

Contains the full text of *Occupational Health and Safety Letter*, published every two weeks, a newsletter on workplace health and safety, covering concerns such as exposure to toxic chemicals and radiation, smoking and indoor air pollution control, drug and alcohol abuse on the job, AIDS, computer ergonomics, crimical regulatory and tort liability and workplace behavioural issues and problems.

Corresponds to *Occupational Health and Safety Letter* newsletter. On DIALOG and Data-Star, this newsletter is available as part of the PTS Newsletter Database.

14:736. Online   Executive Telecom System International, Human Resource Information Network (ETSI/HRIN)

File name	
Start year	1990
Number of records	
Update period	

This database can also be found on:
PTS Newsletter Database

Orphan Drug Database
National Organization for Rare Disorders (NORD)

14:738. Master record

Database type	Directory, Textual
Number of journals	
Sources	Government departments and Pharmacopoeias
Start year	1983
Language	English
Coverage	USA

Number of records	400
Update size	–
Update period	Monthly

Keywords

Rare Diseases; Drugs; Therapeutic Agents

Description

Information on over 400 orphan drugs (that is, therapeutic agents providing treatment for less than 200,000 US residents). Includes US FDA-approved and experimental drugs, giving brand and generic names, indicated diseases and manufacturer data.

14:739. Online   CompuServe Information Service

File name	
Start year	1983
Number of records	400
Update period	Monthly
Price/Charges	Subscription: US$8.95 per month
Downloading is allowed	

OTC Market Report: Update USA

Nicholas Hall & Company

14:740. Master record

Database type	Textual
Number of journals	1
Sources	Newsletter
Start year	1990
Language	English
Coverage	USA and Canada
Number of records	
Update size	–
Update period	Monthly

Keywords

Company Profiles; Health Care Products; Hygiene Products; Marketing; Market Reports

Description

Containing the full text of *OTC Market Report*, a newsletter covering the over-the-counter health and hygiene products market in the USA and Canada. Includes company profiles, product and market reports, new product announcements and 'hard data' dealing with the market size and market share in OTC markets.

Corresponds to *OTC Market Report*: Update USA monthly newsletter. On DIALOG and Data-Star this database is available as part of the PTS Newsletter Database.

This database can be found on:
PTS Newsletter Database

OTC News & Market Report

Nicholas Hall & Company

14:742. Master record

Database type	Textual
Number of journals	1
Sources	
Start year	1989
Language	English
Coverage	Europe

Number of records	
Update size	–
Update period	Monthly

Keywords

Advertising; Company Profiles; Health Care Products; Hygiene Products

Description

Contains the full text of the monthly newsletter covering the over-the-counter health and hygiene products trade in the European market. Includes product reports at a country level, company profiles of industry leaders, new products, company mergers and acquisitions, expansions, financial performance, advertising and strategic direction.

Corresponds to *OTC News & Market Report* monthly newsletter. On DIALOG and Data-Star this newsletter is made available as part of the PTS Newsletter Database.

This database can be found on:
PTS Newsletter Database

P&T Quik

Micromedex Inc

14:744. Master record

Alternative name(s)	Computerized Clinical Information System: P&T Quik; CCIS: P&T Quik
Database type	Textual, Directory
Number of journals	
Sources	
Start year	
Language	English
Coverage	International
Number of records	
Update size	–
Update period	Monthly

Keywords

Drug Therapy; Drugs

Description

Provides a series of monographs on newly approved FDA drugs or other drugs of recent concern being considered for placement on hospital formularies by Pharmacy and Therapeutics Committees. It is available monthly on diskette accompanied by paper copies of each monograph. A compilation of all the P&T Quik monographs is available on CD-ROM.

14:745. Diskette   Micromedex Inc

File name	P&T Quik
Alternative name(s)	Computerized Clinical Information System: P&T Quik; CCIS: P&T Quik
Start year	
Number of records	
Update period	Monthly

Notes

This database is available as a standalone product on diskette, as well as being a part of CCIS, Computerized Clinical Information System.

This database can also be found on:
CCIS

PASCAL

Centre National de la Recherche Scientifique, Institut de l'Information Scientifique et Technique, Science Humaines et Sociales (CNRS/INIST)

14:747. Master record

Alternative name(s)	Programme Applique a la Selection et a la Compilation Automatique de la Litterature
Database type	Bibliographic
Number of journals	8,500
Sources	Books, conference proceedings, dissertations, journals, maps, monographs, patents (biotechnology), reports, technical reports and theses
Start year	1973
Language	English (titles and keywords), French and Spanish (keywords)
Coverage	International
Number of records	9 million
Update size	500,000
Update period	Monthly
Index unit	Articles
Thesaurus	Biomedical Thesaurus in 3 volumes
Database aids	PASCAL User Manual, PASCAL Classification Scheme and PASCAL Dictionary in 3 Volumes (French, English, Spanish): Exact Sciences, Technology, Medicine

Keywords

Bioagriculture; Biomedicine; Biotechnology; Cell Biology; Civil Engineering; Construction; Demography; Electrical Engineering; Epidemiology; Ergonomics; Immunology; Metallurgy; Microbiology; Mineralogy; Nutrition; Parasitology; Patents; Physics; Pollution; Public Health; Travel Medicine; Tropical Medicine

Description

PASCAL is a multidisciplinary and multilingual bibliographic database covering the core of scientific, technical and medical literature worldwide. Subjects covered include: Life sciences – biology, tropical medicine, biomedical engineering, biochemistry, biotechnology, pharmacology, microbiology, ophthalmology, dermatology, anaesthesia, human diseases, animal biology, reproduction, genetics, zoology, plant biology, agronomics, agricultural science, psychology; Earth sciences – mineralogy, mining economics, cristallography, stratigraphy, hydrology, paleontology; Physical sciences physics, information science, computer science, astronomy, electrical engineering, electronics, atoms and molecules, general, physical, analytical, inorganic and organic chemistry; Engineering sciences – energy, metallurgy, pollution, mechanical industries, construction, welding and brazing, civil engineering, building and public works, transportation.

In addition there are specialised subfiles in the following areas: information science, documentation, energy, metallurgy, civil engineering, earth sciences, biotechnology, zoology of invertebrates, agriculture and tropical medicine.

On ESA-IRS, DIALOG and QUESTEL searches can be limited to one of the two subfiles PASCAL: Biotechnologies and PASCAL: Medécine Tropicale dating from 1982 on ESA-IRS and QUESTEL, but on DIALOG from 1986. Each subfile holds over 40,000 records.

Biotechnologies contains citations, with abstracts to the international biotechnology literature, covering biochemistry, cell biology, microbiology and applications of cultured microorganisms and cells in agriculture, energy, food processing, medicine, metallurgy and pollution control. Some patents are included in this area. Corresponds to PASCAL THEMA 215: biotechnologies.

Medécine Tropicale provides citations, with abstracts, to the international literature of tropical medicine, covering human and animal parasites and diseases, the biology and control of vectors, intermediate hosts and reservoirs, ergonomics, nutrition, physical and social demography, public health and medical issues relating to travellers. Corresponds to PASCAL THEMA 235: Médecine Tropicale.

These subfiles are available as part of PASCAL on DIALOG, QUESTEL and ESA-IRS.

PASCAL is the online version of the print publication Bibliographie Internationale (1984 onwards) and corresponds to the publication Bulletin Signaletique (1973–1983). The titles in the PASCAL file are in their original languages and are translated into French and/or English. Approximately fifty per cent of records have abstracts which are in French or English (from 1982 the titles and keywords are also given in English). Journal articles account for approximately ninety-three per cent of the file. 8,500 journals are regularly scanned. Source materials are published in various languages: English 63%, French 12%, Russian 10%, German 8% and other languages 7%.

The controlled terms are in French and also in English for records since 1982 and in Spanish for records since 1977. German controlled terms are also provided in the area of metallurgy.

14:748. Online — CompuServe Information Service

File name	IQUEST File 1284
Alternative name(s)	Programme Applique a la Selection et a la Compilation Automatique de la Litterature
Start year	1973
Number of records	9 million
Update period	Monthly
Price/Charges	Subscription: US$8.95 per month Database entry fee: US$9/search; some databases carry a surcharge ($2–75) Online print: US$10 references free; then $9 per ten; abstracts $3 each

Downloading is allowed

Notes

Accessed via IQUEST or IQMEDICAL, this database is offered by a Questel gateway. IQUEST can either search across all databases, a database of the user's choice or selected multiple databases.

14:749. Online — DIALOG

File name	File 144
Alternative name(s)	Programme Applique a la Selection et a la Compilation Automatique de la Litterature
Start year	1973
Number of records	3,866,245
Update period	Monthly
Price/Charges	Connect time: US$60.00 Online print: US$0.50 Offline print: US$0.50 SDI charge: US$12.00

Notes

DIALINDEX Categories: AGRI, BIOCHEM, BIOSCI, BIOTECH, CHEMLIT, EECOMP, ENERGY, ENERGYP, GEOLOGY, GEOLOGYP, GEOPHYS, MATERIAL, MEDICINE, METALS, PHYSICS, SCITECHB.

14:750. Online — ESA-IRS

File name	File 14
Alternative name(s)	Programme Applique a la Selection et a la Compilation Automatique de la Litterature
Start year	1973
Number of records	8,263,000 (October 1991)
Update period	Monthly
Price/Charges	Subscription: UK£70.29
	Database entry fee: UK£3.51
	Online print: UK£0.07 – 0.56
	Offline print: UK£0.50
	SDI charge: UK£3.51

Notes

QUESTALERT and QUESTORDER are both available on this file. The LIMIT ALL command can be used to limit all subsequent sets. This can be cancelled by entering a new LALL or a BEGIN command.

From 1993 ESA-IRS are charging an annual fee of 100 Accounting Units (c.UK£ 70.29) to all users. This is equivalent to the fee for full documentation and will not be charged to customers already paying for documentation.

Record composition

Abstract /AB; Author AU; Classification Code CC; Classification Number CN; CODEN CO; Controlled Terms (Descriptors) /CT; Controlled Terms in English /KE; Controlled Terms in French /KF; Controlled Terms in Spanish or German /KO; Corporate Source CS; Country/Place of Publication CY; Document Type DT; Domain (Subfile) DO; Generic Controlled Terms (Broader Terms) /CT*; Geographical Coordinates GC; International Patent Classification PC; ISBN BN; ISSN SN; Journal Name JN; Language LA; Language of Summary LS; Location of Document LC; Major Controlled Terms /CT* or /MAJ; Map Type CA; Meeting Date MD; Meeting Location ML; Meeting Title MT; Native Number NN; Report Number RN; Patent Application Number PA; Patent Holder (Corporate) PH; Patent Number PN; Patent Priority PP; Publication Year PY; Publisher PB; Report Number RN; Single Controlled Terms /ST; Source SO; Titles (English) /ET; Titles (French) /FT; Titles (other) /OT and Titles (all) /TI

The titles are in their original language and are translated into French and/or English. The Controlled Terms are in French and also in English for records since 1982, and Spanish for records since 1984. German controlled terms are also provided in the area of metallurgy. Abstracts are in French or English (English especially from 1990 onwards). The EXPAND command can be used to display the PASCAL thesaurus. The basic index includes the following data fields: Abstract, Controlled Terms in any language, Controlled Terms in English, Controlled Terms in French, Controlled Terms in Spanish or German, Generic Controlled Terms, Single Controlled Terms, Titles (English), Titles (French), Titles (Other). The Classification Name is the principal hierarchical category corresponding to the classification code of the record. Some fields are searchable in both French and English. The data field Source may include: monographic source, collective source or title of collection. The prefix 'SO=' corresponds to the information displayed immediately after the title. It does not correspond to the field labelled 'Source Information' in the displayed record. To search for journal names the prefix 'JN=' should be used. Role indicators which are used with substances to identify the role they play in a chemical reaction or process are placed after the

name of the substance with the symbol | as separator in file 205 and the symbol ! as separator in file 204. Role indicators have been used in chemistry-and physics-related records since 1979 and in metallurgy related reocrds since 1980. They are as follows: ENT: Primary material, FIN: End product, ACT: Active product, SUB: Substrate, solvent, etc, ANA: Analytically determined compound, SEC: Secondary material.

14:751. Online — ESA-IRS

File name	File 204
Alternative name(s)	Programme Applique a la Selection et a la Compilation Automatique de la Litterature
Start year	1973 – 1983
Number of records	4,900,000
Update period	Closed File
Price/Charges	Subscription: UK£70.29
	Database entry fee: UK£3.51
	Online print: UK£0.07 – 0.56
	Offline print: UK£0.50
	SDI charge: UK£3.51

Downloading is allowed
Thesaurus is online

Notes

QUESTALERT and QUESTORDER are both available on this file. The LIMIT ALL command can be used to limit all subsequent sets. This can be cancelled by entering a new LALL or a BEGIN command.

From 1993 ESA-IRS are charging an annual fee of 100 Accounting Units (c.UK£ 70.29) to all users. This is equivalent to the fee for full documentation and will not be charged to customers already paying for documentation.

Record composition

Abstract /AB; Author AU; Classification Code CC; Controlled Terms (Descriptors) /CT; Corporate Source CS; Country/Place of Publication CY; Document Type DT; ISBN BN; ISSN SN; Journal Name JN; Language LA; Major Controlled Terms /CT* or /MAJ; Map Type CA; Native Number NN; Report Number RN; Single Controlled Terms /ST; Titles (English) /ET; Titles (French) /FT; Titles (other) /OT and Titles (all) /TI

The EXPAND command can be used to display the PASCAL thesaurus. The basic index includes the following data fields: Abstract, Controlled Terms (Descriptors), Major Controlled Terms, Single Controlled Terms, Titles (English), Titles (French), Titles (other), Titles (all). Examples of documents types in file 204 include: Journal Article (Code TP), Patent (TB), Conference (TC), Book (TL), Map (TM), Miscellaneous (TS), Monography (LM), Thesis (TT), Report (TR). Role indicators which are used with substances to identify the role they play in a chemical reaction or process are placed after the name of the substance with the symbol | as separator in file 205 and the symbol ! as separator in file 204. Role indicators have been used in chemistry-and physics-related records since 1979 and in metallurgy related reocrds since 1980. They are as follows: ENT: Primary material, FIN: End product, ACT: Active product, SUB: Substrate, solvent, etc, ANA: Analytically determined compound, SEC: Secondary material.

14:752. Online — ESA-IRS

File name	File 205
Alternative name(s)	Programme Applique a la Selection et a la Compilation Automatique de la Litterature
Start year	1984

Number of records
Update period   Monthly
Price/Charges   Subscription: UK£70.29
                       Database entry fee: UK£3.51
                       Online print: UK£0.07 – 0.56
                       Offline print: UK£0.50
                       SDI charge: UK£3.51

Downloading is allowed
Thesaurus is online

Notes

QUESTALERT and QUESTORDER are both available on this file. The LIMIT ALL command can be used to limit all subsequent sets. This can be cancelled by entering a new LALL or a BEGIN command.

From 1993 ESA-IRS are charging an annual fee of 100 Accounting Units (c.UK£ 70.29) to all users. This is equivalent to the fee for full documentation and will not be charged to customers already paying for documentation.

Record composition

Abstract /AB; Author AU; Classification Code CC; Classification Number CN; CODEN CO; Controlled Terms (Descriptors) in any language /CT; Controlled Terms in English /KE; Controlled Terms in French /KF; Controlled Terms in Spanish or German /KO; Corporate Source CS; Country of Publication CY; Document Type DT; Domain (Subfile) DO; Generic Controlled Terms (Broader Terms) /CT*; Geographical Coordinates GC; International Patent Classification PC; ISBN BN; ISSN SN; Journal Name JN; Language LA; Language of Summary LS; Location of Document LC; Map Type CA; Meeting Date MD; Meeting Location ML; Meeting Title MT; Native Number NN; Patent Application Number PA; Patent Holder (Corporate) PH; Patent Number PN; Patent Priority PP; Publication Year PY; Publisher PB; Report Number RN; Single Controlled Terms /ST; Source SO and Titles /TI

The basic index includes the following data fields: Abstract, Controlled Terms in any language, Controlled Terms in English, Controlled Terms in French, Controlled Terms in Spanish or German, Generic Controlled Terms, Single Controlled Terms, Titles. The Classification Name is the principal hierarchical category corresponding to the classification code of the record. Some fields are searchable in both French and English. The data field Source may include: monographic source, collective source or title of collection. The prefix 'SO=' corresponds to the information displayed immediately after the title. It does not correspond to the field labelled 'Source Information' in the displayed record. To search for journal names the prefix 'JN=' should be used. Role indicators which are used with substances to identify the role they play in a chemical reaction or process are placed after the name of the substance with the symbol | as separator in file 205 and the symbol ! as separator in file 204. Role indicators have been used in chemistry-and physics-related records since 1979 and in metallurgy related reocrds since 1980. They are as follows: ENT: Primary material, FIN: End product, ACT: Active product, SUB: Substrate, solvent, etc, ANA: Analytically determined compound, SEC: Secondary material.

14:753. Online   Questel

File name   PASC73
Alternative name(s)   Programme Applique a la Selection
                      et a la Compilation Automatique de
                      la Litterature
Start year   1973
Number of records 9 million
Update period

14:754. CD-ROM   Centre National de la Recherche Scientifique, Institut de l'Information Scientifique et Technique, Science Humaines et Sociales (CNRS/INIST)

File name   PASCAL CD-ROM
Alternative name(s)   Programme Applique a la Selection
                      et a la Compilation Automatique de
                      la Litterature; CD-ROM PASCAL
Format notes   IBM
Software   GTI
Start year   1987
Number of records 450,000
Update period   Quarterly
Price/Charges   Subscription: FFr15,000 – 17,790

Notes

Each disc corresponds to one year update of the PASCAL database, that is, approximately 500,000 records. An annual subscription with quarterly updates. Costs 15,000 FFr for current year (1990, 1 disc); 7,500 Ffr for each backfile disc (1987, 1988, 1989, 1 disc each). The full collection with the current year subscription costs 35,000 – 41,150 FFr. Can be used in a LAN network provided the network conforms to the standards required for the MSCDEX extension. Several commercial packages exist to make it possible to operate PASCAL CD-ROM in a suitable network environment.

14:755. Tape   Centre National de la Recherche Scientifique, Institut de l'Information Scientifique et Technique, Science Humaines et Sociales (CNRS/INIST)

File name   PASCAL
Alternative name(s)   Programme Applique a la Selection
                      et a la Compilation Automatique de
                      la Litterature
Format notes   9-track 1,600 or 6,250 BPI magnetic
                   tapes, EBCDIC character set, with
                   or without IBM-OS label
Start year   1987
Number of records 500,000
Update period   Annually
Price/Charges

Notes

Each tape corresponds to one year update of the PASCAL database, that is, approximately 500,000 records.

14:756. Videotex   Minitel

File name   PASCAL 362936011
Alternative name(s)   Programme Applique a la Selection
                      et a la Compilation Automatique de
                      la Litterature
Start year
Number of records
Update period

14:757. Database subset

Online   ESA-IRS

File name   File 37 – Training Pascal
Alternative name(s)   Programme Applique a la Selection
                      et a la Compilation Automatique de
                      la Litterature
Start year   1984–1985
Number of records 48,325(October 1991)
Update period   Not updated

Price/Charges   Connect time: UK£6.99 per hour
Downloading is allowed
Thesaurus is online

Notes

Training database (subfile of PASCAL main file, File 14). Neither QUESTALERT nor QUESTORDER are available. Services such as offline prints are also not available.

Record composition

Abstract /AB; Author AU; Classification Code CC; Classification Name CN; CODEN CO; Controlled terms in any language /CT; Controlled terms in English /KE; Controlled terms in French /KF; Controlled terms in Spanish or German /KO; Corporate Source CS; Country of Publication CY; Document Type DT; Domain DO; Generic controlled terms (broader terms) /CT*; Geographical Coordinates GC; ISBN BN; ISSN SN; Journal Name JN; Language LA; Language of Summary LS; Location of Document LC; Map Type CA; Meeting Title MT; Meeting Date MD; Meeting Location ML; Native Number NN; Patent Application Number PA; Patent Holder (Corporate) PH; Patent Number PN; Patent Priority PP; Publication Year PY; Publisher PB; Report Number RN; Single Controlled Terms /ST; Source SO and Titles /TI

The EXPAND command can be used to display the PASCAL thesaurus. The basic index includes the following data fields: Abstract, Controlled terms in any language, Controlled terms in English, Controlled terms in French, Controlled terms in Spanish or German, Generic controlled terms (broader terms), Single controlled terms, Titles. The classification name is the principal hierarchical category corresponding to the classification code of the record. Some fields are searchable in both French and English. Pascal can be divided into a number of sub-files (domains), a list of which can be obtained by entering the command E DO =. Source (SO=) may include: monographic source, collective source, or title of collection. The 'SO=' field is placed between title and author in the displayed record. To search for journal names the prefix 'JN=' should be used. Role indicators which are used with substances to identify the role they play in a chemical reaction or process are placed after the name of the substance with the symbol | as separator in file 205 and the symbol ! as separator in file 204. Role indicators have been used in chemistry-and physics-related records since 1979 and in metallurgy related reocrds since 1980. They are as follows: ENT: Primary material, FIN: End product, ACT: Active product, SUB: Substrate, solvent, etc, ANA: Analytically determined compound, SEC: Secondary material. The LIMIT ALL command can be used to limit all subsequent sets. The limitation can be cancelled by entering a new LALL or a BEGIN command.

This database can also be found on:
Metropolitan
Medata-ROM

PatentImages

MicroPatent
Chadwyck-Healey

14:759. Master record

Database type	Patents, Image
Number of journals	
Sources	Patents and Gazette

Start year	1976 (1976–1990 backfile to be produced in first six months 1992)
Language	English
Coverage	USA
Number of records	1,000 patents per disc
Update size	52,000
Update period	Weekly
Index unit	Patents

Keywords

Biotechnology; Patents; Patents – Biotechnical; Patents – Chemical; Patents – Electrical; Patents – Mechanical; Patents – Pharmaceutical; Pharmaceuticals

Description

Complete facsimiles of all US patents, complete and exactly as published by the USPTO. Image databases contain facsimiles of entire patent documents, complete with all structures and drawings, with full searchable bibliographic fields. There is comprehensive coverage of US patents since 1976 and databases tailored to specific industries. The subsets from the complete set of US Patents available are: PatentImages – Chemical and Pharmaceutical; and PatentImages – Biotechnology.

Retrieval is based on eleven searchable fields. The software and user-interface used to publish the US Patents is the same as that used at the European Patents Office.

14:760. CD-ROM   Chadwyck-Healey

File name	PatentImages – All Technologies
Format notes	IBM
Software	Patsoft
Start year	1976 (1976–1990 backfile to be produced in first six months 1992)
Number of records	1,000 patents per disc
Update period	Weekly
Price/Charges	Subscription: UK£2,900 – 3,900

Notes

Updated at the rate of one or two discs per week (that is, around 100 discs per year), each containing about one thousand new patents, within two weeks of issue of the patents by the USPTO.

Discount available when taken with the full text FullText and the bibliographic APS (to be renamed CAPS – Claims and Abstracts Patent Searching), which is to be launched under its new name with added data in 1993, featuring exemplary claims in addition to patents abstracts. CAPS complements this image database.

May be purchased as full 15-year set or as one, five or ten year sections. Additionally, a 300-disc, backfile from 1976 is being made available allowing users to make a complete and up-to-date library of of US chemical patents.

Software which allows searchers to retrieve documents from PatentImages and send them to any fax machine without going through Patsoft (PatentImages software) is under development by MicroPatent, to be called PatentPower and scheduled for release in late 1992, priced around £250.

14:761. Database subset
CD-ROM   Chadwyck-Healey

File name	PatentImages – Chemical and Pharmaceutical
Alternative name(s)	Chemical PatentImages; Chemical and Pharmaceutical PatentImages
Format notes	IBM
Software	Patsoft

Start year
Number of records
Update period   Every two weeks
Price/Charges   Subscription: UK£1,700

Notes

A subset of the PatentImages CD-ROM published by Chadwyck Healey. Contains complete facsimiles of US chemical and pharmaceutical patents, complete with all structures and drawings, exactly as published by the USPTO. Subscription provides users with biweekly discs (that is, around 25 discs per year), each containing over 1,000 of the latest chemical patents. Discs are produced at the rate of 1–2 per week, within two weeks of issue of the patents by the USPTO.

The Chemical backfile, being delivered year by year, was due to be complete by the end of 1992, and a complete backfile (from 1976) of 300 discs, will cost UK£ 2,650. Trade-in discounts are available for owners of chemical patent collections on microfilm. This will allow users to make a complete and up-to-date library of US chemical patents.

Patents Preview
Derwent Publications Inc

14:762. Master record

Database type   Bibliographic
Number of journals
Sources
Start year   1993
Language   English, Japanese, French and
                       German
Coverage   USA, Japan, Germany, UK and
                       France
Number of records
Update size   —
Update period   Weekly
Index unit   Patents
Abstract details   Derwent staff

Keywords

Patents – Pharmaceutical; Pharmaceuticals

Description

Alerting service for the latest in pharmaceutical research with abstracts of patents from the USA, Japan, Germany, UK and France plus those issued under the world and European patent agreements. Abstracts include a summary of the patent claims; the generic and specific chemical structures; and the English text from all documents (including those originally in German, French or Japanese).

14:763. Diskette   Derwent Publications Inc

File name   Patents Preview on Diskette
Format notes   IBM
Start year   1993
Number of records
Update period   Weekly
Delay   7 days

Notes

The diskette will combine entries from the seven current Patent Preview printed titles: Central Nervous System; Antimicrobials; Inflammation and Gastrointestinal System; Diagnostic Agents; Immune System; Cardiovascular System; and Cancer Chemotherapy and Endocrine System. It is available to users of Molecular Design Limited's ISIS/Base, Chembase or MACCS-II software: all text fields are searchable

and chemical structures are searchable by complete structure or substructure. A generic structure covering the widest claim plus an exemplified or claimed specific compound is given. Pharmaceutical data includes mode of action, use, advantage, etc. Text and structure searches may be combined for complete flexibility. Default display formats are included but users can develop additional formats to display all or chosen fields.

Record composition

Abstracts; Therapeutic classification; Title; Bibliographic data; Mode of action; Use; Dosage; Clinical data and Advantage

PATSCAN CD-ROM
Optical Storage Systems Inc

14:764. Master record

Database type   Factual, Directory, Textual
Number of journals
Sources
Start year
Language   French and English
Coverage   Canada
Number of records
Update size   —
Update period   Not updated

Keywords

Drugs; Patents

Description

Contains three databases: bibliographic descriptions of Canadian patents 1981–1989; Canadian patent classification schedules; drug reference database (St. Paul's).

14:765. CD-ROM   Optical Storage Systems
Inc

File name   PATSCAN CD-ROM Demo Disc
Format notes   IBM
Software   KAware
Start year
Number of records
Update period   Not updated

Pediatric Infectious Diseases Journal: 1985–1990
CMC ReSearch
Williams and Wilkins

14:766. Master record

Database type   Factual, Textual, Image
Number of journals   1
Sources   Journal
Start year   1985
Language   English
Coverage   International
Number of records
Update size   —
Update period   Annually

Keywords

Drugs; Paediatrics; Infectious Diseases

Description

Full text, tables and images from the 1985 to 1990 issues of Williams and Wilkins journal with review articles and original studies on viral and bacterial illness, plus latebreaking news on diseases, techniques and drugs. Said to provide 'clinically-useful material for the front-line practitioner'.

Equivalent to *Pediatric Infectious Disease Journal*.

14:767. CD-ROM CMC ReSearch

File name	Pediatric Infectious Diseases Journal: 1985–1990
Format notes	IBM, Mac
Software	DiscPassage
Start year	1985
Number of records	
Update period	Annually
Price	UK£250

Notes

May also be purchased as part of a collection at a special price – Microinfo (UK) sell a Pediatric Library comprising: Pediatrics on Disc (1983- June 1991); Pediatric Infectious Disease Journal (1985–1990); Pediatrics in Review & Redbook and Year Book on Disc (1988,1989,1990), available for PC or Macintosh, at a one-time purchase price of £625, with updates available at additional cost.

Optech (also based in UK) also provide a collection of discs at a special discounted price for hospital libraries, research departments and medical organisations – the Pediatric library collection comprises six CMC titles on five discs: Paediatrics on Disc 1983–1990; Wilm's and other Renal Tumours of Children; Paediatric Infectious Diseases Journal; Year Book 1988,1989; Paediatrics in Review and Redbook, at a cost of £699.

Personal Medical Library
EBSCO

14:768. Master record

Database type	Textual, Directory
Number of journals	
Sources	
Start year	
Language	English
Coverage	International
Number of records	
Update size	–
Update period	Not updated

Keywords

Drugs; Nutrition; Paediatrics; Personal Health Care; Pregnancy; Sports Medicine; Surgery

Description

A one-stop reference for personal health care needs. Contains the complete text and images of seven books: *Complete Guide to Sports Injuries; Complete Guide to Symptoms, Illness and Surgery; Complete Guide to Prescription and Non-prescription Drugs; Complete Guide to Pediatric Symptoms, Illness and Medications; Complete Guide to Medical Tests; Complete Guide to Vitamins, Minerals and Supplements;* and *Drugs, Vitamins, Minerals in Pregnancy*. Matches symptoms with illnesses, describes medical tests and procedures, explains and illustrates surgeries and defines vitamin and drug interactions. Includes nearly 800 images from the *Sports Injuries* and *Symptoms,*

Illness and Surgery books, which are accessible from within associated text. Information source is Medical Data Exchange.

Aimed at consumers. A one-time publication.

14:769. CD-ROM EBSCO

File name	Personal Medical Library
Format notes	IBM
Start year	
Number of records	
Update period	Not updated
Price	US$299 – 315

Pharma Marketing Service Datenbank
Ärzte Zeitung Verlagsgesellschaft mbH

14:770. Master record

Alternative name(s)	PMS; DPMS
Database type	Textual, Bibliographic
Number of journals	200
Sources	journals, newspapers and press releases
Start year	December 1987
Language	German
Coverage	International
Number of records	9,000
Update size	5,200
Update period	Weekly
Database aids	Themencodes/Schlagwort-Schluessel, Dreieich, Ärzte Zeitung, 1990

Keywords

Marketing; Pharmaceutical Industry

Description

Pharma Marketing Service is a German language database focusing on all the topics needed in pharmaceutical marketing including advertising, public relations and sales promotion. News is reported on companies, markets, products, health policy, medical science and pharmacology. The database is used by professionals in the pharmaceutical industry as well as in research institutes, trade associations, advertising agencies and consultancies. It also provides valuable data for market development, competitor surveys and market research and reports on pharmaceutical innovations, international legislation and regulations, product development and companies' financial news. The database contains the full text (that is, citations and abstracts) from the hard copy together with titles, information categories and descriptors to facilitate subject searches.

The database corresponds to Pharma Marketing Service weekly newsletter. News from Western Europe accounts for approximately 50% of the citations, USA news for approximately 25%, Eastern European news approximately 15% and Japanese news approximately 5%. A team of editors draws news from 200 international newspapers and scientific and economic journals. In addition, news from the producer's own correspondents, and news from press releases of pharmaceutical companies, government agencies and national and international organizations is included.

German and international newspapers, concentrating on news from Western Europe.

14:771. Online

File name	
Alternative name(s)	PMS; DPMS
Start year	1987
Number of records	
Update period	Weekly

14:772. Online   Data-Star

File name	DPMS
Alternative name(s)	PMS; DPMS
Start year	December 1987
Number of records	9,000
Update period	Weekly (45 times per year)
Database aids	Data-Star Business Manual and Data-Star Online Manual (search for NEWS-DPMS in NEWS)
Price/Charges	Subscription: SFr80.00
	Connect time: SFr274.00
	Online print: SFr1.60
	Offline print: SFr1.88
	SDI charge: SFr7.80

Notes

From June 1993 Data-Star have introduced an annual fee/subscription per contract (that is, not per password) of SFr 80.00 (c.UK£ 32.00) payable every June. For North American customers billed in dollars who also use DIALOG, the DIALOG fee also covers access to Data-Star. Academic customers, 'commitment' customers and customers currently billed in dollars are exempt.

Record composition

Accession Number and Update Code AN; Classification Codes CC; Date of Publication DT; Descriptors DE and Length LE

There are six broad groups of subject categories: A – Arzneimittel (drugs), F- Firmen (companies), G – Gesundheitspolitik (health policy), H – Marketing Mix, M – Maerkte (markets0, W – Medizin (medical science). Classification codes should be used for more specific searches. Descriptors are terms based on the classification codes concepts.

Pharma-Digest

Société Suisse de Pharmacie

14:773. Master record

Database type	
Number of journals	
Sources	
Start year	
Language	English
Coverage	Switzerland
Number of records	
Update size	–
Update period	

Keywords

Drugs; Pharmaceuticals; Surgery

Description

This database in the medical and pharmaceutical field forms part of the MediROM and PharmaROM CD-ROMs, originally intended for Swiss pharmacists.

This database can be found on:
PharmaROM

PharmaBiomed Business Journals

Predicasts International Inc

14:775. Master record

Alternative name(s)	PTPB; Predicasts PharmaBiomed Business Journals
Database type	Factual, Textual
Number of journals	30
Sources	Journals
Start year	1990
Language	English
Coverage	International
Number of records	
Update size	–
Update period	Weekly
Thesaurus	PTS Company Thesaurus
Database aids	PTS User's Manual, 1989 ed.

Keywords

Biotechnology; Health Care; Marketing; Ophthalmology; Pharmaceuticals

Description

PTPB contains the full text of over thirty journals from international trade publications in pharmaceuticals, biotechnology and healthcare, including *Health Business*; *Pharmaceutical Manufacturing Review*; *Japan Report: Medical Technology*; *In Vivo: The Business and Medicine Report*; *Antiviral Agents Bulletin*; and *Ophthalmology Times*. Of use to information professionals, researchers and consultants for information on methods and techniques, business practices, new products, companies, markets, market share, research and development, regulations and applied technology in this field. All documents in the database are full text.

Information is selected from a growing list (currently thirty) of trade journals from the pharmaceutical, biotechnology and healthcare industries.

The database is indexed with Predicasts' Product, Event and Country codes.

14:776. Online   Data-Star

File name	PTPB
Alternative name(s)	Predicasts PharmaBiomed Business Journals
Start year	1990
Number of records	
Update period	Weekly
Price/Charges	Subscription: UK£32.00
	Connect time: UK£80.40
	Online print: UK£0.00 – 0.49
	Offline print: UK£0.10 – 0.73
	SDI charge: UK£4.00

Notes

From June 1993 Data-Star have introduced an annual fee/subscription per contract (that is, not per password) of SFr 80.00 (c.UK£ 32.00) payable every June. For North American customers billed in dollars who

also use DIALOG, the DIALOG fee also covers access to Data-Star. Academic customers, 'commitment' customers and customers currently billed in dollars are exempt.

14:777. Database subset

Online   **Data-Star**

File name	TRPT – PharmaBiomed Business Journals Training database
Alternative name(s)	PTPB; Predicasts PharmaBiomed Business Journals
Start year	1990
Number of records	
Update period	Weekly
Price/Charges	Connect time: Free

Notes

Free training database from Data-Star for PharmaBiomed Business Journals.

Pharmaceutical and Healthcare Industry News Database
Pharmaprojects PJB Publications Ltd

14:778. Master record

Alternative name(s)	PHIND
Database type	Textual
Number of journals	4
Sources	Newsletters
Start year	1980
Language	English
Coverage	International
Number of records	113,270
Update size	—
Update period	Daily
Index unit	Newsletters, articles and reports
Database aids	User guide available from producer

Keywords

Applied Science; Herbicides; Marketing; Medical Diagnostics; Pesticides; Plant Protection; Product Liability

Description

This database contains information on product developments, markets, regulatory affairs of importance to the international pharmaceutical, medical device, veterinary and agrochemical industries. All publications have already been made available online in abstract form, but this is the only database which contains the full-text of every report and the only one which makes these reports available before publication. It includes all the text, pre-publication, current and archival material from four major international industry newsletters:

Scrip World Pharmaceutical News (1/82+, issue number 655) which contains world pharmaceutical news and is the most widely read international pharmaceutical industry newsletter, being used at all levels within pharmaceutical companies, regulatory authorities, financial instituions, service industries and others to gain an insight into significant events throughout the world, paying special attention to product developments, regulatory affairs, market intelligence, company results and personnel;

Clinica World Medical Device News (10/80+, issue number 1) which contains world medical device news and provides a similar service for the device and diagnostic industry;

Animal Pharm World Animal Health News (1/82+,

issue number 1) which contains world animal health news; and

Agrow World Agrochemical News (10/85+, issue number 1) which contains world agrochemical news and is aimed at the herbicide, pesticide, rodenticide and plant growth regulator industries.

All four print publications follow a similar structure and contains sections on: Product and Research News, Company News, International News, People and Conferences, plus regular monitoring ofregulatiory bodies such as the US Food and Drug Administration, the US Environmental Protection Agency, the European Economic Community and the World Health Organisation. Reports are added to a daily and current file within three working days of writing, before publication. Items destined for publication in *Scrip* or *Clinica* are therefore available online days before the printed newsletters will reach users.

Each report has been written on the basis of news gathered from a wide variety of sources, and the range of information available is evaluated for relevance to the major industrial areas covered and is amplified by investigative reporting. They are subsequently moved into the archival file after approximately three weeks. Covers company activities (marketing, mergers, acquisitions, sales), product research and development (clinical trials, launches, approvals, etc), regulatory decisions (labelling changes, pesticide bans, product liability, etc) and notices of conferences, symposia and executive appointments.

The database corresponds to *Agrow World Crop Protection News*, *Animal Pharm World Animal Health News*, *Clinica World Medical Device and Diagnostic News* and *Scrip World Pharmaceutical News*.

14:779. Online   **BRS**

File name	PHID
Alternative name(s)	PHIND
Start year	1980
Number of records	113,270
Update period	Daily
Price/Charges	Connect time: US$145.00/155.00
	Online print: US$3.52/3.60
	Offline print: US$3.60
	SDI charge: US$5.00

Notes

Contains details of company activities and product development on a daily basis before publication of the printed version.

14:780. Online   **BRS**

File name	PHIC
Alternative name(s)	PHIND
Start year	1980
Number of records	113,270
Update period	Daily
Price/Charges	Connect time: US$145.00/155.00
	Online print: US$3.52/3.60
	Offline print: US$3.60
	SDI charge: US$5.00

Notes

This is the current file Pharmaceutical and Healthcare Industry News Database.

14:781. Online   **BRS**

File name	PHIN
Alternative name(s)	PHIND
Start year	1980
Number of records	113,270
Update period	Daily

Price/Charges — Connect time: US$145.00/155.00
Online print: US$0.77/0.85
Offline print: US$1.10

Notes

Pharmaceutical and Healthcare Industry News Database – Backfile: records are removed from the daily and current file into this archival file after approximately three weeks.

14:782. Online — CompuServe Information Service

File name	IQUEST File 2076: SCRIP – Retrospective
Alternative name(s)	PHIND
Start year	1986
Number of records	
Update period	Daily
Price/Charges	Subscription: US$8.95 per month Database entry fee: US$9/search; some databases carry a surcharge ($2–75) Online print: US$10 references free; then $9 per ten; abstracts $3 each

Notes

Accessed via IQUEST or IQMEDICAL, this database is offered by a Data-Star gateway. IQUEST can either search across all databases, a database of the user's choice or selected multiple databases.

This is the archive file of information, removed from SCRIP – CURRENT NEWS and SCRIP – DAILY NEWS files.

14:783. Online — CompuServe Information Service

File name	IQUEST File 2074: SCRIP – Daily News
Alternative name(s)	PHIND
Start year	1986
Number of records	
Update period	Daily
Price/Charges	Subscription: US$8.95 per month Database entry fee: US$9/search; some databases carry a surcharge ($2–75) Online print: US$10 references free; then $9 per ten; abstracts $3 each

Notes

Accessed via IQUEST, this database is offered by a Data-Star gateway. IQUEST can either search across all databases, a database of the user's choice or selected multiple databases.

This is the daily news file of pre-publication material used for daily scanning of reports on topics of particular interest and is included in the SCRIP CURRENT NEWS database. For all information on a particular topic it is necessary to search both SCRIP CURRENT NEWS and SCRIP RETROSPECTIVE.

14:784. Online — CompuServe Information Service

File name	IQUEST File 2075: SCRIP – Current News
Alternative name(s)	PHIND
Start year	1986
Number of records	
Update period	Daily
Price/Charges	Subscription: US$8.95 per month Database entry fee: US$9/search; some databases carry a surcharge ($2–75) Online print: US$10 references free; then $9 per ten; abstracts $3 each

Notes

Accessed via IQUEST, this database is offered by a Data-Star gateway. IQUEST can either search across all databases, a database of the user's choice or selected multiple databases.

This is the file containing current news, including SCRIP – DAILY NEWS, and is used for scanning for recently written reports.

14:785. Online — Data-Star

File name	PHIN – Pharmaceutical & Healthcare Industry News – Archive file
Alternative name(s)	PHIND
Start year	1980 (to circa five weeks ago)
Number of records	113,270
Update period	Daily
Database aids	Data-Star Business and Biomedical Manuals, Berne, Data-Star, 1989 and Online manual (search NEWS-PHIN in NEWS)
Price/Charges	Subscription: SFr80.00 Connect time: SFr263.00 Online print: SFr5.48 Offline print: SFr5.81

Notes

This is the archive file of information, removed from PHID and/or PHIC files. For all information on a particular topic it is necessary to search both PHIN and PHIC.

From June 1993 Data-Star have introduced an annual fee/subscription per contract (that is, not per password) of SFr 80.00 (c.UK£ 32.00) payable every June. For North American customers billed in dollars who also use DIALOG, the DIALOG fee also covers access to Data-Star. Academic customers, 'commitment' customers and customers currently billed in dollars are exempt.

Record composition

Accession Number and Update Code AN; Date of Entry of Report DT; Date of Publication YD; Month of Publication YM; Occurrence Table OC; Source SO; Title TI; Text of Report TX; Update Code UP and Year of Publiction YR

14:786. Online — Data-Star

File name	PHID – Pharmaceutical and Healthcare Industry News – Daily News (pre-publication)
Alternative name(s)	PHIND
Start year	Today only
Number of records	113,270
Update period	Daily
Database aids	Data-Star Business and Biomedical Manuals, Berne, Data-Star, 1989 and Online manual (search NEWS-PHIN in NEWS)
Price/Charges	Subscription: SFr80.00 Connect time: SFr263.00 Online print: SFr5.48 Offline print: SFr5.81

Notes

PHID is the daily news file of pre-publication material used for daily scanning of reports on topics of particular interest. PHID is included in the database PHIC. For all information on a particular topic it is necessary to search both PHIN and PHIC.

From June 1993 Data-Star have introduced an annual fee/subscription per contract (that is, not per password) of SFr 80.00 (c.UK£ 32.00) payable every June. For North American customers billed in dollars who

also use DIALOG, the DIALOG fee also covers access to Data-Star. Academic customers, 'commitment' customers and customers currently billed in dollars are exempt.

Record composition

Accession Number and Update Code AN; Date of Entry of Report DT; Date of Publication YD; Month of Publication YM; Occurrence Table OC; Source SO; Title TI; Text of Report TX; Update Code UP and Year of Publiction YR

14:787. Online   Data-Star

File name	PHIC – Pharmaceutical and Healthcare Industry News – Current news including PHID (up to 5 weeks of data)
Alternative name(s)	PHIND
Start year	Latest four to five weeks
Number of records	113,270
Update period	Daily
Database aids	Data-Star Business and Biomedical Manuals, Berne, Data-Star, 1989 and Online manual (search NEWS-PHIN in NEWS)
Price/Charges	Subscription: SFr80.00
	Connect time: SFr263.00
	Online print: SFr5.48
	Offline print: SFr5.81

Notes

This is the file containing current news, including PHID (up to five weeks of data). PHIC is used for scanning for recently written reports. PHIC includes PHID but PHID and PHIC are not included in PHIN. For all information on a particular topic both PHIN and PHIC must be searched.

From June 1993 Data-Star have introduced an annual fee/subscription per contract (that is, not per password) of SFr 80.00 (c.UK£ 32.00) payable every June. For North American customers billed in dollars who also use DIALOG, the DIALOG fee also covers access to Data-Star. Academic customers, 'commitment' customers and customers currently billed in dollars are exempt.

Record composition

Accession Number and Update Code AN; Date of Entry of Report DT; Date of Publication YD; Month of Publication YM; Occurrence Table OC; Source SO; Title TI; Text of Report TX; Update Code UP and Year of Publiction YR

14:778. Online   DIALOG

File name	File 129
Alternative name(s)	PHIND
Start year	1980
Number of records	179,399
Update period	Weekly
Price/Charges	Connect time: US$150.00
	Online print: US$0.90
	Offline print: US$0.90
	SDI charge: US$5.00

Notes

The Pharmacuetical and Healthcare Industry News Database (PHIND) is divided into two files – daily (File 130) and current information (File 129), which includes some unpublished articles, and archival material dating back to 1980.

14:779. Online   DIALOG

File name	File 130
Alternative name(s)	PHIND

Start year	1980
Number of records	179,399
Update period	Daily
Price/Charges	Connect time: US$150.00
	Online print: US$4.00
	Offline print: US$4.00
	SDI charge: US$5.00 (weekly)/ 2.00 (daily)

Notes

The Pharmaceutical and Healthcare Industry News Database (PHIND) on Dialog is divided into two files – daily (File 130) and current information (File 129), which includes some unpublished articles, and archival material dating back to 1980.

DIALINDEX Categories: BIOBUS, BIOTECH, PHARM, PHARMINA, PHIND.

14:790. Database subset

Online   Data-Star

File name	TRPI – Pharmaceutical and Healthcare Industry News Training File
Alternative name(s)	PHIND
Start year	
Number of records	
Update period	
Database aids	Data-Star Business and Biomedical Manuals, Berne, Data-Star, 1989 and Online manual (search NEWS-PHIN in NEWS)
Price/Charges	Connect time: UK£Free

Record composition

Accession Number and Update Code AN; Date of Entry of Report DT; Date of Publication YD; Month of Publication YM; Occurrence Table OC; Source SO; Title TI; Text of Report TX; Update Code UP and Year of Publiction YR

Pharmaceutical Bibliography

Information Institute of Medical Science and Technology, State Medicine and Drug Administration Bureau

14:791. Master record

Database type	Bibliographic
Number of journals	
Sources	Journals
Start year	1984
Language	Chinese
Coverage	China
Number of records	70,000
Update size	10,000
Update period	Continuously
Index unit	Articles

Keywords

Pharmaceuticals

Description

Contains abstracts and bibliographic citations to articles on the pharmaceutical industry in China. Covers research, production and use of pharmaceuticals in China.

Abstracts are classified. Equivalent to the print *China Pharmaceutical Abstracts*.

14:792. Online   **Information Institute of Medical Science and Technology, State Medicine and Drug Administration Bureau**

File name	Pharmaceutical Bibliography
Start year	1984
Number of records	70,000
Update period	Continuously

Pharmaceutical Business News
Financial Times Business Information

14:793. Master record

Database type	Textual
Number of journals	1
Sources	Newsletter
Start year	Data-Star and FT Profile: 1986; Mead Data Central: 1989
Language	English
Coverage	International
Number of records	
Update size	–
Update period	Twice per month

Keywords

Pharmaceutical Industry; Pharmaceutical Products

Description

Contains the full text of *Pharmaceutical Business News*, a newsletter covering pharmaceutical product development worldwide. Includes news on latest developments in research and pre-clinical trials, legal and regulatory developments and company news, including global reporting and analyses on joint ventures, mergers, acquisitions and financial performance.

Corresponds to the twice monthly publication *Pharmaceutical Business News* newsletter.

14:794. Online   FT Profile

File name	Pharmaceutical Business News
Alternative name(s)	FT Profile – Pharmaceutical Business News
Start year	1986
Number of records	
Update period	Twice per month
Price/Charges	Connect time: UK£2.40 Online print: UK£0.04 – 0.10 per line Offline print: UK£0.01 per line

Notes

Registration fee required, including free documentation and training. Usage charges for access consist of two elements: a connect rate for time online, and a display rate (applies only to lines of file text). There is no charge for blank lines, system messages, menus or help information.

14:795. Online   Mead Data Central (as a NEXIS database)

File name	PBNWS – NEXIS
Alternative name(s)	NEXIS – Pharmaceutical Business News
Start year	1989
Number of records	
Update period	Twice per month

Price/Charges	Subscription: US$1,000 – 3,000 (Depending on needs) Connect time: US$49.00 (Telecomms + connect time) Database entry fee: US$6.00 Online print: US$0.04 per line

Notes

Libraries: CONSUM and WORLD.

A subscription charge which covers all transactional charges, connect time, telecommunications and the small administration charge can take the place of the individual charges. Subscriptions are negotiated with customers and vary according to the number of menus (thus, files) that are to be used – typically a minimum subscription would be about US$ 1,000. All charges include training and a 24-hour help line.

This database can also be found on:
PTS Newsletter Database
NEXIS
FT Profile

Pharmaceutical News Index
University Microfilms International/Data Courier Inc

14:797. Master record

Alternative name(s)	PNI
Database type	Bibliographic
Number of journals	
Sources	Newsletters
Start year	1974
Language	English
Coverage	International
Number of records	400,000
Update size	36,500
Update period	Weekly
Database aids	Search Tools: The Guide to UMI/Data Courier Online $75.00, Source Book (journals list) Free, Capabilities brochure Free and Log/On (Newsletter) Free

Keywords

Cosmetics; Pharmaceutical Industry; Medical Device Industry

Description

PNI contains citations to current news about pharmaceuticals, cosmetics, medical devices, and related health fields. PNI records refer to twenty-one major US and international newsletters on pharmaceutical-related topics such as health legislation and policy making; statistical data; pharmaceutical research; over-the-counter prescription markets; drug and device recalls; litigation and court decisions; market analysis; biotechnology updates; research and development in progress; veterinary pharmaceuticals; livestock disease news; personnel changes; corporate financial information; new drug application approvals; acquisitions and mergers,; government contracts; product successes and failures; health and beauty aids; advertising campaigns; new product development and joint ventures. The newsletters are: *Animal Pharm World; Animal Health News; Applied Genetic News; Biomedical Business International; Biomedical Safety Standards; Biomedical Technology Information Service; Clinica Lab Letter; Clinica World Medical Device News; Radiology & Imaging Letter; Drug*

Research Reports ('The Blue Sheet'); FDC Reports ('The Pink Sheet'), FDC Reports ('The Rose Sheet'), Health Devices; Medical Devices, Diagnostics, and Instrumentation Reports ('The Gray Sheet'); Pharma; PMA Newsletter; Quality Control Reports ('The Gold Sheet'), SCRIP World Pharmaceutical News; Washington Drug and Device Letter; Weekly Pharmacy Reports ('The Green Sheet'), and Technology Reimbursement Reports ('The Beige Sheet'): PNI cites and indexes all articles from these publications on drugs; corporation and industry sales, mergers, acquisitions, etc.; government legislation, regulations, and court action, and requests for proposals, research grant applications, industry speeches, press releases, and other news items.

14:798. Online   BRS

File name	PNII
Alternative name(s)	PNI
Start year	
Number of records	400,000
Update period	Weekly
Price/Charges	Connect time: US$125.00/135.00
	Online print: US$0.22/0.70
	Offline print: US$0.70

Downloading is allowed

14:799. Online   CompuServe Information Service

File name	IQUEST File 1097
Alternative name(s)	PNI
Start year	1985
Number of records	
Update period	Weekly
Price/Charges	Subscription: US$8.95 per month
	Database entry fee: US$9/search; some databases carry a surcharge ($2–75)
	Online print: US$10 references free; then $9 per ten; abstracts $3 each

Downloading is allowed

Notes

Accessed via IQUEST or IQMEDICAL, this database is offered by a DIALOG gateway. IQUEST can either search across all databases, a database of the user's choice or selected multiple databases.

14:800. Online   DIALOG

File name	File 42
Alternative name(s)	PNI
Start year	1974
Number of records	377,550
Update period	Weekly
Price/Charges	Connect time: US$159.00
	Online print: US$0.90
	Offline print: US$0.90
	SDI charge: US$12.95

Notes

DIALINDEX Categories: BIOTECH, PHARM, PHARMINA, PHARMR, REGS.

14:801. Online   ORBIT

File name	PNII – Pharmaceutical News Index
Alternative name(s)	PNI
Start year	1974
Number of records	340,000
Update period	Weekly
Database aids	Quick Reference Guide (9/88) Free (single copy)
Price/Charges	Connect time: UK£135.00
	Online print: UK£0.75/0.75
	Offline print: UK£0.75/0.75
	SDI charge: UK£5.50

Downloading is allowed

Notes

Electronic SDI service is now available within two hours on ORBIT. They can be downloaded and reformatted on a word processor. Results are retrieved in the low cost PRINTS file, $15 per connect hour.

14:802. Online   STN

File name	PNI
Alternative name(s)	PNI
Start year	1974
Number of records	400,000
Update period	Weekly

Downloading is allowed

14:803. Tape   University Microfilms International/Data Courier Inc

File name	PNI – Pharmaceutical News Index
Alternative name(s)	PNI
Format notes	IBM
Start year	1974
Number of records	400,000
Update period	Weekly or monthly depending on subscription. Annual lease is $9,000 (weekly updates), $6,000 (monthly updates), or for the archival files, $2,500 each.
Price/Charges	Subscription: US$2,500 – 9,000

For more details of constituent databases, see:
FDA on CD-ROM

Pharmaceuticals Section
World Health Organisation – Division of Drug Management and Policies

14:804. Master record

Alternative name(s)	UN Consolidated List of Products
Database type	Textual, Factual
Number of journals	
Sources	
Start year	1985
Language	English
Coverage	International
Number of records	3,000
Update size	–
Update period	Daily

Keywords

Pharmaceuticals

Description

A full text and factual database of information on pharmaceutical products whose consumption and/or sale have been banned, withdrawn, severely restricted or not approved by governments worldwide.

Available to UN system organizations; also to external users with restrictions. Printed products: *Pharmaceuticals section (UN consolidated list of products whose consumption and/or sale have been banned, withdrawn, severely restricted or not approved by governments)*. The database is also available as a printout.

14:805. Tape   World Health Organisation – Division of Drug Management and Policies

File name	Pharmaceuticals Section
Alternative name(s)	UN Consolidated List of Products
Format notes	IBM
Software	ADABAS
Start year	1985

Number of records	3,000
Update period	Daily

also use DIALOG, the DIALOG fee also covers access to Data-Star. Academic customers, 'commitment' customers and customers currently billed in dollars are exempt.

Pharmacontacts
Pharmaprojects PJB Publications Ltd

14:806. Master record

Alternative name(s)	Company Directory Database
Database type	Directory
Number of journals	
Sources	Directories
Start year	Current information
Language	German and English
Coverage	International
Number of records	20,000
Update size	–
Update period	Monthly

Keywords

Agrochemicals; Crop Protection; Education – Veterinary Medicine; Regulatory Agencies – Pharmaceuticals; Regulatory Agencies – Agrochemicals; Regulatory Agencies – Veterinary Medicine; Research and Development – Agriculture

Description

Pharmacontacts contains the names and addresses of over 7,000 pharmaceutical companies, agrochemical/crop protection companies and 2,400 animal-related health companies worldwide. In addition, details of 56 pharmaceutical and agrochemical regulatory bodies, research agencies in agrochemicals and veterinary science, 161 veterinary regulatory bodies and 140 veterinary institutions in this area are included. Wherever possible, telephone, telex, and telefax numbers are included.

The database, from the producers of PHIND, has been extensively researched, being based on the *Scrip* directories of pharmaceutical companies, the *Animal Pharm* directory of animal health companies (the *Agrow Directory of Agrochemical Companies*) and, in future, on the *Clinica* directories of device and diagnostic companies.

14:807. Online   BRS

File name	PHCO
Alternative name(s)	Company Directory Database
Start year	Current information
Number of records	20,000
Update period	Weekly
Price/Charges	Connect time: US$145.00/155.00
	Online print: US$1.25/1.35
	Offline print: US$0.82

14:808. Online   Data-Star

File name	PHCO
Alternative name(s)	Company Directory Database
Start year	Current information
Number of records	20,000
Update period	Monthly
Price/Charges	Subscription: UK£32.00
	Connect time: UK£105.20
	Online print: UK£0.88
	Offline print: UK£0.54

Notes

From June 1993 Data-Star have introduced an annual fee/subscription per contract (that is, not per password) of SFr 80.00 (c.UK£ 32.00) payable every June. For North American customers billed in dollars who

Pharmaprojects Discontinued Products
Pharmaprojects PJB Publications Ltd

14:809. Master record

Database type	Textual
Number of journals	
Sources	Company reports, Broker reports, Conference papers, Journals, Monographs, Patents, Database producers, Pharmacopoeias and Direct contacts
Start year	Current information
Language	English
Coverage	International
Number of records	4,000
Update size	–
Update period	Monthly
Index unit	products and patents

Keywords

Biochemistry; Drugs; Pharmaceuticals; Pharmaceutical Industry

Description

Descriptions of pharmaceutical products that are no longer under development and whose entries have been removed from the Pharmaprojects database. DIALOG and STN combine, in one file each, the current and discontinued records of Pharmaprojects.

14:810. Online   BRS

File name	PHAB
Start year	
Number of records	4,000
Update period	Monthly
Price/Charges	Connect time: US$145.00/155.00
	Online print: US$1.51/1.59 (Non subscribers 49.92/50.00)
	Offline print: US$1.75 (Non subscribers 50.00)
	SDI charge: US$25.00

Notes

This is the back file of Pharmaprojects database, containing records which have been transferred from the PHAR file when products are discontinued. Users can search in both PHAB and PHAR via the merged PHAZ file.

Differential charges for subscribers and non-subscribers to Pharmaprojects.

14:811. Online   Data-Star

File name	PHDI – Pharmaprojects Discontinued Drugs
Start year	
Number of records	4,000
Update period	Weekly
Database aids	Data-Star Business Manual and Data-Star Online Manual (search NEWS-PHAR in NEWS)
Price/Charges	Subscription: SFr80.00
	Connect time: SFr263.00
	Online print: SFr2.66 (Non-subscriber 76.00)
	Offline print: SFr2.94(Non-subscriber 76.00)
	SDI charge: Not applicable

Downloading is allowed

Notes

PHDI contains products whose development has been discontinued and have been transferred from Pharmaprojects PHAR file. It also contains products for which there is no evidence of continuing development, these products being transferred from PHAR annually in May. Products which have been launched in all major markets are removed from PHAR every year and are not transferred to PHDI.

Differential charges for subscribers and non-subscribers to Pharmaprojects.

In March 1993, the file was reloaded with new therapeutic activity codes: some codes have changed (for example, A8A5 the old code for Antiobesity has become A8A3 Anoretic/Antiobesity). Both the codes and the descriptions are searchable in the descriptor (DE) field.

From June 1993 Data-Star have introduced an annual fee/subscription per contract (that is, not per password) of SFr 80.00 (c.UK£ 32.00) payable every June. For North American customers billed in dollars who also use DIALOG, the DIALOG fee also covers access to Data-Star. Academic customers, 'commitment' customers and customers currently billed in dollars are exempt.

Pharmaprojects

PJB Publications Ltd

14:812. Master record

Database type	Bibliographic, Factual, Directory, Image, Chemical structures/DNA sequences
Number of journals	
Sources	Company reports, Broker reports, Conference papers, Journals, Monographs, Patents, Direct contacts, Database producers and Pharmacopoeias
Start year	
Language	German and English
Coverage	International
Number of records	5,500
Update size	180
Update period	Monthly
Index unit	products and patents

Keywords

Biochemistry; Drugs; Pharmaceuticals; Pharmaceutical Industry

Description

Pharmaprojects online reports on the progress of new pharmaceutical products, both new chemical entities and biotechnological entities, at all stages of development. The information is taken from the publication *Pharmaprojects*. It covers over 5,000 pharmaceutical products, including biotechnological products, new formulations and combinations currently under development by more than 800 companies worldwide. It can be monitored for new formulations and compounds either associated with given companies or therapeutic activities. Each document in the database is a report on a single product, providing: generic name, synonyms; trade names and research codes; chemical names (soon to conform to CAS index name format) and CAS Registry number; the originating company and licensees; detailed information on its stage of development in 28 countries; standardised therapeutic activity descriptors; descriptive text con-

taining key literature references to relevant literature where appropriate. The text is updated with each stage of the product's development, initially detailing pharmacological, then clinical studies, progressing through registration, joint-development agreements, and finally licensing and marketing. Pharmaprojects uses literature references to compounds as a starting point for direct enquiries to the drugs' developers to provide stage of development information not available elsewhere. The database includes patent numbers supplied by the developers of the new drugs in some monographs. It primarily addresses the information needs of the pharmaceutical industry and closely related fields, but is also of interest to those involved in the evaluation of pharmaceutical company performance. In early 1993, a drug action classification system was added to the file so that drugs which act by a specific pharmacological mechanism can now be located.

The database corresponds to the printed *Pharmaprojects*. Pharmaprojects staff attend major conferences and meetings to report the most up-to-date information, while offers of licensing or joint development agreements are obtained direct from originating companies. Every month some 100–150 new compounds are added to the Pharmaprojects database and major changes are made to around 200 existing products entries. All companies with products appearing in Pharmaprojects are contacted at least annually and are offered the opportunity to comment on the completeness and accuracy of their products' entries. SDI became available on Pharmaprojects in October 1989.

Activity descriptors in the text are not standardised so all reasonable synonyms should be searched. The Country data field contains the status of a given product in a country. The following range of statuses is available: Preclinical; Clinical; Phase 1 Clinical Trials; Phase II Clinical Trials; Phase III Clinical Trials; Pre-registration; Registered (but not yet launched); Launched (with or without launch date). Chemical names are predominantly in CAS Index name format: for precise retrieval it is suggested that the registry number is used.

14:813. Online   BRS

File name	PHAR
Start year	
Number of records	5,500
Update period	Monthly
Price/Charges	Connect time: US$145.00/155.00
	Online print: US$1.51/1.59
	Offline print: US$1.75
	SDI charge: US$25.00

Notes

This is the current file of Pharmaproject database. Records of discontinued products are transferred to the PHAB file (see Pharmaprojects Discontinued Products). Users can search in both PHAB and PHAR via the merged PHAZ file on BRS.

Differential charges for subscribers and non-subscribers to Pharmaprojects.

14:814. Online   BRS

File name	PHAZ
Start year	
Number of records	5,500
Update period	Monthly
Price/Charges	Connect time: US$145.00/155.00
	Online print: US$1.51/1.59
	Offline print: US$1.75
	SDI charge: US$25.00

Notes

This is the merged file of Pharmaproject database. Users can search in both PHAB and PHAR via the merged PHAZ file on BRS. Differential charges for subscribers and non-subscribers to Pharmaprojects.

14:815. Online   Data-Star

File name	PHAR
Start year	
Number of records	5,500
Update period	Monthly
Database aids	Data-Star Business Manual and Data-Star Online Manual (search NEWS-PHAR in NEWS)
Price/Charges	Subscription: SFr80.00
	Connect time: SFr263.00
	Online print:
	SFr2.66(Non-subscriber 76.00)
	Offline print:
	SFr2.94(Non-subscriber 76.00)
	SDI charge: Not applicable

Notes

PHAR is completely reloaded every week, with products whose development has been discontinued being transferred to Pharmaprojects Discontinued Drugs (PHDI). PHDI also contains products for which there is no evidence of continuing development, these products being transferred from PHAR annually in May. Products which have been launched in all major markets (PharmaLaunched – PHLP) are removed from PHAR every year and they are not transferred to PHDI. PHAR and PHDI can be searched simultaneously by using the superfile PHZZ.

Differential charges for subscribers and non-subscribers to Pharmaprojects.

In March 1993, the file was reloaded with new therapeutic activity codes: some codes have changed (for example, A8A5 the old code for Antiobesity has become A8A3 Anoretic/Antiobesity). Both the codes and the descriptions are searchable in the descriptor (DE) field.

From June 1993 Data-Star have introduced an annual fee/subscription per contract (that is, not per password) of SFr 80.00 (c.UK£ 32.00) payable every June. For North American customers billed in dollars who also use DIALOG, the DIALOG fee also covers access to Data-Star. Academic customers, 'commitment' customers and customers currently billed in dollars are exempt.

Record composition

Accession Number and Update Code AN; Company Descriptor CO; Country Descriptor and Status CN; Descriptors DE; Date when entry was last updated ED; Molecular Formula MF; Registry Number RN; Source SO; Synonyms SY; Text TE; Title TI; Update Code UP and Update Information UD

14:816. Online   Data-Star

File name	PHLP – PharmaLaunched
Start year	
Number of records	
Update period	Weekly
Database aids	Data-Star Business Manual and Data-Star Online Manual (search NEWS-PHAR in NEWS)
Price/Charges	Subscription: UK£32.00
	Connect time: UK£105.20
	Online print: UK£30.40
	Offline print: UK£30.40
	SDI charge: UK£8.22

Notes

A file containing all the products that have been launched in major markets. The records are removed from the PHAR file each year and are not transferred to the PHDI file.

Differential charges for subscribers and non-subscribers to Pharmaprojects.

In March 1993, the file was reloaded with new therapeutic activity codes: some codes have changed (for example, A8A5 the old code for Antiobesity has become A8A3 Anoretic/Antiobesity). Both the codes and the descriptions are searchable in the descriptor (DE) field.

From June 1993 Data-Star have introduced an annual fee/subscription per contract (that is, not per password) of SFr 80.00 (c.UK£ 32.00) payable every June. For North American customers billed in dollars who also use DIALOG, the DIALOG fee also covers access to Data-Star. Academic customers, 'commitment' customers and customers currently billed in dollars are exempt.

Record composition

Accession Number and Update Code AN; Company Descriptor CO; Country Descriptor and Status CN; Descriptors DE; Date when entry was last updated ED; Molecular Formula MF; Registry Number RN; Source SO; Synonyms SY; Text TE; Title TI; Update Code UP and Update Information UD

14:817. Online   DIALOG

File name	File 128
Start year	1980
Number of records	12,072
Update period	Monthly
Price/Charges	Connect time: US$180.00
	Online print: US$60.00
	Offline print: US$60.00
	SDI charge: US$13.50

Notes

The database contains data on 5,400 products in active development and 4,700 products whose development has been terminated or is currently in question. File 128 is the public access database and File 928 is available at a reduced rate for subscribers to the print Pharmaprojects.

14:818. Online   DIALOG

File name	File 928
Start year	1980
Number of records	12,072
Update period	Monthly
Price/Charges	Connect time: US$180.00
	Online print: US$2.00
	Offline print: US$2.00
	SDI charge: US$13.50

Notes

The database contains data on 5,400 products in active development and 4,700 products whose development has been terminated or is currently in question. File 128 is the public access database and File 928 is available at a reduced rate for subscribers to the print Pharmaprojects.

14:819. Online   STN

File name	PHAR
Start year	1990

Number of records	14,391
Update period	Monthly
Price/Charges	Connect time: US$150.00
	Online print: US$40.00
	Offline print: US$40.00
	SDI charge: US$10.00

Notes

STN also includes discontinued or non-developed products which have been removed from the current print version.

14:820. Diskette   PJB Publications

File name	Pharmastructures
Start year	1990
Number of records	4,000
Update period	Monthly

Notes

This is equivalent to Pharmaprojects online, but offers graphics of chemical entries. The file includes both active and discontinued projects. It is menu- based and details some 4,000 chemical structures. Two versions are available: Psidom and Chembase, the differences between them including output formatting and the fact that users can search by molecular formula on the Chembase version. A backfile in the process of being added.

The database consists of twenty-one 5.25 inch or eleven 3.5 inch diskettes at an annual cost of UK£1200 for Pharmaprojects subscribers, UK£1700 for non-subscribers. Monthly updates are available and the database is also in print as *Pharmastructures in Print*.

14:821. Database subset

Online   Data-Star

File name	TRPH – Pharmaprojects Training File
Start year	
Number of records	
Update period	
Price/Charges	Connect time: Free

Pharmarom

Pharmarom Institute
CAT Benelux

14:822. Master record

Database type	Factual, Textual
Number of journals	
Sources	
Start year	
Language	
Coverage	
Number of records	—
Update size	
Update period	

Description

Medicine descriptions with availability in Dutch pharmacies.

14:823. CD-ROM   CAT Benelux

File name	
Start year	
Number of records	
Update period	

PharmaROM

OFAC
Bureau van Dijk
Galenica
Médecine et Hygiéne
OVP – Editions du Vidal
Société Suisse de Pharmacie
Telmed
Thieme-Verlag

14:824. Master record

CD-ROM   OFAC

Database type	Factual
Number of journals	
Sources	
Start year	
Language	French, English and German
Coverage	Switzerland
Number of records	
Update size	—
Update period	Twice a year

Keywords

Drugs; Drug Therapy; Pharmaceuticals; Surgery; Travel

Description

Primarily destined for the Swiss pharmacists.

Twelve databases in the pharmaceutical and health care fields, including: Dictionnaire Vidal; Index Nominum; Interactions of the Medical Letter; Interactions de la Société Suisse de Pharmacie; Pharma-Digest; Phytotherapie; Teledoc Galenica; Thermalisme; Vergiftungen; Voyages et Santé. Logical links are possible within the data of some databases.

For more details of constituent databases, see:
Dictionnaire Vidal
Index Nominum
Interactions of the Medical Letter
Interactions de la Société Suisse de Pharmacie
Pharma-Digest
Phytotherapie
Teledoc Galenica
Thermalisme
Vergiftungen
Voyages et Santé

Pharmline

UK National Health Service, Regional
Drug Information Service

14:825. Master record

Database type	Bibliographic
Number of journals	100
Sources	Editorials, journals, letters and reviews
Start year	1978
Language	English
Coverage	
Number of records	62,500
Update size	10,000
Update period	Weekly

Thesaurus	Pharmline Thesaurus, 4th edition, Leicester, Drug Information Pharmacist's Group, 1987.

Keywords

Drugs; Pharmacy Practice

Description

Pharmline is produced by the regional drug information services of the United Kingdom. The aim of the working party is to offer a contextually defined and goal-directed database as well as access to published drug literature through Pharmline. The subject areas of this database include drugs and professional pharmacy practice. Articles containing information on the following topics are consistently included: adverse affects of drugs, clinical pharmacokinetics including metabolism, bioavailability, drug interactions, drug modification of laboratory tests, information science, where relevant to drug information, new drugs, new uses of established drugs, new routes of administration and dosage schedules, pharmaceuticals, pharmacology, pharmacy practice, use of drugs in breast feeding, pregnancy, neonates, liver failure and renal failure. Papers referring principally to animal studies are excluded.

14:826. Online — CompuServe Information Service

File name	IQUEST File 2142
Start year	1978
Number of records	62,500
Update period	Weekly
Price/Charges	Subscription: US$8.95 per month Database entry fee: US$9/search; some databases carry a surcharge ($2–75) Online print: US$10 references free; then $9 per ten; abstracts $3 each
Downloading is allowed	

Notes

Accessed via IQUEST, this database is offered by a Data-Star gateway. IQUEST can either search across all databases, a database of the user's choice or selected multiple databases.

Record composition

Abstract AB; Accession Number and Update Code AN; Article Type AT; Author AU; Descriptors DE; Manufacturer MF; Source SO; Title TI; Update Code UP and Year of publication YR

14:827. Online — Data-Star

File name	LINE – Pharmline
Start year	1978
Number of records	62,500
Update period	Weekly
Database aids	Data-Star Biomedical Manual and Data-Star Online Manual (search NEWS-LINE in NEWS)
Price/Charges	Subscription: SFr80.00 Connect time: SFr140.20 Online print: SFr0.62 Offline print: SFr0.54 SDI charge: SFr6.80
Downloading is allowed	

Notes

From June 1993 Data-Star have introduced an annual fee/subscription per contract (that is, not per password) of SFr 80.00 (c.UK£ 32.00) payable every June. For North American customers billed in dollars who also use DIALOG, the DIALOG fee also covers access to Data-Star. Academic customers, 'commitment' customers and customers currently billed in dollars are exempt.

Record composition

Abstract AB; Accession Number and Update Code AN; Article Type AT; Author AU; Descriptors DE; Manufacturer MF; Source SO; Title TI; Update Code UP and Year of publication YR

Pharmpat
Chemical Abstracts Service

14:828. Master record

Database type	Bibliographic
Number of journals	
Sources	
Start year	1988
Language	German and English
Coverage	International
Number of records	5,000
Update size	—
Update period	Bimonthly

Keywords

Chemical Substances; Drugs; Pharmaceuticals; Patents

Description

Covers worldwide chemical and biochemical patents related to drugs and pharmaceutical chemistry.

14:829. Online — STN

File name	PHARMPAT
Start year	1988
Number of records	5,000
Update period	Bimonthly

Pharmsearch
Institut National de la Propriété Industrielle (INPI)

14:830. Master record

Database type	Bibliographic
Number of journals	
Sources	Patents
Start year	1989
Language	English and French
Coverage	France, USA and Europe
Number of records	46,068
Update size	—
Update period	Twice a month

Keywords

Pharmaceutical Products; Patents

Description

A database of bibliographical details of pharmaceutical patents produced by the French Patent Office. These are accessed as a result of structure searching in MPHARM, a complementary database, by means of Markush DARC software, originally developed in conjunction with Questel and Derwent. Users transfer results from MPHARM to Pharmsearch, the database being linked by compound number. Both databases also cover the older French BSM (Brevets Speciaux de Medicaments) system which ran from 1961–1971. Records are sourced from all US, European and French patents covering pharmaceutical, chemical and biological topics. Covers applications for published French and European licences, as well as American, in the areas of chemistry and pharmaceutical biology. Provides the largest Markush structural background on the market including Peptide patents – over 50,000 patents and 70,000 structures. Contains bibliographic information and specially written abstracts. Patents are added to the database within six to ten weeks of publication date (fourteen weeks for US Patents). The database includes details of patent number, applicant, date of registration, formula, etc. The indexing uses internationally accepted chemical nomenclature and terminology specially adapted for the pharmaceutical industry and the records contain an original summary which highlights all the pharmacological properties and therapeutic instructions, the chemical structure as described in the patent, all the chemical structures covered by the patent, all the compounds covered by the same generic structure, and the precise position of all the groups. Patents found to be equivalent to previously indexed patents do not normally appear in the database. When a patent claiming the same priority as a previously indexed document has a different claim scope, the 'equivalent' patent is indexed without reference to the earlier record. Each record has a short English-language abstract, covering pharmacological, therapeutic and galenic areas, and patent documents in the French language also have a short French-language abstract.

Pharmsearch is designed to make the most of information available from generic structures and can be consulted through simple screen drawing. Coverage will be extended for US and European patents back from 1978, and for French patents from 1961. The French patents are in English and French, all others are in English.

Patent document and priority numbers are indexed for crossfile searching in Derwent format in /XPN and /XPR fields, which do not print in any of the standard formats. Patent title are not given in the record. Th document PN, application AP and priority nymbers and dates of the patent are recorded. Patentee PA names and the country of origin of the patentee are provided, but the names of inventors are not. International Patent Classification codes are searchable IC. INPI's indexers assign uncontrolled terms corresponding to three-letter codes describing therapeutic effects EFF and processes PROC, and numeric Pharmsearh Classification codes PHC. Compound numbers CN correspiond to structure records in the Markush DARC companion file MPHARM. Specific compunds and generic structures from the claims together with examples are indexed topologically, and the structure records are searchable and displayable in the MPHARM file.In Markush DARC, the parent structure is displayed and each variable group for a Markush structure is shown as a separate screen along with the molecular sub-structure to which it is attached. Patents cited as prior art references in the indexed documents are listed RF, but non-patent literature references are not searchable.

14:831. Online　　　　　　　　　Questel

File name	PHARM
Software	Markush DARC

Start year	1989
Number of records	50,000
Update period	Twice a month
Delay	6 weeks

Notes
Pharmsearch can be consulted through simple screen drawing, eliminating the imprecision resulting from chemical names or classification systems. A list of compound numbers retrieved after a Markush DARC search in the MPHARM structure database can be transferred to the PHARM bibliographic database.

Record composition
Accession Number – AN; Compund Number – CN; Document Number – PN; Application – AP; Patentee – PA; Country of Origin of Patent – PAC; International Patent Classification Code – IC; EAB; Uncontrolled Index Term – IT; Processes – PROC; Effects – EFF; Pharmsearch Classification Codes – PHC; Abstract – AB; Priority Number – PR and Prior Art References – RF

Physician's AIDSLINE
National Library of Medicine
National Institute of Allergy and Infectious Diseases (US)

14:832. Master record
CD-ROM　　　　　　　　Macmillan New Media

Alternative name(s)	AIDSLINE, Physician's
Database type	Bibliographic, Textual, Directory
Number of journals	
Sources	
Start year	
Language	
Coverage	
Number of records	
Update size	—
Update period	Annually

Keywords
HIV

Description
Contains three databases: AIDSLINE, AIDSTRIALS and AIDSDRUGS from the National Library of Medicine.

AIDSLINE with nearly 60,000 citations from MEDLINE, CancerLit, CatLine, and Health Planning and Administration databases plus abstracts from the 5th and 6th International Conference on AIDS; and

AIDSTRIALS and AIDSDRUGS, which contain information from the National Institute of Allergy and Infectious Diseases and the NLM describing 321 clinical trials currently in progress and the 101 drugs being tested in the trials.

Aimed at the primary care physician who refers AIDS patients.

Notes

Available from January 1992.

For more details of constituent databases, see:
AIDSLINE
AIDSTRIALS
AIDSDRUGS

Physician's Desk Reference
Medical Economics Company Inc

14:834. Master record

Alternative name(s)	PDR
Database type	Factual
Number of journals	
Sources	Pharmacopoeias and Monographs
Start year	Current information
Language	English
Coverage	USA
Number of records	2,750
Update size	—
Update period	Monthly

Keywords

Drugs; Ophthalmology; Pharmaceutical Products

Description

Contains the complete text of the current year's edition of three important reference works: *Physician's Desk Reference, Physician's Desk Reference for Non-Prescribed Drugs* and *Physicians Desk Reference for Ophthalmology*, together with the entire contents of *PDR's Drug Interactions and Side Effects Index*. Also includes all official FDA-approved labelling in the PDR and companion volumes. Contains full, official prescribing information on prescription and over-the-counter pharmaceuticals plus drug interactions and side effects, as found in the *Drug Interactions and Side Effects Index* and the *Indications Index*.

Corresponds to all five volumes: *Physicians' Desk Reference, Physicians' Desk Reference for Nonprescription Drugs, Physicians' Desk Reference for Ophthalmology, Physicians' Desk Reference Drug Interactions and Side Effects Index*, and *Physicians' Desk Reference Indications Index*.

14:835. Online
Chemical Information Systems Inc (CIS)

File name	Physician's Desk Reference
Alternative name(s)	PDR
Start year	Current information
Number of records	2,750
Update period	Monthly

Notes

Annual subscription of $300 to CIS required.

14:836. CD-ROM
Medical Economics Company Inc

File name	Physician's Desk Reference
Alternative name(s)	PDR
Format notes	IBM
Start year	Current information
Number of records	2,750
Update period	Annually
Price/Charges	Subscription: UK£330 – 595

Notes

Contains the full text of *PDR*, plus all the prescribing information in *PDR for Nonprescription Drugs* and *PDR for Ophthalmology*, and the entire contents of *PDR's Drug Interactions and Side Effects Index* on a single disc, without illustrations. While the print volumes serve as a handy reference work for the health consumer, the CD-ROM is aimed at the health professional. The user is offered a product look-up blank which is the easiest and quickest means of retrieving information on a specific drug. The beginning of each monograph states 'Information based on official labeling in effect date'.

Also features a facility for creating patient files containing treatment regimens, allowing automatic screening for drug interactions.

Features include interactions checks, split-screen comparisons and free-text searching. Prescribing information for trade name pharmaceutical products, over-the-counter products and ophthalmological preparations, including manufacturer, generic description, indications, precautions, interactions, adverse reactions, dosage and administration, overdose management, contraindications and patient instructions. In an overview of general health CD-ROMs, Nicholas Tomaiuolo noted that the major difference between Physicians' Desk Reference and USP DI is that 'the latter is the only published reference work that uses a structured review system contributed to by experts. The PDR contains basically recapitulated drug package inserts provided by pharmaceutical manufacturers' (*CD-ROM World* 8(1) January 1993 p 38–49).

A version additionally containing the *Merck Manual* of diagnosis and therapy is also available, cost is: for annual subscription £595, subscription renewal £530. Searching possible by brand name, generic ingredient, therapeutic category, interaction potential, side effect or manufacturer.

14:837. CD-ROM
Medical Economics Company Inc

File name	Physician's Desk Reference with Merck Manual
Alternative name(s)	PDR
Format notes	IBM
Start year	Current information
Number of records	2,750
Update period	Monthly
Price/Charges	Subscription: US$895

Notes

Contains the full text without illustrations. While the print volumes serve as a handy reference work for the health consumer, the CD-ROM is aimed at the health professional. The user is offered with a product look-up blank which is the easiest and quickest means of retrieving information on a specific drug. The beginning of each monograph states 'Information based on official labeling in effect date'. Enhanced with the *Merck Manual* on the same disc, this version allows users to locate a disorder in Merck and zoom directly to the proper medication entry in PDR.

Also features a facility for creating patient files containing treatment regimens, allowing automatic screening for drug interactions.

Phytotherapie
Telmed

14:838. Master record

Database type	
Number of journals	
Sources	

Start year
Language   French
Coverage   Switzerland
Number of records
Update size   —
Update period

Keywords

Drugs; Pharmaceuticals; Surgery

Description

This database in the medical and pharmaceutical field forms part of the MediROM and PharmaROM CD-ROMs, originally intended for Swiss pharmacists.

This database can be found on:
MediROM
PharmaROM

Pill Book Version 3.0
Yakugyo Jiho Co Ltd

14:840. Master record

Alternative name(s)   EB Pill Book
Database type   Factual, Directory, Textual
Number of journals
Sources
Start year
Language   Japanese
Coverage   Japan
Number of records
Update size   —
Update period   Annually

Keywords

Drugs; Pharmaceuticals

Description

Contains information on 9,000 drugs, covering efficacy and adverse reactions. Designed for general readers interested in prescribed drugs.

14:841. CD-ROM 8cm   Yakugyo Jiho Co Ltd

File name   Pill Book Version 3.0
Alternative name(s)   EB Pill Book
Format notes   Sony, Data, Discman
Software   Proprietary
Start year
Number of records
Update period   Annually
Price   Yen2,900

Plantas Medicinales
Ministerio de Sanidad y Consumo de España, Dirección General de Farmacia y Productos Sanitarios, Servicio de Gestión del Banco de Datos de Medicamentos

14:842. Master record

Alternative name(s)   Herbal Remedies
Database type   Textual
Number of journals
Sources   Pharmacopoeias and Government departments
Start year   1988
Language   Spanish
Coverage   Spain

Number of records   3,100
Update size   —
Update period   Daily, as new data become available

Keywords

Alternative Medicine; Medicinal Plants; Herbal Remedies

Description

Descriptions of medicinal plants registered or awaiting registration for use in Spain, giving name, therapeutic group, active and excipient ingredients, dosage and administration, producing laboratory, price and administrative information.

14:843. Online   Ministerio de Sanidad y Consumo de España, Dirección General de Farmacia y Productos Sanitarios, Servicio de Gestión del Banco de Datos de Medicamentos

File name
Alternative name(s)   Herbal Remedies
Start year   1988
Number of records   3,100
Update period   Daily, as new data become available

Poisindex
Micromedex Inc

14:844. Master record

Alternative name(s)   Computerized Clinical Information System: Poisindex; CCIS: Poisindex
Database type   Factual, Bibliographic, Textual, Directory, Numeric
Number of journals
Sources
Start year
Language   English
Coverage   USA and International
Number of records
Update size   —
Update period   Quarterly

Keywords

Occupational Health and Safety; Pharmaceutical Products; Poisons

Description

The 'standard of care' in the identification and treatment of exposures to potentially toxic agents. A toxicology database with two files designed to identify and provide ingredient information for over 750,000 domestic and foreign commercial, industrial, pharmaceutical, zoological, and botanic substances, as well as warfare agents and nerve gas antidotes.

Substance identification – a file containing information on any of about 360,000 toxic and non-toxic substances. Covers commonly used household products, industrial chemicals and products, pharmaceutical products (prescription, generic and over-the-counter) and biological entities (botanic, zoologicand food poisoning). Users can search by: brand or trade name; manufacturer's name; generic or chemical name;

street or slang terminology; botanic and common name (including phonetic or incorrect spelling).

Management Treatment Protocols – contains over 775 management/treatment protocols for toxic exposure to substances, including drugs, household and industrial products and plants, by ingestion, inhalation or skin/eye contact.

The detailed management/treatment protocols include multi-ingredient substances and diagnostic lists which reflect the experience and expertise of clinical toxicologists, clinical pharmacists and physicians in major poison units and emergency departments worldwide. The file is continuously reviewed by an editorial board which consists of practicing toxicologists, emergency physicians, clinical pharmacists and nurses who are involved in major areas of toxicology. It is republished every quarter to insure that the contents reflect the most current information on toxicology.

Users can search by substance, clinical effects, laboratory methods, case reports, treatment, range of toxicity, kinetics, pharmacology/toxicology and animal poisoning.

A mushroom identification program is included, designed to ask a series of questions which will eventually lead the subscriber to at least a genus description of the mushroom and a brief description of its possible toxicity. Written in layman terminology, this programme allows for the direct questioning of the person calling the poison centre.

14:845. Online   Mead Data Central (as a NEXIS database)

File name	POISON – NEXIS
Alternative name(s)	Computerized Clinical Information System: Poisindex; CCIS: Poisindex
Start year	1974
Number of records	360,000
Update period	Quarterly
Price/Charges	Subscription: US$1,000 – 3,000 (Depending on needs) Connect time: US$49.00 (Telecomms + connect time) Database entry fee: US$24.00 (Search charge) Online print: US$0.04 per line

Notes
Library: GENMED; Group file: MEDEX.

Record composition
Title TITLE; Overview OVERVIEW; Clinical Effects Overview OV-CLEF; Life Support Overview OV-LIFE; Substances Included SUBS; Therapeutic/Toxic Class of Substance CLASS; Geographic Location GEOG; Prevention of Contamination CONT; Summary of Clinical Effects CLEF-SUM; Clinical Effects: Involving the Eyes EYES; Clinical Effects: Cardiovascular CARD; Clinical Effects: Respiratory RESP; Clinical Effects: Neurologic NEUR; Clinical Effects: Gastrointestinal GAST; Clinical Effects: Genitourinary GENT; Clinical Effects: Hematologic HEMA; Clinical Effects: Dermatologic DREM; Clinical Effects: Musculoskeletal MUSC; Clinical Effects: Endocrine System ENDO; Clinical Effects: Psychiatric PSYCH; Clinical Effects: Pregnancy/Breat Milk PREG; Clinical Effects: Immunologic IMMU; Laboratory Processes (Diagnosis) LAB; Diagnosis Laboratory Methods METH; Diagnosis Monitoring Parameters MONIT;

Diagnosis Respiratory Muscle Performance RMP; Diagnosis Radiographic Studies XRAY; Treatment TRMT; Treatment Life Support LIFE; Treatment Summary TRMT-SUM; Range of Toxicity TOX; Pharmacology/Toxicology of Agent TOXICOLOGY; Pharmacology/Toxicology of Agent PHAR; Mechanics of Agent KINETICS; References REFS and Outline of Protocols OUTLINE

14:846. Tape   Micromedex Inc

File name	Poisindex
Alternative name(s)	Computerized Clinical Information System: Poisindex; CCIS: Poisindex
Software	Proprietary
Start year	1973
Number of records	
Update period	Quarterly

Notes
Annual subscription to CCIS required. Identidex is available to subscribers of this database for an additional fee.

This database can also be found on:
CCIS
NEXIS

PolTox I: NLM, CSA, IFIS
National Library of Medicine
Cambridge Scientific Abstracts

14:848. Master record
CD-ROM   Compact Cambridge

Alternative name(s)	PolTox 1: NLM, CSA, IFIS
Database type	Bibliographic
Number of journals	
Sources	
Start year	1981
Language	English
Coverage	International
Number of records	813,000
Update size	23,000
Update period	Quarterly

Description
Collection of pollution and toxicology records from a wide range of sources: the National Library of Medicine's TOXLINE subfile as well as Pollution Abstracts, Toxicology Abstracts, Ecology Abstracts, Health and Safety Science Abstracts, the toxicology section of Food Science and Technology Abstracts and Part 3 of the Aquatic Sciences and Fisheries Abstracts: Aquatic Pollution and Environmental Quality. With PolTox II it seeks to provide the beginnings of a CD-ROM library of environmental pollution and toxic substances. One reviewer especially liked the bringing together of material from so many different sources but pointed out that the drawback comes from the different indexing for the various source databases. He also found it frustrating having to switch between discs.

Lower subscription of UK£870 if only 1985 to present is required. Special discount is available for combined purchase of all three volumes. See also PolTox II and PolTox III.

For more details of constituent databases, see:
TOXLINE
Pollution Abstracts
Toxicology Abstracts
Ecology Abstracts
Health and Safety Science Abstracts
Food Science and Technology Abstracts
Aquatic Sciences and Fisheries Abstracts

PolTox II: Excerpta Medica
Elsevier Science Publishers

14:850. Master record
CD-ROM   **Compact Cambridge**

Alternative name(s)	PolTox 2: Excerpta Medica
Database type	Bibliographic
Number of journals	
Sources	
Start year	1981
Language	
Coverage	
Number of records	260,000
Update size	–
Update period	Quarterly

Keywords
Cosmetics; Environmental Health; Environmental Pollution; Environmental Toxicology; Food Additives; Food Contaminants; Occupational Health and Safety; Pharmaceuticals; Pollution; Toxic Substances; Waste Management

Description
This CD-ROM database contains a subset of EMBASE giving citations and abstracts to the worldwide literature on scientific, industrial and social concerns on toxic items and environmental health. Subjects covered include environmental pollution and toxicology. Pollution-related topics include chemical pollution and its effect on man, animals, plants and micro-organisms; environmental impact of chemical pollution, including measurement, treatment, prevention and control; radiation and thermal pollution; noise and vibration; dangerous goods; wastewater treatment and measurement; meteorological aspects of pollution; and legal and socioeconomic aspects of pollution. Toxicology coverage includes pharmaceutical toxicology; foods, food additives and contaminants; cosmetics, toiletries and household products; occupational toxicology; waste materials in air, soil and water; toxins and venoms; chemical teratogens, mutagens and carcinogens; phototoxicity, toxic mechanisms; predictive toxicology; regulatory toxicology; laboratory methods and techniques; and antidotes and symptomatic treatment.

The database, together with PolTox I, seeks to provide the beginnings of a CD-ROM library on environmental pollution and toxic substances. One reviewer especially liked the bringing together of material from so many different sources but pointed out there are drawbacks in the different indexing for the various source databases and in the frustration of having to switch between discs. See also PolTox I and PolTox

III. Special discount is available for combined purchase of all three volumes.

For more details of constituent databases, see:
EMBASE

PolTox III: CAB
CAB International

14:852. Master record
CD-ROM   **Compact Cambridge**

Alternative name(s)	PolTox 3: CAB
Database type	Bibliographic
Number of journals	
Sources	
Start year	1984
Language	
Coverage	
Number of records	150,000
Update size	–
Update period	Quarterly

Keywords
Drugs; Environmental Health; Food Contaminants; Pollution; Toxic Substances; Waste Management

Description
Database devoted to the agricultural, scientific, industrial and social dimensions of pollution, toxic substances and environmental health. PolTox III covers the agricultural aspects of the two subjects from the CAB ABSTRACTS database. Topics covered include environmental agrochemicals; groundwater contamination, run-off and leaching; heavy metals in soils, crops and animals; reclamation and re-vegetation of polluted sites; environmental impact of farming; waste management, treatment and disposal; toxicology; food contamination; carcinogens; and health hazards of pesticides, drug residues, side effects of drugs, steroids and hormones in animals.

See also PolTox I and PolTox II. Special discount is available for combined purchase of all three volumes.

For more details of constituent databases, see:
CAB Abstracts

Prescription Drugs – A Pharmacist's Guide
Quanta

14:854. Master record

Database type	Directory, Textual, Factual
Number of journals	
Sources	Monograph
Start year	
Language	English
Coverage	International
Number of records	
Update size	–
Update period	
Index unit	Drug

Keywords
Drugs

Description

Descriptions of the 200 most widely-used prescription drugs with details of manufacturer, dosage, side-effects, use in pregnancy, tolerance, overdose, prevalence, generic equivalents, etc. The subtitle, A Pharmacist's Guide, means written by pharmacists for the lay person and not a guide for pharmacists – in fact, Quanta say it is written for secondary school level. Reviewing the product (*CD-ROM Librarian* 7(11) p.62–64), Sheldon Cheney noted that buying any CD-ROM was like buying a pig in a poke – 'you cannot easily peek in the bag to see how full it is . Prescription Drugs – A Pharmacist's Guide is a rather small pig'. It turns out that the material on the disc equates to about 133 pages of the Physicians' Desk Reference (PDR) and that many of the drugs entries repeat information which is found in others. This disc is 'about one-fifteenth of the Product Information section of PDR for over twice the price'. It contains less technical information than PDR so many of the target readers will find it easier to understand. The text of the entries seems to contain both typographical errors and missing word but is easy to read. Despite this and the limited choice of drugs, the reviewer gave the product a middle score and suggested that if Quanta had tidied up the product this would have been higher.

14:855. CD-ROM   Quanta

File name	Prescription Drugs – A Pharmacist's Guide
Format notes	IBM, Mac
Software	SmarTrieve Compton's NewMedia (IBM); TextWare (Mac)
Start year	
Number of records	
Update period	
Price	US$129

Notes

SmarTrieve is not customised for the product so that, for instance, although there is only one database present, there is a drop-down menu which apparently should offer a choice of database presented to the user. Searching can also produce some peculiarities according to Sheldon Cheney (*CD-ROM Librarian* 7(11) p.62–64). Starting with a phrase search for 'poison ivy' produced a screen that asked, 'use 'poison ivy' as a phrase?' – this was tried twice once answered positively and once negatively with the same result. The reviewer tried searching for lyme as in Lyme disease and was met with a window message, 'Select a word to replace 'lyme', ESC to cancel' and a choice of words which could be used to replace lyme – LAAMU, LAMU, LIMA, LIME, LLAMA, LOMA, LOME or LOMWE.' A similar experience when searching for Atrovent ended in a loop where the single choice of replacement was ATTRACTS – which when selected resulted in an identical message with the choice of word again ATTRACTS. The review suggests very strongly that students need to ask the right answer to get the right question and this poor access, added to the high price being charged for a subset of another CD-ROM product, suggests the reviewer's score of three out of five is on the generous side.

14:856. CD-ROM 8cm   Quanta

File name	Prescription Drugs – A Pharmacist's Guide
Format notes	Sony, Data, Discman
Start year	
Number of records	
Update period	
Price	US$144

Principios Activos Farmacologicos Comercializados en España
Consejo General de Colegios Oficiales de Farmaceuticos de España

14:857. Master record

Database type	Textual, Factual
Number of journals	
Sources	Pharmacopoeias, Journals, Monographs and Government documents
Start year	Current information
Language	Spanish
Coverage	Spain
Number of records	6,300
Update size	–
Update period	Monthly

Keywords

Drugs; Neonatal Medicine; Obstetrics; Pharmaceuticals

Description

Information on active ingredients in drugs authorised for use in Spain, giving name, CAS Registry number, type of substance (for example, chemical compound, plant extract, microorganism), clinical action and mechanism, indications and contraindications, precautions, interactions, side effects, posological data, pharmacokinetics and notes on use during pregnancy and lactation.

Corresponds to *Diccionario de Principios Activos en España*.

14:858. Online   Ministerio de Sanidad y Consumo de Espana, Dirección General de Farmacia y Productos Sanitarios, Servicio de Gestión del Banco de Datos de Medicamentos

File name	
Start year	Current information
Number of records	6,300
Update period	Monthly

Notes

Subscription required.

Product Alert
Marketing Intelligence Service Ltd

14:859. Master record

Database type	Textual
Number of journals	1
Sources	
Start year	1988
Language	English
Coverage	USA and Canada
Number of records	16,000
Update size	–
Update period	Weekly

Keywords

Beauty Care; Consumer Products; Health Care Products; Marketing; Packaging; Pets; Product Catalogues

Description

A weekly newsletter providing descriptions of new consumer products introduced in North America. Covers packaged foods and beverages, household products, pet products and health and beauty aids. Includes product description, key ingredients, retail price, packaging information and manufacturer's name and location.

Corresponds to *Product Alert* weekly newsletter. On DIALOG and Data-Star, this newsletter is available as part of the PTS Newsletter Database, supplied by Predicast.

This database can be found on:
PTS Newsletter Database

Product Monographs
IMS AG, International Services Division

14:861. Master record

Database type	Directory, Textual
Number of journals	
Sources	Products
Start year	Current information
Language	English
Coverage	International
Number of records	230,000
Update size	–
Update period	Annually or twice per year, depending on country

Keywords

Pharmaceutical Products; Pharmaceuticals; Drugs

Description

One of the four files in IMSworld Online Service database, Product Monographs contains standardised profiles for about 230,000 pharmaceutical products marketed in 44 countries, giving international product name, brand name, packaging size and description, ingredients, formulation and strength, price, marketing company.

14:862. Online

IMS AG, International Services Division

File name	
Start year	Current information
Number of records	230,000
Update period	Annually or twice per year, depending on country

This database can also be found on:
IMSWorld Online Service

PSTA
International Food Information Service GmbH (IFIS)

14:864. Master record

Alternative name(s)	Packaging Science and Technology Abstracts
Database type	Bibliographic
Number of journals	400+
Sources	Books, conference proceedings, dissertations, grey literature, laws/regulations, patents, periodicals, standards and research reports
Start year	1976
Language	English and German (some titles and abstracts)
Coverage	International

Number of records	34,000
Update size	6,000
Update period	Every two months
Thesaurus	Thesaurus Packaging

Keywords

Marketing; Packaging; Trade

Description

PSTA covers all fields of packaging science and technology, dealing mainly with the packing of food but also other goods such as cosmetics and drugs. It contains citations on packaging from scientific, technical marketing and management literature. Subjects covered included: administration of packaging; aerosols; chemical products; closures; coating; cushioning materials; design; dosing; education; electrotechnical products; environment; filling; foods; handling; labelling; law; machine parts; marketing; materials; packaging process; pharmaceutical products; printing; production; quality control; storage; transport; wrapping. The database also incorporates records sourced from Section F Food Packaging (materials and methods) from FSTA.

The database corresponds to the printed *International Packaging Abstracts* for 1981 and *Packaging Science and Technology Abstracts* from 1982 to date. Approximately 89% of records contain documentation units of which 50% are in German, 34% in English and 5% French. 99% of records contain English abstracts and for German language literature German abstracts are added. Titles are in English and German.

Controlled terms of the *Packaging Thesaurus* have been used since 1984. The *Thesaurus* is hierarchically structured and bilingual. Controlled terms can be searched directly or through free text. Until 1982 IPAB supplied the records for the database (approximately 3,500) and from then onwards they were supplied by PSTA, each using different vocabularies. PSTA documents are assigned single-letter section codes (analogous to FSTA), PAPA documents are assigned numerical ones.

14:865. Online

CISTI, Canadian Online Enquiry Service CAN/OLE

File name	PSTA
Alternative name(s)	Packaging Science and Technology Abstracts
Start year	
Number of records	
Update period	
Price/Charges	Connect time: Canadian $40.00
	Online print: Canadian $0.13 – 0.25
	Offline print: Canadian $0.13 – 0.25

14:866. Online

DIALOG

File name	File 252
Alternative name(s)	Packaging Science and Technology Abstracts
Software	
Start year	1982
Number of records	27,917
Update period	5 times yearly
Price/Charges	Connect time: US$96.00
	Online print: US$0.70
	Offline print: US$0.70
	SDI charge: US$7.00

Notes

DIALINDEX categories: MATERIAL, PKGTECH.

14:867. Online   DIMDI

File name	PS81
Alternative name(s)	Packaging Science and Technology Abstracts
Software	GRIPS
Start year	1981
Number of records	33,934
Update period	Every two months
SDI period	2 months
Database aids	User Manual PSTA and Memocard PSTA
Price/Charges	Connect time: UK£30.78–35.52
	Online print: UK£0.31–0.48
	Offline print: UK£0.22–0.29

Downloading is allowed
Thesaurus is online

Notes

Suppliers of online documents: British Library Document Supply Centre, Boston Spa, England; Bayerische Staatsbiliothek München, München, Germany; Harkers Information Retrieval System, Sydney, Australia; Universitätsbibliothek und TIB, Hannover, Germany. Searches are possible from January 1981.

Record composition

Abstract AB; Abstractor's Initials AI; Abstract Languages AL; Additional Authors AA; Author AU; Author's Annotation AN; Corporate Author CA; Corporate Source CS; Controlled Terms CT; German Abstract ABGERM; German Controlled Terms CTGERM; Document Type DT; Entry Date ED; Freetext (Basic Index) FT; International Standard Book Number SB; ISBN SB; ISSN SS; Journal Title JT; Language LA; Document Number ND; Number of Patent NP; Number of References RN; Patent Country CP; Patent Priority PPR; Publisher PU; Publication Year PY; Section Code SC; Source SO; Subunit SU and Title TI

The unit record contains information about author(s), titles, bibliographic data, subject categories, abstracts (99%). The basic index consists of the following data fields: Title, Controlled Term, German Controlled Term, Abstract, German Abstract.

14:868. Online   ESA-IRS

File name	File 55
Alternative name(s)	Packaging Science and Technology Abstracts; PACKABS
Start year	1976
Number of records	30,200 (October 1991)
Update period	Every two months
Price/Charges	Subscription: UK£70.29
	Database entry fee: UK£3.51
	Online print: UK£0.10 – 0.67
	Offline print: UK£0.65
	SDI charge: UK£2.81

Notes

The PACKABS file is part of the IFIS QUESTCLUSTER (file number 251). The other QUESTCLUSTER component files are FSTA (File 20) and FSTA (VITIS) (File 133). QUESTORDER can be used to order original documents. The default supplier, if no supplier is specified in the ORDER ISSUE command, is Universitaetsbibliothek und TIB.

From 1993 ESA-IRS are charging an annual fee of 100 Accounting Units (c.UK£ 70.29) to all users. This is equivalent to the fee for full documentation and will not be charged to customers already paying for documentation.

Record composition

Abstract /AB; Abstract (English words) /AE; Abstract (German words) /AG; All Title Versions /TI; Author AU; Class Code CC; Controlled Terms /CT; Corporate Source CS; Document Type DT; Journal Name JN; Language LA; Language of Summary LS; Native Accession Number NN; Patent Number PN; Patent Origin PO; Publication Date PD; Publisher PB; Title (English words) /TE; Title (German words) /TG; TItle + Abstract (English words) /EN and Title + Abstract (German words) /GE

14:869. Online   GEM

File name	PSTA
Alternative name(s)	Packaging Science and Technology Abstracts
Start year	
Number of records	
Update period	

14:870. Tape   International Food Information Service GmbH (IFIS)

File name	PSTA
Alternative name(s)	Packaging Science and Technology Abstracts
Format notes	2–9 or ISO 2709 format; 6250 bpi
Start year	1976
Number of records	34,000
Update period	Every two months
Price/Charges	Subscription: DM2,900

PsycINFO
American Psychological Association

14:871. Master record

Alternative name(s)	Psychological Abstracts
Database type	Bibliographic
Number of journals	1,300
Sources	Book reviews (until 1980 only), dissertations, journals, monographs and reports
Start year	1967
Language	English and Original language (titles)
Coverage	International
Number of records	820,000
Update size	48,000
Update period	Monthly
Index unit	Book chapters, Books and articles
Abstract details	Author – edited by PsycINFO staff to house style Journal – edited by PsycINFO staff to house style PsycINFO staff
Thesaurus	Thesaurus of Psychological Index Terms 5th ed. 1988
Database aids	PsycINFO User Manual. Washington: APA, 1992, PsycINFO News (free, quarterly newsletter), Search PsycINFO: Student Workbook, Search PsycINFO: Instructor Guide and Instructional videotape: How to use PsycLIT on CD-ROM (18 minutes; US$ 65.00; VHS/U-Matic/VHS-PAL; from APA). A PsycINFO User Manual is also available by separate purchase, which covers searching on both the online PsycINFO database and the PsycLIT CD-ROM

Keywords

Clinical Psychology; Educational Psychology; Ethology; Linguistics; Neurology; Physiology; Psychometrics; Statistics

Description

PsycINFO contains citations with abstracts, compiled by the American Psychological Association, to the worldwide (from nearly fifty countries in over 25 languages) literature on psychology and the behavioural sciences. Said to be 'probably the most comprehensive source', subjects covered include: psychology, psychiatry, sociology, anthropology, education, pharmacology, physiology and linguistics and related clinical, social and biological disciplines. The database includes information on the behavioural treatment of disease, drug therapy, drug addiction, development psychology, medicine, sociology, law, educational psychology and behavioral aspects of education, as well as such fringe areas as social processes, linguistics, pharmacology, physiology, management and advertising.

The largest part of the database refers to original research, although case studies, literature reviews, surveys and conference reports are also covered. It may be possible to use a term such as 'case report' to limit a search to this kind of material, but results must be examined with some care as they may well include material on the theory of case study! Thus, PsycINFO lays most emphasis on academic and research material while, for instance, Mental Health Abstracts lays more emphasis on clinical psychology and psychiatry. While there is some duplication of records between ERIC and PsycINFO in areas such as educational psychology, a search on the same topic carried out in both files will produce far from identical results – the ERIC titles showing far more material based on practical experience in the classroom. Lengthy abstracts are provided for most documents in the database and every entry since 1984 includes one of three age identifiers: 'childhood', 'adolescence' or 'adulthood' in addition to more specific terms where appropriate. Abstracts of experimental studies include hypotheses, research methods, results and conclusions; abstracts of reviews and theoretical articles contain a statement of purpose, sources and conclusions. Approximately twenty per cent of the items – short journal articles, articles from fringe areas of psychology (such as the pharmacology of lithium with a brief discussion of its implications for the treatment of manic depression), books, book chapters, and announcements of instructional materials – include an annotation rather than an abstract, that is, a one- or two-sentence statement expanding the information found in the title and clarifying the relevance of the document. It is of value to psychologists, researchers, executives, educators and students.

From 1967 to 1979 the database corresponds to the printed *Psychological Abstracts* (first published in 1927). From 1980 onwards it contains more references than the equivalent printed publication (about twenty per cent), notably references drawn from the print *Dissertation Abstracts International*. A PSYCALERT database containing newly received materials not yet fully indexed for PsycINFO, was introduced on DIALOG, but seems to be no longer available. About 44 per cent of material is drawn from non-American sources (about thirty per cent from Europe) and English-language publications account for some ninety per cent of the database. The approximately twenty per cent of records without abstracts or annotations are documents with very explicit titles that require virtually no additional information to relay their content (for example, bibliographies). The file was reloaded on BRS, Data-Star and DIMDI in late 1992/early 1993 with a revised and enlarged classification system.

Each record contains an Index or Key Phrase, written by PsycINFO indexers, containing a brief description of the contents of the document. This phrase appears under each subject term in the Volume Index to Psychological Abstracts. The Index Phrase uses an uncontrolled vocabulary and is constructed according to established indexing rules; it should be used in conjunction with the title for high-precision searching if no subject terms are available. Phrases for experimental studies include information about: independent and dependent variables; subject population (human or animal); and publication type (where available). The subject population is described as precisely as possible including information about sex, age, educational grade, race, special characteristics, and animal type. In three cases, subjects under the age of seventeen, disordered populations and animals, the use of subject terms for subject population is mandatory. In the first case, the most specific term possible is used unless more than three terms are applicable in which case the broader term is used. The type of term used depends on whether the research is school-related or not. If it is, terms appropriate to the age group are used (for example, Preschool Students or High School Students) while for non-school related work, regardless of whether the subject are referred to by grade level, 'children terms' such as Neonates, Infants or Adolescent Mothers are used. For non-experimental articles the Index Phrase may simply be a short description statement. Although child and adolescent populations are indexed so precisely, adult populations are indexed using a wide variety of terms or not at all.

Disordered populations are indexed with a term specifying the disorder – there are two types of term: the name of the disorder (BRAIN DAMAGE) and the population term (BRAIN DAMAGED) – while some disorders are represented by both types of term, most are not. Animal populations have a descriptor for the type of animal: the broadest terms are VERTEBRATES and INVERTEBRATES. The terms HUMAN MALE and HUMAN FEMALE are used only if the sex of the subject population is significant; comparative articles use the term HUMAN SEX DIFFERENCES. The Thesaurus contains the names of many tests – specific test names are used only if the article deals with the psychometric aspect of the test. Up to four authors are included in records; where there are more than four, the term 'et al' is added. The institution of the first-named author is given in the form in which it appears in the source document; this may mean that variant forms appear. The journal title is given in full in the form that is given in the Journal Coverage List except that first words such as 'The' or 'An' are omitted.

14:872. Online   BRS

File name	PSYC
Alternative name(s)	Psychological Abstracts
Start year	1967
Number of records	820,000
Update period	Monthly
Price/Charges	Connect time: US$43.00/53.00
	Online print: US$0.39/0.47
	Offline print: US$0.22
	SDI charge: US$5.85

Notes

BRS also provides a number of saved searches listing terms relevant to concepts: Psychiatric patients/ Mental disorders (PSY1); Substance abuse (PSY2); Learning disabilities (PSY3); Communication/ Language/Speech disorders (PSY4); Racial and ethnic groups (PSY5); Tests and measurement (PSY6); Developing countries (PSY9); Mental health personnel (PSY7); and Talking therapies (PSY8) (Command '.EXEC CL(zzzz)' where zzzz equals abbreviation given above). The file was reloaded in late 1992/early 1993 with a revised and enlarged classification system. The reload features a complete map-back of the expanded PsycINFO classification system and the addition of the SpeedSearch function to several paragraphs (use, for example, PY=). The revised and expanded PsycINFO classification code system, which was mapped back on PsycINFO'2 history tapes in 1992, is now searchable throughout PsycINFO on BRS – back to 1967.

SpeedSearch, which allows accelerated searching of key paragraphs, can now be used for the update, publication year, language, single-word descriptor, human-animal tag, age-group and document type fields.

14:873. Online CompuServe Information Service

File name	PSYCINFO
Alternative name(s)	Psychological Abstracts
Start year	1967
Number of records	820,000
Update period	Monthly
Price/Charges	Subscription: US$8.95 per month
Downloading is allowed	

14:874. Online Data-Star

File name	PSYC
Alternative name(s)	Psychological Abstracts
Start year	1967
Number of records	820,000
Update period	Monthly
SDI period	Monthly
Database aids	Data-Star Biomedical Manual and Online manual (search as NEWS-PSYC in NEWS)
Price/Charges	Subscription: UK£32.00
	Connect time: UK£42.16
	Online print: UK£0.29
	Offline print: UK£0.13
	SDI charge: UK£3.36

Notes

It is possible to search for documents NOT in the print version with 'DBO.AN.' and publication types may be searched by either PT=10 or PT=J both meaning journal; the complete list is given in the online guide. Descriptor codes (SC) are synonyms for the terms in the DE field and are not the same as classification codes. American spellings are used in all except Title and Institution fields where either English or American spelling may be used. Data-Star also provides a number of saved searches listing terms relevant to concepts: Psychiatric patients/Mental disorders (MDIS); Substance abuse (ABUS); Learning disabilities (LDIS); Communication/Language/Speech disorders (CDIS); Racial and ethnic groups (RACE); Tests and measurement (TEST); Developing countries (WRLD); Mental health personnel (MHPR); and Talking therapies (THRP) (Command '.EXEC CL=zzzz' where zzzz equals abbreviation given above). The file was reloaded in late 1992/early 1993 with a revised and enlarged classification system.

From June 1993 Data-Star have introduced an annual fee/subscription per contract (that is, not per password) of SFr 80.00 (c.UK£ 32.00) payable every June. For North American customers billed in dollars who also use DIALOG, the DIALOG fee also covers access to Data-Star. Academic customers, 'commitment' customers and customers currently billed in dollars are exempt.

Record composition

Accession Number AN; Update Code AN; PsycINFO Entry Date ED; Author Names AU; Institution IN; Title TI; Source SO; ISBN or ISSN IS; Language LG; Year of Publication YR; Classification Codes CC; Publication Type PT; Descriptors DE; Major Descriptors (included in DE) MJ; Minor Descriptors (included in DE) MN; Age AG (as, for instance, 'ELDERLY.AG.' but limit as 'ELDER=Y'); Abstract AB; Key Phrase ID; Descriptor Codes SC; Entry Date ED (Limit only); Human H (Limit only – as 'H=Y'); Update Month UP (Limit only) and Update Date UD (Limit only)

14:875. Online DIALOG, Knowledge Index

File name	File 11
Alternative name(s)	Psychological Abstracts
Start year	1967
Number of records	814,843
Update period	Monthly
Price/Charges	Connect time: US$55.00
	Online print: US$0.35
	Offline print: US$0.20
	SDI charge: US$5.95
Thesaurus is online	

Notes

This database is also available to home users during evenings and weekends at a reduced rate on the Knowledge Index service of DIALOG – file name in this case is PsycINFO, and searches are made with simplified commands or menus.

As on other hosts, every entry since 1984 includes one of three age identifiers: 'childhood', 'adolescence' or 'adulthood' in addition to more specific terms where appropriate, but searching for populations on DIALOG is further simplified since the 1990 introduction of of the age group prefix (AG=) which automatically collects together materials, however indexed, in the groupings 'child', 'adolescent', 'adult' and 'elderly' (the latter being a subset of 'adult') DIALOG also provides a number of saved searches listing terms relevant to concepts: Psychiatric patients/Mental disorders (MDIS); Substance abuse (ABUSE); Learning disabilities (LDIS); Communication/Language/Speech disorders (CDIS); Racial and ethnic groups (RACE); Tests and measurement (TEST); Developing countries (WORLD); Mental health personnel (MHPRS); and Talking therapies (THRPY) (Command 'EXS SBzzzz/USER 3471' where zzzz equals abbreviation given above).

In one study (Nahl-Jakobovits and Carol Tenopir. Databases Online and on CD-ROM: How do they compare, let us count the ways. *Database* February 1992 42–50), about seventeen per cent of records retrieved were unique to DIALOG as compared with the PsycLIT CD-ROM; while some of these were due to entry date anomalies, most were due to the inclusion of dissertations which PsycLIT does not presently include.

DIALINDEX Categories: EDUCAT, LANGUAGE, PSYCH, SOCSCI.

14:876. Online DIMDI

File name	PI67
Alternative name(s)	Psychological Abstracts

Start year	1967
Number of records	849,976
Update period	Monthly
SDI period	1 month
Database aids	PsycINFO User Manual, Memocard and DIMDI PsycINFO chapter
Price/Charges	Connect time: UK£12.65–17.39
	Online print: UK£0.33–0.51
	Offline print: UK£0.10–0.17
	SDI charge: UK£0.60

Downloading is allowed

Notes

Menu driven user guidance is available in German and English. 80% of the records contain abstracts. The unit record contains information about author(s), title and other bibliographic data, as well as controlled vocabulary. Searches are possible from January 1967.

Record composition

Abstract AB; Author AU; Controlled Term Code CC; Corporate Source CS; Controlled Term CT; Document Type DT; Document Type Code DTC; Entry Date ED (Search only); Journal Title JT; Language LA; Number of Document ND; Preferred Qualifier PQ; Publication Year PY; Section Code SC; Section Heading SH; Source SO (Display only); ISSN SS; Title TI and Uncontrolled Terms UT

The content of the *Thesaurus of Psychological Index Terms* has been translated into German by the Zentralstelle für psychologische Information und Dokumentation (ZPID): *PSYNDEX Terms, Deskriptoren/Subject Terms zur Datenbank PSYNDEX*. The command 'DISPLAY PPS=?' will show a list of all currently available preprocessed searches which can be included in a search (for example, 'FIND HYPNOTHERAPY AND PPS=CANCER'). The hierarchical nature of the online thesaurus may be exploited to broaden a search and it is recommended as the most specific terms possible are used in the indexing: 'FIND CT=PSYCHOTHERAPY' will only access records indexed using that terms while 'FIND CT DOWN PSYCHOTHERAPY' will access this term plus all records containing one of its 32 narrower terms for specific types of therapy. Controlled Terms (CT) and Section Headings (SH) equivalent to the Content Classification Categories are taken from the Thesaurus of Psychological Index Terms while uncontrolled terms (UT) are short English phrases describing the contents of the document. Free-text searching includes the abstract, controlled term, section heading, title and uncontrolled term fields. The Corporate Source (CS) of the first-named author is given in the form in which it appears in the source document; this may mean that variant forms arise but the field is searchable word by word and not as a phrase. Conversely, the Journal Title (JT) field is indexed as a phrase so that front-end truncation is recommended to deal with names forms such as 'The Journal of . . .'. Languages may be searched as four-letter codes or written in full. Section Headings (SH), which correspond to the Content Classification Categories of the Thesaurus are indexed as phrases and by the individual words of the phrase; DOWN, UP and TREE may be used with the DISPLAY command to show the headings together with their broader and narrower categories as well as their corresponding Section Codes (SC). Titles (TI) and Uncontrolled Terms (UT) are indexed by individual words and thus form a part of the basic index. The file was reloaded in late 1992/early 1993 with a revised and enlarged classification system.

14:877. Online   OCLC EPIC

File name	File 3
Alternative name(s)	Psychological Abstracts
Start year	
Number of records	
Update period	

14:878. Online   OCLC FirstSearch

File name	PsycFIRST
Alternative name(s)	Psychological Abstracts
Start year	1989
Number of records	
Update period	

Notes

Latest three year subset.

14:879. Online   Tech Data

File name	PsycINFO
Alternative name(s)	Psychological Abstracts
Start year	1967
Number of records	820,000
Update period	Monthly

14:880. Online   University of Tsukuba

File name	PsycINFO
Alternative name(s)	Psychological Abstracts
Start year	
Number of records	
Update period	

Notes

Access limited to affiliates of the University of Japan.

14:881. CD-ROM   SilverPlatter

File name	PsycLIT
Alternative name(s)	Psychological Abstracts
Format notes	Mac, IBM
Software	SPIRS/MacSPIRS
Start year	1974 journals; 1987 books
Number of records	570,000
Update period	Quarterly
Delay	2–4 months
Database aids	Instructional videotape: How to use PsycLIT on CD-ROM (18 minutes; US$ 65.00; VHS/U-Matic/VHS-PAL; from APA). A PsycINFO User Manual is also available by separate purchase, which covers searching on both the online PsycINFO database and the PsycLIT CD-ROM
Price/Charges	Subscription: UK£2,460 – 3,690
Thesaurus is online	

Notes

PsycLIT on SilverPlatter, the CD-ROM version of PsycINFO online, holds citations with abstracts to over 1,300 journals in psychology and the behavioural sciences, plus book chapters and book records. A function called HOTLINKS allows users to toggle between chapters in the same book, or between chapters and their parent book. Full book records will include a complete table of contents, a summary of the book's general contents and complete bibliographic information including the ISBN. Archival disc covers the years 1974 to 1986 and the current disc covers 1987 to present day.

In one study about five per cent of records retrieved were unique to the CD-ROM as compared with the DIALOG implementation; however this was generally due to the inclusion on the current disc of articles from outside the label time period and therefore excluded from the DIALOG search. The PsycLIT CD-ROM does not presently include references to dissertations and this accounted for many of the unique DIALOG records. Users should also be aware that according to Nahl-Jakobovits and Carol Tenopir (Databases Online and on CD-ROM: How do they compare, let us count the ways. *Database* February 1992 42–50), 'for PsycLIT it takes four years to enter all the documents of a given publication year into the database. Searchers should be aware that the most current date on the disc label does not mean that all (or even most) of the articles published during that year are on the disc.' According to the database producer who responded to this statement via the editor, the majority of publications enter the database within a range of three to 23 months, with the average being twelve months. Péter Jacsó made the point that the publisher enters records every month onto the database as can be seen from the UD= field, however, this is the date of entry not the date of publication. As the CD-ROM is updated every three months and there is then a production/delivery time lag, the real time-lag for users is two to four months after the date in the UD= field plus the unknown lag between date of publication and date of entry. Journal coverage is from 1974 to the present, and book chapter and book coverage from 1987.

Includes *The Thesaurus of Psychological Index Terms* on disc and a separate tutorial (there are two discs for PsycLIT).

There are differential prices for Psychological Abstracts print subscribers. The regular subscription (with the archival disc) for non-subscribers to PA is UK£2,950 for single users and £4,425 for 2–8 networked users; for PA subscribers the prices (with archival disc) are £2,460 for single users and £3,690 for 2–8 networked users.

14:882. Fixed disk   SilverPlatter

File name	PsycINFO
Alternative name(s)	Psychological Abstracts
Format notes	IBM
Software	SPIRS
Start year	1984
Number of records	
Update period	Monthly
Delay	2–4 months
Database aids	Instructional videotape: How to use PsycLIT on CD-ROM (18 minutes; US$ 65.00; VHS/U-Matic/VHS-PAL; from APA). A PsycINFO User Manual is available by separate purchase, which covers searching on both the online PsycINFO database and the PsycLIT CD-ROM
Price/Charges	Subscription: UK£4,463 – 19,688
Thesaurus is online	

Notes

This database is available only on fixed disk, covering 1984 onwards, with updates supplied on CD-ROM. This means that up to thirty networked users can have access to a single file containing the complete database from 1984. Search speeds are up to ten times faster than CD-ROM searching. Includes *The Thesaurus of Psychological Index Terms* and a separate tutorial.

There are differential costs for subscribers and non-subscribers to Psychological Abstracts: prices are, for PA subscribers – 8 users UK£4,463, 12 users £6,694, 15 users £8,367, 20 users £11,648 and 30 users £18,211. For non-subscribers to PA prices are; for 8 users £5,250, for 12 users £7,875, for 15 users £9,844, for 20 users £13,125 and for 30 users £19,688. There is also a backfile available on hard disk, from 1967–1983.

14:883. Fixed disk   SilverPlatter

File name	PsycINFO
Alternative name(s)	Psychological Abstracts
Format notes	IBM
Software	SPIRS
Start year	1967–1983
Number of records	
Update period	Not updated
Delay	2–4 months
Database aids	Instructional videotape: How to use PsycLIT on CD-ROM (18 minutes; US$ 65.00; VHS/U-Matic/VHS-PAL; from APA). A PsycINFO User Manual is available by separate purchase, which covers searching on both the online PsycINFO database and the PsycLIT CD-ROM
Price/Charges	Subscription: US$10,000
Thesaurus is online	

Notes

This is the backfile of PsycINFO, available only on fixed disk, covering 1967 to 1983, available as a one-time purchase from SilverPlatter. Up to thirty networked users can have access to a single file containing all of the records for those years. Search speeds are up to ten times faster than CD-ROM searching. Includes *The Thesaurus of Psychological Index Terms* and a separate tutorial. One-time charge for the backfile is US$10,000. There is also a current fixed disc available, covering 1984 to the present.

14:884. Tape   American Psychological Association

File name	PsycINFO
Alternative name(s)	Psychological Abstracts
Start year	1984
Number of records	820,000
Update period	Monthly
Price/Charges	Subscription: US$12,500

Notes

A backfile tape (1967–1983) is available for a one-time fee of US$ 10,000.

14:885. Database subset

Online   DIALOG, Knowledge Index

File name	File 212 – ONTAP PsycINFO Training File
Alternative name(s)	Psychological Abstracts
Start year	January to December 1987
Number of records	43,605
Update period	Closed File
Price/Charges	Connect time: US$15.00

Notes

This is the low cost training file containing records from 1987 of File 11, the main PsycINFO file from DIALOG. Offline prints are not available in ONTAP files.

PsyComNet
PsyComNet

14:886. Master record

Database type	Bibliographic
Number of journals	
Sources	
Start year	1960
Language	English
Coverage	USA

Number of records
Update size —
Update period Annually

Keywords

Mental Health; Psychopharmacology; Neuro-psychology; Child Psychiatry

Description

Citations to published literature on mental health and related topics, including psychiatry, psychopharmacology, neuropsychology and child psychiatry. Also offers online conferencing and electronic mail facilities.

14:887. Online   PsyComNet

File name
Start year 1960
Number of records
Update period Annually

PTS Newsletter Database

Predicasts International Inc

14:888. Master record

Alternative name(s)	Predicasts Newsletter Database
Database type	Textual
Number of journals	
Sources	
Start year	1988
Language	German and English
Coverage	International
Number of records	722,656
Update size	63,000
Update period	Daily
Database aids	PTS Users Manual, Cleveland, Ohio, Predicasts
Hosts have included	CORIS (Thomson Financial Network) (Until 1/92)

Keywords

Acid Rain; Advertising; Air Pollution; Alcohol Abuse; Antiviral Drugs; Asbestos; Asbestosis; Automation and Control; Beauty Care; Beauty Care; Beverages; Biotechnology; Biotechnology Industries; Brewing; Cancer; Ceramics; Chemical Industry; Chromatography; Composites; Computer Data Security; Computer Ergonomics; Company Profiles; Consumer Products; Cosmetics; Data Security; Defence Waste Disposal; Diagnosis; Diagnostic Equipment; Diagnostic Products; Drug Abuse; Drug Treatment; Drugs; Education – Cancer; Electrodialysis; Employee Benefits; Environmental Policy; Ergonomics; Explosion; Filtration; Fire; Food and Drink; Food Additives; Food Processing; Food Technology; Genetic Engineering; Greenhouse Effect; Hazardous Chemicals; Hazardous Substances; Hazardous Substances Transport; Hazardous Waste; Health and Safety; Health Care; Health Care Management; Health Care Products; Health Insurance; Health Services; HIV; Household Products; Hygiene Products; Information Services; Information Systems; Legal Liability; Legislation; Liability Insurance; Manufacturing; Marketing; Market Reports; Materials Industry; Medicare; Medical Equipment; Medical Textiles; Medical Waste Management; Membrane Technology; Metals; Nuclear Waste; Occupational Health and Safety; Packaging; Patents; Personal Hygiene; Pesticides; Pets; Pharmaceutical Industry; Pharmaceutical Products; Pharmaceuticals; Pollution; Polymers; Product Catalogues; Product Liability; Prosthetics; Public Health; Radiation; Research and Development; Separation Technology; Smoking; Standards; Textiles; Waste Management; Water Pollution; Water Purification

Description

Produced by Predicasts, PTS Newsletter is a multi-industry database providing concise information on company activities, new technologies, emerging industry trends, government regulations and international trade opportunities. It consists of the full text of over 500 business and industry newsletters covering almost fifty different industries and subject areas. It is international in scope, covering all major economic and political regions of the world, including Eastern and Western Europe, the USA, the Pacific Rim, Latin America, Asia and the Middle East. Facts, figures and analyses are provided on the following industrial and geographical areas: advanced materials, biotechnology, broadcasting and publishing, computers and electronics, chemicals, defense and aerospace, energy, environment, financial services and markets, instrumentation, international trade, general technology, Japan, Middle East, manufacturing, medical and health, materials packaging, research and development, telecommunications and transportation.

Newsletters include *Multinational Service* which covers decisions and policies affecting corporations operating worldwide; and *Europe Report* which offers broad coverage of EC activities relating to economic and monetary affairs, the internal market and legislation and regulations relating to business. Both Newsletters are published by the Europe Information Service of Cooper's & Lybrand Europe. Middle East coverage includes the *Israel High-Tech Report*; *The Middle East News Network*; and *The Middle East Consultants' Newsletter*.

14:889. Online   Data-Star

File name	PTBN
Alternative name(s)	Predicasts Newsletter Database
Start year	January 1988
Number of records	533,000
Update period	Weekly
Database aids	Data-Star Business Manual, Berne and Online manual (search for NEWS-PTBN in NEWS)
Price/Charges	Subscription: UK£32.00
	Connect time: UK£80.40
	Online print: UK£0.28 – 0.55
	Offline print: UK£0.26 – 1.00
	SDI charge: UK£4.00

Also available on FIZ Technik via a gateway from Data-Star

Notes

From June 1993 Data-Star have introduced an annual fee/subscription per contract (that is, not per password) of SFr 80.00 (c.UK£ 32.00) payable every June. For North American customers billed in dollars who also use DIALOG, the DIALOG fee also covers access to Data-Star. Academic customers, 'commitment' customers and customers currently billed in dollars are exempt.

14:890. Online   DIALOG

File name	PTSNL
Alternative name(s)	Predicasts Newsletter Database
Start year	1989
Number of records	722,656
Update period	Daily
Price/Charges	Connect time: US$126.00
	Online print: US$0.90

Notes

PTSNL is a menu-access version of the PTS Newsletter Database. PTSNL provides users with the unique capability to easily retrieve the latest issue (or any available issue) of a newsletter, display a Table of Contents listing articles contained in a selected issue, and print the full text of newsletter articles selected by title. To search newsletters for information on specific subjects, use File 636 (the main PTS file), which utilizes the full range of DIALOG search commands.

14:891. Online   DIALOG

File name	File 636
Alternative name(s)	Predicasts Newsletter Database
Start year	1989
Number of records	722,656
Update period	Daily
Price/Charges	Connect time: US$126.00
	Online print: US$0.90
	Offline print: US$0.90
	SDI charge: US$1.00 (daily) – 3.00 (weekly)

Notes

This is the main file of PTS on DIALOG. There is also a menu access version – PTSNL, which enables the user to retrieve the latest issue of a newsletter, print the full text of newspaper articles, etc. It does not have the full range of DIALOG search commands.

14:892. Online   Dow Jones News/Retrieval

File name	
Alternative name(s)	Predicasts Newsletter Database
Start year	
Number of records	
Update period	Weekly

14:893. Online   FIZ Technik (gateway)

File name	PTBN
Alternative name(s)	Predicasts Newsletter Database
Start year	1988 (January)
Number of records	Volume 1: 159,000
Update period	Weekly
Price/Charges	Connect time: SFr201.00
	Online print: SFr0.61 – 1.22
	Offline print: SFr0.24 – 1.83
	SDI charge: SFr10.00

Available via a gateway to Data-Star

For more details of constituent databases, see:
AIDS Weekly
Air/Water Pollution Report
Alliance Alert – Medical Health
Antiviral Agents Bulletin
Applied Genetics News
Asbestos Control Report
BBI Newsletter
Biomedical Materials
Biomedical Polymers
Cancer Weekly
Cosmetic Insiders' Report
Diagnostics Business-Matters
Environment Week
European Cosmetic Markets
FDA Medical Bulletin
Food Chemical News
Genetic Technology News
Hazmat Transport News
Health Business
Health Daily
Industrial Health and Hazards Update
International Product Alert
Japan Report: Medical Technology
Japan Science Scan
Managed Care Law Outlook

Managed Care Outlook
Managed Care Report
Medical Bulletin
Medical Scan
Medical Waste News
Medical Textiles
Membrane and Separation Technology News
National Report on Computers and Health
Nuclear Waste News
Occupational Health and Safety Letter
OTC Market Report: Update USA
OTC News and Market Report
Pesticide and Toxic Chemical News
Pharmaceutical Business News
Product Alert
PRODUCTSCAN
Report on Defense Plant Wastes
Soviet Bio/Medical Report
Toxic Materials News
Worldwide Biotech

R&D Focus
IMSWorld Publications Ltd

14:896. Master record

Database type	Factual, Textual
Number of journals	
Sources	Newsletter
Start year	1992
Language	English
Coverage	International
Number of records	
Update size	2,200
Update period	Monthly

Keywords

Drugs; Pharmaceuticals

Description

The database monitors drugs from their earliest laboratory or patent report through to their entry onto the marketplace. Provides comprehensive details of each drug's development, including substance and property data, latest news, company and country information, and a summarised table of events. Incorporating Drug License Opportunities, the database consists of five sections: Drug Updates – a monthly service providing a review of new and existing drugs; Drug News – a quick alert news service. A weekly newsletter reports new developments on companies, drugs and healthcare institutions around the world; Meetings Diary – a monthly listing of forthcoming major meetings concentrating on scientific topics; Drug Abstracts – a monthly service which highlights the best scientific literature; and Cumulative Indexes – monthly cumulative indexes enable all information to be accessed by product, therapeutic class or company.

14:897. CD-ROM   IMSWorld Publications Ltd

File name	
Format notes	IBM
Software	Clearview
Start year	1992
Number of records	
Update period	Monthly
Price/Charges	Subscription: UK£3,650

14:898. Database subset

Online	Data-Star
File name	IPMR – IMSWorld R&D Focus Meetings Diary
Start year	Current and future
Number of records	
Update period	Monthly
Database aids	Data-Star Guide to IPMR in Data-Star Business Manual and Data-Star Online Guide in BASE database (search BASE-IPMR)
Price/Charges	Subscription: SFr80.00
	Connect time: SFr152.60
	Online print: SFr1.68
	Offline print: SFr1.96

Downloading is allowed

Notes

Imsworld R&D Focus Meetings Diary contains Imsworld's Medical and Pharmaceutical Meetings Diary which is part of R&D Focus. The database provides international coverage of forthcoming meetings up to the year 2000 likely to be of interest to the pharmaceutical industry. Meetings selected for inclusion are oriented towards biomedical subjects and research and development in these areas. The database is of value to those interested in attending pharma-related meetings, presenting research papers, sponsorship or using company representation at such meetings as part of a promotional campaign. Meetings are classified by therapy areas, utilising the top-level (1-digit) EPhMRA coding. Details of conference name, location, date and contact address, telephone and fax numbers where available are given for each meeting. Each month newly-announced meetings are added and past ones deleted. The database is compiled from a variety of national and international medical, pharmaceutical and information sources including announcements in journals, press releases, trade papers, conference organisers and professional associations. The database is the first of three elements of IMSWorld's R&D Focus service. The other two are the weekly service Drug News and the monthly service of Drug Updates combined with Drug Abstracts. Together these databases provided detailed and timely information on drugs in development worldwide, from earliest laboratory reports through to market.

From June 1993 Data-Star have introduced an annual fee/subscription per contract (that is, not per password) of SFr 80.00 (c.UK£ 32.00) payable every June. For North American customers billed in dollars who also use DIALOG, the DIALOG fee also covers access to Data-Star. Academic customers, 'commitment' customers and customers currently billed in dollars are exempt.

Record composition

Accession number and update code AN; Contact name/address CT; Country name (in LO) CN; Date(s) of meeting DT; Entry date (first listed) (YYMM) ED; Location LO; Publication date (YYMM) PD; Source SO; Telecommunications TL; Therapeutic class codes CC; Title of meeting TI; Update (YYMMDD) UD; Update (YYMM) UP and Year of meeting (YY) YR

The command DOCZ can be used at any time to retrieve the total number of records currently in the database. Data in IPMR is gathered from sources in many countries therefore English/American spelling and word differences may appear in the title paragraph. For example it is necessary to try PEDIATRICS and PAEDIATRICS, ANAESTHETICS and ANES-THESIOLOGY to ensure complete retrieval. The command .ROOT CC can be used at any time in IPMR to see a complete list of the therapeutic class coding for future meetings, and print out the titles of all meetings in a particular field.

Radiolab
Georg Thieme Verlag

14:899. Master record

Database type	
Number of journals	
Sources	
Start year	
Language	German
Coverage	Germany
Number of records	
Update size	–
Update period	Annually

Keywords

Drugs; Drug Therapy; Gynaecology; Internal Medicine; Medical Diagnosis; Rheumatology; Urology

Description

This database enables the user to enter signs and symptoms and the program will then find the corresponding diseases. Full text descriptions of the diseases are available.

This database can be found on:
DIAGNOSIS, Vergiftungen, Radiolab

Reisemedizin

14:901. Master record

Database type	Textual, Factual
Number of journals	
Sources	
Start year	
Language	German
Coverage	Switzerland
Number of records	
Update size	–
Update period	
Hosts have included	AEK (AerzteKasse)

Keywords

Drugs; Pharmaceuticals; Surgery

Description

This is one of ten databases in the medical and pharmaceutical fields on the MediROM database. It is possible to establish logical links between the data of some of the databases.

This database can be found on:
MediROM (AEK)

Reprorisk
Micromedex Inc

14:903. Master record

Alternative name(s)	CCIS: Reprorisk; Computerized Clinical Information System: Reprorisk; Reproductive Risk Information System
Database type	Bibliographic, Textual
Number of journals	
Sources	

Start year	1990
Language	English
Coverage	International
Number of records	
Update size	—
Update period	Quarterly

Keywords

Drugs; Gynaecology; Pregnancy; Teratology

Description

Reprorisk (Teratogen Information System) is developed by the University of Washington in Seattle, Reproductive Risk Information System. Contains several modules addressing the reproductive risk of drugs, chemicals, and physical and environmental agents for females and males. Currently includes the Teratogen Information System (TERIS) developed by the University of Washington which addresses the teratogenicity of over seven hundred drugs and environmental agents that affect the unborn child. Also includes Shepard's *Catalogue of Teratogen Agents* and Reprotext.

14:904. CD-ROM   Micromedex Inc

File name	Reprorisk
Alternative name(s)	CCIS: Reprorisk; Computerized Clinical Information System: Reprorisk; Reproductive Risk Information System
Start year	1990
Number of records	
Update period	Quarterly

Notes

This database is available as a standalone product, as well as being a part of CCIS, Computerized Clinical Information System.

For more details of constituent databases, see:
TERIS – Teratogen Information System
Shepard's Catalogue of Teratogen Agents
Reprotext

This database can also be found on:
CCIS
TOMES Plus

Reprotext
Micromedex Inc

14:907. Master record

Database type	Bibliographic, Textual
Number of journals	
Sources	
Start year	1990
Language	English
Coverage	International
Number of records	
Update size	—
Update period	Quarterly

Description

Part of the Reprorisk database, a supplementary product of the Computerized Clinical Information System (CCIS) from Micromedex, which contains several modules addressing the reproductive risk of drugs, chemicals, and physical and environmental agents for females and males.

This database can be found on:
Reprorisk

Rote Liste
Bundesverband der Pharmazeutischen Industrie eV

14.910. Master record

Database type	
Number of journals	
Sources	
Start year	
Language	German
Coverage	Germany
Number of records	
Update size	—
Update period	

Keywords

Drugs; Pharmaceuticals

Description

One of the databases on the CD-ROM Lauer Mobi-med 3 plus

This database can be found on:
Lauer Mobi-med 3 plus.
CD-ROM Vidal

Scientific American Medicine
Scientific American Inc

14:912. Master record

Alternative name(s)	SAM
Database type	Textual
Number of journals	
Sources	Original material
Start year	Current information
Language	English
Coverage	International
Number of records	
Update size	—
Update period	Monthly

Keywords

Cardiovascular Medicine; Dermatology; Endocrinology; Gastroenterology; Haematology; Immunology; Infectious Diseases; Interdisciplinary Medicine; Internal Medicine; Metabolism; Nephrology; Neurology; Oncology; Respiratory Medicine; Rheumatology

Description

Information for physicians and medical researchers on developments in cardiovascular medicine, dermatology, endocrinology, gastroenterology, haematology, immunology, infectious diseases, interdisciplinary medicine, metabolism, nephrology, neurology, oncology, psychiatry, respiratory medicine and rheumatology. Provides general information on diagnoses, treatments, drug dosages and laboratory values, with summary articles on current medical topics.

Corresponds to *Scientific American Medicine*, a loose-leaf medical text written and edited by leading authorities in internal medicine.

14:913. Online — BRS Online Service, Morning Search, BRS/Colleague

File name	SAMM
Alternative name(s)	SAM
Start year	Current information
Number of records	
Update period	Monthly
Price/Charges	Connect time: US$41.00/51.00
	Online print: US$0.91/0.99
	Offline print: US$0.73

This database can also be found on:
Consult Scientific American Medicine

Scottish Poisons Information Bureau

Royal Infirmary, The Scottish Poisons Information Bureau

14:915. Master record

Database type	Bibliographic, Textual, Factual
Number of journals	
Sources	
Start year	
Language	English
Coverage	
Number of records	10,000
Update size	—
Update period	Irregular

Keywords

Biochemistry

Description

The database contains information on ingredients, toxicity, features and treatment of poisonings for about 10,000 products – drugs, household products, plants, pesticides, chemicals and toiletries. It also contains recent references to clinical toxicology literature.

14:916. Online — Royal Infirmary

File name	SPIB
Start year	
Number of records	10,000
Update period	Irregular

SCRIPTEL

Taylor Nelson Medical

14:917. Master record

Database type	Statistical
Number of journals	
Sources	
Start year	1983
Language	English
Coverage	
Number of records	3,000
Update size	—
Update period	Twice a month

Keywords

Drugs; Marketing

Description

Data, in time series format, on the volume of 3000 prescription drugs dispensed by 300 chemists participating in the survey. Data are stored as grossed four weekly figures in intervals of two weeks.
Corresponds to *Scriptcount 300*.

14:918. Online — Taylor Nelson Medical

File name	SCRIPTEL
Start year	1983
Number of records	
Update period	Twice a month

SEDBASE

Elsevier Science Publishers

14:919. Master record

Alternative name(s)	Meyler's Side Effects of Drugs Database
Database type	Textual, Factual
Number of journals	4,500
Sources	Journals and Books
Start year	Current
Language	English
Coverage	International
Number of records	56,000
Update size	—
Update period	Quarterly
Index unit	Articles
Database aids	SEDBASE User Manual, Amsterdam, Elsevier Science Publishers, 1989

Keywords

Drugs; Pharmaceuticals

Description

SEDBASE is a highly specialised full-text online database that critically analyses the published drug side effect literature on drugs currently in use, giving synopses of clinically relevant drug reactions and interactions reported in the international literature. Some 9,000 articles on adverse drug reactions are published in the scientific literature each year. The goal in SEDBASE is to document every drug known to have a side effect reported in the literature. These articles are identified and collected for SEDBASE from 4,500 journals published in 110 countries using the resources of the Excerpta Medica database, EMBASE. All articles are sent to the recognised authorities who critically assess the information and distill the key elements for inclusion. SEDBASE does not include speculative or unsubstantiated statements on the side effects of ethical drugs. SEDBASE contains data on all drugs used in medical therapy. These data are indexed for side effects and drug names.

SEDBASE is organised by drug class chapters and specific subjects covered include: adverse drug reactions, drug interactions, drug toxicity, special risk situations, and pharmacological or patient-dependent factors associated with the occurrence of side-effects. SEDBASE contains five different record types:

(1)   text records from *Meyler's Side Effects of Drugs*;
(2)   Text records from *Side Effects of Drugs Annuals* (SEDA);
(3)   new SEDBASE texts which are not yet published in the book series;
(4)   9,000 EMBASE citations (mostly with an abstract); and
(5)   book references. SEDBASE acts as a quality filter since its drug class chapters are prepared by recognized authorities.

Sources: SEDBASE is derived from full text, current

1133

information from the last twelve years of: *Meyler's Side Effects of Drugs* (published every 4 years), an encyclopaedia of drug adverse effects and interactions which is widely used all over the world as the standard reference tool in that field; *Side Effects of Drugs Annual* (published every year in between); and *Marler's Pharmacological and Chemical Synonyms*.

A SEDBASE record consists of two parts, the first part comprises a text or reference and the second an indexing part listing the drugs (drug name, interacting drug name) and the side effects discussed in the text/reference. The indexing part consists of one or more SED-indexing-data-blocks describing all the side effects for a given drug or drug combination. The Title field contains name, class number and synonyms for the specific drug, its side effects and any interacting drug. Synonyms are searched using title but are displayed in the synonym paragraph. Class numbers should be used to retrieve whole categories of side effects or drugs. The full classification lists are available from Elsevier Science Publishers.

14:920. Online   BRS

File name	SEDB
Alternative name(s)	Meyler's Side Effects of Drugs Database
Start year	Current
Number of records	56,000
Update period	Quarterly

14:921. Online   Data-Star

File name	SEDB
Alternative name(s)	Meyler's Side Effects of Drugs Database
Start year	Current
Number of records	56,000
Update period	Every three months
Database aids	Data-Star Biomedical Manual, Berne, Data-Star, 1989 and Online manual (search NEWS-SEDB in NEWS)
Price/Charges	Subscription: SFr80.00
	Connect time: SFr135.00
	Online print: SFr5.83
	Offline print: SFr5.71
	SDI charge: Not applicable
Downloading is allowed	

Notes

From June 1993 Data-Star have introduced an annual fee/subscription per contract (that is, not per password) of SFr 80.00 (c.UK£ 32.00) payable every June. For North American customers billed in dollars who also use DIALOG, the DIALOG fee also covers access to Data-Star. Academic customers, 'commitment' customers and customers currently billed in dollars are exempt.

Record composition

Accession Number and Update Code AN; Cited reference from EMBASE CR; Complementary texts from Annuals and previous editions of Meyler T2; Source Statement (display only) SO; Synonyms (display only) SY; Superlabel for T1 and T2 TX; Text from latest edition of 'Meyler's Side Effects of Drugs' T1; Title TI and Update Code UP

14:922. Online   DIALOG

File name	File 70
Alternative name(s)	Meyler's Side Effects of Drugs Database
Start year	Current
Number of records	54,040
Update period	Quarterly reloads

Price/Charges	Connect time: US$90.00
	Online print: US$4.50
	Offline print: US$4.50
Downloading is allowed	

Notes

DIALINDEX Categories: DRUGDIR, PHARM, PHARMR, TOXICOL.

14:923. Online   DIMDI

File name	SD00
Alternative name(s)	Meyler's Side Effects of Drugs Database
Start year	Current
Number of records	56,000
Update period	Quarterly
Price/Charges	
Downloading is allowed	

Record composition

Abstract AB; Author AU; Book Chapter BCH; Book Title BTI; Classification CC; Coden CO; Cross Reference CREF; Corporate Source CS; Country CY; Drug Name DN; Drug Synonym DNS; Editor EDR; Effect Name EFF; Effect Synonym EFFS; Factors of Influence FI; Interacting Drug IDN; Interacting Drug Name Synonym IDNS; Journal Title JT; Language LA; Number of Document ND; Number of Document Embase; Pagination PG; Publisher PU; Publication Year PY; Secondary Source SEC; Source SO; Special Factors FA; Terminology TE; Text TEXT and Title TI

The basic index (FT) comprises Abstract, Book Chapter, Book Title, Cross Reference, Drug Name, Drug Synonym, Effect Name, Effect Synonym, Factors of Influence, Interacting Drug, Interacting Drug Name Synonym, Text and Title. The terminology sections are: Drug Name, Drug Synonym, Interacting Drug and Interacting Drug Name Synonym. To limit the search terms to the same side-effects-of-drugs-indexing-datablock, the qualifier /SAME GROUP is used; to limit the SHOW to only those fields containing the search terms, the following search has to be performed in addition: FIND GROUP WHERE <Table Number>.

14:924. CD-ROM   SilverPlatter

File name	Meyler's Side Effects of Drugs Database
Alternative name(s)	Meyler's Side Effects of Drugs Database
Format notes	IBM, Mac
Software	SPIRS
Start year	
Number of records	44,000
Update period	Twice a year
Price/Charges	Subscription: UK£755 – 1,132

Notes

Regular subscriptions are £755 for single users and £1,132 for 2–8 networked users.

This database can also be found on:
Logo-A Pharmaceutical Products (Discontinued)

Shepard's Catalogue of Teratogen Agents
Micromedex Inc

14:926. Master record

Database type	Bibliographic, Textual
Number of journals	
Sources	

Start year	1990
Language	English
Coverage	International
Number of records	
Update size	–
Update period	Quarterly

Description
Part of the Reprorisk database, a supplementary product of the Computerized Clinical Information System (CCIS) from Micromedex, which contains several modules addressing the reproductive risk of drugs, chemicals, and physical and environmental agents for females and males.

This database can be found on:
Reprorisk

Slcalc
Micromedex Inc

14:928. Master record

Database type	Factual
Number of journals	
Sources	
Start year	
Language	
Coverage	
Number of records	
Update size	–
Update period	Quarterly

Description
Slcalc interconverts S.I. units and traditional units. Le Système International D'Unites (S.I. Units) is a system of measurement for laboratory values (clinical chemistry and drug concentrations) in molar units. Traditional units are measured in mass units (metric and common units). To change from one system to the other, unique conversion factors are used. These conversion factors, which are the basis of an interactive calculator, take into account the molecular weight of the substance, the traditional units, and the S.I. units of measure, Slcalc contains analytes, which are accessible by more than 400 names, synonyms and abbreviations.

14:929. CD-ROM   Micromedex Inc

File name	Slcalc
Start year	
Number of records	
Update period	Quarterly

Smoking and Health
US Department of Health and Human Services

14:930. Master record

Database type	Bibliographic
Number of journals	
Sources	Journals, reports, books, book reviews, monographs and patents
Start year	1960; with some older material
Language	English
Coverage	International

Number of records	43,114
Update size	–
Update period	Quarterly
Index unit	Articles

Keywords
Tobacco; Smoking

Description
Contains bibliographic citations and abstracts to journal articles, reports, and other literature that discusses the effects of smoking on health. Aspects covered include: chemistry, pharmacology and toxicology, mortality and morbidity, neoplastic diseases, non-neoplastic respiratory diseases, cardiovascular diseases, pregnancy and infant health, other diseases and conditions, behavioral and psychological aspects, smoking prevention and intervention, smoking cessation methods, tobacco product additives, tobacco manufacturing and processing, tobacco economics, and legislation.

Corresponds to the print *Smoking and Health Bulletin*.

14:931. Online   CompuServe Information Service

File name	IQUEST File 2224
Start year	1960
Number of records	
Update period	Quarterly
Price/Charges	Subscription: US$8.95 per month Database entry fee: US$9/search; some databases carry a surcharge ($2–75) Online print: US$10 references free; then $9 per ten; abstracts $3 each

Downloading is allowed

Notes
Accessed via IQUEST or IQMEDICAL, this database is offered by a DIALOG gateway. IQUEST can either search across all databases, a database of the user's choice or selected multiple databases.

14:932. Online   DIALOG

File name	File 160
Start year	
Number of records	
Update period	
Price/Charges	Connect time: US$45.00 Offline print: US$0.20

Social Issues Resources Series
Social Issues Resources Series Inc

14:933. Master record

Alternative name(s)	SIRS; Social Issues Resources Series; Social Issues Resource Series Combined Text & Index CD-ROM
Database type	Textual, Factual, Bibliographic
Number of journals	800
Sources	Journals
Start year	1989
Language	English
Coverage	International

Number of records	5,000
Update size	–
Update period	Twice a year (March and September)
Index unit	Articles
Abstract details	SIRS staff

Keywords

HIV; Alcohol Abuse; Crime; Mental Health; Pollution

Description

This CD-ROM combines three of the SIRS publications – *Science Issues*, *Critical Issues* and *Global Perspectives* (material on the latter only since 1991), plus the index. Contains the full text of about ninety per cent of articles and complete bibliographic citations plus abstracts to the remaining ten per cent of over 5,000 full-text articles exploring 34 major social issues and five science disciplines. Three search options are provided – keyword, Library of Congress headings and topical tables of contents. Lois Shumaker, reviewing the product in *CD-ROM Librarian* (7(7) p.44–47) praised both the documentation and the online help – which even gives citation and footnote styles according to both the MLA style guide and Turabian. Shumaker felt that there was room for improvement in a product evidently still in the 'developing mode' citing a number of minor irritations such as the loss of a search history when going back to the initial menu to use the User Guide.

No additional charge for networking. Also available packaged with SIRS CD-ROM LAN III – an expandable multi-user network offering instantaneous data-retrieval and featuring three CD-ROM drives, laser printer, 100 Mbyte fixed disk and three workstations with SVGA colour monitors. Runs under DOS 5.0, Novell Netware 3.11 and CBIS CD-Connection software for US$ 12,250.

Corresponds to looseleaf binders published by SIRS on a variety of subjects – four of the subject series – *Science Issues*, *Critical Issues*, *Social Issues and Global Perspectives* – are available on CD ROM, each with an index. The first disc combines three publications (*Science Issues*, *Critical Issues* and *Global Perspectives*) plus the index; the second is *Science Issues* plus the index; the third, Social Issues, combines *Critical* and *Social Issues* plus the index; the fourth disc contains an index only.

14:934. Database subset

CD-ROM	**Social Issues Resources Series Inc**
File name	SIRS Social Issues Text & Index CD-ROM
Alternative name(s)	SIRS; Social Issues Resources Series
Format notes	IBM
Software	CD-SIRS
Start year	1989
Number of records	3,000
Update period	Annually (March)
Price/Charges	Subscription: US$550

Notes

Contains the full text of about ninety per cent of articles and complete bibliographic citations plus abstracts to the remaining ten per cent of over 3,000 full-text articles published in SIRS *Social Issues* and SIRS *Critical Issues*. Covers issues such as: pollution, work, health, mental health, crime, sexuality, alcohol, atmosphere and family. No additional charge for

networking. Corresponds to looseleaf binders published by SIRS on a variety of subjects – four of the subject series are available on CD-ROM, each with an index.

Software allows the printing of full or partial texts as well as downloading.

Social Work Abstracts
National Association of Social Workers (US)

14:935. Master record

Alternative name(s)	SWAB
Database type	Bibliographic, Textual
Number of journals	450
Sources	Theses, Journals and Books
Start year	July 1977
Language	English
Coverage	USA (primarily) and International (some)
Number of records	25,000
Update size	2,500
Update period	Quarterly
Index unit	Articles

Keywords

Aging; Alcohol Abuse; Drug Abuse; Family; Mental Health; Social Work

Description

Contains abstracts of around 25,000 journal articles (including articles originally published in foreign languages) and citations of social work and related literature dating back to 1977, plus listings of over 600 major social work books. Doctoral theses are also featured. Aging, alcoholism, drug abuse, crime and delinquency, economic security, employment, family and child welfare, health and medical care, housing and urban development, mental health, mental retardation and schools are some of the topics covered. Also encompassed are social policy, social work service methods, social work professional issues and related fields of knowledge such as economics, psychiatry, psychology and sociology. It also includes full-text information on professional standards, US legal regulations, state licensing laws and career information.

14:936. Online

		BRS
File name	SWAB	
Alternative name(s)	SWAB	
Start year	1977	
Number of records	25,000	
Update period	Quarterly	
Price/Charges	Connect time: US$67.00/77.00	
	Online print: US$0.16/0.24	
	Offline print: US$0.42	

Notes

SWRA (Social Work Research and Abstracts) subscribers receive a special discount.

14:937. CD-ROM

		SilverPlatter
File name	Social Work Abstracts Plus	
Alternative name(s)	SWAB	
Format notes	IBM	
Software	SPIRS	
Start year	1977	

Number of records	25,000
Update period	Twice a year
Price/Charges	Subscription: UK£790 – 1,185

Notes

Contains two files – Social Work Abstracts and the complete 1991 NASW Register of Clinical Social Workers.

Social Work Abstracts – bibliographic records on journal literature in the areas of the social work profession, theory and practice, areas of service, social issues and social problems from 1977 to the present.

Register of Clinical Social Workers – a directory of clinical social workers in the United States; gives name, address, telephone, employer, education, employment history.

The cost for single user is UK£790, for 2–8 users on a network the cost would be UK£1,185. SWRA (Social Work Research and Abstracts) subscribers receive a special discount.

Soviet Bio/Medical Report

Newmedia International Japan

14:938. Master record

Database type	Textual
Number of journals	1
Sources	Newsletter
Start year	1991
Language	English
Coverage	Soviet Union
Number of records	
Update size	–
Update period	Monthly

Keywords

Diagnosis; Drug Treatment

Description

Contains the full text of the newsletter *Soviet Bio/Medical Report*. Reviews developments, advances and application of medical treatment, diagnosis, drug treatment and practice in a range of medical specialties in the Soviet Union.

Corresponds to the monthly publication *Soviet Bio/Medical Report* newsletter. Data-Star and DIALOG are supplied with PTS Newsletter Database by Predicast.

This database can be found on:
PTS Newsletter Database

Sozialmedizin

Institut für Documentation und Information über Sozialmedizin und öffentliches Gesundheitswesen – IDIS

14:940. Master record

Alternative name(s)	SOMED
Database type	Bibliographic
Number of journals	700
Sources	Bibliographies, books, dissertations, grey literature, journals, letters and technical reports
Start year	1978
Language	German (all keywords are in German), English and French
Coverage	Germany (primarily), European (primarily) and International (some)
Number of records	263,482
Update size	15–20,000
Update period	Monthly
Index unit	Articles and letters
Abstract details	Authors' abstracts, abstracts compiled by IDIS or signed critical reviews.
Thesaurus	SOMED-Thesaurus

Keywords

Drug Abuse; Environmental Toxicology; Occupational Medicine; Public Health; Social Medicine

Description

SOMED is a bibliographic database containing references covering the whole field of 'social' (non clinical) medicine. Subjects covered include: community medicine; epidemiology; evaluation and quality assurance in public health; health education; health politics; organisation of health care; industrial hygiene; industrial toxicology; vital statistics; medical rehabilitation; preventive medicine; occupational medicine; school health; social pediatrics; social psychology; social medicine; drug abuse and misuse; alcoholism; smoking; environmental toxicology, medicine and hygiene. The database is the online version of: *Dokumentation Sozialmedizin, öffentlicher Gesundheitsdienst, Gesundheitserziehung, Dokumentation Gefährdung durch Alkohol, Rauchen, Drogen, Arzneimittel* and *Documentation Medizin im Umweltschultz*. Approximately 62% of records have abstracts in German, English and French, the average length of which are 800 to 1,000 characters. Languages are mixed, German and English with 45% each, French and others. Older segments of the database (1955-1977) are not online but can be searched at IDIS on request. Input into the database is based on the current selection of journal articles, books and other literatures of the IDIS special library. Search results of retrospective searches in original and secondary literature are also fed back into the SOMED system. The following items are not indexed: book reviews, hospital reports, communications from medical associations and announcements of new pharmaceuticals by the industry. There is no cover to cover indexing and articles are indexed selectively. The journals indexed are published in the IDIS list of journals issued every year. Books and book chapters each account for approximately 5% of all entries and approximately 45% of references to books contain an abstract.

Indexing is based on the descriptors of the *SOMED Thesaurus* which is in German and consists of about 3,800 descriptors and approximately 3,000 synonyms. The Thesaurus is revised annually. Approximately seven to twelve descriptors are assigned to each reference using the most specific descriptors possible but more general terms are also included. For non-specific precoordinated descriptors, one or more descriptors are used in combination to describe a given subject matter. Two to five descriptors describing the main aspects of a citation are given weighted descriptors status and are listed in the SOMED weighted descriptors field. In addtion to the controlled vocabulary SOMED subfile codes assign references to specific SOMED subfiles although are primarily internal markers of IDIS they can be used for limiting searches to qualified literature.

14:941. Online   DIMDI

File name	SM78
Alternative name(s)	SOMED
Software	GRIPS
Start year	1978
Number of records	263,482
Update period	Monthly
Delay	1–12 months
SDI period	1 month
Database aids	Memocard SOMED and DIMDI Online User Manual/SOMED
Price/Charges	Connect time: UK£03.88–08.62
	Online print: UK£0.16–0.34
	Offline print: UK£0.07–0.14

Downloading is allowed
Thesaurus is online

Notes

Searches are possible since January 1978. Approximately 85% of the original literature referred to in SOMED can be obtained via the Idis-Literaturservice (SUPPL=IDIS). Suppliers of online documents: British Library Document Supply Centre, Boston Spa, England; Harkers Information Retrieval System, Sydney, Australia; Institüt für Dokumentation und Information über Sozialmedizin und öffentliches Gesundheitswesen, Bielefeld, Germany; Koninklijke Nederlandse Akademie van Wetenschapen, Amsterdam, The Nederlands.

Record composition

Abstract AB; Author's Affiliation AF; Abstract Source AS; Author AU; Controlled Term CT; Controlled Term Weighted CTW; Decimal Classification DC; Entry Date ED; Editor EDR; Freetext FT; ISBN SB; Journal Title TJ; Language LA; Location LO; Number of Document ND; Publishers' Home and Name PU; Publication Year PY; Section Code SC; Series SE; Source SO and Title TI

STAT!-Ref

Teton Data Systems
Aries Systems Corporation

14:942. Master record

CD-ROM	Teton Data Systems
Database type	Textual, Dictionary, Directory, Factual
Number of journals	
Sources	Journals and Books
Start year	
Language	English
Coverage	USA, Europe, Australasia and Asia
Number of records	
Update size	—
Update period	Quarterly
Index unit	Articles

Keywords

Drugs

Description

A library of twenty full text (plus tables) medical reference textbooks developed by a physician for physicians. Offers instant access to current medical information from a comprehensive range of textbooks, drug references and ten years of selected Clinical MEDLINE abstracts from the National Library of Medicine for either primary care or cardiology.

Contains the full text of twenty leading reference sources for primary care medicine. These include: *Scientific American Medicine* (from Scientific American); *Drug Information* (USP DI Volumes 1 and 2 from US Pharmacopeial Convention Formulary Service); *Current Diagnosis and Treatment – Emergency, Medical, Obstetrics and Gynecology and Surgery* (from Appleton-Lange); *AMA Drug Evaluation; Honsten's Drug Interactions; The Medical Letter; Medical Toxicology; Stedman's Dictionary; New England Journal of Medicine*; and *Journal of the American Medical Association*. Contains the equivalent of 10,000 to 20,000 printed pages.

One disc contains the user's choice of MEDLINE subset and all the books. The subscription starts at US$ 295 for just the Clinical MEDLINE subset and the books range in price from $40 to $350. A subscription to the entire library is $2,500.

For more details of constituent databases, see:
MEDLINE
USP DI Volume 1: Drug Information for the Health Care Professional
AfterCare Instructions: USP DI Drug Information Leaflets

SWEDIS

Socialstyrelsens Läkemedelsavdelning

14:944. Master record

Alternative name(s)	Swedish Drug Information System
Database type	Factual, Textual
Number of journals	
Sources	
Start year	
Language	English and Swedish keywords
Coverage	Sweden
Number of records	
Update size	—
Update period	Daily

Keywords

Pharmaceutical Products

Description

The main topic of interest of the SWEDIS databank is the control of pharmaceutical preparations (läkemedelskontroll). The databank consists of registers of; pharmaceutical products, pharmaceutical speciality products, naturopathic preparations (naturmedel), sterile disposable products and cosmetic and hygienic preparations. There is also information on drug consumption, pharmaceutical postcontrol, statistics of drug sales from 1971 onwards, pharmaceutical substances and how to identify pharmaceutical pellets. SWEDIS is connected to INTDIS (International Drug Information System) at a WHO branch in Uppsala. The SWEDIS material is submitted from the drug department of the Swedish National Social Welfare Board, from WHO, from Apoteksbolaget and from Läkemedelsstatistik AB.

14:945. Online — Socialstyrelsens Läkemedelsavdelning

File name — SWEDIS
Alternative name(s) — Swedish Drug Information System
Start year
Number of records
Update period — Daily

Notes

Subscription fee required.

Swedish Biomedicine

MIC Karolinska Institutets Bibliotek OCH Informationscentral (MIC-KIBIC)

14:946. Master record

Alternative name(s) — SWEMED
Database type — Bibliographic
Number of journals
Sources — Journals, Reports and Dissertations
Start year — 1982
Language — Original language titles, English and Swedish
Coverage — Sweden and Norway
Number of records — 16,000
Update size — 1,000
Update period — Twice a week
Thesaurus — Medical Subject Headings (MeSH)

Keywords

Anatomy; Biomedicine; Nutrition; Pathology; Microbiology

Description

Can be regarded as a Swedish complement to MEDLINE – contains Swedish biomedical literature not covered by MEDLINE. Contains about 5,000 references to Swedish biomedical journals (for example, *Läkartidningen*), reports and dissertations from Swedish and Norwegian universities since 1982. Coverage includes medicine, dentistry, nursing, nutrition, pharmacology.

14:947. Online — MIC/Karolinska Institute Library and Information Center (MIC KIBIC)

File name — Swemed
Alternative name(s) — SWEMED
Start year — 1982
Number of records — 16,000
Update period — Twice a week

Teledoc Galenica

Galenica

14:948. Master record

Database type
Number of journals
Sources
Start year
Language — French
Coverage — Switzerland

Number of records
Update size — —
Update period

Keywords

Drugs; Pharmaceuticals; Surgery

Description

This database in the medical and pharmaceutical field forms part of the PharmaROM CD-ROM, originally intended for Swiss pharmacists.

This database can be found on:
PharmaROM

Telegenline

RR Bowker Company EIC/Intelligence

14:950. Master record

Database type — Bibliographic
Number of journals — 7,000
Sources — Books, conference proceedings, government reports (US), journals, monographs, research reports and symposia
Start year — 1973
Language — English
Coverage — International
Number of records — 25,200
Update size — —
Update period — Closed File
Database aids — EIC/Intelligence Telegenline Search Aid and Telegenline User's Manual
Hosts have included — DIMDI (Until 1.1.92)

Keywords

Genetic Engineering

Description

Telegenline contains information on the entire field of genetic engineering and biotechnology. Subjects covered include: industrial microbiology; fermentation technologies; genetics relating to plants, animals, humans, bacteria, viruses, plasma and computers; gene therapy: research techniques; applications in energy and mining; food processing; chemistry; pharmaceuticals and medicine; agriculture applications; biohazards; pollution control; public health and occupational safety; social impact; military applications; education; finance; international issues, research founding, ethics and values.

The database corresponds to the printed *Telegen Reporter*. Abstracts have been available since March 1983 and are now contained in approximately 85% of documents.

Indexing in TELEGENLINE consists of two stages. First all TELEGENLINE documents are assigned to one of the twenty-one sections of the *Telegen Reports* (the print equivalent of TELEGENLINE) as follows: 01 Business & Economics; 02 Social Impacts and Constraints; 03 Patent and Legal Issues; 04 Policy and Regulatory Issues; 05 General; 06 International; 07 Industrial Microbiology; 08 Chemical Applications; 09 Energy and Mining Applications; 10 Biohazards and Environmental Applications; 11 Food Processing and Production Applications; 12 Crop Applications; 13 Livestock Applications; 14 Pharmaceutical and Medical Applications; 15 Research on Human Genes; 16 Research on Animal Genes; 17 Research on Plant

Genes; 18 Research on Yeast and Fungus Genes; 19 Research on Bacterial Genes; 20 Research on Viral Genes; 21 General Research. Secondly the documents are indexed by Key Terms taken from an alphabetical, non-structured list containing approximately 2,000 terms. The Key Terms are indexed on three levels: Level 1 – primary descriptors; Level 2 – secondary descriptors and Level 3 – tertiary descriptors. The Key Terms are searchable directly as well as through freetext, the data fields section headings and secton codes can only be searched directly and the data fields Title and Abstracts are only searchable through freetext.

14:951. Online   ESA-IRS

File name	File 49
Start year	1976–1990
Number of records	25,477(October 1991)
Update period	No longer updated
Price/Charges	Subscription: UK£70.29
	Database entry fee: UK£3.49
	Online print: UK£0.63
	Offline print: UK£0.60
	SDI charge: UK£3.49

Downloading is allowed
Thesaurus is online

Notes

From 1993 ESA-IRS are charging an annual fee of 100 Accounting Units (c.UK£ 70.29) to all users. This is equivalent to the fee for full documentation and will not be charged to customers already paying for documentation.

Record composition

Abstract /AB; Author AU; Class Code Name CC; Classification Code CC; Controlled Terms /CT; Corporate Source CS; Document Type DT; Major Controlled Terms /CT or /MAJ; Source Data SO and Title /TI

TERIS
Micromedex Inc

14:952. Master record

Alternative name(s)	Teratogen Information System
Database type	Bibliographic, Textual
Number of journals	
Sources	
Start year	
Language	English
Coverage	USA and International
Number of records	
Update size	–
Update period	Quarterly

Keywords

Drugs

Description

Teratogen Information System (TERIS) developed by the University of Washington which addresses the teratogenicity of over seven hundred drugs and environmental agents that affect the unborn child.

Part of the Reprorisk database from Micromedex, which contains several modules addressing the reproductive risk of drugs, chemicals, and physical and environmental agents for females and males. Also part of TOMES Plus.

14:953. Online   TERIS

File name	
Alternative name(s)	Teratogen Information System
Start year	
Number of records	
Update period	Quarterly

This database can also be found on:
Reprorisk
TOMES Plus

Term-X
Electronic Data Expertise
Ouwehand Consultancy
(Ye Olde Hand Consultancy)

14:955. Master record

Database type	Textual, Image, Multimedia, Dictionary
Number of journals	
Sources	
Start year	
Language	Dutch and English
Coverage	Netherlands
Number of records	
Update size	–
Update period	Quarterly

Description

Medical and pharmaceutical term translation system including graphs and pictures, used in combination with databanks online. Will be available in more languages later.

14:956. CD-ROM   Ouwehand Consultancy

File name	Term-X
Format notes	IBM
Software	Term-Connect
Start year	
Number of records	
Update period	Quarterly

Therapeutic Patent Fast-Alert
Current Drugs Ltd

14:957. Master record

Alternative name(s)	TPdb; Current Patents Fast Alert (former name)
Database type	Bibliographic, Factual, Patents
Number of journals	
Sources	Patents and Patents (US)
Start year	July 1989
Language	English
Coverage	International
Number of records	300 patents
Update size	–
Update period	Weekly
Index unit	Patents
Abstract details	Each English language abstract is written by an expert from Current Drugs Ltd abstractors in the specific subject or therapeutic area listed

Keywords

Biotechnology; Cardiology; DNA; Immunology; Molecular Biology; Patents – Agrochemical; Patents – Biotechnical; Patents – Therapeutic; Pharmaceuticals; Therapeutic Medicine; Trademarks

Description

A rapidly-updated biotechnology and therapeutic patent database which can be accessed online or run in-house using MACCS, ISIS/Base or Chembase database software. Therapeutic (formerly Current Patents) Patent Fast-Alert is a database of 'informed summaries' and bibliographic data for agrochemical, biotechnical and pharmaceutical patents in selected therapeutic areas. Contains citations with abstracts to pharmaceutical patents and applications. Subjects covered include: antimicrobial patents (vaccines, antivirals, antifungals, antibacterials, antiparasitics) and cardiovascular patents (cardiovascular chemotherapy, blood products), anti-inflammatory, biotechnology, agrochemicals, anti-allergic, gastro-intestinal, hormone, central nervous system patents including antidepressants, antipsychotics, analgesics, antiepileptics, antimigraines and treatments for Alzheimer's Disease, Parkinson's Disease and stroke, diagnostic and drug delivery anticancer, metabolic disease, plus immunology patent documents, all selected from the UK and the European Patent Office, PCT applications, German (for agrochemicals only) applications, and United States–granted patents, with coverage of the various therapeutic categories beginning at various times since 1989. It also includes patents on herbicides, plant growth regulators, insecticides and fungicides published since late 1990.

Summaries of patents are provided less than ten days after the patents are available to the database producer. In comparison with the European Documentation Abstract Journal which provides patent information with an average time-lag of two to three months, Fast-Alert has a time lag of only two to four weeks. Its great value, according to Dr D Cowan of Helix Biotechnology Ltd, UK, is that it highlights the very latest technology in biotechnology and immunology which ultimately underpin the developments in the more clinical subjects. The sheer pace of development in the field of genetic technologies and the increasing number of important molecular biology techniques and discoveries both make it of particular importance for industrialists and academics to stay up-to-date. Comments provided by the Fast-Alert abstractors are valuable, not the least in demonstrating that the writer has a far greater knowledge of that field than is normally the case with professional abstractors.

Abstracts include a therapeutic classification assigned by Current Drugs and examples of preferred compounds, inventor name and International Patent Classification (IPC). Critical evaluations of selected pharmaceutical patents are later printed in the monthly Current Opinion in Therapeutic Patents which forms the basis of Current Patents Evaluation (See Separate Entry). The focus of these services is to inform the scientific community of advances in drug development, rather than to provide access to patents as legal documents or prior art.

The database corresponds to the following printed weekly bulletins: *Antimicrobial Fast-Alert; Anticancers; Cardiovascular Fast-Alert; CNS Agents Fast-Alert; Anti-inflammatory/Anti-allergic/GI Fast-Alert; Anticancer and Hormone Fast-Alert; Biotechnology and Immunology Fast- Alert; Herbicide and Growth Regulator Fast-Alert; Hormonals and Metabolic Disease Therapy; Respiratory agents; Agrochemicals; Insecticide and Fungicide Fast-Alert.* Fast-Alert maintains an authority list of terms used in a three-tier classification system. Copies are available from Current Drugs Ltd.

Descriptors are uncontrolled terms so searches should be carried out using free-text and qualified to .DE. Designated states are given for PCT (World) and EP (European) patents only.

14:958. Online   Data-Star

File name	CPBM
Alternative name(s)	TPdb; Current Patents Fast Alert (former name)
Start year	Latest six weeks
Number of records	4,000
Update period	Weekly
Database aids	Data-Star Biomedical Manual and Online manual (search as NEWS-CPBM in NEWS)
Price/Charges	Subscription: UK£32.00 Connect time: UK£45.68 Online print: UK£3.81 Offline print: UK£3.81

Notes

CPBM provides comprehensive coverage of biomedical patent information less than ten days after the original patents are available, the current file holding records up to six weeks of data. Discounts are available online to subscribers to the printed Current Drugs bulletins in two or more therapeutic areas.

From June 1993 Data-Star have introduced an annual fee/subscription per contract (that is, not per password) of SFr 80.00 (c.UK£ 32.00) payable every June. For North American customers billed in dollars who also use DIALOG, the DIALOG fee also covers access to Data-Star. Academic customers, 'commitment' customers and customers currently billed in dollars are exempt.

Record composition

Abstract AB; Accession Number and Update Code AN; Annotated Title AT; Descriptor DE; Designated States DS; Filing Date FD; Filing Month FM; International Patent Classification IC; Inventor IN; Patent Assignee PA; Priority Application Date PY; Priority Application Month MP; Publication Date PD; Publication Number PN; Section Code SC; Title TI and Update Code UP

14:959. Online   Data-Star

File name	CPBA
Alternative name(s)	TPdb; Current Patents Fast Alert (former name)
Start year	1989 to six weeks ago
Number of records	4,000+
Update period	Not updated
Database aids	Data-Star Biomedical Manual and Online manual (search as NEWS-CPBM in NEWS)
Price/Charges	Subscription: UK£32.00 Connect time: UK£45.68 Online print: UK£2.13 Offline print: UK£2.13

Notes

CPBA is the archive file, containing data six weeks old and over. Discounts are available online to subscribers to the printed Current Drugs' bulletins in two or more therapeutic areas.

From June 1993 Data-Star have introduced an annual fee/subscription per contract (that is, not per password) of SFr 80.00 (c.UK£ 32.00) payable every June. For North American customers billed in dollars who

also use DIALOG, the DIALOG fee also covers access to Data-Star. Academic customers, 'commitment' customers and customers currently billed in dollars are exempt.

Record composition

Abstract AB; Accession Number and Update Code AN; Annotated Title AT; Descriptor DE; Designated States DS; Filing Date FD; Filing Month FM; International Patent Classification IC; Inventor IN; Patent Assignee PA; Priority Application Date PY; Priority Application Month MP; Publication Date PD; Publication Number PN; Section Code SC; Title TI and Update Code UP

14:960. Online — Internet

File name	
Alternative name(s)	TPdb; Current Patents Fast Alert (former name)
Start year	July 1989
Number of records	300 patents
Update period	Weekly

14:961. Online — ORBIT

File name	CPFA
Alternative name(s)	TPdb; Current Patents Fast Alert (former name)
Start year	1989 (July) to most recent six weeks
Number of records	4,000
Update period	Weekly

Notes

Discounts are available online to subscribers to the printed Current Drugs' bulletins in two or more therapeutic areas. Electronic SDI service is now available within two hours on ORBIT. They can be downloaded and reformatted on a word processor. Results are retrieved in the low cost PRINTS file, $15 per connect hour.

14:962. Online — ORBIT

File name	CPFN
Alternative name(s)	TPdb; Current Patents Fast Alert (former name)
Start year	Most recent six weeks
Number of records	4,000
Update period	Weekly

Notes

Discounts are available online to subscribers to the printed Current Drugs' bulletins in two or more therapeutic areas. Electronic SDI service is now available within 2 hours on ORBIT. They can be downloaded and reformatted on a word processor. Results are retrieved in the low cost PRINTS file, $15 per connect hour.

14:963. Diskette — Current Drugs Ltd

File name	
Alternative name(s)	TPdb; Current Patents Fast Alert (former name)
Format notes	IBM
Start year	July 1989
Number of records	300 patents
Update period	Weekly

14:964. Tape — Current Drugs Ltd

File name	Therapeutic Patent Fast-Alert
Alternative name(s)	TPdb; Current Patents Fast Alert (former name)
Format notes	IBM
Software	MACCS; ISIS/Base; Chembase
Start year	July 1989

Number of records	300 patents
Update period	Weekly

Notes

Software will display structure diagrams.

Thermalisme
Telmed

14:965. Master record

Database type	
Number of journals	
Sources	
Start year	
Language	French
Coverage	Switzerland
Number of records	
Update size	—
Update period	

Keywords

Drugs; Pharmaceuticals; Surgery

Description

This database in the medical and pharmaceutical field forms part of the MediROM and PharmaROM CD-ROMs, originally intended for Swiss pharmacists.

This database can also be found on:
MediROM
PharmaROM

TOMES Plus
Micromedex Inc

14:966. Master record
CD-ROM — Micromedex Inc

Database type	Bibliographic, Directory, Factual, Textual, Numeric
Number of journals	
Sources	Conference papers, government papers, journals and letters
Start year	
Language	English
Coverage	USA (primarily) and International (some)
Number of records	
Update size	—
Update period	Quarterly
Index unit	Articles and letters

Keywords

Air Pollution; Biological Hazards; Cancer; Chemical Hazards; Chemical Substances; Clinical Medicine; Dangerous Chemicals; Drugs; Emergency Medicine; Explosion; Fire; Fire Hazards; First Aid; Food Additives; Gynaecology; Hazardous Chemicals; Hazardous Substances; Hazardous Waste; Health and Safety; Health Hazards; Industrial Hygiene; Legislation; Occupational Health and Safety; Oil Pollution; Pollution; Pregnancy; Teratology; Waste Management; Water Pollution

Description

A reference source (Microinfo say 'a unique collection of toxicology, health and safety and related environmental response data') on medical and hazard information regarding thousands of chemicals used in the industrial setting with in-depth coverage of clinical effects, range of toxicity, workplace standards, kinetics, and physicochemical parameters. The disc consists of completely referenced peer-reviewed data from thirteen individual databases:

(1) Meditext which provides detailed, comprehensive, and referenced protocols for the medical evaluation and treatment of individuals exposed to chemical agents.

(2) Hazardtext which contains protocols for initial response to incidents (fires, spills, leaks) from hazardous materials.

(3) 1st Medical Response which contains protocols for response to injuries and illnesses occurring in the workplace.

(4) Hazardous Substances Data Bank (HSDB) (produced by the National Library of Medicine) which contains reviews on the toxicity, hazards and regulatory status of over 4,400 frequently used chemicals each covered by up to 150 data fields including many regulated by EPA and OSHA. Significant human exposure potential, environmental fate, standards, regulations and other areas are covered in-depth.

(5) OHMTADS (Oil and Hazardous Materials – Technical Assistance Data System) from the US Environmental Protection Agency contains information on the health and environmental effects, with up to 120 data fields for each, of 1,400 chemicals to facilitate rapid effective response to emergency spills and to offer broad support to environmental research and enforcement activities. Chemical identifiers include: name, synonyms, trade names, Accession number, CAS registry number, SIC code, chemical formula and composition. Data areas covered include: physical and chemical properties, reactivity, transportation and storage, detection, fire protection and explosion, environmental fate and chemistry, toxicology, human contact and hazard information, response and disposal advise;

(6) IRIS (Integrated Risk Information System) from the Environmental Protection Agency which deals with health risk assessment information on over 350 chemicals of regulatory interest and is intended to serve as a guide for the hazard identification and dose-response assessment steps of EPA risk assessments.

(7) CHRIS (Chemical Hazard Response Information System) from the US Coast Guard contains reviews on fire hazards, fire fighting recommendations, reactivities, physiochemical properties, health hazards, use of protective clothing and shipping information covering 1,100 key chemicals with up to 94 data fields each and is useful in preparing material safety data sheets and in safety program design and training. It contains detailed information to assist with emergency response, accident prevention and safety procedure design in the transportaton of hazardous chemicals. Chemical identifiers include: name, synonyms, CAS registry number, DOT ID number and class, IMO/UN designation and chemical formula. Data for each chemical includes: labelling, observable characteristics, physical and chemical properties, health hazards, fire hazards, chemical reactivity, water pollution, shipping information, hazard classification and assessment, and summary accident response advice;

(8) Reprorisk (Teratogen Information System) developed by the University of Washington in Seattle provides current, authoritative information on the teratogenic effects following drug ingestion on environmental agent exposure during pregnancy.

(9) DOT Emergency Response Guides prepared by the Department of Transportation is a reference source for initial response to releases, fires or explosions involving over 2,000 frequently transported chemicals.

(10) RTECS (Registry of Toxic Effects on Chemical Substances database) from the National Institute for Occupational Safety and Health (NIOSH) a leading source for basic acute and chronic toxic information. It is a non-bibliographic database and contains identification, toxicity and general information on approximately 110,000 chemical substances and approximately 400,000 compound names. Chemicals are identified by prime name, synonym RETECS accession number, CAS registry number, molecular formula and weight or Wiswesser line notation. Toxic effects data with accompanying bibliographic references are present under five main categories; skin and eye irritation, mutation, reproductive effects, tumorigenic and toxicity data. Information covers type of effects, organ system affected, route of administration, animal species and dose.

(11) The SARATEXT chemical database module offers a complete source of information on the acute and chronic health effects and recommendations for medical treatment for individuals exposed to any of the chemicals listed on the SARA Title III Extremely Hazardous Substances (EHS) list, plus information on medical reporting requirements.

(12) Infotext is a general information module containing regulatory standards, guidelines and listings, along with a a variety of other non-chemical specific documents.

(13) The New Jersey Hazardous Substance Fact Sheets from the New Jersey Department of Health gives employee-oriented exposure risk information for over 700 hazardous substances.

TOMES Plus is the only source for Meditext, Hazardtext, Saratext, Infotext, 1st Medical Response Protocols and Reprorisk documents and, according to Micromedex, provides the only compilation of government and proprietary information available. It enables users to provide quick response to environmental incidents involving hazardous materials, address worker and community right-to-know issues, evaluate chemical exposure to employees and community, retrieve information for MSDS preparation, assist industry and community representatives with personal protection and disaster planning, educate health and safety professionals, and to assist in maintaining regulatory compliance for dealing with chemicals in the workplace.

Any additional discs cost £650. Reprorisk is not included in standard subscription price but may be included on TOMES Plus for an additional price of £230.

For more details of constituent databases, see:
Meditext
Hazardtext Inc
1st Medical Response
HSDB – Hazardous Substances Data Bank
OHM-TADS
IRIS – Integrated Risk Information System
CHRIS
Reprorisk
RTECS

DOT Emergency Response Guides
SARATEXT
Infotext
New Jersey Hazardous Substance Fact Sheets

TOXALL
National Library of Medicine

14:968. Master record

Alternative name(s)	Toxicology Information Online
Database type	Bibliographic
Number of journals	
Sources	Government documents (US), journals, monographs, research projects, Patents, Conference proceedings, Research communications and Symposia
Start year	1940, partly
Language	English
Coverage	International
Number of records	2,500,000
Update size	120,000
Update period	Monthly

Keywords

Aneuploidy; Accident Prevention; Biological Hazards; Chemical Substances; Chromosome Abnormalities; Drugs; Environmental Health; Epidemiology; Ergonomics; Hazardous Substances; Hazardous Waste; Health Physics; Industrial Materials; Industrial Processes; Metabolism; Occupational Health and Safety; Occupational Psychology; Pathology; Pesticides; Pollution; Safety Education; Standards; Vocational Training; Waste Management; Water Treatment

Description

TOXALL/TOXLINE (Toxicology Information Online) is the National Library of Medicine's extensive collection of online bibliographic information covering the toxicological effects of drugs, pesticides and other chemicals. The database contains references to published material and research in progress in areas such as adverse drug reactions, carcinogenesis, mutagenesis, teratogenesis, environmental pollution and food contamination, toxicology, pharmacology, analytical chemistry and occupational safety. Most of the citations include, in addition to the bibliographic information, abstracts and/or indexing term and/or indexing terms and/or CAS Registry numbers.

TOXALL is composed of several database segments of toxicological interest (from CA, BIOSIS Previews and MEDLINE) and of total contents of specialised toxicological data collections. As the data in the different subunits is provided by different producers, there is a relatively great number of duplicates in the database. In addition the structure of the records also varies, for example some include abstracts and some use MeSH Indexing, others do not.

The subfiles are, with starting date of coverage being the publication year shown:

ANEUPL (Aneuploidy file of the Environmental Mutagen Information Center) pre 1950 to the present;
Chemical-Biological Activities – CA (Chemical Abstracts);
CISDOC (International Labour Office) (ILO) Abstracts 1981 to the present;
CRISP (Toxicology Research Projects (RPROJ) 1988 to the present;

EMIC (Environmental Mutagen Information Center File of the Oak Ridge National Laboratory (ORNL) 1950 to the present;
EPIDEM (Epidemiology Information System File of the FDA) 1940 to the present;
ETIC (Environmental Teratology Information Center File of ORNL) 1950 to the present;
Federal Research in Progress (FEDRIP) 1982;
HAPAB (Health Aspects of Pesticides Abstract Bulletin of the Environmental Protection Agency (EPA) (see PESTAB));
HAYES (Hayes File on Pesticides);
HMTC (Abstract Bulletin of the US Army's Hazardous Materials Technical Center) 1982 to the present;
International Pharmaceutical Abstracts (IPA) 1969 to the present;
HEEP – see Toxicological Aspects of Environmental Health;
NIOSH (References of the National Institute for Occupational Safety and Health Technical Information Center (NIOSHTIC) database) 1984 to the present;
NTIS (Toxicology Document and Data Depository (TD3) of the National Technical Information Service (NTIS) 1979 to the present;
PESTAB (Pesticides Abstracts of the EPA (Formerly HAPAB) 1968–1981;
PPBIB (Poisonous Plants Bibliography) pre-1976;
RPROJ (Research Projects Directory);
Toxicological Aspects of Environmental Health (BIOSIS) (formerly BIOSIS/HEEP, Health Effects of Environmental Pollutants) 1970 to the present;
TMIC (Toxic Materials Information Center File);
TOXBIB (Toxicity Bibliography from the MEDLINE file) 1965 to the present;
TSCATS (Toxic Substances Control Act Test Submissions File of the EPA) (all relevant submissions).

References in TOXLINE are from producers that do not require royalty charges; references on toxicology from producers that do require royalty charges are placed in TOXLIT.

The database contains approximately 20,000 citations from between 1940 and 1965, 640,000 from 1965 to 1976, EMIC since 1960 and ETIC since 1965. About 45% of the records added per year are from the TOXBIB subfile, which is derived from MEDLINE. Approximately eighty-two per cent of documents contain abstracts. Some hosts only carry TOXLINE. TOXLIT comprises IPA (International Pharmaceutical Abstracts), CA (Chemical Abstracts) and Toxicological Aspects of Environmental Health (BIOSIS) (formerly BIOSIS/HEEP).

The datafield Controlled Terms contains vocabulary from all of the subunits. The datafields CAS Registry Number, Chemical Abstracts Classification Codes and ILO Classification Codes can only be searched directly. The datafield Controlled Terms can be searched directly as well as through freetext and the data fields Title and Abstract can only be searched through freetext. The following points are recommended for drugs and chemicals: always use Registry numbers when available; for a broad concept search use as many synonyms as possible in title, keywords and abstract; for TOXBIB only use controlled terms from *MeSH*.

14:969. Online   DIMDI

File name	TX65
Start year	1940, partly

Number of records	3,466,353
Update period	Monthly
SDI period	1 month
Price/Charges	Connect time: UK£35.99–39.78
	Online print: UK£0.52–0.70
	Offline print: UK£0.48–0.55

Downloading is allowed

Notes

As TOXALL is composed of several database segments of toxicological interest (from Chemical Abstracts Service, MEDLINE, BIOSIS Previews) and total contents of specialised toxicological data collections, single citations may occur more than once. DIMDI recommends using CHEMLINE for the retrieval of synonyms and CAS Registry Numbers of chemical substances before starting a TOXALL search. It also advises that a search for chemical substances should not be restricted to the CAS Registry Number field because several TOXALL subunits do not contain this field. The TOXALL subunits are pooled to create the subfiles TOXLINE and TOXLIT which can be accessed separately by using their poolkeys. TOXLIT contains the subunits CA, BIOSIS/HEEP (up to July 1985: HEEP) and IPA. TOXLINE contains the other subunits ANEUPL, DART, EMIC, ETIC, FEDRIP, HAYES, HMTC, ILO, NIOSH, PESTAB/HAPAB, PPBIB, RPROJ, TD3, TMIC, TOXBIB, TSCATS. Documents total over 3 million since 1965 (about 20,000 citations from 1940 to 1965, 640,000 from 1965 to 1976, EMIC since 1960, ETIC since 1950).

Suppliers of online documents: British Library Document Supply Centre, Boston Spa, England; Harkers Information Retrieval System, Sydney, Australia; Instituto de Informacion y Documentacion en Ciencia y Tecnologica, Madrid, Spain; State Central Scientific Medical Library Supplier Center, Moscow, USSR. 82% of records contain abstracts. Searches are available from January 1965.

Record composition

Abstract AB; Author AU; BIOSIS Section Heading BISH; Chemical Abstracts Section Code CASC; Chemical Abstracts Section Heading CASH; CAS Reg. No CR; Corporate Source CS; Controlled Term CT; Country CY; Document Date DT; Date Received REC; Entry Month EM; Free Text FT; Gene Symbol GE; International Labour Office Classification Code ILCC; International Labour Organisation Section Heading ILSC; International Pharmaceutical Abstracts Section Code IPSC; International Pharmaceutical Association Section Heading IPSH; ISSN SS; Journal Code JC; Journal Title JT; Language LA; Machine Date MD; Number of Document ND; Number of Supporting Agency NS; Number of Unit Record (DIMDI) NU; Order Number OD; Preprocessed Search PPS; Price PR; Publication Year PY; Qualifier AF; Secondary Source SEC; Source SO; Subunit SU; Supporting Agency SA; Title TI; Toxic Substances Control Act Section Code TSCC; Type of Award TA and ZIP Code ZP

CALL TOXDUP provides the user with a means to define its own hitlist of subunits from TOXALL and its subfiles TOXLINE and TOXLIT and thereby identify duplicate records.

14:970. Database subset

Online   **BLAISE-LINK**

File name	TOXLINE
Start year	
Number of records	
Update period	

14:971. Database subset

Online   **BLAISE-LINK**

File name	TOXLIT
Start year	
Number of records	
Update period	

14:972. Database subset

Online   **BRS**

File name	TOXL
Start year	1965
Number of records	
Update period	Monthly
Price/Charges	Connect time: US$26.00/36.00
	Online print: US$0.07/0.15

Notes

Records from the IPA and BIOSIS subfiles are excluded from this database.

14:973. Database subset

Online   **BRS**

File name	XTOL
Start year	1965
Number of records	
Update period	Monthly
Price/Charges	Connect time: US$26.00/36.00
	Online print: US$0.07/0.15

Notes

This is a subfile of BRS's TOXL database and contains documents from all TOXLINE subfiles except the MEDLINE-derived subfile TOXBIB. It contains approximately thirty per cent of the documents in TOXLINE covering the pharmacological, biomedical, physiological and toxicological effects of drugs and other chemicals. Data from proprietary sources is excluded.

14:974. Database subset

Online   **CompuServe Information Service**

File name	IQUEST File 2576 – TOXLINE
Start year	1965
Number of records	
Update period	Monthly
Price/Charges	Subscription: US$8.95 per month
	Database entry fee: US$9/search; some databases carry a surcharge ($2–75)
	Online print: US$10 references free; then $9 per ten; abstracts $3 each

Downloading is allowed

Notes

Coverage dates vary depending on subfile. Accessed via IQUEST or IQMEDICAL, this database is offered by a DIALOG gateway. IQUEST can either search across all databases, a database of the user's choice or selected multiple databases.

14:975. Database subset

Online   **Data-Star**

File name	TOXX
Start year	Current month
Number of records	1,152,262
Update period	Monthly
Database aids	Data-Star Biomedical Manual and Online Guide (search NEWS-TOXL in NEWS)
Price/Charges	Connect time: SFr78.00
	Online print: SFr0.21–0.24
	Offline print: SFr6.80
	SDI charge: SFr0.24

Notes

The current month file does not include references from Toxicology Research Projects (CRISP); Epidemiology Information System File of the FDA (EPIDEM); the Federal Research in Progress Database (FEDRIP); the Abstracts Bulletin of the US Army's Hazardous Materials Technical Centre (HMTC); or the Toxic Substances Control Act Test Submissions File of the EPA (TSCATS). For TOXBIB use also Medical Subject Headings Annotated Alphabetic List (MeSH) and Tree Structrures (TREE) published annually.

From June 1993 Data-Star have introduced an annual fee/subscription per contract (that is, not per password) of SFr 80.00 (c.UK£ 32.00) payable every June. For North American customers billed in dollars who also use DIALOG, the DIALOG fee also covers access to Data-Star. Academic customers, 'commitment' customers and customers currently billed in dollars are exempt.

Record composition

Abstract AB; Accession number and secondary source ID or by code for faster retrieval AN; Author(s) AU; Availability, Order-ID-number, Prices AV; Award type AW; CAS Registry number(s) RN; Classification code CC; Comment CM; Corporate name CA; Entry month EM; Gene symbol GS; Institution, address IN; Keywords KW; Journal coden CD; Language of original LG; MESH-Descriptors in TOXBIB DE; Publication type PT; Source and ISSN-number in TOXBIBSO; Supporting agency SA; Title TI and Year of publication YR

14:976. Database subset

Online   Data-Star

File name	TOXL
Start year	1981 to date
Number of records	1,152,262
Update period	Monthly
Database aids	Data-Star Biomedical Manual and Online guide (search NEWS-TOXL in NEWS)
Price/Charges	Subscription: SFr80.00
	Connect time: SFr78.00
	Online print: SFr0.21–0.24
	Offline print: SFr6.80
	SDI charge: SFr0.24

Notes

For TOXBIB users should also consult Medical Subject Headings Annotated Alphabet List (MeSH) and Tree Structures (TREE) published annually.

From June 1993 Data-Star have introduced an annual fee/subscription per contract (that is, not per password) of SFr 80.00 (c.UK£ 32.00) payable every June. For North American customers billed in dollars who also use DIALOG, the DIALOG fee also covers access to Data-Star. Academic customers, 'commitment' customers and customers currently billed in dollars are exempt.

Record composition

Abstract AB; Accession number and secondary source ID or by code for faster retrieval AN; Author(s) AU; Availability, Order-ID-number, Prices AV; Award type AW; CAS Registry number(s) RN; Classification code CC; Comment CM; Corporate name CA; Entry month EM; Gene symbol GS; Institution, address IN; Keywords KW; Journal coden CD; Language of original LG; MESH-Descriptors in TOXBIB DE; Publication type PT; Source and ISSN-number in TOXBIBSO; Supporting agency SA; Title TI and Year of publication YR

14:977. Database subset

Online   Data-Star

File name	TO80
Start year	Pre 1965–1980
Number of records	
Update period	Monthly
Database aids	Data-Star Biomedical Manual and Online guide (search NEWS-TOXL in NEWS)
Price/Charges	Subscription: SFr80.00
	Connect time: SFr78.00
	Online print: SFr0.21–0.24
	Offline print: SFr6.80
	SDI charge: SFr0.24

Notes

The Health Aspects of Pesticides Abstracts Bulletin of the Environmental Protection Agency (HAPAB) is only available in the two files which extend back further than 1965 – TO80 and TOZZ – that is before it was renamed Pesticides Abstracts.

This file does not include references from Toxicology Research Projects (CRISP); Epidemiology Information System File of the FDA (EPIDEM); the Federal Research in Progress Database (FEDRIP); the Abstracts Bulletin of the US Army's Hazardous Materials Technical Centre (HMTC); or the Toxic Substances Control Act Test Submissions File of the EPA (TSCATS). For TOXBIB users should also consult Medical Subject Headings Annotated Alphabet List (MeSH) and Tree Structures (TREE) published annually.

From June 1993 Data-Star have introduced an annual fee/subscription per contract (that is, not per password) of SFr 80.00 (c.UK£ 32.00) payable every June. For North American customers billed in dollars who also use DIALOG, the DIALOG fee also covers access to Data-Star. Academic customers, 'commitment' customers and customers currently billed in dollars are exempt.

Record composition

Abstract AB; Accession number and secondary source ID or by code for faster retrieval AN; Author(s) AU; Availability, Order-ID-number, Prices AV; Award type AW; CAS Registry number(s) RN; Classification code CC; Comment CM; Corporate name CA; Entry month EM; Gene symbol GS; Institution, address IN; Keywords KW; Journal coden CD; Language of original LG; MESH-Descriptors in TOXBIB DE; Publication type PT; Source and ISSN-number in TOXBIBSO; Supporting agency SA; Title TI and Year of publication YR

14:978. Database subset

Online   Data-Star

File name	TOZZ
Start year	Pre 1965
Number of records	1,152,262
Update period	Monthly
Database aids	Data-Star Biomedical Manual and Online guide (seacrh NEWS-TOXL in NEWS)
Price/Charges	Subscription: UK£32.00
	Connect time: UK£31.20
	Online print: UK£0.00 – 0.71
	Offline print: UK£0.08 – 0.10
	SDI charge: UK£2.72

Notes

Data-Star recommends the following search tactics in relation to drugs and chemicals: always use Registry numbers when available; for a broad concept search use as many synonyms as possible in title, keyword and abstract, for multi-word names use ADJ or WITH and for TOXBIB only use specific DE-searching using online MeSH and Tree. The Health Aspects of Pesticides Abstracts Bulletin of the Environmental Protection Agency (HAPAB) is only available in the two files which extend back further than 1965 – TO80 and TOZZ – that is before it was renamed Pesticides Abstracts. For TOXBIB users should also consult Medical Subject Headings Annotated Alphabet List (MeSH) and Tree Structures (TREE) published annually.

From June 1993 Data-Star have introduced an annual fee/subscription per contract (that is, not per password) of SFr 80.00 (c.UK£ 32.00) payable every June. For North American customers billed in dollars who also use DIALOG, the DIALOG fee also covers access to Data-Star. Academic customers, 'commitment' customers and customers currently billed in dollars are exempt.

Record composition

Abstract AB; Accession number and secondary source ID or by code for faster retrieval AN; Author(s) AU; Availability, Order-ID-number, Prices AV; Award type AW; CAS Registry number(s) RN; Classification code CC; Comment CM; Corporate name CA; Entry month EM; Gene symbol GS; Institution, address IN; Keywords KW; Journal coden CD; Language of original LG; MESH-Descriptors in TOXBIB DE; Publication type PT; Source and ISSN-number in TOXBIBSO; Supporting agency SA; Title TI and Year of publication YR

14:979. Database subset

Online   Data-Star

File name	TRTO – Training file (TOXLINE)
Start year	
Number of records	
Update period	Monthly
Price/Charges	Connect time: UK£Free
	Online print: UK£Free

Notes

Data-Star recommends the following search tactics in relation to drugs and chemicals: always use Registry numbers when available; for a broad concept search use as many synonyms as possible in title, keyword and abstract, for multi-word names use ADJ or WITH and for TOXBIB only use specific DE-searching For TOXBIB users should also consult Medical Subject Headings Annotated Alphabet List (MeSH) and Tree Structures (TREE) published annually.

Record composition

Abstract AB; Accession number and secondary source ID or by code for faster retrieval AN; Author(s) AU; Availability, Order-ID-number, Prices AV; Award type AW; CAS Registry number(s) RN; Classification code CC; Comment CM; Corporate name CA; Entry month EM; Gene symbol GS; Institution, address IN; Keywords KW; Journal coden CD; Language of original LG; MESH-Descriptors in TOXBIB DE; Publication type PT; Source and ISSN-number in TOXBIBSO; Supporting agency SA; Title TI and Year of publication YR

14:980. Database subset

Online   DIALOG

File name	File 156
Start year	
Number of records	1,647,025
Update period	Monthly
Price/Charges	Connect time: US$66.00
	Online print: US$0.25
	Offline print: US$0.25
	SDI charge: US$7.50

Notes

Coverage dates vary depending on subfile.

14:981. Database subset

Online   DIMDI

File name	TX165
Start year	1940, partly
Number of records	1,196,643
Update period	Monthly
SDI period	1 month
Price/Charges	Connect time: UK£05.20–08.99
	Online print: UK£0.16–0.34
	Offline print: UK£0.09–0.15

Downloading is allowed

Notes

TOXLINE is a TOXALL-subfile containing the following subunits ANEUPL, EMIC, EPIDEM, ETIC, FEDRIP, HAYES, HMTC, ILO, NIOSH, PESTAB/HAPAB, PPBIB, RPROJ, TD3, TMIC, TOXBIB, TSCATS. Public Health Services (USA)-supported research from FEDRIP is not included in TOXLINE because that information is already available in the RPROJ subunit.

Suppliers of online documents: British Library Document Supply Centre, Boston Spa, England; Harkers Information Retrieval System, Sydney, Australia; Instituto de Informacion y Documentacion en Ciencia y Tecnologica, Madrid, Spain; State Central Scientific Medical Library Supplier Center, Moscow, USSR. 82% of records have abstracts.

Record composition

Abstract AB; Author AU; BIOSIS Section Heading BISH; Chemical Abstracts Section Code CASC; Chemical Abstracts Section Heading CASH; CAS Reg. No CR; Corporate SOurce CS; Controlled Term CT; Country CY; Date Project Begins DB; Date Project Ends DE; Date Received REC; Document Date DT; Entry Month EM; Free Text FT; Gene Symbol GE; International Labour Office Section Code ILSC; International Labour Organisation Section Heading ILSC; International Pharmaceutical Abstracts Section Code IPSC; International Pharmaceutical Association Section Heading IPSH; ISSN SS; Journal Code JC; Journal Title JT; Language LA; Machine Date MD; Number of Document ND; Number of Supporting Agency NS; Number of Unit Record (DIMDI) NU; Order Number OD; Preprocessed Search PPS; Price PR; Publication Year PY; Qualifier AF; Secondary Source SEC; Source SO; Subunit SU; Supporting Agency SA; Title TI; Toxic Substances Control Act Section Code TSCC; Type of Awared TA and ZIP Code ZP

14:982. Database subset

Online   DIMDI

File name	T265
Start year	1965

Number of records	2,269,710
Update period	Monthly
SDI period	1 month
Database aids	Online User Manual/TOXALL
Price/Charges	Connect time: UK£33.36–37.15
	Online print: UK£0.53–0.71
	Offline print: UK£0.50–0.56

Downloading is allowed

Notes

TOXLIT is a TOXALL-subfile containing the following subunits BIOSIS/HEEP, CA and IPA. From Chemical Abstracts the following segments are taken: CBAC Chemical/Biological Activities, plus other parts of CA referring to toxicology, pharmacology and biochemistry.

Suppliers of online documents: British Library Document Supply Centre, Boston Spa, England; Harkers Information Retrieval System, Sydney, Australia; Instituto de Informacion y Documentacion en Ciencia y Tecnologica, Madrid, Spain; State Central Scientific Medical Library Supplier Center, Moscow, USSR. Searches are possible from January 1965. 82% of records have abstracts.

Record composition

Abstract AB; Author AU; BIOSIS Section Heading BISH; Chemical Abstracts Section Code CASC; Chemical Abstracts Section Heading CASH; CAS Reg.No CR; Controlled Term CT; Corporate Source CS; Country CY; Date Received REC; Document Date DT; Entry Month EM; Free Text FT; International Labour Office Section Code ILSC; International Labour Office Section Heading ILSH; International Pharmaceutical Abstracts Section Code IPSC; International Pharmaceutical Association Section Heading IPSH; ISSN SS; Journal Code JC; Journal Title JT; Language LA; Machine Date MD; Number of Document ND; Number of Supporting Agency NS; Number of Unit Record (DIMDI) NU; Order Number OD; Preprocessed Search PPS; Price PR; Publication Year PY; Qualifier AF; Source SO; Subunit SU; Supporting Agency SA; Title TI; Toxic Substances Control Act Section Code TSCC; Type of Awared TA and ZIP Code ZP

14:983. Database subset

Online   **Japan Information Center of Science and Technology (JICST)**

File name	TOXLINE
Alternative name(s)	Toxicology Information Online
Start year	
Number of records	
Update period	

14:984. Database subset

Online   **Japan Information Center of Science and Technology (JICST)**

File name	TOXLIT
Alternative name(s)	Toxicology Information Online
Start year	
Number of records	
Update period	

14:985. Database subset

Online   **National Library of Medicine**

File name	TOXLINE
Start year	Varies by file

Number of records	
Update period	Monthly

14:986. Database subset

Online   **National Library of Medicine**

File name	TOXLIT
Start year	1965
Number of records	
Update period	Monthly

14:987. Database subset

Tape   **National Library of Medicine**

File name	TOXLINE
Format notes	IBM
Start year	Varies by file
Number of records	
Update period	Monthly

Notes

Corresponds to the TOXLINE online database. Contact NLM for pricing information.

14:988. Database subset

Tape   **National Library of Medicine**

File name	TOXLIT
Format notes	IBM
Start year	1965
Number of records	
Update period	Monthly

Notes

Corresponds to the TOXLIT online database. Contact NLM for pricing information.

For more details of constituent databases, see:
TOXLIT
TOXLINE

This database can also be found on:
PolTox I: NLM, CSA, IFIS
Toxline on SilverPlatter
Toxline Plus

Toxline on SilverPlatter

National Library of Medicine
National Chemicals Inspectorate of Sweden

14:991. Master record

CD-ROM   **SilverPlatter**

Database type	Bibliographic
Number of journals	
Sources	Journals
Start year	1966
Language	English
Coverage	International
Number of records	1 million
Update size	50,000
Update period	Quarterly

Keywords

Aneuploidy; Chromosome Abnormalities; Drugs; Occupational Health and Safety; Pesticides; Pollution; Water Treatment

Description

Toxline on SilverPlatter provides a collection of toxicological information, the majority supplied by the National Library of Medicine, but also from fifteen other separate sources. Toxline contains references to published material and research in progress in the areas of adverse material and research in progress in the areas of adverse drug reaction, air pollution, carcinogenesis via chemicals, drug toxicity, food contamination, occupational hazards, pesticides and herbicides, toxicological analysis, water treatment and more. Subjects covered include: basic and applied research in all areas of the life, physical, social, behavioural, and engineering sciences. The database contains three sections:

(1) TOXLINE which includes the public domain records in the NLM file from 1981 to the present. Information is taken from eleven sources including CAS, MEDLINE and BIOSIS.

(2) RISKLINE – A secondary bibliographic database from the National Chemicals Inspectorate in Sweden, who provide selected and evaluated material on risk assessment; and

(3) FEDRIP, containing research supported by the US Public Health Service and featuring toxicology-related reports submitted to the National Technical Information Service.

One reviewer thought that while this product covered many of the same topics as the PolTox series, it is not as specific in its focus and does not draw on the same sources although there is some overlap.

Almost all of Toxline's citations include abstracts, indexing terms and CAS Registry Numbers.

Subscription costs are: regular subscriptions (1966+) £900 for single users and £1,1350 for 2–8 networked users; regular subscriptions (1981+) £685 for single users and £1,028 for 2–8 networked users.

For more details of constituent databases, see:
TOXLINE
RISKLINE
FEDRIP

Keywords

Aneuploidy; Chromosome Abnormalities; Drugs; Occupational Health and Safety; Pesticides; Pollution; Water Treatment

Description

Toxline Plus combines:

TOXLINE database (National Library of Medicine database of published material and research in progress relating to drug/chemical effects);
RISKLINE a secondary database from Sweden;
TOXLIT from the Chemical Abstracts Service (CAS) and toxicology related data from BIOSIS and the American Society of Hospital Pharmacists (ASHP) (IPA).

Toxline Plus' initial one million records will include approximately 70,000 from CAS; 37,000 from BIOSIS; 12,000 from ASHP; and 50,000 from NLM and will provide references with abstracts to literature in all areas of toxicology: chemicals; pharmaceuticals; pesticides; environmental pollutants; mutagens; and teratology. CAS will provide interactions of chemical substances with biological systems; BIOSIS will provide industrial medicine, occupational health, pollution and waste disposal; ASHP will provide adverse drug reactions, toxicity, and drug evaluations; and NLM will provide poisoning, adverse or environmental effects of chemicals, hazardous materials management, and health and safety. One reviewer thought that while this product covered many of the same topics as the PolTox series, it is not as specific in its focus and does not draw on the same sources although there is some overlap.

There are five discs with discounts for academic institutions, and costs are: regular subscription for single users £2,500 and £5,000 for 2–8 networked users; for academic institutions cost is £1,875 for single users, £3,750 for 2–8 networked users.

For more details of constituent databases, see:
Toxline
RISKLINE
TOXLIT
BIOSIS
IPA

Toxline Plus

National Library of Medicine
American Society of Hospital Pharmacists
BIOSIS
Chemical Abstracts Service
National Chemicals Inspectorate of Sweden

14:993. Master record
CD-ROM   **SilverPlatter**

Sources	
Start year	1985
Language	English
Coverage	International
Number of records	1.2 million
Update size	170,000
Update period	Quarterly

TOXLINE

National Library of Medicine

14:995. Master record

Database type	Bibliographic, Factual
Number of journals	17,400
Sources	Journals
Start year	1945
Language	English
Coverage	International
Number of records	660,000
Update size	–
Update period	Monthly

Keywords

Aneuploidy; Chromosome Abnormalities; Drugs; Occupational Health and Safety; Pesticides; Pollution; Water Treatment

Description

TOXLINE is a part of TOXALL with references from producers that do not require royalty charges; references on toxicology from producers that do require royalty charges are placed in TOXLIT. The database contains approximately 20,000 citations from between 1940 and 1965, 640,000 from 1965 to 1976, EMIC since 1960 and ETIC since 1965. Approximately eighty-two per cent of documents contain abstracts. Some hosts only carry TOXLINE.

For more details of constituent databases, see:
Aneuploidy
CISDOC
Environmental Mutagens – EMIC
Environmental Teratology – ETIC
Epidemiology Information System – EPIDEM
Federal Research in Progress – FEDRIP
Hayes File on Pesticides – HAYES
Hazardous Materials Technical Center – HMTC
International Pharmaceutical Abstracts – IPA
NIOSHTIC, subset
Pesticides Abstracts – PESTAB (post-1965)
Pesticides Abstracts – HAPAB (pre-1965)
Poisonous Plants Bibliography – PPBIB
Toxic Substances Control Act Test Submissions – TSCATS
MEDLINE, subset – Toxicity Bibliography – TOXBIB
Toxicological Aspects of Environmental Health – BIOSIS (formerly HEEP)
Toxicology/Epidemiology Research Projects – RPROJ – CRISP
Toxicology Document and Data Depository – NTIS
Toxic Materials Information Center File – TMIC

This database can also be found on:
TOXALL
PolTox I: NLM, CSA, IFIS
Toxline on SilverPlatter
Toxline Plus

TOXLIT
National Library of Medicine

14:998. Master record
Database type
Number of journals
Sources
Start year
Language
Coverage
Number of records
Update size   –
Update period

Keywords
Aneuploidy; Chromosome Abnormalities; Drugs; Occupational Health and Safety; Pesticides; Pollution; Water Treatment

Description
TOXLIT is a part of TOXALL with references from producers that require royalty charges; references on toxicology from producers that do not require royalty charges are placed in TOXLINE. The database contains approximately 20,000 citations from between 1940 and 1965, 640,000 from 1965 to 1976, EMIC since 1960 and ETIC since 1965. Approximately eighty-two per cent of documents contain abstracts. Some hosts only carry TOXLINE.

For more details of constituent databases, see:
Chemical Abstracts – CA
Biological Abstracts – BIOSIS
International Pharmaceutical Abstracts – IPA

This database can also be found on:

TOXALL
PolTox I: NLM, CSA, IFIS
Toxline on SilverPlatter
Toxline Plus

USP DI Volume 1: Drug Information for the Health Care Professional
Micromedex Inc
US Pharmacopeial Convention

14:1001. Master record
Alternative name(s)	USP DI Drug Information for the Health Care Professional; Drug Information for the Health Care Professional: USP DI Volume 1; CCIS: USP DI Volume 1
Database type	Factual, Textual
Number of journals	
Sources	Monographs
Start year	1988
Language	English and Spanish
Coverage	USA
Number of records	5,000
Update size	–
Update period	Quarterly

Keywords
Drugs

Description
Published by the US Pharmacopeial Convention, this database provides access to clinically relevant, consensus based, dispensing, prescribing and drug use information, including all medically accepted uses, both labelled and unlabelled, for virtually all US and Canadian medicines. Covers indications, precautions, pharmacology, dosing information and V.A. classifications. It is recognized as a compendium for unlabelled uses, patient counselling, and drug utilisation review in the Medicaid provisions of the Omnibus budget Reconciliation Act of 1990 (OBRA '90). Information is available in Spanish, English and Easy-to-Read (low literacy) versions.

14:1002. CD-ROM   Micromedex Inc
File name	CCIS: USP DI Volume 1
Alternative name(s)	USP DI Drug Information for the Health Care Professional; Drug Information for the Health Care Professional: USP DI Volume 1; CCIS: USP DI Volume 1
Start year	1988
Number of records	5,000
Update period	Quarterly
Price/Charges	Subscription: UK£360

Notes
As part of the CCIS system, this database complements the Drugdex system. The database can be purchased as a standalone product, cost is £360, with a £65 licence fee.

14:1003. CD-ROM   SilverPlatter
File name	USP DI Volume 1: Drug Information for the Health Care Professional
Alternative name(s)	USP DI Drug Information for the Health Care Professional; Drug Information for the Health Care Professional: USP DI Volume 1; CCIS: USP DI Volume 1
Start year	1988

| Number of records | 5,000 |
| Update period | Quarterly |

Notes

From 1993, this database is automatically accompanied by USP DI Volume 2, Advice for the Patient.

This database can also be found on:
STAT!-Ref
CCIS
MAXX

Vergiftungen
Georg Thieme Verlag

14:1005. Master record

Database type	
Number of journals	
Sources	
Start year	
Language	German
Coverage	
Number of records	
Update size	–
Update period	

Keywords

Drugs; Pharmaceuticals; Surgery

Description

Forms part of the DIAGNOSIS database from Medisoft and the MediROM database from AEK.

This database can be found on:
DIAGNOSIS, Vergiftungen, Radiolab
MediROM
PharmaROM

VETDOC
Derwent Publications Ltd

14:1007. Master record

Alternative name(s)	Veterinary Literature Documentation
Database type	Bibliographic
Number of journals	
Sources	Journals
Start year	1968
Language	English
Coverage	International
Number of records	96,000
Update size	4,800
Update period	Quarterly
Index unit	Articles

Keywords

Veterinary Drugs

Description

VETDOC contains citations, with abstracts, to the worldwide journal literature on veterinary drugs, vaccines, growth promotants, toxicology and hormonal control of breeding for domestic and farm animals. Subject areas covered include analysis, biochemistry, chemistry, endocrinology, microbiology, pathology, pharmacology, zoology and management.

The database corresponds to the biweekly *Vetdoc Abstract Journal* and *Associated Classified Editions*. Each record contains indepth keywording and fragmentation codes.

14:1008. Online ORBIT

File name	UDBV
Start year	1983
Number of records	96,000
Update period	Quarterly
SDI period	Monthly
Price/Charges	Connect time: US$60.00
	Online print: US$0.25/0.25
	Offline print: US$0.25/0.25
	SDI charge: US$8.50

Downloading is allowed

Notes

The corresponding file VETD contains records for the years 1968–1982. Electronic SDI service is now available within two hours on ORBIT. They can be downloaded and reformatted on a word processor. Results are retrieved in the low cost PRINTS file, $15 per connect hour. Online access is restricted to VETDOC subscribers.

14:1009. Online ORBIT

File name	VETD
Start year	1968–1982
Number of records	
Update period	Quarterly
SDI period	Monthly
Price/Charges	Connect time: US$60.00
	Online print: US$0.25/0.25
	Offline print: US$0.25/0.25
	SDI charge: US$8.50

Downloading is allowed

Notes

See corresponding file UDBV for records from 1983 onwards. Electronic SDI service is now available within two hours on ORBIT. They can be downloaded and reformatted on a word processor. Results are retrieved in the low cost PRINTS file, $15 per connect hour. Online access is restricted to VETDOC subscribers.

Virginia Disc: VADISC 1
Nimbus Records Ltd
Virginia Polytechnic Institute and State University

14:1010. Master record

Database type	Computer software, Bibliographic, Textual, Factual, Statistical, Image, Cartographic, Multimedia
Number of journals	
Sources	
Start year	
Language	English
Coverage	
Number of records	
Update size	–
Update period	
Database aids	Twelve-page description of software and data and User Agreement

Keywords

Nutrition

Description

The Virginia Disc series was conceived to demonstrate the feasibility of local publishing of CD-ROMs, especially by universities, and to stimulate interest in both CD-ROM and innovative approaches to information storage and retrieval. Manifold data, images, computer science, consumer information and software included in 35 searchable collections.

VADISC 1 contains about 6,000 files totalling about 600 Mbytes and includes over thirty searchable databases and a thirty-minute slide demonstration of the contents. Some data may be downloaded, some may be searched with the software packages included. Major software packages include FoxBASE+ (compiled dBASE III Plus programs); HyperLink (hypertext package); PC-Write (shareware editor/word processor) Personal Librarian (full-text retrieval software with Boolean logic, truncation, wild cards, proximity operators and ranking of search results); Perfect Hash Functions (Software routines which demonstrate the applicability of perfect hashing as a method of accessing data on CD-ROMs); TOPIC (full-text retrieval software incorporating artificial intelligence and fuzzy set concepts supporting reusable topic specifications that can form the kernel of more complex queries); and Window Book Technology (hypertext system).

The data collections included are:

Four collections from the Association for Computing Machinery (use Personal Librarian);
Computer World – a collection of 2351 computer articles (TOPIC);
Electronic Mail Digest Archives (TOPIC);
Inter-American Compendium of Registered Veterinary Drug products (FoxBASE+);
IPIS-Hypertext – the Integrated Preservation Information System (HyperLink);
King James Bible (Personal Librarian);
Rutgers' Information Retrieval Database (Dr Tefko Saracevic) on the elements involved in information seeking, searching and retrieving, particularly relating to the cognitive context and human decisions and interactions involved (Personal Librarian);
University of Melbourne Computer Science Bibliography (Personal Librarian);
University Self Study – survey of last ten years at VPI&SU providing variable information in full-text form (Personal Librarian);
US Department of Agriculture Extension Information – possibly the single most important collection on the disc, including a list of Virginia publication titles (Personal Librarian); general information fact sheets on agriculture, clothing and textiles, gardening, health and nutrition, home and financial management, home economics, pests, rural community development and youth leadership (Personal Librarian); Florida Agricultural Information Retrieval System (FAIRS) with data; Florida Pest Control Guides; Virginia Master Gardener Handbook (Window Book or Personal Librarian); Recipe Nutrition Analysis; Pesticide Spray Bulletine (Personal Librarian);
US Geographical and Population Data (FoxBASE+);
Virginia Genealogical Database (Personal Librarian);
Virginia Tech Faculty Expertise Database (Personal Librarian).

Public Domain data collections include:

Artificial Intelligence List (eMail messages);
Architectural Images (AUTOCAD files requiring VGA or Targa board);
Dual Independent Map Format file of US state boundaries;
Florida Extension Images of flora and fuana native to Florida (require VGA or Targa board);
Information Retrieval List (eMail messages);
Information Retrieval Test Collections including ADI,

CACM, CISI, Cranfield, MEDLINE, NPL, TIME and LISA (Sheffield);
Survey Points in Virginia, Washington DC and Baltimore;
University of Maryland CVL Images – a collection of 200 varied images;
US Geological data of digital elevation models, digital line graph data, land use/land cover data and population/place data.

In addition a DVI directory has files that are usable with Pro750trademark symbol Application Development Platform from Intel or other compatible DVI systems – full motion video sequences, photographic stills and images.

14:1011. CD-ROM   Virginia Polytechnic Institute and State University

File name	VADISC I
Software	Needs MS-DOS V3.3 or above and Microsoft Extensions V2.0 or above.
Start year	
Number of records	
Update period	
Database aids	Twelve-page description of software and data and User Agreement

Vital Signs: the Good Health Resource
Texas Caviar

14:1012. Master record

Alternative name(s)	Vital Signs: a Personal Health Resource
Database type	Textual, Multimedia
Number of journals	
Sources	
Start year	
Language	English and Spanish
Coverage	
Number of records	
Update size	—
Update period	Annually

Keywords

Cancer; Clinical Medicine; Drug Abuse; HIV; Paediatrics; Personal Health Care

Description

A bilingingual multimedia health and fitness reference that contains comprehensive information concerning every facet of personal and family health and well-being. Many topics are covered in Spanish. Discussions deal with current issues of interest to various age and social groups. Can be used as an emergency guide, or to aid health workers discuss issues such as grief with patients. Includes a directory of toll-free telephone numbers users can call for expanded information on subjects such as AIDS, drug abuse and cancer. Also includes interactive record-keeping tools to track prescriptions, inoculations and illnesses. A full CD-Audio sound track is included plus a glossary of medical terms. Has images to help explain medical information, materials developed for consumer understanding, audio presentations, and multimedia instructional modules. Covers ears, eyes, nose, breast, urinary tract and prostate, skin, lymph nodes, extremities, bones, joints, infant/child care and development, child/wife abuse or neglect, fever, tiredness and blood pressure. Assembled by physicians and experienced health providers. Original information source is the Knowledge Resources Corporation, National Centers for Disease Control.

Keyword search capability

14:1013. CD-ROM   Texas Caviar

File name	Vital Signs: the Good Health Resource
Alternative name(s)	Vital Signs: a Personal Health Resource
Format notes	IBM, Mac
Software	Software Mart
Start year	
Number of records	
Update period	Annually
Price/Charges	Subscription: UK£59.38

Voyages et Santé
Telmed

14:1014. Master record

Database type	
Number of journals	
Sources	
Start year	
Language	French
Coverage	Switzerland
Number of records	
Update size	—
Update period	

Keywords

Drugs; Pharmaceuticals; Travel

Description

This database in the medical and pharmaceutical field forms part of the MediROM and PharmaROM CD-ROMs, originally intended for Swiss pharmacists.

This database can be found on:
MediROM
PharmaROM

World Drug Index with structures
Derwent Publications Ltd
Molecular Design Ltd
Chemical Design Ltd

14:1016. Master record

Alternative name(s)	Standard Drug File with Graphics (Previous name); SDF + G (Previous name)
Database type	Factual, Chemical structures
Number of journals	
Sources	
Start year	1983
Language	
Coverage	
Number of records	37,800
Update size	—
Update period	Irregular

Keywords

Drugs

Description

The World Drug Index with structures (formerly Standard Drug File with Graphics, part of the Standard Drug File, which is now Derwent Drug Registry) contains a wider range of drugs than the Derwent Drug Registry, being compiled from a wider range of sources. It is available in three different versions from Derwent: World Drug Index with structures – In-house, produced with Molecular Design Ltd; World Drug Index with structures on CD-ROM (available end April 1993, when the name change of the database occurs); and World Drug Index with structures 3D. All were previously called Standard Drug File with Graphics. In addition to searches on drug names, Chemical Abstracts Registry Numbers, Derwent Registry Names and Medical Concepts, it is possible to search chemical structures and substructures graphically. The database is available to link with any of the commonly-available graphics software packages: MACCS II, DARC-SMS, ORAC, etc. It is not available online.

Derwent have reorganised their collection of drug databases, resulting in three new names: Derwent Drug Registry (formerly Standard Drug File); Derwent Drug File (formerly Ringdoc); and, with the launch of a CD-ROM in Spring 1993, the World Drug Index (formerly the Standard Drug File with Graphics).

14:1017. CD-ROM   Derwent Publications Ltd

File name	World Drug Index with structures CD-ROM
Alternative name(s)	Standard Drug File with Graphics (Previous name); SDF + G (Previous name)
Start year	1983
Number of records	37,800
Update period	Irregular

Notes

The World Drug Index with structures (formerly Standard Drug File with Graphics) contains a wider range of drugs than the Derwent Drug Registry, being compiled from a wider range of sources. In addition to searches on drug names, Chemical Abstracts Registry Numbers, Derwent Registry Names and Medical Concepts, it is possible to search chemical structures and substructures graphically. It is available to link with any of the commonly-available graphics software packages: MACCS II, DARC-SMS, ORAC, etc. This CD-ROM version of the database was available from the end of April 1993, when the name change of the database occurred.

14:1018. Tape   Derwent Publications Ltd

File name	World Drug Index with structures – In-house
Alternative name(s)	Standard Drug File with Graphics (Previous name); SDF + G (Previous name)
Start year	1983
Number of records	37,800
Update period	Irregular

Notes

The World Drug Index with structures (formerly Standard Drug File with Graphics) contains a wider range of drugs than the Derwent Drug Registry, being compiled from a wider range of sources. This is the currently available in-house version from Derwent and Molecular Design Ltd, supplied on tape. In addition to searches on drug names, Chemical Abstracts Registry Numbers, Derwent Registry Names and Medical Concepts, it is possible to search chemical structures and substructures graphically. It is available to link with any of the commonly-available graphics software packages: MACCS II, DARC-SMS, ORAC, etc.

14:1019. Tape   Derwent Publications Ltd

File name   World Drug Index with structures – 3D
Alternative name(s)   Standard Drug File with Graphics (Previous name); SDF + G (Previous name)
Start year   1983
Number of records   37,800
Update period   Irregular

Notes

The World Drug Index with structures (formerly Standard Drug File with Graphics) contains a wider range of drugs than the Derwent Drug Registry, being compiled from a wider range of sources. This version of the database contains three-dimensional representations of the structures, and is available from Chemical Design Ltd. In addition to searches on drug names, Chemical Abstracts Registry Numbers, Derwent Registry Names and Medical Concepts, it is possible to search chemical structures and substructures graphically. It is available to link with any of the commonly-available graphics software packages: MACCS II, DARC-SMS, ORAC, etc.

Worldwide Biotech
Worldwide Videotex

14:1020. Master record

Database type   Textual
Number of journals   1
Sources
Start year   1990
Language   English
Coverage   USA (some) and International (some)
Number of records
Update size   –
Update period   Monthly

Keywords

Biotechnology Industries; Pharmaceutical Industry

Description

A monthly newsletter for the international biotechnology industry, providing news and information on biotechnology as an international industry, reporting on the deals between US biotechnology companies and international pharmaceutical companies. Monitors the European Community market place and the growing interest and deals in the US biotechnology and pharmaceuticals industry.

Corresponds to the monthly *Worldwide Biotech* newsletter. On DIALOG and Data-Star this database is available as part of the PTS Newsletter Database, supplied by Predicasts.

This database can be found on:
PTS Newsletter Database

FORENSIC SCIENCE

AgeLine

American Association of Retired
Persons, National Gerontology
Resource Center (AARP)

15:1. Master record

Database type	Bibliographic
Number of journals	
Sources	Dissertations, Government documents, Journals, Monographs and Reports
Start year	1978 (selected coverage back to 1966)
Language	English
Coverage	USA (primarily) and English-speaking countries (some)
Number of records	30,900
Update size	3,000
Update period	Every two months
Index unit	Articles and Book chapters
Abstract details	AgeLine staff
Thesaurus	Thesaurus of Aging Terminology

Keywords

Aging; Gerontology; Health Care Services; Pathology

Description

AgeLine contains citations, with abstracts, to the literature on social gerontology, the study of aging in social, psychological, health-related and economic contexts. The delivery of health care for the older population and its associated costs and policies is particularly well covered, as are public policy, employment and consumer issues. Subjects covered include: demographics, economics, employment, political action, health and health care services, housing, intergenerational relationships, social and family relationships, psychological aspects, retirement, transportation, consumer aspects and leisure. The literature covered is of interest to researchers, health professionals, service planners, policymakers, employers, older adults and their families and consumer advocates.

Journal citations compose roughly two-thirds of the database with the rest devoted to citations from books, book chapters and reports. An original, informative abstract accompanies each citation. There is no print equivalent of this database.

Journal coverage includes gerontological, social science, health, business and current events periodicals.

15:2. Online   BRS

File name	AARP
Start year	1978 (selected coverage back to 1966)
Number of records	29,297
Update period	Every two months
Price/Charges	Connect time: US$48.00/58.00
	Online print: US$0.32/0.40
	Offline print: US$0.40

15:3. Online   CompuServe Information Service

File name	IQUEST File 1949
Start year	1978
Number of records	29,297
Update period	Every two months
Price/Charges	Subscription: US$8.95 per month
	Database entry fee: US$9/search; some databases carry a surcharge ($2–75)
	Online print: US$10 references free; then $9 per ten; abstracts $3 each
Downloading is allowed	

Notes

Accessed via IQUEST or IQMEDICAL, this database is offered by a BRS gateway. IQUEST can either search across all databases, a database of the user's choice or selected multiple databases.

15:4. Online   DIALOG

File name	File 163
Start year	1978 (selected coverage back to 1966)
Number of records	30,905
Update period	Every two months
Price/Charges	Connect time: US$60.00
	Online print: US$0.25
	Offline print: US$0.25
	SDI charge: US$5.95

Notes

DIALINDEX Categories: PSYCH, SOCISCI

American Medical Association Journals Online

American Medical Association

15:5. Master record

Alternative name(s)	AMAJO
Database type	Textual
Number of journals	10
Sources	Journals
Start year	
Language	English
Coverage	International
Number of records	
Update size	—
Update period	Weekly for JAMA; Monthly for specialty journals

Keywords

Clinical Medicine; Dermatology; Internal Medicine; Laboratory Medicine; Neurology; Ophthalmology; Otolaryngology; Paediatrics; Pathology; Plastic Surgery; Surgery

Description

Contains the full text articles from ten medical journals, including *JAMA*. The medical journals are:

AJDC, American Journal of Diseases of Children, 1982–89, 1991–;

Archives of Dermatology, 1982–89, 1991–;
Archives of General Psychiatry, 1982–89, 1991–;
Archives of Internal Medicine, 1982–89, 1991–;
Archives of Neurology, 1982–89, 1991–;
Archives of Ophthalmology, 1982–89, 1991–;
Archives of Otolaryngology – Head and Neck Surgery, 1982–89, 1991–;
Archives of Pathology and Laboratory Medicine, 1982–89, 1991–;
Archives of Surgery, 1982–89, 1991–;
JAMA, The Journal of the American Medical Association 1982.

15:6. Online   DIALOG

File name	File 442
Alternative name(s)	AMAJO
Start year	
Number of records	
Update period	Weekly for JAMA; Monthly for specialty journals
Price/Charges	Subscription: US$78.00
	Online print: US$1.00
	Offline print: US$1.00
	SDI charge: US$1.50

Notes

This database can also be accessed as a menu-driven option on Medtext, a collection of full text medical journals available on DIALOG.

For more details of constituent databases, see:
American Journal of Diseases of Children
Archives of Dermatology
Archives of General Psychiatry
Archives of Internal Medicine
Archives of Neurology
Archives of Ophthalmology
Archives of Otolaryngology – Head and Neck Surgery
Archives of Pathology and Laboratory Medicine
Archives of Surgery
Journal of the American Medical Association

Analytical Abstracts
Royal Society of Chemistry

15:8. Master record

Database type	Bibliographic
Number of journals	2,000
Sources	Conference proceedings, journals, monographs, Technical reports and standards
Start year	1978
Language	English
Coverage	International
Number of records	150,000+
Update size	15,000
Update period	Monthly
Index unit	Conference papers and articles
Abstract details	RSC – abstracts are written specifically aimed at the analytical user.
Database aids	Analytical Abstracts Online User Manual UK£30 ($50), Analysis Hotline (newletter) Free and Analytical Abstracts Information Pack – Free

Keywords

Analytical Chemistry; Forensic Science; Inorganic Chemistry

Description

Analytical Abstracts is the only abstracting service devoted solely to analytical chemistry. It covers all aspects of analytical chemistry appearing world-wide including applications of analytic techniques in inorganic, organic, agricultural, pharmacy, food chemistry, agriculture, analytical methods, analytical instruments, biochemical, environmental, food and pharmaceutical chemistry. The database contains citations with, since 1984, high quality English-language abstracts enabling the user to assess the analytical relevance of the original paper. Subjects covered include: the application of various analytical techniques, including use of computers and instruments in general, inorganic, organic, biochemical, pharmaceutical, food, agricultural and environmental chemistry. Records include chemical names, trade names, Chemical Abstracts Service (CAS) Registry Numbers and analytical techniques used (for example, gas chromatography).

The data corresponds to the printed *Analytical Abstracts*. Journal articles represent 98% of the file. Items are selected from over 2,000 journals world-wide, originally published in more than twenty languages. The 'core' list of journals totals more than 300 primary titles.

All Analytical Abstracts material has been indexed by the producer to facilitate the retrieval of Analytes (the chemical substances being separated, determined, identified or detected), the Matrix (the medium or type of sample in which the analyte is present) and the Concept (techniques, reagents, apparatus, or fields of study that is anything which is not an analyte or a matrix). Chemical nomenclature is based on that recommended by the International Union of Pure and Applied Chemistry; organic compounds are indexed at the parent compound, followed by substituent groups. Esters and salts of organic acids are indexed under the name of the acid constituent. Colour Index names are used for the names of dyes; enzymes are named according to the approved names of the International Union of Biochemistry; drugs according to the British Pharmacopoeia Commission and pesticides according to the British Standards Institute. CAS Registry Numbers are included for all compounds that are indexed as an ANALYTE or a MATRIX. Note that if the compound of interest is not indexed (that is, it is a solvent, interferent or reagent), or is indexed as a CONCEPT (for example, a novel reagent), CAS Registry Numbers will not help.

Abbreviations for techniques such as gas chromatography and atomic-absorption spectrophotometry are given in the form of capital letters, with no full stops (GC, AAS, etc.) However, references dating from prior to 1986 have an 'old-style' abbreviation viz 'g.c.' or 'a.a.s.' and so proximity operators must be used.

Analytical Abstracts modified its index categorisation in 1991 as a result of editorial changes in its print equivalent. The modifications are in Section and Subsection headings. Cross-reference headings have also changed in format and content. In January 1993, the producers are changing to the American spelling 'Sulfur' rather than the English 'Sulphur' – the change will be implemented on all chemical names containing the term or 'sulp', 'sulph', 'sulpho', 'sulphate', etc. The only exceptions are approved drug and pesticide names. Pre-1993 data will NOT be altered.

15:9. Online   Data-Star

File name	ANAB
Start year	1978

Number of records	126,018
Update period	Monthly
Database aids	Data-Star Chemical Manual, Berne, Data-Star, 1989 and Online manual (search NEWS-ANAB in NEWS)
Price/Charges	Subscription: SFr80.00
	Connect time: SFr200.00
	Online print: SFr2.57
	Offline print: SFr1.56
	SDI charge: SFr15.51

Downloading is allowed

Notes

From June 1993 Data-Star have introduced an annual fee/subscription per contract (that is, not per password) of SFr 80.00 (c.UK£ 32.00) payable every June. For North American customers billed in dollars who also use DIALOG, the DIALOG fee also covers access to Data-Star. Academic customers, 'commitment' customers and customers currently billed in dollars are exempt.

Record composition

Abstract AB; Accession Number and Update Code AN; Author AU; Author Affiliation IN; Availability AV; Coden CD; Conference Data CT; Cross Reference XR; Descriptor superlabel for DA, DC, DM; Descriptor/s: analyte DA; Descriptor/s: concept DC; Descriptor: matrix DM; Language of Article LG; Publication Type PT; Publisher PB; Section Details SC; Source SO; Title TI; Update Code UP; Year YR and Year of Publication PY

15:10. Online   DIALOG, Knowledge Index

File name	File 305
Start year	1980
Number of records	150,000+
Update period	Monthly
Price/Charges	Connect time: US$174.00
	Online print: US$1.30
	Offline print: US$1.30
	SDI charge: US$6.50

Downloading is allowed

Notes

This database is also available to home users during evenings and weekends at a reduced rate on the Knowledge Index service of DIALOG – file name in this case is CHEM2, and searches are made with simplified commands or menus.

Record composition

Accession Number; Title; Author; Corporate Source; Journal; Coden; Publication Date; Language; Abstract; Analyte; Matrix and Section Code

DIALINDEX Categories: BIOCHEM, CHEMLIT, FOODSCI, POLLUT, RNCHEM, RNMED, SCITECHB.

15:11. Online   ORBIT

File name	ANAB
Start year	1980
Number of records	150,000+
Update period	Monthly
Database aids	Quick Reference Guide (1/89) Free (single copy) and Database Manual (1986) $7.50

Price/Charges	Connect time: US$142
	Online print: US$1.05
	Offline print: US$0.70
	SDI charge: US$8.50

Downloading is allowed

Notes

Electronic SDI service is now available within two hours on ORBIT. They can be downloaded and reformatted on a word processor. Results are retrieved in the low cost PRINTS file, $15 per connect hour.

Record composition

Accession Number AN; Title TI; Author AU; Corporate Source OS; Source SO; Language LA; CODEN JC; ISSN NU; Document Type DT; Classification Codes CC; Index Terms IT and Abstract AB

15:12. Online   STN

File name	ANABSTR
Start year	1980
Number of records	159,929
Update period	Monthly
Price/Charges	Connect time: DM220.00
	Online print: DM2.70
	Offline print: DM2.70
	SDI charge: DM18.00

Downloading is allowed

Record composition

Accession Number AN; Title TI; Author AU; Source SO; Document Type DT; Language LA; Abstract AB; Classification Codes CC and Index Terms IT

15:13. CD-ROM   SilverPlatter

File name	Analytical Abstracts
Format notes	IBM, Mac
Software	SPIRS/MacSPIRS
Start year	1980
Number of records	160,000
Update period	Quarterly
Price/Charges	Subscription: UK£885 – 2,212

Downloading is allowed

Notes

Requires a signed subscription and licence agreement. Regular subscription is UK£885 for a single user, £2,212 for 2–8 networked users. Discounts are available to print subscribers – £585 for a single user, £1,462 for 2–8 networked users. Chuck Huber, the reviewer in *CD-ROM Professional* (5(4) p.120–121) thought the SilverPlatter implementation good, the software allowing searching by CAS Registry Number and by the substance's role as either analyte or matrix. He makes the point that with the excellence of the Royal Society's indexing in the print version, the advantages of searching the CD-ROM are reduced but, as the print index does not cumulate annually, there is an advantage to set against the high price differential.

15:14. Database subset

Online   DIALOG

File name	File 385 – ONTAP Analytical Abstracts Training File
Start year	January to June 1987
Number of records	6,041
Update period	Closed File
Price/Charges	Connect time: US$15.00

Notes

The training file for Analytical Abstracts contains records from the January to June updates to File 305, the main Analytical Abstracts file on DIALOG. Offline prints are not available in ONTAP files.

Anatomist
Folkstone Design

15:15. Master record

Database type	Multimedia, Factual
Number of journals	
Sources	
Start year	
Language	English
Coverage	
Number of records	
Update size	–
Update period	

Keywords
Anatomy

Description
Human anatomy in hypermedia format. Material identifies over 2,500 terms with with 500 illustrations, text, and speech giving the correct pronunciations of anatomical terms. Students own notes can be added as desired.

Based on material from the print *Anatomy Coloring Book* by Wynn Kapit and Lawrence Elson with supplementary material from Tortora's *Principles of Human Anatomy*.

15:16. CD-ROM   Folkstone Design

File name	Anatomist
Format notes	Mac
Software	HyperCard
Start year	
Number of records	
Update period	
Price	US$295

Notes
Although well designed and easy to use, the stack contains several spelling errors and omits important command key combinations from the keyboard shortcuts section. According to reviewer, Layne Nordgren (*CD-ROM Professional* 5(6) p146–7), it is also impossible to navigate back to Anatomist without getting an error message and having to restart the application. At the beginning of the program the user is presented with an illustrations window with small circles that are 'hot spots' representing a single anatomical term. When the spot is clicked on, the term is pronounced in a female voice, the entire structure is highlighted in grey and the text of the term is presented. The reviewer ends that, despite the poor quality of some illustrations and the lack of colour, the disc is an excellent resource for supplementing teaching and learning of anatomy. It could also be used in a laboratory as a reference tool. Unfortunately, the price may put it out of reach of many students.

Archives of Pathology and Laboratory Medicine
American Medical Association

15:18. Master record

Database type	Bibliographic, Textual, Factual
Number of journals	
Sources	Newsletter
Start year	1982
Language	English
Coverage	International

Number of records	
Update size	–
Update period	Monthly
Index unit	Articles, letters and reviews

Keywords
Laboratory Medicine; Pathology

Description
Archives of Pathology and Laboratory Medicine chronicles current research developments and clinical topics relevant to the practice of pathology, including clinical applications to diagnosis and laboratory monitoring of therapy. Sections include: Full text of original contributions; Editorials; Book reviews; Clinical notes; Letters to the editor; Photograph essays; Commentaries; Review articles; Case reports.

15:19. Online   Mead Data Central (as a NEXIS database)

File name	ARP – NEXIS
Alternative name(s)	NEXIS – Archives of Pathology and Laboratory Medicine
Start year	1982
Number of records	
Update period	Monthly
Price/Charges	Subscription: US$1,000 – 3,000 (Depending on needs) Connect time: US$49.00 (Telecomms + connect time) Database entry fee: US$24.00 (Search charge) Online print: US$0.04 per line

Notes
Library: GENMED; Group file: JNLS.

A subscription charge which covers all transactional charges, connect time, telecommunications and the small administration charge can take the place of the individual charges. Subscriptions are negotiated with customers and vary according to the number of menus (thus, files) that are to be used – typically a minimum subscription would be about US$ 1,000. All charges include training and a 24-hour help line.

Record composition
Publication; Cite; Date; Section; Length; Title; Source; Author; Abstract (SUM-ABS); Text; Additional information (SUPP-INFO); Reference (BIBLIO-REF); Graphic; Correction; Correction Date; Discussion and Editor's Note

15:20. CD-ROM   CMC ReSearch

File name	Archives of Pathology and Laboratory Medicine on CD-ROM
Format notes	IBM
Software	DiscPassage
Start year	Most recent five years
Number of records	
Update period	Annually
Price/Charges	Subscription: UK£265

Notes
This disc contains five years of the *Archives of Pathology and Laboratory Medicine*. Images from text are included.

BodyWorks
Software Marketing Corporation

15:21. Master record

Database type	Factual, Graphical, Textual
Number of journals	
Sources	

Start year
Language   English
Coverage
Number of records
Update size   —
Update period

Keywords

Anatomy; First Aid

Description

A reference tool for students, institutions and families which lets users explore the systems, structures and functions of the body in colourful, animated detail. Textual information on first aid, fitness, sport injuries and common illnesses as well as graphics which can be zoomed on for greater detail. Buttons give direct access to digestive, circulatory, nervous, reproductive, lymphatic, skeletal and muscular systems.

15:22. Diskette   Software Marketing Corporation

File name   BodyWorks
Format notes   IBM
Start year
Number of records
Update period
Price   UK£80

Notes

The New York Times said, 'The main point of BodyWorks is to serve as a teacher of, and reference to, human anatomy, and it does that strikingly well'.

CAB Abstracts
CAB International

15:23. Master record

Database type   Bibliographic
Number of journals   14,000
Sources   Books, company reports, conference proceedings, dissertations, grey literature, journals, monographs, patents, research reports, standards and theses
Start year   1972
Language   English (original language titles)
Coverage   International
Number of records   2,800,000
Update size   150,000
Update period   Monthly
Abstract details   CAB's own indexers write detailed informative English-language summaries for each record.
Thesaurus   CAB Abstracts Thesaurus
Database aids   CAB Abstracts Online Manual, CAB Serials Checklist, CAB Section Code Lists, CAB International Database News. and IULAS (International Union List of Agricultural Serials)

Keywords

Agricultural Economics; Agrochemicals; Anatomy; Animal Breeding; Animal Diseases; Bioagriculture; Crop Protection; Diet; Entomology; Environmental Health; Forestry; Horticulture; Immunology; Medical Entomology; Medical Immunology; Medical Mycology; Medical Parasitology; Mycology; Nutrition; Paper
and Packaging; Pathology; Pest Management;

Physiology; Plant Diseases; Plant Genetics; Pollution; Public Health; Rural Sociology; Soil Management; Sport; Tourism; Travel; Veterinary Entomology; Veterinary Mycology; Water Management

Description

Contains citations, with abstracts, to the worldwide literature in the agricultural sciences and related areas of applied biology. Subjects covered include agricultural engineering; agricultural entomology; animal breeding; biocontrol; biodeterioration and biodegradation; biotechnology; crop protection; dairy science and technology; economics; engineering; environment; forestry and forest products; genetics; herbicides; helminthology; horticulture; irrigation; leisure, recreation and tourism; medical and veterinary entomology; microbiology; mycology; nutrition (human and animal); parasitology (human and animal); plant breeding and pathology; protozoology; rural development and sociology; soil science and fertilizers and arid lands (1980 to 1982). Coverage of veterinary medicine begins in 1972. Also contains useful material on rural development in third world countries. Animal breeding and production, animal nutrition & dairy science and technology, covers: animals including farm mammals of economic or domestic importance; laboratory mammals; poultry, game and other birds of economic importance; fish, molluscs and crustacea; and certain invertebrates used in genetic studies. Subjects covered include performance traits and products; breeding and genetics; biotechnology; reproduction; nutrition; the dairy industry; housing and equipment for livestock and in aquaculture; and nongenetic effects on animals. Crop protection and pests covers: entomology; plant pathology; nematology and weed science for the full ranges of agricultural, horticultural, plantation and forestry crops. Covers areas of pest taxonomy; biology; ecology; management; and economic and social impact. Environmental health and toxicology covers: environmental agrochemicals (insecticides, fungicides, pesticides, fertilisers); groundwater contamination, runoff and leaching; heavy metals in soil, crops and animals; reclamation and re-vegetation of polluted sites; environmental impact of farming; waste management, treatment and disposal; toxicology (toxic plants, wastes, food poisoning, carcinogens); and steroids and hormones in animals. Forestry covers: silviculture and forestry management; tree biology; forest pests and their control; forest land use; wood properties; timber extraction, conversion and management; wood products; marketing and trade; agroforestry systems and related land use; plant and animal species for agroforestry; environmental and service aspects of agroforestry systems; and sociological, cultural and economic aspects of agroforestry systems. Horticulture covers: literature on temperate tree fruits and nuts; small fruits; viticulture; vegetables; temperate, tropical and greenhouse; ornamental plants; minor industrial crops; subtropical and tropical fruits and plantation crops. Leisure, recreation and tourism covers: leisure industries, travel and transport, marketing of services and products, natural resources and environmental issues, facility management and planning, sport, and leisure and tourism policies. Plant genetics covers: material on breeding; genetic resources; varieties; molecular and general genetics; in vitro culture; cytology and ploidy; reproductive behaviour; evolution and taxonomy; stress tolerance; disease and pest resistance; and quality and yield components. Soil science covers: soil management; crop management; fertilisers and amendments; agricultural meteorology;

pollution; land reclamation; irrigation and drainage; plant nutrition and plant water relations. Veterinary science covers: animals including farm animals; pets; game animals; all animals of economic importance, including farmed fish and shellfish; commercially important wild fish; zoo animals and wild animals. Subjects include viral and bacterial diseases; protozoology; mycology; helminthology; arthropod parasites; toxicology; immunology; pharmacology and therapeutics; physiology; biochemistry and anatomy; zootechny, hygiene and food inspection, and related areas. About 85% of items are abstracted in English with each abstract containing 80–100 words. Sources are published in 74 languages.

Corresponds to the fifty main journals and specialized journals published by the Commonwealth Agricultural Bureaux (CAB) International, an international, intergovernmental organisation registered with the United Nations. Membership is open to all governments wishing to participate. *The International Union List of Agricultural Serials*, a compilation of the serials indexed in AGRICOLA, AGRIS and CAB lists which database indexes a given title. Several hosts have separate subfiles by subject. On all BRS services four subsets are available separately; on agricultural economics, rural development and sociology; on human nutrition; on leisure, recreation and tourism; and on medical and veterinary sciences. On Data-Star, three subsets are available separately: on human nutrition, on human parasitology and mycology; and on medical and veterinary sciences. On DIMDI there are eleven subsets available separately: Animal; Animal Production; Economics; Engineering; Forestry; Human; Nutrition; Plant; Plant Protection; Tourism; and Veterinary Science.

From 1972 to 1983 the Controlled Terms take the form of subject index entries and additional index entries. The number of controlled terms allocated varies from one item/abstract to another. Various collections of uncontrolled, semi-controlled and controlled terms and phrases (keyword units) were used. The Controlled Terms vary between abstract journals. The most strictly controlled list of terms are used in *Index Veterinarius*, which from 1972 to 1976 used *Veterinary Subject Headings* (CAB, 1972) and from 1977 the *Veterinary Multilingual Thesaurus* (there is about 60% agreement between them). The Controlled Terms are the subject index entries used to generate the printed subject indices of the abstract journals, while the additional index entries, where present are used to facilitate retrieval. No hierarchical structure is available for controlled terms. The controlled terms comprise various categories of descriptors and names of organisms are in Latin or in English. Various systems of chemical notation and geographical terms are also used. From 1984 onwards controlled index terms are allocated from the *CAB Thesaurus*. A cumulative, alphabetic list of all Controlled Terms, including the descriptors from 1972/83 plus the descriptors of the *CAB Thesaurus* can be accessed by the DISPLAY-command. Almost every abstract is accompanied by a Section Code except the title-only items in *Index Veterinarius*. Usually the Section Codes are structured hierarchically corresponding to the sections and subsections of the CABI abstract journals. Two types of Section Codes are in use: Primary Sequencing Codes and Cross Reference Codes. Primary Sequencing Codes describe the main topic of an article and place an abstract within a given section of an abstract journal. These sections are often subdivided into several subsections; accordingly the assigned Primary Sequencing Codes are taken from

the lower levels of the hierarchy. One to two Primary Sequencing Codes are allocated to each abstract.

Cross Reference Codes, which do not occur in every abstract, cover the secondary aspects of an article and refer to another relevant journal section. Where allocated, they are taken from the higher levels of the hierarchy. Four to five Cross Reference Codes may be assigned to an abstract. The Section Codes are up to ten characters long, prefixed by a two character abstract journal code. Different codes and headings are used in each abstract journal so two different codes may be allocated. Section Headings refer to chapter headings and are broader terms to the Section Codes which makes it possible to use them for coarse subdivisions of a subject. (See CAB Abstracts Online for further advice).

15:24. Online   BIS

File name	CABA
Start year	
Number of records	
Update period	

15:25. Online   BRS, Morning Search, BRS/Colleague

File name	
Start year	
Number of records	
Update period	Monthly
Price/Charges	Connect time: US$62.00/72.00
	Online print: US$0.47/0.55
	Offline print: US$0.55
	SDI charge: US$12.50
Downloading is allowed	

Notes

Indexing is detailed and comprehensive using a controlled vocabulary.

15:26. Online   CISTI, Canadian Online Enquiry Service CAN/OLE

File name	CAB
Start year	
Number of records	
Update period	
Price/Charges	Connect time: Canadian $40.00
	Online print: Canadian $0.45
	Offline print: Canadian $0.45

Notes

CISTI accessible only in Canada.

15:27. Online   Data-Star

File name	CABI
Start year	1984
Number of records	1,000,000
Update period	Monthly
Database aids	Data-Star Biomedical, Business and Chemical Manuals. and Online manual (search NEWS-CABI in NEWS)
Price/Charges	Subscription: SFr80.00
	Connect time: SFr50.80
	Online print: SFr127.00
	Offline print: SFr1.01
	SDI charge: SFr12.40
Downloading is allowed	
Thesaurus is online	

Notes

From June 1993 Data-Star have introduced an annual fee/subscription per contract (that is, not per password) of SFr 80.00 (c.UK£ 32.00) payable every June. For North American customers billed in dollars who

also use DIALOG, the DIALOG fee also covers access to Data-Star. Academic customers, 'commitment' customers and customers currently billed in dollars are exempt.

Record composition

Abstract AB; Accession Number and Update Code AN; Article Type AT; Author(s) AU; Author Affiliation IN; Descriptors DE; Foreign Title TT; Geographic Descriptor CN; ISBN Number IS; Language of summary in original LS; Original Language LG; Publication Year YR; References AV; Section heading(s) SC; Source SO; Title TI; Update Code UP and Updated Code UD

15:28. Online   DIALOG, Knowledge Index

File name	File 50
Start year	1972 – 1983
Number of records	13,000
Update period	Monthly
Price/Charges	Connect time: US$54.00
	Online print: US$0.90
	Offline print: US$0.90
	SDI charge: US$15.00

Downloading is allowed
Thesaurus is online

Notes

This database is also available to home users during evenings and weekends at a reduced rate on the Knowledge Index service of DIALOG – file name in this case is CAB ABSTRACTS, and searches are made with simplified commands or menus.

DIALINDEX Categories: AGRI, BIOTECH, CAB, ENVIRON, FOODSCI, LEISURE, NUTRIT, VETSCI. The One-Search facility enables the two files of AGRICOLA, the one file of AGRIS and the two files of CAB to be searched simultaneously.

15:29. Online   DIALOG, Knowledge Index

File name	File 53
Start year	1984
Number of records	2,500,000
Update period	Monthly
Price/Charges	Connect time: US$54.00
	Online print: US$0.90
	Offline print: US$0.90

Downloading is allowed

Notes

This database is also available to home users during evenings and weekends at a reduced rate on the Knowledge Index service of DIALOG – file name in this case is CAB ABSTRACTS, and searches are made with simplified commands or menus.

DIALINDEX Categories: AGRI, BIOTECH, CAB, ENVIRON, FOODSCI, LEISURE, NUTRIT, VETSCI.

15:30. Online   DIMDI

File name	CV72
Software	GRIPS
Start year	1972
Number of records	2,842,569
Update period	Monthly
SDI period	1 month
Database aids	Memocard CAB ABSTRACTS and User Manual CAB ABSTRACTS
Price/Charges	Connect time: UK£18.74–22.53
	Online print: UK£0.40–0.58
	Offline print: UK£0.33–0.40

Downloading is allowed
Thesaurus is online

Notes

Contains all citations included in the abstract journals of the CAB. Abstracted records are 82% of the total. The unit record contains information about author(s), title and other bibliographic data as well as institutions, keywords, subunit(s) and abstracts (eighty-four per cent). More complex subjects or clearly defined subject areas are represented in the following DIMDI subfiles consisting of one or several subunits which can be used like individual databases: CAB Ado; CAB Animal; CAB Animal Products; CAB Economics; CAB Engineering; CAB Forestry; CAB Human; CAB Nutrition; CAB Plant; CAB Plant Protection; CAB Leisure Recreation Tourism; CAB Veterinary Science.

Suppliers of online documents: British Library Document Supply Centre, Boston Spa, England; Harkers Information Retrieval System, Sydney, Australia; Instituto de Informacion y Documentacion en Ciencia y Tecnologia, Madrid, Spain; Universitätsbibliothek und TIB, Hannover, Germany; Zentralbibliothek der Landbauwissenschaft, Bonn, Germany.

Record composition

Additional Author AA; Abstract AB; Abstractor's Initials AI; Abstract Language AL; Author AU; Author's Variants AV; Classification Code CC; Corporate Author CA; Corporate Source CS; Controlled Terms CT; Decimal Code DC; Document Type DT; Entry Date ED; Entry Month EM; Free Text FT; Geographical Codes GC; Geographical Heading GH; Journal Title JT; Language LA; Abstract Number NA; Document Number ND; Cross Reference Number NX; Original Field OF; Order Number OD; Publisher's Name PU; Preprocessed Searches PPS; Publication Year PY; ISBN SB; Section Code SC; Subfile SF; Section Headings SH; Source SO; Secondary Journal Source SSO; Subunit SU and Title TI

The Basic Index includes the data fields: Title, Abstract, Controlled Term, Section Heading, Geographical Heading. Controlled Terms from 1984 correspond to the polyhierarchic structured CAB thesaurus; prior to 1984: mixture of terms. Access points with Producer's equivalent name in brackets: Subunits (SU) (Abstract Journals); Section Codes (SC) (Sequencing Code Numbers); Section Headings (SH) (Section Headings); Decimal Codes (DC) (Decimal Codes); Geographical Codes (GC) (Geographical Codes); Controlled Terms (CT) Subject Index Entries; Geographical Headings (GH) Countries.

15:31. Online   ESA-IRS

File name	File 124
Start year	1986+
Number of records	760,000
Update period	Monthly
Price/Charges	Subscription: UK£70.29
	Database entry fee: UK£3.51
	Online print: UK£0.07 – 0.60
	Offline print: UK£0.64
	SDI charge: UK£2.46

Downloading is allowed
Thesaurus is online

Notes

From 1993 ESA-IRS are charging an annual fee of 100 Accounting Units (c.UK£ 70.29) to all users. This is equivalent to the fee for full documentation and will not be charged to customers already paying for documentation.

Record composition

Abstract /AB; Abstract Journal AJ; Author AU; Bureau Bees Decimal Code (1) BD; CAB Record No. NR; Classification Code CC; Classification Name CN; Controlled Terms /CT; Corporate Source CS; Fertilizer Decimal Code (1) SD; Journal Announcement (Updates) UP; Journal Name JN; Language LA; Native Number NN; Publication Year PY; Publisher PB; Summary Language SL; Title /TI and UDC Number UC

15:32. Online   ESA-IRS

File name	File 132
Start year	1972+
Number of records	2,600,000
Update period	Monthly
Price/Charges	Subscription: UK£70.29
	Database entry fee: UK£3.51
	Online print: UK£0.07 – 0.60
	Offline print: UK£0.64
	SDI charge: UK£2.46

Downloading is allowed
Thesaurus is online

Notes

From 1993 ESA-IRS are charging an annual fee of 100 Accounting Units (c.UK£ 70.29) to all users. This is equivalent to the fee for full documentation and will not be charged to customers already paying for documentation.

Record composition

Abstract /AB; Abstract Journal AJ; Author AU; Bureau Bees Decimal Code (1) BD; CAB Record No. NR; Classification Code CC; Classification Name CN; Controlled Terms /CT; Corporate Source CS; Fertilizer Decimal Code (1) SD; Journal Announcement (Updates) UP; Journal Name JN; Language LA; Native Number NN; Publication Year PY; Publisher PB; Summary Language SL; Title /TI and UDC Number UC

15:33. Online   ESA-IRS

File name	File 16
Start year	1972–1985
Number of records	1,900,000
Update period	Closed File
Price/Charges	Subscription: UK£70.29
	Database entry fee: UK£3.51
	Online print: UK£0.07 – 0.60
	Offline print: UK£0.64
	SDI charge: UK£2.46

Downloading is allowed
Thesaurus is online

Notes

From 1993 ESA-IRS are charging an annual fee of 100 Accounting Units (c.UK£ 70.29) to all users. This is equivalent to the fee for full documentation and will not be charged to customers already paying for documentation.

Record composition

Abstract /AB; Abstract Journal AJ; Author AU; Bureau Bees Decimal Code (1) BD; CAB Record No. NR; Classification Code CC; Classification Name CN; Controlled Terms /CT; Corporate Source CS; Fertilizer Decimal Code (1) SD; Journal Announcement (Updates) UP; Journal Name JN; Language LA; Native Number NN; Publication Year PY; Publisher PB; Summary Language SL; Title /TI and UDC Number UC

15:34. Online   Japan Information Center of Science and Technology (JICST)

File name	CABA
Start year	1979
Number of records	1,590,000
Update period	Monthly
Price/Charges	Connect time: US$55.00
	Online print: US$0.20
	Offline print: US$0.20
	SDI charge: US$11.48

Downloading is allowed

Record composition

Abstract AB; Accession Number AN; Author AU; Broader Terms BT; Classification Codes CC; Controlled Terms CT; Corporate Source CS; Country of Publication CY; Document Type DT; Language LA; Source SO and Title TI

15:35. Online   STN

File name	CABA
Start year	1979
Number of records	1,900,000
Update period	Monthly
Price/Charges	Connect time: DM85.00
	Online print: DM1.34
	Offline print: DM1.42
	SDI charge: DM17.57

Also available on JICST.

15:36. Online   University of Tsukuba

File name	CAB Abstracts
Start year	
Number of records	
Update period	

Notes

Access through University of Tsukuba limited to affiliates of the University of Japan.

15:37. CD-ROM   SilverPlatter

File name	CABCD Vol.1 1984–86
Format notes	IBM, Mac, NEC
Software	SPIRS
Start year	1984–1986
Number of records	
Update period	Annually
Database aids	Silverplatter CAB User Manual, Quick Reference Cards and SPIRS User Manual
Price/Charges	Subscription: UK£1,425–2,850

Thesaurus is online

Notes

Nearly sixty-five per cent of the records are drawn from English language sources, the remainder from articles in over 75 languages. Approximately ninety-five per cent of records have an English language abstract. CABCD has 930,000 records in total, with 130,000 records being added each year. It is available in separate discs as four volumes to date, dating from 1984 through to 1995. There are various price ranges depending on number of volumes purchased. Vol.1, 1984–1986, costs UK£ 1,425 for single users, £2,850 for 2–8 networked users.

Record composition

English language title; foreign language title (where appropriate); author; author's address; source title; citation details; publication year; publication type; language of original document; summary language; abstract; subject index terms; geographic index terms and subfile codes (CABI Abstract Journal code)

The Index command can be used to provide access to a list of all words, descriptors and hyphenated phrases which have been indexed in the free-text fields. The index excludes information present in the limit fields, such as language and date. The index is arranged alphabetically word by word, and can be browsed and terms selected which are then searched for automatically using the OR operator. Use of the Index shows up inevitable spelling mistakes

15:38. CD-ROM   SilverPlatter

File name	CABCD Vol.2 1987–89
Format notes	IBM, Mac, NEC
Software	SPIRS
Start year	1987–1989
Number of records	
Update period	Annually
Database aids	Silverplatter CAB User Manual, Quick Reference Cards and SPIRS User Manual
Price/Charges	Subscription: UK£2,850 5,700
Thesaurus is online	

Notes

Nearly sixty-five per cent of the records are drawn from English language sources, the remainder from articles in over 75 languages. Approximately ninety-five per cent of records have an English language abstract. This is the second volume of CABCD. CABCD has 930,000 records in total, with 130,000 records being added each year. It is available in separate discs as four volumes to date, dating from 1984 through to 1995. There are various price ranges depending on number of volumes purchased: Vol.2, 1987–1989, £2,850 for single users, £5,700 for 2–8 networked users.

Record composition

English language title; foreign language title (where appropriate); author; author's address; source title; citation details; publication year; publication type; language of original document; summary language; abstract; subject index terms; geographic index terms and subfile codes (CABI Abstract Journal code)

The Index command can be used to provide access to a list of all words, descriptors and hyphenated phrases which have been indexed in the free-text fields. The index excludes information present in the limit fields, such as language and date. The index is arranged alphabetically word by word, and can be browsed and terms selected which are then searched for automatically using the OR operator. Use of the Index shows up inevitable spelling mistakes

15:39. CD-ROM   SilverPlatter

File name	CABCD Vol.3 1990–92
Format notes	IBM, Mac, NEC
Software	SPIRS
Start year	1990–92
Number of records	
Update period	Annually
Database aids	Silverplatter CAB User Manual, Quick Reference Cards and SPIRS User Manual
Price/Charges	Subscription: UK£1,710–9,000
Thesaurus is online	

Notes

Nearly sixty-five per cent of the records are drawn from English language sources, the remainder from articles in over 75 languages. Approximately ninety-five per cent of records have an English language abstract. CABCD has 930,000 records in total, with

130,000 records being added each year. This is the third volume of CABCD. It is available in separate discs as four volumes to date, dating from 1984 through to 1995. There are various price ranges depending on number of volumes purchased: Vol.3, 1990–1992, £3,845 for single users, £7,690 for 2–8 networked users; Vol.3 1992 renewal purchase £1,710 for single users, £3,420 for 2- 8 networked users.

Record composition

English language title; foreign language title (where appropriate); author; author's address; source title; citation details; publication year; publication type; language of original document; summary language; abstract; subject index terms; geographic index terms and subfile codes (CABI Abstract Journal code)

The Index command can be used to provide access to a list of all words, descriptors and hyphenated phrases which have been indexed in the free-text fields. The index excludes information present in the limit fields, such as language and date. The index is arranged alphabetically word by word, and can be browsed and terms selected which are then searched for automatically using the OR operator. Use of the Index shows up inevitable spelling mistakes

15:40. CD-ROM   SilverPlatter

File name	CABCD Vol.4 1993–95
Format notes	IBM, Mac, NEC
Software	SPIRS
Start year	1993–95
Number of records	
Update period	Annually
Database aids	Silverplatter CAB User Manual, Quick Reference Cards and SPIRS User Manual
Price/Charges	Subscription: UK£4,500 – 9,000
Thesaurus is online	

Notes

Nearly sixty-five per cent of the records are drawn from English language sources, the remainder from articles in over 75 languages. Approximately ninety-five per cent of records have an English language abstract. This is the prospective fourth volume of CABCD. CABCD has 930,000 records in total, with 130,000 records being added each year. It is available in separate discs as four volumes to date, dating from 1984 through to 1995. There are various price ranges depending on number of volumes purchased: Vol.4 1993–1995 £4,500 for single users, £9,000 for 2- 8 networked users. Prices on application for purchase of Vol.4 1993.

Record composition

English language title; foreign language title (where appropriate); author; author's address; source title; citation details; publication year; publication type; language of original document; summary language; abstract; subject index terms; geographic index terms and subfile codes (CABI Abstract Journal code)

The Index command can be used to provide access to a list of all words, descriptors and hyphenated phrases which have been indexed in the free-text fields. The index excludes information present in the limit fields, such as language and date. The index is arranged alphabetically word by word, and can be browsed and terms selected which are then searched for automatically using the OR operator. Use of the Index shows up inevitable spelling mistakes

15: 41. Diskette   CAB International

File name	CABI Abstract Journals on Floppy Disk
Format notes	IBM
Start year	
Number of records	
Update period	Same as for printed journal
Price/Charges	

Notes

Any one of the CAB International Abstract Journals may be received on floppy disk, according to the purchaser's requirements. Update frequency is the same as for the particular printed journal (monthly, bimonthly or quarterly). Price is double the cost of the equivalent printed journal. The diskettes are supplied without retrieval software, but the subscriber has the choice of three formats – comma delimited, CDS-ISIS or Pro-Cite – to enable use with most commercial database management software, with Micro CDS-ISIS or with Pro-Cite.

15:42. Database subset

Online   BRS Online Service, Morning Search, BRS/Colleague

File name	CAB: Veterinary and Medical
Start year	1980–1990
Number of records	8,200
Update period	Monthly
Price/Charges	Connect time: US$62.00/72.00
	Online print: US$0.47/0.55
	Offline print: US$0.55
	SDI charge: US$12.50

Downloading is allowed

Notes

A subset of CAB Abstracts containing all documents from: *Index Veterinarius*; *Veterinary Bulletin*; *Reviews of Applied Entomology, Series B*; *Review of Medical and Veterinary Mycology*; *Nutrition Abstracts and Reviews, Series B*; *Helminthology Abstracts, Series A*; *Animal Disease Occurrence* (ceased publication 1989) and *Small Animal Abstracts* (ceased publication in 1989).

15:43. Database subset

Online   Data-Star

File name	PARA – CAB: Medical Parasitology & Mycology
Start year	1984
Number of records	60,000
Update period	Monthly
Database aids	Data-Star Biomedical Manual
Price/Charges	Subscription: SFr80.00
	Connect time: SFr127.00
	Online print: SFr1.01
	Offline print: SFr1.04
	SDI charge: SFr12.40

Downloading is allowed
Thesaurus is online

Notes

PARA is a source of information on human parasitic organisms, their biology, transmission and control and investigation techniques. It contains informative abstracts of journal articles, conference reports, theses and other literature on helminths, protozoans, arthropods and fungi of medical significance. The database includes: interaction of organisms with humans, including epidemiology, pathogenesis and pathology, immunology, serology and resistance, allergies, toxicology and poisoning; biology of organisms, including ecology, life history, behaviour, physi-

ology, biochemistry, evolution and genetics; biology of vectors and intermediate hosts of parasites; prevention, control and treatment of diseases caused by the organisms, including biological and environmental methods, vaccines and therapeutic agents and chemical control by means of anthelmintics, anti-protozoal drugs, insecticides and anti-fungal agents; investigation technqiues, including diagnosis, research methods and equipment and animal models. The database takes all human-related material from: *Helminthological Abstracts*, *Protozoological Abstracts*, *Review of Medical and Veterinary Entomology* and *Review of Medical and Veterinary Mycology*.

From June 1993 Data-Star have introduced an annual fee/subscription per contract (that is, not per password) of SFr 80.00 (c.UK£ 32.00) payable every June. For North American customers billed in dollars who also use DIALOG, the DIALOG fee also covers access to Data-Star. Academic customers, 'commitment' customers and customers currently billed in dollars are exempt.

Record composition

Abstract AB; Accession Number and Update Code AN; Article Type AT; Author AU; Author Affiliation IN; Description DE; Foreign Title TT; Geographic Descriptor CN; ISSN Number IS; Language of Original Summary; Original Language LG; Publication Year YR; Section code and heading SC; Source SO; Title TI and Update Code UP

15:44. Database subset

Online   Data-Star

File name	VETS – CAB: Veterinary Science/Medicine
Start year	1984
Number of records	150,000
Update period	Monthly
Database aids	Data-Star Biomedical Manual
Price/Charges	Subscription: SFr80.00
	Connect time: SFr127.00
	Online print: SFr1.01
	Offline print: SFr1.04
	SDI charge: SFr12.40

Downloading is allowed
Thesaurus is online

Notes

A bibliographic source of information on all aspects of veterinary science and medicine. Documents comprising bibliographic details with or without an abstract are included for literature on all aspects of veterinary medicine. Subjects covered include: diseases of livestock, poultry, pets, laboratory animals, zoo animals, farmed fish and shellfish and certain wild animals; anatomy, physiology, biochemistry, pharmacology, surgery, radiography, toxicology, immunology and immunogenetics of domestic animals; bacteriology, virology, mycology, protozoology, helminthology and entomology related to animal diseases; zoonoses; meat inspection and economics of animal diseases. Abstracts sources include: *Veterinary Bulletin*, *Index Veterinarius* and *Small Animal Abstracts* and, in part, *Helminthological Abstracts*, *Review of Medical and Veterinary Entomology*; *Protozoological Abstracts*, *Review of Medical and Veterinary Mycology*, *Animal Breeding Abstrats*, *Diary Science Abstracts* and *Nutrition Abstracts and Reviews Series B, Livestock Feeds and Feeding*.

From June 1993 Data-Star have introduced an annual fee/subscription per contract (that is, not per password) of SFr 80.00 (c.UK£ 32.00) payable every June.

For North American customers billed in dollars who also use DIALOG, the DIALOG fee also covers access to Data-Star. Academic customers, 'commitment' customers and customers currently billed in dollars are exempt.

Record composition
Abstract AB; Accession Number and Update Code AN; Article Type AT; Author AU; Author Affiliation IN; Description DE; Foreign Title TT; Geographic Descriptor CN; ISBN Number IS; Language of Original Summary; Original Language LG; Publication Year YR; Section code and heading SC; Source SO; Title TI and Update Code UP

15:45. Database subset
Online   **DIALOG, Knowledge Index**

File name	File 250 – ONTAP CAB Abstracts Training File
Start year	January – March 1985
Number of records	34,388
Update period	Closed File
Price/Charges	Connect time: US$15.00

Notes
The low-cost training file containing records from the January to March 1985 updates to File 50, the main CAB Abstracts file on DIALOG. Offline prints are not available in ONTAP files.

15:46. Database subset
Online   **DIMDI**

File name	C773 – CAB ANIMAL PRODUCTS
Start year	1972
Number of records	541,364
Update period	Monthly
SDI period	1 month
Price/Charges	Connect time: UK£18.74–22.53
	Online print: UK£0.40–0.58
	Offline print: UK£0.33–0.40

Downloading is allowed

Notes
Contains the relevant citaions on animal breeding and production from CAB Abstracts. Journals referenced: *Animal Breeding Abstracts*; *Dairy Science Abstracts*; *Nutrition Abstracts and Reviews (B. Livestock Feeds and Feeding)*; *Nutrition Abstracts (1973–1976)*; *Poultry Abstracts*; *Pig News and Information*. Searches are possible from January 1973. 95% of thte records have abstracts.

CAB ANIMAL PROD is defined as subfile to CAB ABASTRACTS with: FIND SU=(0A;0D;0N;1N;2N; 7A;7D).

15:47. Database subset
Online   **DIMDI**

File name	C872 – CAB VETERINARY SCIENCE
Start year	1972
Number of records	678,064
Update period	Monthly
SDI period	1 month
Price/Charges	Connect time: UK£18.74–22.53
	Online print: UK£0.40–0.58
	Offline print: UK£0.33–0.40

Downloading is allowed

Notes
Contains citations on veterinary science from CAB Abstracts. Journals referenced: *Helminothological Abstracts (A. Animal and Human)*; *Index Veterinarius*; *Review of Applied Entomology (B. Medical and Veterinary)*; *Review of Medical and Veterinary Mycology*; *Veterinary Bulletin*; *Protozoological Abstracts* (from 1977); *Animal Disease Occurrence* (from 1980); *Small Animal Abstracts* (from 1984).Searches are possible from January 1972. 95% of the records have abstracts.

CAB VET SCIENCE is defined as subfile to CAB ABSTRACTS with: FIND SU= (0H;0I;0L;0V;0Y; 2V;7V).

15:48. Database subset
Online   **DIMDI**

File name	C980 – CAB ADO
Alternative name(s)	Animal Disease Occurrence
Start year	1980
Number of records	
Update period	Twice a year
Price/Charges	Connect time: UK£18.74–22.53
	Online print: UK£0.40–0.58
	Offline print: UK£0.33–0.40

Downloading is allowed

Notes
Equivalent to the printed *Animal Disease Occurrence*. Covers epidemiology of animal diseases. Contains records on the incidence of animal diseases worldwide. Data include the country of occurrence, number of animals affected, duration of the disease, number of deaths, and economic effects. Each record includes a citation to the source publication. All documents have abstracts. Approximately ninety per cent of the ADO documents are also published in the Veterinary Bulletin but without additional factual data.

Record composition
Animal Species ANI

15:49. Database subset
Online   **DIMDI**

File name	CX72 – CAB ANIMAL
Start year	1972
Number of records	1,629,488
Update period	Monthly
SDI period	1 month
Price/Charges	Connect time: UK£18.74–22.53
	Online print: UK£0.40–0.58
	Offline print: UK£0.33–0.40

Downloading is allowed

Notes
Contains the animal relevant documents of CAB Abstracts. Journals referenced: *Animal Breeding Abstracts*; *Apicultural Abstracts*; *Dairy Science Abstracts*; *Helminthological Abstracts (A. Animal and Human)*; *Index Veterinarius*; *Review of Applied Entomology (B. Medical and Veterinary)*; *Review of Applied Entomology (B. Medical and Veterinary)*; *Review of Medical and Veterinanry Mycology*; *Nutrition Abstracts and Reviews (A. Human and Experimental)* (from 1977); *World Agricultural Economics and Rural Sociology Abstracts*; *Nutrition Abstracts and Reviews (A. Human and Experimental)*; *Veterinary Bulletin*; *Protozoological Abstracts* (from 1977); *Nutrition Abstracts (1973–1976)*; *Rural Extension, Education and Training Abstracts* (from 1978); *Rural Development Abstracts*; *Animal Disease Occurence*; *Leisure, Recreation and Tourism Abstracts*; *Poultry Abstracts*; *Pig News and Information*; *Biocontrol News and Information*; *Biodeterioration Abstracts*; *Small Animal Abstracts*; *Agricultural Engineering Abstracts*. Searches are possible from January 1972. 70% of the records have abstracts.

15:50. Database subset

Online — DIMDI

File name	CZ73 – CAB HUMAN
Start year	1972
Number of records	547,742
Update period	Monthly
SDI period	1 month
Price/Charges	Connect time: UK£18.74–22.53
	Online print: UK£0.40–0.58
	Offline print: UK£0.33–0.40

Downloading is allowed

Notes

Contains the human nutrition and parasitology documents of CAB Abstracts. Journals referenced: *Helminthological Abstracts (A. Animal and Human)*; *Review of Applied Entomology (B. Medical and Veterinary)*; *Review of Medical and Veterinary Mycology*; *Nutrition Abstracts and Reviews (A. Human and Experimental)*; *Protozoological Abstracts*; *Nutrition Abstracts*. 95% of the records have abstracts. Searches are available from January 1973. (CAB HUMAN is defined as subfile to CAB ABSTRACTS with: FIND SU= (0H;0J;0L;0U;0Y; 1N;2N).

15:51. Database subset

Online — ESA-IRS

File name	File 112 – Training CAB Abstracts
Start year	1984/5
Number of records	28,000
Update period	None
Thesaurus is online	

Notes

Training file and subset of the full CAB Abstracts file which has the file numbers 16 (1972–1985), 124 (1986 to date) and 132 (1972 to date). It is available at a low access fee for user training. Services such as offline prints, automatic current awareness and document ordering are not available with the training file.

Record composition

Abstract /AB; Abstract Journal AJ; Author AU; CAB Record Number NR; Classification Codes CC; Classification Names CN; Controlled Terms /CT; Corporate Source CS; Journal Announcement (Updates) UP; Journal Name JN; Language LA; Native Accession Number NN; Publication Year PY; Publisher PB; Summary Language SL; Title /TI and UDC Numbers UC

15:52. Database subset

CD-ROM — SilverPlatter

File name	VetCD (CAB Spectrum series)
Alternative name(s)	CABVetCD (CAB Spectrum series)
Format notes	IBM, Mac, NEC
Software	SPIRS/MacSPIRS
Start year	1973
Number of records	300,000
Update period	Annually
Price	UK£3,980 – 7,960
	Subscription: UK£1,155 – 2,310

Notes

Covers veterinary science and relevant records from CAB Abstracts database in such areas as protozoology; mycology; helminthology; and applied entomology. Contains abstracts and citations published in the following CABI abstract journals: *Index Veterinarius* (1933-), *Veterinary Bulletin* (1931–), *Helminthological Abstracts, Protozoological Abstracts, Review of Medical and Veterinary Entomology* and *Review of Medical and Veterinary Mycology*. Animals covered include farm animals, pets and game animals; all animals of economic importance including farmed fish and shellfish; commercially important wild fish; zoo animals and wild animals. Other subjects covered include: viral and bacterial diseases, arthropod parasites, toxicology, immunology, pharmacology, biochemistry, food inspection and other related areas.

Archival disc covering 1973–1991 is available for outright purchase at UK£ 3,980 for single users, £7,960 for 2–8 networked users (member country). Annual renewals cost UK£ 1,155 for single users, £2,310 for 2–8 networked users. There are various journals options and print/updates prices on application to CAB or SilverPlatter. There is also a VETCD/BEASTCD combined set available: full set £5,495 for single users, £10,990 for 2–8 networked users; annual renewal £1,655 for single users, £3,310 for 2–8 networked users.

In-depth indexing using controlled terms from the *CAB Thesaurus*.

This database can also be found on:
Human Nutrition on CD-ROM

Cambridge Scientific Abstracts Life Sciences

Cambridge Scientific Abstracts

15:54. Master record

Alternative name(s)	CSAL
Database type	Bibliographic
Number of journals	
Sources	Journals, Books, Conference papers, Technical reports, Patents, Theses and Dissertations
Start year	1978
Language	English
Coverage	International
Number of records	1,164,810
Update size	–
Update period	Monthly

Keywords

Acute Poisoning; Aging; Air Pollution; Algology; Amino-Acids; Anatomy; Antibiotics; Aquaculture; Atmospheric Science; Bacteriology; Behavioural Ecology; Bioengineering; Biological Membranes; Biotechnology; Bone Disease; Calcium Metabolism; Chemoreception; Chronic Poisoning; Clinical Medicine; Clinical Toxicology; DNA; Drugs; Ecology; Ecosystems; Endocrinology; Entomology – Agricultural; Entomology – Applied; Entomology – Human; Entomology – Veterinary; Environmental Biology; Ethology; Genetic Engineering; Hazardous Substances; HIV; Histology; Human Ecology; Immune Disorders; Immunology; Infectious Diseases; Land Pollution; Marine Biotechnology; Marine Engineering; Microbiology; Molecular Biology; Molecular Neurobiology; Mycology; Naval Engineering; Noise Pollution; Oceanography; Neurology; Neuropharmacology; Neurophysiology – Animal; Neuroscience; Nucleic Acids; Nutrition; Oncology; Occupational Health and Safety; Osteoporosis; Osteomalacia; Pathology; Peptides; Pharmaceuticals; Pheromones; Physiology; Pollution; Proteins; Protozoology; Psychophysics;

Public Health; Radiation; Rhinology; RNA; Sleep; Smoking; Substance Abuse; Taste Perception; Thermal Pollution; Viral Genetics; Water; Water Pollution

Description

A superfile providing access to the following abstracting services:

Life Sciences Collection;
Aquatic Sciences and Fisheries Abstracts;
Oceanic Abstracts;
Pollution Abstracts.

Covers the worldwide technical literature on medical and biological disciplines from journals, books, conference papers, technical reports, patents, theses and dissertations.

15:55. Online   BRS

File name	Cambridge Scientific Abstracts Life Sciences
Alternative name(s)	CSAL
Start year	1978
Number of records	1,164,810
Update period	Monthly

Notes

A superfile providing access to the following abstracting services: the Life Science Collection, Aquatic Sciences and Fisheries Abstracts, Oceanic Abstracts and Pollution Abstracts.

For more details of constituent databases, see:
Life Sciences Collection
Aquatic Sciences and Fisheries Abstracts
Oceanic Abstracts
Pollution Abstracts

Cancerlit
National Cancer Institute, US National Institutes of Health

15:57. Master record

Alternative name(s)	Cancer Literature Online
Database type	Bibliographic
Number of journals	3,500+
Sources	Conference proceedings, dissertations, government publications, journals, meeting abstracts, monographs, reports, symposia, technical reports and theses
Start year	1963
Language	English
Coverage	International
Number of records	778,000+
Update size	100,000
Update period	Monthly
Index unit	Articles
Abstract details	Authors
Thesaurus	Medical Subject Headings (MeSH) (from 1980); annual editions
Database aids	MeSH Tree Structures; annual editions, MeSH Permuted Terms; annual editions and Gene Symbols (from 1991)

Keywords

Cancer; Oncology; Immunology; Pathology

Description

Contains citations, with abstracts, to the worldwide literature on oncological epidemiology, pathology, treatment, and research. The database covers the treatment of cancer as well as information on epidemiology, pathogenesis and immunology. Another important aspect is chemical, physical and viral carcinogenesis. Subject coverage within oncology: biochemistry, biology, carcinogenesis (viral, chemical, other), epidemiology, genetics, growth factors, immunology, mutagents – mutagenicity, pathology, physiology, physiopathology, pathogenesis and prevention. Approximately eighty per cent of references are stored with an English abstract, all documents between 1963 and 1983 having abstracts. Since 1977 proceedings of meetings, monographs, theses and Government and symposia reports have been included. The database contains information from approximately seventy countries.

References are included from: *Cancer Therapy Abstracts* (formerly *Cancer Chemotherapy Abstracts* 1967–80) and *Carcinogenesis Abstracts* from 1963–1976. From 1977 citations are taken only from primary publications. From June 1983 all citations from MEDLINE with an oncological content are automatically transferred to CANCERLIT. They are marked in the data field SEC with SEC=MEDL and SEC =L. From June 1983 85% of the citations are from MEDLINE. As the rate of abstracts is approximately 60% in MEDLINE, a decline in the rate of abstracts is expected. All non-MEDLINE-derived documents still have 100% English abstracts. Databases providing citations: MEDLINE; Carcinogenesis Abstracts – CARC (only up to 1979); Cancer Therapy Abstracts (only up to 1979); Herner & Company (as from 1982 – some meeting abstracts) International Cancer Research Data Bank Program (most non-MEDLINE derived records); Oncology Abstracts, the print equivalent has been available since 1986. Biomedical journals account for approximately eighty-six per cent of sources, reports twelve per cent, monographs one per cent and these one per cent. Cancerlit contains documents in about forty languages.

Before 1980 documents were not indexed with any vocabulary. From 1980, *MeSH* is used for indexing and the hierarchical structure of *MeSH* makes it possible to search for a whole group of related descriptors in one step. Since January 1985 new records have been indexed with chemical names and CAS Registry/EC numbers. Corresponds in part to the printed *Index Medicus*.

15:58. Online   BLAISE-LINK

File name	CANCERLIT
Alternative name(s)	Cancer Literature On-Line
Start year	1963
Number of records	
Update period	Monthly

15:59. Online   BRS, BRS After Dark, BRS/Colleague

File name	CANR
Alternative name(s)	Cancer Literature On-Line
Start year	
Number of records	
Update period	Monthly
Price/Charges	Connect time: US$26.00/36.00
	Online print: US$0.07/0.15
	Offline print: US$0.20
	SDI charge: US$5.60

15:60. Online — CISTI MEDLARS

File name	CANCERLIT
Alternative name(s)	Cancer Literature On-Line
Start year	1963
Number of records	625,000+
Update period	Monthly

15:61. Online — CompuServe Information Service

File name	IQUEST File 1931
Alternative name(s)	Cancer Literature On-Line
Start year	1980
Number of records	
Update period	Monthly
Price/Charges	Subscription: US$8.95 per month Database entry fee: US$9/search; some databases carry a surcharge ($2–75) Online print: US$10 references free; then $9 per ten; abstracts $3 each

Downloading is allowed

Notes

Accessed via IQUEST or IQMEDICAL, this database is offered by a BRS gateway. IQUEST can either search across all databases, a database of the user's choice or selected multiple databases.

15:62. Online — Data-Star

File name	CANC
Alternative name(s)	Cancer Literature On-Line
Start year	1983+
Number of records	
Update period	Monthly
Database aids	Data-Star Biomedical Manual and Online manual (search NEWS-CANC in NEWS)
Price/Charges	Subscription: SFr80.00 Connect time: SFr78.00 Online print: SFr0.00–0.18 Offline print: SFr0.21–0.24 SDI charge: SFr6.80

Downloading is allowed
Thesaurus is online

Notes

From June 1993 Data-Star have introduced an annual fee/subscription per contract (that is, not per password) of SFr 80.00 (c.UK£ 32.00) payable every June. For North American customers billed in dollars who also use DIALOG, the DIALOG fee also covers access to Data-Star. Academic customers, 'commitment' customers and customers currently billed in dollars are exempt.

Record composition

Abstract AB; Accession Number AN; Author(s) AU; Author Affiliation IN; CAS Registry Number or Enzyme Commission Number RN; Comment CM; Descriptors DE; Entry Month EM; Gene symbol GE; Journal Code JC; Journal Subset SB; Language of Original LG; Original Language Title TT; Publication Type PT; Secondary Source Identifier SI; Source SO; Title TI and Year of Publication YR

15:63. Online — Data-Star

File name	CANX
Alternative name(s)	Cancer Literature On-Line
Start year	Latest month
Number of records	
Update period	Monthly
Database aids	Data-Star Biomedical Manual

Price/Charges	Subscription: SFr80.00 Connect time: SFr78.00 Online print: SFr0.00–0.18 Offline print: SFr0.21–0.24 SDI charge: SFr6.80

Downloading is allowed
Thesaurus is online

Notes

From June 1993 Data-Star have introduced an annual fee/subscription per contract (that is, not per password) of SFr 80.00 (c.UK£ 32.00) payable every June. For North American customers billed in dollars who also use DIALOG, the DIALOG fee also covers access to Data-Star. Academic customers, 'commitment' customers and customers currently billed in dollars are exempt.

Record composition

Abstract AB; Accession Number AN; Author(s) AU; Author Affiliation IN; CAS Registry Number or Enzyme Commission Number RN; Comment CM; Descriptors DE; Entry Month EM; Gene symbol GE; Journal Code JC; Journal Subset SB; Language of Original LG; Original Language Title TT; Publication Type PT; Secondary Source Identifier SI; Source SO; Title TI and Year of Publication YR

15:64. Online — Data-Star

File name	CAZZ
Alternative name(s)	Cancer Literature On-Line
Start year	1963
Number of records	778,662
Update period	Monthly
Database aids	Data-Star Biomedical Manual and Online manual (search NEWS-CANC in NEWS)
Price/Charges	Subscription: SFr80.00 Connect time: SFr78.00 Online print: SFr0.00–0.18 Offline print: SFr0.21–0.24 SDI charge: SFr6.80

Downloading is allowed
Thesaurus is online

Notes

From June 1993 Data-Star have introduced an annual fee/subscription per contract (that is, not per password) of SFr 80.00 (c.UK£ 32.00) payable every June. For North American customers billed in dollars who also use DIALOG, the DIALOG fee also covers access to Data-Star. Academic customers, 'commitment' customers and customers currently billed in dollars are exempt.

Record composition

Abstract AB; Accession Number AN; Author(s) AU; Author Affiliation IN; CAS Registry Number or Enzyme Commission Number RN; Comment CM; Descriptors DE; Entry Month EM; Gene symbol GE; Journal Code JC; Journal Subset SB; Language of Original LG; Original Language Title TT; Publication Type PT; Secondary Source Identifier SI; Source SO; Title TI and Year of Publication YR

15:65. Online — DIALOG, Knowledge Index

File name	File 159
Alternative name(s)	Cancer Literature On-Line
Start year	1963
Number of records	823,103
Update period	Monthly
Price/Charges	Connect time: US$36.00 Online print: US$0.12 Offline print: US$0.12 SDI charge: US$5.25

Notes

This database is also available to home users during evenings and weekends at a reduced rate on the Knowledge Index service of DIALOG – file name in this case is Cancerlit, and searches are made with simplified commands or menus.

DIALINDEX Categories: MEDICINE, RNMED

15:66. Online DIMDI

File name	CL63
Alternative name(s)	Cancer Literature On-Line
Software	GRIPS
Start year	1963–1979
Number of records	194,832
Update period	Not updated
SDI period	1 month
Database aids	Memocard CANCERLIT and User Manual MEDLINE, AIDSLINE, BIOETHICSLINE, CANCERLIT, HEALTH
Price/Charges	Connect time: UK£5.84–10.58
	Online print: UK£0.17–0.35
	Offline print: UK£0.09–0.15

Downloading is allowed
Thesaurus is online

Notes

File CL63 covers records for the period 1963–1979. 100% of the records have abstracts. Suppliers of online documents: British Library Document Supply Centre, Boston Spa, England; Bayerische Stattsbibliothek München, München, Germany; Harkers Information Retrieval System, Sydney, Australia; Institute for Scientific Information, Philadelphia, USA; Koninklikjke Nederlandse Akademie van Wetenschapen, Amsterdam, The Nederlands; Zentralbibliothek der Medizin, Köln, Germany.

German author names with a dipthong (ä,ö,ü) are treated differently from MEDLINE (in MEDLINE ae;oe;ue). In CANCERLIT the 'e' of the umlaut is usually deleted and it is recommended to use the truncation symbol (#). For example Alfred Müller (F AU=MULLER A OR AU = MUELLER A, or F AU = MU#LLER (preferable). For Number of Document, from June 1983 the three letter standardised NLM-codes for journals are used. Prior to June 1983, five letter codes were used. Deviating from MEDLINE, the numerical code carries a prefix in CANCERLIT indicating the secondary source of a citation. The Number of Report is the Cancergram identification number, available from 1978. Cancergrams are monthly current awareness publications of the Naitonal Cancer Institute with over sixty different subject related bulletins. Articles are selected by scientists. The first four characters identify the Cancergram series and the last four digits identify the publication month and year of the particular Cancergram issue. Approximately one-third of records carry one or more Cancergram Numbers which are assigned to records annually in January. The Secondary Source Identifier is the secondary supplier or source of a citation. Deviating from MEDLINE, AIDSLINE and HEALTH, only the following abbreviations without numerical codes are used in CANCERLIT: CARTH – Carcinogenesis Abstracts; CATH – Cancer Therapy Abstracts; HERN – Herner & Company; ICDB – International Cancer Research Data Bank Program.

Record composition

Abstract AB; Abstract Source AS; Author AU; Classification Code CC; CAS-Reg.No. CR; Corporate Source CS; Controlled Term CT; Document Type DT; Entry Date ED; Enzyme Code EZ; Gene Symbol GE;

ITTRI/Franklin Number IF; Journal Title Code JC; Journal Title JT; Language LA; Last Revision Date LR; Number of Contract NC; Number of Document ND; Notes NO; Number of Report NR; Publication Year PY; Qualifier QF; Secondary Source Identifier SEC; Source SO; ISSN SS; Terminology TE and Title TI

The Basic Index includes the data fields Title, Abstract, Controlled Term, Gene Symbols and Terminology. All citations are indexed at least with one Document Type.

15:67. Online DIMDI

File name	CL80
Alternative name(s)	Cancer Literature On-Line
Software	GRIPS
Start year	1980
Number of records	786,183
Update period	Monthly
SDI period	1 month
Database aids	Memocard CANCERLIT and User Manual MEDLINE, AIDSLINE, BIOETHICSLINE, CANCERLIT, HEALTH
Price/Charges	Connect time: UK£5.84–10.58
	Online print: UK£0.17–0.35
	Offline print: UK£0.09–0.15

Downloading is allowed
Thesaurus is online

Notes

File CL80 covers the period 1980 to date. Suppliers of online documents: British Library Document Supply Centre, Boston Spa, England; Bayerische Statts-bibliothek München, München, Germany; Harkers Information Retrieval System, Sydney, Australia; Institute for Scientific Information, Philadelphia, USA; Koninklikjke Nederlandse Akademie van Wetenschapen, Amsterdam, The Nederlands; Zentral-bibliothek der Medizin, Köln, Germany. German author names with a dipthong (ä,ö,ü) are treated differently from MEDLINE (in MEDLINE ae;oe;ue). In CANCERLIT the 'e' of the umlaut is usually deleted and it is recommended to use the truncation symbol (#). For example, Alfred Müller (F AU=MULLER A OR AU = MUELLER A, or F AU = MU#LLER (preferable). Deviating from MEDLINE, the numerical code carries a prefix in CANCERLIT indicating the secondary source of a citation. The Number of Report is the Cancergram identification number, available from 1978. Cancergrams are monthly current awareness publications of the National Cancer Institute with over sixty different subject related bulletins. Articles are selected by scientists. The first four characters identify the Cancergram series and the last four digits identify the publication month and year of the particular Cancergram issue. Approximately one-third of records carry one or more Cancergram Numbers which are assigned to records annually in January. The Secondary Source Identifier is the secondary supplier or source of a citation. Deviating from MEDLINE, AIDSLINE and HEALTH, only the following abbreviations without numerical codes are used in CANCERLIT: CARTH – Carcinogenesis Abstracts; CATH – Cancer Therapy Abstracts; HERN – Herner & Company; ICDB – International Cancer Research Data Bank Program.

Record composition

Abstract AB; Abstract Source AS; Author AU; Classification Code CC; CAS-Reg.No. CR; Corporate Source CS; Controlled Term CT; Document Type DT; Entry Date ED; Enzyme Code EZ; Gene Symbol GE; ITTRI/Franklin Number IF; Journal Title Code JC;

Journal Title JT; Language LA; Last Revision Date LR; Number of Contract NC; Number of Document ND; Notes NO; Number of Report NR; Publication Year PY; Qualifier QF; Secondary Source Identifier SEC; Source SO; ISSN SS; Terminology TE and Title TI

15:68. Online   Japan Information Center of Science and Technology (JICST)

File name	
Alternative name(s)	Cancer Literature On-Line
Start year	
Number of records	
Update period	

15:69. Online   MIC/Karolinska Institute Library and Information Center (MIC KIBIC)

File name	CANCERLIT
Alternative name(s)	Cancer Literature On-Line
Start year	1963
Number of records	680,000
Update period	Monthly

Notes

Online ordering and SDI service available.

15:70. Online   National Library of Medicine

File name	Cancerlit
Alternative name(s)	Cancer Literature On-Line
Start year	
Number of records	
Update period	

15:71. Online   University of Tsukuba

File name	
Alternative name(s)	Cancer Literature On-Line
Start year	
Number of records	
Update period	

Notes

Access through University of Tsukuba limited to affiliates of the University of Japan.

15:72. CD-ROM   Aries Systems Corporation

File name	Cancerlit – Knowledge Finder
Format notes	Mac, IBM
Software	Knowledge Finder 2.0
Start year	1985
Number of records	650,000
Update period	Quarterly

Notes

Corresponds in part to the Cancerlit online database.

15:73. CD-ROM   CD Plus

File name	CD Plus/Cancerlit
Format notes	Mac, Unix, IBM
Software	OVID 3.0
Start year	1984
Number of records	128,992
Update period	Monthly
Price/Charges	Subscription: UK£845

Notes

Covers 1984 to present on one disc. Offers the ability to limit by local journal holdings. For the experienced searcher, the software offers MeSH explodes, 'personal pre-explodes' for frequently exploded terms, SDIs and Save Searches, enhanced MeSH tree structures, and emulation of National Library of Medicine and dot-dot syntax.

Record composition

Author; Institution; Title; Personal Names as Subjects; Original Titles; Grant Numbers and Comments

This database has an index of all searchable terms together with the online *MeSh Thesaurus* which offers mapping from natural language to MeSH – a facility which should give significantly improved precision for the inexperienced searcher. The on-screen help provides scope notes, definitions and task descriptors.

15:74. CD-ROM   Compact Cambridge

File name	Cancerlit
Format notes	NEC, 9800, Mac, IBM
Software	SearchLITE
Start year	Most recent five years.
Number of records	190,000
Update period	Quarterly
Price/Charges	Subscription: UK£635

Notes

Contains a four year backfile, plus the current year. May be combined with PDQ – Physicians Data Query on a single disc at UK£930.

This database can also be found on:
AIDSLINE
Cancer-CD
Oncodisc

For more details of constituent databases, see:
MEDLINE

Clinical Protocols

National Cancer Institute, US National Institutes of Health

15:77. Master record

Alternative name(s)	Clinical Cancer Protocols; CLINPROT
Database type	Factual, Textual
Number of journals	
Sources	Clinical trial protocols
Start year	1960s
Language	English
Coverage	International
Number of records	
Update size	–
Update period	

Keywords

Cancer; Clinical Oncology; Pathology

Description

The database comprises summaries of clinical trials of anticancer drugs and treatment modalities. All records contain a detailed abstract. Gives patient entry criteria, therapy regimen and special study parameters. Includes open (active) and closed protocols. Investigators' names and addresses are given, together with the supporting agency. The data is of special interest to clinical oncologists who are actively engaged in the development and evaluation of clinical therapy methods.

The US National Cancer Institute ceased production

of CLINPROT in June 1991 as the content is duplicated within Physician's Data Query (PDQ) database. On some hosts the protocol file is accessible separately.

Colleague Mail
BRS Online Service, BRS/Colleague

15:78. Master record

Alternative name(s)	MEDLINK
Database type	Directory, Textual, Computer software
Number of journals	1
Sources	Journal, Airlines, Database producers, Electronic media and Original material
Start year	
Language	English
Coverage	USA
Number of records	
Update size	—
Update period	Current six to eight months
Index unit	Classified advertisements

Keywords
Molecular Biology; HIV; Travel; Air Travel; Anaesthesia; Personal Computers; HIV; Pathology; Surgery; Gastroenterology; Intensive Care; Proctology; Dermatology; Geriatrics; Gerontology; Genetics – Human; Immunology; Health Care Administration; Neurology; Cancer; Oncology; Ophthalmology; Sickle-Cell Disease

Description
Contains a number of services for medical professionals, including classified advertisements from the *New England Journal of Medicine*, a calendar of medical events, electronic mail, gateway access to Official Airlines Guide (OAG) Electronic Edition Travel Service (see separate entry), American Airlines EASY Sabre (see separate entry) and other databases available through BT Tymnet Dialcom Service. There are also a number of bulletin boards available, operated by physician-editors: AIDS/HIV, Anesthesia Safety and Technology, Cellforum (pathology, cell biology, molecular biology), Clinical Drug Information, Colon & Rectal Surgery, Critical Care, Dermatology, Geriatrics and Gerontology, Hackers' Forum (microcomputer products and applications), Materia Eclectica, Medical Ethics, MEDLINK Help & Tips, Neurology, Oncology, Ophthalmology, Sickle-Cell Disease.

Partially equivalent to *New England Journal of Medicine* (classified advertisements).

15:79. Online   BRS, BRS/Colleague

File name	
Alternative name(s)	MEDLINK
Start year	
Number of records	
Update period	current six to eight months

For more details of constituent databases, see:
American Airlines EAASY SABRE
OAG Electronic Edition Travel Service

COMETT
Commission of the European Communities (CEC)
Hamburg Educational Partnership

15:81. Master record

Database type	Textual, Courseware, Multimedia
Number of journals	
Sources	
Start year	
Language	
Coverage	Europe
Number of records	
Update size	—
Update period	

Keywords
Cardiology; Pathology; Radiography

Description
A multimedia training programme for: hydraulic instruments; X-ray devices; technical instruments; a programme containing CD-ROM and videodisc (Tate Gallery); and a programme for pathology and cardiology with illustrations and animation. Information is provided by the University of Milan, Danish Computer Centre, British Broadcasting Corporation and Fachhochschule Hamburg, four partners of the European Community's Program in Education and Training in Technology.

15:82. CD-ROM and   Fachhochschule
Videodisc   Hamburg
combined

File name	COMETT
Format notes	IBM, Mac
Start year	
Number of records	
Update period	

Comprehensive Core Medical Library
BRS

15:83. Master record

Database type	Textual
Number of journals	
Sources	Journals and monographs
Start year	Textbooks, current editions; journals, see Description
Language	English
Coverage	English-speaking countries (primarily)
Number of records	
Update size	—
Update period	Weekly
Index unit	Articles, book chapters, book reviews, editorials and letters to the editor

Keywords
HIV; Anatomy

Description
CCML contains full text of major medical textbooks and over seventy medical journals. The database is designed to help both information and medical professionals obtain the full text of authoritative medical information quickly and efficiently. It can be used to

locate contextual references, additional references from bibliographies and footnotes, and access the full text of articles, chapters, letters to the editor, editorials and book reviews. Retrospective coverage and updating varies by source. It includes the *American College of Obstetricians and Gynecologists' Precis III* and *Standards for Obstetric-Gynecologic Services* (6th edition); Berkow's *The Merck Manual*; Blacklow's *MacBryde's Signs and Symptoms*; Boucek's *Coronary Artery Disease, Pathological and Clinical Assessment*; Cohen's *Emergencies in Obstetrics & Gynecology*; Griffith's *Instructions for Patients*; Hollingworth's *Pregnancy, Diabetes, and Birth*; Kaplan's *Comprehensive Textbook of Psychiatry*; Karliner's *Coronary Care*; Mandell, Douglas, and Bennett's *Principles & Practice of Infectious Diseases* (2nd edition); Margulies and Thaler's *The Physician's Book of Lists*; Ogilvie's *Birch's Emergencies in Medical Practice*; Parillo's *Major Issues in Critical Care Medicine*; Percival's *Holland and Brews Manual of Obstetrics*; Rakel's *Conn's Current Therapy* (1985, 1986, 1987, 1988); Rowland's *Merritt's Textbook of Neurology*; Sabiston's *Texbook of Surgery* (12th edition); Schiff's *Diseases of the Liver*; Schwartz's *Principles and Practice of Emergency Medicine* (2nd edition); Williams' *Gray's Anatomy*; and Wyngaarden's *Cecil Textbook of Medicine*. Publishers include Churchill Livingstone, J.B. Lippincott, and W.B. Saunders. Also includes the serials *Cardiology Clinics*, *Emergency Medicine Clinics of North America*, and *Medical Clinics of North America*, published by W.B. Saunders. The complete list of journals and yearbooks covered as at 12/92 follows:

Journals:
ACOG Technical Bulletin (3/73–)
Age and Ageing (7/86–)
AIDS: Papers from Science (1/82–12/85)
American Family Physician (7/91–)
American Heart Journal (1/86–)
American Journal of Cardiology (1/86–)
American Journal of Medicine (5/86–)
American Journal of Obstetrics and Gynaecology (1/86–)
American Journal of Physical Medicine and Rehabilitation (4/91–)
American Journal of Psychiatry (8/85–)
American Journal of Public Health (7/85–)
American Journal of Roentgenology (11/90–)
American Journal of Surgery (2/86–)
Anesthesia and Analgesia (1/88–)
Anesthesiology (8/86–)
Annals of Internal Medicine (8/84–)
Annals of Neurology (9/86–)
Annals of Rheumatic Diseases (1/87–11/88)
Annals of Surgery (2/85–)
Annals of Thoracic Surgery (1/91–)
Archives of Disease in Childhood (7/85–)
Arteriosclerosis (1/86–)
Arthritis and Rheumatism (1/86–)
British Heart Journal (1/86–)
British Journal of Diseases of the Chest (1/87–7/88)
British Journal of Obstetrics and Gynaecology (1/87–)
British Journal of Rheumatology (2/86–)
British Journal of Surgery (5/86–)
British Journal of Urology (7/87–)
British Medical Journal (7/83–)
Canadian Medical Association Journal (11/86–)
Cancer Treatment Reports (1/85–12/87)
Circulation (7/87–)
Circulation Research (7/88–)
Clinical Chemistry (6/92–)
Clinical Diabetes (1/86–)
Clinical Orthopaedics (5/85–)

Clinical Pediatrics (6/85–5/90)
Clinical Pharmacology and Therapeutics (7/85–)
Critical Care Medicine (11/90–)
Diabetes (1/86–)
Diabetes Care (1/86–)
Emergency Medicine Reports (11/85–10/86)
Fertility and Sterility (3/86–4/89)
Gastroenterology (7/91–)
Genitournary Medicine (4/88–)
Gut (4/86–)
Harvard Medical School Health Letter (11/85–)
Heart and Lung (1/86–1/89)
Hypertension and Arteriosclerosis (7/88–)
Journal of Allergy and Clinical Immunology (1/86–)
Journal of American Board of Family Practice (1/88–)
Journal of the American College of Cardiology (1/89–)
Journal of American Medical Association (1/92–)
Journal of Bone and Joint Surgery (7/85–)
Journal of Clinical Chemistry (6/92–)
Journal of Clinical Investigation (7/86–)
Journal of Clinical Pathology (1/86–)
Journal of Laboratory and Clinical Medicine (1/86–)
Journal of Neurology, Neurosurgery and Psychiatry (2/86–)
Journal of Pediatrics (1/86–)
Journal of Reconstructive Surgery (11/90–)
Journal of the National Cancer Institute (1/85–3/88)
Journal of Trauma (11/90–)
Journal of Urology (10/90–)
Lancet (7/83–)
Medical Letter (8/82–)
Medical Science Research (1/87–5/88)
Medicine (11/85–)
Morbidity and Mortality Weekly Report (6/85–9/90)
Nature (10/85–9/89)
Neurology (1/87–)
New England Journal of Medicine (1/83–)
Obstetrical and Gynecological Survey (1/86–)
Obstetrics and Gynaecology (1/88–)
Pediatrics (7/85–)
Physical Therapy (3/86–)
Quarterly Journal of Medicine (5/86–8/88)
Seminars in Liver Disease (2/86–8/87)
Seminars in Neurology (3/86–3/88)
Seminars in Respiratory Medicine (7/85–10/88)
Sexually Transmitted Diseases (4/85–)
Stroke (7/88–)
Thorax (1/86–1/89)

Year Books:
Year Book of Anesthesia
Year Book of Cancer
Year Book of Cardiology
Year Book of Critical Care Medicine
Year Book of Dentistry
Year Book of Dematology
Year Book of Diagnostic Radiology
Year Book of Digestive Diseases
Year Book of Drug Therapy
Year Book of Emergency Medicine
Year Book of Endocrinology
Year Book of Family Practice
Year Book of Hand Surgery
Year Book of Hematology
Year Book of Infectious Diseases
Year Book of Medicine
Year Book of Neurology and Neurosurgery
Year Book of Nuclear Medicine
Year Book of Obstetrics and Gynaecology
Year Book of Ophtalmology
Year Book of Orthapaedics
Year Book of Otolaryngology
Year Book of Patology
Year Book of Pediatrics

Year Book of Plastic Surgery
Year Book of Podiatric Medicine
Year Book of Perinatal/Neonatal Medicine
Year Book of Psychiatry
Year Book of Pulmonary Disease
Year Book of Rehabilitation
Year Book of Sports Medicine
Year Book of Surgery
Year Book of Urology
Year Book of Vascular Surgery.

15:84. Online   BRS

File name	CCML
Alternative name(s)	CCML
Start year	
Number of records	
Update period	Weekly
Price/Charges	Connect time: US$41.00/51.00
	Online print: US$0.91/0.99
	Offline print: US$0.99
	SDI charge: US$10.30

15:85. Database subset

Online   BRS

File name	JOUR
Start year	
Number of records	
Update period	Weekly
Price/Charges	Connect time: US$41.00/51.00
	Online print: US$0.91/0.99
	Offline print: US$0.99

Notes

This database contains the full text of all the medical journals included in the Comprehensive Core Medical Library.

15:86. Database subset

Online   BRS

File name	MEDB
Start year	Concurrent with publication of new editions
Number of records	
Update period	Varies
Price/Charges	Connect time: US$41.00/51.00
	Online print: US$0.91/0.99
	Offline print: US$0.99

Notes

This database contains the full text of the medical textbooks and reference works included in the Comprehensive Core Medical Library.

15:87. Database subset

Online   BRS

File name	PCTJ – Comprehensive Core Medical Library Practice File
Alternative name(s)	CCML
Start year	
Number of records	
Update period	
Price/Charges	Connect time: Free/US$10.00
	Online print: Free

Notes

The training file for CCML.

For more details of constituent databases, see:
American Family Physician
American Journal of Psychiatry
American Journal of Public Health
Annals of Internal Medicine
Annals of Neurology
British Journal of Surgery
British Medical Journal

Canadian Medical Association Journal
Cancer Treatment Reports
Clinical Pediatrics
Critical Care Medicine
Journal of American Medical Association
Morbidity and Mortality Weekly Report
New England Journal of Medicine
Obstetrics and Gynaecology
Pediatrics
Sexually Transmitted Diseases

Criminal Justice Periodical Index
University Microfilms International

15:89. Master record

Database type	Bibliographic
Number of journals	120
Sources	Journals and Newsletters
Start year	1975
Language	English
Coverage	Canada, UK and USA
Number of records	182,778
Update size	12,000
Update period	Monthly
Index unit	Articles

Keywords

Forensic Science; Child Abuse; Computer Crime; Drug Abuse

Description

The Criminal Justice Periodical Index database provides cover-to-cover indexing of over 100 journals, newsletters, and law reporters. Contains citations to articles in magazines, journals, newsletters, and law reporting publications on the administration of justice and law enforcement. Subjects covered include abortion, arrest (police methods), child abuse, the justice system, penology, commercial crime, computer crime, court reform, crime prevention, drug abuse, due process of law, evidence, family law, fingerprinting, forensic science, jail administration, judges, juvenile offenders, legal aid, narcotics trafficking, negligence, environmental and industrial crime, political and social crime, organized crime, parole officers prisons, recidivism, security forces, victimless crimes, violence, and more.

Corresponds to *Criminal Justice Periodical Index*.

15:90. Online   DIALOG

File name	File 171
Start year	1975
Number of records	182,778
Update period	Monthly
Price/Charges	Subscription: US$66.00
	Online print: US$0.25
	Offline print: US$0.25
	SDI charge: US$7.95

EMBASE
Elsevier Science Publishers

15:91. Master record

Alternative name(s)	Excerpta Medica
Database type	Bibliographic
Number of journals	4,700
Sources	Case studies, clinicians, journals, monographs, research communications, reviews, surveys and symposia
Start year	1974
Language	English
Coverage	International

Forensic Science
EMBASE

Number of records	4,950,000+
Update size	350,000
Update period	Weekly
Index unit	Articles
Abstract details	Adaptations of the authors' summaries and selected on the basis of content and length by an international group of practicing medical and other qualified specialists and when necessary modified, shortened or extended to obtain the optimal information value. A group of over 2,000 biomedical specialists assist with the preparation of abstracts in particular subject areas and articles in non-Western European languages
Thesaurus	EMTREE Thesaurus METAGS
Database aids	Guide to the Classification and Indexing System, MALIMET (available online and on microfiche), Mini-Malimet, MECLASE Drug Trade Names (DN) and EMBASE List of Journals Abstracted

Keywords

HIV; Anaesthesia; Anatomy; Anthropology; Bioengineering; Biotechnology; Cancer; Cardiology; Clinical Medicine; Clinical Neurology; Cosmetics; Drugs; Environmental Health; Environmental Pollution; Environmental Toxicology; Epilepsy; Food Additives; Food Contaminants; Forensic Medicine; Forensic Science; Gastroenterology; Gynaecology; Immunology; Industrial Medicine; Nephrology; Neuroscience; Neuromuscular Disorders; Nuclear Medicine; Obstetrics; Occupational Health and Safety; Patents; Pathology; Pharmaceuticals; Pollution; Public Health; Radiology; Toxic Substances; Waste Management

Description

EMBASE is the trademark for the English language Excerpta Medica database. Excerpta Medica was founded as a non-profit making organisation in 1946 with the goal of improving the availability and dissemination of medical knowledge through the publication of a series of abstract journals. The database contains citations, with abstracts, to the worldwide biomedical literature on human medicine and areas of biological sciences related to human medicine with an emphasis on the pharmacological effects of drugs and chemicals. The four main categories of primary literature sources are: specialist medical publications; general biomedicine publications; specialist non-medical publications and general scientific publications. Subjects covered include: anatomy; anesthesiology (including resuscitation and intensive care medicine); anthropology; pharmacology of anesthetic agents, spinal, epidural and caudal anesthesia and acupuncture (as anesthetic); autoimmunity; biochemistry; bioengineering; cancer; dangerous goods; dermatology; developmental biology; drug adverse reactions; drug dependence; drug effects; endocrinology; environmental health and pollution control (covering chemical pollution and its effect on man, animals, plants and microorganisms; measurement, treatment, prevention and control); exocrine pancreas; forensic science; gastroenterology (including diseases and disorders of: digestive systems; mouth; pharynx and more); genetics; gerontology and geriatrics; health economics; hematology; hepatobiliary system; hospital management; immunology (including immunity; hypersensitivity; histocompatibility and all aspects of the immune system); internal medicine; legal and socioeconomic aspects; mesentary; meteorological aspects; microbiology; nephrology (covering diagnosis; treatment; epidemiology; prevention; infections; glomerular and tubular disorders; blood purification; dialysis; kidney transplantation; toxic nephropathy and including important clinical abstracts with epidemiological studies and major clinical trials, with particular emphasis on hypertension and diabetes); neurosciences (especially clinical neurology and neurosurgery, epilepsy and neuromuscular disorders but also covering nonclinical articles on neurophysiology and animal models for human neuropharmacology); noise and vibration; nuclear medicine; obstetrics and gynaecology (including endocrinology and menstrual cycle, infertility, prenatal diagnosis and fetal monitoring, anticonceptions, breast cancer diagnosis, sterilisation and psychosexual problems and neonatal care of normal children); occupational health and industrial medicine; opthalmology; otorhinolaryngology; paediatrics; pathology (including general pathology and organ pathology, pathological physiology and pathological anatomy, as well as laboratory methods and techniques used in pathology. General pathology topics range from cellular pathology, fetal and neonatal pathology, including congenital disorders, injury (both chemical and physical), inflammation and infection, immuno-pathology, collagen diseases and cancer pathology); peritoneum; pharmacology (including the effects and use of all drugs; experimental aspects of pharmacokinetics and pharmacodynamics; drug information); physiology; psychiatry and psychology (including addiction; alcoholism; sexual behaviour; suicide; mental deficiency and the clinical use or abuse of psychotropic and psychomimetic agents); public health; radiation and thermal pollution; radiology (including radiodiagnosis, radiotherapy and radiobiology, ultrasound diagnosis, thermography, adverse reactions to radiotherapy and techniques and apparatus, radiobiology of radioisotopes, aspects of radiohygiene, new labelling techniques and tracer applications); rehabilitation; surgery; toxicology (including pharmaceutical toxicology; foods, food additives, and contaminants; cosmetics, toiletries, and household products; occupational toxicology; waste material in air, soil and water; toxins and venoms; chemical teratogens, mutagens, and carcinogens; phototoxicity; regulatory toxicology; laboratory methods and techniques; and antidotes and symptomatic treatment); urology; wastewater treatment and measurement. The database is particularly strong in drug-related literature, where records include manufacturers and drug trade names and generic names. Information on veterinary medicine, nursing and dentistry is generally excluded.

Excerpta Medica is extremely current as articles are indexed within thirty days of receipt and are online very soon after that. Approximately 900 journals (the Rapid Input Processing (RIP)) are processed with priority which means that within eleven weeks of the receipt
of the original document, the completely-indexed records are available. More than 100,000 records are given this priority treatment. Some hosts have companion databases giving training or details of the indexing vocabularies and thesauri.

EMBASE concentrates on journal articles although about 1,000 books per annum were indexed between 1975 and 1980. The source journals include all forty-six sections of *Excerpta Medica*, the *Drug Literature Index* and *Adverse Reactions Titles*. New titles are added and old titles deleted at a rate of about 200–300 per year. The database covers sources from 110 countries with the following geographical scope: North America 36%, Western Europe 35%, United Kingdom 14%, USSR and Eastern Europe 7%, Asia 6%, Central and South America 1%, Austalia & South Pacific 1%, Africa and Middle East 1%. Approximately 50% of the citations are from drug and pharmaceutical literature and approximately 40% of citations added to the database each year do not appear in the corresponding printed abstract journals and indexes. Approximately 65% of the citations contain abstracts of on average 200 words with a maximum of 800 words which indicate the content of the articles and are not intended to summarise the results or express opinions. This makes free-text searching of the abstracts, titles and other searchable elements of the citation valuable. This compares with approximately sixty-five per cent of the records in MEDLINE and fifty-four per cent in BIOSIS. The records of the other leading bioscience database, SciSearch, now do contain abstracts. Approximately 75% of the articles are in the English language. Of the other leading bioscience databases, approximately eighty-eight per cent of articles on SciSearch are in English, eighty-six per cent of articles on BIOSIS and seventy-four per cent on MEDLINE. In addition approximately thirty-seven per cent of records with non-English sources contain English-language abstracts online. This compares with sixty-seven per cent on BIOSIS and twenty-six per cent on MEDLINE. SciSearch does now contain abstracts. Important publications NOT indexed in EMBASE include Meyler's *Side Effects of Drugs*, 1972–1980 published by Excerpta Medica and *Side Effects of Drugs Annual*, 1981 to the present, published by Elsevier.

A core collection of 3,500 biomedical journals supplemented by journals in the areas of agriculture, technology, economics, chemistry, environmental protection and sociology. General criteria used for selection are first that the document should be of potential relevance to medicine and secondly the information should be of lasting value for which reasons news items and comments are generally excluded.

EMBASE section headings are based on medical specialities; a total of forty-seven subfiles group together citations on topics such as anatomy, paediatrics, opthalmology, gastroenterelogy, cancer, plastic surgery, occupational health. Each subfile or section has its own hierarchical scheme. The thesaurus *MALIMET (Master List of Medical Terms)* is used which contains more than 250,000 preferred terms and 255,000 synonyms which are mapped to the preferred terms when used. It is used for indexing highly specific concepts such as names of drugs and chemicals; diseases and syndromes; anatomical and physiological aspects and diagnostic and therapeutic methods. *MALIMET* is growing at a rate of over 12,000 descriptors per annum, mainly through drug names and names of chemical compounds. The size of the complete *MALIMET* thesaurus for EMBASE (more than 250,000 preferred terms compared to 15,000 in *MeSH*) may indicate its tendency to provide a greater variety of possible terms and therefore, less consistent application in indexing. In 1993, all non-drug *MeSH* terms were included in the thesaurus mapped to *MALIMET* terms so that a search strategy can be transferred from MEDLINE.

Indexing incorporates the following rules: natural word order (acute leukemia, not leukemia acute); American spelling (tumor, not tumour), singular noun forms and not plural or adjectival forms (stomach tumor, not gastric tumors, but optic nerve, not eye nerve); the most specific term must be used. Since 1979,

MALIMET terms have been weighted. Class A terms (weighted) indicate the main concepts while Class B terms (not weighted) indicate the less important concepts of a document. In addition to *MALIMET* broad concepts are indexed with EMCLAS and EMTAGS. EMCLAS is a poly-hierarchical decimal classification scheme of the forty-six subject subfiles which make up the sections of the printed Excerpta Medica containing approximately 6,500 entries. It is then further subdivided into a five level hierarchy of sub-categories. Indexing is performed by medical specialists and scientists whose specialism corresponds to the subject areas forming the major subdivisions of EMCLAS. The indexing builds up sequentially as the article is indexed by each of the sections for which it is relevant. On average each document is indexed for 3.5 different sections.

EMTAGS is a group of approximately 220 codes which represent general concepts such as groups, gender, organ systems, experimental animals and article type. In January 1991 about 10% of the terms were changed including important descriptors such as CANCER or BENIGN NEOPLASM.

EMBASE editors also add 'uncontrolled' drug terms to augment MALIMET descriptors in selected records. EMBASE provides a hierarchical classification system (EMTREES) reflecting fifteen broad facets of biomedicine. From January 1991 a new version of EMTREE went online comprising 35,000 terms. New descriptors and changes in the hierarchy were made in the following areas: anatomy of the eye; diseases; drugs; techniques; biological phenomea and document types. Prior to 1988 Section Headings based on medical speciality areas were used instead of EMTREES to index EMBASE citations. In both classification schemes, codes are constructed to facilitate broad concept retrieval through truncation. In addition three uncontrolled vocabularies are used: Medical Secondary Text; Drug (Trade Names) and Manufacturers' Names are used. Medical Secondary Text consists of free-text words, numbers and phrases, describing concepts which are not fully covered by the controlled terms, for example quantiative information such as the number of patients or experimental animals. Drug (Trade) Names consists of trade names of drugs referred to in an original document with the main aspect of biological effects of compounds listed. Manufacturers' Names lists the names of drug manufacturers. The value of controlled indexing is important when searching for topics where a subject population has been specified.

Relatively few bioscience databases provide consistent indexing for subject populations (that is, humans or specific test animals) and related characteristics commonly requested such as age groups, gender, occupation and racial or ethnic groups. EMBASE provides extensive consistent indexing for the identification of test animals and age groups with a less consistent approach for the indexing of humans, occupational groups, racial/ethnic groups and gender. In addition, in most bioscience files a form of pharmaceutical nomenclature exists. For EMBASE the preferred search terms are generic name, classification by action/use and CAS Registry Number although restrictions by date, subfile and vendor may apply to the latter and vendor documentation should be consulted for guidelines. The search terms Enzyme Commission Number, investigational code, chemical name and trade name should be cross-referenced to the preferred terminology in the thesaurus. In 1993, improved CAS Registry Numbers mean that there is a single Number assigned for every substance.

15:92. Database subset

Online   DIMDI

File name	E374 – EMFORENSIC
Alternative name(s)	Excerpta Medica
Software	GRIPS
Start year	1974
Number of records	66,341
Update period	Weekly
Delay	1–5 months
SDI period	1 week
Database aids	User Manual EMBASE and Memocard EMBASE
Price/Charges	Connect time: UK£08.06- 16.35
	Online print: UK£0.41–0.59
	Offline print: UK£0.34–0.41

Thesaurus is online

Notes

This is a subfile of EMBASE. EMFORENSIC contains citations to the worldwide literature on forensic sciences. It corresponds to the Forensic Sciences Abstracts section of *Excerpta Medica* and to the citations from that section contained in EMBASE. Approximately 58% of records contain abstracts. The corresponding file E483 contains records covering the period 1983 to date. Searches are possible from January 1974. The EMBASE subfiles have different groupings for costing – EMFORENSIC is in Group 1, with EMHEALTH, EMCANCER and EMTOX.

Record composition

Abstract AB; Abstract Language AL; ADONIS Number ANR; Author AU; Classification Code CC; Conference CF; Coden CO; CAS-Reg No CR; Corporate Source CS; Controlled Terms CT; Qualifier /QF; Weighting /W1; Country CY; Drug Trade Name DN; Document Name DT; EMCLAS Code EC; Entry Date ED; Editor EDR; EMCLAS Term ET; EMTAGS-Code IC; EMTAGS-Term IT; CY/JT JC; Journal Title JT; Language LA; Manufacturer's Name MN; Number of Document ND; Publisher PU; Publication Year PY; Qualifier QF; ISBN-NO SB; Source SO; ISSN-NO and Title TI

Hedges or limit capabilities are provided to limit to (pps=) human; adverse drug reactions; AIDS; animals, birds; animals, cold-blooded; animals, vertebrate; cancer; developing countries; and ecotoxicity. The basic Index includes the data fields: Abstract, Controlled Term, Drug Trade Name, EMTAGS-Term, Manufacturer's Name, Title. EMFORENSIC is defined as subfile to EMBASE with: FIND EC DOWN 49.

15:93. Database subset

Online   DIMDI

File name	E383 – EMFORENSIC
Alternative name(s)	Excerpta Medica
Software	GRIPS
Start year	1983
Number of records	37,284
Update period	Weekly
Delay	1–5 months
SDI period	1 week
Database aids	User Manual EMBASE and Memocard EMBASE
Price/Charges	Connect time: UK£08.06- 16.35
	Online print: UK£0.41–0.59
	Offline print: UK£0.34–0.41

Downloading is allowed
Thesaurus is online

Notes

This is a subfile of EMBASE. EMFORENSIC contains citations to the worldwide literature on forensic sciences. It corresponds to the 'Forensic Sciences Abstracts' section of *Excerpta Medica* and to the citations from that section contained in EMBASE. Approximately 61% of records contain abstracts. The corresponding file E474 contains records covering the period 1974 to date. The EMBASE subfiles have different groupings for costing – EMFORENSIC is in Group 1, with EMHEALTH, EMCANCER and EMTOX.

Record composition

Abstract AB; Abstract Language AL; ADONIS Number ANR; Author AU; Classification Code CC; Conference CF; Coden CO; CAS-Reg No CR; Corporate Source CS; Controlled Terms CT; Qualifier /QF; Weighting /W1; Country CY; Drug Trade Name DN; Document Name DT; EMCLAS Code EC; Entry Date ED; Editor EDR; EMCLAS Term ET; EMTAGS-Code IC; EMTAGS-Term IT; CY/JT JC; Journal Title JT; Language LA; Manufacturer's Name MN; Number of Document ND; Publisher PU; Publication Year PY; Qualifier QF; ISBN-NO SB; Source SO; ISSN-NO and Title TI

Hedges or limit capabilities are provided to limit to (pps=) human; adverse drug reactions; AIDS; animals, birds; animals, cold-blooded; animals, vertebrate; cancer; developing countries; and ecotoxicity. The basic Index includes the data fields: Abstract, Controlled Term, Drug Trade Name, EMTAGS-Term, Manufacturer's Name, Title. EMFORENSIC is defined as subfile to EMBASE with: FIND EC DOWN 49.

15:94. Database subset

CD-ROM   SilverPlatter

File name	Excerpta Medica – Pathology
Alternative name(s)	Excerpta Medica
Format notes	IBM, Mac
Software	SPIRS/MacSPIRS
Start year	1980
Number of records	266,000
Update period	Quarterly
Price/Charges	Subscription: UK£755 – 1,132

Notes

One of the Elsevier speciality *Excerpta Medica* range, this CD-ROM database is a subset of EMBASE covering pathology. Subjects covered include general pathology and organ pathology, pathophysiology, pathological anatomy and laboratory methods and techniques used in pathology. General pathology topics range from cellular pathology, foetal and neonatal pathology including congenital disorders, injury (both chemical and physical), inflammation and infection, immunopathology, collagen diseases and cancer pathology. Relevant abstracts from other clinical and basic disciplines are also included.

Prices are: for single users UK£755, for 2–8 networked users £1,132.

This database can also be found on:
Eyenet
Cancer-CD
Medata-ROM
Logo-A Pharmaceutical Products (Discontinued)

Expert and the Law
National Forensic Center

15:96. Master record

Database type	Textual
Number of journals	1
Sources	Newsletters

Start year	1981 (December 7)
Language	English
Coverage	USA (primarily) and International (some)
Number of records	—
Update size	—
Update period	Within 2 weeks after receipt of new materials

Keywords
Forensic Science

Description
Contains full text of *The Expert and the Law*, a newsletter covering the application of scientific, medical, and technical knowledge to litigation. Includes news about the use of consultants by attorneys and feature articles on the effective use of experts and consultants (for example, ethical considerations when expert witnesses incur out-of-pocket expenses).

15:97. Online   Mead Data Central (as a NEXIS database)

File name	EXPTLW – NEXIS
Alternative name(s)	NEXIS – Expert and the law
Start year	1981 (December 7)
Number of records	
Update period	Within 2 weeks after receipt of new materials
Price/Charges	Subscription: US$1,000 – 3,000 (Depending on needs)
	Connect time: US$49.00 (Telecomms + connect time)
	Database entry fee: US$6.00
	Online print: US$0.04 per line

Notes
Libraries: GENFED, HEALTH, LEGNEW, MEDMAL AND PRLIAB; Group files: ALLLEG, NWLTRS, CURRNT, ARCHIV, OMNI and LGLNEW.

A subscription charge which covers all transactional charges, connect time, telecommunications and the small administration charge can take the place of the individual charges. Subscriptions are negotiated with customers and vary according to the number of menus (thus, files) that are to be used – typically a minimum subscription would be about US$ 1,000. All charges include training and a 24-hour help line.

Record composition
Body (BODY); Byline (BYLINE); Correction; Correction Date; date; Graphic; Headline; Headline and Lead (HLEAD); Lead; Length; Publication and Section

This database can also be found on:
NEXIS

Expertnet
ExpertNet Ltd

15:99. Master record

Database type	Directory
Number of journals	
Sources	

Start year	Current information
Language	English
Coverage	USA
Number of records	1,300
Update size	—
Update period	Monthly
Host have included	Dialcom

Keywords
Forensic Science

Description
Contains biographical profiles for over a thousand medical experts, each of whom has signed an agreement with ExpertNet Ltd. indicating a willingness to participate in medicolegal consultation and serve as expert witnesses or consultants to attorneys. All geographic areas are represented as well as virtually all medical specialties. Virtually all of the experts are physicians in active practices. Although many of these experts have medicolegal experience, 'professional witnesses' are discouraged from participation in ExpertNet. In addition, the database contains user-friendly menu screens designed to assist the searcher in identifying the appropriate medical areas and terminology to use in locating an expert(s). Each profile contains information about the expert's medical specialties, education and clinical training, past experience and current positions. Provides state of residence and first three digits of ZIP code, age, professional experience, state licence and date of board certification, and hourly fee. Also includes general remarks, for example, research, publications, awards, medical/legal experience); willingness to consult for plaintiffs, defendants or either; willingness to testify; typical hourly fees; and any geographic limitations on travel. Name, address, and telephone number are available upon request. This database is not searchable by name or address; however, access points include state of residence, state of licensure, geographic limitation and past experience.

15:100. Online   ABA/net (as a private network on iNet America)

File name	
Start year	Current information
Number of records	
Update period	

Notes
Subscription to ABA/net required.

15:101. Online   DIALOG

File name	File 183
Start year	Current information
Number of records	1,300
Update period	5/6 times yearly
Price/Charges	Connect time: US$60.00
	Online print: US$0.30 – 120.00 (full text)
	Offline print: US$0.30 – 120.00 (full text)

Notes
DIALINDEX Categories: None.

15:102. Online   West Publishing Company

File name	EXPNET
Start year	Current information

Number of records
Update period

Notes

Subscription to West Publishing Company required.

Family Doctor, The
CMC ReSearch

15:103. Master record

Database type	Textual, Image, Directory, Factual
Number of journals	
Sources	
Start year	1991
Language	English
Coverage	
Number of records	1,500 questions; 1,600 drugs.
Update size	—
Update period	Varies

Keywords

Anatomy; Drugs; Home Health Care

Description

Written and edited by Dr Allen H Bruckheim – a US nationally-recognised physician and medical expert, this is a medical guide for do-it-yourself diagnosis and advice consisting of colour illustrations and text covering common diseases, symptoms, medical procedures, and human anatomy. It brings together a substantial amount of medical information written in plain English for lay users. Includes a wide-ranging question-and-answer section – over a thousand commonly asked questions covering subjects as diverse as ultrasound scans and why limbs swell in aeroplanes. Health update booklets provide answers in further detail on selected subjects, inlcuding the heart, ageing, arthritis, diabetes, colon cancer and cholesterol control.

Also includes details of support groups, photographs to help identify medications and data on a large number of drugs commonly prescribed for everyday ailments: the comprehensive *Consumer Guide to Prescription Drugs* – the equivalent of a 992-page book providing detailed information on over 1,600 brand name products, including: brand names, type of drug, ingredients, dosage forms, storage, uses, treatment, side effects, interactions and warnings, common abbreviations and over two hundred images to assist in drug identification.

Dr Bruckheim was awarded the Vincent Downing Award by the metropolitan New York Chapter of the American Medical Writers Association for this product in 1992. Previous winners have been the originator of the *Merck Manual* and the author of the *Complete Guide to Prescription and Nonprescription Drugs*.

Full-text word searching, browsing, or table of contents.

15:104. CD-ROM CMC ReSearch

File name	Family Doctor, The
Format notes	IBM, Mac
Software	DiscPassage
Start year	1991
Number of records	1,500 questions; 1,600 drugs.
Update period	Varies
Price	UK£80

15:105. CD-ROM 8cm CMC ReSearch

File name	Portable Family Doctor, The
Format notes	Sony, Data, Discman
Start year	1991
Number of records	1,500 questions; 1,600 drugs.
Update period	Varies
Price	US$49.95

Forensic Science Database
Home Office Forensic Science Service – HOFSS

15:106. Master record

Database type	Bibliographic
Number of journals	300
Sources	Conference proceedings, government documents, grey literature, journals, monographs and reports
Start year	1976, with some earlier materials
Language	English
Coverage	International
Number of records	35,000
Update size	—
Update period	Nine times per year
Thesaurus	Thesaurus of Forensic Science, 3rd ed., Aldermaston, HOFSS
Database aids	FORS Users Guide, Aldermaston, HOFSS

Keywords

Biotechnology; Drugs; Forensic Science; Pathology

Description

Forensic Science Database contains citations, with abstracts, to the worldwide literature on forensic sciences. The database is multidisciplinary and covers literature relevant to the examination of evidential materials, analytical methods and the presentation and interpretation of findings. Subjects covered include: drugs and toxicology, forensic biology, forensic chemistry, documents and firearms examination, safety and management aspects of running a Forensic Science Service, pathology, case law, information management and use of computers and the management of forensic science laboratories and programmes. The database also covers techniques and problems which are also encountered in many analytical laboratories, especially areas of toxicology and body fluid identification. The database is a valuable infomation tool for forensic scientists and other professionals involved in crime investigation and the provision of expert testimony to the Courts.

Sources include about 300 journals and over 1,500 books, periodicals, conference proceedings, technical reports, government documents, and grey literature together with a series of abstracting and bibliographic services.

15:107. Online CompuServe Information Service

File name	IQUEST File 2657
Start year	1977
Number of records	35,000
Update period	Monthly
Price/Charges	Subscription: US$8.95 per month
	Database entry fee: US$9/search; some databases carry a surcharge ($2–75)
	Online print: US$10 references free; then $9 per ten; abstracts $3 each

Downloading is allowed

Notes

Accessed via IQUEST or IQMEDICAL, this database is offered by a Data-Star gateway. IQUEST can either search across all databases, a database of the user's choice or selected multiple databases.

Record composition

Abstract AB; Accession Number and Update Code AN; Author AU; Author Affiliation IN; Availability of Original Article AV; Descriptors DE; Language of article LG; Source SO; Title TI; Update Code and Year of Publication YR

The data field, Title, deals with conference proceedings by listing the title of the paper, the collective title of the proceedings and the name, location and date of the conference.

15:108. Online   Data-Star

File name	FORS
Start year	1976, with some earlier materials
Number of records	35,000
Update period	Nine times per year
Database aids	Data-Star Biomedical Manual, Berne, Data-Star, 1989 and Online manual (search NEWS-FORS in NEWS)
Price/Charges	Subscription: SFr80.00
	Connect time: SFr101.20
	Online print: SFr0.42
	Offline print: SFr0.65

Downloading is allowed

Notes

From June 1993 Data-Star have introduced an annual fee/subscription per contract (that is, not per password) of SFr 80.00 (c.UK£ 32.00) payable every June. For North American customers billed in dollars who also use DIALOG, the DIALOG fee also covers access to Data-Star. Academic customers, 'commitment' customers and customers currently billed in dollars are exempt.

Record composition

Abstract AB; Accession Number and Update Code AN; Author AU; Author Affiliation IN; Availability of Original Article AV; Descriptors DE; Language of article LG; Source SO; Title TI; Update Code and Year of Publication YR

The data field title deals with conference proceedings by listing the title of the paper, the collective title of the proceedings and the name, location and date of the conference.

Forensic Services Directory
National Forensic Center

15:109. Master record

Database type	Directory
Number of journals	
Sources	
Start year	Current information
Language	English
Coverage	USA (primarily), Canada (primarily) and International (some)
Number of records	
Update size	–
Update period	Three to four times per year

Keywords

Forensic Science

Description

Contains the names of thousands of scientific, medical, and technical experts available to serve as expert trial witnesses or consultants to attorneys, corporations, and the government. Also lists translators, testing laboratories, investigators, and other specialists providing trial support services. Also includes resources available from specialized libraries, organisations, and agencies.

Corresponds to *Forensic Services Directory*.

15:110. Online   Mead Data Central (as a NEXIS database)

File name	EXPERT – NEXIS
Alternative name(s)	NEXIS – Forensic Services Directory
Start year	Current information
Number of records	
Update period	Three to four times per year
Price/Charges	Subscription: US$1,000 – 3,000 (Depending on needs)
	Connect time: US$49.00 (Telecomms + connect time)
	Database entry fee: US$11.00 (Search charge)
	Online print: US$0.04 per line

Notes

Library: LEXREF.

A subscription charge which covers all transactional charges, connect time, telecommunications and the small administration charge can take the place of the individual charges. Subscriptions are negotiated with customers and vary according to the number of menus (thus, files) that are to be used – typically a minimum subscription would be about US$ 1,000. All charges include training and a 24-hour help line.

15:111. Online   West Publishing Company (FSD)

File name	FSD
Start year	Current information
Number of records	
Update period	Three to four times per year

Notes

Subscription to West Publishing Company required.

This database can also be found on:
NEXIS

Gastrointestinal Absorption Database
US Environmental Protection Agency (EPA), Office of Pesticides and Toxic Substances

15:113. Master record

Alternative name(s)	GIABS
Database type	Bibliographic
Number of journals	
Sources	Reports and Journals
Start year	1967 to December 1987
Language	English
Coverage	International
Number of records	12,000+
Update size	–
Update period	Varies

Keywords

Chemical Substances; Pathology; Physiology

Description

Contains citations to the worldwide literature on experiments in gastrointestinal absorption, distribution, metabolism, and excretion of orally administered chemical substances. Covers reports on test conditions (for example, substance tested, test animal) in more than 4,900 studies involving more than 3,100 chemical substances administered to laboratory animals or human subjects.

New data are to be added when Environmental Protection Agency Funds become available.

15:114. Online
Chemical Information Systems Inc (CIS)

File name	
Alternative name(s)	GIABS
Start year	1967 to December 1987
Number of records	12,000+
Update period	Varies

Notes

Annual subscription fee of $300 to Chemical Information Systems required. Chemical Information Systems is a subsidiary of Fein-Marquart Associates.

IDIS Drug File
Iowa Drug Information Service

15:115. Master record

Database type	Bibliographic
Number of journals	160
Sources	Journals
Start year	1966
Language	English
Coverage	International
Number of records	300,000
Update size	—
Update period	Monthly
Index unit	Articles
Database aids	Drug and disease cross-reference lists with the IDIS controlled vocabulary terms are available from the producer.

Keywords

Drug Therapy; Pathology

Description

IDIS Drug File presents an online index to the IDIS drug literature microfilm file, which contains some 240,000 articles, relating to drugs and drug therapy in humans published since 1965 in over 160 biomedical journals. Subjects covered include age group of study population, study design, treatment efficacy, dosage administration technique, pharmacokinetics, pharmaceutics, incompatibilities, drug interactions, toxicology and side effects. Animal studies are not included. Each record contains title, author(s), bibliographic details.

Articles are taken from over 140 of the top English language medical and pharmaceutical journals.

Documents are extensively indexed with terms for drugs, diseases and type of information. The corresponding microfilm number is also given, directing users to the microfilmed journal article, which is available from the producer as IDIS Drug Literature Microfilm File. There may be multiple index documents for the same journal article to reflect a group of concepts presented within the article. Drug and dis-

ease cross-reference lists with the IDIS controlled vocabulary terms are available from the producer.

Drug indexing terms are adapted from the United States Adapted Names; Disease indexing terms are adapted from the International Classification of Diseases, 9th Revision, Clinical Modification.

15:116. Online
BRS

File name	IDIS
Start year	1966
Number of records	300,000
Update period	Monthly
Price/Charges	Connect time: US$42.00/52.00
	Online print: US$0.27/0.35
	Offline print: US$0.45
	SDI charge: US$6.95

Downloading is allowed

15:117. Online
Data-Star

File name	IOWA
Start year	1966
Number of records	336,000
Update period	Monthly
Database aids	Data-Star Biomedical Manual, Berne, Data-Star, 1988 and Online Manual (search in NEWS for NEWS-IOWA)
Price/Charges	Subscription: SFr80.00
	Connect time: SFr87.80
	Online print: SFr0.63
	Offline print: SFr0.79
	SDI charge: SFr8.40

Downloading is allowed

Notes

From June 1993 Data-Star have introduced an annual fee/subscription per contract (that is, not per password) of SFr 80.00 (c.UK£ 32.00) payable every June. For North American customers billed in dollars who also use DIALOG, the DIALOG fee also covers access to Data-Star. Academic customers, 'commitment' customers and customers currently billed in dollars are exempt.

Record composition

Accession Number and Update Code AN; Author(s) AU; Descriptors DE; Microfilm Number MF; Publication Type PT; Source SO; Title TI; Update Code UP and Year of Publication YR

INTOX
Technische Universitët München, Toxikologishe Abteilung
DIMDI

15:118. Master record

Alternative name(s)	Datenbank über Vergiftungsfälle; Database on Poisoning
Database type	Factual
Number of journals	
Sources	Case studies
Start year	1975
Language	German
Coverage	Germany
Number of records	259,638
Update size	20,000
Update period	Monthly

Keywords

Clinical Toxicology; Drugs; Poisons; Forensic Science

Description

INTOX is a non-bibliographic database containing data on individual cases of poisoning from German poison control centres and clinical-toxicological departments of hospitals. Subjects covered include: epidemiology of poisoning; clinical toxicology; forensic medicine and drug dependence. Records of poison control centres and institutes of forensic medicine in the Federal Republic of Germany are evaluated. Information on individual cases of poisoning given includes the name of the poison, the year of poisoning, the age group of the patient, the degree of severity, etiology, poisoning symptoms, therapy, outcome and analytical data. In addition almost all records contain data on toxicological analytics which is the determination of poisons and their metabolites in body fluids and tissues.

None of the records contain abstracts. Institutions supplying INTOX data include: Toxikologishe Abteilung (Giftnotruf), Klinikum rechts der Isar, Technical University, Munich, Giftinformationszentrale, Land Baden-Württemberg, Universitäts-Kinderklinik, Mathildenstr.1, Freiburg, the Department of Clinical Toxicology of the Municipal Hospital Friedrichshain, Berlin and the Reanimation Centre of the Rudolf Virchow Medical School, Charlottenburg, Berlin.

15:119. Online   DIMDI

File name	GI00
Alternative name(s)	Datenbank über Vergiftungsfälle; Database on Poisoning
Start year	1975
Number of records	259,638
Update period	Monthly
Price/Charges	Connect time: UK£03.88–08.62
	Online print: UK£0.16–0.34
	Offline print: UK£0.07–0.14
	SDI charge: UK£None
Downloading is allowed	

Notes

DIMDI's aim is to extend the number of institutions supplying data for INTOX to create an instrument for representative evaluations on cases of poisoning in Germany.

Life Sciences Collection
Cambridge Scientific Abstracts

15:120. Master record

Alternative name(s)	LSC; CSA Life Sciences Collection
Database type	Bibliographic
Number of journals	5,000
Sources	Journals, books, serial monographs, conference proceedings, patents (US), patents (UK), patents (Japanese) and reports
Start year	1978
Language	English
Coverage	International
Number of records	1,500,000
Update size	98,000
Update period	Monthly

Keywords

Acute Poisoning; Aging; Algology; Amino-Acids; Anatomy; Antibiotics; Aquaculture; Bacteriology; Behavioural Ecology; Bioengineering; Biological Membranes; Biotechnology; Bone Disease; Calcium Metabolism; Chemoreception; Chronic Poisoning; Clinical Medicine; Clinical Toxicology; DNA; Drugs; Ecology; Ecosystems; Endocrinology; Entomology – Agricultural; Entomology – Applied; Entomology – Human; Entomology – Veterinary; Environmental Biology; Ethology; Genetic Engineering; Hazardous Substances; HIV; Histology; Human Ecology; Immune Disorders; Immunology; Infectious Diseases; Marine Biotechnology; Microbiology; Molecular Biology; Molecular Neurobiology; Mycology; Neurology; Neuropharmacology; Neurophysiology – Animal; Neuroscience; Nucleic Acids; Nutrition; Oncology; Occupational Health and Safety; Osteoporosis; Osteomalacia; Pathology; Peptides; Pharmaceuticals; Pheromones; Physiology; Pollution; Proteins; Protozoology; Psychophysics; Public Health; Radiation; Rhinology; RNA; Sleep; Smoking; Substance Abuse; Taste Perception; Viral Genetics

Description

Life Sciences Collection contains abstracts of information in the fields of (and corresponding to abstract journals from CSA): animal behaviour; biochemistry-amino-acid, peptide and protein; biochemistry – nucleic acids; biochemistry-biological membranes; biotechnology research (from 1984 to date); calcified tissue; chemoreception; ecology; endocrinology; entomology; genetics; human genomes; basic research and clinical applications; immunology, marine biotechnology, microbiology- algology, mycology and protozoology; microbiology-bacteriology; microbiology-industrial & applied microbiology; oncology-oncogenes and growth factors; neurosciences (from 1983 to date); toxicology; virology and AIDS. AIDS is covered in depth. The worldwide coverage is of journal articles, books, conference proceedings, report literature, patents, theses and dissertations.

Corresponds to the series of abstracting journals published by CSA: *Animal Behavior Abstracts*; *Biochemistry Abstracts-Amino-acid, Peptide and Protein*; *Biochemistry Abstracts-Biological Membranes*; *Biochemistry Abstracts-Nucleic Acids*; *Calcified Tissue Abstracts*; *Biotechnology Research Abstracts* (from 1984 to date); *Chemoreception Abstracts*; *Ecology Abstracts*; *Endocrinology Abstracts*; *Entomology Abstracts*; *Genetics Abstracts*; *Human Genome Abstracts*; *Basic Research and Clinical Applications*; *Immunology Abstracts*; *Marine Biotechnology Abstracts*; *Microbiology Abstracts-Algology, Mycology & Protozoology*; *Microbiology Abstracts-Bacteriology*; *Microbiology Abstracts-Industrial & Applied Microbiology*; *Neurosciences Abstracts* (from 1983 to date); *Oncogenes and Growth Factors Abstracts*; *Toxicology Abstracts*; *Virology and AIDS Abstracts*. Most recently added were *Marine Biotechnology Abstracts* and *Oncogenes and Growth Factors Abstracts*. Also includes *Oncology Abstracts* and *Feeding, Weight and Obesity Abstracts* for the period they were published.

15:121. Online   BIOSIS Life Science Network

File name	Life Sciences Collection
Start year	1978
Number of records	1,500,000
Update period	Monthly
Price/Charges	Connect time: US$9.00
	Online print: US$6.00 per 10; 2.25 per abstract; 3.50 per full text article

Also available via the Internet by telnetting to LSN.COM.

Notes

On Life Science Network users can search this database or they can scan a group of subject-related databases. There is a charge of $2.00 per scan of subject-related databases. To search one database and display up to ten citations costs $6.00. Most charges are for information retrieved. There are no charges if there are no results and no charge to transfer results to a printer or diskette. Articles may also be ordered via an online document delivery request. A telecommunications software package is also available, costing $12.95, providing an automatic connection to Life Science Network for heavy users of the service, with capability to transfer to print or disk and customised colour options.

15:122. Online   DIALOG

File name	File 76
Start year	1978
Number of records	1,392,381
Update period	Monthly
Price/Charges	Connect time: US$90.00
	Online print: US$0.75
	Offline print: US$0.75
	SDI charge: US$9.50

15:123. Online   STN

File name	LIFESCI
Start year	1978
Number of records	1,500,000
Update period	Monthly

15:124. CD-ROM   Compact Cambridge

File name	Life Sciences Collection
Alternative name(s)	LSC; CSA Life Sciences Collection
Format notes	NEC, 9800, IBM
Start year	1982
Number of records	
Update period	Quarterly
Price	UK£1,165 – 2,985 (Initial with backfiles)
	Subscription: UK£985

Notes

Contains eighteen subject orientated subfiles in the life and biosciences field, covering some 5,000 core journals, books, serial monographs, etc. Over 98,000 abstracts are added each year. Subscribers to CSA's life sciences print journals receive a £500 credit towards the first year's subscription to LSC CD-ROM 1982-present or 1985-present.

15:125. Tape   Cambridge Scientific Abstracts

File name	Life Sciences Collection on Magnetic Tape
Alternative name(s)	LSC; CSA Life Sciences Collection
Format notes	9-track, unlabelled, 1600 bpi, EBCDIC.
Start year	1982
Number of records	
Update period	Monthly
Price/Charges	Subscription: US$13,950

Notes

The series of abstracting journals published by CSA are available on this tape as a collection. They are also available separately as tape subsets of the Life Sciences Collection, the online database to which this tape corresponds.

Price for the current year tape is $13,950; single-year archival file is $7,100.

15:126. Database subset
Tape   Cambridge Scientific Abstracts

File name	Calcified Tissue Abstracts on Magnetic Tape
Format notes	9-track, unlabelled, 1600 bpi, EBCDIC
Start year	1978
Number of records	
Update period	Quarterly

Notes

A subset of the Life Sciences Collection. Contains citations, with abstracts, to the worldwide literature on the metabolism of calcium and related minerals. Covers intestinal absorption of calcium, phosphorous and magnesium; osteoporosis, osteomalacia and other bone diseases; and effects of pregnancy, menopause, aging and metabolism on bone structure and calcium metabolism. Corresponds to *Calcified Tissue Abstracts* and in part to the Life Science Collection online database. Contact Cambridge Scientific Abstracts for pricing information.

15:127. Database subset
Tape   Cambridge Scientific Abstracts

File name	Entomology Abstracts on Magnetic Tape
Format notes	9-track, unlabelled, 1600 bpi, EBCDIC.
Start year	1982
Number of records	
Update period	Monthly

Notes

A subset of the Life Sciences Collection. Contains citations, with abstracts, to the worldwide literature on insects, arachnids, myriapods, onychophorans and terrestrial isopods. Covers geographic distribution, nomenclature, new species, techniques and methodology, morphology of all life cycle stages, physiology, anatomy, histology, biochemistry, toxicology and resistance, ecology, behaviour, and medical, veterinary, agricultural and applied entomology. Corresponds to *Entomology Abstracts* and in part to the Life Sciences Collection online database. Contact CSA for pricing information.

This database can also be found on:
Cambridge Scientific Abstracts Life Sciences
Human Nutrition on CD-ROM

Medical Science Research Database
Medical Science Research Elsevier Science Publishers

15:128. Master record

Database type	Textual
Number of journals	
Sources	
Start year	1982
Language	English
Coverage	
Number of records	57,000
Update size	600
Update period	Bimonthly

Keywords

Physiology; Pathology; Anatomy

Description

The Medical Science Research database (formerly IRCS Medical Science database) consists of the full text, including tables, or peer-reviewed research articles published in Medical Science Research (incorporating IRCS Medical Science journals). Articles are approximately 1,000 words long and are concise but complete accounts of research with full methodological and result information. Coverage includes all areas of clinical and biomedical science, with major coverage in the following areas: alimentary system, anatomy and human biology, biochemistry, biomedical technology, cardiovascular system, cell and membrane biology, clinical medicine, clinical pharmacology and therapeutics, connective tissue, skin and bone, dentistry and oral biology, developmental biology and medicine, drug metabolism and toxicology, endocrine system, environmental biology and medicine, experimental animals, the eye, haematology, immunology and allergy, metabolism and nutrition, microbiology, parasitology and infectious diseases, nervous system, pathology, physiology, psychology and psychiatry, reproduction, obstetrics and gynaecology, social and occupational medicine, surgery and transplantation, techniques and methods.

This database appears to be no longer available.

MEDLINE
National Library of Medicine

15:129. Master record

Database type	Bibliographic
Number of journals	3,500
Sources	Conference proceedings, journals, monographs and reviews
Start year	1964
Language	English
Coverage	International
Number of records	7,500,000
Update size	370,000
Update period	Weekly except January and February which are updated monthly.
Index unit	Biographies, case studies, comparative studies, editorials, letters, news releases, obituaries, reviews, articles, book chapters and interview
Abstract details	Author abstracts (since 1975) are available for approximately 70% of the citations
Thesaurus	Medical Subject Headings (MeSH)
Database aids	MeSH Tree Structures, Permuted MeSH, MeSH Supplementary Chemical Records with CAS Registration Numbers or Enzyme Codes (from June 1980), Gene Symbols from January 1991), List of Serials Indexed for Online Users, includes NLM Journal codens, List of Journals Indexed in Index Medicus includes subject order serials index and Indexing Manual

Keywords

HIV; Anaesthesia; Anatomy; Applied Science; Biochemistry; Biotechnology; Cancer; Cardiology; Cardiovascular Diseases; Chemical Substances; Clinical Medicine; Forensic Science; Geriatrics; Gynaecology; Handicapped; Health and Safety; Immunology; Infectious Diseases; Medical History; Mental Health; Microbiology; Obstetrics;

Occupational Health and Safety; Orthopaedics; Paediatrics; Patents; Pathology; Physiology; Pollution; Public Health; Radiology; Social Services; Toxicology

Description

MEDLINE (MEDlars (MEDical Literature ANalysis and Retrieval System) onLINE) is a vast source of medical information covering the whole field of medicine and health science information. It is the most current file and includes the current year and at least two additional years depending on the host utilised. MEDLINE backfiles are segmented and are available back to 1966. Subjects covered include (1) basic sciences/research in medicine such as bacteriology, biochemistry, environmental research, genetics, immunology, microbiology, parasitology, physiology and virology; and (2) applied sciences/clinical medicine such as anatomy, biomedical technology, clincial medicine, communication disorders, dental medicine, dermatology, environmental medicine, experimental medicine, forensic medicine, gerontology, gynaecology, health care services, hospital administration, immunology, medical education, medical psychology, medical technology, neurology, nutrition, occupational medicine, nursing oncology, opthalmology, orthopedics, parasitology, paramedical professions, pathology, pharmacy, pharmacology, physiology, policy issues, population, psychiatry, psychology, rehabilitation, research, social science medicine; social medicine, sport medicine, toxicology and veterinary medicine.

MEDLINE corresponds to the printed publications: *Index Medicus*, *Index to Dental Literature*, *International Nursing Index* and various other bibliographies. Author abstracts are provided for approximately seventy per cent of items in the database. The database also covers chapters and articles from selected monographs from 1976 to 1981. About 74% of citations are to English-language sources and the remaining citations represent over 40 other languages. This compares with 88% English- language sources on SciSearch, 86% on BIOSIS and 75% in EMBASE, the other leading bioscience databases. 50% of records were added after January 1975. More than 90% of journals are evaluated cover to cover. The database contains 304,354 citations for the years 1964/5 but as the controlled vocabulary and retrieval is different from the later years, these years are often offered as a separate file. Citations are automatically transferred from MEDLINE to other NLM-databases, therefore many of the journals indexed are also found in CANCERLIT (approximately 85% overlap with MEDLINE), HEALTH (approximately 80% overlap with MEDLINE) and AIDSLINE (approximately 75% overlap with MEDLINE). For BIOETHICSLINE no automatic transfer takes place but many MEDLINE-journals related to biomedical ethics are also evaluated for BIOETHICSLINE. Journals are categorised on three different levels of priority. Those on the third level are indexed in less depth than journals on levels one and two. The time lag between the appearance of the publication and availability on magnetic tape is usually shorter for priority one and two than for priority three journals. Journals to be considered for MEDLINE are selected by an advisory committee of physicians, scientists, librarians and publishers of medical journals appointed by the NLM. Journal information which is not indexed includes abstracts on congresses, book reviews, hospital reports, communications from medical associations, announcements of new drugs by pharmaceutical companies. Regarding the length of abstracts, between 1975 and 1977 there was no limitation regarding the length of abstracts. Between 1977 and 1980 no abstract longer than 200 words and between 1981 and 1983 no abstract longer than 250 words was stored. Due to these limitations only 45% of the citations contain abstracts for this period of input. From 1984 onwards, abstracts exceeding 250 words or 400 words for abstracts of articles ten pages or more in length are included but truncated and these abstracts have the message 'ABSTRACTS TRUNCATED AT 250/400 WORDS' at their end. From 1984, 65% of the citations contain an abstract. This compares with 60% in EMBASE and 54% in BIOSIS. Records of the other leading bioscience database, SciSearch, now also contains abstracts. Since 1980, 26% of MEDLINE records with non-English sources contain English-language abstracts online. This compares with 67% on BIOSIS and 37% on EMBASE. Abstracts from articles from journal titles of priority three have only been stored since Spring 1989.

MEDLINE's Tree Structures classification is the most detailed alphanumeric scheme developed for online searching. It is directly related to the controlled vocabulary in the database. It is necessary to use the hardcopy search aids produced – MeSH annotated alphabetic list, TREE structures, Permuted terms etc. to obtain successful search results, and, as they are re-edited and published by NLM each year, to use the latest edition only, as new terminology is included annually. Generally, new sets become available in December for use in the following year. The MeSH descriptors have check tags for gender, age groups, human, animal, article type and can also be subdivided using standard subheadings. A two-tier level of indexing is used with an average of twelve descriptors assigned, of which three to five descriptors are major or primary headings which appear in Index Medicus or other print sources. In addition to the controlled vocabulary terms, textwords or free-text terms may be used for retrieval from the title, abstract, authors address and other parts of the citation. Exploded treewords, which are the hierarchical arrangement of Medical Subject Headings can also be used for retrieval of broad categories of information.

Every Medical Subject Heading has at least one corresponding alpha-numeric code or tree number which determines its location in the hierarchically arranged Tree Structures. Some headings have more than one tree number because they are located in more than one tree. There are a total of fifteen broad subject categories or trees as follows: A. Anatomical Terms; B. Organisms; C. Diseases; D. Chemicals and Drugs; E. Analytical, Diagnostic and Therapeutic Technics and Equipment; F. Psychiatry and Psychology; G. Biological Sciences; H. Physical Sciences; I. Anthropology, Education, Sociology and Social Phenomena; J. Technology, Industry, Agriculture, Food; K. Humanities; L. Information Science and Communications; M. Named Groups of Persons; N. Health Care; and Z. Geographicals. These broad categories are then broken down into narrower subcategories. The hardcopy thesaurus indicates when narrower terms are available under a code.

In addition to numerous cross-references MeSH precoordinates frequently searched concepts, for example, PREGNANCY IN DIABETES. It also contains history notes indicating starting dates for consistent usage of indexer- added terms online and hints for retrospective searching on topics where preferred terminology has changed over time, for example ROBOTICS (87) search AUTOMATION 1966–86. MEDLINE also permits indexers to identify concepts

lacking adequate descriptors in MeSH. Since June 1980 its identifier field has been used to index chemicals discussed in the full text of source documents ensuring access to names or numbers of compounds whether or not they are included among MeSH descriptors. Registry Numbers have been assigned in MEDLINE records since June 1980. MEDLINE also consistently adds Enzyme Commission (EC) numbers to records for sources which discuss enzymes.

The datafield Document Type was introduced to MEDLINE in 1991, Prior to this some of the Document Types had been MeSH-Terms for example historial article, review. Most of these MeSH terms have been deleted and replaced by a corresponding Document Type retrospectively. Indexing with MeSH is performed by specially trained staff in indexing institutes in the USA. The value of controlled vocabulary is important when searching for topics where a subject population has been specified. Relatively few bioscience databases provide consistent indexing for subject populations (ie humans or specific test animals) and related characteristics commonly requested such as age groups, gender, occupation and racial or ethnic groups. In comparison with BIOSIS, EMBASE and SciSearch MEDLINE provides the most extensive consistent indexing for the subject population groups, humans, test animals, racial/ethnic groups, gender and age groups but provides less consistent indexing of occupational gropus, where fewer controlled terms are augmented with natural language keywords in strategies. A study on indexing consistency in MEDLINE has shown an average consistency for central concept main heading (equivalent to MeSH term-/MAJOR; that is, *Toxicology in records) identification of 61.1% for central concept subheadings (for example, *MeSH term-TOXICITY), of 54.9% and for central main heading/subheading combinations (for example, *Skin Drug Effects) of 43.1%. In most bioscience files a form of pharmaceutical nomenclature exists. For MEDLINE the preferred search terms are generic name, classification by action/use and CAS Registry Number although restrictions by date, subfile and vendor may apply to the latter and vendor documentation should be consulted for guidelines. Restrictions also apply for the search term Enzyme Commission Number and vendor documentations should again be consulted for guidelines. For the search terms investigational code, chemical name and trade name, the terminology is inconsistent and alternative names should be used in search strategies. Retrospective searching however may require the entry of other names used for the same substance at earlier stages in its development life cycle. The use of synonyms is advisable when searching compounds yet to be added as controlled MeSH descriptors.

In 1993, after the annual reload, there are some new features available: new file labels; page, issue and volume numbers in the source paragraph are now searchable, it is now possible to retrieve articles where the user has incomplete information, for example, an article written by Schellenberg., published in a journal on Page 668; review articles are now searchable with a .LIMIT-command; 94 descriptors have been replaced by more up-to-date terminology; 421 new and updated MeSH terms and new publication types in the PT field.

15:130. Database subset

CD-ROM	Aries Systems Corporation
File name	PathLine
Format notes	IBM, Mac
Software	Knowledge Finder 2.0

Start year | Most recent nine years.
Number of records |
Update period | Quarterly
Price/Charges | Subscription: US$395

Notes

Archival MEDLINE subset of pathology citations and abstracts.

This database can also be found on:
Online Journal of Current Clinical Trials
Developmental and Reproductive Toxicology
BiblioMed Cardiology
BiblioMed Infectious Diseases
AIDS Compact Library
Compact Library: Viral Hepatitis
OnDisc Discovery Training Toolkit
Lancet
British Medical Journal
New England Journal of Medicine
Annals of Internal Medicine
Morbidity and Mortality Weekly Report
American Journal of Public Health
Infectious Diseases – Personal MEDLINE
Obstetrics & Gynecology – Personal MEDLINE
Journal of the American Medical Association
Pediatrics – Personal MEDLINE
Family Practice – Personal MEDLINE
Critical Care Medicine – Personal MEDLINE
Emergency Medicine – Personal MEDLINE
Gastroenterology and Hepatology Medicine – Personal Medline
Canadian Medical Association Journal
Human Nutrition on CD-ROM
Oxford Database of Perinatal Trials
Entrez: Sequences
STAT!-Ref
Medata-ROM
AIDSLINE
Bioethicsline
NEXIS
TOXLINE
MAXX

National Medical Slide Bank

Chadwyck-Healey

15:132. Master record

Alternative name(s) | UK National Medical Slide Bank
Database type | Image
Number of journals |
Sources |
Start year |
Language |
Coverage |
Number of records | 12,440
Update size | –
Update period |
Thesaurus | World Health Organisation International Classification of Diseases (9th edition)

Keywords

Pathology

Description

Contains colour images covering the visual manifestations of a wide range of diseases and injuries and aspects of medical treatment and healthcare practice. It includes the best slides from the specialist photographic libraries of the leading medical schools and teaching hospitals. The images are arranged in 77 chapters according to the World Health Organisation *International Classification of Diseases* (9th edition).

Indexed according to the International Statistical Classification of Diseases, Injuries, and Causes of Death.

15:133. VideoDisc   Chadwyck-Healey

File name | National Medical Slide Bank
Alternative name(s) | UK National Medical Slide Bank
Format notes | IBM
Start year |
Number of records |
Update period |
Price/Charges | Subscription: UK£950

Notes

The videodisc of images is accompanied by a detailed printed catalogue and a free-text searchable index on diskette which can provide immediate access to any image. Interactive software can be used with the database to create computer-assisted learning programmes.

Pathology and Radiology

Eidetic
Elsevier Science Publishers

15:134. Master record

Database type | Various data formats included
Number of journals |
Sources |
Start year |
Language | English
Coverage |
Number of records |
Update size | –
Update period |

Keywords

Pathology; Radiology

Description

Images plus text (Titles to be announced).

15:135. CD-ROM   Elsevier Science Publishers

File name | Pathology and Radiology
Format notes | IBM
Start year |
Number of records |
Update period |

Physician Data Query

National Cancer Institute, US National Institutes of Health

15:136. Master record

Alternative name(s) | PDQ
Database type | Bibliographic, Directory, Textual
Number of journals |
Sources | Clinicians, directories, research reports and textbooks
Start year | Current
Language | English
Coverage | USA (primarily) and International (some)
Number of records | Variable
Update size | Variable
Update period | Monthly

Keywords

Cancer; Pathology

Description

Physician Data Query is an English-language factual database produced by the National Cancer Institute (NCI) and its PDQ Editorial Board and is designed to assist physicians in the treatment and referral of cancer patients. The database is composed of three interrelated files: (1) the Cancer Information File (2) the Protocol File and (3) the Directory File.

(1)   The Cancer Information File contains full-text information on about eighty cancer types provided, reviewed and updated by an Editorial Board of experts both inside and outside the US National Cancer Institute. It contains information on patients with descriptions, stage explanations and general treatment options and on prognosis, cellular classification, stage information and treatment by cell type/stage. Literature citations with abstracts on the key medical literature on the individual oncological aspects are also included. When there is no effective treatment for a particular cancer, the file describes current investigative approaches under evaluation in clinical trials. An editorial board of 72 oncologists is responsible for the currency and accuracy of the information.

(2)   The Protocol File contains information on over 7,700 active and closed treatment protocols on new methods of cancer treatment; it includes clinical research objectives, special study parameters, treatment regimens and schedules, patient entry criteria and participating institutions. Each protocol provides detailed information on drug dosage, schedule and dosage modification organised into tables. It also includes most data from the NCI database CLINPROT, which was discontinued in March 1991. The file also contains approximately forty descriptors of approved standard therapies, revised by the PDQ Editorial Board.

(3)   The Directory File contains a listing of the names, addresses, telephone numbers of 17,000 physicians and surgeons (mainly North American, but also European and Latin American), and 2,400 organizations and institutions (mainly in the United States of America) devoted to the care of cancer patients. It also details their medical speciality and professional affiliation. European organisations and physicians are listed in PDQ when they participate in programmes such as the EORTC (European Organisation for Research and Treatment of Cancer), or when they are members of the major oncologic societies in the United States, such as the American Society of Clinical Oncology. PDQ also contains full-text information on supportive care in neoplatic diseases, early detection guidelines and design of clincial trials

15:137. Online   BLAISE-LINK

File name	PDQ
Alternative name(s)	PDQ
Start year	
Number of records	
Update period	Continuously

15:138. Online   CISTI MEDLARS

File name	Physician Data Query
Alternative name(s)	PDQ
Start year	
Number of records	
Update period	Monthly

15:139. Online   DIMDI

File name	PQ00
Alternative name(s)	PDQ
Start year	Current
Number of records	33,633
Update period	Monthly
Database aids	PDQ User Guide
Price/Charges	Connect time: UK£03.88–08.62
	Online print: UK£0.16–0.34
	Offline print: UK£0.07–0.14

Downloading is allowed

Notes

PDQ is available on DIMDI only via a menu-driven interface to provide a simple and effective handling for physicians with no previous knowledge of the GRIPS command language and database structure.

15:140. Online   National Library of Medicine

File name	Physician Data Query
Alternative name(s)	PDQ
Start year	
Number of records	
Update period	

15:141. CD-ROM   Compact Cambridge

File name	PDQ
Alternative name(s)	PDQ
Format notes	NEC, 9800, IBM
Software	SearchLITE
Start year	
Number of records	
Update period	Quarterly
Price/Charges	Subscription: UK£605

Notes

Provides easy access to state-of-the-art cancer treatment. PDQ and Cancerlit from Compact Cambridge are available on one disc, price £930.

15:142. CD-ROM   SilverPlatter

File name	PDQ
Alternative name(s)	PDQ
Format notes	IBM
Software	SearchLITE
Start year	
Number of records	
Update period	Quarterly
Price/Charges	Subscription: UK£685 – 1,028

Notes

The CD-ROM includes all three component files of PDQ. Contains treatment recommendations for 85 types of cancer in two formats. One for patient information and one – more detailed – for clinicians. Subscription costs are: £685 for single users, £1,028 for 2–8 networked users.

PDQ is accessed by SearchLITE software developed by I.S. Grupe. It can best exploit the full text contained in PDQ and is ideal for novice users.

15:143. Database subset

Online	BRS
File name	PDQB
Alternative name(s)	PDQ
Start year	
Number of records	
Update period	Monthly
Price/Charges	Connect time: US$39.00/49.00
	Online print: US$0.14/0.22
	Offline print: US$0.22

Notes

This database contains information on clinical trials that are no longer accepting patients. Protocols with the status 'closed' will not be reopened. Protocols with the status 'temporarily closed' have been closed while the investigators analyse results of the trials or for other reasons. A 'temporarily closed' protocol may be reopened in the future. All protocols contain detailed information on objectives, patient entry criteria and details of the treatment regimen. Each record retains the same information as it had while in the active protocol file with two exceptions: only the name of the lead investigator and the lead organisation are retained; and a closing date has been added.

15:144. Database subset

Online **BRS**

File name	PDQC
Alternative name(s)	PDQ
Start year	
Number of records	
Update period	Monthly
Price/Charges	Connect time: US$39.00/49.00
	Online print: US$0.14/0.22
	Offline print: US$0.22

Notes

This database contains comprehensive information on more than eighty types of cancer. It includes up to date information on prognosis, staging, cellular classification, standard and investigational treatments together with references to medical literature. An editorial board of 72 oncologists is responsible for the currency and accuracy of the information.

15:145. Database subset

Online **BRS**

File name	PDQD
Alternative name(s)	PDQ
Start year	
Number of records	
Update period	Monthly
Price/Charges	Connect time: US$39.00/49.00
	Online print: US$0.14/0.22
	Offline print: US$0.22

Notes

This database contains the names, addresses and telephone numbers of more than 15,000 physicians and almost 2,000 organisations devoted to the care of cancer patients. The information on individual physicians is primarily gathered from the membership directories of more than fifteen professional societies and associations.

15:146. Database subset

Online **BRS**

File name	PDQI
Alternative name(s)	PDQ
Start year	
Number of records	
Update period	Monthly
Price/Charges	Connect time: US$39.00/49.00
	Online print: US$0.14/0.22
	Offline print: US$0.22

Notes

This database contains descriptions of types of cancer, stage explanations and treatment options for patients and other laypersons dealing with cancer.

15:147. Database subset

Online **BRS**

File name	PDQP
Alternative name(s)	PDQ
Start year	
Number of records	
Update period	Monthly

Price/Charges	Connect time: US$39.00/49.00
	Online print: US$0.14/0.22
	Offline print: US$0.22

Notes

This database contains information on more than 1,300 active cancer treatment protocols. All clinical trials directly supported by the National Cancer Institute (NCI) as well as those voluntarily submitted by other investigators, are included. Documents contain detailed information on objectives, patient entry criteria, details of the treatment regimen, and participating organisations.

15:148. Database subset

Online **BRS**

File name	PDQS
Alternative name(s)	PDQ
Start year	
Number of records	
Update period	
Price/Charges	Connect time: US$39.00/49.00
	Online print: US$0.14/0.22
	Offline print: US$0.22

Notes

Supportive care subset.

15:149. Database subset

Online **CompuServe Information Service**

File name	IQUEST File 1956 – Physician Data Query Patient Information File
Alternative name(s)	PDQ
Start year	
Number of records	
Update period	Monthly
Price/Charges	Subscription: US$8.95 per month
	Database entry fee: US$9/search; some databases carry a surcharge ($2–75)
	Online print: US$10 references free; then $9 per ten; abstracts $3 each
Downloading is allowed	

Notes

This database contains descriptions of types of cancer, stage explanations and treatment options for patients and other laypersons dealing with cancer. Accessed via IQUEST or IQMEDICAL, this database is offered by a BRS gateway. IQUEST can either search across all databases, a database of the user's choice or selected multiple databases.

15:150. Database subset

Online **CompuServe Information Service**

File name	IQUEST File 1957 – Physician Data Query Directory File
Alternative name(s)	PDQ
Start year	
Number of records	
Update period	Monthly
Price/Charges	Subscription: US$8.95 per month
	Database entry fee: US$9/search; some databases carry a surcharge ($2–75)
	Online print: US$10 references free; then $9 per ten; abstracts $3 each
Downloading is allowed	

Notes

This database contains the names, addresses and telephone numbers of more than 15,000 physicians and almost 2,000 organisations devoted to the care of cancer patients. The information on individual physicians is primarily gathered from the membership directories of more than fifteen professional societies and associations.

Accessed via IQUEST or IQMEDICAL, this database is offered by a BRS gateway. IQUEST can either search across all databases, a database of the user's choice or selected multiple databases.

15:151. Database subset

Online   CompuServe Information Service

File name	IQUEST File 1958 – Physician Data Query Protocol File
Alternative name(s)	PDQ
Start year	
Number of records	
Update period	Monthly
Price/Charges	Subscription: US$8.95 per month Database entry fee: US$9/search; some databases carry a surcharge ($2–75) Online print: US$10 references free; then $9 per ten; abstracts $3 each

Downloading is allowed

Notes

This database contains information on more than 1,300 active cancer treatment protocols. All clinical trials directly supported by the National Cancer Institute (NCI) as well as those voluntarily submitted by other investigators, are included. Documents contain detailed information on objectives, patient entry criteria, details of the treatment regimen, and participating organisations.

Accessed via IQUEST or IQMEDICAL, this database is offered by a BRS gateway. IQUEST can either search across all databases, a database of the user's choice or selected multiple databases.

15:152. Database subset

Online   CompuServe Information Service

File name	IQUEST File 2604 – Physician Data Query Cancer Information File
Alternative name(s)	PDQ
Start year	
Number of records	
Update period	Monthly
Price/Charges	Subscription: US$8.95 per month Database entry fee: US$9/search; some databases carry a surcharge ($2–75) Online print: US$10 references free; then $9 per ten; abstracts $3 each

Downloading is allowed

Notes

This database contains comprehensive information on more than eighty types of cancer. It includes up to date information on prognosis, staging, cellular classification, standard and investigational treatments together with references to medical literature. An editorial board of 72 oncologists is responsible for the currency and accuracy of the information.

Accessed via IQUEST or IQMEDICAL, this database is offered by a BRS gateway. IQUEST can either search across all databases, a database of the user's choice or selected multiple databases.

15:153. Database subset

Online   Mead Data Central (as a NEXIS database)

File name	PERSON – NEXIS
Alternative name(s)	PDQ
Start year	
Number of records	13,000
Update period	Monthly
Price/Charges	Subscription: US$1,000 – 3,000 (Depending on needs) Connect time: US$49.00 (Telecomms + connect time) Database entry fee: US$14.00 (Search charge) Online print: US$0.04 per line

Notes

Library GENMED; Group file: DIRECT.

The PDQ file on NEXIS is divided into six separate files: PROTOC (cancer protocol information); STATE (state-of-the-art cancer information); PIF (patient information); TERMS (general terms, cancer names, drug names); PERSON (index of physician names); and ORGA (index of organisations that sponsor cancer-related programs). A group file exists for PERSON and ORGA called DIRECT.

The PERSON file contains a Physician Directory, a listing of over 13,000 physicians involved with cancer treatment and research. Each listing contains name, address, telephone numbers, affiliation and PDQ the term number designated for each individual physician. All the physicians listed are protocol partners and/or members of one or more of the following professional societies: American College of Mohs Micrographic Surgery and Cutaneous Oncology; American Society for Therapeutic Radiology and Oncology; American Society of Pediatric Hematology and Oncology; American Society of Colon and Rectal Surgery; American Society for Head and Neck Surgery; American Society of Clinical Oncology; American Urological Association Inc; Society of Gynecologic Oncologists; Society of Head and Neck Surgeons; American Academy of Dermatology; American Society of Hematology; Society of Surgical Oncology; Society of Urologic Oncology; American College of Surgeons; Society of Pelvic Surgeons; and American Radium Society. The Physician Directory is not necessarily comprehensive, nor does inclusion or exclusion of a particular individual physician constitute an endorsement or a judgement of professional competence.

A subscription charge which covers all transactional charges, connect time, telecommunications and the small administration charge can take the place of the individual charges. Subscriptions are negotiated with customers and vary according to the number of menus (thus, files) that are to be used – typically a minimum subscription would be about US$ 1,000. All charges include training and a 24-hour help line.

Record composition

Board Certification BOARD-CERTIF; Contact Organisation CONTACT-ORG/COOR; Location LOCATION/LOCA; Subject's Medical Speciality MED-SPECIALITY/SPEC; Name, Address and Telephone Number of Subject NAME-ADDR-TELE/NADT; Name and Term Number NAME; PDQ Status PDQ-STATUS/PDQS; Name of Primary and Secondary Affiliations PERSON-AFFIL/PEAF; Type of Position Held PERSON-TYPE/TYPE and Subject's Name PNAM

All documents in the PIF file contain PDQ term numbers. These identify the cancer name, drug names, physicians and organisations. The format of the number is xxx/xxxxx.

15:154. Database subset

Online	Mead Data Central (as a NEXIS database)
File name	PIF – NEXIS
Alternative name(s)	PDQ
Start year	
Number of records	
Update period	Monthly
Price/Charges	Subscription: US$1,000 – 3,000 (Depending on needs) Connect time: US$49.00 (Telecomms + connect time) Database entry fee: US$14.00 (Search charge) Online print: US$0.04 per line

Notes

Library GENMED.

The PDQ file on NEXIS is divided into six separate files: PROTOC (cancer protocol information); STATE (state-of-the-art cancer information); PIF (patient information); TERMS (general terms, cancer names, drug names); PERSON (index of physician names); and ORGA (index of organisations that sponsor cancer-related programs). A group file exists for PERSON and ORGA called DIRECT.

This file, Patient Information (PIF), is one of two which provide detailed summaries of prognosis, staging, cellular classification and treatment of over 75 types of cancer. The PIF file is designed to provide cancer information to patients in layman's language that is very basic and easy to understand. The easy-to-follow explanations are of cancer type, various disease stages and treatment options of the disease. Throughout the file and documents are instructions for patients to consult their physician or other members of the medical staff for additional information and/or explanations.

A subscription charge which covers all transactional charges, connect time, telecommunications and the small administration charge can take the place of the individual charges. Subscriptions are negotiated with customers and vary according to the number of menus (thus, files) that are to be used – typically a minimum subscription would be about US$ 1,000. All charges include training and a 24-hour help line.

Record composition

Cancer Name CANCER-NAME/CNAM/NAME; Prognosis PROG/PROGNOSIS; Developmental Stage STAGING/STGE and Treatment options TREAT-OPTIONS/TREAT-OVERVIEW/TOOV/TROP All documents in the PIF file contain PDQ term numbers. These identify the cancer name, drug names, physicians and organisations. The format of the number is xxx/xxxxx.

15:155. Database subset

Online	Mead Data Central (as a NEXIS database)
File name	PROTOC – NEXIS
Alternative name(s)	PDQ
Start year	
Number of records	
Update period	Monthly

Price/Charges	Subscription: US$1,000 – 3,000 (Depending on needs) Connect time: US$49.00 (Telecomms + connect time) Database entry fee: US$14.00 (Search charge) Online print: US$0.04 per line

Notes

Library GENMED.

The PDQ file on NEXIS is divided into six separate files: PROTOC (cancer protocol information); STATE (state-of-the-art cancer information); PIF (patient information); TERMS (general terms, cancer names, drug names); PERSON (index of physician names); and ORGA (index of organisations that sponsor cancer-related programs). A group file exists for PERSON and ORGA called DIRECT.

This file, Cancer Treatment Protocols (PROTOC), covers descriptions of 1,300 active clinical trials in the United States, Canada and Western Europe as well as standard treatment regimens of proven efficiency. Protocol summaries include the title, identification number, chairman, study objectives, patient eligibility criteria, details of treatment and the names and addresses of physicians participating in the trial. The file may be searched by free text or by diagnosis and stage of disease, phase of trial, therapeutic agent, treatment modality, patient age or geographic location of theparticipating physicians. Each protocol includes detailed information on the administration of the treatment program.

About eighty per cent of the protocols are clinical trials sponsored by the National Cancer Institute (NCI) which have been reviewed and approved by the NCI's Cancer Therapy Evaluation Program. The balance of the protocols are voluntary submissions from cancer research institutions throughout the United States and Canada which are reviewed and approved by the PDQ Editorial Board. The International Cancer Information Center encourages investigators to voluntarily submit protocols not funded by NCI for inclusion.

A subscription charge which covers all transactional charges, connect time, telecommunications and the small administration charge can take the place of the individual charges. Subscriptions are negotiated with customers and vary according to the number of menus (thus, files) that are to be used – typically a minimum subscription would be about US$ 1,000. All charges include training and a 24-hour help line.

Record composition

Criteria for Entering protocol ENTRY-CRITERIA/ CRIT; Drug Forms DFOR; Drug Dosage and Modality DMKY; Drug Modification Guidelines DMGD; Combines dmky and dmgd DOSAGE-MOD/DMOD; Drug Dosage Scedules DSCH; Study Endpoints STUDY-ENDPOINTS/ENDP; Cancer Entities ENTY; Keywords KEYWORDS; Protocol Name PROTOCOL-NAME/NAME/PRNM; Protocol Objectives OBJEC-TIVES/POBJ; Organisations ORGANIZATIONS/ ORGA; Protocol Outline PROTOCOL-OUTLINE/ OUTL; Study Parameters STUDY-PARAMETERS/ PARA; Participating Organisation PART; Dates of Protocol PROTOCOL-DATES/PDAT; Phase of Cancer Study PHASE-OF-STUDY/PHAS; Primary Organisation PORG; Protocol Details PROTOCOL-DETAILS; Protocol Type PROTOCOL-TYPE/TYPE; Protocol Status STATUS/STAT; Criteria for Participant Stratification STRATIFICATION/STRA;

Therapy Modality THERAPY-MODALITY/THER and Warning WARNING

All documents in the PIF file contain PDQ term numbers. These identify the cancer name, drug names, physicians and organisations. The format of the number is xxx/xxxxx.

15:156. Database subset

Online **Mead Data Central (as a NEXIS database)**

File name	STATE – NEXIS
Alternative name(s)	PDQ
Start year	
Number of records	
Update period	Monthly
Price/Charges	Subscription: US$1,000 – 3,000 (Depending on needs) Connect time: US$49.00 (Telecomms + connect time) Database entry fee: US$14.00 (Search charge) Online print: US$0.04 per line

Notes

Library GENMED.

The PDQ file on NEXIS is divided into six separate files: PROTOC (cancer protocol information); STATE (state-of-the-art cancer information); PIF (patient information); TERMS (general terms, cancer names, drug names); PERSON (index of physician names); and ORGA (index of organisations that sponsor cancer-related programs). A group file exists for PERSON and ORGA called DIRECT.

This file, State-of-the-Art Cancer Information Statements for Physicians (STATE), is one of two which provide detailed summaries of the prognosis, staging, cellular classification and treatment for over 75 types of cancer. The STATE file contains current, detailed, prognostic information and descriptions of cancer staging. Treatments are listed within each statement according to stage and/or cell type. The information in STATE is reviewed monthly or as new clinical data becomes available by an editorial board composed of 27 prominent oncologists and sixty associate editors. Each document in the STATE file references medical literature. These references are listed within the document along with a PDQ reference number which can be used in the REFS file to obtain abstracts for most references.

A subscription charge which covers all transactional charges, connect time, telecommunications and the small administration charge can take the place of the individual charges. Subscriptions are negotiated with customers and vary according to the number of menus (thus, files) that are to be used – typically a minimum subscription would be about US$ 1,000. All charges include training and a 24-hour help line.

Record composition

Cancer Name CANCER-NAME/CNAM/NAME; Cellular Classification CELLULAR-CLASS/CELL; Prognosis PROGNOSIS/PROG; Staging STAGING/STGE; Treatment Options Overview TREAT-OVERVIEW/TROV and Treatment procedures TREAT-PROCS/TRPR

All documents in the PIF file contain PDQ term numbers. These identify the cancer name, drug names, physicians and organisations. The format of the number is xxx/xxxxx.

15:157. Database subset

Online **Mead Data Central (as a NEXIS database)**

File name	TERMS – NEXIS
Alternative name(s)	PDQ
Start year	
Number of records	
Update period	Monthly
Price/Charges	Subscription: US$1,000 – 3,000 (Depending on needs) Connect time: US$49.00 (Telecomms + connect time) Database entry fee: US$14.00 (Search charge) Online print: US$0.04 per line

Notes

Library GENMED.

The PDQ file on NEXIS is divided into six separate files: PROTOC (cancer protocol information); STATE (state-of-the-art cancer information); PIF (patient information); TERMS (general terms, cancer names, drug names); PERSON (index of physician names); and ORGA (index of organisations that sponsor cancer-related programs). A group file exists for PERSON and ORGA called DIRECT.

The TERMS file contains a listing of PDQ terms which have been classified into various categories and assigned term numbers and which can be used as separate search terms when searching the other PDQ files. The TERMS file provides a listing of various cancer terms along with closely related clinical diagnosis terms, broader terms, narrower terms and PDQ term numbers.

A subscription charge which covers all transactional charges, connect time, telecommunications and the small administration charge can take the place of the individual charges. Subscriptions are negotiated with customers and vary according to the number of menus (thus, files) that are to be used – typically a minimum subscription would be about US$ 1,000. All charges include training and a 24-hour help line.

Record composition

Broader Terms BROADER-TERMS/BTRM; Cancer Name CANCER-NAME/CTNM; Similar/closest Diagnoses CLOSEST-DIAG/CRCD; Cancer Name and Other Name NAME; Narrower Terms NARROWER-TERMS/NTRM; Other Names OTHER-NAME/ONAM; Related terms RELATED-TERMS/RTRM and Subject Classification TERM-TYPE/TYPE

All documents in the PIF file contain PDQ term numbers. These identify the cancer name, drug names, physicians and organisations. The format of the number is xxx/xxxxx.

15:158. Database subset

Online **Mead Data Central (as a NEXIS database)**

File name	ORGA – NEXIS
Alternative name(s)	PDQ
Start year	
Number of records	1,600
Update period	Monthly
Price/Charges	Subscription: US$1,000 – 3,000 (Depending on needs) Connect time: US$49.00 (Telecomms + connect time) Database entry fee: US$14.00 (Search charge) Online print: US$0.04 per line

Notes

Library GENMED: Group file: DIRECT.

The PDQ file on NEXIS is divided into six separate files: PROTOC (cancer protocol information); STATE (state-of-the-art cancer information); PIF (patient information); TERMS (general terms, cancer names, drug names); PERSON (index of physician names); and ORGA (index of organisations that sponsor cancer-related programs). A group file exists for PERSON and ORGA called DIRECT. The Organisation Directory (ORGA) is a listing of over 1,600 hospitals and clinics with organised programmes for cancer care. The information includes PDQ term numbers, names, addresses and telephone numbers of health care organisations as well as parent organisations, suborganisations and affiliated organisations where applicable. The information is updated continuously and the listing for each organisation is verified at least once each year. A subscription charge which covers all transactional charges, connect time, telecommunications and the small administration charge can take the place of the individual charges. Subscriptions are negotiated with customers and vary according to the number of menus (thus, files) that are to be used – typically a minimum subscription would be about US$ 1,000. All charges include training and a 24-hour help line.

Record composition

Contact Person CONTACT-PERSON/CPER; Location LOCATION/LOCA; Name, Address and Telephone Number NAME-ADDR-TELE/NADT; Official Name and Alternative Names of Organisation ORG-NAME/ONAM; Organisation's Affiliation ORG-AFFIL/ORAF; Organisation Type ORG-TYPE/TYPE; Parent Organisation PAOR; PDQ Status PDQ-STATUS/PDQS and Suborganisations SUOR

All documents in the PIF file contain PDQ term numbers. These identify the cancer name, drug names, physicians and organisations. The format of the number is xxx/xxxxx.

This database can also be found on:
Oncodisc
NEXIS

Public Health and Tropical Medicine

Bureau of Hygiene and Tropical Diseases

15:159. Master record

Alternative name(s)	PHTM
Database type	Bibliographic
Number of journals	1,100
Sources	Bibliographies, books, conference proceedings, grey literature, journals, dissertations, research reports, reports, standards and patents
Start year	1984
Language	English and Original language titles
Coverage	International
Number of records	70,000
Update size	12,000
Update period	Monthly
Abstract details	BHTD academic staff or authorised outside scientists

Keywords

Epidemiology; HIV; Immunology; Legionnaires' Disease; Public Health; Pathology; Tropical Medicine; Virology

Description

PHTM contains selected references from abstract journals published by BHTD on all aspects of communicable diseases, including tropical diseases, AIDS and HIV infections. Subjects covered include bacterial, viral, fungal and protozoal infections and helminthiases (including AIDS and Legionnaires' disease); toxicology and industrial health; cancer epidemiology; medical entomology; community health – primary health care.

Equivalent to the three printed products: Abstracts of Hygiene and Communicable Diseases; Tropical Diseases Bulletin; AIDS and Retroviruses Update. Corresponding to these printed products, all documents in the database are assigned to three subunits: 1T – Abstracts on Hygiene and Communicable Diseases; 2T – Tropical Diseases Bulletin; 3T – AIDS and Retroviruses Update. A single document may be assigned to several subunits.

Items are selected for inclusion on the basis of newness, importance and relevance.

Apart from a semi-controlled vocabulary, which is to be elaborated into a thesaurus later, this is a free text database.

15:160. Online — CompuServe Information Service

File name	IQUEST File 2137
Alternative name(s)	PHTM
Start year	1982
Number of records	
Update period	Monthly
Price/Charges	Subscription: US$8.95 per month Database entry fee: US$9/search; some databases carry a surcharge ($2–75) Online print: US$10 references free; then $9 per ten; abstracts $3 each

Downloading is allowed

Notes

About thirty per cent of references carry an indicative abstract. Accessed via IQUEST or IQMEDICAL, this database is offered by a Data-Star gateway. IQUEST can either search across all databases, a database of the user's choice or selected multiple databases.

15:161. Online — DIMDI

File name	AZ84
Alternative name(s)	PHTM
Start year	1984
Number of records	87,744
Update period	Monthly
SDI period	1 month
Database aids	DIMDI's Online User Manual
Price/Charges	Connect time: UK£14.11–29.09 Online print: UK£0.45–0.63 Offline print: UK£0.37–0.43

Downloading is allowed
Thesaurus is online

Notes

PHTM contains all citations included in the abstract journals Tropical Diseases Bulletin, Abstracts on Hygiene and Communicable Diseases and Current AIDS literature. Subjects include AIDS and

Legionnaire's disease. All documents of the producer's subunit 3T form the subfile AIDS, file A184 on DIMDI. Suppliers of online documents: British Library Document Supply Centre, Boston Spa, England; Harkers Information Retrieval System, Sydney, Australia; Zentralbibliothek der Medizin, Köln, Germany.

Record composition

Abstract AB; Additional Author(s) AA; Abstract Language AL; Author(s) AU; Author's Variants AV; Corporate Author(s) CA; Corporate Source CS; Controlled Term CT; Document Type DT; Entry Date ED; Free Text FT; Geographical Heading GH; (I)SBN-(International) Standard Book Number SB; Journal Title JT; Language LA; Number of Abstract NA; Number of Document ND; Notes NO; Publisher's Name PN; Publication Year PY; Secondary Source SSO; Section Code SC; Source SO; Subfile SF; Subunit SU and Title TI

Approximately 74% of records contain abstracts. Documents are indexed in four stages. First subunits are selected by the appropriate reference publication; secondly the appropriate section code is allocated; thirdly descriptors are assigned using a semi-controlled vocabulary followed by the assignment of geographical headings (which do not indicate the country of publication). The unit record contains information about author(s), title and other bibliographic data as well as institutions, keywords and abstracts.

15:162. CD-ROM — Bureau of Hygiene and Tropical Diseases

File name	Public Health and Tropical Medicine
Alternative name(s)	PHTM
Format notes	IBM
Start year	
Number of records	
Update period	

15:163. Database subset

Online — BIOSIS Life Science Network

File name	AIDS Abstracts
Alternative name(s)	PHTM
Start year	1983
Number of records	14,000
Update period	Monthly
Price/Charges	Connect time: US$9.00
	Online print: US$6.00 per 10; 2.25 per abstract; 3.50 per full text article

Downloading is allowed
Also available via the Internet by telnetting to LSN.COM.

Notes

This is a subfile of the Public Health and Tropical Medicine database, containing all the citations included in the abstract journal Current AIDS Literature. Contains bibliographic information with annotations to indicate nature, scope and content and critically evaluated abstracts of papers on all viruses in the HIV/HTLV family and AIDS-related retroviruses and associated infections. Coverage includes public health, social aspects, health education, developing country issues, clinical aspects, treatment, etiology, pathology, serology, immunology, virology, epidemiology, seroepidemiology, transmission, control and safety. The main source of information contained in AIDS is the joint collection of journals, proceeedings, reports and books of the Bureau of Hygiene and Tropical Diseases (BHTD); altogether some 1,400 journal titles are scanned. A list of publications is

available from BHTD. These are supplemented with material from other bibliographic sources in London and elsewhere. The database corresponds in part to Abstracts on Hygiene and Communicable Diseases and Current AIDS Literature (formerly AIDS and Retroviruses Update). An English language title is always provided. Non-English references that carry an abstract will also give the original title in brackets.

On Life Science Network users can search this database or they can scan a group of subject-related databases. There is a charge of $2.00 per scan of subject-related databases. To search one database and display up to ten citations costs $6.00. Most charges are for information retrieved. There are no charges if there are no results and no charge to transfer results to a printer or diskette. Articles may also be ordered via an online document delivery request. A telecommunications software package is also available, costing $12.95, providing an automatic connection to Life Science Network for heavy users of the service, with capability to transfer to print or disk and customised colour options.

A controlled vocabulary is assigned to most but not all documents by the database producer.

15:164. Database subset

Online — BRS

File name	AIDD
Alternative name(s)	PHTM
Start year	1983
Number of records	11,846
Update period	Monthly
Price/Charges	Connect time: US$56.00/66.00
	Online print: US$0.62/0.70
	Offline print: US$0.70

Notes

This is a subfile of the Public Health and Tropical Medicine database, containing all the citations included in the abstract journal Current AIDS Literature. Contains bibliographic information with annotations to indicate nature, scope and content and critically evaluated abstracts of papers on all viruses in the HIV/HTLV family and AIDS-related retroviruses and associated infections. Coverage includes public health, social aspects, developing country issues, clinical aspects, treatment, etiology, pathology, serology, immunology, virology, epidemiology, seroepidemiology, transmission, control and safety. The main source of information contained in AIDS is the joint collection of journals, proceeedings, reports and books of the Bureau of Hygiene and Tropical Diseases (BHTD); altogether some 1,400 journal titles are scanned. A list of publications is available from BHTD. These are supplemented with material from other bibliographic sources in London and elsewhere. The database corresponds in part to Abstracts on Hygiene and Communicable Diseases and Current AIDS Literature (formerly AIDS and Retroviruses Update). An English language title is always provided. Non-English references that carry an abstract will also give the original title in brackets.

A controlled vocabulary is assigned to most but not all documents by the database producer.

15:165. Database subset

Online — Data-Star

File name	AIDS
Alternative name(s)	PHTM
Start year	1984

Number of records	11,846
Update period	Monthly
Database aids	Data-Star Biomedical Manual and Online manual (search NEWS-AIDS in NEWS)
Price/Charges	Connect time: SFr131.00
	Online print: SFr1.14
	Offline print: SFr1.04
	SDI charge: SFr6.80

Notes

This is a subfile of the Public Health and Tropical Medicine database, containing all the citations included in the abstract journal *Current AIDS Literature*. The main source of information contained in AIDS is the joint collection of journals, proceedings, reports and books of the Bureau of Hygiene and Tropical Diseases (BHTD); altogether some 1,400 journal titles are scanned. A list of publications is available from BHTD. These are supplemented with material from other bibliographic sources in London and elsewhere. The database corresponds in part to *Abstracts on Hygiene and Communicable Diseases* and *Current AIDS Literature* (formerly *AIDS and Retroviruses Update*). An English language title is always provided. Non-English references that carry an abstract will also give the original title in brackets. About thirty per cent of references carry an indicative abstract.

From June 1993 Data-Star have introduced an annual fee/subscription per contract (that is, not per password) of SFr 80.00 (c.UK£ 32.00) payable every June. For North American customers billed in dollars who also use DIALOG, the DIALOG fee also covers access to Data-Star. Academic customers, 'commitment' customers and customers currently billed in dollars are exempt.

Record composition

Abstract AB; Accession Number Update Code AN; Author AU; Author Affiliation IN; Classification Code CC; Corporate Author CA; Cross References XR; Country Name(s) CN; Descriptors DE; Language LG; Notes NT; Source SO; Title TI; Update Code UP and Year of Publication YR

A controlled vocabulary is assigned to most but not all documents by the database producer.

15:166. Database subset

Online   **DIMDI**

File name	A184 – AIDS and Retroviruses
Alternative name(s)	PHTM
Software	GRIPS
Start year	1984
Number of records	20,597
Update period	Monthly
SDI period	1 month
Price/Charges	Connect time: UK£14.11–29.09
	Online print: UK£0.45–0.63
	Offline print: UK£0.37–0.43

Downloading is allowed

Notes

This a subfile of the PHTM database and contains all citations included in the abstract journal *Current AIDS Literature*. Searches are possible from January 1984. Suppliers of online documents: British Library Document Supply Centre, Boston Spa, England; Bayerische Staatsbibliothek München, München, Germany; Harkers Information Retrieval System, Sydney. The main source of information contained in AIDS is the joint collection of journals, proceedings, reports and books of the Bureau of Hygiene and Tropical Diseases (BHTD); altogether some 1,400

journal titles are scanned. A list of publications is available from BHTD. These are supplemented with material from other bibliographic sources in London and elsewhere. The database corresponds in part to *Abstracts on Hygiene and Communicable Diseases* and *Current AIDS Literature* (formerly *AIDS and Retroviruses Update*). An English language title is always provided. Non-English references that carry an abstract will also give the original title in brackets.

A controlled vocabulary is assigned to most but not all documents by the database producer.

This database can also be found on:
AIDS Compact Library

Swedish Biomedicine

MIC Karolinska Institutets Bibliotek OCH Informationscentral (MIC-KIBIC)

15:168. Master record

Alternative name(s)	SWEMED
Database type	Bibliographic
Number of journals	
Sources	Journals, Reports and Dissertations
Start year	1982
Language	Original language titles, English and Swedish
Coverage	Sweden and Norway
Number of records	16,000
Update size	1,000
Update period	Twice a week
Thesaurus	Medical Subject Headings (MeSH)

Keywords

Anatomy; Biomedicine; Nutrition; Pathology; Microbiology

Description

Can be regarded as a Swedish complement to MEDLINE – contains Swedish biomedical literature not covered by MEDLINE. Contains about 5,000 references to Swedish biomedical journals (for example, *Läkartidningen*), reports and dissertations from Swedish and Norwegian universities since 1982. Coverage includes medicine, dentistry, nursing, nutrition, pharmacology.

15:169. Online   MIC/Karolinska Institute Library and Information Center (MIC KIBIC)

File name	Swemed
Alternative name(s)	SWEMED
Start year	1982
Number of records	16,000
Update period	Twice a week

Talking Dictionary of Medical Terminology (Anatomy & Physiology)

TBTG Footscray Institute of Technology

15:170. Master record

Database type	Multimedia, Courseware
Number of journals	
Sources	

Start year
Language   English
Coverage
Number of records
Update size   –
Update period

Keywords
Anatomy; Physiology

Description
Interactive audio teaching programme: definitions, use and graphics; aimed at the introductory level for paramedical or physical education students.

15:171. CD-ROM   **TBTG Footscray Institute of Technology**

File name
Format notes   IBM
Start year
Number of records
Update period
Price   Australian $550

Wonders of Learning CD-ROM Library: The Human Body
National Geographic Society
Discis Knowledge Research

15:172. Master record
Alternative name(s)   The Human Body
Database type   Multimedia, Factual, Courseware
Number of journals
Sources

Start year
Language   English and Spanish
Coverage   International
Number of records
Update size   –
Update period

Keywords
Anatomy

Description
A part of the Wonders of Learning CD-ROM Library in which 23 separate books are contained on five CD-ROMs, the disc is suitable for home or school use. For teachers, the series includes activity guides that can easily be accessed and printed.

Each disc includes more than 600 photographs, originally-scored background music, and animal sound effects. Users can slow down the narration, insert a time delay between phrases, pause to learn the meaning of words and hear words translated into Spanish. The text's font, size, style and line spacing can be altered to suit needs.

15:173. CD-ROM   **National Geographic Society**

File name   The Human Body
Alternative name(s)   The Human Body
Format notes   Mac
Start year
Number of records
Update period
Price   US$99.95

Notes
Educational discount reduces cost to $89.95.

HOSPITAL ADMINISTRATION

Advanced Medical Information Services
AMS Corporation

16:1. Master record

Database type	Bibliographic, Textual, Factual
Number of journals	
Sources	Press releases, News releases, Journals and Reports
Start year	1985 (June)
Language	Japanese
Coverage	Japan
Number of records	350,000+
Update size	—
Update period	Continuously/Weekly/Monthly
Index unit	Drug and articles

Description
Contains news, literature references, and other information and electronic services for physicians, hospital administrators and public health officials in Japan.

News: Contains full text of news stories related to medicine and health care. Also includes press releases from public agencies, infectious disease surveillance alerts, adverse drug reaction reports, health care product recalls, and other news items of interest of interest to health care providers.

AMS Database: Contains approximately 190,000 citations to Japanese medical literature. Also provides information on approximately 160,000 therapeutic drugs.

News is updated continuously, throughout the day. AMS Database citations are updated weekly; drug information updated monthly. Other information services include bulletin boards, classified advertisements, electronic mail, a directory of users, and access to databases available through AMA/NET and BRS/Colleague.

16:2. Online   AMS Corporation

File name	Advanced Medical Information Services
Start year	1985 (June)
Number of records	350,000+
Update period	Continuously/Weekly/Monthly

Notes
Monthly subscription required.

AgeLine
American Association of Retired Persons, National Gerontology Resource Center (AARP)

16:3. Master record

Database type	Bibliographic
Number of journals	
Sources	Dissertations, Government documents, Journals, Monographs and Reports
Start year	1978 (selected coverage back to 1966)
Language	English
Coverage	USA (primarily) and English-speaking countries (some)
Number of records	30,900
Update size	3,000
Update period	Every two months
Index unit	Articles and Book chapters
Abstract details	AgeLine staff
Thesaurus	Thesaurus of Aging Terminology

Keywords
Aging; Gerontology; Health Care Services; Pathology

Description
AgeLine contains citations, with abstracts, to the literature on social gerontology, the study of aging in social, psychological, health-related and economic contexts. The delivery of health care for the older population and its associated costs and policies is particularly well covered, as are public policy, employment and consumer issues. Subjects covered include: demographics, economics, employment, political action, health and health care services, housing, intergenerational relationships, social and family relationships, psychological aspects, retirement, transportation, consumer aspects and leisure. The literature covered is of interest to researchers, health professionals, service planners, policymakers, employers, older adults and their families and consumer advocates.

Journal citations compose roughly two-thirds of the database with the rest devoted to citations from books, book chapters and reports. An original, informative abstract accompanies each citation. There is no print equivalent of this database.

Journal coverage includes gerontological, social science, health, business and current events periodicals.

16:4. Online   BRS

File name	AARP
Start year	1978 (selected coverage back to 1966)
Number of records	29,297
Update period	Every two months
Price/Charges	Connect time: US$48.00/58.00
	Online print: US$0.32/0.40
	Offline print: US$0.40

16:5. Online — CompuServe Information Service

File name	IQUEST File 1949
Start year	1978
Number of records	29,297
Update period	Every two months
Price/Charges	Subscription: US$8.95 per month
	Database entry fee: US$9/search; some databases carry a surcharge ($2–75)
	Online print: US$10 references free; then $9 per ten; abstracts $3 each

Downloading is allowed

Notes

Accessed via IQUEST or IQMEDICAL, this database is offered by a BRS gateway. IQUEST can either search across all databases, a database of the user's choice or selected multiple databases.

16:6. Online — DIALOG

File name	File 163
Start year	1978 (selected coverage back to 1966)
Number of records	30,905
Update period	Every two months
Price/Charges	Connect time: US$60.00
	Online print: US$0.25
	Offline print: US$0.25
	SDI charge: US$5.95

Notes

DIALINDEX Categories: PSYCH, SOCISCI

16:7. CD-ROM — SilverPlatter

File name	AgeLine
Format notes	IBM, Mac
Start year	1978
Number of records	29,297
Update period	Three times per year
Price/Charges	

AMA/NET Medical Procedure Coding and Nomenclature
American Medical Association

16:9. Master record

Database type	Directory
Number of journals	
Sources	
Start year	Current
Language	English
Coverage	USA
Number of records	6,000+
Update size	—
Update period	Annually

Keywords

Medical Codes; Medical Insurance

Description

Provides identification codes and descriptions of procedures in the areas of medicine, surgery, and diagnostic services. Codes can be used by physicians to report medical services and procedures on patient bills and by insurance companies in processing claims.

Corresponds to current edition or *Physicians' Current Procedural Terminology*.

16:10. Online — AMA/NET

File name	
Start year	Current
Number of records	6,000+
Update period	Annually

Notes

Initiation fee of $30 for AMA members or $50 for non-members to AMA/NET required.

AMA/NET Social and Economic Aspects of Medicine
American Medical Association

16:11. Master record

Database type	Bibliographic
Number of journals	700
Sources	Journals, Newspapers, Monographs, Legal papers and Reports
Start year	1981
Language	English
Coverage	
Number of records	
Update size	—
Update period	Monthly
Index unit	Articles

Keywords

Public Health; Sociology; Medical Insurance; Practice Management

Description

Contains citations to articles on the non-clinical aspects of health care, including economics, education, ethics, international relations, legislation, political science, psychology, public health, medical practices, and sociology. Includes such topics as cost containment, insurance reimbursement, medical staff relations, and practice management. Covers legislative reports, monographs, newspapers and over 700 journals.

16:12. Online — AMA/NET

File name	
Start year	1981
Number of records	
Update period	Monthly

Notes

Initiation fee of $30 for AMA members or $50 for non-members to AMA/NET required.

Australian Government Publications
National Library of Australia

16:13. Master record

Alternative name(s)	AGP
Database type	Bibliographic
Number of journals	
Sources	Monographs, Journals, Pamphlets and Government documents
Start year	1983 – 1987
Language	English
Coverage	Australia

Number of records	54,000+
Update size	–
Update period	Not updated

Keywords

Health Services; Public Services Administration

Description

Contains citations to publications produced by the government of the Commonwealth of Australia and its states and territories. Covers all subjects within the scope of government activity, including agriculture, economics and financial institutions, small business, trade and export, law and legislation, health services, public service administration, transportation engineering, technology, and the environment. Also covers compilations of parliamentary debates, transcripts of proceedings of parliamentary committees, and proceedings of courts and tribunals.

Corresponds to Australian Government Publications.

16:14. Online OZLINE (formerly National Library of Australia)

File name	
Alternative name(s)	AGP
Start year	1983 – 1987
Number of records	54,000+
Update period	Not updated

AVLINE

National Library of Medicine

16:15. Master record

Alternative name(s)	AudioVisuals onLINE
Database type	Library catalogue/cataloguing aids, Bibliographic
Number of journals	
Sources	National Library of Medicine and A-V material
Start year	1975
Language	English
Coverage	USA
Number of records	18,000
Update size	1,200
Update period	Weekly

Keywords

Surgery

Description

Contains citations to audiovisual and other non-print teaching materials catalogued by the National Library of Medicine (NLM). Primarily clinical in scope, covers items used for health sciences education and for continuing education of practitioners. Selected records added prior to July 31, 1981 may contain critical appraisals resulting from peer reviews conducted (until March 1982) by the Association of American Medical Colleges. Information for obtaining each item is also included.

It is possible to search for particular types of media or to specify the running time. NLM classmarks on all items are useful for searching or for cataloguing. Some records have abstracts.

16:16. Online BLAISE-LINK

File name	AVLINE
Alternative name(s)	AudioVisuals onLINE
Start year	1976

Number of records	
Update period	Weekly

16:17. Online CISTI MEDLARS

File name	AVLINE
Alternative name(s)	AudioVisuals onLINE
Start year	1975
Number of records	18,000
Update period	Weekly

Notes

Charges depend on amount and type of usage.

16:18. Online National Library of Medicine

File name	AVLINE
Alternative name(s)	AudioVisuals onLINE
Start year	1975
Number of records	18,000
Update period	Weekly

16:19. Tape National Library of Medicine

File name	AVLINE
Alternative name(s)	AudioVisuals onLINE
Start year	1975
Number of records	18,000
Update period	Weekly

Notes

Corresponds to the AVLINE online database. Contact NLM for pricing information.

This database can also be found on:
AIDSLINE

CINAHL

CINAHL

16:22. Master record

Alternative name(s)	Cumulative Index to Nursing and Allied Health Literature; Nursing and Allied Health
Database type	Bibliographic
Number of journals	300
Sources	Journals, monographs, dissertations and A-V material
Start year	1983
Language	English
Coverage	International
Number of records	99,000
Update size	21,000
Update period	Monthly
Index unit	Articles and book
Thesaurus	CINAHL Thesaurus (MeSH-based)
Database aids	CINAHL Subject Heading List, 1993 (available from producer), CINAHL Database Search Guide, 1993 (available from producer) and CINAHL Teaching Guide, 1993 (available from producer)

Keywords

Physical Therapy; Cardiopulmonary Therapy; Laboratory Technology; Paramedicine; Respiratory Therapy; Occupational Therapy; Radiology; Emergency Health Care; Medical Records; Medical Social Work; Medical Librarianship; Surgical Nursing; Health Education; Management

Description

The nursing and allied health (CINAHL) database is a comprehensive and authoritative source of literature refences aimed at nurses, allied health professionals and others interested in health care administration.

Contains the complete Nursing and Allied Health database, including references to periodical literature in nursing and allied health, with abstracts from over one third of those articles; books from over thirty health care publishers, nursing dissertations and abstracts and references to the publications of the American Nurses Association and the National League of Nursing. Covers all aspects of nursing and allied health disciplines. Although the emphasis is primarily nursing, 35% of references relate to allied health disciplines such as cardiopulmonary technology, occupational therapy, physical therapy and rehabilitation, medical and laboratory technology, radiologic technology, emergency services and social services in health care, medical records, health sciences librarianship, medical assisting, the physician's assistant, surgical technology, and health education. Also includes relevant articles from management, psychological and popular journals. Also lists new books in nursing and allied health fields. Audiovisual materials as well as library science journals for nursing and allied health are also included. The vast majority of records are unique to CINAHL, although there is some overlap in journal coverage with *Excerpta Medica* (EMBASE) and MEDLINE.

Corresponds to the printed *Cumulative Index to Nursing and Allied Health Literature*. Since 1986 abstracts from approximately forty nursing journals have been included in the file. Books included since 1984.

Virtually all English-language nursing journals are included.

The CINAHL thesaurus is based on *MeSH*, but is tailor-made for the fields of nursing and allied health. Major and minor descriptors and free text searching are available. An extremely useful feature is the inclusion of more than twenty-four identifiers or document types which help to limit retrieval for specific concepts such as books, statistics, computer programs, research articles etc. The See also references from the printed index and the number of references in the citations are also included. The 1993 Subject Heading List contains 6,900 terms, 2,000 of which are not found on any other database.

16:23. Online   BRS, Morning Search, BRS/Colleague

File name	NAHL
Alternative name(s)	Nursing and Allied Health; CINAHL
Start year	
Number of records	
Update period	Monthly
Price/Charges	Connect time: US$37.00/47.00
	Online print: US$0.20/0.28
	Offline print: US$0.28
	SDI charge: US$7.25

16:24. Online   CompuServe Information Service

File name	IQUEST File 1278
Alternative name(s)	Nursing and Allied Health; CINAHL
Start year	1983
Number of records	
Update period	Monthly
Price/Charges	Subscription: US$8.95 per month
	Database entry fee: US$9/search; some databases carry a surcharge ($2–75)
	Online print: US$10 references free; then $9 per ten; abstracts $3 each

Downloading is allowed

Notes
Accessed via IQUEST or IQMEDICAL, this database is offered by a BRS gateway. IQUEST can either search across all databases, a database of the user's choice or selected multiple databases.

16:25. Online   Data-Star

File name	NAHL
Alternative name(s)	Nursing and Allied Health; CINAHL
Start year	1983
Number of records	103,799
Update period	Monthly
Database aids	Biomedical manual and Online manual (search NEWS-NAHL in NEWS)
Price/Charges	Subscription: SFr80.00
	Connect time: SFr107
	Online print: SFr0.42
	Offline print: SFr0.37
	SDI charge: SFr6.80

Thesaurus is online

Notes
Four subsets have been created to help narrow a search. Users can limit retrieval to articles from nursing journals as 'Nursing.SB.', Core nursing journals as 'Core with nursing.SB.', Allied health journals as 'Allied with health.SB.' and journals published in the USA and Canada as 'USA with Canada.'

From June 1993 Data-Star have introduced an annual fee/subscription per contract (that is, not per password) of SFr 80.00 (c.UK£ 32.00) payable every June. For North American customers billed in dollars who also use DIALOG, the DIALOG fee also covers access to Data-Star. Academic customers, 'commitment' customers and customers currently billed in dollars are exempt.

Record composition
Author AU; Title TI; Source SO; Language LG; Publication type PT; Descriptors (MeSH) DE; Year of publication YR; Subset SB; Major desriptors MJ; Minor descriptors MN and UMI order number UMI

16:26. Online   DIALOG, Knowledge Index

File name	File 218
Alternative name(s)	CINAHL; Nursing and Allied Health
Start year	1983
Number of records	123,290
Update period	Monthly
Price/Charges	Connect time: US$54.00
	Online print: US$0.15
	Offline print: US$0.25
	SDI charge: US$6.95

Notes
This database is also available to home users during evenings and weekends at a reduced rate on the Knowledge Index service of DIALOG – file name in this case is MEDI14, and searches are made with simplified commands or menus.

16:27. CD-ROM   CD Plus

File name	CD Plus/CINAHL-CD
Alternative name(s)	Nursing and Allied Health; CINAHL
Format notes	Mac, Unix, IBM
Software	OVID 3.0
Start year	1983
Number of records	100,000
Update period	Monthly
Price/Charges	Subscription: UK£685

Notes

One disc. Offers the ability to limit by local journal holdings. For the experienced searcher, the software offers MeSH explodes, 'personal pre-explodes' for frequently exploded terms, SDIs and Save Searches, enhanced MeSH tree structures, and emulation of National Library of Medicine and dot-dot syntax.

Record composition

Author; Title; Source; Abstract; Subject Heading and Instrumentation

This database has an index of all searchable terms together with the online MeSh Thesaurus which offers mapping from natural language to MeSH – a facility which should give significantly improved precision for the inexperienced searcher. The on-screen help provides scope notes, definitions and task descriptors.

16:28. CD-ROM   Compact Cambridge

File name	CINAHL-CD
Alternative name(s)	CINAHL; Nursing and Allied Health
Format notes	NEC, 9800, Mac, IBM
Start year	1983
Number of records	100,000+
Update period	Monthly
Price/Charges	Subscription: UK£700

16:29. CD-ROM   SilverPlatter

File name	Nursing & Allied Health (CINAHL)-CD
Alternative name(s)	Nursing and Allied Health; CINAHL
Format notes	Mac, IBM
Software	SPIRS/MacSPIRS
Start year	1983
Number of records	140,000
Update period	Every two months
Price/Charges	Subscription: UK£790 – 1,186.5
Thesaurus is online	

Notes

One disc. The CD includes an on-screen equivalent to CINAHL's print thesaurus. Prices are: regular subscription £790 for single users, £1,186.5 for 2–8 networked users.

Tree explosions, major and minor assignments of descriptors, the use of sub-headings, and free text searching are available.

16:30. Fixed disk   SilverPlatter

File name	Nursing & Allied Health (CINAHL)-CD
Alternative name(s)	Nursing and Allied Health; CINAHL
Format notes	IBM, Mac
Software	SPIRS/MacSPIRS
Start year	1983
Number of records	140,000
Update period	Every two months
Price/Charges	Subscription: UK£1,028 – 1,713
Thesaurus is online	

Notes

Contains the entire database, with an on-screen equivalent of CINAHL's print thesaurus, on a fixed disk with updates supplied on CD-ROM. This means that up to thirty networked users can have access to a single file containing the complete database. Search speeds are up to ten times faster than CD-ROM searching.

Prices are: £1,028 for 2–8 networked users, £1,370 for 9–16 users and £1,713 for 17–24 users. Hard disk fee is US$1,500.

Tree explosions, major and minor assignments of descriptors, the use of sub-headings, and free text searching are available.

Colleague Mail
BRS Online Service, BRS/Colleague

16:31. Master record

Alternative name(s)	MEDLINK
Database type	Directory, Textual, Computer software
Number of journals	1
Sources	Journal, Airlines, Database producers, Electronic media and Original material
Start year	
Language	English
Coverage	USA
Number of records	
Update size	–
Update period	Current six to eight months
Index unit	Classified advertisements

Keywords

Molecular Biology; HIV; Travel; Air Travel; Anaesthesia; Personal Computers; HIV; Pathology; Surgery; Gastroenterology; Intensive Care; Proctology; Dermatology; Geriatrics; Gerontology; Genetics – Human; Immunology; Health Care Administration; Neurology; Cancer; Oncology; Ophthalmology; Sickle-Cell Disease

Description

Contains a number of services for medical professionals, including classified advertisements from the *New England Journal of Medicine*, a calendar of medical events, electronic mail, gateway access to Official Airlines Guide (OAG) Electronic Edition Travel Service (see separate entry), American Airlines EASY Sabre (see separate entry) and other databases available through BT Tymnet Dialcom Service. There are also a number of bulletin boards available, operated by physician-editors: AIDS/HIV, Anesthesia Safety and Technology, Cellforum (pathology, cell biology, molecular biology), Clinical Drug Information, Colon & Rectal Surgery, Critical Care, Dermatology, Geriatrics and Gerontology, Hackers' Forum (microcomputer products and applications), Materia Eclectica, Medical Ethics, MEDLINK Help & Tips, Neurology, Oncology, Ophthalmology, Sickle-Cell Disease.

Partially equivalent to *New England Journal of Medicine* (classified advertisements).

16:32. Online   BRS, BRS/Colleague

File name	
Alternative name(s)	MEDLINK
Start year	
Number of records	
Update period	current six to eight months

For more details of constituent databases, see:
American Airlines EAASY SABRE
OAG Electronic Edition Travel Service

Conquest Marketing Information System

Donnelley Marketing Information
Services

16:34. Master record

Database type	Factual, Statistical, Textual, Numeric, Cartographic, Directory, Mapped statistical, Computer software, Organisational/Biographical
Number of journals	
Sources	
Start year	1970
Language	English
Coverage	USA and Canada
Number of records	
Update size	—
Update period	Annually

Keywords

Demography; Health Care Market; Hospital Facilities; Physicians; Product Catalogues; Shopping Centres (US); Television

Description

A US consumer information database with more than 25 files offering access to current year demographic estimates and five years of data on key demographic variables. Includes details of 1980 and 1970 US Census data; 30,000 shopping centres; more than 7.5 million commercial businesses; sales potentials for 21 types of retail stores; retail sales estimates; consumer lifestyles; product usage and median data; business statistics and listings; financial deposit and location data; shopping centres; grocery stores; geographic boundaries and streets.

There is also access to ClusterPLUS, the only updated life style segmentation system. Industry packages include Conquest/Financial, Conquest/ Advertising, Conquest/Canada, TV Conquest, Conquest/Health Care, and Cable Conquest.

16:35. Database subset

CD-ROM   **Donnelley Marketing Information Services**

File name	Conquest Health Care Market Profile
Start year	
Number of records	
Update period	Annually

Notes

Contains data on health care products and service usage patterns categorised by the 47 ClusterPlus lifestyle grouping. Includes information on: Wellness/Fitness centres; Home health care; Maternity services; Outpatient non-surgery; Physician referral; etc. Part of Conquest Marketing Information System.

16:36. Database subset

CD-ROM   **Donnelley Marketing Information Services**

File name	Conquest Hospital Facilities
Start year	

Number of records	
Update period	Annually
Price/Charges	Subscription: US$1,000

Notes

Contains descriptive and operational data on over 7,000 US hospitals. Information includes: Name; Address; Number of beds; Discharges; Inpatient days; Average length of stay; Financial data. Part of Conquest Marketing Information System

DHSS-Data

Department of Health and Social
Security

16:37. Master record

Alternative name(s)	Department of Health and Social Security – Data
Database type	Bibliographic, Library catalogue/cataloguing aids
Number of journals	2,000+
Sources	Administrative circulars, government documents, journals, monographs, official publications, pamphlets and reports
Start year	1983 (October); earliest data from 1961
Language	English
Coverage	UK (primarily) and International (some)
Number of records	84,691
Update size	13,000
Update period	Weekly
Index unit	Articles
Thesaurus	DHSS-Data Thesaurus, new edition in preparation

Keywords

Building; Child Care; Health Care; Public Administration; Social Services; Standards

Description

DHSS-DATA contains citations, with some abstracts (approximately 40%) to the long-established abstracting and current awareness bulletins from the library of the Departments of Health and Social Security in London. The core subjects covered by the database are health service and hospital administration including: planning, design, construction and maintenance of health service buildings; medical equipment and supplies; public health, nursing and primary care; occupational diseases, social policy, social welfare, social security, social services for children, families, the handicapped and old people; and social security and occupational pensions. The database currently focuses on new holdings; references to older holdings are to be added in the future. An important feature of the database is the inclusion of full details, including sources of supply, of Department of Health and Department of Social Security publications.

Source documents are available as an inter-library loan.

Government publications originate primarily in the United Kingdom, the United States, and with the World Health Organisation.

From 1986 Tags enable a search to be restricted to specific sectors of the Health or Social Services such as Health, Social Services, Social Security, Pensions and Health Buildings. In late 1992, the database was restructured to provide more up-to-date and better quality records, with increased coverage of official publications.

16:38. Online — CompuServe Information Service

File name	IQUEST File 2141
Alternative name(s)	Department of Health and Social Security – Data
Start year	1983
Number of records	84,691
Update period	Weekly
Price/Charges	Subscription: US$8.95 per month Database entry fee: US$9/search; some databases carry a surcharge ($2–75) Online print: US$10 references free; then $9 per ten; abstracts $3 each

Downloading is allowed

Notes

Accessed via IQUEST or IQMEDICAL, this database is offered by a Data-Star gateway. IQUEST can either search across all databases, a database of the user's choice or selected multiple databases.

Record composition

Abstract AB; Accession Number and Update Code AN; Author(s) AU; Corporate Author(s) CA; Descriptor(s) DE; Notes NT; Publication Type PT; Publication Year YR; Publication Year (Archive) YA; Source SO; Title TI and Update Code UP

16:39. Online — Data-Star

File name	DHSS
Alternative name(s)	Department of Health and Social Security – Data
Start year	1983 (October); earliest data from 1961
Number of records	84,691
Update period	Weekly
Database aids	Data-Star Biomedial Manual and Online manual (search NEWS-DHSS in NEWS)
Price/Charges	Subscription: SFr80.00 Connect time: SFr127.20 Online print: SFr0.39 Offline print: SFr0.80 SDI charge: SFr6.80

Downloading is allowed

Notes

The Superlabel DHZZ can be used to search DHSS-DHSS and DHMT-MEDTEH simultaneously. The following tags, appearing on records from 1986, enable a search to be restricted to specific sectors of the Health or Social Services: YYH Health, YYQ Social Services, YYS Social Security, YYP Pensions, YYB Health Buildings.

From June 1993 Data-Star have introduced an annual fee/subscription per contract (that is, not per password) of SFr 80.00 (c.UK£ 32.00) payable every June. For North American customers billed in dollars who also use DIALOG, the DIALOG fee also covers access to Data-Star. Academic customers, 'commitment' customers and customers currently billed in dollars are exempt.

Record composition

Abstract AB; Accession Number and Update Code AN; Author(s) AU; Corporate Author(s) CA; Descriptor(s) DE; Notes NT; Publication Type PT; Publication Year YR; Publication Year (Archive) YA; Source SO; Title TI and Update Code UP

DRI Health Care Cost Forecasting
Data Resources Inc (DRI)

16:40. Master record

Database type	Statistical
Number of journals	
Sources	Databases
Start year	4-year forecasts, with historical series from 1976
Language	
Coverage	USA
Number of records	100
Update size	–
Update period	Quarterly

Keywords

Health Care Costs; Medical Equipment; Pharmaceuticals

Description

Contains quarterly forecast indexes of United States health care costs. Covers labour, food, utilities, medical equipment, supplies, pharmaceuticals, physician services, and capital. Also provides forecasts of the 'market basket' indexes developed by the United States Health Care Financing Administration (HCFA) for hospitals, nursing homes, and home health- care agencies. Some series are available at a regional level.

Sources include DRI data banks and models, and the Health Care Financing Administration.

16:41. Online — Data Resources Inc (DRI)

File name	
Start year	4-year forecasts, with historical series from 1976
Number of records	100
Update period	Quarterly

Notes

Subscription to DRI required.

DSI
Dansk Sygehus Institut

16:42. Master record

Alternative name(s)	Dansk Sygehus Institut
Database type	Bibliographic
Number of journals	
Sources	Books, Reports and Journals
Start year	1977
Language	Danish
Coverage	
Number of records	18,000
Update size	–
Update period	Daily
Index unit	Articles

Description

DSI contains references to literature on hospitals, nursing and health services. Disciplines covered are: Medicine, nursing, pharmacology, economics, management, building, technology, law, sociology etc. Document types indexed are: Books, reports, serials and articles.

16:43. Online   DSI

File name	DSI
Alternative name(s)	Dansk Sygehus Institut
Start year	1977
Number of records	18,000
Update period	Daily

Esculap

Helsingborgs sjukvårdsdistrikt, Lasarettet (Helsingborg Heath Care District)

16:44. Master record

Alternative name(s)	Helsingborgs sjukvårdsdistrikts databas; Helsingborg Health Care District
Database type	Bibliographic
Number of journals	
Sources	Reports
Start year	1987
Language	Swedish
Coverage	International
Number of records	1,800
Update size	700
Update period	Irregular
Index unit	Reports

Keywords
Clinical Medicine

Description

This database contains citations to the documents acquired since 1987 by the Helsingborg Health Care District in the fields of medicine, with an emphasis on the clinical aspect, and other areas relating to health care. It also includes reports issued by the District Authority. Subjects covered include: medicine; health care; nursing; hospitals and hospital administration.

16:45. Online   Bibliotekstjänst AB (Btj)

File name	Esculap
Alternative name(s)	Helsingborgs sjukvårdsdistrikts databas; Helsingborg Health Care District
Start year	1987
Number of records	1,800
Update period	Irregular

EURODOC

World Health Organisation – Regional Office for Europe

16:46. Master record

Database type	Bibliographic
Number of journals	
Sources	

Start year	1988
Language	English
Coverage	Europe
Number of records	3,000
Update size	–
Update period	Daily
Thesaurus	MeSH-based

Keywords
Health Services

Description

A bibliographical database dealing with health and health services in Europe.

Available to UN system organisations and World Health Organisation Member States. Also available as a printout.

Indexing terms are drawn from *Medical Subject Headings (MeSH)* of the US National Library of Medicine.

16:47. Online   World Health Organisation – Health Documentation Service

File name	EURODOC
Format notes	Wang, VS7310
Software	MIMER/IR
Start year	1988
Number of records	3,000
Update period	Daily

Faculty of Public Health Medicine's Part Two Theses, 1991

Health Care Evaluation Unit, University of Bristol

16:48. Master record

Database type	Bibliographic
Number of journals	
Sources	Theses
Start year	1991
Language	English
Coverage	UK
Number of records	1,300+
Update size	–
Update period	

Description

Bibliographic references plus abstracts to theses lodged with the Faculty at the University of Bristol. User-definable choice of fields to display.

16:49. Diskette   Health Care Evaluation Unit, University of Bristol

File name	Faculty of Public Health Medicine's Part Two Theses, 1991
Format notes	IBM
Software	Cardbox
Start year	1991

Number of records   1,300+
Update period

Notes

Software not supplied.

FDC Reports

FDC Reports Inc

16:50. Master record

Database type   Textual
Number of journals   3
Sources   Conference reports, courts, direct
                       contacts, government documents
                       (US), journals, laws/regulations,
                       ministry reports, newsletters, press
                       releases, reports and trade journals
Start year   1984
Language   English
Coverage   USA (primarily) and International
                       (some)
Number of records   22,767
Update size   —
Update period   Weekly
Index unit   Articles and trademarks

Keywords

Applied Science; Beauty Care; Biomedical Research;
Cosmetics; Dermatology; Drugs; Health Care
Management; Marketing; Perfumes;
Pharmaceuticals; Skin Care

Description

FDC Reports contains the full text of five related
paramedical newsletters: Prescription and OTC
Pharmaceuticals (*The Pink Sheet*), Medical Devices,
Diagnostics and Instrumentation Reports (*The Gray
Sheet*), and Toiletries, Fragrances and Skin Care (*The
Rose Sheet*), health policy and biomedical research
(*The Blue Sheet*) and pharmaceuticals (*The Green
Sheet*).

Together the newsletters provide up-to-date information about companies, product development, marketing, packaging, scientific news, personnel, retailing
and advertising, trade association news, United
States Food and Drug Administration regulatory activities, and corporate news, including financial operations, mergers and acquisitions, marketing and
licensing agreements, legal news and market share of
importance to the worldwide health care industry. *The
Pink Sheet* focuses on the pharmaceutical industry
and includes over-the-counter drugs as well as prescription products. New products are profiled through
all phases of the approval process, from early investigational stages through marketing. Personnel
changes, marketing/licensing agreements, and
mergers/acquisitions are covered regularly. Activities
of major trade associations and regulatory bodies
such as the Food and Drug Administration are
reported. *The Gray Sheet* provides varied and
detailed information pertinent to the costmetics
industry, including toiletries, fragrances and skin care.
Coverage includes marketing information, new product introductions, line extensions, promotions and
advertising activities at retail. A Trademark Review is
also provided which is a compilation of cosmetics-
related product trademarks registered and filed for
opposition with the US Patent and Trademark Office.
The Rose Sheet also includes descriptions of cosmetics trademarks registered and filed for opposition with
the United States Patent and Trademark Office. The

database contains six types of records: full-text journal
articles, FDA Recalls & Court Actions, Weekly
Trademark Review records, Medical Device
Approvals, New Drug Approvals and Abbreviated New
Drug Approvals. *The Blue Sheet* deals with news and
information concerning health policy and biomedical
research topics including government funding and
legal issues. *The Green Sheet* is particularly valuable
in tracking the latest developments in drug sales and
marketing.

Sources for all newsletters include new product
announcements, market research reports, press releases, sales and earnings reports, United States
Securities and Exchange Commission filings, government and trade association reports, reports from conferences, meetings, and conventions, and interviews
with industry leaders. News coverage is focused primarily on US and multi-national activities and
accounts for approximately eighty five per cent of the
database. Approximately ten per cent is focused on
Europe and five per cent on Japan and other
countries.

The accession numbers field contains volume number, publication code, issue number and article number. The source field contains five options: pink-sheet,
gray-sheet, green-sheet, blue-sheet and rose-sheet.

16:51. Online   BRS

File name   FDCR
Start year   1984
Number of records   22,767
Update period   Weekly
Price/Charges   Connect time: US$110.00/120.00
                       Online print: US$0.92/1.00
                       Offline print: US$1.00
                       SDI charge: US$10.00

Notes

Contains the entire text of the following FDC Report
publications: *The Pink Sheet, The Gray Sheet* and
The Rose Sheet.

16:52. Online   Data-Star

File name   FDCR
Start year   January 1988
Number of records   620+ documents
Update period   Weekly
Database aids   Data-Star Business Manual and
                       Data-Star Online Manual (search
                       for NEWS-FDCR in NEWS)
Price/Charges   Subscription: SFr80.00
                       Connect time: SFr187.00
                       Online print: SFr1.64
                       Offline print: SFr1.89
                       SDI charge: SFr10.00
Downloading is allowed

Notes

From June 1993 Data-Star have introduced an annual
fee/subscription per contract (that is, not per password) of SFr 80.00 (c.UK£ 32.00) payable every June.
For North American customers billed in dollars who
also use DIALOG, the DIALOG fee also covers
access to Data-Star. Academic customers, 'commitment' customers and customers currently billed in
dollars are exempt.

Record composition

Accession Number and Update Code AN; Date of
Publication DT; Month of Publication YM; Occurence
Table OC; Source SO; Text of article TX; Title TI;
Update Code UP and Year of Publication YR

16:53. Online   **DIALOG**

File name	File 187
Start year	1987
Number of records	31,232
Update period	Weekly
Price/Charges	Connect time: US$120.00
	Online print: US$1.20
	Offline print: US$1.50
	SDI charge: US$3.95

Notes

DIALINDEX Categories: BIOBUS, PHARMINA, REGS.

16:54. Online   **Mead Data Central**
(as a NEXIS database)

File name	FDC – NEXIS
Alternative name(s)	NEXIS – FDC Reports
Start year	1984
Number of records	
Update period	Weekly
Price/Charges	Subscription: US$1,000 – 3,000
	(Depending on needs)
	Connect time: US$49.00
	(Telecomms + connect time)
	Database entry fee: US$24.00
	(Search charge)
	Online print: US$0.04 per line

Notes

Library: GENMED. FDC is the Group File containing all five reports: *Blue, Gray, Green, Pink* and *Rose*.

A subscription charge which covers all transactional charges, connect time, telecommunications and the small administration charge can take the place of the individual charges. Subscriptions are negotiated with customers and vary according to the number of menus (thus, files) that are to be used – typically a minimum subscription would be about US$ 1,000. All charges include training and a 24-hour help line.

16:55. Database subset
Online   **Mead Data Central**
(as a NEXIS database)

File name	BLUE – NEXIS
Alternative name(s)	NEXIS – FDC Reports
Start year	1984
Number of records	
Update period	Weekly
Price/Charges	Subscription: US$1,000 – 3,000
	(Depending on needs)
	Connect time: US$49.00
	(Telecomms + connect time)
	Database entry fee: US$14.00
	(Search charge)
	Online print: US$0.04 per line

Notes

Library: GENMED; Group File: FDC.

The full text of the weekly newsletter, *The Blue Sheet*, on health policy and research which provides professionals with news and information concerning health policy and biomedical research covering topics such as government funding, legislative proposals, legal issues and research developments. Documents display in reverse chronological order by date and then in ascending order by page number.

A subscription charge which covers all transactional charges, connect time, telecommunications and the small administration charge can take the place of the individual charges. Subscriptions are negotiated with customers and vary according to the number of menus (thus, files) that are to be used – typically a minimum subscription would be about US$ 1,000. All charges include training and a 24-hour help line.

Record composition

Publication; Cite; Date; Section; Length; Title; Author; Text; Reference (BIBLIO-REF); Graphic; Correction; Correction Date and Editor's Note

This database can also be found on:
NEXIS

Francis
Centre National de la Recherche Scientifique, Institut de l'Information Scientifique et Technique, Science Humaines et Sociales (CNRS/INIST)

16:57. Master record

Database type	Bibliographic, Textual
Number of journals	7,500
Sources	Journals, Books, Reports, Dissertations, Conference proceedings and Research communications
Start year	1972
Language	French (keywords), English (keywords), Spanish (keywords) and Others
Coverage	France (primarily), Europe and International
Number of records	1,500,000+
Update size	80,000
Update period	Quarterly; Files 603 and 616 twice a year
Index unit	Articles

Keywords

Anthropology; Applied Linguistics; Chemical Substances; Computers and Law; Demography; Descriptive Linguistics; Environmental Health; Epidemiology; Ergonomics; Ethnolinguistics; Forensic Science; Health Care Management; Health Economics; History of Education; History of Medicine; History of Science; History of Technology; Human Ecology; Information Technology; Language Biology; Language Pathology; Linguistics; Mathematical Linguistics; Medical Education; Occupational Psychology; Occupational Medicine; Pharmaceutical Industry; Philosophy; Philosophy of Education; Psycholinguistics; Public Health; Semiotics; Social Medicine; Social Psychology; Social Services; Sociolinguistics; Sociology of Education; Vocational Training; Testing Methods

Description

Francis is a collection of twenty multidisciplinary bibliographic databases. It contains news and information, covering the core literature in: humanities, social sciences, economic sciences, computer processing, legal sciences, energy economics, health and medicine. There is especially good coverage of European and French research, with exhaustive coverage of fields where research is most active or which correspond to French national priorities. Most of the references also contain an analysis. The records include keywords for searching. Over 9,000 periodicals, books, reports, dissertations, etc. are indexed.

Databases included are:

Art and Archaeology (Near East, Asia, America) (File 526);

International Bibliography of Administrative Science (File 528);

Ethnology (File 529);

History of Science and Technology (Histoire des Sciences et des Techniques (File 522) containing citations, half with abstracts, to literature on the history of science and technology, including the exact sciences, earth sciences, life sciences, medicine and pharmacology. Corresponds to *Bulletin Signaletique Sciences Humaines: Section Histoire des Sciences et des Techniques* (522). There are 74,600 records dating from 1972, with 4,000 additions quarterly;

History of Literature and Literary Sciences (File 523);

History of Religion and Religious Sciences (File 527);

Information Technology and the Law (File 603);

Philosophy (File 519);

Prehistory and Protohistory (File 525);

Index of Art and Archaeology; Educational Sciences (Sciences de l'Education) (File 520) Contains citations, about half with abstracts, to the worldwide literature on education. Covers history and philosophy of education; education and psychology; sociology of education; planning and economics; educational research; teaching methods; testing and guidance; school life; vocational training; and adult education and employment. Corresponds to the *Bulletin Signaletique Sciences Humaines; Section Sciences de l'Education* (520). Records, approximately 40,000, date from 1979 and are updated quarterly with 4,000 additions each quarter;

Linguistic Sciences (Sciences du Langue) (File 524) contains citations, with some abstracts, to the international journal literature on linguistics, including language biology and pathology, psycholinguistics, sociolinguistics, ethnolinguistics, historical linguistics, descriptive studies, linguistics and mathematics, semiotics and communications, discursive semiotics and applied linguistics. Corresponds to *Bulletin Signaletique Sciences Humaines: Section Sciences du Langue* (524). There are 62,500 records on the file, dating from 1972, updated quarterly with 3,200 additions;

Sociology (Sociologie) (File 521) contains citations, most with abstracts, to the worldwide periodical and other literature in the field of sociology. Covers social psychology; social organization and structure; social problems; human ecology; demography; rural and urban sociology; economic and political sociology; sociology of knowledge, religion, education, art, communication, leisure, organisations, health, law, and work; and social work. The 68,000 records date from 1972, with 4,000 additions quarterly. Corresponds to the *Bulletin Signaletique Sciences Humaines: Section Sociologie* (521).

DOGE (Management) (File 616);

ECODOC (General Economics) (File 617);

Energy Economics (File 731);

Employment and Training (File 600);

RESHUS (Health-related Humanities) (Reseau documentaire en Sciences Humaines de la Santé) (File 610). A sectorial database on health economy, epidemiology, health and development, health organisation, health socio-economic aspects, medical ethic. Contains citations, with abstracts, to selected French literature from 1978 in the fields of health sciences: economics, sociology, legislation, geography, epidemiology, history, research and teaching, demography; human aspects of health:

childbirth, death and illness, health developments, risk factors in failing health, ethics, health and society; health intervention systems: health organizations and politics; status, prevention and care unit management and structure, expenses and financing; and evaluation of health performances. There are 16,000 records updated quarterly with 1,300 additions per quarter. 84.5% of the documents indexed are French, 15% English and 0.5% are in other languages. 81% of references are journal articles, the other 19% coming from books, dissertations, proceedings and so on. All documents are fully analysed. Corresponds to the quarterly bulletin *RESHUS* and File 610 of *Bulletin Signaletique Sciences Humaines: Section Reseau Documentaire en Sciences Humaines de la Santé*.

Latin America (File 533);

International Geographical Bibliography (File 531); and two new releases,

Cognisciences (File 90) and

Spécial Préhistoire (File 47).

An index to author and source is cumulated annually. 7,500 periodical titles are covered, comprising 90% of the references, plus research reports, proceedings, and French dissertations.

Some of the databases can be purchased as combinations – File 521 (Sociology) and 529 (Ethnology) can be purchased as File 946; File G22 is a combination of File 525 (Prehistory and Special Prehistory (new release). Bibliographic publications are produced quarterly as hard copy, corresponding to the subject areas covered in the Francis database, Computer Science and the Law being published only twice a year.

There is very good coverage of French periodicals.

Francis has one lexicon (alphabetical list of subject terms used to index the information found in the database) per subject field. There are thesauri for the Energy Economics, Administrative Science, Geography and RESHUS databases. There are trilingual keywords English-French-Spanish or English-French-German in some files, and a bilingual English-French classification scheme.

16:58. Online Européenne de Données

File name	Francis
Start year	1972
Number of records	1,500,000+
Update period	Quarterly; Files 603 and 616 twice a year
Database aids	Francis User Manual (French) for Européenne de Données users

16:59. Online Questel

File name	Francis
Start year	1972
Number of records	1,500,000+
Update period	Quarterly; Files 603 and 616 twice a year
Database aids	Francis User Manual (French or English) for Questel users

16:60. CD-ROM Centre National de la Recherche Scientifique, Institut de l'Information Scientifique et Technique, Science Humaines et Sociales (CNRS/INIST)

File name	Francis
Format notes	IBM
Software	GTI
Start year	1984

Number of records	500,000
Update period	Annually
Price/Charges	Subscription: FFr4,000 – 17,500

Notes

The first CD-ROM produced covers the years 1984–90. Additional discs will be produced each year – 6,000 FFr for current year (1991, 1 disc); 17,500 French francs for retrospective disc 1984–1990.

16:61. Tape — Centre National de la Recherche Scientifique, Institut de l'Information Scientifique et Technique, Science Humaines et Sociales (CNRS/INIST)

File name	Francis
Format notes	9-track 1,600 or 6,250 BPI magnetic tapes, EBCDIC character set, with or without IBM-OS label
Start year	1972
Number of records	1,500,000+
Update period	Quarterly; Files 603 and 616 twice a year

16:62. Videotex — Centre National de la Recherche Scientifique, Institut de l'Information Scientifique et Technique, Science Humaines et Sociales (CNRS/INIST)

File name	Francis
Start year	1972
Number of records	1,500,000+
Update period	Quarterly; Files 603 and 616 twice a year

16:63. Videotex — Minitel

File name	Francis (36293601)
Start year	1972
Number of records	1,500,000+
Update period	Quarterly; Files 603 and 616 twice a year

Notes

Available directly via Minitel by dialling 36.29.36.01.

16:64. Database subset

Online — Européenne de Données

File name	RESH
Alternative name(s)	Reseau documentaire en Sciences Humaines de la Santé; RESHUS
Start year	1978
Number of records	16,000
Update period	Quarterly

Notes

A subfile of the multidisciplinary Francis database, RESHUS is a sectorial database on health economy, epidemiology, health and development, health organisation, health socio-economic aspects, medical ethic. Contains citations, with abstracts, to selected French literature from 1978 in the fields of health sciences: economics, sociology, legislation, geography, epidemiology, history, research and teaching, demography; human aspects of health: childbirth, death and illness, health developments, risk factors in failing health, ethics, health and society; health intervention systems: health organizations and politics; status, prevention and care unit management and structure, expenses and financing; and evaluation of health performances. There are 16,000 records updated quarterly with 1,300 additions per quarter. 84.5% of the documents indexed are French, 15% English and

0.5% are in other languages. 81% of references are journal articles, the other 19% coming from books, dissertations, proceedings and so on. All documents are fully analysed. Corresponds to the quarterly bulletin *RESHUS* and File 610 of *Bulletin Signaletique Sciences Humaines: Section Reseau Documentaire en Sciences Humaines de la Santé.*

16:65. Database subset

Online — Questel

File name	Francis: RESHUS
Alternative name(s)	Reseau documentaire en Sciences Humaines de la Santé; RESHUS
Start year	1978
Number of records	16,000
Update period	Quarterly

Notes

A subfile of the multidisciplinary Francis database, RESHUS is a sectorial database on health economy, epidemiology, health and development, health organisation, health socio-economic aspects, medical ethic. Contains citations, with abstracts, to selected French literature from 1978 in the fields of health sciences: economics, sociology, legislation, geography, epidemiology, history, research and teaching, demography; human aspects of health: childbirth, death and illness, health developments, risk factors in failing health, ethics, health and society; health intervention systems: health organizations and politics; status, prevention and care unit management and structure, expenses and financing; and evaluation of health performances. There are 16,000 records updated quarterly with 1,300 additions per quarter. 84.5% of the documents indexed are French, 15% English and 0.5% are in other languages. 81% of references are journal articles, the other 19% coming from books, dissertations, proceedings and so on. All documents are fully analysed. Corresponds to the quarterly bulletin *RESHUS* and File 610 of *Bulletin Signaletique Sciences Humaines: Section Reseau Documentaire en Sciences Humaines de la Santé.*

There is a thesaurus for this database.

Frost & Sullivan Market Research Reports
Frost & Sullivan Inc

16:66. Master record

Alternative name(s)	F & S Market Research Reports
Database type	Textual
Number of journals	
Sources	Research reports, Company reports, Journals, EEC statistics, Government statistics (US) and OECD statistics
Start year	1990
Language	English
Coverage	USA, Europe and Scandinavia
Number of records	1,500
Update size	—
Update period	Monthly

Keywords

Automotive Industry; Biotechnology; Chemical Substances; Data Processing; Electromedical Instrumentation; Defence; Electronics; Marketing; Manufacturing; Machinery; Packaging; Paper and Packaging; Plastics; Textiles

Description

The full text Frost and Sullivan market research report database providing comprehensive analyses of European and US industrial markets. Analysis of industrial markets is by product-group, end-user application and country. Market size, forecasts for a five year period, key suppliers and their market shares, plus current legislative issues are covered. Proprietary market information is provided on many specialist topics and product groups. Industrial areas analysed include chemicals, electromedical instrumentation, medical devices, pharmaceuticals, data processing, electronic components and test equipment, industrial automation, communications, defence, instrumentation and controls, plant and machinery, biotechnology, energy, environment, the automotive industries, paper, packaging, textiles and plastics.

The research reports are chiefly wrtten by independent industry consultants and are chiefly based on proprietary market research, supplemented by EEC and Government statistics, OECD statistics, company reports and journals. Much of this information is not covered by any other publisher. Reports are added to this database four months after publication in hard copy. Coverage is 50% USA and 50% Pan-European (including all EC countries, Scandinavia and other European countries).

16:67. Online — Data-Star

File name	FSMR
Alternative name(s)	F & S Market Research Reports
Start year	1990
Number of records	1,500
Update period	Monthly
Price/Charges	Subscription: UK£32.00
	Connect time: UK£68.40
	Online print: UK£3.33

Notes

From June 1993 Data-Star have introduced an annual fee/subscription per contract (that is, not per password) of SFr 80.00 (c.UK£ 32.00) payable every June. For North American customers billed in dollars who also use DIALOG, the DIALOG fee also covers access to Data-Star. Academic customers, 'commitment' customers and customers currently billed in dollars are exempt.

Frost & Sullivan Market Research Reports Summaries

Frost & Sullivan Inc

16:68. Master record

Alternative name(s)	F & S Market Research Reports Summaries
Database type	Bibliographic
Number of journals	
Sources	Research reports
Start year	Current 2–3 years
Language	English
Coverage	International
Number of records	409 documents
Update size	—
Update period	Monthly

Keywords

Chemical Substances; Defence; Electronics; Data Processing; Transport; Food and Drink; Manufacturing; Marketing; Machinery; Instrumentation; Pharmaceuticals; Drugs

Description

Contains citations, with detailed abstracts, to Frost & Sullivan market research reports. Reports provide analyses and forecasts of market size and share by product and company. Industries analysed include chemicals, communications, consumer products, data processing, defense, electronics, food, health, instrumentation, machinery and transportation. Includes forecasts by country for a five year period plus appraisal of technological developments and applications. Reports are written by consultants who are experts within their field.

The database contains only references to the full published Frost and Sullivan Market Research reports. Original reports may be obtained from Frost and Sullivan; each document records the report number and price information for the original report.

16:69. Online — Data-Star

File name	FSFS
Alternative name(s)	F & S Market Research Reports Summaries
Start year	Current 2–3 years
Number of records	409 documents
Update period	Monthly
Database aids	Data-Star Business Manual, Berne, Data-Star and Online manual (search NEWS-FSFS in NEWS)
Price/Charges	Subscription: UK£32.00
	Connect time: UK£40.00
	Online print: UK£0.30
	Offline print: UK£0.20

Notes

From June 1993 Data-Star have introduced an annual fee/subscription per contract (that is, not per password) of SFr 80.00 (c.UK£ 32.00) payable every June. For North American customers billed in dollars who also use DIALOG, the DIALOG fee also covers access to Data-Star. Academic customers, 'commitment' customers and customers currently billed in dollars are exempt.

General Practitioner

Haymarket Marketing Publications Ltd

16:70. Master record

Database type	Textual
Number of journals	3
Sources	Journals and newspapers
Start year	January 1987
Language	English
Coverage	International
Number of records	22,174
Update size	—
Update period	Varies with publication

Keywords

Clinical Medicine; General Practice; Primary Health Care

Description

General Practitioner contains the full text of three publications of interest to general practitioners and others involved in primary health care, nursing, or administration.

(1) *GP-General Practitioner* is the best-read newspaper for Britain's family doctors. It includes news coverage of medico-political matters, medical scientific developments and financial affairs and is seen as

a principal source of clinical, business and general news for GPs. *GP-General Practitioner* on GPGP is updated weekly.

(2)   *Mims Magazine* is the leading fortnightly journal for GPs and concentrates on issues relating to pharmaceutical developments, prescription trends, therapeutics and detection and analysis of side effects. It contains news items about new products together with indications and side-effects by outside experts including GPS. The journal is currently looking at the many issues concerned with prescribing under the GP contract and in particular is performing a systematic analysis of the cost-effectiveness of drugs in major therapeutic areas. *Mims Magazine* on GPGP is updated every fortnight.

(3)   *Medeconomics* is a journal covering the business, management, finance and organisational aspects of general practice within the British National Health Service. Subjects relate to the business efficiency of GPs practices and cover: taxation, pensions, control of practice expenses, accounting in the practice, computers, personal finance, surgery premises and the implications for the GP of major changes in government legislation. *Medeconomics* on GPGP is updated on a monthly basis.

16:71. Online   Data-Star

File name	GPGP
Start year	1987
Number of records	22,174
Update period	Varies with publication
Database aids	Data-Star Biomedical Manual and Data-Star Online Manual (search NEWS-GPGP in NEWS)
Price/Charges	Subscription: SFr80.00
	Connect time: SFr101.20
	Online print: SFr0.77
	Offline print: SFr1.58
	SDI charge: SFrNot applicable

Downloading is allowed

Notes

The special features paragraph lists additional pictorial and graphical information available in the original article but not reproduced online. The following special features are available: Charts, Figures, Illustrations, Photographs, Drawings, Graphs, Maps, Tables.

From June 1993 Data-Star have introduced an annual fee/subscription per contract (that is, not per password) of SFr 80.00 (c.UK£ 32.00) payable every June. For North American customers billed in dollars who also use DIALOG, the DIALOG fee also covers access to Data-Star. Academic customers, 'commitment' customers and customers currently billed in dollars are exempt.

Record composition

Accession Number and Update Code AN; Author(s) AU; Length of Document LE; Publication Date YD; Publication Month YM; Publication Year YR; Source SO; Special Feature(s) SF; Text TE; Title TI and Update Code UP

Health Care Competition Week
Capitol Publications Inc

16:72. Master record

Database type	Textual
Number of journals	1
Sources	Newsletters and Conference reports

Start year	1988
Language	English
Coverage	USA
Number of records	
Update size	—
Update period	Weekly

Keywords

Health Care Management

Description

Contains full text of *Health Care Competition Week*, a newsletter covering proven administrative and marketing strategies for hospitals, health maintenance organizations, and other health care providers to help them remain competitive in a rapidly changing market. Includes concise coverage of corporate developments and financial performance, issues in health care cost containment, industry statistics, cost-saving and money- making ideas for product lines, in depth conference reports, columns from health care experts, legislative news and earnings reports.

Corresponds to the weekly *Health Care Competition Week Newsletter*.

16:73. Online   CompuServe Information Service

File name	IQUEST File 2309
Start year	Current year
Number of records	
Update period	Weekly
Price/Charges	Subscription: US$8.95 per month Database entry fee: US$9/search; some databases carry a surcharge ($2–75) Online print: US$10 references free; then $9 per ten; abstracts $3 each

Downloading is allowed

Notes

Accessed via IQUEST or IQMEDICAL, this database is offered by a NewsNet gateway. IQUEST can either search across all databases, a database of the user's choice or selected multiple databases.

16:74. Online   NewsNet Inc

File name	
Start year	1988
Number of records	
Update period	Weekly

Notes

Monthly subscription to NewsNet required; differential charges for subscribers and non-subscribers to Health Care Competition Week.

This database can also be found on:
PTS Newsletter Database

Health Care Reform Week

16:79. Master record

Database type	Factual, Textual
Number of journals	
Sources	
Start year	
Language	English
Coverage	USA
Number of records	
Update size	—
Update period	Weekly

Keywords

Medicare; Health Care

Description

Focuses on policy making in Congress, Health and Human Services, and the Health Care Financing Administration, with a special emphasis on Medicare.

16:80. Online   CompuServe Information Service

File name	IQUEST File 3129
Start year	Current year
Number of records	
Update period	Weekly
Price/Charges	Subscription: US$8.95 per month
	Database entry fee: US$9/search;
	some databases carry a surcharge
	($2–75)
	Online print: US$10 references free;
	then $9 per ten; abstracts $3 each

Downloading is allowed

Notes

Accessed via IQUEST or IQMEDICAL, this database is offered by a NewsNet gateway. IQUEST can either search across all databases, a database of the user's choice or selected multiple databases.

16:81. Online   NewsNet Inc

File name	
Start year	
Number of records	
Update period	Weekly

Health Care
Mosgorsprawka

16:82. Master record

Database type	Reference
Number of journals	
Sources	
Start year	
Language	English
Coverage	USSR
Number of records	
Update size	–
Update period	

Keywords

Public Health

Description

General index of health care organisation in the USSR.

16:83. Diskette   Mosgorsprawka

File name	
Start year	
Number of records	
Update period	

Health Industry Research Reports
JA Micropublishing Inc

16:84. Master record

Database type	Bibliographic
Number of journals	
Sources	Reports and Research communications
Start year	1982
Language	English
Coverage	International

Number of records	6,000
Update size	–
Update period	Quarterly

Description

Contains citations, with abstracts, to research reports issued by about seventy security and investment firms on the health industry and individual industry firms. Covers hospital management, pharmaceuticals, medical hardware, life insurance, hospitals, and health care. Citations include title, author, publisher, date, and for companies, geographic location and product listings. Each abstract contains a description of the type of statistical data to be found in the original article.

Users can order full text of documents online.

16:85. Online   BRS, Morning Search, BRS/Colleague

File name	HIRR
Start year	1982
Number of records	6,000
Update period	Quarterly

Health Planning and Administration
National Library of Medicine American Hospital Association

16:86. Master record

Database type	Bibliographic
Number of journals	225
Sources	Book chapters, databases (NLM), journals, monographs, reports and theses
Start year	1975
Language	English
Coverage	International
Number of records	623,372
Update size	40,000
Update period	Monthly
Abstract details	Author
Thesaurus	Medical Subject Headings (MeSH)
Database aids	MeSH Tree Structures, Permuted MeSH and List of Serials Indexed for Online Users (LSIOU).

Keywords

Health Care Administration; Management

Description

Health Planning and Administration database, which is produced by the National Library of Medicine in co-operation with the American Hospital Association, contains citations to the worldwide literature on the non-clinical aspects of health care planning. Subjects covered within this field include health care administration and facilities, health insurance, financial management, personnel administration, quality issues, manpower planning, legal aspects, licensure, accreditation and health maintenance organisations (HMOs) and related topics. According to the Data-Star manual the database can be used to: ascertain the financial impact of AIDS on health care systems since 1987; discover what training programs are available for hospital administrators; monitor recent developments in home-care services; establish budgeting guidelines in specialist clinics and plan 3-year manpower requirements for new medical departments.

Printed sources include: *Hospital Literature Index* (1975–), this being the hard-copy counterpart of Health Planning and Administration; *Index Medicus*; *International Nursing Index*; *Index To Dental Literature*; *Weekly Government Abstracts: Health Planning Series* (produced by the National Health Planning Information Center (NHPIC))(1975–1981). Approximately eighty per cent of references are drawn from the MEDLINE database (from 1975 onwards) and the structure, indexing rules and search strategy are therefore almost identical with MEDLINE. MeSH Supplementary Chemical Records (TE,CR,EZ) and Gene Symbols (GE) are not used in HEALTH. Approximately fifty per cent of the citations contain abstracts prepared by authors. The database includes about 400 English-language periodicals of the Special Health List evaluated by the American Hospital Association as well as some records of English-language periodicals evaluated by the Association of American Medical Colleges (prior to 1979). Documents (9,451 records 1975–1981) from the National Health Planning Information Center (NHPIC) were added in May 1983 covering documents such as monographs, technical reports and dissertations but not periodicals and these account for about two per cent of all citations. These citations have additional fields which are marked NHPIC only. The Noted field is used in references derived from NHPIC to refer to related documents, or the presence of identification numbers. In MEDLINE-derived records this field is used to note the presence of a comment to an article published in the same journal. A secondary source field is composed of an abbreviation for the secondary supplier: MED/ (MEDLINE); AHA/ (American Hospital Association); NP/ (National Health Planning Information Centre); and AAMC/ (Association of American Medical Colleges). Records which are duplicated in MEDLINE can be eliminated by combining the last search statement with those articles unique to the Health database. On DIALOG this is done by SF=HEALTH and on BRS by using H.LI. On NLM search as H(LI) or AHA (SI) for the Hospital Literature Index citations and NP (SI) for the NHPIC citations.

Sources include journals covered in MEDLINE (see); journals reviewed for the American Hospital Association's *Hospital Literature Index* back to 1975; and since 1983 monographs, monograph chapters, theses, and technical reports supplied by the National Health Planning Information Center from *Weekly Government Abstracts: Health Planning Series*, plus additional journals of special importance to the health field.

16:87. Online — Australian MEDLINE Network

File name	Health Planning and Administration
Start year	
Number of records	
Update period	

16:88. Online — BLAISE-LINK

File name	HEALTH
Start year	1975
Number of records	
Update period	Monthly

16:89. Online — BRS, Morning Search, BRS/Colleague

File name	HLTH
Start year	1975
Number of records	623,372
Update period	Monthly

Price/Charges	Connect time: US$26.00/36.00
	Online print: US$0.07/0.15
	Offline print: US$0.20
	SDI charge: US$5.10

Notes

It is possible to discover records which are unique to the HEALTH database and eliminate those which duplicate MEDLINE records by using H.LI.

16:90. Online — CISTI MEDLARS

File name	Health Planning and Administration
Start year	1975
Number of records	623,372
Update period	Monthly

16:91. Online — CompuServe Information Service

File name	IQUEST File 1234
Start year	1975
Number of records	623,372
Update period	Monthly
Price/Charges	Subscription: US$8.95 per month
	Database entry fee: US$9/search; some databases carry a surcharge ($2–75)
	Online print: US$10 references free; then $9 per ten; abstracts $3 each

Downloading is allowed

Notes

Accessed via IQUEST or IQMEDICAL, this database is offered by a BRS gateway. IQUEST can either search across all databases, a database of the user's choice or selected multiple databases.

16:92. Online — Data-Star

File name	HLPA
Start year	1975
Number of records	623,372
Update period	Monthly
Database aids	Tree Structures, Permuted MeSH and Data-Star Guide to HLPA in Data-Star Biomedical Manual

Thesaurus is online

Notes

HLPA is offered on behalf of and in co-operation with the Swiss Academy of Medical Sciences and its documentation service DOKDI. The command DOCZ will retrieve the total number of documents currently on the database; documents with abstracts can be located by AB=AB. Qualify single source names to .SO., but use the hyphenated NLM journal abbreviation to search multi-word sources. Use .ROOT to locate abbreviations or search on ISSN. The NHPIC subfile contains non-journal sources and users should search free text within this subset.

From June 1993 Data-Star have introduced an annual fee/subscription per contract (that is, not per password) of SFr 80.00 (c.UK£ 32.00) payable every June. For North American customers billed in dollars who also use DIALOG, the DIALOG fee also covers access to Data-Star. Academic customers, 'commitment' customers and customers currently billed in dollars are exempt.

Record composition

Abstract AB; Accession Number and Secondary Source identification AN; Author(s) AU; Country of Publication ZN; Descriptors (MeSH subheadings) DE; Entry Date on NLM Computer ED; Index Month IM; Institution IN; Journal Code JC; Journal Subset SB; Language LG; Major Descriptor Term MJ; Minor

Descriptor Term MN; Personal Name as Source PN; Publication Type PT; Secondary Source SI; Source SO; Special List Indicator LI; Title of Article TI; Transliterated Title TT and Year of Publication YR

16:93. Online   DIALOG, Knowledge Index

File name	File 151
Start year	1975
Number of records	569,202
Update period	Monthly
Price/Charges	Connect time: US$36.00
	Online print: US$0.12
	Offline print: US$0.12
	SDI charge: US$5.25

Notes

This database is also available to home users during evenings and weekends at a reduced rate on the Knowledge Index service of DIALOG – file name in this case is Health Planning and Administration, and searches are made with simplified commands or menus.

It is possible to discover records which are unique to the HEALTH database and eliminate those which duplicate MEDLINE records by using SF=HEALTH.

16:94. Online   DIMDI

File name	HE75
Start year	1975
Number of records	629,357
Update period	Monthly
SDI period	1 month
Database aids	User Manual, List of Serials Indexed for Online Users and Memocard Health
Price/Charges	Connect time: UK£05.84–10.58
	Online print: UK£0.17–0.35
	Offline print: UK£0.09–0.15

Downloading is allowed
Thesaurus is online

Notes

There is menu-driven guidance available in German and English.

Record composition

Abstract AB; Abstract Source AS; Author AU; Book Title BTI; Classification Code CC; Corporate Source CS; Controlled Term CT; Country CY; Document Type DT; Entry Date ED; Freetext FT; Gene Symbol GE (from 1991); Index Medicus Date IMD; Journal Title Code JC; Journal Title JT (abbreviation); Language LA; Last Revision Date LR; Number of Document ND; Number of Grant NG; Notes NO; Order Number OD; Procurement Source PC; Personal Name as Subject PS; Publisher PU; Publication Year PY; Qualifier QF; Number of References RN; Supporting Agency SA; Secondary Source SEC; Source SO; ISSN SS; Subunit SU; Type of Award TA and Title TI

The DIMDI implimentation of the *MeSH thesaurus* allows bilingual access and the hierarchical structure makes it possible to search for a whole group of related descriptors in one step. The Source field is a composite containing the journal title, the volume and issue number, publication year, etc.

Documents may be ordered online from the British Library Document Supply Centre, Zentralbibliothek der Medizin, Köln, Bayerische Staatsbibliothek München, and Koninklijke Nederlandse Akademie van Wetenschapen, Amsterdam. The basic index includes the fields: Title, Abstract and Controlled Term.

16:95. Online   National Library of Medicine

File name	Health Planning and Administration
Start year	1975
Number of records	623,372
Update period	Monthly

Notes

It is possible to discover records which are unique to the HEALTH database and eliminate those which duplicate MEDLINE records by using H(LI) or AHA(SI) for the Hospital Literature Index citations and NP(SI) for the NHPIC citations.

16:96. CD-ROM   CD Plus

File name	CD Plus/Health Planning and Administration
Format notes	IBM
Software	OVID 3.0
Start year	1975
Number of records	569,202
Update period	Monthly
Price/Charges	Subscription: UK£845

Downloading is allowed

Notes

Offers the ability to limit by local journal holdings. For the experienced searcher, the software offers *MeSH* explodes, 'personal pre-explodes' for frequently exploded terms, SDIs and Save Searches, enhanced MeSH tree structures, and emulation of National Library of Medicine and dot-dot syntax.

Record composition

Author; Institution; Title; Sponsoring Agencies; Original Titles and Grant Numbers

This database has an index of all searchable terms together with the online *MeSh Thesaurus* which offers mapping from natural language to MeSH – a facility which should give significantly improved precision for the inexperienced searcher. The on-screen help provides scope notes, definitions and task descriptors.

16:97. CD-ROM   Compact Cambridge

File name	Health: Planning and Administration
Format notes	IBM
Start year	Most recent ten years
Number of records	350,000
Update period	Quarterly
Price/Charges	Subscription: UK£515

Thesaurus is online
The disc includes a thesaurus of MeSH terms.

16:98. CD-ROM   EBSCO

File name	Health Planning and Administration/EBSCO CD
Format notes	IBM
Start year	1975
Number of records	475,000
Update period	Quarterly
Price/Charges	Subscription: US$795

Notes

Searching is performed by a fill-in-the-blanks screen called a Query Profile which supports full Boolean logic. Search SDIs can be stored for reuse and local titles can be flagged so that these a highlighted on a display of records following a search. The software also monitors journal usage and numbers of searches performed to aid in the management of user collections.

16:99. CD-ROM — SilverPlatter

File name	HealthPLAN-CD
Format notes	IBM, Mac
Software	SPIRS/MacSPIRS
Start year	1981
Number of records	432,000
Update period	Quarterly
Database aids	Quick Reference Card and SilverPlatter Manual
Price/Charges	Subscription: UK£685 – 1,025
Thesaurus is online	

Notes

Like MEDLINE on SilverPlatter, HealthPLAN supports explodable thesaurus terms (broader headings plus their narrower related terms); the only shortcoming of the system is that HealthPLAN does not automatically map search terms to the preferred term. Nicholas G Tomaiuolo reviewed HealthPLAN (CD-ROM World 8(4) 1993 77–81) and felt that the disc would be a natural complement to the SilverPlatter MEDLINE database, the more especially as it has the ability when searching to exclude MEDLINE references. He gave a rating of four (very good) out of five and noted the principal shortcomings as its 'redundant method of searching (where each stage of a search query receives a number with postings) and the inconvenient manner of changing defaults during browsing and printing routines. Pluses include super easy installation, handy online thesaurus tools, very good technical support and SilverPlatter's cooperative and helpful customer service and sales department.'

The regular subscription for the CD-ROM is £685 for single users and £1,028 for 2–8 networked users. It is also available for loading on to a hard disc – cost is £1,028 for 2–8 netorked users, £1,370 for 9–16 users, £1,713 for 17–24 users. The fee for the hard disc is US$2,000.

This CD-ROM database has an index of all searchable terms together with the online MeSh Thesaurus which contains three tools: an alphabetical list of permuted terms, selected term detail and MeSH trees.

16:100. Fixed disk — SilverPlatter

File name	HealthPLAN
Format notes	IBM
Software	SPIRS
Start year	1975
Number of records	432,000
Update period	Quarterly
Database aids	Quick Reference Card and SilverPlatter Manual
Price/Charges	Subscription: UK£1,028 – 1,713

Notes

Contains the entire database. This database is available on fixed disk, with updates supplied on CD-ROM. This means that up to thirty networked users can have access to a single file containing the complete database – cost is £1,028 for 2–8 networked users, £1,370 for 9–16 users, £1,713 for 17–24 users. The fee for the hard disk is US$2,000. Search speeds are up to ten times faster than CD-ROM searching.

This database has an index of all searchable terms together with the online MeSh Thesaurus which contains three tools: an alphabetical list of permuted terms, selected term detail and MeSH trees.

16:101. Tape — National Library of Medicine

File name	Health Planning and Administration
Start year	1975
Number of records	623,372
Update period	Monthly

Notes

It is possible to discover records which are unique to the HEALTH database and eliminate those which duplicate MEDLINE records by using H(LI) or AHA(SI) for the Hospital Literature Index citations and NP(SI) for the NHPIC citations.

Corresponds to the Health Planning and Administration online database.

For more details of constituent databases, see:
MEDLINE

Healthcare Evaluation System
National Planning Data Corporation

16:104. Master record

Database type	Directory, Statistical
Number of journals	
Sources	
Start year	Current year
Language	English
Coverage	USA
Number of records	
Update size	—
Update period	Varies (see notes)

Description

Contains information on health care facilities, including hospitals, nursing homes, home health agencies, health maintenance organizations (HMOs), outpatient and ambulatory care facilities, and freestanding emergency clinics (FECs). Provides facility name and address; number of beds; number of patients, including Medicare and Medicaid patients; average length of stay; types of services offered; and the number and types of surgical procedures performed. Also includes information on approval and accreditation and type of control (for example, non-profit/church owned, county government, investor-owned). Information can be retrieved for individual facilities and for all facilities by ZIP code or county.

Source of data is SMG Marketing Group Inc. Updating: Hospital data, quarterly; HMO, FEC, ambulatory care facility, and home health agency data, annually; nursing home data, periodically, as new data become available.

16:105. Online — National Planning Data Corporation

File name	
Start year	Current year
Number of records	
Update period	Varies (see notes)

Healthcare Financial Management
Healthcare Financial Management Association

16:106. Master record

Database type	Textual, Factual
Number of journals	1
Sources	Journal

Start year 1989
Language English
Coverage USA (primarily)
Number of records
Update size —
Update period Monthly
Index unit Articles and Reviews

Keywords

Hospital Management

Description

Covers the administrative and financial procedures of hospital management.

IAC editorial criteria for the database include feature articles listed in the table of contents plus book reviews of 200 words or more.

16:107. Online Mead Data Central (as a NEXIS database)

File name HLTFIN – NEXIS
Start year 1989
Number of records
Update period Monthly
Delay 2–5 weeks
Price/Charges Subscription: US$1,000 – 3,000 (Depending on needs) Connect time: US$49.00 (Telecomms + connect time) Database entry fee: US$6.00 (Search charge) Online print: US$0.04 per line

Notes

Libraries: INSURE and NEXIS; Group files: ALLINS, MAGS, FIN, CURRNT, ARCHIV, OMNI and ASAP.

On NEXIS, this journal is available as a part of ASAP Publications.

A subscription charge which covers all transactional charges, connect time, telecommunications and the small administration charge can take the place of the individual charges. Subscriptions are negotiated with customers and vary according to the number of menus (thus, files) that are to be used – typically a minimum subscription would be about US$ 1,000. All charges include training and a 24-hour help line.

Record composition

Publication PUBLICATION; Subject SUBJECT; Date DATE; Section SECTION; Terms TERMS; Type TYPE; Body BODY; Byline BYLINE; Company COMPANY; Geographic GEOGRAPHIC; Graphic GRAPHIC; Headline HEADLINE; Headline and Lead HLEAD; Lead LEAD; Length LENGTH; Name NAME and Product Name PRODUCT-NAME

This database can also be found on:
NEXIS

HECLINET

Deutsches Krankenhausinstitut eV (DKI)

Technische Universitaet Berlin, Institut für Krankenhausbau (IFK)

16:109. Master record

Alternative name(s) Health Care Literature Information Network
Database type Bibliographic
Number of journals
Sources Bibliographies, conference proceedings, dissertations, grey literature, journals, monographs, newspapers, reports, standards and theses
Start year 1969
Language Original language (titles), Original language (abstracts), English (abstracts), English (titles), German (abstracts), German (titles), English (index terms) and German (index terms)
Coverage International
Number of records 97,879
Update size 4,500
Update period Every two months
Abstract details HECLINET staff
Thesaurus Thesaurus Krankenhauswesen (1988, 6th revision)
Database aids Kompendium HELCINETInformationsdienst Krankenhauswesen/Health Care Information Service

Keywords

Health Economics; Health Services; Hospital Hygiene

Description

HECLINET contains citations, with abstracts, to the worldwide literature on hospital administration and non-clinical aspects of health services. 80% of the records derive from journals. Subjects in the area of hospital literature covered include hospital architecture; hospital planning; hospital operation and organisation; accounting; hospital information systems; hospital technology; hospital financing; hospital hygiene and sanitation. Subjects within the non-clinical literature in the neighbouring areas of health care include education and training; regional planning; organisation and management; health economics; health policy; hospital insurance; planning; law and jurisdiction.

The database corresponds in part to *Informationsdienst Krankenhauswesen (Health Care Information Service)* which is produced every two months. Up to 1980, 90% of all entries in the database were available in the printed version but after 1981 this was reduced to 60%. The database is produced in co-operation with the hospital institutes of Austria, Denmark, Sweden and Switzerland and the following institutions which belong to the HECLINET network participate in the evaluation of the sources: Dansk Sygehus Institut (DSI); Österreichishes, Bundesinstitut für Gesundheitswesen (OEBIG); Schweizerisches Institut für Gesundheitsund Krankenhauswesen (SKI); Sjukvardens och socialvardens planerings och rationaliseringsinstitut (SPRI); Centrum Medyczne Ksztalcenia Podyplomowego (CMW). Approximately 34% of the records contain an abstract of between 100 and 500 words. An additional 20% of the records contain an annotation consisting of a one or two sentence statement augmenting the information contained in the title or elaborating on the relevance of the documents. The annotations have three main purposes: (1) they give more precise hospital descriptions including the number of beds, spaces or specialisations; (2) they provide references to a conference if the item concerned is a copy of a lecture; (3) they indicate continuations and secondary or supplementary publications. The sources evaluated for inclusion include: 300 journals on hospital and health care (a shortened version of the list of journals appears annually in the first issue of *Informationsdienst Krankenhauswesen*); 200 journals on architecture, city planning and construction engineering (the reference section on documentation on Dokumentation Gebäudelehre of the Universitätsbibliothek of the Technische Universität Berlin provides a special referral service for these journals); twenty journals from the area of Operations Research, selected by the Betriebswirtschaftliche Institut der Universität Erlangen/Nürnberg and 600 economic journals examined and made available by the Wirtschaftswissenschaftliche Documentation der Technischen Universität Berlin. Approximately 50% of the records are in German, 30% in English, 5.6% in French, 3.5% in Scandinavian languages and 2.5% in Dutch. The accepted form of journal title is provided in the list of original citations in the Kompensium Heclinet together with the original publication place. For non-German/English titles a translation is given in parentheses preceded by an abbreviated form of the original language title.

Covers journals in the fields of health care, economics, architecture, and operations research.

The unit record contains bibliographic data including author(s), title architect, plus controlled vocabulary terms, geographic terms, additional subject information and an abstract. The *Thesaurus Krankenhauswesen* which is used for indexing is a comprehensive, hierarchically structured dictionary and contains approximately 1,100 descriptors and 2,500 cross-references. 71 of the descriptors serve individually or in combination as sorting aids and are used for the general content structuring of the printed version of the *Informationsdienst Krankenhauswesen/Health Care Information Service*. Certain descriptor groups can be expanded with numerical additions. For example most of the subcategories of the descriptor hospital give the number of beds and some descriptors can be augmented by the year. The Annual Indexers' Conference of the HECLINET Network determines additions, deletions or alterations to the descriptors and these are put into effect in the following volume of the Informationsdienst Krankenhauswesen except in cases of urgency when they are carried out via round-robin correspondence coordinated by the Institut für Krankenhausbau. Only original documents (primary sources) are selected and evaluated and the indexing is carried out by professional specialists in the respective fields such as architects, economists and planners. The leading professional journals from each country are given priority in the evaluation procedure.

16:110. Online   DIMDI

File name	HN69
Alternative name(s)	Health Care Literature Information Network
Software	GRIPS
Start year	1969
Number of records	97,879
Update period	Every two months
Delay	2–4 months
SDI period	2 months
Price/Charges	Connect time: UK£15.80–20.55
	Online print: UK£0.32–0.50
	Offline print: UK£0.23–0.30

Downloading is allowed
Thesaurus is online

Notes

Suppliers of online documents: British Library Document Supply Centre, Boston Spa, England; Bayerische Staatsbibliothek München, München, Germany; Harkers Information Retrieval System, Sydney, Australia; Zentralbibliothek und TIB, Hannover, Germany. Menu driven guidance is available in German and English. Searches are possible from January 1969.

Record composition

Abstract AB; Abstract Language AL; Additional Source Information ASI; Architect AR; Author AU; Classification Code CC; Controlled Term CT; Document Type DT; Entry Date ED; Free Text FT; Geographical Heading GH; Journal Title JT; Language LA; Location LO; Location0 LO0; Number of Document ND; Number of Document, Identifier NDI; Publication Place PP; Publication Year PY; Qualifier QF; Subject Heading SH; Source SO and Title TI

The unit record contains bibliographic data including author(s), title architect, plus controlled vocabulary terms, geographic terms, additional subject information and an abstract. The *Thesaurus Krankenhauswesen* is available online from DIMDI in both German and English. The Subject Headings consist of individual descriptors or combinations of two descriptors and are used in the general content structuring of the printed version of the *Informationsdienst Krankenhauswesen/Health Care Information Service* and can also be used for online searching. The Geographical Headings refer to the geographical designations which are treated or referred to in the corresponding document and can consist of continents, parts of continents, countries, regional subdivisions or cities. The Additional Source Information includes illustrations, tables, diagrams and other aids included in the text. The basic index includes the data fields: Title, Abstract, Controlled Term, Controlled Term German, Section Heading, Section Heading German, Geographical Heading and Geographical Heading German. Freetext searches can be conducted in German or English.

Hospital Admissions Records for Canada
Health & Welfare Canada

16:111. Master record

Database type	Statistical
Number of journals	
Sources	Medical Records
Start year	
Language	English
Coverage	Canada
Number of records	
Update size	—
Update period	

Description

Contains about 70% of all hospital admissions records in Canada during the last ten years. Used for internal disease surveillance research.

16:112. CD-ROM   Health & Welfare Canada

File name	Hospital Admissions Records for Canada
Format notes	IBM

Start year
Number of records
Update period

Notes
Currently on a set of six discs.

Hospital Database
Urban Decision Systems Inc (UDS)

16:113. Master record
Database type	Directory, Factual, Textual, Numeric
Number of journals	
Sources	
Start year	Current information
Language	English
Coverage	USA
Number of records	
Update size	—
Update period	Periodically, as new data become available.

Description
Contains information on US hospitals and their utilisation. Gives hospital name, address and phone number, manager's name, type of hospital, type of control (for example, investor-owned, county) and approval and accreditation. Utilisation data include admissions and emergency visits, inpatient and outpatient surgical procedures, bed occupancy rate, average length of stay per patient, beds per ward (for example, paediatric, cardiac, cancer), and staffed versus unstaffed beds. Also includes data on each facility's market area demographics, including population, age distribution, sex and income.

Corresponds in part to *Hospital Market Atlas*, published by SMG Marketing Group Inc.

16:114. Online   STSC Inc
File name	
Start year	Current information
Number of records	
Update period	Periodically, as new data become available.

Notes
Monthly minimum subscription of $5 to STSC required.

Hospital Morbidity
Innotech
Health & Welfare Canada

16:115. Master record
Database type	Textual, Statistical
Number of journals	
Sources	Government documents
Start year	1989–1990
Language	English
Coverage	Canada
Number of records	
Update size	—
Update period	Annually

Description
Contains patient records from the Health Protection branch for statistical analysis.

16:116. CD-ROM   Innotech
File name	Hospital Morbidity
Format notes	IBM, Mac
Software	FindIt
Start year	1989–1990
Number of records	
Update period	Annually

Hospitals
American Hospital Publishing Inc

16:117. Master record
Alternative name(s)	Journal of American Hospital Association
Database type	Textual, Factual
Number of journals	1
Sources	Newsletter
Start year	1983
Language	English
Coverage	International
Number of records	
Update size	—
Update period	Twice per week
Index unit	Articles

Keywords
Hospital Management; Marketing; Health Care Management

Description
Hospitals, formerly the *Journal of American Hospital Association*, is written for health care executives. The newsletter focuses on practice and problems in health care management. It also covers all aspects of hospital management, including legislation, finance, marketing, long-term care, service management, technology, policy and planning and information management. Articles focus on the economic aspects of medical quality, business management and medical care.

16:118. Online   CompuServe Information Service
File name	IQUEST File 7135
Alternative name(s)	Journal of American Hospital Association
Start year	1983
Number of records	
Update period	Twice per week
Price/Charges	Subscription: US$8.95 per month Database entry fee: US$9/search; some databases carry a surcharge ($2–75) Online print: US$10 references free; then $9 per ten; abstracts $3 each

Downloading is allowed

Notes
Accessed via IQUEST or IQMEDICAL, this database is offered by a DIALOG gateway; on DIALOG it forms a part of the Trade and Industry ASAP database. IQUEST can either search across all databases, a database of the user's choice or selected multiple databases.

16:119. Online   Mead Data Central (as a NEXIS database)
File name	HOSPTL – NEXIS
Alternative name(s)	Journal of American Hospital Association
Start year	1983

Number of records	
Update period	Twice per week
Delay	2–5 weeks
Price/Charges	Subscription: US$1,000 – 3,000
	(Depending on needs)
	Connect time: US$49.00
	(Telecomms + connect time)
	Database entry fee: US$6.00
	(Search charge)
	Online print: US$0.04 per line

Notes

Library: NEXIS; Group files: BUS, CURRNT, ARCHIV, OMNI and ASAP

On NEXIS, this journal is available as a part of ASAP Publications.

A subscription charge which covers all transactional charges, connect time, telecommunications and the small administration charge can take the place of the individual charges. Subscriptions are negotiated with customers and vary according to the number of menus (thus, files) that are to be used – typically a minimum subscription would be about US$ 1,000. All charges include training and a 24-hour help line.

Record composition

Publication PUBLICATION; Subject SUBJECT; Date DATE; Section SECTION; Terms TERMS; Type TYPE; Body BODY; Byline BYLINE; Company COMPANY; Geographic GEOGRAPHIC; Graphic GRAPHIC; Headline HEADLINE; Headline and Lead HLEAD; Lead LEAD; Length LENGTH; Name NAME and Product Name PRODUCT-NAME

This database can also be found on:
NEXIS

JCAH Perspectives
Joint Commission on Accreditation of Hospitals

16:121. Master record

Alternative name(s)	Joint Commission on Accreditation of Hospitals Perspectives
Database type	Textual, Factual, Bibliographic
Number of journals	1
Sources	Newsletter
Start year	1984
Language	English
Coverage	USA
Number of records	
Update size	—
Update period	Twice per month

Keywords

Standards; Medical Education

Description

The official bi-monthly newsletter of the Joint Commission on Accreditation of Hospitals provides up-to-date information about JCAH and its accreditation programmes, including changes in standards, policies and procedures. Also featured are explanations of surveys and accreditation procedures and any announcements concerning JCAH's publications and education programmes.

16:122. Online — Mead Data Central (as a NEXIS database)

File name	PERS – NEXIS
Alternative name(s)	Joint Commission on Accreditation of Hospitals Perspectives
Start year	1984

Number of records	
Update period	Twice per month
Delay	2–3 weeks
Price/Charges	Subscription: US$1,000 – 3,000
	(Depending on needs)
	Connect time: US$49.00
	(Telecomms + connect time)
	Database entry fee: US$20.00
	(Search charge)
	Online print: US$0.04 per line

Notes

Library: HEALTH; Group file: JCAHO.

A subscription charge which covers all transactional charges, connect time, telecommunications and the small administration charge can take the place of the individual charges. Subscriptions are negotiated with customers and vary according to the number of menus (thus, files) that are to be used – typically a minimum subscription would be about US$ 1,000. All charges include training and a 24-hour help line.

Record composition

Publication; Cite; Date; Section; Length; Title; Source; Author; Series; Abstract (SUM-ABS); Text; Additional information (SUPP-INFO); Reference (BIBLIO-REF); Graphic; Correction and Correction Date

This database can also be found on:
NEXIS

Journal of Health Care Marketing
American Marketing Association

16:124. Master record

Database type	Textual, Factual
Number of journals	1
Sources	Journal
Start year	1991
Language	English
Coverage	International
Number of records	
Update size	—
Update period	Quarterly

Keywords

Health Care Marketing; Health Care Management

Description

The *Journal of Health Care Marketing* is one of the leaders in this highly specialised and dynamic industry. It provides its users with the latest examples of research and practice, techniques and applications in the health services profession. In addition, it provides a forum for practitioners and academics to discuss the numerous ideas that can enhance and improve upon increased profitability of health care institutions and the job performance of the professional. Information is presented that will contribute to the marketing knowledge by: providing the strategic planning framework to enhance the marketing mix; present creative and practical applications of marketing techniques to health care issues; and offers current and respected research and discussions of health care professionals.

The *Journal of Health Care Marketing* is the official publication of the Academy of Health Services Marketing; a wholly-owned subsidiary of the American Marketing Association.

16:125. Online   Mead Data Central (as a NEXIS database)

File name   JNLHCM – NEXIS
Start year   1991
Number of records
Update period   Quarterly
Delay   Within 30 days
Price/Charges   Subscription: US$1,000 – 3,000
(Depending on needs)
Connect time: US$49.00
(Telecomms + connect time)
Database entry fee: US$6.00
(Search charge)
Online print: US$0.04 per line

Notes

Libraries: MARKET and NEXIS; Group files: ALLMKT, CURMKT, OMNI, CURRNT, MAGS and BUS.

A subscription charge which covers all transactional charges, connect time, telecommunications and the small administration charge can take the place of the individual charges. Subscriptions are negotiated with customers and vary according to the number of menus (thus, files) that are to be used – typically a minimum subscription would be about US$ 1,000. All charges include training and a 24-hour help line.

Record composition

Publication; Date; Section; Length; Headline; Byline; Highlight; Lead; Body; Graphic; Correction; Correction Date and Bibliography

This database can also be found on:
NEXIS

LabNet
IMS America Ltd, Hospital/Laboratory/Veterinary Database Division

16:127. Master record

Database type   Textual
Number of journals
Sources
Start year   Current 6 years
Language   English
Coverage   Continental US
Number of records
Update size   —
Update period   Hospital purchase, monthly; private lab purchase, quarterly

Keywords

Diagnostic Products; Marketing

Description

Contains sales data on diagnostic products (for example, test kits, reagents) purchased by about 350 hospitals and 220 private laboratories. Includes projected nationwide product sales in dollars and units, average price per unit, product market share and sales trends.

Corresponds to *IMS Diagnostic Market-Hospital and Private Labs*.

16:128. Online   IMS America Ltd

File name   LabNet (IMS)
Start year   Current 6 years

Number of records
Update period   Hospital purchase, monthly; private lab purchase, quarterly

Notes

Subscription to *IMS Diagnostic Market-Hospital and Private Labs* required.

Lithium Consultation
University of Wisconsin-Madison, Department of Psychiatry, Lithium Information Center

16:129. Master record

Database type   Textual, Computer software
Number of journals
Sources
Start year   Current information
Language   English
Coverage   International
Number of records
Update size   —
Update period   Periodically, as new data become available

Keywords

Biochemistry; Lithium – Pharmacology; Patient Management

Description

Contains information to help physicians select patients suitable for treatment with lithium and to help in patient management. Patient data are input and information is retrieved on the patient's suitability for treatment, expected responsiveness, possible contraindications, procedures for initiating lithium therapy, managing side-effects and alternative treatments.

16:130. Online   University of Wisconsin-Madison, Department of Psychiatry, Lithium Information Center

File name
Start year   Current information
Number of records
Update period   Periodically, as new data become available

Managed Care Law Outlook
Capitol Publications Inc

16:131. Master record

Database type   Bibliographic, Textual
Number of journals   1
Sources   Newsletter
Start year   1989
Language   English
Coverage   USA
Number of records
Update size   —
Update period   Monthly

Keywords

Health Insurance; Health Care Management

Description

Features briefings and analysis of important legal issues affecting health maintenance organisations (HMOs), preferred provider organizations (PPOs) and benefit options, along with coverage of important court cases, decisions and legal and legislative trends involving management care systems. Also includes a calendar of events.

Corresponds to the monthly newsletter *Managed Care Law Outlook*. DIALOG and Data-Star are available on PTS Newsletter Database, supplied by Predicasts.

Notes

Monthly subscription to NewsNet required; differential charges for subscribers and non-subscribers to the printed newsletter.

16:132. Online   NewsNet Inc

File name	
Start year	l989
Number of records	
Update period	Monthly

Notes

Monthly subscription to NewsNet required; differential charges for subscribers and non-subscribers to the printed newsletter.

This database can also be found on:
PTS Newsletter Database

Managed Care Outlook
Capitol Publications Inc

16:134. Master record

Database type	Bibliographic, Textual
Number of journals	1
Sources	Newsletter, Conference proceedings and Case studies
Start year	1988 (Jan 8)
Language	English
Coverage	USA
Number of records	
Update size	—
Update period	Every two weeks
Index unit	Articles

Keywords

Health Care Management; Information Systems

Description

Contains the full text of *Managed Care Outlook*, a newsletter which provides health care executives with business briefing on all aspects of the managed health care industry. Covers health maintenance organizations (HMOs), preferred provider organizations (PPOs) triple E-option plans, utilisation reviews, information systems and contracting. Also covers mergers and acquisitions, industry trends, regional, legal and policy news, conferences coverage, case studies and employer evaluations of health plans.

Corresponds to the twice monthly publication *Managed Care Outlook*. DIALOG and Data-Star are available on PTS Newsletter Database, supplied by Predicasts.

16:135. Online   NewsNet Inc

File name	
Start year	1988 (Jan 8)

Number of records	
Update period	Every two weeks

Notes

Monthly subscription to NewsNet required; differential charges for subscribers and non-subscribers to *Managed Care Outlook*.

This database can also be found on:
PTS Newsletter Database

Managed Care Report
Atlantic Information Services Inc
Predicasts International Inc

16:137. Master record

Database type	Bibliographic, Textual
Number of journals	1
Sources	Newsletter
Start year	Data-Star and DIALOG 1988; NewsNet Aug 1988
Language	English
Coverage	USA
Number of records	
Update size	—
Update period	Monthly

Keywords

Employee Benefits; Health Care Management

Description

Contains full text of *Managed Care Report*, a newsletter on the prepaid health care industry, covering news of business developments and federal compliance activities of HMOs (health maintenance organisations, PPOs (preferred provider organisations), and other managed care companies. It focuses on federal managed care laws and regulations developed in the US Congress and at HCFA, OMB, DOD and OPM. Also covered are case studies of cost-effective programs, impact of programs on employee benefit plans and managed care news of employers, insurers and providers.

Corresponds to *Managed Care Report* newsletter. DIALOG and Data-Star are available on PTS Newsletter Database, supplied by Predicasts.

16:138. Online   NewsNet Inc

File name	
Start year	1988
Number of records	
Update period	Monthly

Notes

Monthly subscription to NewsNet required; differential charges for subscribers and non-subscribers *Managed Care Report*

This database can also be found on:
PTS Newsletter Database

Medical and Psychological Previews
BRS Information Technologies

16:140. Master record

Database type	Bibliographic
Number of journals	240
Sources	Journals

Start year
Language English
Coverage
Number of records 19,500
Update size 7,000
Update period
Hosts have included BRS (until 30.9.92.)

Description

Gives bibliographic citations from 240 core medical journals prior to their appearance in MEDLINE. Covers: clinical medicine, psychology, psychiatry, nursing, hospital administration. Includes editorials, notes and letters. Covers the last four months.

BRS discontinued this database at the end of September 1992.

Ministerie WVC

Netherlands Ministry of Welfare, Health and Cultural Affairs

16:141. Master record

Database type Bibliographic
Number of journals
Sources Books, Reports, Government publications and Periodicals
Start year 1982
Language Dutch
Coverage Netherlands (primarily) and International (some)
Number of records 67,000
Update size 8,000
Update period Daily

Keywords

Elderly; Hospitals; Welfare; Social Services; Recreation; Libraries; Sport; Museums; Health Care; Emergency Services

Description

Citations, with abstracts, to the international literature on social services, health care, recreation and culture in the Netherlands, services to youth, the elderly, minority groups and handicapped people, veterinary and human medicine, hospitals, emergency services, sports, leisure, performing and fine arts, libraries and museums.

Corresponds to *WVC Documentatie*, with additional information online.

16:142. Online   Rijks Computer Centrum

File name
Start year 1982
Number of records 67,000
Update period Daily

National Report on Computers & Health

United Communications Group

16:143. Master record

Database type Textual
Number of journals 1
Sources Newsletter, Government departments and Companies
Start year 1988
Language English
Coverage USA

Number of records
Update size –
Update period Daily

Keywords

Computer Data Security; Data Security; Health Care Management; Medicare

Description

A newsletter covering new computer and communications hardware and software, aimed at chief information officers, MIS directors and DP managers in the health care industry. Includes coverage of of the impact on health care providers of vendor mergers and acquisitions, data security strategies, Medicare regulations on hospital data processing, medical computing and new product announcements.

Corresponds to *The National Report on Computers and Health* newsletter. On DIALOG and Data-Star, this newsletter is available as part of the PTS Newsletter Database.

This database can be found on:
PTS Newsletter Database

Nebraska HealthNetwork

Nebraska Department of Health, Nebraska HealthNetwork

16:145. Master record

Alternative name(s) NHN
Database type Directory, Textual, Statistical
Number of journals
Sources Government departments, Universities and Institutions
Start year 1985
Language English
Coverage USA (Nebraska, primarily)
Number of records
Update size –
Update period Weekly

Keywords

Physicians; Hospitals; Nursing Homes; Health Care Education; Medical Education

Description

An information service for health care professionals. Includes directories of physicians (by location and specialty), hospitals and nursing homes (by location, type, licensee and administrator), health care education programmes (by type and degree offered), state senators (by address, district and committee), media (by type, location and contact), seminar announcements, continuing medical education programmes and toll-free phone numbers for health information. Also includes medical alerts and press releases from the Nebraska Department of Health and health data from the University of Nebraska Medical Center, Creighton University Medical Center and Nebraska Hospital Association, abstracts of health-related news items, the most recent vital statistics report from the Nebraska Department of Health and an electronic mail service.

Corresponds in part to *Better Health* newsletter from the Nebraska Department of Health.

16:146. Online — Nebraska Department of Health, Nebraska HealthNetwork

File name	
Alternative name(s)	NHN
Start year	1985
Number of records	
Update period	Weekly

PAHO Document Retrieval System Online

World Health Organisation – Pan American Health Organization

16:147. Master record

Alternative name(s)	PAHOLINE
Database type	Bibliographic, Textual
Number of journals	
Sources	Monographs, Projects, Government documents, Grey literature and Journals
Start year	1978
Language	English, French, Portuguese and Spanish
Coverage	International
Number of records	24,000
Update size	–
Update period	Daily
Thesaurus	Medical Subject Headings (MeSH); PAHOLINE thesaurus

Keywords

Health Services; Health Care Planning; Medical Education; Infectious Diseases; Public Health; Legislation

Description

A bibliographic and textual database of citations and information from Pan American Health Organization holdings, covering most aspects of health, and health planning and education, including legislation, projects, monographs and training material from PAHO.

Available to UN system organisations; also to external users. Printed products include: *PAHODOC*; *PAHOSTC*; *PAHO nutrition*; *PAHO disaster preparedness*; specialised subject bibliographies; *PAHO disaseter update*; *PAHO-MEET*; *TABCONT*. The database is also available on microfiche.

Indexing terms are taken from *Medical Subject Headings (MeSH)* of the US National Library of Medicine and *PAHOLINE thesaurus*.

16:148. Online — MDC

File name	PAHOLINE
Alternative name(s)	PAHOLINE
Start year	1978
Number of records	24,000
Update period	Daily

16:149. Online — National Library of Medicine

File name	PAHOLINE
Alternative name(s)	PAHOLINE
Start year	1978
Number of records	24,000
Update period	Daily

16:150. Online — World Health Organisation – Pan American Health Organization

File name	PAHOLINE
Alternative name(s)	PAHOLINE
Software	ADABAS
Start year	1978
Number of records	24,000
Update period	Daily

16:151. Online — World Health Organisation – Pan American Health Organization

File name	PAHOLINE – BIRS file
Alternative name(s)	PAHOLINE
Start year	1978
Number of records	24,000
Update period	Daily

16:152. Tape — World Health Organisation – Pan American Health Organization

File name	PAHOLINE
Alternative name(s)	PAHOLINE
Start year	1978
Number of records	24,000
Update period	Daily

Plans and Projects Monitor

IGA Ltd

16:153. Master record

Database type	Factual, Textual
Number of journals	
Sources	Reports
Start year	1983
Language	English
Coverage	International
Number of records	15,000
Update size	–
Update period	Fortnightly

Keywords

Civil Engineering; Telecommunications; Construction; Regional Studies; Third World

Description

Details on future capital projects and development plans, particularly in the Third World. Project areas include energy, mining, petrochemicals, telecommunications, heavy engineering, civil engineering, public works, hospitals, agriculture, schools, harbours. Information includes procurement plans, sources of funds, analyses of national, sectoral and supranational economic plans.

Corresponds in part to *Plans and Projects Monitor*

16:154. Online — FT Profile

File name	
Start year	1983
Number of records	15,000
Update period	Fortnightly
Price/Charges	Connect time: UK£2.40
	Online print: UK£0.04 – 0.10 per line
	Offline print: UK£0.01 per line

Notes

Registration fee required, including free documentation and training. Usage charges for access consist of two elements: a connect rate for time online, and a display rate (applies only to lines of file text). There is no charge for blank lines, system messages, menus or help information.

PTS Newsletter Database

Predicasts International Inc

16:155. Master record

Alternative name(s)	Predicasts Newsletter Database
Database type	Textual
Number of journals	
Sources	
Start year	1988
Language	German and English
Coverage	International
Number of records	722,656
Update size	63,000
Update period	Daily
Database aids	PTS Users Manual, Cleveland, Ohio, Predicasts
Hosts have included	CORIS (Thomson Financial Network) (Until 1/92)

Keywords

Acid Rain; Advertising; Air Pollution; Alcohol Abuse; Antiviral Drugs; Asbestos; Asbestosis; Automation and Control; Beauty Care; Beauty Care; Beverages; Biotechnology; Biotechnology Industries; Brewing; Cancer; Ceramics; Chemical Industry; Chromatography; Composites; Computer Data Security; Computer Ergonomics; Company Profiles; Consumer Products; Cosmetics; Data Security; Defence Waste Disposal; Diagnosis; Diagnostic Equipment; Diagnostic Products; Drug Abuse; Drug Treatment; Drugs; Education – Cancer; Electrodialysis; Employee Benefits; Environmental Policy; Ergonomics; Explosion; Filtration; Fire; Food and Drink; Food Additives; Food Processing; Food Technology; Genetic Engineering; Greenhouse Effect; Hazardous Chemicals; Hazardous Substances; Hazardous Substances Transport; Hazardous Waste; Health and Safety; Health Care; Health Care Management; Health Care Products; Health Insurance; Health Services; HIV; Household Products; Hygiene Products; Information Services; Information Systems; Legal Liability; Legislation; Liability Insurance; Manufacturing; Marketing; Market Reports; Materials Industry; Medicare; Medical Equipment; Medical Textiles; Medical Waste Management; Membrane Technology; Metals; Nuclear Waste; Occupational Health and Safety; Packaging; Patents; Personal Hygiene; Pesticides; Pets; Pharmaceutical Industry; Pharmaceutical Products; Pharmaceuticals; Pollution; Polymers; Product Catalogues; Product Liability; Prosthetics; Public Health; Radiation; Research and Development; Separation Technology; Smoking; Standards; Textiles; Waste Management; Water Pollution; Water Purification

Description

Produced by Predicasts, PTS Newsletter is a multi-industry database providing concise information on company activities, new technologies, emerging industry trends, government regulations and international trade opportunities. It consists of the full text of over 500 business and industry newsletters covering almost fifty different industries and subject areas. It is international in scope, covering all major economic and political regions of the world, including Eastern and Western Europe, the USA, the Pacific Rim, Latin America, Asia and the Middle East. Facts, figures and analyses are provided on the following industrial and geographical areas: advanced materials, biotechnology, broadcasting and publishing, computers and electronics, chemicals, defense and aerospace, energy, environment, financial services and markets, instrumentation, international trade, general technology, Japan, Middle East, manufacturing, medical and health, materials packaging, research and development, telecommunications and transportation.

Newsletters include *Multinational Service* which covers decisions and policies affecting corporations operating worldwide; and *Europe Report* which offers broad coverage of EC activities relating to economic and monetary affairs, the internal market and legislation and regulations relating to business. Both Newsletters are published by the Europe Information Service of Cooper's & Lybrand Europe. Middle East coverage includes the *Israel High-Tech Report*; *The Middle East News Network*; and *The Middle East Consultants' Newsletter*.

16:156. Online — Data-Star

File name	PTBN
Alternative name(s)	Predicasts Newsletter Database
Start year	January 1988
Number of records	533,000
Update period	Weekly
Database aids	Data-Star Business Manual, Berne and Online manual (search for NEWS-PTBN in NEWS)
Price/Charges	Subscription: UK£32.00
	Connect time: UK£80.40
	Online print: UK£0.28 – 0.55
	Offline print: UK£0.26 – £1.00
	SDI charge: UK£4.00

Also available on FIZ Technik via a gateway from Data-Star

Notes

From June 1993 Data-Star have introduced an annual fee/subscription per contract (that is, not per password) of SFr 80.00 (c.UK£ 32.00) payable every June. For North American customers billed in dollars who also use DIALOG, the DIALOG fee also covers access to Data-Star. Academic customers, 'commitment' customers and customers currently billed in dollars are exempt.

16:157. Online — DIALOG

File name	PTSNL
Alternative name(s)	Predicasts Newsletter Database
Start year	1989
Number of records	722,656
Update period	Daily
Price/Charges	Connect time: US$126.00
	Online print: US$0.90

Notes

PTSNL is a menu-access version of the PTS Newsletter Database. PTSNL provides users with the unique capability to easily retrieve the latest issue (or any available issue) of a newsletter, display a Table of Contents listing articles contained in a selected issue, and print the full text of newsletter articles selected by title. To search newsletters for information on specific subjects, use File 636 (the main PTS file), which utilizes the full range of DIALOG search commands.

16:158. Online   DIALOG

File name	File 636
Alternative name(s)	Predicasts Newsletter Database
Start year	1989
Number of records	722,656
Update period	Daily
Price/Charges	Connect time: US$126.00
	Online print: US$0.90
	Offline print: US$0.90
	SDI charge: US$1.00 (daily) – 3.00 (weekly)

Notes

This is the main file of PTS on DIALOG. There is also a menu access version – PTSNL, which enables the user to retrieve the latest issue of a newsletter, print the full text of newspaper articles, etc. It does not have the full range of DIALOG search commands.

16:159. Online   Dow Jones News/Retrieval

File name	
Alternative name(s)	Predicasts Newsletter Database
Start year	
Number of records	
Update period	Weekly

16:160. Online   FIZ Technik (gateway)

File name	PTBN
Alternative name(s)	Predicasts Newsletter Database
Start year	1988 (January)
Number of records	Volume 1: 159,000
Update period	Weekly
Price/Charges	Connect time: SFr201.00
	Online print: SFr0.61 – 1.22
	Offline print: SFr0.24 – 1.83
	SDI charge: SFr10.00

Available via a gateway to Data-Star

For more details of constituent databases, see:
AIDS Weekly
Air/Water Pollution Report
Alliance Alert – Medical Health
Antiviral Agents Bulletin
Applied Genetics News
Asbestos Control Report
BBI Newsletter
Biomedical Materials
Biomedical Polymers
Cancer Weekly
Cosmetic Insiders' Report
Diagnostics Business-Matters
Environment Week
European Cosmetic Markets
FDA Medical Bulletin
Food Chemical News
Genetic Technology News
Hazmat Transport News
Health Business
Health Daily
Industrial Health and Hazards Update
International Product Alert
Japan Report: Medical Technology
Japan Science Scan
Managed Care Law Outlook
Managed Care Outlook
Managed Care Report
Medical Bulletin
Medical Scan
Medical Waste News
Medical Textiles
Membrane and Separation Technology News
National Report on Computers and Health
Nuclear Waste News
Occupational Health and Safety Letter

OTC Market Report: Update USA
OTC News and Market Report
Pesticide and Toxic Chemical News
Pharmaceutical Business News
Product Alert
PRODUCTSCAN
Report on Defense Plant Wastes
Soviet Bio/Medical Report
Toxic Materials News
Worldwide Biotech

Quality Review Bulletin
Joint Commission on Accreditation of Hospitals

16:161. Master record

Database type	Textual, Factual
Number of journals	1
Sources	Journal
Start year	1984
Language	English
Coverage	USA (primarily)
Number of records	
Update size	–
Update period	Monthly
Index unit	Articles, Editorials and Letters

Keywords

Patient Care; Hospital Management

Description

The *Quality Review Bulletin* offers practical assistance on quality assurance activities and patient care evaluation techniques. Articles address quality assurance/utilisation review approaches, activity, theory and research. All features are critiqued by at least two outside experts in the health care field.

16:162. Online   Mead Data Central (as a NEXIS database)

File name	QRB – NEXIS
Start year	1984
Number of records	
Update period	Monthly
Delay	2–3 weeks
Price/Charges	Subscription: US$1,000 – 3,000 (Depending on needs)
	Connect time: US$49.00 (Telecomms + connect time)
	Database entry fee: US$14.00 (Search charge)
	Online print: US$0.04 per line

Notes

Library: HEALTH; Group file: JCAHO.

Regular sections include: articles, editorials and letters; specific exclusions are progress notes, tables of contents, meetings calendar.

A subscription charge which covers all transactional charges, connect time, telecommunications and the small administration charge can take the place of the individual charges. Subscriptions are negotiated with customers and vary according to the number of menus (thus, files) that are to be used – typically a minimum subscription would be about US$ 1,000. All charges include training and a 24-hour help line.

Record composition

Publication; Cite; Date; Section; Length; Title; Source; Author; Abstract (SUM-ABS); Text; Additional information (SUPP-INFO); Reference (BIBLIO-REF); Graphic; Correction; Correction Date; Discussion and Editor's Note

This database can also be found on:
NEXIS

SANTECOM
Hopital Charles-Lemoyne

16:163. Master record

Database type	Bibliographic
Number of journals	
Sources	Journals, Government departments and Conference proceedings
Start year	1977
Language	English and French
Coverage	Canada
Number of records	4,000
Update size	1,800
Update period	Monthly
Index unit	Articles

Keywords

Nutrition; Perinatal Health Care; Occupational Health; Health Care Management; Women's Health; Home Health Care; Infectious Diseases; Legislation; Gerontology; Mental Health; Paediatrics; Community Health; Public Health

Description

Citations, with abstracts, to Canadian community health literature, including adolescent, environmental, handicapped, mental, occupational and women's health, gerontology, home care, infectious diseases, law, management, nutrition, perinatality and preventive dentistry.

16:164. Online   Services Documentaires Multimedia Inc (SDM)

File name	
Start year	1977
Number of records	4,000
Update period	Monthly

Spriline
Planning and Rationalization Institute for the Health and Social Services
Spri Bibliotek och utredningsbanken Stiftelsen Stockholms läna Äldrecentrum

16:165. Master record

Alternative name(s)	Spri Library and Research Report Bank
Database type	Bibliographic, Textual
Number of journals	350
Sources	Journals, Research reports and Grey literature
Start year	1988
Language	Swedish (primarily) and English
Coverage	International
Number of records	16,000
Update size	3,000
Update period	Irregular

Keywords

Health Care Planning

Description

Concerns the area of health and medical care, with the exception of medical literature of a purely scientific character. Spri stands for Sjukvardens och socialvardens planerings-och rationaliseringsinstitut. Spriline consists of two parts: the library collections and journal articles from about 350 journals which are mainly Swedish; Spri's Research Report Bank (Spri's utredningsbank) that is, unpublished research reports from the health care sector in Sweden and in other Scandinavian countries.

The Spri Library and Research Bank offers a complete document delivery service. Other products – Spri litteraturtjänst, Nytt fran Spris utredninngsbank, Utredninsgbankens jkatalog, Fou-primavard.

Terms in Swedish from an inhouse thesaurus. Retrieval from all fields of the reference.

16:166. Online   MIC/Karolinska Institute Library and Information Center (MIC KIBIC)

File name	Spriline
Alternative name(s)	Spri Library and Research Report Bank
Start year	1988
Number of records	16,000
Update period	Irregular

Notes

Online ordering available.

NURSING

ASSIA
Bowker-Saur Ltd

17:1. Master record

Alternative name(s)	Applied Social Sciences Index and Abstracts
Database type	Bibliographic, Textual
Number of journals	550
Sources	Journals and Newspapers
Start year	1987
Language	English
Coverage	International
Number of records	68,000
Update size	18,000
Update period	Every two months
Index unit	Articles
Abstract details	Subject specialists
Database aids	ASSIA Thesaurus, Bowker-Saur UK£53

Keywords
HIV; Child Abuse; Child Development; Child Psychiatry; Criminology; Drug Abuse; Dyslexia; Ethnic Problems; Geriatrics; Health Services; Housing; Immigration; Industrial Relations; Legislation; Pensions; Pollution; Prison Services; Probation; Public Administration; Race Relations; Riots; Rural Studies; Social Welfare; Television; Unemployment; Urban Studies

Description
Citations, with abstracts, to the international English-language literature on applied social science. Covers the information needs of all those engaged in the caring services and the core sociology which supports these services. Aspects of law, business, national politics as well as nursing and health sciences, social studies, communication and, in particular, local government are included. It has a strong emphasis on the applied aspects of the social sciences. About 40% of ASSIA's coverage is on the United Kingdom, 45% on North America and 15% on the rest of the world. Coverage is of both theoretical and practical articles. Covers child development, industrial relations, social welfare, criminology, politics, child abuse, pollution, geriatrics, immigration, housing, child psychiatry, probation, prison services, nervous disorders, European regulations, unemployment, social effects of television, dyslexia, public administration, drug problems, AIDS, health services retirement pensions, riots, race relations, manpower, inner city problems, rural depredation and ethnic problems.

Corresponds to bi-monthly *Applied Social Sciences Index and Abstracts*. The print version of *Applied Social Science Index and Abstracts* has been described variously as 'one of the most useful of the many databases in the social sciences'; 'an essential resource'; and 'an excellent source of information . . . with highly developed and accurate indexing'.

Non-selective coverage of core journals; coverage of all major social sciences and related media. About 80% abstracted from cover-to-cover, 20% selectively. Cross references, synonym references and related headings. All documents contain a short informative abstract, full bibliographic details and index terms which facilitate both general and specific subject searches. Bowker-Saur have produced a thesaurus containing around 8,259 terms which have appeared in ASSIA since its first publication. Its coverage is comprehensive, embracing social science in the widest sense.

17:2. Online   Data-Star

File name	ASSI
Alternative name(s)	Applied Social Sciences Index and Abstracts
Start year	1987
Number of records	68,000
Update period	Every two months
Database aids	Data-Star Biomedical Manual, Berne, Data-Star, 1990 and Online manual (search for NEWS-ASSI in NEWS)
Price/Charges	Subscription: UK£32.00 Connect time: UK£45.68 Online print: UK£0.55 Offline print: UK£0.62 SDI charge: UK£3.76

Notes
From June 1993 Data-Star have introduced an annual fee/subscription per contract (that is, not per password) of SFr 80.00 (c.UK£ 32.00) payable every June. For North American customers billed in dollars who also use DIALOG, the DIALOG fee also covers access to Data-Star. Academic customers, 'commitment' customers and customers currently billed in dollars are exempt.

17:3. CD-ROM   Bowker-Saur Ltd

File name	ASSIA Plus
Alternative name(s)	Applied Social Sciences Index and Abstracts
Format notes	IBM
Software	Bowker Plus
Start year	1987
Number of records	100,000
Update period	Quarterly
Price/Charges	Subscription: UK£1,150

AVLINE
National Library of Medicine

17:5. Master record

Alternative name(s)	AudioVisuals onLINE
Database type	Library catalogue/cataloguing aids, Bibliographic
Number of journals	
Sources	National Library of Medicine and A-V material
Start year	1975
Language	English
Coverage	USA
Number of records	18,000
Update size	1,200
Update period	Weekly

Keywords
Surgery

Description

Contains citations to audiovisual and other non-print teaching materials catalogued by the National Library of Medicine (NLM). Primarily clinical in scope, covers items used for health sciences education and for continuing education of practitioners. Selected records added prior to July 31, 1981 may contain critical appraisals resulting from peer reviews conducted (until March 1982) by the Association of American Medical Colleges. Information for obtaining each item is also included.

It is possible to search for particular types of media or to specify the running time. NLM classmarks on all items are useful for searching or for cataloguing. Some records have abstracts.

17:6. Online   BLAISE-LINK

File name	AVLINE
Alternative name(s)	AudioVisuals onLINE
Start year	1976
Number of records	
Update period	Weekly

17:7. Online   CISTI MEDLARS

File name	AVLINE
Alternative name(s)	AudioVisuals onLINE
Start year	1975
Number of records	18,000
Update period	Weekly

Notes

Charges depend on amount and type of usage.

17:8. Online   National Library of Medicine

File name	AVLINE
Alternative name(s)	AudioVisuals onLINE
Start year	1975
Number of records	18,000
Update period	Weekly

17:9. Tape   National Library of Medicine

File name	AVLINE
Alternative name(s)	AudioVisuals onLINE
Start year	1975
Number of records	18,000
Update period	Weekly

Notes

Corresponds to the AVLINE online database. Contact NLM for pricing information.

This database can also be found on:
AIDSLINE

BiblioMed Cardiology
National Library of Medicine

17:12. Master record
CD-ROM   **Healthcare Information Services Inc**

Database type	Bibliographic, Textual
Number of journals	280
Sources	Monographs and journals
Start year	Most recent ten years
Language	English
Coverage	International
Number of records	400,000
Update size	—
Update period	Quarterly

Keywords

Cardiology

Description

Selected subset of MEDLINE, for last ten years, with full abstracts.

Also contains full text of the *Yearbook of Cardiology*, as well as Giuliani's *Cardiology: Fundamentals and Practices.*

For more details of constituent databases, see:
MEDLINE
Yearbook of Cardiology

Birth Defects Encyclopedia Online
Center for Birth Defects Information Services Inc

17:14. Master record

Database type	Textual, Encyclopedia
Number of journals	
Sources	
Start year	
Language	English
Coverage	International
Number of records	2,000
Update size	
Update period	

Description

Comprises a comprehensive, systematic knowledgebase of the biomedical sciences as they relate to human anomalies of clinical relevance, with special attention to the application of that knowledge to patient care. Contains more than two thousand articles on specific birth defect conditions and complex syndromes, arranged under some ten thousand established names and terms.

17:15. Online   BRS

File name	BDEO
Format notes	IBM
Start year	
Number of records	2,000
Update period	
Price/Charges	Connect time: US$40.00/50.00
	Online print: US$0.42/0.50
	Offline print: US$0.60

Cancer Treatment Symposia
US Department of Health and Human Services

17:16. Master record

Database type	Textual, Factual
Number of journals	1
Sources	Newsletter
Start year	1983
Language	English
Coverage	International
Number of records	
Update size	—
Update period	
Index unit	Articles

Keywords

Cancer; Drugs; Surgery

Description

The publication chronicles symposia in any of the following topical areas of investigation: surgery, radiotherapy, chemotherapy, biologic response modification, supportive care, pharmacology, cell biology and kinetics, mechanisms of drug action and medicinal chemistry. Cancer Treatment Symposia also contains information addressing scientific, educational, ethical and humanistic issues.

17:17. Online — Mead Data Central (as a NEXIS database)

File name	CTS – NEXIS
Alternative name(s)	NEXIS – Cancer Treatment Symposia
Start year	1983–1985
Number of records	
Update period	
Price/Charges	Subscription: US$1,000 – 3,000 (Depending on needs)
	Connect time: US$49.00 (Telecomms + connect time)
	Database entry fee: US$24.00 (Search charge)
	Online print: US$0.04 per line

Notes

Library name: GENMED; Group files: ARCJNL.

A subscription charge which covers all transactional charges, connect time, telecommunications and the small administration charge can take the place of the individual charges. Subscriptions are negotiated with customers and vary according to the number of menus (thus, files) that are to be used – typically a minimum subscription would be about US$ 1,000. All charges include training and a 24-hour help line.

Record composition

Publication; Cite; Section; Length; Title; Author; Abstract (SUM-ABS); Text; Additional information (SUPP-INFO); Reference (BIBLIO-REF); Graphic; Correction and Correction Date

This database can also be found on:
NEXIS

CATLINE
National Library of Medicine

17:19. Master record

Alternative name(s)	CATalog onLINE
Database type	Bibliographic, Library catalogue/cataloguing aids
Number of journals	
Sources	Government publications, journals, monographs and National Library of Medicine
Start year	1400
Language	English
Coverage	International
Number of records	699,000
Update size	12,000
Update period	Every two months
Thesaurus	Medical Subject Headings (MeSH)
Database aids	MeSH Annotated Alphabetic List, MeSH Tree Structures and Permuted MeSH.

Keywords

Physiology

Description

This database contains bibliographic records of books and first issues of serials in the biomedical sciences in the National Library of Medicine catalogue. Subjects covered: anthropology; biochemistry; bioengineering; biology (medical aspects); biophysics; dental medicine; environmental health; forensic medicine; geriatrics; gerontology; health education; hospital service; human medicine; legal medicine; medical education; medical technology; nursing; occupational medicine; pharmacy; pharmacology; physiology; psychiatry; psychology (medical aspects); rehabilitation; social medicine; sports medicine; veterinary medicine.

CATLINE is used primarily for authoritative cataloguing, ordering and interlibrary loan information but can also be used to compile online bibliography of books and/or serials on a given subject.

The unit record contains information about author(s), title and other bibliographic data base as well as controlled vocabulary (MeSH terms). Titles are present in the original language (approximately 50% foreign language items) and searchable via free text vocabulary. Approximately 1% of records contain abstracts.

The structure of CATLINE corresponds largely to MEDLINE with regard to indexing and search strategy. Indexed by aid of the MeSH thesaurus which is hierarchically structured. There are three basic differences to MEDLINE. First MeSH Supplementary Chemical Records cannot be used in CATLINE; secondly the weighting of MeSH-descriptors is not possible in CATLINE and thirdly CATLINE has additional subheadings. The MEDLINE qualifiers or subheadings are called 'topical subheadings' in CATLINE. CATLINE has three further types of subheadings: form-subheadings, language-subheadings and geographical subheadings. Form-subheadings describe the form of a catalogued subject, for example biography. Language-subheadings, which are used only in combination with MeSH-terms or form-subheadings, describe dictionaries or similiar material. Geographical subheadings are used to index when the geographical regions referred to in text and are also used for historical countries. CATLINE has further additional 'topical subheadings' which replace the CHECK TAGS of the MEDLINE database. Instead of the 'age group checktags' (for example, INFANT, CHILD, ADULT, etc) CATLINE has the following topical subheadings: in infancy and childhood; in adolescence; in adulthood; in middle age; in old age; in pregnancy. These subheadings are used in the same way as the other topical subheadings and are used for the MeSH categories C (Diseases), E (Analytical, Diagnostic and Therapeutic Technics and Equipment), F (Psychiatry and Psychology) and G (Biological Sciences).

17:20. Online — Australian MEDLINE Network

File name	CATLINE
Alternative name(s)	CATalog onLINE
Start year	
Number of records	
Update period	

17:21. Online — BLAISE-LINK

File name	CATLINE
Alternative name(s)	CATalog onLINE
Start year	

Number of records
Update period   Weekly

17:22. Online   CISTI MEDLARS
File name   CATLINE
Alternative name(s)   CATalog onLINE
Start year   1801
Number of records
Update period   Weekly

17:23. Online   DIMDI
File name   CA79
Alternative name(s)   CATalog onLINE
Software   GRIPS
Start year   1400
Number of records   699,073
Update period   Monthly
SDI period   1 month
Price/Charges   Connect time: UK£03.88–08.62
                               Online print: UK£0.16–0.34
                               Offline print: UK£0.07–0.14

Downloading is allowed
Thesaurus is online

Notes
Suppliers of online documents: British Library Document Supply Centre, Boston Spa, England; Harkers Information Retrieval System, Sydney, Australia; Zentralbibliothek der Medizin, Köln, Germany. Titles are present in the original language (approximately 50% foreign language items) and searchable via free text vocabulary.

Record composition
Abstract AB; Abstract Language AL; Authorship Statement AST; Author AU; Bibliography Note BIN; Corporate Author CA; Classification Code CC; Conference Name CNA; Collation COL; Controlled Term CT; Country CY; Dashed-on-Entry DO; Document Type DT; Entry Date ED; First/Last Issue FL; Form-Subheading FS; Freetext FT; Geographic Sub-heading GS; History Note HN; ISBN-NO SB; ISSN-NO SS; Issuing Body IB; Keyword KW; Language LA; Language, Primary LP; Langue Subheading LS; Numeric/Chronologic Desig. Note NCD; Personal Name of Subject PS; Publishing Place PP; Publisher PU; Publication Year PY; Qualifier QF; Series Title SE; Title Coninuation TC; Title TI; Topical Sub-heading TS and Uniform Title UNT

The unit record contains information about author(s), title and other bibliographic details as well as controlled vocabulary terms (MeSH terms).

17:24. Online   National Library of Medicine
File name   CATLINE
Alternative name(s)   CATalog onLINE
Start year
Number of records
Update period

17:25. Tape   National Library of Medicine
File name   CATLINE
Alternative name(s)   CATalog onLINE
Format notes   9-track, IBM standard labels or
                               unlabelled, 1600 or 6250 bpi,
                               EBCDIC
Start year   1400
Number of records   699,000
Update period   Every two months

Notes
Corresponds to the CATLINE online database. Contact NLM for pricing information.

This database can also be found on:
AIDSLINE
Bioethicsline

CINAHL
CINAHL

17:27. Master record
Alternative name(s)   Cumulative Index to Nursing and
                               Allied Health Literature; Nursing
                               and Allied Health
Database type   Bibliographic
Number of journals   300
Sources   Journals, monographs, dissertations
                               and A-V material
Start year   1983
Language   English
Coverage   International
Number of records   99,000
Update size   21,000
Update period   Monthly
Index unit   Articles and book
Thesaurus   CINAHL Thesaurus (MeSH-based)
Database aids   CINAHL Subject Heading List, 1993
                               (available from producer), CINAHL
                               Database Search Guide, 1993
                               (available from producer) and
                               CINAHL Teaching Guide, 1993
                               (available from producer)

Keywords
Physical Therapy; Cardiopulmonary Therapy; Laboratory Technology; Paramedicine; Respiratory Therapy; Occupational Therapy; Radiology; Emergency Health Care; Medical Records; Medical Social Work; Medical Librarianship; Surgical Nursing; Health Education; Management

Description
The nursing and allied health (CINAHL) database is a comprehensive and authoritative source of literature refences aimed at nurses, allied health professionals and others interested in health care administration. Contains the complete Nursing and Allied Health database, including references to periodical literature in nursing and allied health, with abstracts from over one third of those articles; books from over thirty health care publishers, nursing dissertations and abstracts and references to the publications of the American Nurses Association and the National League of Nursing. Covers all aspects of nursing and allied health disciplines. Although the emphasis is primarily nursing, 35% of references relate to allied health disciplines such as cardiopulmonary technology, occupational therapy, physical therapy and rehabilitation, medical and laboratory technology, radiologic technology, emergency services and social services in health care, medical records, health sciences librarianship, medical assisting, the physician's assistant, surgical technology, and health education. Also includes relevant articles from management, psychological and popular journals. Also lists new books in nursing and allied health fields. Audiovisual materials as well as library science journals for nursing and allied health are also included. The vast majority of records are unique to CINAHL, although there is some overlap in journal coverage with *Excerpta Medica* (EMBASE) and MEDLINE.

Corresponds to the printed *Cumulative Index to Nursing and Allied Health Literature*. Since 1986 abstracts from approximately forty nursing journals have been included in the file. Books included since 1984.

Virtually all English-language nursing journals are included.

The CINAHL thesaurus is based on *MeSH*, but is tailor-made for the fields of nursing and allied health. Major and minor descriptors and free text searching are available. An extremely useful feature is the inclusion of more than twenty-four identifiers or document types which help to limit retrieval for specific concepts such as books, statistics, computer programs, research articles, etc. The See also references from the printed index and the number of references in the citations are also included. The 1993 Subject Heading List contains 6,900 terms, 2,000 of which are not found on any other database.

17:28. Online — BRS, Morning Search, BRS/Colleague

File name	NAHL
Start year	
Number of records	
Update period	Monthly
Price/Charges	Connect time: US$37.00/47.00
	Online print: US$0.20/0.28
	Offline print: US$0.28
	SDI charge: US$7.25

17:29. Online — CompuServe Information Service

File name	IQUEST File 1278
Start year	1983
Number of records	
Update period	Monthly
Price/Charges	Subscription: US$8.95 per month
	Database entry fee: US$9/search; some databases carry a surcharge ($2–75)
	Online print: US$10 references free; then $9 per ten; abstracts $3 each

Downloading is allowed

Notes

Accessed via IQUEST or IQMEDICAL, this database is offered by a BRS gateway. IQUEST can either search across all databases, a database of the user's choice or selected multiple databases.

17:30. Online — Data-Star

File name	NAHL
Start year	1983
Number of records	103,799
Update period	Monthly
Database aids	Biomedical manual and Online manual (search NEWS-NAHL in NEWS)
Price/Charges	Subscription: SFr80.00
	Connect time: SFr107
	Online print: SFr0.42
	Offline print: SFr0.37
	SDI charge: SFr6.80

Thesaurus is online

Notes

Four subsets have been created to help narrow a search. Users can limit retrieval to articles from nursing journals as 'Nursing.SB.', Core nursing journals as 'Core with nursing.SB.', Allied health journals as 'Allied with health.SB.' and journals published in the USA and Canada as 'USA with Canada'.

From June 1993 Data-Star have introduced an annual fee/subscription per contract (that is, not per password) of SFr 80.00 (c.UK£ 32.00) payable every June. For North American customers billed in dollars who also use DIALOG, the DIALOG fee also covers access to Data-Star. Academic customers, 'commitment' customers and customers currently billed in dollars are exempt.

Record composition

Author AU; Title TI; Source SO; Language LG; Publication type PT; Descriptors (MeSH) DE; Year of publication YR; Subset SB; Major desriptors MJ; Minor descriptors MN and UMI order number UMI

17:31. Online — DIALOG, Knowledge Index

File name	File 218
Start year	1983
Number of records	123,290
Update period	Monthly
Price/Charges	Connect time: US$54.00
	Online print: US$0.15
	Offline print: US$0.25
	SDI charge: US$6.95

Notes

This database is also available to home users during evenings and weekends at a reduced rate on the Knowledge Index service of DIALOG – file name in this case is MEDI14, and searches are made with simplified commands or menus.

17:32. CD-ROM — CD Plus

File name	CD Plus/CINAHL-CD
Format notes	Mac, Unix, IBM
Software	OVID 3.0
Start year	1983
Number of records	100,000
Update period	Monthly
Price/Charges	Subscription: UK£685

Notes

One disc. Offers the ability to limit by local journal holdings. For the experienced searcher, the software offers *MeSH* explodes, 'personal pre-explodes' for frequently exploded terms, SDIs and Save Searches, enhanced *MeSH* tree structures, and emulation of National Library of Medicine and dot-dot syntax.

Record composition

Author; Title; Source; Abstract; Subject Heading and Instrumentation

This database has an index of all searchable terms together with the online *MeSh Thesaurus* which offers mapping from natural language to *MeSH* – a facility which should give significantly improved precision for the inexperienced searcher. The on-screen help provides scope notes, definitions and task descriptors.

17:33. CD-ROM — Compact Cambridge

File name	CINAHL-CD
Format notes	NEC, 9800, Mac, IBM
Start year	1983
Number of records	100,000+
Update period	Monthly
Price/Charges	Subscription: UK£700

17:34. CD-ROM — SilverPlatter

File name	Nursing & Allied Health (CINAHL)-CD
Format notes	Mac, IBM
Software	SPIRS/MacSPIRS
Start year	1983
Number of records	140,000
Update period	Every two months
Price/Charges	Subscription: UK£790 – 1,186.5

Thesaurus is online

Notes

One disc. The CD-ROM includes an on-screen equiv-alent to CINAHL's print thesaurus. Prices are: regular subscription £790 for single users, £1,186.5 for 2–8 networked users.

Tree explosions, major and minor assignments of descriptors, the use of sub-headings, and free text searching are available.

17:35. Fixed disk   SilverPlatter

File name	Nursing & Allied Health (CINAHL)-CD
Format notes	IBM, Mac
Software	SPIRS/MacSPIRS
Start year	1983
Number of records	140,000
Update period	Every two months
Price/Charges	Subscription: UK£1,028 – 1,713
Thesaurus is online	

Notes

Contains the entire database, with an on-screen equivalent of CINAHL's print thesaurus, on a fixed disk with updates supplied on CD-ROM. This means that up to thirty networked users can have access to a single file containing the complete database. Search speeds are up to ten times faster than CD-ROM searching.

Prices are: £1,028 for 2–8 networked users, £1,370 for 9–16 users and £1,713 for 17–24 users. Hard disk fee is US$1,500.

Tree explosions, major and minor assignments of descriptors, the use of sub-headings, and free text searching are available.

DHSS-Data
Department of Health and Social Security

17:36. Master record

Alternative name(s)	Department of Health and Social Security – Data
Database type	Bibliographic, Library catalogue/cataloguing aids
Number of journals	2,000+
Sources	Administrative circulars, government documents, journals, monographs, official publications, pamphlets and reports
Start year	1983 (October); earliest data from 1961
Language	English
Coverage	UK (primarily) and International (some)
Number of records	84,691
Update size	13,000
Update period	Weekly
Index unit	Articles
Thesaurus	DHSS-Data Thesaurus, new edition in preparation

Keywords

Building; Child Care; Health Care; Public Administration; Social Services; Standards

Description

DHSS-DATA contains citations, with some abstracts (approximately 40%) to the long-established abstracting and current awareness bulletins from the library of the Departments of Health and Social Security in London. The core subjects covered by the database are health service and hospital administration includ-ing: planning, design, construction and maintenance of health service buildings; medical equipment and supplies; public health, nursing and primary care; occupational diseases, social policy, social welfare, social security, social services for children, families, the handicapped and old people; and social security and occupational pensions. The database currently focuses on new holdings; references to older holdings are to be added in the future. An important feature of the database is the inclusion of full details, including sources of supply, of Department of Health and Department of Social Security publications.

Source documents are available as an inter-library loan.

Government publications originate primarily in the United Kingdom, the United States, and with the World Health Organization.

From 1986 Tags enable a search to be restricted to specific sectors of the Health or Social Services such as Health, Social Services, Social Security, Pensions and Health Buildings. In late 1992, the database was restructured to provide more up-to-date and better quality records, with increased coverage of official publications.

17:37. Online   CompuServe Information Service

File name	IQUEST File 2141
Alternative name(s)	Department of Health and Social Security – Data
Start year	1983
Number of records	84,691
Update period	Weekly
Price/Charges	Subscription: US$8.95 per month Database entry fee: US$9/search; some databases carry a surcharge ($2–75) Online print: US$10 references free; then $9 per ten; abstracts $3 each
Downloading is allowed	

Notes

Accessed via IQUEST or IQMEDICAL, this database is offered by a Data-Star gateway. IQUEST can either search across all databases, a database of the user's choice or selected multiple databases.

Record composition

Abstract AB; Accession Number and Update Code AN; Author(s) AU; Corporate Author(s) CA; Descriptor(s) DE; Notes NT; Publication Type PT; Publication Year YR; Publication Year (Archive) YA; Source SO; Title TI and Update Code UP

17:38. Online   Data-Star

File name	DHSS
Alternative name(s)	Department of Health and Social Security – Data
Start year	1983 (October); earliest data from 1961
Number of records	84,691
Update period	Weekly
Database aids	Data-Star Biomedial Manual and Online manual (search NEWS-DHSS in NEWS)
Price/Charges	Subscription: SFr80.00 Connect time: SFr127.20 Online print: SFr0.39 Offline print: SFr0.80 SDI charge: SFr6.80
Downloading is allowed	

Notes

The Superlabel DHZZ can be used to search DHSS-DHSS and DHMT-MEDTEH simultaneously. The following tags, appearing on records from 1986, enable a search to be restricted to specific sectors of the Health or Social Services: YYH Health, YYQ Social Services, YYS Social Security, YYP Pensions, YYB Health Buildings.

From June 1993 Data-Star have introduced an annual fee/subscription per contract (that is, not per password) of SFr 80.00 (c.UK£ 32.00) payable every June. For North American customers billed in dollars who also use DIALOG, the DIALOG fee also covers access to Data-Star. Academic customers, 'commitment' customers and customers currently billed in dollars are exempt.

Record composition

Abstract AB; Accession Number and Update Code AN; Author(s) AU; Corporate Author(s) CA; Descriptor(s) DE; Notes NT; Publication Type PT; Publication Year YR; Publication Year (Archive) YA; Source SO; Title TI and Update Code UP

DRI Health Care Cost Forecasting
Data Resources Inc (DRI)

17:39. Master record

Database type	Statistical
Number of journals	
Sources	Databases
Start year	4-year forecasts, with historical series from 1976
Language	
Coverage	USA
Number of records	100
Update size	—
Update period	Quarterly

Keywords
Health Care Costs; Medical Equipment; Pharmaceuticals

Description
Contains quarterly forecast indexes of United States health care costs. Covers labour, food, utilities, medical equipment, supplies, pharmaceuticals, physician services, and capital. Also provides forecasts of the 'market basket' indexes developed by the United States Health Care Financing Administration (HCFA) for hospitals, nursing homes, and home health-care agencies. Some series are available at a regional level.

Sources include DRI data banks and models, and the Health Care Financing Administration.

17:40. Online   Data Resources Inc (DRI)

File name	
Start year	4-year forecasts, with historical series from 1976
Number of records	100
Update period	Quarterly

Notes
Subscription to DRI required.

DSI
Dansk Sygehus Institut

17:41. Master record

Alternative name(s)	Dansk Sygehus Institut
Database type	Bibliographic
Number of journals	
Sources	Books, Reports and Journals

Start year	1977
Language	Danish
Coverage	
Number of records	18,000
Update size	—
Update period	Daily
Index unit	Articles

Description
DSI contains references to literature on hospitals, nursing and health services. Disciplines covered are: medicine, nursing, pharmacology, economics, management, building, technology, law, sociology etc. Document types indexed are: books, reports, serials and articles.

17:42. Online   DSI

File name	DSI
Alternative name(s)	Dansk Sygehus Institut
Start year	1977
Number of records	18,000
Update period	Daily

Esculap
Helsingborgs sjukvårdsdistrikt, Lasarettet (Helsingborg Heath Care District)

17:43. Master record

Alternative name(s)	Helsingborgs sjukvårdsdistrikts databas; Helsingborg Health Care District
Database type	Bibliographic
Number of journals	
Sources	Reports
Start year	1987
Language	Swedish
Coverage	International
Number of records	1,800
Update size	700
Update period	Irregular
Index unit	Reports

Keywords
Clinical Medicine

Description
This database contains citations to the documents acquired since 1987 by the Helsingborg Health Care District in the fields of medicine, with an emphasis on the clinical aspect, and other areas relating to health care. It also includes reports issued by the District Authority. Subjects covered include: medicine; health care; nursing; hospitals and hospital administration.

17:44. Online   Bibliotekstjänst AB (Btj)

File name	Esculap
Alternative name(s)	Helsingborgs sjukvårdsdistrikts databas; Helsingborg Health Care District
Start year	1987
Number of records	1,800
Update period	Irregular

General Practitioner
Haymarket Marketing Publications Ltd

17:45. Master record

Database type	Textual
Number of journals	3
Sources	Journals and newspapers

Start year   January 1987
Language   English
Coverage   International
Number of records 22,174
Update size   —
Update period   Varies with publication

Keywords

Clinical Medicine; General Practice; Primary Health Care

Description

General Practitioner contains the full text of three publications of interest to general practitioners and others involved in primary health care, nursing, or administration.

(1) *GP-General Practitioner* is the best-read newspaper for Britain's family doctors. It includes news coverage of medico- political matters, medical scientific developments and financial affairs and is seen as a principal source of clinical, business and general news for GPs. *GP-General Practitioner* on GPGP is updated weekly.
(2) *Mims Magazine* is the leading fortnightly journal for GPs and concentrates on issues relating to pharmaceutical developments, prescription trends, therapeutics and detection and analysis of side effects. It contains news items about new products together with indications and side-effects by outside experts including GPS. The journal is currently looking at the many issues concerned with prescribing under the GP contract and in particular is performing a systematic anaysis of the cost-effectiveness of drugs in major therapeutic areas. *Mims Magazine* on GPGP is updated every fortnight.
(3) *Medeconomics* is a journal covering the business, management, finance and organisational aspects of general practice within the British National Health Service. Subjects relate to the business efficiency of GPs practices and cover: taxation, pensions, control of practice expenses, accounting in the practice, computers, personal finance, surgery premises and the implications for the GP of major changes in government legislation. *Medeconomics* on GPGP is updated on a monthly basis.

17:46. Online   Data-Star

File name   GPGP
Start year   1987
Number of records 22,174
Update period   Varies with publication
Database aids   Data-Star Biomedical Manual and
                  Data-Star Online Manual (search
                  NEWS-GPGP in NEWS)
Price/Charges   Subscription: SFr80.00
                  Connect time: SFr101.20
                  Online print: SFr0.77
                  Offline print: SFr1.58
                  SDI charge: SFrNot applicable
Downloading is allowed

Notes

The special features paragraph lists additional pictorial and graphical information available in the original article but not reproduced online. The following special features are available: Charts, Figures, Illustrations, Photographs, Drawings, Graphs, Maps, Tables.

From June 1993 Data-Star have introduced an annual fee/subscription per contract (that is, not per password) of SFr 80.00 (c.UK£ 32.00) payable every June. For North American customers billed in dollars who also use DIALOG, the DIALOG fee also covers access to Data-Star. Academic customers, 'commitment' customers and customers currently billed in dollars are exempt.

Record composition

Accession Number and Update Code AN; Author(s) AU; Length of Document LE; Publication Date YD; Publication Month YM; Publication Year YR; Source SO; Special Feature(s) SF; Text TE; Title TI and Update Code UP

Health Planning and Administration
National Library of Medicine
American Hospital Association

17:47. Master record

Database type   Bibliographic
Number of journals 225
Sources   Book chapters, databases (NLM),
                  journals, monographs, reports and
                  theses
Start year   1975
Language   English
Coverage   International
Number of records 623,372
Update size   40,000
Update period   Monthly
Abstract details Author
Thesaurus   Medical Subject Headings (MeSH)
Database aids   MeSH Tree Structures, Permuted
                  MeSH and List of Serials Indexed
                  for Online Users (LSIOU).

Keywords

Health Care Administration; Management

Description

Health Planning and Administration database, which is produced by the National Library of Medicine in co-operation with the American Hospital Association, contains citations to the worldwide literature on the non-clinical aspects of health care planning. Subjects covered within this field include health care administration and facilities, health insurance, financial management, personnel administration, quality issues, manpower planning, legal aspects, licensure, accreditation and health maintenance organisations (HMOs) and related topics. According to the Data-Star manual the database can be used to: ascertain the financial impact of AIDS on health care systems since 1987; discover what training programs are available for hospital administrators; monitor recent developments in home-care services; establish budgeting guidelines in specialist clinics and plan three-year manpower requirements for new medical departments.

Printed sources include: *Hospital Literature Index* (1975-), this being the hard-copy counterpart of Health Planning and Administration; *Index Medicus*; *International Nursing Index*; *Index To Dental Literature*; *Weekly Government Abstracts: Health Planning Series* (produced by the National Health Planning Information Center (NHPIC))(1975–1981). Approximately eighty per cent of references are drawn from the MEDLINE database (from 1975 onwards) and the structure, indexing rules and search strategy are therefore almost identical with MEDLINE. MeSH Supplementary Chemical Records (TE,CR,EZ) and Gene Symbols (GE) are not used in HEALTH.

Approximately fifty per cent of the citations contain abstracts prepared by authors. The database includes about 400 English-language periodicals of the Special Health List evaluated by the American Hospital Association as well as some records of English-language periodicals evaluated by the Association of American Medical Colleges (prior to 1979). Documents (9,451 records 1975–1981) from the National Health Planning Information Center (NHPIC) were added in May 1983 covering documents such as monographs, technical reports and dissertations but not periodicals and these account for about two per cent of all citations. These citations have additional fields which are marked NHPIC only. The Noted field is used in references derived from NHPIC to refer to related documents, or the presence of identification numbers. In MEDLINE-derived records this field is used to note the presence of a comment to an article published in the same journal. A secondary source field is composed of an abbreviation for the secondary supplier: MED/ (MEDLINE); AHA/ (American Hospital Association); NP/ (National Health Planning Information Centre); and AAMC/ (Association of American Medical Colleges). Records which are duplicated in MEDLINE can be eliminated by combining the last search statement with those articles unique to the Health database. On DIALOG this is done by SF=HEALTH and on BRS by using H.LI. On NLM search as H(LI) or AHA (SI) for the Hospital Literature Index citations and NP (SI) for the NHPIC citations.

Sources include journals covered in MEDLINE (see); journals reviewed for the American Hospital Association's *Hospital Literature Index* back to 1975; and since 1983 monographs, monograph chapters, theses, and technical reports supplied by the National Health Planning Information Center from *Weekly Government Abstracts: Health Planning Series*, plus additional journals of special importance to the health field.

17:48. Online — Australian MEDLINE Network

File name	Health Planning and Administration
Start year	
Number of records	
Update period	

17:49. Online — BLAISE-LINK

File name	HEALTH
Start year	1975
Number of records	
Update period	Monthly

17:50. Online — BRS, Morning Search, BRS/Colleague

File name	HLTH
Start year	1975
Number of records	623,372
Update period	Monthly
Price/Charges	Connect time: US$26.00/36.00
	Online print: US$0.07/0.15
	Offline print: US$0.20
	SDI charge: US$5.10

Notes

It is possible to discover records which are unique to the HEALTH database and eliminate those which duplicate MEDLINE records by using H.LI.

17:51. Online — CISTI MEDLARS

File name	Health Planning and Administration
Start year	1975

Number of records	623,372
Update period	Monthly

17:52. Online — CompuServe Information Service

File name	IQUEST File 1234
Start year	1975
Number of records	623,372
Update period	Monthly
Price/Charges	Subscription: US$8.95 per month
	Database entry fee: US$9/search; some databases carry a surcharge ($2–75)
	Online print: US$10 references free; then $9 per ten; abstracts $3 each

Downloading is allowed

Notes

Accessed via IQUEST or IQMEDICAL, this database is offered by a BRS gateway. IQUEST can either search across all databases, a database of the user's choice or selected multiple databases.

17:53. Online — Data-Star

File name	HLPA
Start year	1975
Number of records	623,372
Update period	Monthly
Database aids	Tree Structures, Permuted MeSH and Data-Star Guide to HLPA in Data-Star Biomedical Manual

Thesaurus is online

Notes

HLPA is offered on behalf of and in co-operation with the Swiss Academy of Medical Sciences and its documentation service DOKDI. The command DOCZ will retrieve the total number of documents currently on the database; documents with abstracts can be located by AB=AB. Qualify single source names to .SO., but use the hyphenated NLM journal abbreviation to search multi-word sources. Use .ROOT to locate abbreviations or search on ISSN. The NHPIC subfile contains non-journal sources and users should search free text within this subset.

From June 1993 Data-Star have introduced an annual fee/subscription per contract (that is, not per password) of SFr 80.00 (c.UK£ 32.00) payable every June. For North American customers billed in dollars who also use DIALOG, the DIALOG fee also covers access to Data-Star. Academic customers, 'commitment' customers and customers currently billed in dollars are exempt.

Record composition

Abstract AB; Accession Number and Secondary Source identification AN; Author(s) AU; Country of Publication ZN; Descriptors (MeSH subheadings) DE; Entry Date on NLM Computer ED; Index Month IM; Institution IN; Journal Code JC; Journal Subset SB; Language LG; Major Descriptor Term MJ; Minor Descriptor Term MN; Personal Name as Source PN; Publication Type PT; Secondary Source SI; Source SO; Special List Indicator LI; Title of Article TI; Transliterated Title TT and Year of Publication YR

17:54. Online — DIALOG, Knowledge Index

File name	File 151
Start year	1975
Number of records	569,202
Update period	Monthly
Price/Charges	Connect time: US$36.00
	Online print: US$0.12
	Offline print: US$0.12
	SDI charge: US$5.25

Notes

This database is also available to home users during evenings and weekends at a reduced rate on the Knowledge Index service of DIALOG – file name in this case is Health Planning and Administration, and searches are made with simplified commands or menus.

It is possible to discover records which are unique to the HEALTH database and eliminate those which duplicate MEDLINE records by using SF=HEALTH.

17:55. Online   DIMDI

File name	HE75
Start year	1975
Number of records	629,357
Update period	Monthly
SDI period	1 month
Database aids	User Manual, List of Serials Indexed for Online Users and Memocard Health
Price/Charges	Connect time: UK£05.84–10.58 Online print: UK£0.17–0.35 Offline print: UK£0.09–0.15
Downloading is allowed	
Thesaurus is online	

Notes

There is menu-driven guidance available in German and English.

Record composition

Abstract AB; Abstract Source AS; Author AU; Book Title BTI; Classification Code CC; Corporate Source CS; Controlled Term CT; Country CY; Document Type DT; Entry Date ED; Freetext FT; Gene Symbol GE (from 1991); Index Medicus Date IMD; Journal Title Code JC; Journal Title JT (abbreviation); Language LA; Last Revision Date LR; Number of Document ND; Number of Grant NG; Notes NO; Order Number OD; Procurement Source PC; Personal Name as Subject PS; Publisher PU; Publication Year PY; Qualifier QF; Number of References RN; Supporting Agency SA; Secondary Source SEC; Source SO; ISSN SS; Subunit SU; Type of Award TA and Title TI

The DIMDI implimentation of the *MeSH* thesaurus allows bilingual access and the hierarchical structure makes it possible to search for a whole group of related descriptors in one step. The Source field is a composite containing the journal title, the volume and issue number, publication year, etc.

Documents may be ordered online from the British Library Document Supply Centre, Zentralbibliothek der Medizin, Köln, Bayerische Stattsbibliothek Munchen, and Koninklijke Nederlandse Akademie van Wetenschapen, Amsterdam. The basic index includes the fields: Title, Abstract and Controlled Term.

17:56. Online   National Library of Medicine

File name	Health Planning and Administration
Start year	1975
Number of records	623,372
Update period	Monthly

Notes

It is possible to discover records which are unique to the HEALTH database and eliminate those which duplicate MEDLINE records by using H(LI) or AHA(SI) for the Hospital Literature Index citations and NP(SI) for the NHPIC citations.

17:57. CD-ROM   CD Plus

File name	CD Plus/Health Planning and Administration
Format notes	IBM
Software	OVID 3.0
Start year	1975
Number of records	569,202
Update period	Monthly
Price/Charges	Subscription: UK£845
Downloading is allowed	

Notes

Offers the ability to limit by local journal holdings. For the experienced searcher, the software offers *MeSH* explodes, 'personal pre-explodes' for frequently exploded terms, SDIs and Save Searches, enhanced MeSH tree structures, and emulation of National Library of Medicine and dot-dot syntax.

Record composition

Author; Institution; Title; Sponsoring Agencies; Original Titles and Grant Numbers

This database has an index of all searchable terms together with the online *MeSh Thesaurus* which offers mapping from natural language to *MeSH* – a facility which should give significantly improved precision for the inexperienced searcher. The on-screen help provides scope notes, definitions and task descriptors.

17:58. CD-ROM   Compact Cambridge

File name	Health: Planning and Administration
Format notes	IBM
Start year	Most recent ten years
Number of records	350,000
Update period	Quarterly
Price/Charges	Subscription: UK£515
Thesaurus is online	

17:59. CD-ROM   EBSCO

File name	Health Planning and Administration/EBSCO CD
Format notes	IBM
Start year	1975
Number of records	475,000
Update period	Quarterly
Price/Charges	Subscription: US$795

Notes

Searching is performed by a fill-in-the-blanks screen called a Query Profile which supports full Boolean logic. Search SDIs can be stored for reuse and local titles can be flagged so that these a highlighted on a display of records following a search. The software also monitors journal usage and numbers of searches performed to aid in the management of user collections.

17:60. CD-ROM   SilverPlatter

File name	HealthPLAN-CD
Format notes	IBM, Mac
Software	SPIRS/MacSPIRS
Start year	1981
Number of records	432,000
Update period	Quarterly
Database aids	Quick Reference Card and SilverPlatter Manual
Price/Charges	Subscription: UK£685 – 1,025
Thesaurus is online	

Notes

Like MEDLINE on SilverPlatter, HealthPLAN supports explodable thesaurus terms (broader headings plus their narrower related terms); the only shortcoming of the system is that HealthPLAN does not automatically map search terms to the preferred term. Nicholas G Tomaiuolo reviewed HealthPLAN (*CD-ROM World* 8(4) 1993 77–81) and felt that the disc would be a natural complement to the SilverPlatter MEDLINE database, the more especially as it has the ability when searching to exclude MEDLINE references. He gave a rating of four (very good) out of five and noted the principal shortcomings as its 'redundant method of searching (where each stage of a search query receives a number with postings) and the inconvenient manner of changing defaults during browsing and printing routines. Pluses include super easy installation, handy online thesaurus tools, very good technical support and SilverPlatter's cooperative and helpful customer service and sales department.'

The regular subscription for the CD is £685 for single users and £1,028 for 2–8 networked users. It is also available for loading on to a hard disc – cost is £1,028 for 2–8 netorked users, £1,370 for 9–16 users, £1,713 for 17–24 users. The fee for the hard disc is US$2,000.

This CD-ROM database has an index of all searchable terms together with the online *MeSh Thesaurus* which contains three tools: an alphabetical list of permuted terms, selected term detail and *MeSH* trees.

17:61. Fixed disk — SilverPlatter

File name	HealthPLAN
Format notes	IBM
Software	SPIRS
Start year	1975
Number of records	432,000
Update period	Quarterly
Database aids	Quick Reference Card and SilverPlatter Manual
Price/Charges	Subscription: UK£1,028 – 1,713

Notes

Contains the entire database. This database is available on fixed disk, with updates supplied on CD-ROM. This means that up to thirty networked users can have access to a single file containing the complete database – cost is £1,028 for 2–8 networked users, £1,370 for 9–16 users, £1,713 for 17–24 users. The fee for the hard disc is US$2,000. Search speeds are up to ten times faster than CD-ROM searching.

This database has an index of all searchable terms together with the online *MeSh Thesaurus* which contains three tools: an alphabetical list of permuted terms, selected term detail and *MeSH* trees.

17:62. Tape — National Library of Medicine

File name	Health Planning and Administration
Start year	1975
Number of records	623,372
Update period	Monthly

Notes

It is possible to discover records which are unique to the HEALTH database and eliminate those which duplicate MEDLINE records by using H(LI) or AHA(SI) for the Hospital Literature Index citations and NP(SI) for the NHPIC citations.

Corresponds to the Health Planning and Administration online database.

For more details of constituent databases, see:
MEDLINE

HECLINET
Deutsches Krankenhausinstitut eV (DKI)
Technische Universitaet Berlin, Institut für Krankenhausbau (IFK)

17:65. Master record

Alternative name(s)	Health Care Literature Information Network
Database type	Bibliographic
Number of journals	
Sources	Bibliographies, conference proceedings, dissertations, grey literature, journals, monographs, newspapers, reports, standards and theses
Start year	1969
Language	Original language (titles), Original language (abstracts), English (abstracts), English (titles), German (abstracts), German (titles), English (index terms) and German (index terms)
Coverage	International
Number of records	97,879
Update size	4,500
Update period	Every two months
Abstract details	HECLINET staff
Thesaurus	Thesaurus Krankenhauswesen (1988, 6th revision)
Database aids	Kompendium HELCINETInformationsdienst Krankenhauswesen/Health Care Information Service

Keywords

Health Economics; Health Services; Hospital Hygiene

Description

HECLINET contains citations, with abstracts, to the worldwide literature on hospital administration and non-clinical aspects of health services. 80% of the records derive from journals. Subjects in the area of hospital literature covered include hospital architecture; hospital planning; hospital operation and organisation; accounting; hospital information systems; hospital technology; hospital financing; hospital hygiene and sanitation. Subjects within the non-clinical literature in the neighbouring areas of health care include education and training; regional planning; organisation and management; health economics; health policy; hospital insurance; planning; law and jurisdiction.

The database corresponds in part to *Informationsdienst Krankenhauswesen (Health Care Information Service)* which is produced every two months. Up to 1980, 90% of all entries in the database were available in the printed version but after 1981 this was reduced to 60%. The database is produced in co-operation with the hospital institutes of Austria, Denmark, Sweden and Switzerland and the following institutions which belong to the HECLINET network participate in the evaluation of the sources: Dansk Sygehus Institut (DSI); österreichishes, Bundesinstitut für Gesundheitswesen (OEBIG); Schweizerisches Institut für Gesundheitsund Krankenhauswesen (SKI); Sjukvardens och socialvardens planerings och rationaliseringsinstitut (SPRI); Centrum Medyczne Ksztalcenia Podyplomowego (CMW). Approximately 34% of the records contain an abstract of between

100 and 500 words. An additional 20% of the records contain an annotation consisting of a one or two sentence statement augmenting the information contained in the title or elaborating on the relevance of the documents. The annotations have three main purposes: (1) they give more precise hospital descriptions including the number of beds, spaces or specialisations; (2) they provide references to a conference if the item concerned is a copy of a lecture; (3) they indicate continuations and secondary or supplementary publications. The sources evaluated for inclusion include: 300 journals on hospital and health care (a shortened version of the list of journals appears annually in the first issue of *Informationsdienst Krankenhauswesen*); 200 journals on architecture, city planning and construction engineering (the reference section on documentation on Dokumentation Gebäudelehre of the Universitätsbibliothek of the Technische Universität Berlin provides a special referral service for these journals); twenty journals from the area of Operations Research, selected by the Betriebswirtschaftliche Institut der Universität Erlangen/Nürnberg and 600 economic journals examined and made available by the Wirtschaftswissenschaftliche Documentation der Technischen Universität Berlin. Approximately 50% of the records are in German, 30% in English, 5.6% in French, 3.5% in Scandinavian languages and 2.5% in Dutch. The accepted form of journal title is provided in the list of original citations in the Kompensium Heclinet together with the original publication place. For non-German/English titles a translation is given in parentheses preceded by an abbreviated form of the original language title.

Covers journals in the fields of health care, economics, architecture, and operations research.

The unit record contains bibliographic data including author(s), title architect, plus controlled vocabulary terms, geographic terms, additional subject information and an abstract. The *Thesaurus Krankenhauswesen* which is used for indexing is a comprehensive, hierarchically structured dictionary and contains approximately 1,100 descriptors and 2,500 cross-references. 71 of the descriptors serve individually or in combination as sorting aids and are used for the general content structuring of the printed version of the *Informationsdienst Krankenhauswesen/Health Care Information Service*. Certain descriptor groups can be expanded with numerical additions. For example most of the subcategories of the descriptor hospital give the number of beds and some descriptors can be augmented by the year. The Annual Indexers' Conference of the HECLINET Network determines additions, deletions or alterations to the descriptors and these are put into effect in the following volume of the *Informationsdienst Krankenhauswesen* except in cases of urgency when they are carried out via round-robin correspondence coordinated by the Institut für Krankenhausbau. Only original documents (primary sources) are selected and evaluated and the indexing is carried out by professional specialists in the respective fields such as architects, economists and planners. The leading professional journals from each country are given priority in the evaluation procedure.

17:66. Online   DIMDI

File name	HN69
Alternative name(s)	Health Care Literature Information Network
Software	GRIPS
Start year	1969

Number of records	97,879
Update period	Every two months
Delay	2–4 months
SDI period	2 months
Price/Charges	Connect time: UK£15.80–20.55
	Online print: UK£0.32–0.50
	Offline print: UK£0.23–0.30

Downloading is allowed
Thesaurus is online

Notes

Suppliers of online documents: British Library Document Supply Centre, Boston Spa, England; Bayerische Staatsbibliothek München, München, Germany; Harkers Information Retrieval System, Sydney, Australia; Zentralbibliothek und TIB, Hannover, Germany. Menu driven guidance is available in German and English. Searches are possible from January 1969.

Record composition

Abstract AB; Abstract Language AL; Additional Source Information ASI; Architect AR; Author AU; Classification Code CC; Controlled Term CT; Document Type DT; Entry Date ED; Free Text FT; Geographical Heading GH; Journal Title JT; Language LA; Location LO; Location0 LO0; Number of Document ND; Number of Document, Identifier NDI; Publication Place PP; Publication Year PY; Qualifier QF; Subject Heading SH; Source SO and Title TI

The unit record contains bibliographic data including author(s), title architect, plus controlled vocabulary terms, geographic terms, additional subject information and an abstract. The *Thesaurus Krankenhauswesen* is available online from DIMDI in both German and English. The Subject Headings consist of individual descriptors or combinations of two descriptors and are used in the general content structuring of the printed version of the *Informationsdienst Krankenhauswesen/Health Care Information Service* and can also be used for online searching. The Geographical Headings refer to the geographical designations which are treated or referred to in the corresponding document and can consist of continents, parts of continents, countries, regional subdivisions or cities. The Additional Source Information includes illustrations, tables, diagrams and other aids included in the text. The basic index includes the data fields: Title, Abstract, Controlled Term, Controlled Term German, Section Heading, Section Heading German, Geographical Heading and Geographical Heading German. Freetext searches can be conducted in German or English.

Home Reference Library
Ellis Enterprises

17:67. Master record

Database type	Encyclopedia, Almanac
Number of journals	
Sources	
Start year	
Language	English
Coverage	
Number of records	
Update size	—
Update period	Semiannually

Description

Contains: Encyclopedias; Almanacs; Reference works; Selected information from Nurse's Library, Bible Library, and Physician's Library.

17:68. CD-ROM   Ellis Enterprises

File name	Home Reference Library
Format notes	IBM
Start year	
Number of records	
Update period	Semiannually
Price/Charges	Subscription: US$895

For more details of constituent databases, see:
Nurse Library
Physician Library
Bible Library

Medical and Psychological Previews

BRS Information Technologies

17:70. Master record

Database type	Bibliographic
Number of journals	240
Sources	Journals
Start year	
Language	English
Coverage	
Number of records	19,500
Update size	7,000
Update period	
Hosts have included	BRS (until 30.9.92.)

Description

Gives bibliographic citations from 240 core medical journals prior to their appearance in MEDLINE. Covers: clinical medicine, psychology, psychiatry, nursing, hospital administration. Includes editorials, notes and letters. Covers last 4 months.

BRS discontinued this database at the end of September 1992.

MEDLINE

National Library of Medicine

17:71. Master record

Database type	Bibliographic
Number of journals	3,500
Sources	Conference proceedings, journals, monographs and reviews
Start year	1964
Language	English
Coverage	International
Number of records	7,500,000
Update size	370,000
Update period	Weekly except January and February which are updated monthly
Index unit	Biographies, case studies, comparative studies, editorials, letters, news releases, obituaries, reviews, articles, book chapters and interview
Abstract details	Author abstracts (since 1975) are available for approximately 70% of the citations
Thesaurus	Medical Subject Headings (MeSH)
Database aids	MeSH Tree Structures, Permuted MeSH, MeSH Supplementary Chemical Records with CAS Registration Numbers or Enzyme Codes (from June 1980), Gene Symbols from January 1991), List of Serials Indexed for Online Users, includes NLM Journal codens, List of Journals Indexed in Index Medicus includes subject order serials index and Indexing Manual

Keywords

HIV; Anaesthesia; Anatomy; Applied Science; Biochemistry; Biotechnology; Cancer; Cardiology; Cardiovascular Diseases; Chemical Substances; Clinical Medicine; Forensic Science; Geriatrics; Gynaecology; Handicapped; Health and Safety; Immunology; Infectious Diseases; Medical History; Mental Health; Microbiology; Obstetrics; Occupational Health and Safety; Orthopaedics; Paediatrics; Patents; Pathology; Physiology; Pollution; Public Health; Radiology; Social Services; Toxicology

Description

MEDLINE (MEDlars (MEDical Literature ANalysis and Retrieval System) onLINE) is a vast source of medical information covering the whole field of medicine and health science information. It is the most current file and includes the current year and at least two additional years depending on the host utilised. MEDLINE backfiles are segmented and are available back to 1966. Subjects covered include (1) basic sciences/research in medicine such as bacteriology, biochemistry, environmental research, genetics, immunology, microbiology, parasitology, physiology and virology; and (2) applied sciences/clinical medicine such as anatomy, biomedical technology, clincial medicine, communication disorders, dental medicine, dermatology, environmental medicine, experimental medicine, forensic medicine, gerontology, gynaecology, health care services, hospital administration, immunology, medical education, medical psychology, medical technology, neurology, nutrition, occupational medicine, nursing oncology, opthalmology, orthopedics, parasitology, paramedical professions, pathology, pharmacy, pharmacology, physiology, policy issues, population, psychiatry, psychology, rehabilitation, research, social science medicine; social medicine, sport medicine, toxicology and veterinary medicine.

MEDLINE corresponds to the printed publications: *Index Medicus, Index to Dental Literature, International Nursing Index* and various other bibliographies. Author abstracts are provided for approximately seventy per cent of items in the database. The database also covers chapters and articles from selected monographs from 1976 to 1981. About 74% of citations are to English-language sources and the remaining citations represent over 40 other languages. This compares with 88% English-language sources on SciSearch, 86% on BIOSIS and 75% in EMBASE, the other leading bioscience databases. 50% of records were added after January 1975. More than 90% of journals are evaluated cover to cover. The database contains 304,354 citations for the years 1964/5 but as the controlled vocabulary and retrieval is different from the later years, these years are often offered as a separate file. Citations are automatically transferred from MEDLINE to other NLM-databases, therefore many of the journals indexed are also found in CANCERLIT (approximately 85% overlap with MEDLINE), HEALTH (approximately 80% overlap with MEDLINE) and AIDSLINE (approximately 75% overlap with MEDLINE). For BIOETHICSLINE no automatic transfer takes place but many MEDLINE-journals related to biomedical ethics are also evaluated for BIOETHICSLINE. Journals are categorised on three different levels of priority. Those on the third level are indexed in less depth than journals on levels one and two. The time lag between the appearance of the publication and availability on magnetic tape is usually shorter for priority one and two than for priority three journals. Journals to be considered for MEDLINE are selected by an advisory committee of physicians, scientists, librarians and publishers of medical journals appointed by the NLM. Journal information which is not indexed includes abstracts on congresses, book reviews, hospital reports, communications from medical associations, announcements of new drugs by pharmaceutical companies. Regarding the length of abstracts, between 1975 and 1977 there was no limitation regarding the length of abstracts. Between 1977 and 1980 no abstract longer than 200 words and between 1981 and 1983 no abstract longer than 250 words was stored. Due to these limitations only 45% of the citations contain abstracts for this period of input. From 1984 onwards, abstracts exceeding 250 words or 400 words for abstracts of articles 10 pages or more in length are included but truncated and these abstracts have the message 'ABSTRACTS TRUNCATED AT 250/400 WORDS' at their end. From 1984, 65% of the citations contain an abstract. This compares with 60% in EMBASE and 54% in BIOSIS. Records of the other leading bioscience database, SciSearch, now also contains abstracts. Since 1980, 26% of MEDLINE records with non-English sources contain English-language abstracts online. This compares with 67% on BIOSIS and 37% on EMBASE. Abstracts from articles from journal titles of priority three have only been stored since Spring 1989.

MEDLINE's Tree Structures classification is the most detailed alphanumeric scheme developed for online searching. It is directly related to the controlled vocabulary in the database. It is necessary to use the hardcopy search aids produced – MeSH annotated alphabetic list, TREE structures, Permuted terms etc. to obtain successful search results, and, as they are re-edited and published by NLM each year, to use the latest edition only, as new terminology is included annually. Generally, new sets become available in December for use in the following year. The MeSH descriptors have check tags for gender, age groups, human, animal, article type and can also be subdivided using standard subheadings. A two tier level of indexing is used with an average of twelve descriptors assigned, of which three to five descriptors are major or primary headings which appear in Index Medicus or other print sources. In addition to the controlled vocabulary terms, textwords or free-text terms may be used for retrieval from the title, abstract, authors address and other parts of the citation. Exploded treewords, which are the hierarchical arrangement of Medical Subject Headings can also be used for retrieval of broad categories of information.

Every Medical Subject Heading has at least one corresponding alpha-numeric code or tree number which determines its location in the hierarchically arranged Tree Structures. Some headings have more than one tree number because they are located in more than one tree. There are a total of fifteen broad subject categories or trees as follows: A. Anatomical Terms; B. Organisms; C. Diseases; D. Chemicals and Drugs; E. Analytical, Diagnostic and Therapeutic Technics and Equipment; F. Psychiatry and Psychology; G. Biological Sciences; H. Physical Sciences; I. Anthropology, Education, Sociology and Social Phenomena; J. Technology, Industry, Agriculture, Food; K. Humanities; L. Information Science and Communications; M. Named Groups of Persons; N. Health Care; and Z. Geographicals. These broad categories are then broken down into narrower subcate-

gories. The hardcopy thesaurus indicates when narrower terms are available under a code.

In addition to numerous cross-references MeSH pre-coordinates frequently searched concepts for example PREGNANCY IN DIABETES. It also contains history notes indicating starting dates for consistent usage of indexer-added terms online and hints for retrospective searching on topics where preferred terminology has changed over time, for example ROBOTICS (87) search AUTOMATION 1966–86. MEDLINE also permits indexers to identify concepts lacking adequate descriptors in MeSH. Since June 1980 its identifier field has been used to index chemicals discussed in the full text of source documents ensuring access to names or numbers of compounds whether or not they are included among MeSH descriptors. Registry Numbers have been assigned in MEDLINE records since June 1980. MEDLINE also consistently adds Enzyme Commission (EC) numbers to records for sources which discuss enzymes).

The datafield Document Type was introduced to MEDLINE in 1991, Prior to this some of the Document Types had been MeSH-Terms for example historial article, review. Most of these MeSH terms have been deleted and replaced by a corresponding Document Type retrospectively. Indexing with MeSH is performed by specially trained staff in indexing institutes in the USA. The value of controlled vocabulary is important when searching for topics where a subject population has been specified. Relatively few bioscience databases provide consistent indexing for subject populations (that is, humans or specific test animals) and related characteristics commonly requested such as age groups, gender, occupation and racial or ethnic groups. In comparison with BIOSIS, EMBASE and SciSearch MEDLINE provides the most extensive consistent indexing for the subject population groups, humans, test animals, racial/ethnic groups, gender and age groups but provides less consistent indexing of occupational gropus, where fewer controlled terms are augmented with natural language keywords in strategies. A study on indexing consistency in MEDLINE has shown an average consistency for central concept main heading (equivalent to MeSH term/MAJOR; that is, *Toxicology in records) identification of 61.1% for central concept subheadings (for example, *MeSH term- TOXICITY), of 54.9% and for central main heading/subheading combinations (for example, *Skin Drug Effects) of 43.1%. In most bioscience files a form of pharmaceutical nomenclature exists. For MEDLINE the preferred search terms are generic name, classification by action/use and CAS Registry Number although restrictions by date, subfile and vendor may apply to the latter and vendor documentation should be consulted for guidelines. Restrictions also apply for the search term Enzyme Commission Number and vendor documentations should again be consulted for guidelines. For the search terms investigational code, chemical name and trade name, the terminology is inconsistent and alternative names should be used in search strategies. Retrospective searching however may require the entry of other names used for the same substance at earlier stages in its development life cycle. The use of synonyms is advisable when searching compounds yet to be added as controlled MeSH descriptors.

In 1993, after the annual reload, there are some new features available: new file labels; page, issue and volume numbers in the source paragraph are now searchable, it is now possible to retrieve articles where the user has incomplete information eg. an article written by Schellenberg., published in a journal on Page 668; review articles are now searchable with a .LIMIT-command; 94 descriptors have been replaced by more up-to-date terminology; 421 new and updated *MeSH* terms and new publication types in the PT field.

17:72. Database subset

CD-ROM   **EBSCO**

File name	Core MEDLINE
Format notes	IBM
Software	EBSCO-CD
Start year	Most recent three years.
Number of records	
Update period	Quarterly
Price/Charges	Subscription: US$830
Thesaurus is online	

Notes

A single-disc subset of MEDLINE, containing references from all titles covered in the Abridged Index Medicus and all MEDLINE titles from the three Brandon and Hill lists. The title list is clinically oriented and contains most English-language nursing and psychology titles indexed for MEDLINE.

Searching is performed by a fill-in-the-blanks screen called a Query Profile which supports full Boolean logic. Search SDIs can be stored for reuse and local titles can be flagged so that these a highlighted on a display of records following a search. The software also monitors journal usage and numbers of searches performed to aid in the management of user collections.

17:73. Database subset

CD-ROM   **Knowledge Access**

File name	Nursing Indisc
Format notes	IBM
Software	KAware
Start year	1963
Number of records	200,000
Update period	Quarterly
Price/Charges	Subscription: US$399

Notes

MEDLINE subset containing references to the world-wide literature on nursing and nursing research from 517 journals. Includes references to AIDS treatment, drug abuse, cholesterol, fibre, and nutrition, and so on. Corresponds to the printed publication *International Nursing Index*, and, consequently, in part to the MEDLINE database.

This database can also be found on:
Online Journal of Current Clinical Trials
Developmental and Reproductive Toxicology
BiblioMed Cardiology
BiblioMed Infectious Diseases
AIDS Compact Library
Compact Library: Viral Hepatitis
OnDisc Discovery Training Toolkit
Lancet
British Medical Journal
New England Journal of Medicine
Annals of Internal Medicine
Morbidity and Mortality Weekly Report
American Journal of Public Health
Infectious Diseases – Personal MEDLINE
Obstetrics & Gynecology – Personal MEDLINE
Journal of the American Medical Association
Pediatrics – Personal MEDLINE
Family Practice – Personal MEDLINE
Critical Care Medicine – Personal MEDLINE
Emergency Medicine – Personal MEDLINE

Gastroenterology and Hepatology Medicine – Personal MEDLINE
Canadian Medical Association Journal
Human Nutrition on CD-ROM
Oxford Database of Perinatal Trials
Entrez: Sequences
STAT!-Ref
Medata-ROM
AIDSLINE
Bioethicsline
NEXIS
TOXLINE
MAXX

Nurse Library
Ellis Enterprises

17:75. Master record

Database type	Factual, Textual
Number of journals	
Sources	Books
Start year	
Language	
Coverage	
Number of records	
Update size	–
Update period	Annually

Description

Contains the full text of selected specialty and subspecialty medical and nursing text books, and nursing manuals.

17:76. CD-ROM   **Ellis Enterprises**

File name	Nurse Library
Format notes	IBM
Start year	
Number of records	
Update period	Annually
Price/Charges	Subscription: US$895

This database can also be found on:
Home Reference Library

Physician Data Query
National Cancer Institute, US National Institutes of Health

17:77. Master record

Alternative name(s)	PDQ
Database type	Bibliographic, Directory, Textual
Number of journals	
Sources	Clinicians, directories, research reports and textbooks
Start year	Current
Language	English
Coverage	USA (primarily) and International (some)
Number of records	Variable
Update size	Variable
Update period	Monthly

Keywords

Cancer; Pathology

Description

Physician Data Query is an English-language factual database produced by the National Cancer Institute (NCI) and its PDQ Editorial Board and is designed to assist physicians in the treatment and referral of cancer patients. The database is composed of three interrelated files: (1) the Cancer Information File (2) the Protocol File and (3) the Directory File.

(1) The Cancer Information File contains full-text information on about eighty cancer types provided, reviewed and updated by an Editorial Board of experts both inside and outside the US National Cancer Institute. It contains information on patients with descriptions, stage explanations and general treatment options and on prognosis, cellular classification, stage information and treatment by cell type/stage. Literature citations with abstracts on the key medical literature on the individual oncological aspects are also included. When there is no effective treatment for a particular cancer, the file describes current investigative approaches under evaluation in clinical trials. An editorial board of 72 oncologists is responsible for the currency and accuracy of the information.

(2) The Protocol File contains information on over 7,700 active and closed treatment protocols on new methods of cancer treatment; it includes clinical research objectives, special study parameters, treatment regimens and schedules, patient entry criteria and participating institutions. Each protocol provides detailed information on drug dosage, schedule and dosage modification organised into tables. It also includes most data from the NCI database CLINPROT, which was discontinued in March 1991. The file also contains approximately forty descriptors of approved standard therapies, revised by the PDQ Editorial Board.

(3) The Directory File contains a listing of the names, addresses, telephone numbers of 17,000 physicians and surgeons (mainly North American, but also European and Latin American), and 2,400 organisations and institutions (mainly in the United States of America) devoted to the care of cancer patients. It also details their medical speciality and professional affiliation. European organisations and physicians are listed in PDQ when they participate in programmes such as the EORTC (European Organisation for Research and Treatment of Cancer), or when they are members of the major oncologic societies in the United States, such as the American Society of Clinical Oncology. PDQ also contains full-text information on supportive care in neoplatic diseases, early detection guidelines and design of clincial trials.

17:78. Database subset

Online   **BRS**

File name	PDQS
Alternative name(s)	PDQ
Start year	
Number of records	
Update period	
Price/Charges	Connect time: US$39.00/49.00
	Online print: US$0.14/0.22
	Offline print: US$0.22

Notes
Supportive care subset.

Postgraduate Medicine
McGraw-Hill Inc

17:79. Master record

Database type	Textual
Number of journals	1
Sources	

Start year	1990
Language	English
Coverage	International
Number of records	
Update size	—
Update period	Monthly

Keywords
Clinical Medicine

Description
A magazine covering the diagnosis and treatment of general medical problems, including clinical articles of interest to physicians, nurses, dentists and other health care professionals.

Corresponds to *Postgraduate Medicine* magazine. On DIALOG, NEXIS and Dow Jones News/Retrieval, this database is available as part of the McGraw-Hill Publications Online database.

17:80. Online   **NewsNet Inc**

File name	
Start year	1990
Number of records	
Update period	Monthly

This database can also be found on:
McGraw-Hill Publications Online

Serline
National Library of Medicine

17:82. Master record

Alternative name(s)	Serials Online
Database type	Bibliographic, Library catalogue/cataloguing aids
Number of journals	
Sources	A-V material, conference reports, journals and serials
Start year	Current
Language	English and Original language (titles)
Coverage	International
Number of records	79,010
Update size	24,000
Update period	Monthly
Index unit	Serials
Thesaurus	Medical Subject Headings (MeSH)

Keywords
Physiology

Description
SERLINE is a database of bibliographic records of serials held, on order or in process by the US National Library of Medicine in the areas of medicine, health, nursing, physiology, psychology, dentistry. The documents in SERLINE mainly refer to titles indexed in one of the NLM databases – MEDLINE, Aidsline, Cancerlit and Toxline. In addition to full, abbreviated, added or changed titles SERLINE provides information on ISSN and CODEN, publishing place, publisher, publisher's address, indexing by NLM, microfilming of journal volumes by NLM and the paper quality of journals. SERLINE can be used to find: the full name of a journal abbreviation from MEDLINE; the abbreviation of a journal for an online search; the journals which make up the core cancer journals; all journals indexed for nursing information; all journals indexed in Chemical Abstracts; all journals in French. The official

serial cataloguing information can be found in the NLM database CATLINE.

Corresponds in part to the microfiche publication *Health Sciences Serials*. Approximately forty per cent of the titles are published in the USA. Approximately 51,000 documents are marked 'closed' indicating that the title has changed or that publication has ceased. If the title has changed, the new title shown under the data field NOTE. Both English and American spellings are used in the database.

The controlled vocabulary *Medical Subject Headings (MeSH)* is used to index items which have been catalogued since 1965. Descriptors and section headings are also used for indexing, both of which are directly inverted and freetext searchable. Section headings identify the general subject of a series and are used for series grouping in the NLM *List of Journals Indexed in INDEX MEDICUS*.

17:83. Online — Australian MEDLINE Network

File name	SERLINE
Alternative name(s)	Serials Online
Start year	
Number of records	
Update period	

17:84. Online — BLAISE-LINK

File name	SERLINE
Alternative name(s)	Serials Online
Start year	Titles from the 1660s to date
Number of records	
Update period	Monthly

17:85. Online — CISTI MEDLARS

File name	SERLINE
Alternative name(s)	Serials Online
Start year	
Number of records	79,010
Update period	Monthly

17:86. Online — Data-Star

File name	SERL
Alternative name(s)	Serials Online
Start year	Current
Number of records	79,010
Update period	Monthly
Database aids	Data-Star Biomedical Manual and Online guide (search NEWS-SERL in NEWS)
Price/Charges	Subscription: SFr80.00
	Connect time: SFr78.00
	Online print: SFr0.18
	Offline print: SFr0.24
	SDI charge: SFrNone
Downloading is allowed	
Thesaurus is online	

Notes

From June 1993 Data-Star have introduced an annual fee/subscription per contract (that is, not per password) of SFr 80.00 (c.UK£ 32.00) payable every June. For North American customers billed in dollars who also use DIALOG, the DIALOG fee also covers access to Data-Star. Academic customers, 'commitment' customers and customers currently billed in dollars are exempt.

Record composition

Accession Number and Update Code AN; NLM Call Number; Coden CD; Descriptor DE; First/Last Issue FL; Frequency of Publication FR; Index Authority Date IA; Indexing Status XS; ISSN Number IS; Journal Coden JC; Journal Subset (INDEX MEDICUS titles only) SB; Language LG; List of Journals Indexed – Subject Headings JD; Major Revision Date MR; MESH Tree Number ZN; Notes and Indexing NT; Title and Abbreviation TI and Title Search Key

17:87. Online — DIMDI

File name	SE00
Alternative name(s)	Serials Online
Start year	Current
Number of records	79,499
Update period	Monthly
Price/Charges	Connect time: UK£03.88–08.62
	Online print: UK£0.16–0.34
	Offline print: UK£0.07–0.14
	SDI charge: UK£None
Downloading is allowed	

Record composition

Added Journal Title AJT; Controlled Terms CT; Country of Publication CY; First Publication Year Y1; Frequency FR; Full Journal Titles JT; Journal Code CO; Journal Titles JA; Language LA; Last Publication Year Y2; Open/closed Indicator OC; Publisher PU; Publisher's Address ADR; Publisher's Name PN; Publishing Place PP and Section Headings SH

17:88. Online — National Library of Medicine

File name	SERLINE
Alternative name(s)	Serials Online
Start year	Current
Number of records	79,010
Update period	Monthly

17:89. Tape — National Library of Medicine

File name	SERLINE
Alternative name(s)	Serials Online
Format notes	IBM
Start year	Current
Number of records	79,010
Update period	Monthly

Notes

Corresponds to the SERLINE online database. Contact NLM for pricing information.

Swedish Biomedicine
MIC Karolinska Institutets Bibliotek OCH Informationscentral (MIC-KIBIC)

17:90. Master record

Alternative name(s)	SWEMED
Database type	Bibliographic
Number of journals	
Sources	Journals, Reports and Dissertations
Start year	1982
Language	Original language titles, English and Swedish
Coverage	Sweden and Norway
Number of records	16,000
Update size	1,000
Update period	Twice a week
Thesaurus	Medical Subject Headings (MeSH)

Keywords

Anatomy; Biomedicine; Nutrition; Pathology; Microbiology

Description

Can be regarded as a Swedish complement to MEDLINE – contains Swedish biomedical literature not covered by MEDLINE. Contains about 5,000 references to Swedish biomedical journals (for example, *Läkartidningen*), reports and dissertations from Swedish and Norwegian universities since 1982. Coverage includes medicine, dentistry, nursing, nutrition, pharmacology.

17:91. Online

MIC/Karolinska Institute Library and Information Center (MIC KIBIC)

File name	Swemed
Alternative name(s)	SWEMED
Start year	1982
Number of records	16,000
Update period	Twice a week

MEDICAL DEVICES

21CFR Online
Diogenes

18:1. Master record

Database type	Textual
Number of journals	
Sources	Laws/regulations
Start year	Current information
Language	English
Coverage	USA
Number of records	7,000
Update size	–
Update period	Monthly
Database aids	21CFR Online Users Guide 1991, Rockville, DIOGENES

Description

Contains the full text of Title 21 of the *Code of Federal Regulations (CFR)* – official regulations from two US government departments: the Food and Drug Administration (FDA), concerned with administering food and drugs; and the Drug Enforcement Agency (DEA), involved in drug enforcement. Covers drugs, food, cosmetics, medical devices and veterinary products.

Title 21 is divided into two chapters:

Chapter I: Food and Drug Administration (Department of Health and Human services) –
Subchapter A: General, covering general regulations, hearings, patent term restoration and colour additives.
Subchapter B: Food for Human Consumption, covering food labelling, quality standards, infant formula, general and specific food standards, food additives and seafood inspection.
Subchapter C: Drugs, General, covering drug labelling and advertising, Good Manufacturing Practices, controlled drugs and manufacturer registration.
Subchapter D: Drugs for Human Use, covering approval applications, and requirements for specific drug and antibiotic categories.
Subchapter E: Animal Drugs, Feeds, and Related Products, covering animal food labelling and packaging, and new animal drug and antibiotic approval applications.
Subchapter F: Biologics, covering licensing, standards and Good Manufacturing Practices for biological products.
Subchapter G: Cosmetics, covering labelling, establishment registration and experience reporting for cosmetics.
Subchapter H: Medical Devices, covering labelling, manufacturer registration, device classes, adverse experience reporting and premarket approvals for medical devices.
Subchapter I: Reserved.
Subchapter J: Radiological Health, covering general requirements, records and reports and performance standards for radiological health products.
Subchapter K: Reserved.
Subchapter L: Regulations Under certain Other Acts Administered by the Food and Drug Administration, covering Federal Import Milk Act, Tea Importation Act, Federal Caustic Poisin Act, communicable diseases, interstate conveyance sanitation.

Chapter II: Drug Enforcement Administration (Department of Justice) – covering manufacturer registration, labelling, prescriptions, schedules and import/export of controlled substances.

18:2. Online   BRS

File name	CF21
Start year	
Number of records	
Update period	
Price/Charges	Connect time: US$89.00/99.00
	Online print: US$0.91/0.99
	Offline print: US$0.99

18:3. Online   Data-Star

File name	CF21
Start year	Current information
Number of records	7,000
Update period	Monthly
Database aids	Data-Star Business and Biomedical Manuals, Berne, Data-Star and Online guide (search NEWS-CF21 in NEWS)
Price/Charges	Subscription: UK£32.00
	Connect time: UK£60.00
	Online print: UK£0.60
	Offline print: UK£0.90
	SDI charge: UK£5.12

Notes

From June 1993 Data-Star have introduced an annual fee/subscription per contract (that is, not per password) of SFr 80.00 (c.UK£ 32.00) payable every June. For North American customers billed in dollars who also use DIALOG, the DIALOG fee also covers access to Data-Star. Academic customers, 'commitment' customers and customers currently billed in dollars are exempt.

This database can also be found on:
FDA on CD-ROM

Abledata
Newington Children's Hospital,
Adaptive Equipment Center

18:5. Master record

Database type	Directory
Number of journals	
Sources	Equipment catalogues and suppliers
Start year	Current
Language	English
Coverage	USA and Canada
Number of records	16,000
Update size	2,400
Update period	Monthly
Index unit	Products
Hosts have included	BRS (until 31.10.92)

Keywords

Rehabilitation Aids; Disabled

Description

ABLEDATA is designed for the use of therapists, rehabilitation specialists and other medical personnel and contains descriptions of more than 17,000 rehabilitation aids and equipment for the disabled from over 2,000 companies. Subjects covered include: personal care, therapeutic, sensory, educational, vocational, transport and other technical items; giving generic and brand names, model number, manufacturer's name, address and telephone number, availability, cost, user comments, contraindications and formal evaluations, where available.

The database was formerly produced by National Rehabilitation Information Centers as NARIC Abledata.

18:6. CD-ROM — Trace Research and Development Center, Newington Children's Hospital

File name	Hyper-ABLEDATA
Format notes	IBM, Mac
Software	Hyper-ABLEDATA
Start year	
Number of records	17,000
Update period	Semiannually
Price/Charges	Subscription: US$50

Notes

Descriptions are accompanied by pictures and sound samples (such as voice output devices for the blind) for some items. Products can be located by name, company name or by the functions they perform.

Aldrich Catalogue
Aldrich Chemical Co Inc

18:7. Master record

Database type	Catalogue, Directory
Number of journals	
Sources	
Start year	
Language	English
Coverage	USA
Number of records	19,000 chemicals; 8,000 equipment.
Update size	—
Update period	Annually
Index unit	Chemicals and products

Description

Details of over 19,000 chemicals and 8,000 laboratory equipment items listed in the *Aldrich Catalog/Handbook*.

Includes Aldrich catalogue number, name and synonyms, molecular formula and structure, molecular weight, density, boiling point, melting point, flash point, refractive index, CAS registry number, RTECS number, Beilstein reference, Merck Index reference, Sigma-Aldrich safety book reference, Fleser reference, and FT-IR, IR and NMR references.

Searchable by catalogue number, CAS registry number, molecular formula, and name/synonym.

18:8. CD-ROM — Aldrich Chemical Co Inc

File name	Aldrich Catalogue
Format notes	IBM
Start year	

Number of records	19,000 chemicals; 8,000 equipment.
Update period	Annually
Price/Charges	Subscription: US$25

Notes

Products can be added to a printed purchase order.

Aldrichem DataSearch
Aldrich Chemical Co Inc

18:9. Master record

Database type	Directory, Catalogue
Number of journals	
Sources	
Start year	
Language	English
Coverage	USA
Number of records	50,000 chemicals; 8,000 equipment.
Update size	—
Update period	Annually
Index unit	Chemicals and products

Description

Database of 50,000 chemicals and 8,000 laboratory equipment products listed in the *Aldrich Catalog/Handbook*.

Versatile search capabilities allow user to find suitable starting materials, identify unknown compounds, locate reference information, publish chemical structures and print technical data with structures.

Searchable by Aldrich catalogue number, name and synonyms, name fragment, molecular formula and structure, molecular weight, density, boiling point, melting point, flash point, refractive index, CAS registry number, Merck Index reference, FT-IR, IR and NMR references.

18:10. CD-ROM — Aldrich Chemical Co Inc

File name	Aldrichem DataSearch
Format notes	IBM, Mac
Software	Proprietary
Start year	
Number of records	50,000 chemicals; 8,000 equipment.
Update period	Annually
Price/Charges	Subscription: US$875

Arthur D Little/Online
Arthur D Little Decision Resources

18:11. Master record

Database type	Bibliographic, Factual, Textual
Number of journals	
Sources	Own publications
Start year	1977
Language	English
Coverage	USA (primarily) and International (some)
Number of records	2,300
Update size	—
Update period	Bimonthly
Index unit	Books

Keywords

Applied Science; Telecommunications

Description

Arthur D. Little Online is derived from the publications of Arthur D. Little Decision Resources, plus the non-exclusive publications of Arthur D. Little Inc., its divisions and subsidiaries. Influential industry forecasts, product and market reviews, technology, corporate profiles, opinion research, product and market overviews, public opinion surveys and management commentaries are included. Industries and technologies include information processing, telecommunications, electronics, especially office automation, computers, equipment manufacturere and services; topics covered include: health care, medical equipment, chemicals including speciality chemicals, petrochemicals, packaging, diagnostic products, plastics, fibres, transport, energy, food processing, biotechnology and environmental issues. In addition to indexing and document availability information, most records contain the Table of Contents and List of Tables and Figures from the print document. Most records prior to 1989 contain the complete text of reports. From 1989 forward records contain extensive summaries of the research report.

Indexes or full text for Arthur D. Little publications, including full text of executive summaries of *Industry Outlook Reports, Research Letters, Public Opinion Index Reports.*

18:12. Online · DIALOG

File name	File 192
Start year	1977
Number of records	2,300
Update period	Bimonthly
Price/Charges	Connect time: US$114.00
	Online print: US$1.00
	Offline print: US$0.50

ASTM

National Standards Association Inc American Society for Testing and Materials

18:13. Master record

Database type	Textual, Image
Number of journals	
Sources	
Start year	
Language	English
Coverage	USA
Number of records	8,000
Update size	—
Update period	Monthly

Keywords

Standards

Description

Contains over 8,000 standards for testing methods, definitions, practices and classifications. Covers metals, construction, petroleum products, textiles, paints, plastics, rubber, electrical insulation and electronics, energy sources and medical devices.

18:14. CD-ROM · National Standards Association Inc

File name	ASTM on SPECMASTER
Format notes	IBM
Start year	

Number of records	8,000
Update period	Monthly
Price/Charges	Subscription: UK£3,900

BEFO

Fachinformationszentrum Technik (FIZ Technik)

18:15. Master record

Alternative name(s)	Management and Organization
Database type	Bibliographic, Textual
Number of journals	
Sources	Databases
Start year	1974
Language	German (primarily) and English (titles only)
Coverage	International
Number of records	114,000
Update size	8,000
Update period	Weekly

Keywords

Biomedical Engineering; Construction; Electrical Engineering; Electronic Engineering; Ergonomics; Logistics; Mechanical Engineering; Industrial Health and Safety; Industrial Medicine; Quality Control

Description

Contains citations, with abstracts, to the worldwide literature on management and business organisation of engineering projects. Covers a variety of topics related to mechanical, electrical, electronic, and bio-medical engineering. Includes project planning techniques; organizational aspects of production, quality control, and maintenance; materials supply and logistics; industrial medicine, ergonomics, and human engineering; and industrial health and safety.

Sources of information include DOMA, Meditec and ZDE.

18:16. Online · FIZ Technik

File name	BEFO
Alternative name(s)	Management and Organization
Start year	1974
Number of records	156,000
Update period	Weekly
Price/Charges	Connect time: DM264.00
	Online print: DM0.30 – 2.00
	Offline print: DM2.30
	SDI charge: DM18.00

BioBusiness

BIOSIS

18:17. Master record

Database type	Bibliographic
Number of journals	500
Sources	Conference proceedings, journals, monographs, newsletters, research reports and patents (US)
Start year	1985
Language	English
Coverage	International

Number of records	480,000
Update size	42,000
Update period	Monthly
Database aids	BioBusiness Search Guide, Philadelphia, BIOSIS, How to search BioBusiness,Philadelphia, BIOSIS and Newsletters: BioSearch, BioScene.

Keywords

Cosmetics; Fishing; Forestry; Genetic Engineering; Immunology

Description

BioBusiness is a bibliographic database which focuses specifically on the business applications of biomedical research. It contains citations, with abstracts, to the worldwide periodical literature on business applications of biological and biomedical research. Subjects covered include: agriculture and forestry, animal production, biomass conversion, crop production, diet and nutrition, fermentation, food technology, cosmetics, genetic engineering, health care, industrial microbiology, pharmaceutical products, medical technology, medical diagnostics, medical instrumentation, occupational health, pesticides, pharmaceuticals, protein production, toxicology, veterinary science, waste treatment, energy and the environment, and other industries affected by biotechnological developments. Also covers patents in such areas as immunological testing, food processes, and fishing. For each patent record, includes inventor's name and address, patent title and number, patent classes, date granted, and assignee. BioBusiness can be used to discover: the latest legislation and regulatory controls affecting implementation of biotechnology research; the impact of economic fluctuations on price and production forecasts for agricultural commodities; the financial effects of recycling programs on business; the increased use of natural ingredients in cosmetic and personal care products; the applications of bioengineering in pharmaceuticals; trends in the development and marketing of food products; etc.

A broad spectrum of life science, business and management journals are scanned. Abstracts are included for approximately 55–60% of the records.

Both controlled and uncontrolled terms are used for indexing. The concept codes used are different from the BIOSIS concept codes.

18:18. Online   BIOSIS Life Science Network

File name	
Start year	1985
Number of records	480,000
Update period	Monthly
Price/Charges	Connect time: US$9.00
	Online print: US$6.00 per 10; 2.25 per abstract; 3.50 per full text article

Downloading is allowed
Also available via the Internet by telnetting to LSN.COM.

Notes

On Life Science Network users can search this database or they can scan a group of subject-related databases. There is a charge of $2.00 per scan of subject-related databases. To search one database and display up to ten citations costs $6.00. Most charges are for information retrieved. There are no charges if there are no results and no charge to transfer results to a printer or diskette. Articles may also be ordered via an online document delivery request. A telecommunications software package is also avail-

able, costing $12.95, providing an automatic connection to Life Science Network for heavy users of the service, with capability to transfer to print or disk and customised colour options.

18:19. Online   BRS

File name	BBUS
Start year	1985
Number of records	480,000
Update period	Weekly
Price/Charges	Connect time: UK£88.00/98.00
	Online print: UK£0.46/0.54
	Offline print: UK£0.52

Downloading is allowed

18:20. Online   CISTI, Canadian Online Enquiry Service CAN/OLE

File name	
Start year	1985
Number of records	480,000
Update period	Monthly

Downloading is allowed

18:21. Online   Data-Star

File name	BBUS
Start year	1985
Number of records	277,972
Update period	Weekly
Database aids	Data-Star Business Manual and Online manual (search NEWS-BBUS in NEWS)
Price/Charges	Subscription: UK£32.00
	Connect time: UK£63.60
	Online print: UK£0.41
	Offline print: UK£0.36
	SDI charge: UK£3.94

Downloading is allowed

Notes

From June 1993 Data-Star have introduced an annual fee/subscription per contract (that is, not per password) of SFr 80.00 (c.UK£ 32.00) payable every June. For North American customers billed in dollars who also use DIALOG, the DIALOG fee also covers access to Data-Star. Academic customers, 'commitment' customers and customers currently billed in dollars are exempt.

Record composition

Abstract AB; Accession Number and Update Code AN; Author AU; Author Affliation IN; Company Name CO; Concept Codes CC; Descriptors DE; Language of Article LG; Named Person(s) NA; Publication Details PU; Source SO; Title TI; Update Codes UP and Year of Publication YR

18:22. Online   DIALOG

File name	File 285
Start year	1985
Number of records	371,575
Update period	Weekly
Price/Charges	Connect time: US$126.00
	Online print: US$0.85
	Offline print: US$0.85
	SDI charge: US$10.50

Downloading is allowed

Notes

DIALINDEX Categories: AGRIBUS, BIOBUS, BIOTECH, PHARMINA.

18:23. Online   ESA-IRS

File name	File 137
Start year	1985
Number of records	372,000 (October 1991)
Update period	Weekly

Price/Charges	Subscription: UK£70.29
	Database entry fee: UK£3.49
	Online print: UK£0.74
	Offline print: UK£0.79
	SDI charge: UK£3.49

Downloading is allowed

Notes

The default supplier of original document is British Library Documentation Supply Centre.

From 1993 ESA-IRS are charging an annual fee of 100 Accounting Units (c.UK£ 70.29) to all users. This is equivalent to the fee for full documentation and will not be charged to customers already paying for documentation.

Record composition

Abstract /AB; Additional Source Information NT; Author AU; Concept Code CC; Concept Code Name CN; Corporate Source CS; ISBN BN; Journal Name JN; Language LA; Named Company NM; Named Person SP; Native Number NN; Patent Assignee PH; Patent Number PN; Publication Year PY; Subfile (1) SF; Title /TI; Uncontrolled Terms /UT and US Patent Classification PC

18:24. Online   STN

File name	BIOBUS
Start year	1985
Number of records	480,000
Update period	Weekly

Downloading is allowed

18:25. Tape   BIOSIS

File name	
Format notes	9-track, 800, 1600 or 6250 bpi, variable length records, variable block size.
Start year	1985
Number of records	480,000
Update period	Monthly

Notes

Corresponds to the BioBusiness online database. Annual lease price is $2,350 plus additional usage charges; contact BIOSIS for archival tape prices.

BIOCAS

BIOSIS
Chemical Abstracts Service

18:26. Master record

Alternative name(s)	BIOSIS/CAS Registry Number Concordance
Database type	Directory
Number of journals	
Sources	
Start year	1969–1985
Language	English
Coverage	International
Number of records	1.2 million
Update size	—
Update period	Quarterly

Keywords

Animal Sciences; Bioengineering; Biophysics; Fishing; Immunology; Patents; Plant Sciences

Description

Contains references to citations common to both CA Search and BIOSIS Previews. Each record currently includes the BIOSIS Document Number, the equivalent CA Search Abstract Number and, for approxi-mately 78 percent of the references, CAS Registry Numbers (see Registry Nomenclature and Structure Service). In subsequent updates, CAS Registry Numbers will be available for the remaining BIOSIS citations.

18:27. Online   STN

File name	BIOCAS
Alternative name(s)	BIOSIS/CAS Registry Number Concordance
Start year	
Number of records	
Update period	

BIOLIS

Informationzentrum für Biologie am Forschungsinstitut Senckenberg

18:28. Master record

Alternative name(s)	Biologische Literaturinformation Senckenberg
Database type	Bibliographic
Number of journals	
Sources	Periodicals and serials
Start year	1970
Language	German and English
Coverage	Germany, Switzerland and Austria
Number of records	53,3532,214
Update size	6,000
Update period	Every two months
Index unit	Articles

Keywords

Animal Sciences; Bioengineering; Biophysics; Fishing; Immunology; Patents; Plant Sciences

Description

BIOLIS is a bilingual (German/English) database in the field of biology. It is intended as a supplement to the American database BIOSIS Previews. Subjects covered include: biology; botany; zoology; ecology; environmental protection and paleontology. Each record contains details of authors, title and other bibliographic data as well as free key words and the codes and terms of the BIOSIS classification system.

Sources are publications in the Federal Republic of Germany, Switzerland or Austria which are not listed in BIOSIS Previews.

Articles from serials and periodicals which are published in the Federal Republic of Germany, Switzerland and Austria.

18:29. Online   DIMDI

File name	BS70
Alternative name(s)	Biologische Literaturinformation Senckenberg
Start year	1970
Number of records	53,353
Update period	Every two months
SDI period	2 months
Price/Charges	Connect time: UK£10.55–13.39
	Online print: UK£0.30–0.48
	Offline print: UK£0.23–0.30

Downloading is allowed

Notes

Suppliers of online documents: British Library Document Supply Centre, Boston Spa, England; Harkers Information Retrieval System, Sydney, Australia.

The unit record contains information about author(s), title, and other bibliographic data as well as free key words and the codes and terms of the BIOSIS classification system. At present there are no abstracts.

Searches are possible from January 1970. The English biosystematic names in BIOLIS are associated to the Latin biosystematic names in BIOSIS Previews. BIOLIS is the only database into which Latin biosystematic names have been introduced.

Biomedical Engineering Citation Index with Abstracts
Institute for Scientific Information

18:30. Master record

Database type	Bibliographic, Citation
Number of journals	7,250
Sources	
Start year	
Language	English
Coverage	International
Number of records	30,000
Update size	30,000
Update period	Six times per year
Abstract details	Authors' own abstracts

Description
Abstracted citation index offering complete coverage of significant published literature in biomedical engineering. Covers all areas of engineering as they are applied to medicine and healthcare, including instrumentation, surgical tools, treatment and imaging techniques, implantable devices and organs, artificial limbs and prostheses, as well as biomaterials, biocompatibility, rehabilitation engineering, biosensors, and computer applications in medicine, chemical engineering, materials science, orthopedics, electronic engineering.

All ISI databases have a linked service known as The Genuine Article which can deliver the full text of located articles by mail, facsimile transmission or courier. Orders can be placed via the host service in use, mail, facsimile transmission, telephone or telex. Diskette products have a single-keystroke order information facility. The minimum charge is US$ 11.25 within USA and Canada and US$ 12.20 elsewhere.

18:31. CD-ROM   Institute for Scientific Information

File name	Biomedical Engineering Citation Index with Abstracts
Format notes	IBM, Mac, NEC
Start year	
Number of records	
Update period	Six times per year
Price/Charges	Subscription: US$1,950

Notes
A particular feature of the CD-ROM is ISI's unique Related Records search facility which provides access to records with cited references in common, allowing documents on similar subjects to be easily retrieved and browsed.

A record with a bibliography that is retrieved from any type of search may share identical references with another record. The software identifies those records linked by identical cited references and adds them to the search result display as related records. in this way, related records expand search results. It is a practical and easy way to locate additional information from a single search and is especially useful when searching a broad concept or vaguely defined subject area as there is no need for an complex search strategy. When viewing related records, a reminder of the 'parent record' stays at the top of the screen. A parent record can have a maximum of twenty different related records but the related records can, in turn have related records which may be traced up to five levels of relationship.

Each issue is a year-to-date cumulation ending with the final annual cumulation. Back years are available to 1991.

Biomedical Materials
Elsevier Advanced Technology Publications

18:32. Master record

Database type	Textual
Number of journals	1
Sources	Newsletter
Start year	Jan 1989
Language	English
Coverage	International
Number of records	
Update size	—
Update period	Daily or weekly, as new data are added

Keywords
Ceramics; Composites; Metals; Polymers

Description
Monthly newsletter on research, development and applications of materials used for medical purposes, including ceramics, composites, metals and polymers.

Equivalent to *Biomedical Materials* monthly, which now incorporates Biomedical Polymers newsletter. On DIALOG and Data-Star, Biomedical Materials is available as part of the PTS Newsletter database.

This database can be found on:
PTS Newsletter Database

Biosis Previews Vocabulary
BIOSIS

18:34. Master record

Database type	Factual, Directory, Thesaurus
Number of journals	
Sources	
Start year	
Language	English
Coverage	
Number of records	
Update size	—
Update period	Irregular

Keywords
Immunology; Fishing; Animal Sciences; Plant Sciences; Bioengineering; Biophysics; Patents

Description

Contains the meaning of the numeric code in natural language.

Corresponds to the *Alphabetic Directory of Concept Headings*.

18:35. Online   Data-Star

File name	BVOC VOCABULARY
Start year	
Number of records	
Update period	
Price/Charges	Subscription: SFr80.00
	Connect time: SFr147.00
	Online print: SFr0.00
	Offline print: SFr0.83

Notes

From June 1993 Data-Star have introduced an annual fee/subscription per contract (that is, not per password) of SFr 80.00 (c.UK£ 32.00) payable every June. For North American customers billed in dollars who also use DIALOG, the DIALOG fee also covers access to Data-Star. Academic customers, 'commitment' customers and customers currently billed in dollars are exempt.

BIOSIS Previews
BIOSIS

18:36. Master record

Alternative name(s)	Biological Abstracts
Database type	Bibliographic
Number of journals	9,300
Sources	Bibliographies, conference proceedings, government documents, journals, letters, meeting abstracts, monographs, notes, patents, reviews, reports, research communications, symposia and theses
Start year	1969
Language	English
Coverage	International
Number of records	7,826,768
Update size	535,000
Update period	Weekly
Index unit	Articles, book chapters, letters, meeting abstracts, reports and reviews
Database aids	BIOSIS Previews Search Guide, BIOSCENE BIOSEARCH, BIOSIS Previews Search Guide Master Index and Discovering BIOSIS Previews: An Interactive Disk (IBM-compatible CAL software US$ 45.00)

Keywords

Animal Sciences; Bioengineering; Biophysics; Fishing; Immunology; Patents; Plant Sciences

Description

BIOSIS Previews, the world's largest English language indexing and abstracting service for biology and biomedicine, contains citations, with abstracts, to the worldwide literature on research in the life sciences: microbiology; plant and animal science; experimental medicine; agriculture; pharmacology; ecology; biochemistry; bioengineering; biophysics; including the basic biological disciplines of zoology, genetics, botany; related interdisciplinary fields including food science, veterinary medicine and research medicine, and associated areas of life sciences such as instrumentation.

It covers original research reports, reviews of original research, history and philosophy of biology and biomedicine, and documentation and retrieval of biological information, including references to accounts of field, laboratory, clinical, experimental and theoretical work. The database presents research findings and literature references on all living things and emphasizes their identification (taxonomy), their life processes, environments and applications. From 1986 to 1989 the database covers selective US patents in such areas as immunological testing, food processes, and fishing. For each patent record, the database includes the inventor's name and address, patent title and number, patent classes, date granted, and assignee.

The database corresponds in coverage to *Biological Abstracts (BA)* (1969+) and *Biological Abstracts/RRM (Reports, Reviews, Meetings) (BA/RRM)* (1980+) and *BioResearch Index (BioI)*, the major publications of BIOSIS (*BA/RRM* is the successor to BioI beginning in 1980). *Biological Abstracts* includes approximately 275,000 accounts of original research yearly and *Biological Abstracts/RRM* includes 260,000 citations yearly. As to the origin or sources, approximately fifty per cent of the items in the database originate from Europe and Middle East, twenty-six per cent from North America, fifteen per cent from Asia and Australia, six per cent from Central and South America and three per cent from Africa. Approximately forty-five per cent of database records relate to non-journal literature which means that of the leading bioscience databases, BIOSIS offers the most extensive coverage of this type of literature, EMBASE and MEDLINE both having ceased coverage of non-journal literature in 1980 and 1981 respectively. The references to non-journal literature do not contain abstracts but title keywords augmented by natural language descriptors provide access to scientific communications not found in many other life science databases. Approximately eighty-six per cent of records contain citations to English language sources. This compares to seventy five per cent in EMBASE, seventy four per cent in MEDLINE and eighty-eight per cent in SciSearch. In addition fifty-four per cent of records contain abstracts (from 1986 onwards). This compares with sixty- five per cent of records in MEDLINE and sixty per cent in Embase. The other leading bioscience database, SciSearch, now does contain abstracts. In BIOSIS sixty-seven per cent of records with non-English sources contain English-language abstracts online. This compares with thirty-seven per cent on EMBASE and twenty six per cent on MEDLINE (since 1980). In the UK, the Royal Society of Chemistry operates an SDI service against the tapes of the latest two weeks of BIOSIS and Chemical Abstracts under the name of BIOSCAN. Results are mailed on diskette ready for use with most PC-based searching packages. Printed output is also available. Abstracts from July 1976 to date (from BA on Tape) are available online through BRS, Data-Star, DIALOG, DIMDI, ESA-IRS, and STN International. Abstracts from 1982 to date are available through CISTI.

Most BIOSIS Previews descriptors are natural language terms added by editors to enrich or claify information provided in titles, identifying such factors as: specific scientific or common names or organisms discussed in a source if not included in the citationtitle; virus names; organ systems or tissues used or affected; diseases discussed; geographic location, if pertinent and instrumentation, apparatus methodology. Three data elements are indexed: Keywords, Cross Codes and Biosystematic Codes. The free-text file comprises two data fields: title and added keywords or uncontrolled terms. The added keywords are a data element of indexing whereas the title is a bibliographic data element and is taken from the original publication. The following categories of keywords are added to explain or supplement the title: Descriptors describing the type of the work eg Review, Book, Letter, Abstract; Organisms; Virus-affiliation terms; organs, tracts, tissues; geographic terms; drugs and their affiliation terms; chemical substances and their affiliation terms; enzymes; instrumentation, apparatus, methods; diseases; topics and purposes of a publication. Organisms: each organism is indexed twice – by a keyword and by a Biosystematic code. Categories of keywords used for organism-related concepts include scientific and/or colloquial names, depending on how they appear in the article; abbreviations which characterise the taxonomical classification of an organism (for example SP for species, VAR for variety); pathogenic organisms as causes of diseases and keywords characterising the sex and/or age groups for human beings and animals. Drugs and their affiliation terms: the name of a drug is taken from the publication in the form in which it is given, that is as a commercial or generic name. For each drug mentioned in the title or in the added keywords one or more drug affiliation terms are indexed. Chemical substances and their affiliation terms: for every chemical substance mentioned in the title or added to the title as a keyword, BIOSIS indexes an affiliation term if the effect of the substance is described in the article (herbicide, insecticide). Enzymes: are only indexed with their Enzyme Commission Number (EC) when the EC-number is mentioned in the article. Spelling: prior to 1985 BIOSIS used word segmentation for some biological, anatomical, chemical and enzyme terms in title and added descriptors. This segmentation was dropped from January 1985 to standardise spelling in the freetext sections. Hyphenated words: in the title and added keywords field the words which form a logical unit are linked by a hyphen. This spelling is not used in the abstract. Concept Headings: there are more than 500 concept headings used to index according to broader concepts. These are hierarchically ordered with the section names in the hierarchy corresponding to the section headings in the printed issues. The Concept Headings are weighted into three categories according to the emphasis of an aspect of an article: primary level for the main aspect of an article, secondary level for important aspects and teritary level for incidental aspects.

The availability of weighted indexing is useful as it provides a method for reducing output while maintaining high precision. Biosystematic Codes are also used to denote concept terms and groups of organisms which removes the need to list individually all the items and their synonyms within a group and automatically produces a context of further, more specific queries within that category. Strategy Recommendations (See References) are also given as part of the scope notes on concept codes, providing pointers towards other areas of possibly fruitful examination. The Biosystematic Codes group organisms by accepted taxonomic rules which make it possible to search references to large taxonomic groupings. New Biosystematic Codes for bacteria, based primarily on Bergey's *Manual of Systematic Bacteriology*, were effective from the first update of 1992. 140 new Biosystematic Codes (BCs) for bacteria replaced the 81 codes in use up to the end of

1991. To avoid incorrect use the names of the respective BCs have been supplemented with the years of their validity, for example BS:RHODOSPIRILLACEAE (1979–91). As there was a comparable change with viruses in 1979 respective in 1981, these BCs have been supplemented in the same way, for example BS : COMOVIRUS (1979-). The group known as the blue-green algae or Cyanophyta or Cyanobacteria, indexed till the end of 1991 as algae (BS : CYANOPHYTA, BC : 13900) will now be indexed as bacteria (BS : CYANOBACTERIA (1992-), BC : 09200). Entering the new text version of Biosystematic Codes for viruses and bacteria may cause errors and the use of the numeric version of BC is therefore recommended.

According to Snow in Chapter Five of the *Manual of Online Search Strategies* (2nd Ed. Aldershot: Ashgate, 1992) the Master Index in the *BIOSIS Previews Search Guide* should not be regarded as an authority list or thesaurus, since it does not include all words or concepts that are searchable as indexer-added keywords in the online database. Snow also points out the value of controlled vocabulary when searching for topics where a subject population has been specified. Relatively few bioscience databases provide consistent indexing for subject populations (for example humans or specific test animals) and related characteristics commonly requested such as age groups, gender, occupation and racial or ethnic groups. BIOSIS provides consistent indexing for the identification of humans and test animals with less consistent indexing of occupational groups and racial/ethnic groups and uses a natural language approach for the identification of gender. She also notes that American spellings are used as standard. In most bioscience files a form of pharmaceutical nomenclature exists. For BIOSIS the preferred terminology consists of generic names, classification by use/action and CAS Registry Numbers although certain restrictons apply to the latter (for example date, subfile or vendor restrictions). The use of enzyme commission number, investigational code, chemical name or trade name is inconsistent and it is recommended that alternative names should be used in search strategies. In addition retrospective searching may require entry of other names used for the same substance at earlier stages in its development life cycle.

Review articles can be retrieved by adding the word 'review', restricted to title and added keywords, to a search strategy.

18:37. Online   BRS, Morning Search, BRS/Colleague

File name	BIOL
Alternative name(s)	Biological Abstracts
Start year	1976
Number of records	
Update period	Monthly
Price/Charges	Connect time: US$53.00/83.00
	Online print: US$0.44/0.52
	Offline print: US$0.52
	SDI charge: US$10.75

Notes

Users can search in BIOZ, the merged file for both the current file BIOL and the back file BIOB. Abstracts from July 1976 to date are available.

18:38. Online   BRS, Morning Search, BRS/Colleague

File name	BIOB
Alternative name(s)	Biological Abstracts
Start year	1976

Number of records
Update period   Monthly
Price/Charges   Connect time: US$53.00/83
                       Online print: US$0.44/0.52
                       Offline print: US$0.52
                       SDI charge: US$10.75

Notes

Users can search in BIOZ, the merged file for both the current file BIOL and the back file BIOB. Abstracts from July 1976 to date are available.

18:39. Online   BRS, Morning Search, BRS/Colleague

File name   BIOZ
Alternative name(s)   Biological Abstracts
Start year   1976
Number of records
Update period   Monthly
Price/Charges   Connect time: US$53.00/83
                       Online print: US$0.44/0.52
                       Offline print: US$0.52
                       SDI charge: US$10.75

Notes

Users can search in BIOZ, the merged file for both the current file BIOL and the back file BIOB. Abstracts from July 1976 to date are available.

18:40. Online   CISTI, Canadian Online Enquiry Service CAN/OLE

File name   BA69
Alternative name(s)   Biological Abstracts
Start year   1969–1984
Number of records   4,267,300
Update period   Closed File
Price/Charges   Connect time: Canadian $40.00
                       Online print: Canadian $0.275 – 0.33
                       Offline print: Canadian $0.275 – 0.33

Notes

Abstracts from 1982 to date are available. CISTI is accessible only in Canada.

18:41. Online   CISTI, Canadian Online Enquiry Service CAN/OLE

File name   BA85
Alternative name(s)   Biological Abstracts
Start year   1985–1991
Number of records   3,532,472
Update period   Closed File
Price/Charges   Connect time: Canadian $40.00
                       Online print: Canadian $0.275 – 0.33
                       Offline print: Canadian $0.275 – 0.33

Notes

Abstracts from 1982 to date are available. CISTI is accessible only in Canada.

18:42. Online   CISTI, Canadian Online Enquiry Service CAN/OLE

File name   BA92
Alternative name(s)   Biological Abstracts
Start year   1992
Number of records   185,400
Update period   48 per year

Price/Charges   Connect time: Canadian $40.00
                       Online print: Canadian $0.275 – 0.33
                       Offline print: Canadian $0.275 – 0.33

Notes

Abstracts from 1982 to date are available. CISTI is accessible only in Canada.

18:43. Online   CompuServe Information Service

File name   IQUEST File 1182
Alternative name(s)   Biological Abstracts
Start year   1969
Number of records   7,713,784
Update period   Twice per month
Price/Charges   Subscription: US$8.95 per month
                       Database entry fee: US$9/search; some databases carry a surcharge ($2–75)
                       Online print: US$10 references free; then $9 per ten; abstracts $3 each
Downloading is allowed

Notes

Accessed via IQUEST or IQMEDICAL, this database is offered by a DIALOG gateway. IQUEST can either search across all databases, a database of the user's choice or selected multiple databases.

18:44. Online   Council of Scientific Research

File name
Alternative name(s)   Biological Abstracts
Start year
Number of records
Update period

18:45. Online   Data-Star

File name   BIOL
Alternative name(s)   Biological Abstracts
Start year   1985
Number of records   6,000,000
Update period   Fortnightly
Database aids   Data-Star Biomedical Manual and Data-Star Online Manual (search for NEWS-BIOL in NEWS)
Price/Charges   Subscription: SFr80.00
                       Connect time: SFr147.00
                       Online print: SFr0.40–1.03
                       Offline print: SFr0.90
                       SDI charge: SFr4.94

Notes

Abstracts are provided for about two-thirds of the database.

From June 1993 Data-Star have introduced an annual fee/subscription per contract (that is, not per password) of SFr 80.00 (c.UK£ 32.00) payable every June. For North American customers billed in dollars who also use DIALOG, the DIALOG fee also covers access to Data-Star. Academic customers, 'commitment' customers and customers currently billed in dollars are exempt.

Record composition

Abstract AB; Accession Number or and Update Code AN; Authors AU; Author Affiliation IN; Biosystematic Codes BC; Coden CD; Concept Codes CC; Keywords KW; Language LG; Supertaxa ST; Source SO; Title TI and Year of Publication YR

18:46. Online — Data-Star

File name	BI84
Alternative name(s)	Biological Abstracts
Start year	1970–1984
Number of records	
Update period	
Database aids	Data-Star Biomedical Manual and Data-Star Online Manual (search NEWS-BIOL in NEWS)
Price/Charges	Subscription: SFr80.00
	Connect time: SFr147.00
	Online print: SFr0.40–1.03
	Offline print: SFr0.90
	SDI charge: SFr4.94

Notes

Abstracts from July 1976 are available.

From June 1993 Data-Star have introduced an annual fee/subscription per contract (that is, not per password) of SFr 80.00 (c.UK£ 32.00) payable every June. For North American customers billed in dollars who also use DIALOG, the DIALOG fee also covers access to Data-Star. Academic customers, 'commitment' customers and customers currently billed in dollars are exempt.

Record composition

Abstract AB; Accession Number or and Update Code AN; Authors AU; Author Affiliation IN; Biosystematic Codes BC; Coden CD; Concept Codes CC; Keywords KW; Language LG; Supertaxa ST; Source SO; Title TI and Year of Publication YR

18:47. Online — Data-Star

File name	BIZZ
Alternative name(s)	Biological Abstracts
Start year	1970+
Number of records	6 million
Update period	Every two weeks
Database aids	Data-Star Biomedical Manual and Data-Star Online Manual
Price/Charges	Subscription: SFr80.00
	Connect time: SFr147.00
	Online print: SFr0.40–1.03
	Offline print: SFr0.90
	SDI charge: SFr4.94

Notes

Abstracts from July 1976 to date are available. Abstracts are provided for about two-thirds of the database.

From June 1993 Data-Star have introduced an annual fee/subscription per contract (that is, not per password) of SFr 80.00 (c.UK£ 32.00) payable every June. For North American customers billed in dollars who also use DIALOG, the DIALOG fee also covers access to Data-Star. Academic customers, 'commitment' customers and customers currently billed in dollars are exempt.

Record composition

Abstract AB; Accession Number or and Update Code AN; Authors AU; Author Affiliation IN; Biosystematic Codes BC; Coden CD; Concept Codes CC; Keywords KW; Language LG; Supertaxa ST; Source SO; Title TI and Year of Publication YR

18:48. Online — DIALOG

File name	File 5
Alternative name(s)	Biological Abstracts
Start year	1969
Number of records	7,713,784 Files 5, 55
Update period	Weekly
Price/Charges	Connect time: US$90.00
	Online print: US$0.75
	Offline print: US$0.75
	SDI charge: US$10.50 (biweekly)/14.95 (monthly)

Notes

Abstracts from July 1976 to date are available and for book synopses in BA/RRM from 1985. Most BA/RRM records do not contain abstracts; no Biol records contain abstracts. On DIALOG there are two files – File 5 covers 1969 to the present, File 55 1985 to the present.

DIALINDEX categories: AGRI, BIOCHEM, BIOSCI, BIOTECH, ENRION, FOODSCI, MARINE, MEDENG, MEDICINE, NUTRIT, PHARM, PHARMR, SAFETY, TOXICOL, VETSCI.

18:49. Online — DIALOG

File name	File 55
Alternative name(s)	Biological Abstracts
Start year	1985
Number of records	
Update period	
Price/Charges	Connect time: US$90.00
	Online print: US$0.75
	Offline print: US$0.75
	SDI charge: US$10.50 (biweekly)/14.95 (monthly)

Notes

Abstracts from July 1976 to date are available and for book synopses in BA/RRM from 1985. Most BA/RRM records do not contain abstracts and no Biol records contain abstracts. On DIALOG there are two files – File 5 covers 1969 to the present, File 55 1985 to the present.

DIALINDEX categories: AGRI, BIOCHEM, BIOSCI, BIOTECH, ENRION, FOODSCI, MARINE, MEDENG, MEDICINE, NUTRIT, PHARM, PHARMR, SAFETY, TOXICOL, VETSCI.

18:50. Online — DIMDI

File name	BA70
Alternative name(s)	Biological Abstracts
Software	GRIPS
Start year	1970–1982
Number of records	8,033,918
Update period	Monthly
Database aids	User Manual BIOSIS Previews and Memocard Biosis Previews
Price/Charges	Connect time: UK£23.42–32.18
	Online print: UK£0.37–0.55
	Offline print: UK£0.29–0.36

Downloading is allowed
Thesaurus is online

Notes

Abstracts (52% of the records) are available from July 1976 to date. Searches are possible from January 1970. The Basic Index includes the data fields: Title, Abstract, Uncontrolled Terms. Suppliers of online documents: British Library Document Supply Centre, Boston Spa, England; Bayerishe Staatsbibliothek München, München, Germany; Harkers Information Retrieval System, Sydney, Australia; Koninklijke Nederlandse Akademie van Wetenschapen, Amsterdam, The Netherlands.

Record composition

Abstract AB; Author AU; Biosystematic Code BC; Biosystematic Code-New /NEW; Biosystematic Heading BS; Biosystematic Heading-New /NEW; Coden CD; Corporate Source CS; Entry Date ED;

Free Text FT; Index Term IT; Journal Title JT; Language LA; Document Number ND; Publication Year PY; Subject Code SC; Subject Heading SH; Source SO; Title TI and Uncontrolled Terms UT

18:51. Online   DIMDI

File name	BA83
Alternative name(s)	Biological Abstracts
Software	GRIPS
Start year	1983
Number of records	4,681,303
Update period	Monthly
SDI period	1 month
Database aids	User Manual BIOSIS Previews and Memocard Biosis Previews
Price/Charges	Connect time: UK£23.42–32.18
	Online print: UK£0.37–0.55
	Offline print: UK£0.29–0.36

Downloading is allowed
Thesaurus is online

Notes

Abstracts are available from July 1976 to date. The Basic Index includes the data fields: Title, Abstract, Uncontrolled Terms. Suppliers of online documents: British Library Document Supply Centre, Boston Spa, England; Bayerishe Staatsbibliothek München, München, Germany; Harkers Information Retrieval System, Sydney, Australia; Koninklijke Nederlandse Akademie van Wetenschapen, Amsterdam, The Netherlands.

Record composition

Abstract AB; Author AU; Biosystematic Code BC; Biosystematic Code-New /NEW; Biosystematic Heading BS; Biosystematic Heading-New /NEW; Coden CD; Corporate Source CS; Entry Date ED; Free Text FT; Index Term IT; Journal Title JT; Language LA; Document Number ND; Publication Year PY; Subject Code SC; Subject Heading SH; Source SO; Title TI and Uncontrolled Terms UT

18:52. Online   ESA-IRS

File name	File 7
Alternative name(s)	Biological Abstracts
Start year	1970
Number of records	7,517,000 (October 1991)
Update period	Every two weeks

Downloading is allowed

Notes

From 1973–84 the records contain terms physically split into their components for example PHOSPHO LIPID (not PHOSPHOLIPID). From 1984 the splitting has been interrupted by the Biosis producer. Abstracts from July 1976 to date are available. BIOSIS on ESA-IRS from February 1992 includes new biosystematic codes.

From 1993 ESA-IRS are charging an annual fee of 100 Accounting Units (c.UK£ 70.29) to all users. This is equivalent to the fee for full documentation and will not be charged to customers already paying for documentation.

Record composition

Author AU; Biosystematic Codes BC; Biosystematic Code Name BN; CODEN CO; Concept Codes CC; Concept Code Name CN; Descriptors /UT; Journal Name JN and Title /TI

18:53. Online   Japan Information Center of Science and Technology (JICST)

File name	BIOSIS
Alternative name(s)	Biological Abstracts
Start year	1969
Number of records	6,800,000
Update period	
SDI period	Monthly/bi-weekly
Database aids	Thesaurus Translation List: Japanese-English 1987: English-Japanese 1987.
Price/Charges	Connect time: US$85.00
	Online print: US$0.32
	Offline print: US$0.38
	SDI charge: US$6.10

18:54. Online   OCLC EPIC; OCLC FirstSearch

File name	BIOSIS Previews
Alternative name(s)	Biological Abstracts
Start year	1976
Number of records	
Update period	

18:55. Online   STN

File name	BIOSIS Previews/RN
Alternative name(s)	Biological Abstracts
Start year	1969
Number of records	8,334,568
Update period	Weekly
Price/Charges	Connect time: DM139.00
	Online print: DM1.32
	Offline print: DM1.40
	SDI charge: DM10.70

Downloading is allowed

Notes

Abstracts from July 1976 to date are available.

CAS Registry Numbers, derived from a computer check for chemical names in the title and added keyword fields are present for citations from July 1980 onwards. There is an online thesaurus for for the Biosystematic Code Superterms (/BC) field.

18:56. Online   University of Tsukuba

File name	
Alternative name(s)	Biological Abstracts
Start year	
Number of records	
Update period	

Notes

Access through University of Tsukuba is limited to affiliates of the University of Japan.

18:57. Tape   BIOSIS

File name	BIOSIS Previews
Alternative name(s)	Biological Abstracts
Start year	1969
Number of records	7,826,768
Update period	4 times a month
Price/Charges	Subscription: US$9,125

Notes

Two tapes correspond to *Biological Abstracts* and two tapes correspond to *Biological Abstracts/Reports, Reviews, Meeting literature (BA/RRM)* (formerly *BioResearch Index*), and to the BIOSIS Previews online database.

Annual licence fee is $9,125 plus additional usage charges; contact BIOSIS for archival tape prices.

18:58. Database subset

Online   **CISTI, Canadian Online Enquiry Service CAN/OLE**

File name	ABC3
Alternative name(s)	Biological Abstracts
Start year	1989
Number of records	47,138
Update period	Closed File

Notes

Static training file for BIOSIS Previews enabling users to practice searching using free-text terms, Concept Codes, Biosystematic Codes, Super Taxonomic Codes and bibliographic information.

18:59. Database subset

Online   **Data-Star**

File name	TRBI – Biosis Training File
Alternative name(s)	Biological Abstracts
Start year	1984
Number of records	100,000
Update period	Fortnightly
Database aids	Data-Star Biomedical Manual and Data-Star Online Manual (search for NEWS-BIOL in NEWS)
Price/Charges	Connect time: UK£Free

Notes

Static training file for BIOSIS Previews enabling users to practice searching using free-text terms, Concept Codes, Biosystematic Codes, Super Taxonomic Codes and bibliographic information. Records are taken from 1984, 1990 and 1992 from both the Biological Abstracts and the Biological Abstracts/RRM subfiles of the database.

Record composition

Abstract AB; Accession Number or and Update Code AN; Authors AU; Author Affiliation IN; Biosystematic Codes BC; Coden CD; Concept Codes CC; Keywords KW; Language LG; Supertaxa ST; Source SO; Title TI and Year of Publication YR

18:60. Database subset

Online   **DIALOG**

File name	File 205 – ONTAP BIOSIS Previews Training File
Alternative name(s)	Biological Abstracts
Start year	January 1986 updates to File 5, BIOSIS Previews
Number of records	43,406
Update period	Closed File
Price/Charges	Connect time: US$15.00

Notes

The training file from the January updates of File 5, the main BIOSIS Preview file on DIALOG. It includes records from both Biological Abstracts and Biological Abstracts/Reports, Reviews, Meetings. Allows for low-cost practice using the BISOIS biosystematic and concept codes for searching. Offline prints are not available in ONTAP files.

18:61. Database subset

Online   **ESA-IRS**

File name	File 209 – Training Biosis
Alternative name(s)	Biological Abstracts
Start year	References from 1970, 1980, 1986
Number of records	40,000
Update period	Not updated

Notes

A fixed subset of the main BIOSIS database (File 7), enabling the user to practise ESA-QUEST at low cost. Services such as offline prints, auomatic current awareness and document ordering are not available.

Record composition

Author AU; Biosystematic Codes BC; Biosystematic Code Name BN; CODEN CO; Concept Codes CC; Concept Code Name CN; Descriptors /UT; Journal Name JN and Title /TI

18:62. Database subset

CD-ROM   **SilverPlatter**

File name	BA on CD
Alternative name(s)	Biological Abstracts
Format notes	Mac, IBM
Software	SPIRS v.2.0/MacSPIRS
Start year	1985
Number of records	280,000
Update period	Quarterly
Database aids	The SilverPlatter Users' Manual and Quick Reference Card
Price/Charges	Subscription: UK£1,647 – 6,762

Notes

When combined with BA/RRM on CD, BA on CD forms the equivalent of the online database BIOSIS Previews, incorporating the concept codes, biosystematic codes and super taxonomical codes used by searchers of the online database. On its own this CD-ROM version includes only *Biological Abstracts* whereas BIOSIS online includes *Biological Abstracts* and *Biological Abstract/RRM (Reports, Reviews, Meetings)*. This version only provides initials to authors' first and middle names. According to Condic (Condic, K.S. *CD-ROM Librarian* 6(3) 1991 29–33) each year of the database will appear on a separate CD-ROM, making searching cumbersome for multiple-year access.

In early 1993, SilverPlatter prices for BA on CD were: regular subscriptions UK£5,880 for single users, £6,762 for 2–8 networked users. Prices for those who subscribe to the print or microfilm version – for single users £1,489 and £3,797 for 2–8 networked users. For subscribers to the cumulative index £1,647 for single users and £2,529. For the collection starting with the calendar year 1993 (1985–88, 1989, 1990, 1991 and 1992) prices vary, depending on the user's current subscriptions – prices on application. There are now available back files to 1985. BA on CD requires a signed subscription and licence agreement.

Record composition

Abreviated Journal Title AJ; Abstract AB; Author AU; Biosystematic Codes; Coden CO; Concept Codes CC; Corporate Source CS; Descriptors DE; Journal Anouncement JA; Language of Article LA; Language of Summary LS; Major Concept Codes MJCC; Minor Concept Codes MNCC; Publication Year PY; Source Journal SO; Super Taxa ST; Title TI and Update Code UD

Subject access is via concept codes, biosystematic codes, super taxonomic groups and descriptors. The disc contains over 600 concept codes from the BIOSIS Search Guides. Articles have from one to ten codes assigned to them which are divided into major and minor categories resembling major or minor descriptors found in other databases. Most articles also have one to twelve biosystematic codes assigned to them. Supertaxonomic groups consist of related groups of biosystematic codes which search the English names of groups of animals. Descriptors consist of natural language or controlled vocabulary terms.

18:63. Database subset

CD-ROM   SilverPlatter

File name	BA/RRM on CD
Alternative name(s)	Biological Abstracts
Format notes	IBM, Mac
Software	SPIRS
Start year	1989
Number of records	260,000
Update period	Quarterly
Database aids	Software Manual, Database Manual and Quick Reference Cards
Price/Charges	Subscription: UK£841 – 6,762

Notes

Most records in this database do not contain abstracts as abstracts are included only in the form of book synopses. Equivalent to the printed *Biological Abstracts/RRM (Reports, Reviews and Meetings)*, previously entitled *BioResearch Index*. Records in the database cover notes, short communications, technical reports, bibliographies and taxonomic keys. Books are also included as are abstracts from meetings. When combined with BA on CD, forms the equivalent of the online database BIOSIS Previews. According to Shirley Cousin's review (*CD-ROM Information Products: The Evaluative Guide* 1993 4(1) p.1–12), the majority of records are from Europe and the Middle East (48%) with a further 28 per cent from North America, 16 per cent from Asia and Australia, 6 per cent from South and Central American and the final 2 per cent from Africa.

Pricing, as of January 1993 is: for regular subscribers, single user UK£3,021, and for 2–8 networked users £3,903; Discounts are available for subscribers to the print or microfilm versions of BA – £1,480 for single users, £2,362 for 2–8 networked users; for cumulative index subscribers prices are £841 for single users and £1,723 for 2–8 networked users. For the collection starting with the calendar year 1993 (1985–88, 1989, 1990, 1991 and 1992) prices vary, depending on the user's current subscriptions – prices on application. BA on CD requires asigned subscription and licence agreement.

18:64. Database subset

Tape   BIOSIS

File name	BAT – Biological Abstracts on Tape
Alternative name(s)	Biological Abstracts
Format notes	9-track, 800, 1600, or 6250 bpi, variable length record, variable block size.
Start year	1976
Number of records	
Update period	Twice a month
Price/Charges	Subscription: US$11,000

Notes

Contains abstracts of the worldwide literature on research in the life sciences. Covers articles from over 9,000 periodicals cited in BIOSIS Previews. Corresponds to the abstracts appearing in *Biological Abstracts*, and in part to the BIOSIS Previews online database.

Annual licence fee $11,000 plus additional usage charges; contact BIOSIS for archival tape prices.

This database can also be found on:
TOXLIT
BA/RRM on CD
Foods Intelligence on CD
Toxline Plus

CD-CHROM
Preston Publications

18:66. Master record

Database type	Bibliographic
Number of journals	
Sources	Journals, books, meeting papers, government documents, reports, theses and patents
Start year	1951 (gas); 1984 (liquid).
Language	English
Coverage	International
Number of records	80,000
Update size	–
Update period	Annually

Keywords
Chromatography

Description
Contains citations and abstracts to literature on the subject of gas and liquid chromatography.

18:67. CD-ROM   Preston Publications

File name	CD-CHROM
Format notes	IBM
Software	SearchLITE
Start year	1951 (gas); 1984 (liquid).
Number of records	80,000
Update period	Annually
Price/Charges	Subscription: UK£725

CINAHL
CINAHL

18:68. Master record

Alternative name(s)	Cumulative Index to Nursing and Allied Health Literature; Nursing and Allied Health; CINAHL
Database type	Bibliographic
Number of journals	300
Sources	Journals, monographs, dissertations and A-V material
Start year	1983
Language	English
Coverage	International
Number of records	99,000
Update size	21,000
Update period	Monthly
Index unit	Articles and book
Thesaurus	CINAHL Thesaurus (MeSH-based)
Database aids	CINAHL Subject Heading List, 1993 (available from producer), CINAHL Database Search Guide, 1993 (available from producer) and CINAHL Teaching Guide, 1993 (available from producer)

Keywords
Physical Therapy; Cardiopulmonary Therapy; Laboratory Technology; Paramedicine; Respiratory Therapy; Occupational Therapy; Radiology; Emergency Health Care; Medical Records; Medical Social Work; Medical Librarianship; Surgical Nursing; Health Education; Management

Description

The nursing and allied health (CINAHL) database is a comprehensive and authoritative source of literature refences aimed at nurses, allied health professionals and others interested in health care administration. Contains the complete Nursing and Allied Health database, including references to periodical literature in nursing and allied health, with abstracts from over one third of those articles; books from over thirty health care publishers, nursing dissertations and abstracts and references to the publications of the American Nurses Association and the National League of Nursing. Covers all aspects of nursing and allied health disciplines. Although the emphasis is primarily nursing, 35% of references relate to allied health disciplines such as cardiopulmonary technology, occupational therapy, physical therapy and rehabilitation, medical and laboratory technology, radiologic technology, emergency services and social services in health care, medical records, health sciences librarianship, medical assisting, the physician's assistant, surgical technology, and health education. Also includes relevant articles from management, psychological and popular journals. Also lists new books in nursing and allied health fields. Audiovisual materials as well as library science journals for nursing and allied health are also included. The vast majority of records are unique to CINAHL, although there is some overlap in journal coverage with *Excerpta Medica* (EMBASE) and MEDLINE.

Corresponds to the printed *Cumulative Index to Nursing and Allied Health Literature*. Since 1986 abstracts from approximately forty nursing journals have been included in the file. Books included since 1984.

Virtually all English-language nursing journals are included.

The CINAHL thesaurus is based on *MeSH*, but is tailor-made for the fields of nursing and allied health. Major and minor descriptors and free text searching are available. An extremely useful feature is the inclusion of more than twenty-four identifiers or document types which help to limit retrieval for specific concepts such as books, statistics, computer programs, research articles, etc. The See also references from the printed index and the number of references in the citations are also included. The 1993 *Subject Heading List* contains 6,900 terms, 2,000 of which are not found on any other database.

18:69. Online — BRS, Morning Search, BRS/Colleague

File name	NAHL
Start year	
Number of records	
Update period	Monthly
Price/Charges	Connect time: US$37.00/47.00
	Online print: US$0.20/0.28
	Offline print: US$0.28
	SDI charge: US$7.25

18:70. Online — CompuServe Information Service

File name	IQUEST File 1278
Start year	1983
Number of records	
Update period	Monthly
Price/Charges	Subscription: US$8.95 per month
	Database entry fee: US$9/search; some databases carry a surcharge ($2–75)
	Online print: US$10 references free; then $9 per ten; abstracts $3 each

Downloading is allowed

Notes

Accessed via IQUEST or IQMEDICAL, this database is offered by a BRS gateway. IQUEST can either search across all databases, a database of the user's choice or selected multiple databases.

18:71. Online — Data-Star

File name	NAHL
Start year	1983
Number of records	103,799
Update period	Monthly
Database aids	Biomedical manual and Online manual (search NEWS-NAHL in NEWS)
Price/Charges	Subscription: SFr80.00
	Connect time: SFr107
	Online print: SFr0.42
	Offline print: SFr0.37
	SDI charge: SFr6.80

Thesaurus is online

Notes

Four subsets have been created to help narrow a search. Users can limit retrieval to articles from nursing journals as 'Nursing.SB.', Core nursing journals as 'Core with nursing.SB.', Allied health journals as 'Allied with health.SB.' and journals published in the USA and Canada as 'USA with Canada'.

From June 1993 Data-Star have introduced an annual fee/subscription per contract (that is, not per password) of SFr 80.00 (c.UK£ 32.00) payable every June. For North American customers billed in dollars who also use DIALOG, the DIALOG fee also covers access to Data-Star. Academic customers, 'commitment' customers and customers currently billed in dollars are exempt.

Record composition

Author AU; Title TI; Source SO; Language LG; Publication type PT; Descriptors (MeSH) DE; Year of publication YR; Subset SB; Major desriptors MJ; Minor descriptors MN and UMI order number UMI

18:72. Online — DIALOG, Knowledge Index

File name	File 218
Start year	1983
Number of records	123,290
Update period	Monthly
Price/Charges	Connect time: US$54.00
	Online print: US$0.15
	Offline print: US$0.25
	SDI charge: US$6.95

Notes

This database is also available to home users during evenings and weekends at a reduced rate on the Knowledge Index service of DIALOG – file name in this case is MEDI14, and searches are made with simplified commands or menus.

18:73. CD-ROM — CD Plus

File name	CD Plus/CINAHL-CD
Format notes	Mac, Unix, IBM
Software	OVID 3.0
Start year	1983
Number of records	100,000
Update period	Monthly
Price/Charges	Subscription: UK£685

Notes

One disc. Offers the ability to limit by local journal holdings. For the experienced searcher, the software offers *MeSH* explodes, 'personal pre-explodes' for frequently exploded terms, SDIs and Save Searches, enhanced *MeSH* tree structures, and emulation of National Library of Medicine and dot-dot syntax.

Record composition

Author; Title; Source; Abstract; Subject Heading and Instrumentation

This database has an index of all searchable terms together with the online *MeSh Thesaurus* which offers mapping from natural language to *MeSH* – a facility which should give significantly improved precision for the inexperienced searcher. The on-screen help provides scope notes, definitions and task descriptors.

18:74. CD-ROM Compact Cambridge

File name	CINAHL-CD
Format notes	NEC, 9800, Mac, IBM
Start year	1983
Number of records	100,000+
Update period	Monthly
Price/Charges	Subscription: UK£700

18:75. CD-ROM SilverPlatter

File name	Nursing & Allied Health (CINAHL)-CD
Format notes	Mac, IBM
Software	SPIRS/MacSPIRS
Start year	1983
Number of records	140,000
Update period	Every two months
Price/Charges	Subscription: UK£790 – 1,186.5
Thesaurus is online	

Notes

One disc. The CD-ROM includes an on-screen equivalent to CINAHL's print thesaurus. Prices are: regular subscription £790 for single users, £1,186.5 for 2–8 networked users.

Tree explosions, major and minor assignments of descriptors, the use of sub-headings, and free text searching are available.

18:76. Fixed disk SilverPlatter

File name	Nursing & Allied Health (CINAHL)-CD
Format notes	IBM, Mac
Software	SPIRS/MacSPIRS
Start year	1983
Number of records	140,000
Update period	Every two months
Price/Charges	Subscription: UK£1,028 – 1,713
Thesaurus is online	

Notes

Contains the entire database, with an on-screen equivalent of CINAHL's print thesaurus, on a fixed disk with updates supplied on CD-ROM. This means that up to thirty networked users can have access to a single file containing the complete database. Search speeds are up to ten times faster than CD-ROM searching.

Prices are: £1,028 for 2–8 networked users, £1,370 for 9–16 users and £1,713 for 17–24 users. Hard disk fee is US$1,500.

Tree explosions, major and minor assignments of descriptors, the use of sub-headings, and free text searching are available.

COMETT

Commission of the European
   Communities (CEC)
Hamburg Educational Partnership

18:77. Master record

Database type	Textual, Courseware, Multimedia
Number of journals	
Sources	

Start year	
Language	
Coverage	Europe
Number of records	
Update size	—
Update period	

Keywords

Cardiology; Pathology; Radiography

Description

A multimedia training programme for: hydraulic instruments; X-ray devices; technical instruments; a programme containing CD-ROM and videodisc (Tate Gallery); and a programme for pathology and cardiology with illustrations and animation. Information is provided by the University of Milan, Danich Computer Centre, British Broadcasting Corporation and Fachhochschule Hamburg, four partners of the European Community's Program in Education and Training in Technology.

18:78. CD-ROM and Videodisc combined Fachhochschule Hamburg

File name	COMETT
Format notes	IBM, Mac
Start year	
Number of records	
Update period	

COMLINE: Japan News Wire

COMLINE Business Data Inc

18:79. Master record

Alternative name(s)	Japan News Wire: COMLINE; COMLINE Daily News; COMLINE Daily
Database type	Factual, Textual, Bibliographic, Directory
Number of journals	130
Sources	Companies, Press releases, Newspapers and Trade journals
Start year	Data-Star: 1986; SIS: 1989; NewsNet: 1990
Language	English
Coverage	Japan (primarily)
Number of records	75,000
Update size	15,000
Update period	Daily

Keywords

Bioreactors; Biotechnology; Cancer; Computer Technology; HIV; Medical Equipment; Physics; Telecommunications

Description

The database provides detailed English language summaries, abstracted from over 130 Japanese publications, plus exclusive interviews and research giving information on commercially important Japanese product and technology news covering corporate, industrial, financial, economic affairs as well as information on high-techology developments and research and development. Extensive interviews are conducted by qualified writers and researchers to uncover information that is often exclusive to the Comline database. Data is re-confirmed by fact-checkers, while American and English editors ensure proper, standard and understandable use of English. The activities of Japanese companies in Europe, the US and elsewhere, are also covered. Japan News Wire is the only English language daily business and technical news service from Japan. Subject areas covered include: electronics, biotechnology, medical technology, chemicals and materials, industrial automation, physics, computers, telecommunications, transportation, agriculture, environment, economy, defence and construction. The database does not include political or socio-economic issues.

The database contains original material collected and indexed by COMLINE.

Sourced from major Japanese financial and industrial newspapers and trade journals – all Japanese publications.

18:80. Online   FT Profile

File name	COMLINE Daily
Alternative name(s)	COMLINE: Japan News Wire; COMLINE Daily News
Start year	1991 (January)
Number of records	
Update period	Daily
Price/Charges	Connect time: UK£2.40 Online print: UK£0.04 – 0.10 per line Offline print: UK£0.01 per line

Notes

A Japanese business information source which combines the Daily News Service (Industrial Monitor) with the Tokyo Financial Wire and 100 Japanese language publications.

Registration fee required, including free documentation and training. Usage charges for access consist of two elements: a connect rate for time online, and a display rate (applies only to lines of file text). There is no charge for blank lines, system messages, menus or help information.

18:81. Online   NewsNet Inc

File name	
Alternative name(s)	Japan News Wire: COMLINE; COMLINE Daily News
Start year	1990
Number of records	
Update period	Daily
Database aids	Comline Data Descriptor Table

Notes

This is the daily update version of Japan News Wire database.

18:82. CD-ROM   SilverPlatter

File name	COMLINE
Alternative name(s)	Japan News Wire: COMLINE; COMLINE Daily News; COMLINE
Format notes	IBM
Software	SPIRS
Start year	1986
Number of records	75,000
Update period	6 times per year
Price/Charges	Subscription: UK£719 – 1,150

Notes

Annual subscription price for first time subscribers is reduced to UK £719 for single users, £1,150 for networked users. Subscribers may retain previous disc on update.

18:83. Database subset

Online   NewsNet Inc

File name	COMLINE Daily News: Biotechnology and Medical Technology
Alternative name(s)	Japan News Wire: COMLINE; COMLINE Daily News; COMLINE
Start year	1990
Number of records	
Update period	Daily

Notes

A subset of the Japan News Wire: Comline database, giving summaries of biotechnology industry news and information from Japanese publications. Covers new pharmaceuticals, medical equipment, agricultural science developments, industrial applications of bioreactors and research on anti-cancer and anti-AIDS agents. Gives citations to sources and some contact numbers for further information.

Monthly subscription required, with differential charges to subscribers and non-subscribers to Comline Japan Daily.

Corporate Technology Database

Corporate Technology Information Services

18:86. Master record

Database type	Directory
Number of journals	
Sources	Direct contacts
Start year	Current information
Language	English
Coverage	USA
Number of records	35,000
Update size	–
Update period	Quarterly
Database aids	CorpTech Technology Classification System Manual $45, CorpTech TCS Manual (with 1 year of updates) $95 and CorpTech Products Listing Free

Keywords

Chemical Industry; Defence; Manufacturing; Marketing; Medical Technology; Pharmaceuticals; Telecommunications

Description

The database is a directory of public and private American corporations and operating units of large corporations in all areas of high technology design, development, manufacture, production and marketing. It is a comprehensive source of company information on over 35,000 US manufacturers for market analysis, sales prospecting, mergersd and acquisitions, recruiting and new business developing. Ninety per cent of the listed companies are private or operating units of larger corporations. The products include factory automation, biotechnology, chemicals, computer hardware, the defence industrires, energy and environment, advanced materials, medical technology, pharmaceuticals, photonics, computer software, subassemblies and components, test and measurement, telecommunications and transport, robotics and artificial intelligence. The descriptive information includes company and alternate name, address and contact numbers icluding fax, names and titles of executive officers, annual sales, export activities, number of employees, rate of growth, ownership (for example, public, private, foreign parent), subsidiaries and divisions, year founded, company description, 4-digit Standard Industrial Classification (SIC) codes, and product lists classified by the producer's proprietary high-technology classification system.

Print equivalent is *Corporate Technology Directory, Regional Sales Guide to High-Tech Companies*; *Fast 5,000 Company Locator*. Information is obtained direct from company sources by telephone interviews followed by written verification. The database contains entirely original data collected and indexed by CorpTech.

18:87. Online   Data-Star

File name	CTCO
Start year	Current information
Number of records	35,000
Update period	Quarterly
Database aids	Data-Star Business Manual, Berne and Online manual (search NEWS-CTCO in NEWS)
Price/Charges	Subscription: SFr80.00
	Connect time: SFr123.33
	Online print: SFr2.40
	Offline print: SFr2.88

Notes
From June 1993 Data-Star have introduced an annual fee/subscription per contract (that is, not per password) of SFr 80.00 (c.UK£ 32.00) payable every June. For North American customers billed in dollars who also use DIALOG, the DIALOG fee also covers access to Data-Star. Academic customers, 'commitment' customers and customers currently billed in dollars are exempt.

18:88. Online   ORBIT

File name	CORP
Start year	Current information
Number of records	35,000
Update period	Quarterly
Database aids	Quick Reference Guide (6/89) Free (single copy) and Database Manual (1990) $15
Price/Charges	Subscription: US$7,500

18:89. CD-ROM   Corporate Technology Information Services

File name	CorpTech
Start year	Current information
Number of records	35,000
Update period	Quarterly
Price/Charges	Subscription: US$7,500

Current Contents Search Bibliographic Database
Institute for Scientific Information

18:90. Master record

Database type	Bibliographic
Number of journals	1,300
Sources	Journals
Start year	Most recent twelve months
Language	English
Coverage	International
Number of records	1,547,676
Update size	728,000
Update period	Weekly
Index unit	Articles, reviews, letters, notes and Editorials

Keywords
Applied Science; Atmospheric Science; Clinical Medicine; Immunology; Inorganic Chemistry; Molecular Biology; Neuroscience; Organic Chemistry; Polymers; Statistics; Astrophysics; Spectroscopy; Pathology; Physics; Water Supply

Description
Contains citations to articles listed in the tables of content of leading journals in the sciences, social sciences, and arts and humanities. There are seven subsets:

Clinical medicine (CLIN): Covers a broad range of disciplines including: allergy, anaesthesiology, biomethods, cardiology, clinical and medicinal chemistry, clinical psychiatry and psychology, dentistry, dermatology, epidemiology, family medicine, gastroenterology and hepatology, general and internal medicine, geriatrics and gerontology, hematology, infectious diseases, medical technology and laboratory medicine, neurology, oncology, ophthalmology, orthopedics, otorhinolaryngology, paediatrics, pharmacy, physical medicine and rehabilitation, radiology and nuclear medicine, reproductive systems, respiratory medicine, sports sciences, surgery, and urology.

Life sciences (LIFE): Covers anatomy, biochemistry, biophysics, cytology, endocrinology, experimental medicine, experimental biology, genetics, gerontology, hematology, histology, immunology, microbiology, molecular biology, neuroscience, parasitology, pathology, pharmaceutical chemistry, pharmacology, physiology, radiology and nuclear medicine, toxicology and virology.

Arts and humanities (ARTS).

Engineering, technology, and applied sciences (ENG).

Social and behavioural sciences (BEHA): Covers business, economics, education, geography, history, law, library and information science, management, planning and development, political science, psychiatry, psychology, public health, rehabilitation, sociology.

Agriculture, biology, and environmental sciences (AGRI): Covers agricultural chemistry, economics, engineering, agronomy, animal behaviour, animal husbandry, applied microbiology, biotechnology, botany, conservation, crop science, dairy science, ecology, entomology, environmental sciences, fishery science and technology, forestry, horticulture, marine biology, mycology, nutrition, oceanology, orinthology, pest control, soil science, taxonomy, veterinary medicine and pathology, water research and engineering, wildlife management and zoology.

Physical, chemical, and earth sciences (PHYS): Covers analytical chemistry, applied physics, astronomy, astrophysics, atmospheric sciences, chemical physics, chemistry, condensed matter, crystallography, geology and geophysics, inorganic and nuclear chemistry, mathematics, meteorology, nuclear physics, organic chemistry, paleontology, physical chemistry, physics, polymer chemistry, spectroscopy, statistics and probability.

Includes title, authors, bibliographic data, abstracts and keywords, and, when available, reprint authors' addresses.

Current Contents Search is the online version of ISI's popular *Current Contents* series of publications. *Current Contents* is a weekly service that reproduces the tables of contents from current issues of leading journals in the sciences, social sciences, and arts and humanities. All ISI databases have a linked service known as The Genuine Article which can deliver the full text of located articles by mail, facsimile transmission or courier. Orders can be placed via the host service in use, mail, facsimile transmission, telephone or telex. Diskette products have a single-keystroke order information facility. The minimum charge is US$ 11.25 within USA and Canada and US$ 12.20 elsewhere.

Leading journals in the sciences, social sciences, and arts and humanities.

Keywords supplied by the author are included. In addition, ISI adds Keywords Plus which are generated by analysis of titles of articles that appear in the list of citations.

18:91. Database subset

Online   BRS, Morning Search, BRS/Colleague

File name	CLIN
Alternative name(s)	CBIB: Clinical Medicine
Start year	
Number of records	
Update period	
Price/Charges	Connect time: US$85.00/95.00
	Online print: US$0.57/0.65
	Offline print: US$0.65

Notes

A special print format, CONT, allows the user to print a Table of Contents format that closely mirrors the print product.

18:92. Database subset

Online   DIMDI

File name	I383 – SCICLIN
Software	GRIPS
Start year	1983
Number of records	1,569,589
Update period	Weekly
SDI period	1 week
Database aids	User Manual SCISEARCH/SOCIAL SCISEARCH and Memocard SCISEARCH
Price/Charges	Connect time: UK£14.41–20.32 (Group I); 15.57–23.24 (Group II); 18.50–43.71 (Group III)
	Online print: UK£0.39–0.57
	Offline print: UK£0.31–0.37

Downloading is allowed

Notes

SCICLIN corresponds to the Current Contents edition Clinical Practice. Approximately eight per cent of records contain abstracts. Searches are possible from January 1983.

There are preferential costs for subscribers to the printed product. Groups shown for pricing refer to: 1. Users in the Federal Republic of Germany active in the field of biosciences, with the exception of private companies. Under temporary federal grant there is a rebate for this group of users; 2. Other users who are subscribers of the equivalent printed product. These users have to inform ISI that they wish this preferential rate; 3. Other users who are not subscribers of the equivalent printed product.

Record composition

Abstract AB; Abstract Indicators AI; Author AU; Author's Keywords IT; Cluster Code CC; Cluster Term CT; Cluster Weight /W; Corporate Country CCO; Corporate Source CS; Document Type DT; Entry Date

ED; Free Text FT; Journal Title JT; Keywords Plus UT; Language LA; Number of Document ND; Number of References RN; Publication Year PY; Reference RF; Referenced Journal RJ; Referenced Patent No. RP; Subject Code SC; Subject Heading SH; Source SO; Subunit SU and Title TI

The basic index includes the following data fields: Title, Controlled Term, Index Term, Uncontrolled Term and Abstract.

18:93. Database subset

Diskette   Institute for Scientific Information

File name	Current Contents on Diskette with Abstracts – Clinical Medicine
Format notes	IBM, NEC, Mac
Software	Proprietary Vn.3.0
Start year	
Number of records	
Update period	Weekly
Price/Charges	Subscription: US$750

Notes

Contains citations with abstracts to articles listed in the tables of contents of journals and book series in clinical medicine.

Equivalent in part to the Current Contents Search online database.

Reduced subscription for print subscribers. The latest version of the software (August 1992) allows search profiles to be run against six issues at one time; better file compression to use less hard disk space; expanded online, context sensitive help; better truncation (including left-hand) facilities; and new output options. KeyWords Plus (tm) provides users with search terms taken from an article's bibliography: in this way users should identify many more articles. KeyWords Plus (tm) also allows users to determine on inspection how closely the article pertains to their area of interest. Users are now also able to transfer multiple search terms from the dictionaries to search statements.

Record composition

ISBN; ISSN; Publisher; Author keywords; Key Words Plus; Bibliographic details and Abstracts

18:94. Database subset

Diskette   Institute for Scientific Information

File name	Current Contents on Diskette – Clinical Medicine
Format notes	IBM, NEC, Mac
Software	Proprietary Vn.3.0
Start year	
Number of records	
Update period	Weekly
Price/Charges	Subscription: US$427

Notes

Contains citations to articles listed in the tables of contents of journals and book series in clinical medicine. Equivalent in part to the Current Contents Search online database.

Reduced subscription for print subscribers. The latest version of the software (August 1992) allows search profiles to be run against six issues at one time; better file compression to use less hard disk space; expanded online, context sensitive help; better truncation (including left-hand) facilities; and new output options. KeyWords Plus (tm) provides users with search terms taken from an article's bibliography: in this way users should identify many more articles. KeyWords Plus (tm) also allows users to determine on inspection how closely the article pertains to their area of interest. Users are now also able to transfer multiple search terms from the dictionaries to search statements.

Record composition
ISBN; ISSN; Publisher; Author keywords; Key Words Plus and Bibliographic details

18:95. Database subset

Tape	Institute for Scientific Information
File name	CC Search/Clinical Medicine
Start year	Current
Number of records	
Update period	Weekly
Price/Charges	Subscription: US$15,000 – 18,750

Notes
Contains citations to articles listed in the tables of contents of journals and book series in clinical medicine. Equivalent in part to the Current Contents Search online database.

Reduced subscription for print subscribers. The latest version of the software (August 1992) allows search profiles to be run against six issues at one time; better file compression to use less hard disk space; expanded online, context sensitive help; better truncation (including left-hand) facilities; and new output options. KeyWords Plus (tm) provides users with search terms taken from an article's bibliography: in this way users should identify many more articles. KeyWords Plus (tm) also allows users to determine on inspection how closely the article pertains to their area of interest. Users are now also able to transfer multiple search terms from the dictionaries to search statements.

Annual lease is $15,000 (academic), $18,750 (corporate).

Record composition
ISBN; ISSN; Publisher; Author keywords; Key Words Plus and Bibliographic details

Dechema Equipment Suppliers Databank
DECHEMA Deutsche Gesellschaft für Chemisches Apparatewesen

18:96. Master record

Alternative name(s)	DEQUIP
Database type	Directory, Textual
Number of journals	
Sources	Suppliers
Start year	Current information
Language	English, French and German
Coverage	International
Number of records	50,000
Update size	–
Update period	Reloaded annually
Index unit	Products

Keywords
Bioengineering; Chemical Engineering

Description
Supplies information on manufacturers of apparatus and technical equipment in the fields of chemical engineering and biotechnology. Contains descriptions of products, including protected trade names, available in the Federal Republic of Germany for the chemical engineering and biotechnology industries from over 3,000 companies worldwide. Covers product categories for computer-aided engineering hardware and software; general and specialized analysis and testing equipment; laboratory instruments and chemicals; pumps, compressors, valves, and fittings; process instrumentation, control, and automation equipment; and equipment for use in mechanical and thermal processes, nuclear and radio-chemical applications, materials handling and storage, and safety engineering. Includes manufacturer's name, address, and products. 8,000 product groups and 3,441 companies are listed.

Corresponds in part to ACHEMA Yearbook (Volume 3), 1988. Supplied by FIZ Chemie GmbH. Company names, addresses, and a full text product description are searchable in English. Product names, descriptions and classification information are searchable in English, French and German.

18:97. Online   STN

File name	DEQUIP
Alternative name(s)	DEQUIP
Start year	Current information
Number of records	50,000
Update period	Reloaded annually
Price/Charges	Connect time: DM180.00
	Online print: DM2.80

Diagnostics Business-Matters
Fortia Marketing Consultants Ltd

18:98. Master record

Database type	Textual
Number of journals	1
Sources	Newsletters
Start year	1988
Language	English
Coverage	International
Number of records	
Update size	–
Update period	Daily
Index unit	Articles

Keywords
Company Profiles; Diagnostic Products; Marketing; Research and Development

Description
A monthly newsletter on companies that develop and market medical diagnostic products. Provides business intelligence on the companies involved, along with information on the latest trends and events in research, development, markets, product introduction, joint ventures and merger and acquisition activity. Also features company profile articles. On DIALOG and Data-Star this newsletter is part of the PTS Newsletter Database.

Full text of the monthly Diagnostics Business-Matters newsletter.

This database can be found on:
PTS Newsletter Database

Diogenes

Diogenes
FOI Services
Washington Business Information Inc

18:99. Master record

Database type	Bibliographic, Textual
Number of journals	
Sources	Grey literature, laws/regulations, letters, newsletters, press releases, reports and speeches
Start year	Varies by source, earliest data from 1938
Language	English
Coverage	USA
Number of records	320,000+
Update size	–
Update period	Weekly

Keywords

Pharmaceutical Products; Drugs

Description

DIOGENES contains citations to unpublished US Food and Drug Administration (FDA) regulatory documents covering pharmaceuticals and over-the-counter drugs and medical devices (for example, sunlamps and pacemakers). It is made up of three major types of information:

(1) Unpublished Food and Drug Administration (FDA) documents acquired under the Freedom of Information Act. These documents include: Advisory Committee Minutes, Drug and Device Approval information, Regulatory Letters, Establishment Inspections Reports, Industry/FDA correspondence, and many others. Many of the more timely or substantive documents are included full-text online.

(2) Newsletters published by Washington Business Information Inc. and FDA. These include: *Washington Drug Letter, The GMP Letter, Washington Health Costs Letter, The Food & Drug Letter, Devices & Diagnostics Letter, The Drug Bulletin* and *The Radiological Health Bulletin* which are all online full-text.

(3) Other FDA documentation full-text online includes: Federal Register Notice summaries, complete listings of FDA-approved drugs and devices, *Enforcement Reports, Medical Device Report* incident summaries, press releases and talk papers.

The following publications are included in the database are: (FT denotes full text; coverage and update schedule is given): *Advisory Committees (ADV)* – *Advisory Committee Minutes* (selected; as available); *Advisory Committee Manuscripts* (selected; as available). *Medical Devices (DEV)* – *FDA Premarket Approval List* (PMAs) (all, 1976+; quarterly); *FDA 510(k) List* (all, 1976+; quarterly); *Device Approvals* from *FDA Drug & Device Product Approvals* (all, 1984+; monthly); *Medical Device Reports* (MDRs) (FT; all, 1985+; quarterly); *FDA Medical Devices Bulletin* (FT; all, 1986+; irregularly, as published); *FDA Radiological Health Bulletin* (FT; all, 1986+; irregularly, as published); *Device Documentation* (510(k) Notices) (selected; as available); *Device Documentation* (PMA Summaries) (selected; as available). *Drug (DRG)* – *FDA New Drug Application List* (all, 1938+; quarterly); *Drug Approvals from FDA Drug & Device Product Approvals* (all, 1984+; monthly); *FDA Drug Bulletin* (FT; all, 1985+; irregularly, as published); *FOI Services Drug*

Documentation (SBOAs, Reviews, etc.) (selected; as available). *Establishment Inspection Report (EIR)* – *Establishment Inspection Reports* (selected; as available). *Federal Register (FED)* – *Federal Register Notice Summaries* (FT; all, 1985+; weekly). *Guidelines (GLS)* – *Guidelines* (selected; as available). Letters, Meetings & Telecoms (LTR & MTG) – Correspondence (selected; as available). *Newsletter (NEW)* – *Newsletters* (FT; all, 1981+; weekly). Press Releases & Talk Papers (PRL & TLP) – Press Releases (FT; all, 1984+; as available) and Talk Papers (FT; all, 1984+; as available). Speech (SPE) – Speeches (selected; as available). Regulatory Action (REG) – FDA Enforcement Report (FT; all, 1984+; weekly); Warning (Regulatory) Letters (FT; all, 1984+; weekly); Recall Documentation (selected; as available).

18:100. Online   BRS

File name	DIOG
Start year	Varies by source, earliest data from 1938
Number of records	320,000+
Update period	Weekly
Price/Charges	Connect time: US$104.00/114.00
	Online print: US$1.96/2.04
	Offline print: US$2.08
	SDI charge: US$6.50

18:101. Online   CompuServe Information Service

File name	IQUEST File 1945
Start year	Varies by source, earliest data from 1938
Number of records	
Update period	Weekly
Price/Charges	Subscription: US$8.95 per month
	Database entry fee: US$9/search; some databases carry a surcharge ($2–75)
	Online print: US$10 references free; then $9 per ten; abstracts $3 each

Downloading is allowed

Notes

Accessed via IQUEST, this database is offered by a BRS gateway. IQUEST can either search across all databases, a database of the user's choice or selected multiple databases.

18:102. Online   Data-Star

File name	DIOG
Start year	Unpublished documents 1976+; Newsletters 1981+; Drug approval listings 1938+;
Number of records	320,000+
Update period	Weekly
Database aids	Data-Star Biomedical Manual and Online Manual (search NEWS-DIOG in NEWS)
Price/Charges	Subscription: SFr80.00
	Connect time: SFr195.00
	Online print: SFr2.38
	Offline print: SFrNot applicable
	SDI charge: SFrNot applicable

Notes

From June 1993 Data-Star have introduced an annual fee/subscription per contract (that is, not per password) of SFr 80.00 (c.UK£ 32.00) payable every June. For North American customers billed in dollars who also use DIALOG, the DIALOG fee also covers access to Data-Star. Academic customers, 'commitment' customers and customers currently billed in dollars are exempt.

Record composition

Accession Number and Update Code; Advisory Committee/Speaker AU; Company Name CO; Descriptors DE; Drug/device number or FDA number NU; Generic/Trade/name/s PH; Occurence Paragraph OC; Publication Type PT; Source SO; Text TX; Title TI; Year YR; Year/month YM; Year/date YD; Year of publication or occurrence YR and Update Code UP

18:103. Online DIALOG

File name	File 158
Start year	1976
Number of records	1,196,482
Update period	Weekly
Price/Charges	Connect time: US$129.00
	Online print: US$2.25
	Offline print: US$4.95
	SDI charge: US$3.50

Notes

DIALINDEX Categories: BIOTECH, CHEMBUS, MEDENG, PHARMINA, PHARM, PHARMR, REGS.

DISOD
NPO 'Rubin'

18:104. Master record

Database type	Bibliographic, Factual
Number of journals	
Sources	
Start year	
Language	English
Coverage	
Number of records	36,000
Update size	–
Update period	

Description

Personnel data of NPO 'Rubin', scientific equipment producer.

18:105. Diskette NPO 'Rubin'

File name	
Start year	
Number of records	36,000
Update period	

DRI Health Care Cost Forecasting
Data Resources Inc (DRI)

18:106. Master record

Database type	Statistical
Number of journals	
Sources	Databases
Start year	4-year forecasts, with historical series from 1976
Language	
Coverage	USA

Number of records	100
Update size	–
Update period	Quarterly

Keywords

Health Care Costs; Medical Equipment; Pharmaceuticals

Description

Contains quarterly forecast indexes of United States health care costs. Covers labour, food, utilities, medical equipment, supplies, pharmaceuticals, physician services, and capital. Also provides forecasts of the 'market basket' indexes developed by the United States Health Care Financing Administration (HCFA) for hospitals, nursing homes, and home health-care agencies. Some series are available at a regional level.

Sources include DRI data banks and models, and the Health Care Financing Administration.

18:107. Online Data Resources Inc (DRI)

File name	
Start year	4-year forecasts, with historical series from 1976
Number of records	100
Update period	Quarterly

Notes

Subscription to DRI required.

Electronic MRI Manual
Aries Systems Corporation
UCLA School of Medicine

18:108. Master record

Database type	Factual, Textual
Number of journals	
Sources	Monograph
Start year	
Language	English
Coverage	
Number of records	
Update size	–
Update period	

Keywords

Biotechnology; Magnetic Resonance Imaging; Radiology

Description

Contains the full text of the *MRI Manual* on magnetic resonance imaging written by Robert F. Lufkin, M.D., at the UCLA School of Medicine. Consists of a condensation of presentations made at the UCLA Department of Radiology visiting fellowship programme in MRI. Includes MRI considerations in a variety of radiology subspecialities, including orthopedics, chest, cardiovascular, neurology, head and neck.

Equivalent to the print *MRI Manual*.

18:109. CD-ROM Aries Systems Corporation

File name	Electronic MRI Manual
Format notes	Mac, IBM
Software	Knowledge Finder 2.0
Start year	

Number of records
Update period
Price   US$195 – 495

EMBASE
Elsevier Science Publishers

18:110. Master record

Alternative name(s)	Excerpta Medica
Database type	Bibliographic
Number of journals	4,700
Sources	Case studies, clinicians, journals, monographs, research communications, reviews, surveys and symposia
Start year	1974
Language	English
Coverage	International
Number of records	4,950,000+
Update size	350,000
Update period	Weekly
Index unit	Articles
Abstract details	Adaptations of the authors' summaries and selected on the basis of content and length by an international group of practicing medical and other qualified specialists and when necessary modified, shortened or extended to obtain the optimal information value. A group of 2,000 biomedical specialists assist with the preparation of abstracts in particular subject areas and articles in non-Western European languages.
Thesaurus	EMTREE Thesaurus METAGS
Database aids	Guide to the Classification and Indexing System, MALIMET (available online and on microfiche), Mini-Malimet, MECLASE Drug Trade Names (DN) and EMBASE List of Journals Abstracted

Keywords

HIV; Anaesthesia; Anatomy; Anthropology; Bioengineering; Biotechnology; Cancer; Cardiology; Clinical Medicine; Clinical Neurology; Cosmetics; Drugs; Environmental Health; Environmental Pollution; Environmental Toxicology; Epilepsy; Food Additives; Food Contaminants; Forensic Medicine; Forensic Science; Gastroenterology; Gynaecology; Immunology; Industrial Medicine; Nephrology; Neuroscience; Neuromuscular Disorders; Nuclear Medicine; Obstetrics; Occupational Health and Safety; Patents; Pathology; Pharmaceuticals; Pollution; Public Health; Radiology; Toxic Substances; Waste Management

Description

EMBASE is the trademark for the English language Excerpta Medica database. Excerpta Medica was founded as a non-profit making organisation in 1946 with the goal of improving the availability and dissemination of medical knowledge through the publication of a series of abstract journals. The database contains citations, with abstracts, to the worldwide biomedical literature on human medicine and areas of biological sciences related to human medicine with an emphasis on the pharmacological effects of drugs and chemicals. The four main categories of primary literature sources are: specialist medical publications; general biomedicine publications; specialist non-medical publications and general scientific publications. Subjects covered include: anatomy; anesthesiology (including resuscitation and intensive care medicine); anthropology; pharmacology of anesthetic agents, spinal, epidural and caudal anesthesia and acupuncture (as anesthetic); autoimmunity; biochemistry; bioengineering; cancer; dangerous goods; dermatology; developmental biology; drug adverse reactions; drug dependence; drug effects; endocrinology; environmental health and pollution control (covering chemical pollution and its effect on man, animals, plants and microorganisms; measurement, treatment, prevention and control); exocrine pancreas; forensic science; gastroenterology (including diseases and disorders of: digestive systems; mouth; pharynx and more); genetics; gerontology and geriatrics; health economics; hematology; hepatobiliary system; hospital management; immunology (including immunity; hypersensitivity; histocompatibility and all aspects of the immune system); internal medicine; legal and socioeconomic aspects; mesentary; meteorological aspects; microbiology; nephrology (covering diagnosis; treatment; epidemiology; prevention; infections; glomerular and tubular disorders; blood purification; dialysis; kidney transplantation; toxic nephropathy and including important clinical abstracts with epidemiological studies and major clinical trials, with particular emphasis on hypertension and diabetes); neurosciences (especially clinical neurology and neurosurgery, epilepsy and neuromuscular disorders but also covering non-clinical articles on neurophysiology and animal models for human neuropharmacology); noise and vibration; nuclear medicine; obstetrics and gynaecology (including endocrinology and menstrual cycle, infertility, prenatal diagnosis and fetal monitoring, anti-conceptions, breast cancer diagnosis, sterilisation and psychosexual problems and neonatal care of normal children); occupational health and industrial medicine; opthalmology; otorhinolaryngology; paediatrics; pathology (including general pathology and organ pathology, pathological physiology and pathological anatomy, as well as laboratory methods and techniques used in pathology. General pathology topics range from cellular pathology, fetal and neonatal pathology, including congenital disorders, injury (both chemical and physical), inflammation and infection, immuno-pathology, collagen diseases and cancer pathology); peritoneum; pharmacology (including the effects and use of all drugs; experimental aspects of pharmacokinetics and pharmacodynamics; drug information); physiology; psychiatry and psychology (including addiction; alcoholism; sexual behaviour; suicide; mental deficiency and the clinical use or abuse of psychotropic and psychomimetic agents); public health; radiation and thermal pollution; radiology (including radiodiagnosis, radiotherapy and radiobiology, ultrasound diagnosis, thermography, adverse reactions to radiotherapy and techniques and apparatus, radiobiology of radioisotopes, aspects of radiohygiene, new labelling techniques and tracer applications); rehabilitation; surgery; toxicology (including pharmaceutical toxicology; foods, food additives, and contaminants; cosmetics, toiletries, and household products; occupational toxicology; waste material in air, soil and water; toxins and venoms; chemical teratogens, mutagens, and carcinogens; phototoxicity; regulatory toxicology; laboratory methods and techniques; and antidotes and symptomatic treatment); urology; wastewater treatment and measurement. The database is particularly strong in drug-related literature, where records include manufacturers and drug trade names and generic names. Information on veterinary medicine, nursing and dentistry is generally excluded.

Excerpta Medica is extremely current as articles are

indexed within thirty days of receipt and are online very soon after that. Approximately 900 journals (the Rapid Input Processing (RIP)) are processed with priority which means that within eleven weeks of the receipt of the original document, the completely-indexed records are available. More than 100,000 records are given this priority treatment. Some hosts have companion databases giving training or details of the indexing vocabularies and thesauri.

EMBASE concentrates on journal articles although about 1,000 books per annum were indexed between 1975 and 1980. The source journals include all forty-six sections of *Excerpta Medica*, the *Drug Literature Index* and *Adverse Reactions Titles*. New titles are added and old titles deleted at a rate of about 200–300 per year. The database covers sources from 110 countries with the following geographical scope: North America 36%, Western Europe 35%, United Kingdom 14%, USSR and Eastern Europe 7%, Asia 6%, Central and South America 1%, Austalia & South Pacific 1%, Africa and Middle East 1%. Approximately 50% of the citations are from drug and pharmaceutical literature and approximately 40% of citations added to the database each year do not appear in the corresponding printed abstract journals and indexes. Approximately 65% of the citations contain abstracts of on average 200 words with a maximum of 800 words which indicate the content of the articles and are not intended to summarise the results or express opinions. This makes free-text searching of the abstracts, titles and other searchable elements of the citation valuable. This compares with approximately sixty-five per cent of the records in MEDLINE and fifty-four per cent in BIOSIS. The records of the other leading bioscience database, SciSearch, now do contain abstracts. Approximately 75% of the articles are in the English language. Of the other leading bioscience databases, approximately eighty-eight per cent of articles on SciSearch are in English, eighty-six per cent of articles on BIOSIS and seventy-four per cent on MEDLINE. In addition approximately thirty-seven per cent of records with non-English sources contain English-language abstracts online. This compares with sixty-seven per cent on BIOSIS and twenty-six per cent on MEDLINE. SciSearch does now contain abstracts. Important publications NOT indexed in EMBASE include Meyler's *Side Effects of Drugs*, 1972–1980 published by Excerpta Medica and *Side Effects of Drugs Annual*, 1981 to the present, published by Elsevier.

A core collection of 3,500 biomedical journals supplemented by journals in the areas of agriculture, technology, economics, chemistry, environmental protection and sociology. General criteria used for selection are first that the document should be of potential relevance to medicine and secondly the information should be of lasting value for which reasons news items and comments are generally excluded.

EMBASE section headings are based on medical specialities; a total of forty-seven subfiles group together citations on topics such as anatomy, paediatrics, opthalmology, gastroenterelogy, cancer, plastic surgery, occupational health. Each subfile or section has its own hierarchical scheme. The thesaurus *MALIMET (Master List of Medical Terms)* is used which contains more than 250,000 preferred terms and 255,000 synonyms which are mapped to the preferred terms when used. It is used for indexing highly specific concepts such as names of drugs and chemicals; diseases and syndromes; anatomical and physiological aspects and diagnostic and therapeutic

methods. *MALIMET* is growing at a rate of over 12,000 descriptors per annum, mainly through drug names and names of chemical compounds. The size of the complete *MALIMET* thesaurus for EMBASE (more than 250,000 preferred terms compared to 15,000 in *MeSH*) may indicate its tendency to provide a greater variety of possible terms and therefore, less consistent application in indexing. In 1993, all non-drug *MeSH* terms were included in the thesaurus mapped to *MALIMET* terms so that a search strategy can be transferred from MEDLINE.

Indexing incorporates the following rules: natural word order (acute leukemia, not leukemia acute); American spelling (tumor, not tumour), singular noun forms and not plural or adjectival forms (stomach tumor, not gastric tumors, but optic nerve, not eye nerve); the most specific term must be used. Since 1979, *MALIMET* terms have been weighted. Class A terms (weighted) indicate the main concepts while Class B terms (not weighted) indicate the less important concepts of a document. In addition to *MALIMET* broad concepts are indexed with EMCLAS and EMTAGS. EMCLAS is a poly-hierarchical decimal classification scheme of the forty-six subject subfiles which make up the sections of the printed *Excerpta Medica* containing approximately 6,500 entries. It is then further subdivided into a five level hierarchy of sub-categories. Indexing is performed by medical specialists and scientists whose specialism corresponds to the subject areas forming the major subdivisions of EMCLAS. The indexing builds up sequentially as the article is indexed by each of the sections for which it is relevant. On average each document is indexed for 3.5 different sections.

EMTAGS is a group of approximately 220 codes which represent general concepts such as groups, gender, organ systems, experimental animals and article type. In January 1991 about 10% of the terms were changed including important descriptors such as CANCER or BENIGN NEOPLASM.

EMBASE editors also add 'uncontrolled' drug terms to augment MALIMET descriptors in selected records. EMBASE provides a hierarchical classification system (EMTREES) reflecting fifteen broad facets of biomedicine. From January 1991 a new version of EMTREE went online comprising 35,000 terms. New descriptors and changes in the hierarchy were made in the following areas: anatomy of the eye; diseases; drugs; techniques; biological phenomea and document types. Prior to 1988 Section Headings based on medical speciality areas were used instead of EMTREES to index EMBASE citations. In both classification schemes, codes are constructed to facilitate broad concept retrieval through truncation. In addition three uncontrolled vocabularies are used: Medical Secondary Text; Drug (Trade Names) and Manufacturers' Names are used. Medical Secondary Text consists of free-text words, numbers and phrases, describing concepts which are not fully covered by the controlled terms, for example quantiative information such as the number of patients or experimental animals. Drug (Trade) Names consists of trade names of drugs referred to in an original document with the main aspect of biological effects of compounds listed. Manufacturers' Names lists the names of drug manufacturers. The value of controlled indexing is important when searching for topics where a subject population has been specified.

Relatively few bioscience databases provide consistent indexing for subject populations (that is, humans or specific test animals) and related characteristics commonly requested such as age groups, gender, occupation and racial or ethnic groups. EMBASE provides extensive consistent indexing for the identification of test animals and age groups with a less consistent approach for the indexing of humans, occupational groups, racial/ethnic groups and gender. In addition, in most bioscience files a form of pharmaceutical nomenclature exists. For EMBASE the preferred search terms are generic name, classification by action/use and CAS Registry Number although restrictions by date, subfile and vendor may apply to the latter and vendor documentation should be consulted for guidelines. The search terms Enzyme Commission Number, investigational code, chemical name and trade name should be cross-referenced to the preferred terminology in the thesaurus. In 1993, improved CAS Registry Numbers mean that there is a single Number assigned for every substance.

18:111. Database subset

CD-ROM   **SilverPlatter**

File name	Excerpta Medica – Radiology and Nuclear Medicine
Alternative name(s)	Excerpta Medica
Format notes	IBM, Mac
Software	SPIRS/MacSPIRS
Start year	1980
Number of records	356,000
Update period	Quarterly
Price/Charges	Subscription: UK£755 – 1,132

Notes

One of the Elsevier speciality *Excerpta Medica* range, this CD-ROM database is a subset of EMBASE and covers information on radiology and nuclear medicine. Radiology subjects covered include radiodiagnosis, radiotherapy and radiobiology, ultrasound diagnosis, thermography, adverse reactions to radiotherapy and techniques and apparatus. Nuclear medicine subjects covered include diagnostic and therapeutic applications of radioisotopes in biomedicine, the radiobiology of radioisotopes, aspects of radiohygiene, new labelling techniques and tracer applications. Relevant abstracts from other clinical and basic disciplines are also included.

Prices are: for single users UK£755, for 2–8 networked users £1,132.

This database can also be found on:
Eyenet
Cancer-CD
Medata-ROM
Logo-A Pharmaceutical Products (Discontinued)

Eyenet
American Society of Contemporary Ophthalmology (ASCO)

18:113. Master record

Database type	Bibliographic, Directory, Textual
Number of journals	
Sources	Journals, Suppliers and Monographs
Start year	Current information; Literature Search, 1983
Language	English
Coverage	International

Number of records	
Update size	–
Update period	Varies by file
Index unit	Articles, Book reviews, Editorials, Letters to the editor, Classified advertisements, News items, Product announcements, Calendar, Drug and products

Keywords

Eye Disorders; Ophthalmic Instruments; Ophthalmology; Pharmaceuticals

Description

Contains five files of information for opthalmologists and physicians on eye disorders and their treatment.

Electronic Eye Journal Monthly. Contains full text of selected articles, book reviews, editorials, letters to the editor, and classified advertisements to be published in *Annals of Ophthalmology, Glaucoma*, and *Journal of Ocular Therapy and Surgery*. Also contains news bulletins, product announcements and warnings, and a calendar of conferences and meetings. Updated monthly; bulletins and product news updated daily.
Eye Disorders. Contains information on disorders of the eye (for example, of the eyelid, cornea, optic nerve) and preferred and alternate treatments.
Pharmaceuticals. Provides information on drugs by brand name. Includes manufacturer, form of application (for example, ointment), and concentration.
Instruments. Provides descriptions of about 3,000 instruments, lenses, and other equipment used in the practice of ophthalmology. Descriptions include manufacturer and price.
Literature Search. Provides citations from *Excerpta Medica* to the worldwide literature in the field of opthalmology (see EMBASE).

Database no longer maintained.

18:114. Online   General Electric Information Services Company

File name	Eyenet
Start year	Current information; Literature Search, 1983
Number of records	
Update period	Varies by file

Notes

Access limited to ophthalmologists, physicians, and the ophthalmic industry; monthly maintenance fee to ASCO required. Database no longer maintained.

FDA Electronic Bulletin Board
Food and Drug Administration

18:115. Master record

Database type	Bibliographic, Textual, Directory
Number of journals	
Sources	Speeches, Reports, Press releases, Journals, Trade journals, Newsletters and Laws/regulations
Start year	Current month
Language	English
Coverage	USA

Number of records	
Update size	—
Update period	Daily
Index unit	Articles, Drug and products

Description

Contains full text of reports, press releases, articles, speeches, and other items issued by the FDA. Includes the weekly enforcement report of FDA-regulated products under recall; citations to articles and full text of selected articles from the monthly FDA Consumer magazine; the monthly list of drug and device product approvals; citations to FDA Federal Register announcements; newsletters of interest to physicians and other health professionals; prepared speeches delivered by the FDA Commissioner and Deputy Commissioner; prepared statements delivered by FDA officials at congressional oversight meetings; and a schedule of upcoming FDA-sponsored meetings and conferences.

18:116. Online · Dialcom Inc

File name	FedNews
Start year	Current month
Number of records	
Update period	Daily

FDA on CD-ROM
FD Inc
US Food and Drug Administration

18:117. Master record

Database type	Textual, Factual
Number of journals	
Sources	Laws/regulations, law reports, speeches, press releases, reports, manuals and government documents (US)
Start year	1938
Language	English
Coverage	USA
Number of records	
Update size	—
Update period	Monthly

Keywords

Cosmetics; Drugs; Health Care

Description

Full text of the law relating to US food and drug administration. Federal Statutes, regulations, *FDA Manuals* and Judicial decisions on CD-ROM including over twenty Federal Statutes, *9 CFR* and *21 CFR* updated since last publication, Judicial decisions from 1938 to 1991, and the Food and Drug Administration's staff manual guides, regulatory procedures manual, compliance policy guide, compliance program guidance manual, inspection operations manual and import alerts relating to foods, drugs, cosmetics and medical devices. Also monthly updates of FDA talk papers, press releases, speeches, congrssional testimony of FDA officials, enforcement reports, new and proposed statutes and regulations and FDA-related Federal Register notices, Congressional record entries and changes in FDA guides and manuals.

18:118. CD-ROM · FD Inc

File name	FDA on CD-ROM
Format notes	IBM
Start year	1938

Number of records	
Update period	Monthly
Price/Charges	Subscription: US$2,300

This database can also be found on:
21CFR Online

FDC Reports
FDC Reports Inc

18:120. Master record

Database type	Textual
Number of journals	3
Sources	Conference reports, courts, direct contacts, government documents (US), journals, laws/regulations, ministry reports, newsletters, press releases, reports and trade journals
Start year	1984
Language	English
Coverage	USA (primarily) and International (some)
Number of records	22,767
Update size	—
Update period	Weekly
Index unit	articles and trademarks

Keywords

Applied Science; Beauty Care; Biomedical Research; Cosmetics; Dermatology; Drugs; Health Care Management; Marketing; Perfumes; Pharmaceuticals; Skin Care

Description

FDC Reports contains the full text of five related paramedical newsletters: Prescription and OTC Pharmaceuticals (*The Pink Sheet*), Medical Devices, Diagnostics and Instrumentation Reports (*The Gray Sheet*), and Toiletries, Fragrances and Skin Care (*The Rose Sheet*), health policy and biomedical research (*The Blue Sheet*) and pharmaceuticals (*The Green Sheet*).

Together the newsletters provide up-to-date information about companies, product development, marketing, packaging, scientific news, personnel, retailing and advertising, trade association news, United States Food and Drug Administration regulatory activities, and corporate news, including financial operations, mergers and acquisitions, marketing and licensing agreements, legal news and market share of importance to the worldwide health care industry. *The Pink Sheet* focuses on the pharmaceutical industry and includes over-the-counter drugs as well as prescription products. New products are profiled through all phases of the approval process, from early investigational stages through marketing. Personnel changes, marketing/licensing agreements, and mergers/acquisitions are covered regularly. Activities of major trade associations and regulatory bodies such as the Food and Drug Administration are reported. *The Gray Sheet* provides varied and detailed information pertinent to the costmetics industry, including toiletries, fragrances and skin care. Coverage includes marketing information, new product introductions, line extensions, promotions and advertising activities at retail. A Trademark Review is also provided which is a compilation of cosmetics-related product trademarks registered and filed for opposition with the US Patent and Trademark Office. *The Rose Sheet* also includes descriptions of cosmetics trademarks registered and filed for opposition with the United States Patent and Trademark Office. The database contains six types of records: full-text journal articles, FDA Recalls & Court Actions, Weekly Trademark Review records, Medical Device Approvals, New Drug Approvals and Abbreviated New Drug Approvals. *The Blue Sheet* deals with news and information concerning health policy and biomedical research topics including government funding and legal issues. *The Green Sheet* is particularly valuable in tracking the latest developments in drug sales and marketing.

Sources for all newsletters include new product announcements, market research reports, press releases, sales and earnings reports, United States Securities and Exchange Commission filings, government and trade association reports, reports from conferences, meetings, and conventions, and interviews with industry leaders. News coverage is focused primarily on US and multi-national activities and accounts for approximately eighty five per cent of the database. Approximately ten per cent is focused on Europe and five per cent on Japan and other countries.

The accession numbers field contains volume number, publication code, issue number and article number. The source field contains five options: pink-sheet, gray-sheet, green-sheet, blue-sheet and rose-sheet.

18:121. Online   BRS

File name	FDCR
Start year	1984
Number of records	22,767
Update period	Weekly
Price/Charges	Connect time: US$110.00/120.00
	Online print: US$0.92/1.00
	Offline print: US$1.00
	SDI charge: US$10.00

Notes
Contains the entire text of the following FDC Report publications: *The Pink Sheet*, *The Gray Sheet* and *The Rose Sheet*.

18:122. Online   Data-Star

File name	FDCR
Start year	January 1988
Number of records	620+ documents
Update period	Weekly
Database aids	Data-Star Business Manual and Data-Star Online Manual (search for NEWS-FDCR in NEWS)
Price/Charges	Subscription: SFr80.00
	Connect time: SFr187.00
	Online print: SFr1.64
	Offline print: SFr1.89
	SDI charge: SFr10.00

Downloading is allowed

Notes
From June 1993 Data-Star have introduced an annual fee/subscription per contract (that is, not per password) of SFr 80.00 (c.UK£ 32.00) payable every June. For North American customers billed in dollars who also use DIALOG, the DIALOG fee also covers access to Data-Star. Academic customers, 'commitment' customers and customers currently billed in dollars are exempt.

Record composition
Accession Number and Update Code AN; Date of Publication DT; Month of Publication YM; Occurence Table OC; Source SO; Text of article TX; Title TI; Update Code UP and Year of Publication YR

18:123. Online   DIALOG

File name	File 187
Start year	1987
Number of records	31,232
Update period	Weekly
Price/Charges	Connect time: US$120.00
	Online print: US$1.20
	Offline print: US$1.50
	SDI charge: US$3.95

Notes
DIALINDEX Categories: BIOBUS, PHARMINA, REGS.

18:124. Online   Mead Data Central
                                    (as a NEXIS database)

File name	FDC – NEXIS
Alternative name(s)	NEXIS – FDC Reports
Start year	1984
Number of records	
Update period	Weekly
Price/Charges	Subscription: US$1,000 – 3,000 (Depending on needs)
	Connect time: US$49.00 (Telecomms + connect time)
	Database entry fee: US$24.00 (Search charge)
	Online print: US$0.04 per line

Notes
Library: GENMED. FDC is the Group File containing all five reports: Blue, Gray, Green, Pink and Rose.

A subscription charge which covers all transactional charges, connect time, telecommunications and the small administration charge can take the place of the individual charges. Subscriptions are negotiated with customers and vary according to the number of menus (thus, files) that are to be used – typically a minimum subscription would be about US$ 1,000. All charges include training and a 24-hour help line.

18:125. Database subset

Online   Mead Data Central
                                    (as a NEXIS database)

File name	GRAY – NEXIS
Alternative name(s)	NEXIS – FDC Reports
Start year	1984
Number of records	
Update period	Weekly
Price/Charges	Subscription: US$1,000 – 3,000 (Depending on needs)
	Connect time: US$49.00 (Telecomms + connect time)
	Database entry fee: US$24.00 (Search charge)
	Online print: US$0.04 per line

Notes
Library: GENMED; Group File: FDC.

The full text of the weekly newsletter, *The Gray Sheet*, on the medical devices, diagnostic and instrumentation industry. Written specifically for executives, physicians and other professionals concerned with the medical device industry, the newsletter provides regulatory news and useful business or related information. Topics include news of new products, product research, marketing and advertising, government regulation and oversight, legal issues and corporate and industry performance. A regular feature of the newsletter is an index to the Food and Drug Administration's monthly report of premarket approvals and their supplements.

A subscription charge which covers all transactional charges, connect time, telecommunications and the small administration charge can take the place of the individual charges. Subscriptions are negotiated with customers and vary according to the number of menus (thus, files) that are to be used – typically a minimum subscription would be about US$ 1,000. All charges include training and a 24-hour help line.

Record composition

Publication; Cite; Date; Section; Length; Title; Text; Correction; Correction Date; Discussion and Editor's Note

This database can also be found on:
NEXIS

Friginter
International Institute of Refrigeration (IIR)

18:127. Master record

Database type	Bibliographic
Number of journals	
Sources	Monographs, Journals, Reports and Conference proceedings
Start year	1981
Language	English and French
Coverage	International
Number of records	17,000+
Update size	2,700
Update period	Every two months

Keywords

Cryobiology; Refrigeration

Description

Contains citations, with abstracts, to the worldwide literature on refrigeration techniques and applications. Covers air conditioning, cryobiology, cryoengineering, cryophysics, food science and technology, freeze-drying, gas liquefaction and separation, heat pumps and energy recovery, medical applications, refrigerated storage and transport, refrigerating machinery, thermodynamics, and transport processes.

Corresponds in part to the *Bulletin of the IIR*.

18:128. Online   International Institute of Refrigeration

File name	
Start year	1981
Number of records	17,000+
Update period	Every two months

Notes

Deposit of 1,500 French francs required.

Frost & Sullivan Market Research Reports Summaries
Frost & Sullivan Inc

18:129. Master record

Alternative name(s)	F & S Market Research Reports Summaries
Database type	Bibliographic
Number of journals	
Sources	Research reports

Start year	Current 2–3 years
Language	English
Coverage	International
Number of records	409 documents
Update size	–
Update period	Monthly

Keywords

Chemical Substances; Defence; Electronics; Data Processing; Transport; Food and Drink; Manufacturing; Marketing; Machinery; Instrumentation; Pharmaceuticals; Drugs

Description

Contains citations, with detailed abstracts, to Frost & Sullivan market research reports. Reports provide analyses and forecasts of market size and share by product and company. Industries analysed include chemicals, communications, consumer products, data processing, defense, electronics, food, health, instrumentation, machinery and transportation. Includes forecasts by country for a five year period plus appraisal of technological developments and applications. Reports are written by consultants who are experts within their field.

The database contains only references to the full published Frost and Sullivan Market Research reports. Original reports may be obtained from Frost and Sullivan; each document records the report number and price information for the original report.

18:130. Online   Data-Star

File name	FSFS
Alternative name(s)	F & S Market Research Reports Summaries
Start year	Current 2–3 years
Number of records	409 documents
Update period	Monthly
Database aids	Data-Star Business Manual, Berne, Data-Star and Online manual (search NEWS-FSFS in NEWS)
Price/Charges	Subscription: UK£32.00
	Connect time: UK£40.00
	Online print: UK£0.30
	Offline print: UK£0.20

Notes

From June 1993 Data-Star have introduced an annual fee/subscription per contract (that is, not per password) of SFr 80.00 (c.UK£ 32.00) payable every June. For North American customers billed in dollars who also use DIALOG, the DIALOG fee also covers access to Data-Star. Academic customers, 'commitment' customers and customers currently billed in dollars are exempt.

Handicapped Users Database
Georgia Griffith

18:131. Master record

Database type	Factual, Textual
Number of journals	
Sources	
Start year	Current information
Language	English
Coverage	USA
Number of records	
Update size	–
Update period	Six times per month

Description

Contains information on products and services available to handicapped persons, with an emphasis on uses of microcomputers and related devices (for example, Kurzweil readers). Also includes articles of interest to handicapped and non-handicapped (for example, teachers, parents) persons, information on for-profit and non-profit service organisations, relevant news, and an electronic bulletin board for the exchange of ideas.

18:132. Online — CompuServe Information Service

File name	HUD
Start year	Current information
Number of records	
Update period	Six times per month
Price/Charges	Subscription: US$8.95 per month
Downloading is allowed	

HAP
Hamburg Educational Partnership

18:133. Master record

Alternative name(s)	Hamburg Educational Partnership
Database type	Courseware, Multimedia
Number of journals	
Sources	
Start year	
Language	German
Coverage	Germany
Number of records	
Update size	—
Update period	

Keywords

Radiography

Description

Multimedia training programme, including technical and medical packages on: X-ray devices, magnetic resonance imaging, Lufthansa turbine presentations, Lufthansa hydraulics course unit, theory of automation, C language learning, and thin-film technology. Totals seven educational packages.

18:134. CD-ROM — Hamburg Educational Partnership

File name	HAP
Alternative name(s)	Hamburg Educational Partnership
Format notes	IBM, Mac
Start year	
Number of records	
Update period	

Health Devices Alerts
ECRI

18:138. Master record

Database type	Factual, Textual
Number of journals	
Sources	Government documents (US) and Reports
Start year	1977
Language	English
Coverage	USA

Number of records	120,000
Update size	—
Update period	Weekly
Thesaurus	Universal Medical Device Nomenclature System (UMDNS)

Description

A comprehensive database developed by ECRI, a nonprofit agency and independent evaluator of health technology. It warns and informs of reported medical device problems, hazards, recalls, evaluations, and updates. The selections derive from an extensive review of the medical, legal, and technical literature, various national reporting networks and government sources, and ECRI's own international problem reporting network, abstracts from technical literature on medical device problems; and the complete *Medical Device Reports* from the FDA. Covers reports of problems with diagnostic and therapeutic medical equipment and related materials, ranging from sutures to magnetic resonance imaging units, including implanted devices and related accessories, disposable medical products, clinical laboratory reagents, and selected hospital furniture, casework, and systems. The database has potential for clinicians, purchasing departments, biomedical engineers, and all in health-care concerned with medical device reliability; attorneys or lawyers; and manufacturers of devices.

Consists of four subfiles:

Action Items containing confirmed hazards and recalls investigated by ECRI;

Abstracts of reported problems, device evaluations, comparisons, and technical assessments from the medical, legal and technical literature;

MDRs, the US Food and Drug Administration's (FDA) Medical Device complete Report indexed and reformatted by ECRI; and

PRPs, the FDA's Problem Reporting Program reports indexed by ECRI.

Corresponds to the weekly cumulative *Health Devices Alerts*.

Each entry is indexed using ECRI's internationally endorsed Universal Medical Device Nomenclature System (UMDNS). An online thesaurus is available as an aid in locating broader, narrower and related product names. Most entries have abstracts.

18:139. Online — CompuServe Information Service

File name	IQUEST File 2577
Start year	1977
Number of records	171,602
Update period	Weekly
Price/Charges	Subscription: US$8.95 per month Database entry fee: US$9/search; some databases carry a surcharge ($2–75) Online print: US$10 references free; then $9 per ten; abstracts $3 each
Downloading is allowed	

Notes

Accessed via IQUEST or IQMEDICAL, this database is offered by a DIALOG gateway. IQUEST can either search across all databases, a database of the user's choice or selected multiple databases.

18:140. Online — DIALOG

File name	File 198
Start year	1977

Number of records	171,602
Update period	Weekly
Price/Charges	Connect time: US$75.00 – 105.00
	Online print: US$1.00
	Offline print: US$1.00

Notes

A complete directory of medical devices and manufacturers is available in a companion database, File 188, Health Devices Sourcebook, from ECRI. Differential connect time charges for subscribers and non-subscribers.

18:141. CD-ROM　　　　　　DIALOG OnDisc

File name	Health Devices Alerts
Format notes	Mac, IBM
Software	DIALOG OnDisc Manager
Start year	1977
Number of records	135,000
Update period	Quarterly
Price/Charges	Subscription: UK£1,360

Notes

Price for annual subscription includes $400 online time.

Health Devices Sourcebook
ECRI
Biomedical Engineering Decision Support Systems

18:142. Master record

Database type	Directory
Number of journals	
Sources	Suppliers
Start year	Current information
Language	English
Coverage	USA (primarily) and International (some)
Number of records	8,400
Update size	—
Update period	Annually

Description

This database is a directory file containing current address and marketing information on the North American manufacturers, distributors and importers of over 4,000 classes of medical devices. It includes service companies that buy, sell and repair used equipment. Information provided includes product name, code, and typical price range for all diagnostic and therapeutic medical devices and materials, clinical laboratory equipment and reagents, casework, systems and instrumentation for testing clinical equipment, and selected hospital furniture. Three types of records are contained: product records (49% of the file), manufacturer records (44%), and service records (6%). About 98% of the records relate to United States manufacturers, products, and services, although ECRI plans to add more international coverage in the future. Product records also contain references, if available, to brand-name evaluations or product specifications in other ECRI publications. Manufacturer information includes organization name and type, contact information, product names and codes, trade names, and names of executive officers. Service records contain organisation name, contact information, service category (for example, clinical laboratory, nuclear medicine), type of service offered

(for example, sales, parts, repairs), locations served, and names of service management personnel. The database includes tens of thousands of trade names and more than 6,000 manufacturers, distributors, importers and service companies.

The database corresponds to the monthly *Health Devices Sourcebook*.

Utilises ECRI's internationally endorsed medical device thesaurus and numerical coding system (UMDNS) for product classification. An online thesaurus is available to assist in locating broader, narrower and related product names.

18:143. Online　　　　　　　　　DIALOG

File name	File 188
Start year	Current
Number of records	8,400
Update period	Annually
Price/Charges	Connect time: US$66.00 – 99.00
	Online print: US$1.50
	Offline print: US$1.50

Thesaurus is online

Notes

There is a companion database also produced by ECRI, the Health Devices Alerts Database, File 198 on DIALOG, which lists the products. Differential pricing for subscribers and non-subscribers.

DIALINDEX Categories: PRODUCTS, TRADENMS, USCO.

Health Industry Research Reports
JA Micropublishing Inc

18:144. Master record

Database type	Bibliographic
Number of journals	
Sources	Reports and Research communications
Start year	1982
Language	English
Coverage	International
Number of records	6,000
Update size	—
Update period	Quarterly

Description

Contains citations, with abstracts, to research reports issued by about seventy security and investment firms on the health industry and individual industry firms. Covers hospital management, pharmaceuticals, medical hardware, life insurance, hospitals, and health care. Citations include title, author, publisher, date, and for companies, geographic location and product listings. Each abstract contains a description of the type of statistical data to be found in the original article.

Users can order full text of documents online.

18:145. Online　　　BRS, Morning Search, BRS/Colleague

File name	HIRR
Start year	1982

Number of records	6,000
Update period	Quarterly

Health News Daily
FDC Reports Inc

18:146. Master record

Alternative name(s)	Health Daily (formerly)
Database type	Textual
Number of journals	1
Sources	Government committee meetings, Government reports, Meeting papers, Newsletters, Press releases, Press conferences, Trade association meetings and Direct contacts
Start year	1988
Language	English
Coverage	USA
Number of records	4,400+
Update size	—
Update period	Daily

Keywords
Cosmetics; Pharmaceuticals

Description
Health News Daily Online contains the full text of *Health News Daily*, a daily newsletter on health care delivery. Subjects covered include: policy and legislation, insurance, funding, manufacturing and new technology, medical breakthroughs and treatments, pharmaceuticals and pharmacy, medical devices and diagnostics, biomedical research, cosmetics, health policy, provider payment policies and cost-containment. Using the FDC reports' staff of thirty reporters and editors, each issue provides up-to-date information about companies, products, markets, personnel, regulatory and legislative activities, financial performances and scientific and legal developments. Regular departments include: Product News, People, Litigation, Legislative News, Industry News, Research, Regulatory News, Financings, Reimbursement and Public Health. 'Washington This Week' lists scheduled congressional hearings, agency meetings and industry conferences in the DC area. 'Calendar' presents notices of forthcoming meetings, conferences and seminars around the USA. 'Legislative Roundup' tracks recently introduced bills, committee activities and congressional votes on health care legislation.

Corresponds to the FDC daily publication *Health News Daily*. Formerly produced by Warren Publishing, Inc. Primary news sources include: press conferences, government committee and panel meetings, briefings to financial analysts, company annual meetings, trade association annual meetings and conventions, activities of scientific and standards-setting groups, legislative and regulatory testimony in Congress, professional organizations and direct interviews with industry newsmakers. In addition, the following secondary sources are utilised: new product announcements, market research reports, press releases, consultant studies, wire services, sales and earnings reports, Securities and Exchange Commission (SEC) filings, and government reports.

18:147. Online   BRS

File name	HNDY
Alternative name(s)	Health Daily (formerly)
Start year	1988
Number of records	4,400+
Update period	Daily

Price/Charges	Connect time: US$120.00/130.00
	Online print: US$1.92/2.00
	Offline print: US$2.10

18:148. Online   Data-Star

File name	HNDO
Alternative name(s)	Health Daily (formerly)
Start year	March 1989
Number of records	4,400
Update period	Daily
Database aids	Data-Star Business Manual and Data-Star Online Manual (search for NEWS-FDCR or NEWS-HNDO in NEWS)
Price/Charges	Subscription: SFr80.00
	Connect time: SFr212.60
	Online print: SFr3.25
	Offline print: SFr3.42
	SDI charge: SFr10.00

Downloading is allowed

Notes
This file contains the latest day's update plus the archive from March 1989.

From June 1993 Data-Star have introduced an annual fee/subscription per contract (that is, not per password) of SFr 80.00 (c.UK£ 32.00) payable every June. For North American customers billed in dollars who also use DIALOG, the DIALOG fee also covers access to Data-Star. Academic customers, 'commitment' customers and customers currently billed in dollars are exempt.

Record composition
Accession Number AN; Date of Publication DT; Month of Publication YM; Occurence table OC; Source SO; Text of article (in full) TX; Title TI; Update Code UP and Year of Publication YR

18:149. Online   Data-Star

File name	HNDD
Alternative name(s)	Health Daily (formerly)
Start year	Current – latest day's update
Number of records	
Update period	Daily
Database aids	Data-Star Business Manual and Data-Star Online Manual (search for NEWS-FDCR or NEWS-HNDO in NEWS)
Price/Charges	Subscription: SFr80.00
	Connect time: SFr212.60
	Online print: SFr3.25
	Offline print: SFr3.42
	SDI charge: SFr10.00

Downloading is allowed

Notes
From June 1993 Data-Star have introduced an annual fee/subscription per contract (that is, not per password) of SFr 80.00 (c.UK£ 32.00) payable every June. For North American customers billed in dollars who also use DIALOG, the DIALOG fee also covers access to Data-Star. Academic customers, 'commitment' customers and customers currently billed in dollars are exempt.

Record composition
Accession Number AN; Date of Publication DT; Month of Publication YM; Occurence table OC; Source SO; Text of article (in full) TX; Title TI; Update Code UP and Year of Publication YR

18:150. Online   NewsNet Inc

File name	Health News Daily
Alternative name(s)	Health Daily (formerly)
Start year	1988

Number of records
Update period

Notes

Monthly subscription to NewsNet required; differential charges for subscribers and non-subscribers to Health News Daily.

This database can also be found on:
PTS Newletter

Healthcare Product Comparison System
DIALOG
ECRI

18:152. Master record

Database type	Factual, Directory, Textual
Number of journals	
Sources	
Start year	
Language	English
Coverage	USA
Number of records	
Update size	—
Update period	Quarterly
Index unit	Products

Keywords

Dental Equipment; Health Care Products; Medical Equipment

Description

Provides objective brand-name product comparisons of all types of medical and healthcare equipment from laboratory instruments to x-ray units and surgical lasers. Products covered include dental and surgical equipment, home care devices, hospital furniture, implanted devices, materials management products, obstetrics/gynaecological devices, ophthalmologic, orthopaedic and radiological devices and physical medicine equipment. Each report includes product descriptions and a complete explanation of how the equipment is used, specifications, warranty information, pricing and manufacturer contact information. Includes tables for side-by-side comparisons of products. Sourced from three of ECRI's print Product Comparison Systems – *Clinical Laboratory, Diagnostic Imaging and Radiology*, and *Hospital*.

18:153. CD-ROM   DIALOG OnDisc

File name	Healthcare Product Comparison System
Format notes	Mac, IBM
Software	DIALOG OnDisc Manager
Start year	Current information
Number of records	
Update period	Quarterly
Database aids	DIALOG OnDisc Discovery User's Guide and Data sheets for the DIALOG OnDisc databases
Price/Charges	Subscription: UK£2,150

Notes

Networking price is £2,150 for 1–10 users.

Hearing Impaired Forum
Robert Colbert

18:154. Master record

Database type	Directory, Textual
Number of journals	
Sources	

Start year	
Language	English
Coverage	USA
Number of records	
Update size	—
Update period	Periodically, as new data become available

Keywords

Legislation; Hearing Impairment; Sign Language; Special Education; Telecommunications

Description

News and information on products and services for the hearing impaired, including TV adapters, telecommunications devices, captioned film and video rentals, sign language teaching, the effects of hearing loss, related legislation, educational facilities, organisations, interpreters and an electronic bulletin board.

18:155. Online   General Videotex Corporation, Delphi

File name	
Start year	1986
Number of records	
Update period	Periodically, as new data become available

Information Service in Mechanical Engineering
Cambridge Scientific Abstracts

18:156. Master record

Alternative name(s)	ISMEC
Database type	Bibliographic, Factual
Number of journals	750
Sources	Journals, Monographs, Reports and Conference proceedings
Start year	1973
Language	English
Coverage	International
Number of records	220,000
Update size	9,600
Update period	Every two months
Database aids	CSA User Guide

Keywords

Management; Mechanical Engineering

Description

ISMEC (Information Service In Mechanical Engineering) indexes significant articles in all aspects of mechanical engineering, production engineering, and engineering management from approximately 750 journals published throughout the world. Contains approximately 220,000 citations, with abstracts (from 1982). In addition, books, reports, and conference proceedings are indexed. The primary emphasis is on comprehensive coverage of leading international journals and conferences on mechanical engineering subjects. The principal areas covered are mechanical, nuclear, electrical, electronic, civil, optical, medical, and industrial process engineering; mechanics; production processes; energy and power sources; transport, maintenance and handling; and applications of mechanical engineering.

Corresponds to *ISMEC Abstracts Journal*.

18:157. Online   DIALOG

File name	File 14
Alternative name(s)	ISMEC
Start year	1973
Number of records	235,489
Update period	Every two months
Price/Charges	Connect time: US$90.00
	Online print: US$0.75
	Offline print: US$0.75

18:158. Online   ESA-IRS

File name	File 10
Alternative name(s)	ISMEC
Start year	1973
Number of records	238,500
Update period	Every two months

Notes

QUESTALERT and QUESTORDER are available. Hard Sciences, File 25 on ESA, covers recent years of ISMEC (1982 to date) with searchable abstracts.

From 1993 ESA-IRS are charging an annual fee of 100 Accounting Units (c.UK£ 70.29) to all users. This is equivalent to the fee for full documentation and will not be charged to customers already paying for documentation.

18:159. Online   STN

File name	ISMEC
Alternative name(s)	ISMEC
Start year	1973
Number of records	250,000
Update period	Twice a month

18:160. Tape   STN

File name	ISMEC: Mechanical Engineering Abstracts on Magnetic Tape
Alternative name(s)	ISMEC
Start year	1973
Number of records	220,000
Update period	Every two months
Price/Charges	Subscription: US$7,100

Notes

Corresponds to *ISMEC: Mechanical Engineering Abstracts* and the ISMEC online database. Costs are: current year $7,100; single-year archival file 3,600.

Instrument Making
MoldNIINTI

18:161. Master record

Database type	Bibliographic
Number of journals	
Sources	
Start year	1988
Language	English
Coverage	
Number of records	20,000
Update size	—
Update period	

Description

Bibliographic information in instrument making.

18:162. Diskette   MoldNIINTI

File name	
Start year	1988

Number of records	20,000
Update period	

Investext
Thomson Financial Networks Inc

18:163. Master record

Database type	Textual, Bibliographic
Number of journals	
Sources	Reports
Start year	1982
Language	English
Coverage	USA, Canada, European Community and Japan
Number of records	320,000
Update size	125,000 pages per year
Update period	Weekly
Hosts have included	CORIS (Thomson Financial Network) (Until 1/92)

Keywords

Aerospace; Automotive Industry; Banking Industry; Broadcasting; Chemical Industry; Computer Industry; Insurance Industry; Metals Industry; Pharmaceutical Industry; Social Policy; Telecommunications; Transport; Utilities Industry

Description

The world's largest database of full-text, company, industry research, geographical and topical reports produced by professional research analysts at almost 200 top international brokers and investment bankers in major investment banking and financial research firms in the United States, Australia, Canada, Europe and Japan. This is the largest, long-running database covering investment research information. It provides hard-to-find information on companies and industries – information that is not available from any other source, according to Sharon Ladner in her review of the product (*CD-ROM Professional* 5(4) p. 77–83). Information includes all tabular data plus indexing and abstracts.

Gives historical analyses of firms, together with short and long-term forecasts of sales, financial information, prospects, earnings, research and development expenditures, market share, production and distribution, consumer spending, etc. Industries covered include aerospace, automotive, banking, broadcasting, computers, insurance, metals, pharmaceuticals, telecommunications, utilities.

Company information covers sales, stock prices, balance sheets, financial results, cash flow, capital expenditure. Includes material on 21,000 companies internationally, and 53 industry groups, covering high tech industries, chemical and medical areas as wellas consumer goods and trade. Investext can be used for a wide range of business intelligence activities, including competitive analysis, market research, evaluation of companies for acquisition, corporate planning, sales planning, etc. Each analyst report has on average eight pages. Information covered is originally produced as investment advice for the clients of the investment houses and financial advisers. It is placed on the database after a delay, and recommendations should no longer be considered as investment recommendations. The information remains useful for analytical purposes. Covers 53 industries with good coverage of smaller, regional companies. Most of the recent growth in the Investext database comes by including reports from foreign and regional brokerage firms – as of September 1991, Investext listed 198 contributors to its database – more than half from outside the United States and 35 from outside of New York City.

The archive covers the current twelve months of supplied material. During 1992, the Europe Information Service of Cooper's & Lybrand Europe added their bulletins on the EC to the service. Each bulletin provides detailed coverage of debates, projects and agreements relating to the EC through the bi-weekly European Report and a series of monthly and bi-monthly titles looking at specific areas such as transport, energy and social policy.

US sources for Investext reports written by professional analysts within such investment houses as: Bear Stearns & Co.; J.C. Bradford & Co.; Alex. Brown & Sons Inc.; Butcher & Singer Inc.; Cable Howse & Ragen; Craig- Hallum Inc.; Dain Bosworth Inc.; Dean Witter Reynolds Inc.; Dillon Read & Company Inc.; Donaldson, Lufkin & Jenrette Securities Corp.; Drexel Burnham Lambert Inc.; Eberstadt Fleming Inc.; First Boston Corp.; Fitch Investors Service Inc.; Fox-Pitt, Kelton; Hibbard Brown & Company; E.F. Hutton & Company Inc.; Interstate Securities Corp.; Janney Montgomery Scott inc.; Kidder Peabody and Co. Inc.; C.J. Lawrence, Morgan Grenfell Inc.; Mabon, Nugent & Company; Market Guide Inc.; Merrill Lynch, Pierce, Fenner & Smith Inc.; Morgan Stanley & Co. Inc; Moseley Securities Corporation; The New York Society of Security Analysts; Nomura Securities international Inc.; Oppenheimer & Co. Inc.; Paine webber Inc.; Pershing; Piper, Jaffray & Hopwood Inc.; Prudential-Bache Securities; Rauscher Pierce Refsnes Inc.; Salomon Brothers inc.; Sanyo Securities America Inc.; Stephens Inc.; Tucker, Anthony and R.L.Day Inc.; and Van Kasper & Company.

Other sources of financial research in major industrial countries worldwide include: Algemene Bank Nederland N.V.; Banca Commerciale Italiana; Citicorp Scrimgour Vickers; DAFSA; DEGAB; Kredietbank N.V.; Phillips and Drew Ltd. (Member UBS group); Richardson Greenshields of Canada Limited; Roach Tilley Grice Inc.; Sutro & Company; McLeod Young Weir Limited; Union Bank of Switzerland; Barclays de Zoete Wedd and Yamaichi Research Institute of Securities and Economics Inc.

Complete presentation-style, laser-printed reports corresponding to the individual analyses are available from Investext.

Significant research reports from major investment research institutions willing to make their material publicly available once it has outlived its utility for investment purposes.

18:164. Online   BRS, BRS/Colleague

File name	
Start year	1982
Number of records	320,000
Update period	Weekly

Notes

On this host Investext includes the Market Guide Data Base

18:165. Online   CompuServe Information Service

File name	
Start year	1982

Number of records	200,000
Update period	Weekly
Price/Charges	Subscription: US$8.95 per month
Downloading is allowed	

Notes

Apparently Market Guide Data Base is not included in Investext on this host.

18:166. Online   Data-Star

File name	INVE
Start year	January 1987
Number of records	263,000
Update period	Weekly (Daily in 1992)
Database aids	Data-Star Smart Search Guide to Investext, Investext Product Terms Plus Directory: available free from Data-Star,, Data-Star Business Manual, Berne, Data-Star, and Online guide (search NEWS-INVE in NEWS)
Price/Charges	Subscription: UK£32.00
	Connect time: UK£76.00
	Online print: UK£0.53 – 3.52
	Offline print: UK£0.56 – 3.81

Also available on FIZ Technik via a gateway from Data-Star

Notes

From June 1993 Data-Star have introduced an annual fee/subscription per contract (that is, not per password) of SFr 80.00 (c.UK£ 32.00) payable every June. For North American customers billed in dollars who also use DIALOG, the DIALOG fee also covers access to Data-Star. Academic customers, 'commitment' customers and customers currently billed in dollars are exempt.

On this host Investext includes the Market Guide Data Base

18:167. Online   Data-Star

File name	IV86
Start year	1982 to 1986
Number of records	137,800
Update period	Weekly (Daily in 1992)
Database aids	Data-Star Smart Search Guide to Investext, Investext Product Terms Plus Directory: available free from Data-Star,, Data-Star Business Manual, Berne, Data-Star, and Online guide (search NEWS-INVE in NEWS)
Price/Charges	Subscription: UK£32.00
	Connect time: UK£76.00
	Online print: UK£0.53 – 3.52
	Offline print: UK£0.56 – 3.81

Also available on FIZ Technik via a gateway from Data-Star

Notes

On this host Investext includes the Market Guide Data Base.

From June 1993 Data-Star have introduced an annual fee/subscription per contract (that is, not per password) of SFr 80.00 (c.UK£ 32.00) payable every June. For North American customers billed in dollars who also use DIALOG, the DIALOG fee also covers access to Data-Star. Academic customers, 'commitment' customers and customers currently billed in dollars are exempt.

18:168. Online   Data-Star

File name	IVZZ
Start year	July 1982

Number of records	401,000
Update period	Weekly (Daily in 1992)
Database aids	Data-Star Smart Search Guide to Investext, Investext Product Terms Plus Directory: available free from Data-Star,, Data-Star Business Manual, Berne, Data-Star, and Online guide (search NEWS-INVE in NEWS)
Price/Charges	Subscription: UK£32.00
	Connect time: UK£76.00
	Online print: UK£0.53 – 3.81
	Offline print: UK£0.56 – 3.81

Also available on FIZ Technik via a gateway from Data-Star

Notes

On this host Investext includes the Market Guide Data Base. From June 1993 Data-Star have introduced an annual fee/subscription per contract (that is, not per password) of SFr 80.00 (c.UK£ 32.00) payable every June. For North American customers billed in dollars who also use DIALOG, the DIALOG fee also covers access to Data-Star. Academic customers, 'commitment' customers and customers currently billed in dollars are exempt.

18:169. Online   DIALOG

File name	File 545
Start year	1982 (July)
Number of records	1,742,965 representing 283,096 reports
Update period	Weekly
Price/Charges	Connect time: US$96.00
	Online print: US$5.50
	Offline print: US$5.50
	SDI charge: US$4.00

Notes

There may be differences between search results on the CD-ROM and on the DIALOG online file: one review (*CD-ROM Professional* 5(4)p.77–83) reported that 'during the 12-month review period, InfoTrac Investext did not include reports published by Market Guide, a financial research firm which specialises in smaller publicly owned companies. More recent InfoTrac CD-ROM discs do include Market Guide Reports . . .' while the DIALOG file does. Because names of subsidiaries of public companies are not included in the Subject Index, searches for information on subsidiaries result in 'no hits' even though the data on these corporate forms is often included in the investment reports.

18:170. Online   Dow Jones

File name	
Start year	1982
Number of records	320,000
Update period	Weekly

Notes

Annual fee of $12 to Dow Jones required On this host Investext includes the Market Guide Data Base.

18:171. Online   FIZ Technik (gateway)

File name	INVE
Start year	1987
Number of records	263,000
Update period	Weekly (Daily in 1992)

Database aids	Data-Star Smart Search Guide to Investext, Investext Product Terms Plus Directory: available free from Data-Star,, Data-Star Business Manual, Berne, Data-Star, and Online guide (search NEWS-INVE in NEWS)
Price/Charges	Connect time: SFr190.00
	Online print: SFr1.33 – 8.80 (per paragraph)
	Offline print: SFr1.41 – 9.52 (per paragraph)

Available via Data-Star on a gateway

Notes

On this host Investext includes the Market Guide Data Base.

18:172. Online   FIZ Technik (gateway)

File name	IV89
Start year	1982 to 1989
Number of records	137,800
Update period	Weekly (Daily in 1992)
Database aids	Data-Star Smart Search Guide to Investext, Investext Product Terms Plus Directory: available free from Data-Star,, Data-Star Business Manual, Berne, Data-Star, and Online guide (search NEWS-INVE in NEWS)
Price/Charges	Connect time: SFr190.00
	Online print: SFr1.33 – 8.80 (per paragraph)
	Offline print: SFr1.41 – 9.52 (per paragraph)

Available via Data-Star on a gateway

Notes

On this host Investext includes the Market Guide Data Base.

18:173. Online   FIZ Technik (gateway)

File name	IVZZ
Start year	1987
Number of records	401,000
Update period	Weekly (Daily in 1992)
Database aids	Data-Star Smart Search Guide to Investext, Investext Product Terms Plus Directory: available free from Data-Star,, Data-Star Business Manual, Berne, Data-Star and Online guide (search NEWS-INVE in NEWS)
Price/Charges	Connect time: SFr190.00
	Online print: SFr1.33 – 8.80 (per paragraph)
	Offline print: SFr1.41 – 9.52 (per paragraph)

Available via Data-Star on a gateway

Notes

On this host Investext includes the Market Guide Data Base.

18:174. Online   FT Profile

File name	INV
Start year	Current information only
Number of records	
Update period	
Delay	Reports are generally available online on FT Profile within four to six weeks of publication.
Price/Charges	Connect time: UK£2.40
	Online print: UK£0.04 – 0.10 per line
	Offline print: UK£0.01 per line

Notes

Registration fee required, including free documentation and training. Usage charges for access consist of two elements: a connect rate for time online, and a display rate (applies only to lines of file text). There is no charge for blank lines, system messages, menus or help information.

18:175. Online   Mead Data Central
                           (as a NEXIS database)

File name	INTL
Start year	1982
Number of records	200,000
Update period	Daily
Delay	Varies but usually within thirty days of printed source.

Notes

Libraries: COMPNY and INVEST which have all Investext reports; other libraries have selected reports (for example, transportation industry reports in TRAN). Also: ASIAPC, MDEAFR, NSAMER and WORLD.

Investext sources are listed (with their addresses) in the documentation; individual file names can be used for each source (given in parenthesis with coverage start date):

A.G. Edwards and Sons (AGE 10/88); ABN AMRO Bank NV Advest Inc. (ADV 5/84); Alex Brown and Sons Inc. (AB 1/84); Altman Brenner & Wasserman Inc. (ABW 6/90); Argus Research Corporation (ARG 12/90); B. Metzler Seel (BMS 5/91); Bain Securities Inc. (BSI 10/90); Baird, Patrick & Co. Inc. (BDP 6/90); Balis & Zorn Inc. (BZG 10/88); Banca Commerciale Italiana Piazza (BCI 6/83); Bank in Liechtenstein (BIL 2.91); Barclays de Zoete Wedd Securities Ltd. (BZW 2/90); Bateman Eichler, Hill Richards Inc. (BEH 4/90); Bayerische Vereinsbank AG (BVB 7/91); BDMI Limited (BDM 8/90); Bear Stearns & Co. (BDS 4/83); Beeson Gregory Ltd. (BSG 7/91); Bell Lawrie White & Co (BLL 4/89); Boettcher & Company (BOE 5/89); Booz- Allen & Hamilton (BAH 2/89); B.W.D. Rensburg Ltd. (BWD 1/90); C.J. Lawrence Inc (CJL 1/83); CCF Elysees Bourse (CCF 1/90); Charterhouse Tilney (CHT 11/89); Coburn & Meredith Inc. (CMI 4/90); Coopers & Lybrand Europe (CLE 5/90); County NatWest Securities Asia Ltd (CNA 7/90); County NatWest Securities Japan Ltd. (CNJ 2/91); Craig-Hallum Inc. (CH 4/88); Credit-Lyonnais Securities (Japan) (CLJ 5/91); Credit Suisse First Boston Ltd. (CSF 7/90); Crowell, Weedon & Co. (CRW 12/90); DAFSA (DAF 2/82); Dain Bosworth Inc. (DB 1/83); Daiwa Institute of Research Europe Ltd. (DIR 4/92); Daiwa Securities Co., Ltd. (DAI 10/90); Dean Witter Reynolds Inc. (DW 3/88) Decision Resources Inc. (ADL 2/87); DEGAB (DGB 3/82); Deloitte & Touche Europe Services (DRT 4/91); Dillon Read & Company Inc. (DR 11/88); Donaldson, Lufkin & Jenrette Securities Corp. (DLJ 3/83); Duff & Phelps Inc. (DNP 12/90); Fahnestock/B.C. Christopher (FHN 6/91); First Boston Corp. (FB 7/86); Fitch Investors Service Inc. (FIT 9/84); Fox-Pitt, Kelton (FOX 7/84); FT Analysis Corporation (PLC 3/90); George K. Baum & Co. (GKB 9/90); Gerard Klauer Mattison (GKM 9/90); H.C. Wainwright & Co. (HCW 8/90); Hambrecht & Quist Inc. (HMQ 6/90); Hanifen Imhoff Inc. (HAN 8/91); Henderson Crosthwaite Inst. Brokers Ltd. (HCR 3/90); Henry Cooke, Lumsden (HCL 11/89); Hibbard Brown & Company (HBC 10/88); Hoare Govett Investment Research Ltd. (HGV 1/90); Interstate/ Johnson Lane (INT 5/83); J.C. Bradford & Co. (JCB

11/83); James Capel & Co. Ltd. (JCC 2/90); Janney Montgomery Scott Inc. (JMS 8/88); Jesup, Josephthal & Co. (JSJ 9/90); Johnson Rice & Co. (JR 1/89); Johnston, Lemon & Co. (JL 5/89); Kankaku Securities Co. (KKS 3/91); Kemper Securities Group (KSG 3/91); Kenneth, Jerome & Co. (KJR 9/90); Kidder Peabody and Co. Inc. (KP 1/83); Kredietbank NV (KB 9/83); Ladenburg, Thalman (LDB 9/90); Loewen, Ondaatje, McCutcheon & Co. (LOM 1/91); Mabon Securities Corp. (MNC 10/86); MacDonald, Grippo & Riely (MGR 12/90); Matheson Securities Ltd. (MTH 8/91); McDonald & Company Securities Inc. (MCD 11/89); McIntosh & Company Ltd. (MIH 7/90); Merrill Lynch Capital Markets (MER 9/88); Morgan Stanley & Co. (MRG 6/86); New York Society of Security Analysts (NYSSA 1/84); Oppenheim Finanzanalyse GmbH (OFA 9/90); Oppenheimer & Co. (OPP 12/84); Paine Webber Inc. (PNW 4/85); Panmure Gordon & Co. (PMG 8/89); Paribas Capital Markets (PAR 2/91); Pasfin Sevizi Finanzzziari (PSF 7/90); Pauli & Company Inc. (PLI 1/91); Pershing Division (PER 8/83); Peterbroeck, Van Campenhout & CIE (PCM 8/90); Piper, Jaffray & Hopwood Inc. (PJH 4/83); PNC Institutional Investment Service (PNB 11/88); Prudential-Bache Securities (PB 9/83); Raffensperger, Hughes (RPH 12/89); Rauscher Pierce Refsnes Inc. (RPR 11/83); Research Capital Corporation (RCC 7/91); Riada & Co. (RDA 4/91); Richardson Greenshields (RG 9/83); Robert W. Baird & Co. (RWB 5/90); Rothschild Inc. (RTH 7/91); Rowan Dartington & Co. (RDT 9/90); S.G. Warburg Securities (SGW 6/91); Salomon Brothers Inc. (SB 8/88); Sanford C. Bernstein (SCB 3/89); Sanwa McCarthy Limited (SMC 6/91); SBCI Hong Kong Limited (SBC 6/91); Schroder Securities (Japan) Ltd. (SHJ 4/91); Scotia McLeod Inc. (MYW 2/83); Scott & Stringfellow Investment Corporation (SCT 9/89); Securities Data Company (SDC 1/90); Shearson Lehman Brothers Holdings Inc. (SLH 2/88); Sheppards (SHE 1/90); Smith Barney, Harris Upham & Co. (SBH 6/82); Smith New Court Far East Limited (SFE 12/89); Smith New Court Securities plc (SNC 6/91); SNL Securities (SNL 6/91); Societé General Strauss Turnbull (STN 9/90); Stephens Inc. (SI 5/87); Sun Hung Kai Research (SHK 6/90); Sutro & Company Inc. (STR 6/88); Svenska Handelsbanken (SVK 10/90); The Chicago Corporation (CHC 10/90); The Principal/Eppler, Guerin & Turner, Inc. (EGT 1/90); The Robinson-Humphrey Company Inc. (RHC 10/89); The Stuart-James Co. (STJ 6/90); Thomas James Associates (TJA 2/89); Thomson BankWatch (KBW 1/89); Tucker, Anthony and R.L.Day Inc. (TAD 10/85); UBS Phillips & Drew Global Research Group (PDI 5/84); UBS Phillips & Drew International Ltd. (UPJ 5/91); Union Bank of Switzerland (UBS 9/82); Van Kasper & Company (VNK 1/84); Vereins- und Westbank AG (VWB 10/89); W.I. Carr (Far East) Ltd. (WIC 4/90); Wedbush Morgan Securities Inc. (WDM 9/89); Wertheim Schroder & Co. (WRS 2/89); Wheat First Securities (BUS 6/83); William Blair & Co. (WBC 3/90); Wise Speke Ltd. (WSD 4/91); and Yamaichi Research Institute (YAM 10/82).

Apparently Market Guide Data Base is not included in Investext on this host. The index segments include the following: Company Index lists all companies that are identified at the page level of the report with page references; Subject Index contains subject terms assigned to specific pages, again with page numbers; Product Index contains a list of products reported with references; SIC Index contains the four-digit codes that relate to products reported; and the Associated Industry Index contains a list of industries that are associated with the SIC Codes.

Format FULL2 displays complete report including index segments and FULL3 displays the full report except for the Table of Contents and index segments.

A subscription charge which covers all transactional charges, connect time, telecommunications and the small administration charge can take the place of the individual charges. Subscriptions are negotiated with customers and vary according to the number of menus (thus, files) that are to be used – typically a minimum subscription would be about US$ 1,000. All charges include training and a 24-hour help line.

Record composition

Source SOURCE; Date DATE; Company CO; Ticker Symbols TS; Hierarchical Geographic Company Location GEOCO/GEOREG/GEOSRC; Name NAME; Title TITLE; Type TYPE; Length LENGTH; Analyst ANALYST; Report Number REPORT-NO; Industry INDUSTRY; Abstract ABSTRACT; Contents CONTENTS; Company Index COMPANY-INDEX; Subject Index SUBJECT-INDEX; Product Index PRODUCT-INDEX; SIC Index SIC-INDEX; Associated Industry Index ASSOC-IND-INDEX; Text TEXT; Tables TABLES and Body BODY

18:176. Online   NewsNet Inc

File name	
Start year	1982 (July)
Number of records	234,000
Update period	Weekly (Daily in 1992)

Notes

Monthly subscription to NewsNet required On this host Investext includes the Market Guide Data Base.

18:177. Online   SOURCE, The

File name	
Start year	1982
Number of records	234,000
Update period	Weekly

Notes

Monthly minimum of $10 to THE SOURCE required. On this host Investext includes the Market Guide Data Base.

18:178. CD-ROM   Information Access Company (IAC)

File name	Investext on InfoTrac
Format notes	IBM
Software	Proprietary InfoTrac
Start year	1984
Number of records	289,400
Update period	Monthly
Price/Charges	Subscription: US$7,000

Notes

There may be differences between search results on the CD-ROM and on the DIALOG online file: one review (*CD-ROM Professional* 5(4)p.77–83) reported that 'during the 12-month review period, InfoTrac Investext did not include reports published by Market Guide, a financial research firm which specializes in smaller publicly owned companies More recent InfoTrac CD-ROM discs do include Market Guide Reports .'. Because names of subsidiaries of public companies are not included in the Subject Index, searches for information on subsidiaries result in 'no hits' even though the data on these corporate forms is often included in the investment reports. Sharyn Ladner, in the above-mentioned review, states that InfoTrac Investext is both simple to use and more

cost-effective than online searching on DIALOG for its intended users. The search software is not intended for – and indeed the product is not available to – corporate analysts, but even so it does have some shortcomings (for instance, searching lacks precision and reports can only be printed in full) which might upset some its intended users. Despite this, she has no reservations in recommending the product to academic and public libraries as excellent.

It provides hard-to-find information on companies and industries – information that is not available from any other source.

Subscription includes 386 IBM PC workstation. (Without workstation: $6,000). Due to IAC contractual arrangements with Thomson, this disc is only sold to academic and public libraries.

18:179. Database subset

Online   **Data-Star**

File name	TRST – Investext Training File
Start year	
Number of records	
Update period	Closed file
Price/Charges	Connect time: UK£Free

18:180. Database subset

Online   **DIALOG**

File name	File 277 – ONTAP Investext Training File
Start year	Selected record from 1988 and 1991
Number of records	50,000
Update period	Closed File
Price/Charges	Connect time: US$15.00

Notes

The low-cost training file contains selected records from File 545, the main Investxt file on DIALOG. Offline prints are not available in ONTAP files.

Japan Report: Medical Technology

Business Information & Solutions Ltd, Japan Report Division
Newmedia International Japan

18:182. Master record

Database type	Textual
Number of journals	1
Sources	Newsletter
Start year	1988
Language	English
Coverage	Japan
Number of records	
Update size	—
Update period	Monthly

Keywords

Diagnostic Equipment; Prosthetics

Description

The full text of a newsletter on Japanese medical technology and the production of medical diagnostic equipment and materials, therapeutic substances and prosthetics. Covers new developments and activities in Japan dealing with medical diagnostic reagents, instrumentation and artificial products, production and processes.

Corresponds to *Japan Report: Medical Technology* monthly newsletter. On DIALOG, and Data-Star this newsletter is made available as part of the PTS Newsletter Database.

This database can be found on:
PTS Newsletter Database

LabNet
IMS America Ltd,
    Hospital/Laboratory/Veterinary
    Database Division

18:184. Master record

Database type	Textual
Number of journals	
Sources	
Start year	Current 6 years
Language	English
Coverage	Continental US
Number of records	
Update size	—
Update period	Hospital purchase, monthly; private lab purchase, quarterly

Keywords
Diagnostic Products; Marketing

Description
Contains sales data on diagnostic products (for example, test kits, reagents) purchased by about 350 hospitals and 220 private laboratories. Includes projected nationwide product sales in dollars and units, average price per unit, product market share and sales trends.

Corresponds to *IMS Diagnostic Market-Hospital and Private Labs*.

18:185. Online   IMS America Ltd

File name	LabNet (IMS)
Start year	Current 6 years
Number of records	
Update period	Hospital purchase, monthly; private lab purchase, quarterly

Notes
Subscription to *IMS Diagnostic Market-Hospital and Private Labs* required.

Materials Science Citation Index with Abstracts
Institute for Scientific Information

18:186. Master record

Database type	Bibliographic, Citation
Number of journals	7,250
Sources	
Start year	
Language	English
Coverage	International
Number of records	90,000
Update size	90,000
Update period	Six times per year
Abstract details	Authors' own abstracts

Description
Abstracted citation index offering complete coverage of significant published literature in materials science. Covers all areas including applied physics, ceramics, composites, metals and metallurgy, polymer engineering, semiconductors, and thin films, as well as biomaterials, dental technology and optics.

All ISI databases have a linked service known as The Genuine Article which can deliver the full text of located articles by mail, facsimile transmission or courier. Orders can be placed via the host service in use, mail, facsimile transmission, telephone or telex. Diskette products have a single-keystroke order information facility.

The minimum charge is US$ 11.25 within USA and Canada and US$ 12.20 elsewhere.

18:187. CD-ROM   Institute for Scientific Information

File name	Materials Science Citation Index with Abstracts
Format notes	IBM, Mac, NEC
Start year	
Number of records	
Update period	Six times per year
Price/Charges	Subscription: US$1,950

Notes
A particular feature of the CD-ROM is ISI's unique Related Records search facility which provides access to records with cited references in common, allowing documents on similar subjects to be easily retrieved and browsed.

A record with a bibliography that is retrieved from any type of search may share identical references with another record. The software identifies those records linked by identical cited references and adds them to the search result display as related records. in this way, related records expand search results. It is a practical and easy way to locate additional information from a single search and is especially useful when searching a broad concept or vaguely defined subject area as there is no need for an complex search strategy. When viewing related records, a reminder of the 'parent record' stays at the top of the screen. A parent record can have a maximum of twenty different related records but the related records can, in turn have related records which may be traced up to five levels of relationship.

Each issue is a year-to-date cumulation ending with the final annual cumulation. Back years are available to 1991.

Medical Bulletin
US Food and Drug Administration

18:188. Master record

Database type	Textual
Number of journals	1
Sources	Newsletter and Government departments
Start year	1988
Language	English
Coverage	USA
Number of records	
Update size	—
Update period	Quarterly

Keywords
Drugs; Food Additives

Description

A newsletter, updated quarterly, covering clinical drug testing, approvals of new drugs and medical devices by the US FDA, and information on food additives and food preparation processes.

Corresponds to *Medical Bulletin* quarterly newsletter. On DIALOG and Data-Star, this newsletter is available as part of the PTS Newsletter Database.

This database can be found on:
PTS Newsletter Database

Medical Devices on CD-ROM

FD Inc
US Food and Drug Administration

18:190. Master record

Database type	Textual, Factual
Number of journals	
Sources	Laws/regulations, Government documents (US) and reports
Start year	
Language	English
Coverage	USA
Number of records	
Update size	–
Update period	Quarterly

Description

Full text of laws, regulations, policy and procedures related to the Medical Device regulation. Contains the complete text of the *Food, Drug and Cosmetics Act* with 1990 Amendments, *Federal Regulations* (Title 211, Parts 800–1299); *Medical Device Regulatory Requirements Manuals*; *Guidance Memoranda* (Blue Book and others) – over 50 key documents; Advisory Committees' Guides, and over 100 reports and publications on specific products or processes.

18:191. CD-ROM   FD Inc

File name	Medical Devices on CD-ROM
Format notes	IBM
Software	Proprietary
Start year	
Number of records	
Update period	Quarterly
Price/Charges	Subscription: US$1,485

Medical Instruments and Equipment

Informpribor

18:192. Master record

Database type	Bibliographic
Number of journals	
Sources	
Start year	1988
Language	English
Coverage	
Number of records	2,000
Update size	–
Update period	

Description

Industrial and scientific evaluation of medical equipment.

18:193. Other media   Informpribor

File name	
Start year	1988
Number of records	2,000
Update period	

Medical Scan

Market Intelligence Research Company (MIRC)

18:194. Master record

Alternative name(s)	Medical Market Scan
Database type	Textual
Number of journals	
Sources	Newsletter
Start year	1988
Language	English
Coverage	USA (primarily) and International (some)
Number of records	
Update size	–
Update period	Monthly

Keywords

Health Care; Medical Equipment; Pharmaceutical Industry

Description

Contains the full text of *Medical Scan*, a monthly newsletter on the medical electronics and pharmaceutical industries. Covers market analyses, legal and regulatory developments and business news. Focuses on developing medical technology and treatments and the emerging markets in medical equipment and health care. Provides in-depth analysis of trends in the medical industry and the competitive environment for medical products, equipment and health services.

Corresponds to the monthly *Medical Scan* newsletter. The newsletter on DIALOG and Data-Star is available on PTS Newsletter Database, supplied by Predicasts.

This database can be found on:
PTS Newsletter Database

Medical Textiles

Elsevier Advanced Technology Publications

18:196. Master record

Database type	Textual
Number of journals	1
Sources	Newsletter
Start year	1988
Language	English
Coverage	International
Number of records	
Update size	–
Update period	Monthly

Keywords

Medical Textiles; Textiles

Description

A newsletter on new applications of textiles in medical care.

Corresponds to *Medical Textiles* monthly newsletter. Available on DIALOG and Data-Star as part of the PTS Newsletter Database.

This database can also be found on:
PTS Newsletter Database

MEDITEC Biomedical Engineering
Fachinformationszentrum Technik (FIZ Technik)

18:198. Master record

Alternative name(s)	Medizinische Technik
Database type	Bibliographic
Number of journals	
Sources	Books, conference proceedings, journals, patents and reports
Start year	1968
Language	German, English, French (titles) and Original language (titles)
Coverage	International
Number of records	112,500
Update size	7,200
Update period	Weekly
Abstract details	The author if available and if written in English, French or German, otherwise the producer.
Thesaurus	Thesaurus Medizintechnik; Fachordnung Technik

Keywords
Bioengineering

Description

MEDITEK contains citations with abstracts, to the worldwide literature on biomedical technology and the related areas of biology, biochemistry and medicine, with an emphasis on European and German literature. Subjects covered include: biological sciences including biomechanics, biophysics, biochemistry, biocybernetics; biomedical measurements including the recording, processing and evaluation of bioelectric signals, biomechanic signals, the electrode measuring of organ functions, optical and thermic measurement and investigation; clinical engineering; dental instrumentation; medical diagnostics including electrodiagnostics, X-ray diagnostics, ultrasonic diagnostics and nuclear-medical diagnostics; image processing; data processing in medicine; laboratory diagnostics; therapeutic technology including electrotherapy, ultrasonic therapy and radiation therapy; artificial organs and functions including orthopedics, aids for disabled persons and biomaterials; equipment for rehabilitation; hospital administration and hospital technology. It is the only German-language database in this special field of medicine.

All of the records include abstracts of approximately 1,500 characters in either German or English with a few in French, but mainly German. A translation for other languages is made. Journals account for 80% of all sources, conference proceedings 17.5%, books 1% and patents 0.5%.

From 1986 onwards the controlled terms have been taken exclusively from the *Medical Technology Thesaurus* and consist of 9,500 terms with 11,700 descriptors and references to synonyms (in German and in English), broader terms, narrower terms, cross references, collective terms, related terms, annotations and in part scope notes. They include the names of individuals, organisations and countries. Before then the index terms were taken from the *DZF Precision Technique Thesaurus (DZF Thesaurus Feinwerktechnik)* which contained approximately 1,700 descriptors. An average of ten descriptors is assigned to each record and at most four subject area classes are assigned. In contrast to most databases containing patent information, the indexing International Patent Classification Number is recorded without spaces and hypens. In MEDITEC the main/subgroup is indicated without leading zeros, without spaces and hpyens and is affixed to the subclass.

18:199. Online　　　　　　　　　　DIMDI

File name	MT68
Alternative name(s)	Medizinische Technik
Start year	1968
Number of records	112,500
Update period	Monthly
SDI period	1 month
Database aids	Online User Manual MEDITEC and Memocard MEDITEC
Price/Charges	Connect time: UK£33.68–38.43
	Online print: UK£0.24–0.42
	Offline print: UK£0.15–0.22

Downloading is allowed
Thesaurus is online

Notes

The original title of an article appears followed by its translated title in parentheses. Titles are always available in both German and English. If the title is in another language only its English translation is included with the German translation in parentheses. Abstracts are in German and English and a few in French. All words in the title can be searched in their original language. Suppliers of online documents: British Library Document Supply Centre, Boston Spa, England; Harkers Information Retrieval System, Sydney, Australia; Instituto de Informacion y Documentacion en Ciencia y Tecnologia, Madrid, Spain; Universitätbibliothek und TIB, Hannover, Germany; Zentralbibliothek der Medizin, Köln, Germany. Searches are possible from January 1968. Menu driven user guidance is available in German and English.

Record composition

Abstract AB; Author AU; Corporate Source CS; Controlled Term CT; Document Type DT; Entry Date ED; ISBN SB; Journal Code JC; Journal Title JT; Journal TItle Full JTF; Language LA; Number of Document ND; Number of References RN; Number of Report NR; Publication Availability PA; Number of Paper PP; Publisher PU; Publication Year PY; Section Codes SC; Section Heading SH; Source SO; Title TI; Type of Subject Information TSI; Title of Superordinate Publication TSP and Uncontrolled Term UT

The basic index includes the fields abstract, controlled terms, subject headings, title and uncontrolled terms. Each document record contains one to four subject headings with a code of up to four letters corresponding to the printed Subject List Technology (Fachordnung Technik). The sixteen main subject areas are indicated using one letter, the subgroup areas (according to the hierarchical levels) with two to four letters. The sixteen main subject areas are: A. Operational Management/Organisation; B. Natural Sciences; D. Medical Technology; E. Energy Technology; G. Construction Elements; H. Data Processing; K. Communications Technology; M.

Measurement and Automatic Control Technology; N. Technical Materials; P. Machine Components; R. Production Technology, Tooling Machiner; T. Materials Extraction and Processing; U. Conveyor/ Transportation Technology, Construction Machines; W. Fluid/Aerodynamic Machines, Piston Machine; X. Automotive Technolgoy and Z. Further Areas of Technology.

18:200. Online   FIZ Technik

File name	MEDI
Alternative name(s)	Medizinische Technik
Start year	1968
Number of records	115,000
Update period	Weekly
Price/Charges	Connect time: DM264.00
	Online print: DM0.30 – 2.00
	Offline print: DM2.30
	SDI charge: DM18.00

18:201. Online   Hoechst

File name	MEDI
Alternative name(s)	Medizinische Technik
Start year	
Number of records	
Update period	

National Report on Computers & Health
United Communications Group

18:202. Master record

Database type	Textual
Number of journals	1
Sources	Newsletter, Government departments and Companies
Start year	1988
Language	English
Coverage	USA
Number of records	
Update size	–
Update period	Daily

Keywords
Computer Data Security; Data Security; Health Care Management; Medicare

Description
A newsletter covering new computer and communications hardware and software, aimed at chief information officers, MIS directors and DP managers in the health care industry. Includes coverage of of the impact on health care providers of vendor mergers and acquisitions, data security strategies, Medicare regulations on hospital data processing, medical computing and new product announcements.

Corresponds to *The National Report on Computers and Health* newsletter. On DIALOG and Data-Star, this newsletter is available as part of the PTS Newsletter Database.

This database can be found on:
PTS Newsletter Database

Obstetrics and Gynaecology
Elsevier Science Publishers
CMC ReSearch

18:204. Master record

Database type	Factual, Textual, Image
Number of journals	1
Sources	Journal

Start year	1985
Language	English
Coverage	
Number of records	
Update size	–
Update period	Annually

Keywords
Gynaecology; Obstetrics

Description
Full text of five years of the Elsevier journal with tables and images. Includes: Medical and surgical treatment of female conditions; Obstetric management; Clinical evaluation of drugs and instruments; etc. Covers 1985 – 1990.

18:205. CD-ROM   CMC ReSearch

File name	Obstetrics and Gynaecology on Disc 1985–1990
Format notes	IBM
Software	DiscPassage
Start year	1985
Number of records	
Update period	Annually
Price	UK£265

This database can also be found on:
Comprehensive Core Medical Library

Optics (Dom Optiki)
Dom Optiki

18:207. Master record

Database type	Bibliographic
Number of journals	
Sources	
Start year	
Language	English
Coverage	
Number of records	341,000
Update size	–
Update period	

Keywords
Physics

Description
Bibliographic information on optical instrumentation.

18:208. Diskette   Dom Optiki

File name	
Start year	
Number of records	341,000
Update period	

Optics
NPO 'Optika'

18:209. Master record

Alternative name(s)	NPO 'Optika'
Database type	Bibliographic
Number of journals	
Sources	
Start year	
Language	English
Coverage	

Number of records   28,600
Update size   –
Update period

Keywords

Physics

Description

Information system on all aspects of optics.

18:210. Diskette   NPO

File name
Alternative name(s)   NPO 'Optika'
Start year
Number of records   28,600
Update period

Pharmaceutical and Healthcare Industry News Database

Pharmaprojects PJB Publications Ltd

18:211. Master record

Alternative name(s)   PHIND
Database type   Textual
Number of journals   4
Sources   Newsletters
Start year   1980
Language   English
Coverage   International
Number of records   113,270
Update size   –
Update period   Daily
Index unit   Newsletters, articles and reports
Database aids   User guide available from producer

Keywords

Applied Science; Herbicides; Marketing; Medical Diagnostics; Pesticides; Plant Protection; Product Liability

Description

This database contains information on product developments, markets, regulatory affairs of importance to the international pharmaceutical, medical device, veterinary and agrochemical industries. All publications have already been made available online in abstract form, but this is the only database which contains the full-text of every report and the only one which makes these reports available before publication. It includes all the text, pre-publication, current and archival material from four major international industry newsletters:

Scrip World Pharmaceutical News (1/82+, issue number 655) which contains world pharmaceutical news and is the most widely read international pharmaceutical industry newsletter, being used at all levels within pharmaceutical companies, regulatory authorities, financial instituions, service industries and others to gain an insight into significant events throughout the world, paying special attention to product developments, regulatory affairs, market intelligence, company results and personnei;
Clinica World Medical Device News (10/80+ issue number 1) which contains world medical device news and provides a similar service for the device and diagnostic industry;
Animal Pharm World Animal Health News (1/82+,

issue number 1) which contains world animal health news; and
Agrow World Agrochemical News (10/85+, issue number 1) which contains world agrochemical news and is aimed at the herbicide, pesticide, rodenticide and plant growth regulator industries.

All four print publications follow a similar structure and contain sections on: Product & Research News, Company News, International News, People and Conferences, plus regular monitoring ofregulatiory bodies such as the US Food and Drug Administration, the US Environmental Protection Agency, the European Economic Community and the World Health Organisation. Reports are added to a daily and current file within three working days of writing, before publication. Items destined for publication in *Scrip* or *Clinica* are therefore available online days before the printed newsletters will reach users.

Each report has been written on the basis of news gathered from a wide variety of sources, and the range of information available is evaluated for relevance to the major industrial areas covered and is amplified by investigative reporting. They are subsequently moved into the archival file after approximately three weeks. Covers company activities (marketing, mergers, acquisitions, sales), product research and development (clinical trials, launches, approvals, etc), regulatory decisions (labelling changes, pesticide bans, product liability, etc) and notices of conferences, symposia and executive appointments.

The database corresponds to *Agrow World Crop Protection News*, *Animal Pharm World Animal Health News*, *Clinica World Medical Device and Diagnostic News* and *Scrip World Pharmaceutical News*.

18:212. Online   BRS

File name   PHID
Alternative name(s)   PHIND
Start year   1980
Number of records   113,270
Update period   Daily
Price/Charges   Connect time: US$145.00/155.00
    Online print: US$3.52/3.60
    Offline print: US$3.60
    SDI charge: US$5.00

Notes

Contains details of company activities and product development on a daily basis before publication of the printed version.

18:213. Online   BRS

File name   PHIC
Alternative name(s)   PHIND
Start year   1980
Number of records   113,270
Update period   Daily
Price/Charges   Connect time: US$145.00/155.00
    Online print: US$3.52/3.60
    Offline print: US$3.60
    SDI charge: US$5.00

Notes

This is the current file Pharmaceutical and Healthcare Industry News Database.

18:214. Online   BRS

File name   PHIN
Alternative name(s)   PHIND
Start year   1980
Number of records   113,270
Update period   Daily

Price/Charges   Connect time: US$145.00/155.00
Online print: US$0.77/0.85
Offline print: US$1.10

Notes

Pharmaceutical and Healthcare Industry News Database – Backfile: records are removed from the daily and current file into this archival file after approximately three weeks.

18:215. Online   CompuServe Information Service

File name	IQUEST File 2076: SCRIP – Retrospective
Alternative name(s)	PHIND
Start year	1986
Number of records	
Update period	Daily
Price/Charges	Subscription: US$8.95 per month Database entry fee: US$9/search; some databases carry a surcharge ($2–75) Online print: US$10 references free; then $9 per ten; abstracts $3 each

Notes

Accessed via IQUEST or IQMEDICAL, this database is offered by a Data-Star gateway. IQUEST can either search across all databases, a database of the user's choice or selected multiple databases.

This is the archive file of information, removed from SCRIP – CURRENT NEWS and SCRIP – DAILY NEWS files.

18:216. Online   CompuServe Information Service

File name	IQUEST File 2074: SCRIP – Daily News
Alternative name(s)	PHIND
Start year	1986
Number of records	
Update period	Daily
Price/Charges	Subscription: US$8.95 per month Database entry fee: US$9/search; some databases carry a surcharge ($2–75) Online print: US$10 references free; then $9 per ten; abstracts $3 each

Notes

Accessed via IQUEST, this database is offered by a Data-Star gateway. IQUEST can either search across all databases, a database of the user's choice or selected multiple databases.

This is the daily news file of pre-publication material used for daily scanning of reports on topics of particular interest and is included in the SCRIP CURRENT NEWS database. For all information on a particular topic it is necessary to search both SCRIP CURRENT NEWS and SCRIP RETROSPECTIVE.

18:217. Online   CompuServe Information Service

File name	IQUEST File 2075: SCRIP – Current News
Alternative name(s)	PHIND
Start year	1986
Number of records	
Update period	Daily
Price/Charges	Subscription: US$8.95 per month Database entry fee: US$9/search; some databases carry a surcharge ($2–75) Online print: US$10 references free; then $9 per ten; abstracts $3 each

Notes

Accessed via IQUEST, this database is offered by a Data-Star gateway. IQUEST can either search across all databases, a database of the user's choice or selected multiple databases.

This is the file containing current news, including SCRIP – DAILY NEWS, and is used for scanning for recently written reports.

18:218. Online   Data-Star

File name	PHIN
Alternative name(s)	PHIND
Start year	1980 (to circa five weeks ago)
Number of records	113,270
Update period	Daily
Database aids	Data-Star Business and Biomedical Manuals, Berne, Data-Star, 1989 and Online manual (search NEWS-PHIN in NEWS)
Price/Charges	Subscription: SFr80.00 Connect time: SFr263.00 Online print: SFr5.48 Offline print: SFr5.81

Notes

This is the archive file of information, removed from PHID and/or PHIC files. For all information on a particular topic it is necessary to search both PHIN and PHIC.

From June 1993 Data-Star have introduced an annual fee/subscription per contract (that is, not per password) of SFr 80.00 (c.UK£ 32.00) payable every June. For North American customers billed in dollars who also use DIALOG, the DIALOG fee also covers access to Data-Star. Academic customers, 'commitment' customers and customers currently billed in dollars are exempt.

Record composition

Accession Number and Update Code AN; Date of Entry of Report DT; Date of Publication YD; Month of Publication YM; Occurrence Table OC; Source SO; Title TI; Text of Report TX; Update Code UP and Year of Publiction YR

18:219. Online   Data-Star

File name	PHID
Alternative name(s)	PHIND
Start year	Today only
Number of records	113,270
Update period	Daily
Database aids	Data-Star Business and Biomedical Manuals, Berne, Data-Star, 1989 and Online manual (search NEWS-PHIN in NEWS)
Price/Charges	Subscription: SFr80.00 Connect time: SFr263.00 Online print: SFr5.48 Offline print: SFr5.81

Notes

PHID is the daily news file of pre-publication material used for daily scanning of reports on topics of particular interest. PHID is included in the database PHIC. For all information on a particular topic it is necessary to search both PHIN and PHIC.

From June 1993 Data-Star have introduced an annual fee/subscription per contract (that is, not per password) of SFr 80.00 (c.UK£ 32.00) payable every June. For North American customers billed in dollars who

also use DIALOG, the DIALOG fee also covers access to Data-Star. Academic customers, 'commitment' customers and customers currently billed in dollars are exempt.

Record composition

Accession Number and Update Code AN; Date of Entry of Report DT; Date of Publication YD; Month of Publication YM; Occurrence Table OC; Source SO; Title TI; Text of Report TX; Update Code UP and Year of Publiction YR

18:220. Online — Data-Star

File name	PHIC
Alternative name(s)	PHIND
Start year	Latest four to five weeks
Number of records	113,270
Update period	Daily
Database aids	Data-Star Business and Biomedical Manuals, Berne, Data-Star, 1989 and Online manual (search NEWS-PHIN in NEWS)
Price/Charges	Subscription: SFr80.00 Connect time: SFr263.00 Online print: SFr5.48 Offline print: SFr5.81

Notes

This is the file containing current news, including PHID (up to five weeks of data). PHIC is used for scanning for recently written reports. PHIC includes PHID but PHID and PHIC are not included in PHIN. For all information on a particular topic both PHIN and PHIC must be searched.

From June 1993 Data-Star have introduced an annual fee/subscription per contract (that is, not per password) of SFr 80.00 (c.UK£ 32.00) payable every June. For North American customers billed in dollars who also use DIALOG, the DIALOG fee also covers access to Data-Star. Academic customers, 'commitment' customers and customers currently billed in dollars are exempt.

Record composition

Accession Number and Update Code AN; Date of Entry of Report DT; Date of Publication YD; Month of Publication YM; Occurrence Table OC; Source SO; Title TI; Text of Report TX; Update Code UP and Year of Publiction YR

18:221. Online — Data-Star

File name	TRPI – Pharmaceutical and Healthcare Industry News Training File
Alternative name(s)	PHIND
Start year	
Number of records	
Update period	
Database aids	Data-Star Business and Biomedical Manuals, Berne, Data-Star, 1989 and Online manual (search NEWS-PHIN in NEWS)
Price/Charges	Connect time: UK£Free

Record composition

Accession Number and Update Code AN; Date of Entry of Report DT; Date of Publication YD; Month of Publication YM; Occurrence Table OC; Source SO; Title TI; Text of Report TX; Update Code UP and Year of Publiction YR

18:222. Online — DIALOG

File name	File 129
Alternative name(s)	PHIND

Start year	1980
Number of records	179,399
Update period	Weekly
Price/Charges	Connect time: US$150.00 Online print: US$0.90 Offline print: US$0.90 SDI charge: US$5.00

Notes

The Pharmacuetical and Healthcare Industry News Database (PHIND) is divided into two files – daily (File 130) and current information (File 129), which)includes some unpublished articles, and archival)material dating back to 1980.

18:223. Online — DIALOG

File name	File 130
Alternative name(s)	PHIND
Start year	1980
Number of records	179,399
Update period	Daily
Price/Charges	Connect time: US$150.00 Online print: US$4.00 Offline print: US$4.00 SDI charge: US$5.00 (weekly)/ 2.00 (daily)

Notes

The Pharmaceutical and Healthcare Industry News Database (PHIND) on Dialog is divided into two files – daily (File 130) and current information (File 129), which includes some unpublished articles, and archival material dating back to 1980.

DIALINDEX Categories: BIOBUS, BIOTECH, PHARM, PHARMINA, PHIND.

Pharmaceutical News Index

University Microfilms International/Data Courier Inc

18:224. Master record

Alternative name(s)	PNI
Database type	Bibliographic
Number of journals	
Sources	Newsletters
Start year	1974
Language	English
Coverage	International
Number of records	400,000
Update size	36,500
Update period	Weekly
Database aids	Search Tools: The Guide to UMI/Data Courier Online $75.00, Source Book (journals list) Free, Capabilities brochure Free and Log/On (Newsletter) Free

Keywords

Cosmetics; Pharmaceutical Industry; Medical Device Industry

Description

PNI contains citations to current news about pharmaceuticals, cosmetics, medical devices, and related health fields. PNI records refer to twenty-one major US and international newsletters on pharmaceutical-related topics such as health legislation and policy making; statistical data; pharmaceutical research; over-the-counter prescription markets; drug and device recalls; litigation and court decisions; market analysis; biotechnology updates; research and development in progress; veterinary pharmaceuticals; livestock disease news; personnel changes; corporate financial information; new drug application approvals; acquisitions and mergers,; government contracts; product successes and failures; health and beauty aids; advertising campaigns; new product development and joint ventures. The newsletters are: *Animal Pharm World*; *Animal Health News*; *Applied Genetic News*; *Biomedical Business International*; *Biomedical Safety Standards*; *Biomedical Technology Information Service*; *Clinica Lab Letter*, *Clinica World Medical Device News*; *Radiology & Imaging Letter*; *Drug Research Reports ('The Blue Sheet')*; *FDC Reports ('The Pink Sheet')*, *FDC Reports ('The Rose Sheet')*, *Health Devices*; *Medical Devices, Diagnostics, and Instrumentation Reports ('The Gray Sheet')*; *Pharma*; *PMA Newsletter*; *Quality Control Reports ('The Gold Sheet')*, *SCRIP World Pharmaceutical News*; *Washington Drug and Device Letter*; *Weekly Pharmacy Reports ('The Green Sheet')*, and *Technology Reimbursement Reports ('The Beige Sheet')*: PNI cites and indexes all articles from these publications on drugs; corporation and industry sales, mergers, acquisitions, etc.; government legislation, regulations, and court action, and requests for proposals, research grant applications, industry speeches, press releases, and other news items.

18:225. Online — BRS

File name	PNII
Alternative name(s)	PNI
Start year	
Number of records	400,000
Update period	Weekly
Price/Charges	Connect time: US$125.00/135.00
	Online print: US$0.22/0.70
	Offline print: US$0.70

Downloading is allowed

18:226. Online — CompuServe Information Service

File name	IQUEST File 1097
Alternative name(s)	PNI
Start year	1985
Number of records	
Update period	Weekly
Price/Charges	Subscription: US$8.95 per month
	Database entry fee: US$9/search; some databases carry a surcharge ($2–75)
	Online print: US$10 references free; then $9 per ten; abstracts $3 each

Downloading is allowed

Notes
Accessed via IQUEST or IQMEDICAL, this database is offered by a DIALOG gateway. IQUEST can either search across all databases, a database of the user's choice or selected multiple databases.

18:227. Online — DIALOG

File name	File 42
Alternative name(s)	PNI
Start year	1974
Number of records	377,550
Update period	Weekly
Price/Charges	Connect time: US$159.00
	Online print: US$0.90
	Offline print: US$0.90
	SDI charge: US$12.95

Notes
DIALINDEX Categories: BIOTECH, PHARM, PHARMINA, PHARMR, REGS.

18:228. Online — ORBIT

File name	PNII
Alternative name(s)	PNI
Start year	1974
Number of records	340,000
Update period	Weekly
Database aids	Quick Reference Guide (9/88) Free (single copy)
Price/Charges	Connect time: UK£135.00
	Online print: UK£0.75/0.75
	Offline print: UK£0.75/0.75
	SDI charge: UK£5.50

Downloading is allowed

Notes
Electronic SDI service is now available within two hours on ORBIT. They can be downloaded and reformatted on a word processor. Results are retrieved in the low cost PRINTS file, $15 per connect hour.

18:229. Online — STN

File name	PNI
Alternative name(s)	PNI
Start year	1974
Number of records	400,000
Update period	Weekly

Downloading is allowed

18:230. Tape — University Microfilms International/Data Courier Inc

File name	PNI
Alternative name(s)	PNI
Format notes	IBM
Start year	1974
Number of records	400,000
Update period	Weekly or monthly depending on subscription. Annual lease is $9,000 (weekly updates), $6,000 (monthly updates), or for the archival files, $2,500 each.
Price/Charges	Subscription: US$2,500 – 9,000

For more details of constituent databases, see:
FDA on CD-ROM.

PTS Newsletter Database
Predicasts International Inc

18:231. Master record

Alternative name(s)	Predicasts Newsletter Database
Database type	Textual
Number of journals	
Sources	
Start year	1988
Language	German and English
Coverage	International
Number of records	722,656
Update size	63,000
Update period	Daily
Database aids	PTS Users Manual, Cleveland, Ohio, Predicasts
Hosts have included	CORIS (Thomson Financial Network) (Until 1/92)

Keywords
Acid Rain; Advertising; Air Pollution; Alcohol Abuse; Antiviral Drugs; Asbestos; Asbestosis; Automation and Control; Beauty Care; Beauty Care; Beverages; Biotechnology; Biotechnology Industries; Brewing; Cancer; Ceramics; Chemical Industry; Chromato-

graphy; Composites; Computer Data Security; Computer Ergonomics; Company Profiles; Consumer Products; Cosmetics; Data Security; Defence Waste Disposal; Diagnosis; Diagnostic Equipment; Diagnostic Products; Drug Abuse; Drug Treatment; Drugs; Education – Cancer; Electrodialysis; Employee Benefits; Environmental Policy; Ergonomics; Explosion; Filtration; Fire; Food and Drink; Food Additives; Food Processing; Food Technology; Genetic Engineering; Greenhouse Effect; Hazardous Chemicals; Hazardous Substances; Hazardous Substances Transport; Hazardous Waste; Health and Safety; Health Care; Health Care Management; Health Care Products; Health Insurance; Health Services; HIV; Household Products; Hygiene Products; Information Services; Information Systems; Legal Liability; Legislation; Liability Insurance; Manufacturing; Marketing; Market Reports; Materials Industry; Medicare; Medical Equipment; Medical Textiles; Medical Waste Management; Membrane Technology; Metals; Nuclear Waste; Occupational Health and Safety; Packaging; Patents; Personal Hygiene; Pesticides; Pets; Pharmaceutical Industry; Pharmaceutical Products; Pharmaceuticals; Pollution; Polymers; Product Catalogues; Product Liability; Prosthetics; Public Health; Radiation; Research and Development; Separation Technology; Smoking; Standards; Textiles; Waste Management; Water Pollution; Water Purification

Description

Produced by Predicasts, PTS Newsletter is a multi-industry database providing concise information on company activities, new technologies, emerging industry trends, government regulations and international trade opportunities. It consists of the full text of over 500 business and industry newsletters covering almost 50 different industries and subject areas. It is international in scope, covering all major economic and political regions of the world, including Eastern and Western Europe, the USA, the Pacific Rim, Latin America, Asia and the Middle East. Facts, figures and analyses are provided on the following industrial and geographical areas: advanced materials, biotechnology, broadcasting and publishing, computers and electronics, chemicals, defense and aerospace, energy, environment, financial services and markets, instrumentation, international trade, general technology, Japan, Middle East, manufacturing, medical and health, materials packaging, research and development, telecommunications and transportation.

Newsletters include *Multinational Service* which covers decisions and policies affecting corporations operating worldwide; and *Europe Report* which offers broad coverage of EC activities relating to economic and monetary affairs, the internal market and legislation and regulations relating to business. Both Newsletters are published by the Europe Information Service of Cooper's & Lybrand Europe. Middle East coverage includes the *Israel High-Tech Report*; *The Middle East News Network*; and *The Middle East Consultants' Newsletter*.

18:232. Online   Data-Star

File name	PTBN
Alternative name(s)	Predicasts Newsletter Database
Start year	January 1988
Number of records	533,000
Update period	Weekly
Database aids	Data-Star Business Manual, Berne and Online manual (search for NEWS-PTBN in NEWS)
Price/Charges	Subscription: UK£32.00
	Connect time: UK£80.40
	Online print: UK£0.28 – 0.55
	Offline print: UK£0.26 – 1.00
	SDI charge: UK£4.00

Also available on FIZ Technik via a gateway from Data-Star

Notes

From June 1933 Data-Star have introduced an annual fee/subscription per contract (that is, not per password) of SFr 80.00 (c.UK£ 32.00) payable every June. For North American customers billed in dollars who also use DIALOG, the DIALOG fee also covers access to Data-Star. Academic customers, 'commitment' customers and customers currently billed in dollars are exempt.

18:233. Online   DIALOG

File name	PTSNL
Alternative name(s)	Predicasts Newsletter Database
Start year	1989
Number of records	722,656
Update period	Daily
Price/Charges	Connect time: US$126.00
	Online print: US$0.90

Notes

PTSNL is a menu-access version of the PTS Newsletter Database. PTSNL provides users with the unique capability to easily retrieve the latest issue (or any available issue) of a newsletter, display a Table of Contents listing articles contained in a selected issue, and print the full text of newspaper articles selected by title. To search newsletters for information on specific subjects, use File 636 (the main PTS file), which utilises the full range of DIALOG search commands.

18:234. Online   DIALOG

File name	File 636
Alternative name(s)	Predicasts Newsletter Database
Start year	1989
Number of records	722,656
Update period	Daily
Price/Charges	Connect time: US$126.00
	Online print: US$0.90
	Offline print: US$0.90
	SDI charge: US$1.00 (daily) – 3.00 (weekly)

Notes

This is the main file of PTS on DIALOG. There is also a menu access version – PTSNL, which enables the user to retrieve the latest issue of a newsletter, print the full text of newspaper articles etc. It does not have the full range of DIALOG search commands.

18:235. Online   Dow Jones News/Retrieval

File name	
Alternative name(s)	Predicasts Newsletter Database
Start year	
Number of records	
Update period	Weekly

18:236. Online   FIZ Technik (gateway)

File name	PTBN
Alternative name(s)	Predicasts Newsletter Database
Start year	1988 (January)

Number of records Volume 1: 159,000
Update period Weekly
Price/Charges Connect time: SFr201.00
Online print: SFr0.61 – 1.22
Offline print: SFr0.24 – 1.83
SDI charge: SFr10.00
Available via a gateway to Data-Star

For more details of constituent databases, see:
AIDS Weekly
Air/Water Pollution Report
Alliance Alert – Medical Health
Antiviral Agents Bulletin
Applied Genetics News
Asbestos Control Report
BBI Newsletter
Biomedical Materials
Biomedical Polymers
Cancer Weekly
Cosmetic Insiders' Report
Diagnostics Business-Matters
Environment Week
European Cosmetic Markets
FDA Medical Bulletin
Food Chemical News
Genetic Technology News
Hazmat Transport News
Health Business
Health Daily
Industrial Health and Hazards Update
International Product Alert
Japan Report: Medical Technology
Japan Science Scan
Managed Care Law Outlook
Managed Care Outlook
Managed Care Report
Medical Bulletin
Medical Scan
Medical Waste News
Medical Textiles
Membrane and Separation Technology News
National Report on Computers and Health
Nuclear Waste News
Occupational Health and Safety Letter
OTC Market Report: Update USA
OTC News and Market Report
Pesticide and Toxic Chemical News
Pharmaceutical Business News
Product Alert
PRODUCTSCAN
Report on Defense Plant Wastes
Soviet Bio/Medical Report
Toxic Materials News
Worldwide Biotech

REHADAT
Institut der Deutschen Wirtschaft

18:237. Master record

Database type	Bibliographic, Textual, Factual
Number of journals	
Sources	
Start year	
Language	German
Coverage	Europe
Number of records	
Update size	–
Update period	Twice per year

Keywords
Vocational Training; Rehabilitation

Description
A database about the vocational rehabilitation of disabled people which includes case studies, details of aids to the disabled, training courses, and citations with abstracts.

The institute is widening the scope beyond Europe and translating its current information into English (1/93).

18:238. CD-ROM
REHADAT

File name	Institut der Deutschen Wirtschaft
Format notes	IBM
Start year	
Number of records	
Update period	Twice per year

Notes
This CD-ROM is available free.

Scientific Instruments
Informpribor

18:239. Master record

Database type	Bibliographic
Number of journals	
Sources	
Start year	1984
Language	English
Coverage	International
Number of records	68,000
Update size	–
Update period	

Keywords
Physics

Description
Bibliography on international scientific equipment.

18:240. Diskette
Informpribor

File name	
Start year	1984
Number of records	68,000
Update period	

Siemens X-Ray CD-ROM
Siemens AG
BCB Bertelsmann Computer
Beratungsdienst

18:241. Master record

Database type	Directory, Textual, Image
Number of journals	
Sources	
Start year	
Language	German, French and English
Coverage	International
Number of records	5,166
Update size	–
Update period	

Description
Contains pictures of X-ray machine spare parts with the relevant textual information.

For use by Siemens technicians worldwide.

18:242. CD-ROM   Siemens AG

File name   Siemens X-Ray CD-ROM
Format notes   IBM
Software   Cobra
Start year
Number of records   5,166
Update period

Notes

Designed to be run on a laptop computer with in-built CD-ROM drive; technicians can make graphic searches. Is to be distributed to Siemens technicians worldwide. Networking not available.

Spriline

Planning and Rationalization Institute for the Health and Social Services Spri Bibliotek och utredningsbanken Stiftelsen Stockholms Iäna Äldrecentrum

18:243. Master record

Alternative name(s)   Spri Library and Research Report Bank
Database type   Bibliographic, Textual
Number of journals   350
Sources   Journals, Research reports and Grey literature
Start year   1988
Language   Swedish (primarily) and English
Coverage   International
Number of records   16,000
Update size   3,000
Update period   Irregular

Keywords

Health Care Planning

Description

Concerns the area of health and medical care, with the exception of medical literature of a purely scientific character. Spri stands for Sjukvardens och socialvardens planerings-och rationaliseringsinstitut. Spriline consists of two parts: the library collections and journal articles from about 350 journals which are mainly Swedish; Spri's Research Report Bank (Spri's utredningsbank), that is, unpublished research reports from the health care sector in Sweden and in other Scandinavian countries.

The Spri Library and Research Bank offers a complete document delivery service. Other products – Spri litteraturtjänst, Nytt fran Spris utredninngsbank, Utredninsgbankens jkatalog, Fou-primavard.

Terms in Swedish from an inhouse thesaurus. Retrieval from all fields of the reference.

18:244. Online   MIC/Karolinska Institute Library and Information Center (MIC KIBIC)

File name   Spriline
Alternative name(s) Spri Library and Research Report Bank
Start year   1988

Number of records   16,000
Update period   Irregular

Notes

Online ordering is available.

SWEDIS

Socialstyrelsens Läkemedelsavdelning

18:245. Master record

Alternative name(s)   Swedish Drug Information System
Database type   Factual, Textual
Number of journals
Sources
Start year
Language   English and Swedish keywords
Coverage   Sweden
Number of records
Update size   –
Update period   Daily

Keywords

Pharmaceutical Products

Description

The main topic of interest of the SWEDIS databank is the control of pharmaceutical preparations (läkemedelskontroll). The databank consists of registers of; pharmaceutical products, pharmaceutical speciality products, naturopathic preparations (naturmedel), sterile disposable products and cosmetic and hygienic preparations. There is also information on drug consumption, pharmaceutical postcontrol, statistics of drug sales from 1971 onwards, pharmaceutical substances and how to identify pharmaceutical pellets. SWEDIS is connected to INTDIS (International Drug Information System) at a WHO branch in Uppsala. The SWEDIS material is submitted from the drug department of the Swedish National Social Welfare Board, from WHO, from Apoteksbolaget and from Läkemedelsstatistik AB.

18:246. Online   Socialstyrelsens Läkemedelsavdelning

File name   SWEDIS
Alternative name(s) Swedish Drug Information System
Start year
Number of records
Update period   Daily

Notes

Subscription fee is required.

TECHHULP

Informatievoorziening Gehandicapten NL stichting

18:247. Master record

Database type   Reference
Number of journals
Sources
Start year   1990
Language   Dutch
Coverage
Number of records   10,000
Update size   –
Update period   Quarterly

18:248. CD-ROM — Informatievoorziening Gehandicapten NL stichting

File name	
Start year	1990
Number of records	10,000
Update period	Quarterly

18:249. Diskette — Informatievoorziening Gehandicapten NL stichting

File name	
Start year	1990
Number of records	10,000
Update period	Quarterly

World Textiles

Elsevier Science Publishers
Shirley Institute

18:250. Master record

Database type	Bibliographic
Number of journals	500
Sources	Journals, Patents (US), Patents (UK), Standards (US), Standards (UK), Standards (International), Books, Pamphlets, Technical reports, Conference proceedings and Statistical publications
Start year	1970
Language	English
Coverage	International
Number of records	181,275
Update size	—
Update period	Monthly

Keywords

Medical Textiles; Occupational Health and Safety; Pollution; Textiles

Description

World Textiles covers scientific, technological and business aspects of textiles. References are provided to articles from over 500 international periodicals; UK, US and European patents; UK, US and international standards; technical leaflets and brochures, books and directories, monographs and reports, etc. Subjects covered include: chemistry and physics of fibre forming polymers and fibrous materials, chemicals used in the textile industry (dyes, coatings, flameproofing agents, etc), manufacturing processes, chemical and mechanical treatments; pollution, safety and health hazards; energy conservation; application and performance of materials in industrial textiles, composites, geotextiles, medical textiles, civil engineering, etc, test methods, quality control and monitoring of textile processes.

Print equivalent is *World Textile Abstracts*.

18:251. Online — DIALOG

File name	File 67
Start year	1970
Number of records	181,275
Update period	Monthly
Price/Charges	Subscription: US$66.00
	Online print: US$0.40
	Offline print: US$0.40

18:252. Online — DIALOG

File name	File 67
Start year	1970
Number of records	181,275
Update period	Monthly
Price/Charges	Connect time: US$66.00
	Online print: US$0.40
	Offline print: US$0.40

X-RAY

Brookhaven National Laboratory, Protein Data Bank
DNAStar

18:253. Master record

Database type	Chemical structures/DNA sequences
Number of journals	
Sources	
Start year	
Language	English
Coverage	
Number of records	
Update size	—
Update period	Quarterly

Keywords

DNA; RNA; Radiography

Description

Contains 600 crystallographic structures of proteins, RNAs, polynucleotides and polysaccharides in 3-D. Includes backbone, sidechains and secondary structures of each molecule. Molecules can be rotated to view any angle.

18:254. CD-ROM — DNAStar

File name	X-RAY
Format notes	IBM
Software	X-Ray
Start year	
Number of records	
Update period	Quarterly
Price	US$1,500
	Subscription: US$275

VETERINARY MEDICINE

21CFR Online
Diogenes

19:1. Master record

Database type	Textual
Number of journals	
Sources	Laws/regulations
Start year	Current information
Language	English
Coverage	USA
Number of records	7,000
Update size	–
Update period	Monthly
Database aids	21CFR Online Users Guide 1991, Rockville, DIOGENES

Description

Contains the full text of Title 21 of the Code of Federal Regulations (CFR) – official regulations from two US government departments: the Food and Drug Administration (FDA), concerned with administering food and drugs; and the Drug Enforcement Agency (DEA), involved in drug enforcement. Covers drugs, food, cosmetics, medical devices and veterinary products.

Title 21 is divided into two chapters:

Chapter I: Food and Drug Administration (Department of Health and Human services) –
Subchapter A: General, covering general regulations, hearings, patent term restoration and colour additives.
Subchapter B: Food for Human Consumption, covering food labelling, quality standards, infant formula, general and specific food standards, food additives and seafood inspection.
Subchapter C: Drugs, General, covering drug labelling and advertising, Good Manufacturing Practices, controlled drugs and manufacturer registration.
Subchapter D: Drugs for Human Use, covering approval applications, and requirements for specific drug and antibiotic categories.
Subchapter E: Animal Drugs, Feeds, and Related Products, covering animal food labelling and packaging, and new animal drug and antibiotic approval applications.
Subchapter F: Biologics, covering licensing, standards and Good Manufacturing Practices for biological products.
Subchapter G: Cosmetics, covering labelling, establishment registration and experience reporting for cosmetics.
Subchapter H: Medical Devices, covering labelling, manufacturer registration, device classes, adverse experience reporting and premarket approvals for medical devices.
Subchapter I: Reserved.
Subchapter J: Radiological Health, covering general requirements, records and reports and performance standards for radiological health products.
Subchapter K: Reserved.
Subchapter L: Regulations Under certain Other Acts Administered by the Food and Drug Administration, covering Federal Import Milk Act, Tea Importation Act, Federal Caustic Poisin Act, communicable diseases, interstate conveyance sanitation.

Chapter II: Drug Enforcement Administration (Department of Justice) – covering manufacturer registration, labelling, prescriptions, schedules and import/export of controlled substances.

19:2. Online   BRS

File name	CF21
Start year	
Number of records	
Update period	
Price/Charges	Connect time: US$89.00/99.00
	Online print: US$0.91/0.99
	Offline print: US$0.99

19:3. Online   Data-Star

File name	CF21
Start year	Current information
Number of records	7,000
Update period	Monthly
Database aids	Data-Star Business and Biomedical Manuals, Berne, Data-Star and Online guide (search NEWS-CF21 in NEWS)
Price/Charges	Subscription: UK£32.00
	Connect time: UK£60.00
	Online print: UK£0.60
	Offline print: UK£0.90
	SDI charge: UK£5.12

Notes

From June 1993 Data-Star have introduced an annual fee/subscription per contract (that is, not per password) of SFr 80.00 (c.UK£ 32.00) payable every June. For North American customers billed in dollars who also use DIALOG, the DIALOG fee also covers access to Data-Star. Academic customers, 'commitment' customers and customers currently billed in dollars are exempt.

This database can also be found on:
FDA on CD-ROM

Acubase
Bibliotheque Interuniversitaire Section Medecine

19:5. Master record

Database type	Bibliographic
Number of journals	
Sources	Journals, Conference reports, Theses and Dissertations
Start year	1985
Language	French
Coverage	
Number of records	2,000
Update size	–
Update period	Monthly
Index unit	Articles

Keywords

Acupuncture; Alternative Medicine

Description

Precise and complete references with a keyword analysis of articles, conference reports, theses and dissertations on acupuncture. Aimed at participants, students, teachers and researchers (doctors, surgeons, dentists, vets).

19:6. Online   SUNIST

File name	Acubase
Start year	1985
Number of records	2,000
Update period	Monthly

Aesculapius Project – WHO

ETI SpA
IKONA Srl
World Health Organisation

19:7. Master record

Database type	Bibliographic, Textual, Image
Number of journals	
Sources	Monographs
Start year	1986
Language	English and French
Coverage	International
Number of records	
Update size	—
Update period	Quarterly

Keywords

Immunology

Description

Contains the full text and graphics of six years (1986–1991) of the *WHO Technical Support Series, WHO Bulletin, WHO Weekly Epidemiological* and other selected WHO monographs.

19:8. CD-ROM   IKONA Srl

File name	Aesculapius Project – WHO
Format notes	IBM
Software	Proprietary
Start year	1986
Number of records	
Update period	Quarterly
Price/Charges	Subscription: US$6,000

Agrar Forschungsvorhaben

Zentralstelle für Agrardokumentation
und Information (ZADI)

19:9. Master record

Alternative name(s)	FOHA
Database type	Factual, Directory
Number of journals	
Sources	Research projects
Start year	Current research of one year
Language	German and English Titles
Coverage	Germany
Number of records	6,500
Update size	—
Update period	Annually

Keywords

Forestry; Nutrition; Regional Studies

Description

Contains the current research projects carried out by German Government research institutions, regional authorities, institutes and private research institutions in the agricultural sector. Covers: plant production; agricultural and horticultural engineering and structures; rural building; economics; sociology; environment; agriculture and horticulture in foreign countries; animal production; veterinary science; food science and nutrition; forestry; timber industry.

Print equivalent is *Forschungsvorhaben Im Bereich Der Landbau-, Ernährungs-, Forst- Und Holzwirtschaftswissenschaften sowie der Veterinärmedizin.*

19:10. Online   DIMDI

File name	AV00
Alternative name(s)	FOHA
Start year	Current research of one year
Number of records	6,500
Update period	Annually
Database aids	Word list, Memocard and DIMDI Agrar Forschungsvorhaben Chapter
Price/Charges	Connect time: UK£03.24–07.03
	Online print: UK£0.15–0.33
	Offline print: UK£0.07–0.14

Record composition

Author AU; Corporate Source CS; Date Project Begins DB; Date Project Ends DE; Descriptors CT; Document Type DT; Number of Document ND; Subject Headings SH; Title TI and Special Descriptors (Uncontrolled Terms) UT

Every unit record includes data on author(s), project leader, title and other bibliographic data, institution name, controlled terms, sponsor. Research projects are indexed with Subject Headings (SH), Descriptors (CT) and Special Descriptors (UT). Each title has an English translation which can be searched by using the field identifier ENGL.

AGREP

Commission of the European
Communities (CEC)

19:11. Master record

Alternative name(s)	Agricultural Research Projects; Permanent Inventory of Agricultural Research Projects in the EC
Database type	Textual, Directory
Number of journals	
Sources	Project descriptions
Start year	1975
Language	English (with titles also in original languages)
Coverage	European Community
Number of records	25,000
Update size	5,000
Update period	Quarterly
Thesaurus	Classification Scheme of Agricultural and Forestry Research

Keywords

Agricultural Economics; Rural Sociology

Description

Contains descriptions of current agricultural research projects in member countries of the European Community (EC). Covers conservation and natural resources, land use and development, animal production, veterinary medicine, food and nutrition, fisheries, forestry, agricultural economics and rural sociology. The information is collected nationally by Member States under the sponsorship of the Standing Committee of Agricultural Research (SCAR) and under the management of the Commission of the European Commission. According to the *Manual of Online Search Strategies* (1st Edition 1988) it is useful for European research but compared with the American equivalent database, CRIS/USDA, size and coverage is relatively small. Also AGREP is an inventory file whereas CRIS/USDA is a current file updated monthly and purged annually so only currently active and recently completed projects appear. The unit record contains information about author, title and other bibliographic data as well as research organisation, subject heading and abstract (approximately 14%). Projects are deleted when they are terminated (average lifetime of each project is five years).

Corresponds to the printed *Permanent Inventory of Agricultural Research Projects*.

AGREP documents are described with the classification scheme *Classification Scheme of Agricultural and Forestry Research*.

19:12. Online   Datacentralen

File name	AGREP
Alternative name(s)	Permanent Inventory of Agricultural Research Projects in the EC; Agricultural Research Projects
Start year	1972
Number of records	25,000
Update period	Quarterly

Also accessible from many Danish networks and hosts.

Notes

Charges are according to use.

19:13. Online   DIMDI

File name	AP75
Alternative name(s)	Agricultural Research Projects; Permanent Inventory of Agricultural Research Projects in the EC
Start year	1975
Number of records	24,500+
Update period	Irregular
Database aids	Memocard and DIMDI AGREP Chapter
Price/Charges	Connect time: UK£03.24–07.03 Online print: UK£0.15–0.33 Offline print: UK£0.07–0.14

Downloading is allowed

Record composition

Author AU; Author's Country AC; Corporate Source CS; Facet Codes FC; Facet Headings FH; Language LA; Original Title OT; Number of References RN; Status of Tests STA and Title TI

The classification scheme *Classification Scheme of Agricultural and Forestry Research* is available online and is subdivided into four main groups: 1.Activities (A1100-A8900) which indicates the general line of research (for example, A3100 Biology of plants and animals). 2.Subject Areas (B100-B9900) within which research projects are indexed using groups of objects (eg B4200 Sheep). 3.Fields of Science (C1100-C9000) which indicates the discipline of research (eg C2320 Analytical chemistry); 4.Fields of Research D1100-D9900 which describes the application of research (for example, D3200 Animal nutrition). The

different groups may occur more than once in the documents.

This database can also be found on:
Agrisearch

Agricola
US Department of Agriculture, National Agricultural Library

19:15. Master record

Alternative name(s)	Agricultural Online Access; CAIN (former name)
Database type	Bibliographic
Number of journals	2,120
Sources	A-V material, Book chapters, Government documents, Grey literature, Journals, Monographs, Patents, Technical reports, Software, Theses, Translations and Pamphlets
Start year	1970
Language	English (with titles also in original languages)
Coverage	International
Number of records	2,800,000
Update size	150,000
Update period	Monthly
Index unit	Articles and Book chapters
Thesaurus	CAB-Thesaurus (Commonwealth Agricultural Bureaux, 1982)
Database aids	Agricola User's Guide

Keywords

Agricultural Engineering; Water Supply; Agricultural Economics; Rural Sociology; Pesticides; Fertilizers; Nutrition

Description

Contains citations to the literature in agriculture and related areas that have been acquired by the National Agricultural Library (NAL), as well as citations contributed by cooperating institutions. It is the most comprehensive source of bibliographic citations covering US agriculture and life science information. Topics covered: agricultural economics, engineering and production, rural sociology, animal sciences, aquatic sciences and fisheries, chemistry, entomology, food and human nutrition, forestry, pollution, natural resources, human parasitology, pesticides, plant science, soils and fertilizers, veterinary medicine and water resources. Also covers related areas such as biology and biotechnology, botany, ecology and natural history. The unit record contains information about author(s), title and other bibliographic data as well as institution, keywords and subject headings. Approximately ten per cent of its records contain abstracts but these exist only in the documents of the subunits American Agricultural Economics Documentation Centre and Food and Nutrition Documentation Centre. Used by USDA to produce the *Bibliography of Agriculture* and the *National Agricultural Library Catalog*.

Contributing agencies include land grant institutions, State Agricultre Experiment Stations and Extension Services, the FAO of the United Nations, the NAL Food and Nutrition Information Center (abstracts available from 1973 onwards), the Arid Lands Information Center and the American Agricultural Economics Documentation Center. Corresponds in part to *Bibliography of Agriculture* of the NAL and also to the Food and Agriculture Organisation's *AgrIndex*.

Since 1985 eighty-five per cent of the file is indexed using *CAB Thesaurus* as the controlled vocabulary. Fifteen per cent of the file is indexed using US Library of Congress Subject Headings. From 1983 the whole database is classified by the Agricola Subject Category Codes and the Geographical Codes from the AGRIS Classification Scheme (FAO-AGRIS–3) Amendment No 1, February 1980. The free-text dictionary includes the words from titles, notes, conferences, abstracts and controlled terms.

19:16. Online   BIS

File name	Agricola
Alternative name(s)	Agricultural Online Access; CAIN (former name)
Start year	
Number of records	
Update period	

19:17. Online   BRS, Morning Search, BRS/Colleague

File name	CAIB
Alternative name(s)	Agricultural Online Access; CAIN (former name)
Start year	1970
Number of records	2,700,000
Update period	Monthly
Price/Charges	Connect time: US$27.00/37.00
	Online print: US$0.15/0.23
	Offline print: US$0.23
	SDI charge: US$6.00

Notes

The backfile of Agricola on BRS.

19:18. Online   BRS, Morning Search, BRS/Colleague

File name	CAIN
Alternative name(s)	Agricultural Online Access; CAIN (former name)
Start year	1970
Number of records	2,700,000
Update period	Monthly
Price/Charges	Connect time: UK£27.00/37.00
	Online print: UK£0.15/0.23
	Offline print: UK£0.23
	SDI charge: UK£6.00

Notes

The current file of Agricola on BRS.

19:19. Online   DIALOG, Knowledge Index

File name	File 10
Alternative name(s)	Agricultural Online Access; CAIN (former name)
Start year	1979
Number of records	2,826,702
Update period	Monthly
Price/Charges	Connect time: US$45.00
	Online print: US$0.30
	Offline print: US$0.30
	SDI charge: US$7.25

Thesaurus is online

Notes

File 10 contains citations for the years 1979 to the present. File 110 contains the citations for the years 1970 to 1978. Both files have a similar format and identical coverage and pricing.

This database is also available to home users during

evenings and weekends at a reduced rate on the Knowledge Index service of DIALOG – file name in this case is AGRICOLA, and searches are made with simplified commands or menus.

19:20. Online   DIALOG, Knowledge Index

File name	File 110
Alternative name(s)	Agricultural Online Access; CAIN (former name)
Start year	1970–1978
Number of records	2,700,000
Update period	Monthly
Price/Charges	Connect time: US$45.00
	Online print: US$0.30
	Offline print: US$0.30
	SDI charge: US$7.25

Thesaurus is online

Notes

File 110 contains the citations for the years 1970 to 1978. File 10 contains citations for the years 1979 to the present. Both files have a similar format and identical coverage and pricing.

This database is also available to home users during evenings and weekends at a reduced rate on the Knowledge Index service of DIALOG – file name in this case is AGRICOLA, and searches are made with simplified commands or menus.

19:21. Online   DIMDI

File name	AL83
Alternative name(s)	Agricultural Online Access; CAIN (former name)
Start year	1983
Number of records	1,104,555
Update period	Monthly
SDI period	1 month
Database aids	DIMDI User Manual Agricola
Price/Charges	Connect time: UK£06.75–10.54
	Online print: UK£0.17–0.35
	Offline print: UK£0.10–0.17

Downloading is allowed
Thesaurus is online

Notes

Suppliers of online documents: British Library Document Supply Centre, Boston Spa, England; Harkers Information Retrieval System, Sydney, Australia; The Information Store, San Fransisco, USA; Zentralbibliothek der Landbauwissenschaft, Bonn, Germany.

Record composition

Abstract AB; Abstract Language AL; Author Au; Bibliograhical Level BL; Call Number CN; Coden (serials) CO; Corporate Source CS; Controlled Term CT; Document Type DT; Entry Date ED; Entry Magnetic Tape EM; Free Text FT; Geographic Code GC; Geographic Heading GH; Journal Title JT; Conference KN; Language LA; Number of Document ND; Notes NO; Publication Place PP; Publisher PU; Publication Year PY; ISBN SB; Subject Code SC; Subject Heading SH; Source Level SL; Source SO; ISSN SS; Subunit SU and Title TI

19:22. CD-ROM   Quanta

File name	Agricola
Alternative name(s)	Agricultural Online Access; CAIN (former name)
Format notes	IBM
Start year	
Number of records	
Update period	Quarterly
Price/Charges	Subscription: UK£65

19:23. CD-ROM   Quanta

File name	Agricola Backfile
Alternative name(s)	Agricultural Online Access; CAIN (former name)
Format notes	IBM, Mac
Software	Romware
Start year	
Number of records	
Update period	
Price	US$495

19:24. CD-ROM   SilverPlatter

File name	Agricola
Alternative name(s)	Agricultural Online Access; CAIN (former name)
Format notes	Mac, IBM
Software	SPIRS/MacSPIRS
Start year	1970
Number of records	3 million+
Update period	Quarterly
Price/Charges	Subscription: UK£540–1,066

Notes

Pricing – Current disc (1984+) UK£540; Current disc with archival set (1970+) UK£1,066; Archival set purchase (1970–1984) UK£625. Four discs – complete starter kit, including 2 current discs (start 1985) with quarterly updates and 2 archival discs 1970–1984, is priced at UK£890.

Index contains an alphabetical list of all words and hyphenated phrases from searchable fields. All fields except Citation Notes can be searched but, in some cases (such as intellectual level), this is done by using the LIMIT command rather than by a direct search. A small number of stop words (listed on a Help Screen) have not been indexed.

19:25. Database subset

Online   **DIALOG, Knowledge Index**

File name	File 210 – ONTAP Agricola Training File
Alternative name(s)	Agricultural Online Access; CAIN (former name)
Start year	January to April 1985
Number of records	24,200
Update period	Closed File
Price/Charges	Connect time: US$15.00

Notes

The training file for Agricola on DIALOG, containing records taken from File 10, the main Agricola file on DIALOG. Offline prints are not available in ONTAP files.

AGRIS

Food and Agriculture Organization of the United Nations (FAO)

19:26. Master record

Alternative name(s)	Agricultural Information System; International Information System for the Agricultural Sciences and Technology

Database type	Bibliographic
Number of journals	3,000
Sources	Journals, Conference proceedings, Monographs, Theses, Patents, Maps, Technical reports, Standards, Films and Computer media
Start year	1975
Language	English, French (index terms, starting 1986), Spanish (index terms, starting 1986) and Original language titles
Coverage	International
Number of records	2,700,000
Update size	130,000
Update period	Monthly
Index unit	Articles
Thesaurus	Agrovoc Thesaurus
Database aids	AGRIS Categorization Scheme FAO-AGRIS 3 (Rev.4) 1983 and AGRIS Classification Scheme (inc. Amendment 1) FAO-AGRIS (Rev.3) 1980

Keywords

Aquatic Sciences; Food Science; Forestry; Nutrition; Pollution; Rural Sociology; Statistics

Description

This database is assembled by the Food and Agriculture Organization of the the United Nation. It contains citations, about ten per cent with abstracts (from 1979), to the worldwide literature on all aspects of agriculture. Topics covered include research methods; geography and history; legislation; education, extension and advisory work; economics, development, marketing, and rural sociology; plant production; protection of plants and stored products; forestry; animal production; veterinary medicine; aquatic sciences and fisheries; machinery and buildings; natural resources; water resources; irrigation and drainage; food science and food processing; human nutrition; home economics; and pollution; mathematics and statistics. Produced from the collected input of over one hundred and thirty five national and multinational centres worldwide. According to the *Manual of Online Search Strategies* (2nd ed) none of these centres is in the US so there is a definite bias against US material. This is useful to the searcher as it militates against duplication with Agricola which provides extensive coverage of US material and also gives it a relative strength in for example tropical or third world agricultural questions. It includes unique material such as unpublished scientific and technical reports and theses. All non-English references carry an English translated title. The unit record contains information about author(s), title and other bibliographic data as well as institutions, keywords, subject headings and abstracts. Descriptor fields appear in a proportion of its references.

Corresponds to the monthly *Agrindex*. Approval of the Liaison Office in user's country may be required; contact FAO for complete list of participating countries and addresses of Liaison Offices or consult current issue of *Agrindex*.

Subject access by AGRIS/CARIS Categorisation scheme. Subject categories from 1975 to date, commodity and geographical codes from 1975 to 1985. From 1986 documents are indexed in English, French and Spanish. The *Agrovoc* trilingual thesaurus was used to index fifteen per cent of documents from 1982 and from 1986 it was used to index all of them.

19:27. Online   DIALOG

File name	File 203
Alternative name(s)	Agricultural Information System; International Information System for the Agricultural Sciences and Technology
Start year	1975
Number of records	1,291,330
Update period	Monthly
Price/Charges	Connect time: US$60.00
	Online print: US$0.20
	Offline print: US$0.35

Notes

On DIALOG, only citations to non-US documents are available (that is, sixty-six per cent of the database). US entries are omitted to avoid duplication with Agricola. Dialindex categories: AGRI, VETSCI. Corresponds in part to AgrIndex, published monthly by the Fodd and Agriculture Organization (FAO) of the United Nations.

19:28. Online   DIMDI

File name	AG75
Alternative name(s)	Agricultural Information System; International Information System for the Agricultural Sciences and Technology
Start year	1975–1985
Number of records	1,182,290
Update period	Not Updated
SDI period	1 month
Price/Charges	Connect time: UK£03.24–07.03
	Online print: UK£0.15–0.33
	Offline print: UK£0.07–0.14

Downloading is allowed
Thesaurus is online

Notes

The file has been subdivided into two files by date (1985/6). File AG75 contains records covering the period 1975–1985 and AG86 contains the post-1986 records. Suppliers of online documents: British Library Document Supply Centre, Boston Spa, England; Harkers Information Retrieval System, Sydney, Australia; Zentralbibliothek der Landbauwissenschaft, Bonn, Germany.

Record composition

Abstract AB; Author AU; Bibliographical Level BL; Classification Terms CX; Commodity/Classification Codes CC; Conference Names KN; Corporate Source CS; Document Type DT; Entry Date ED; Geographical Codes GC; Geographical Heading GH; Language LA; Number of Document ND; Section Headings SH; Source SO; Subject Codes SC; Title TI and Uncontrolled Terms UT

AG75 contains the following indexing data elements: Subject Categories, Commodity Codes, Geographical Codes, Uncontrolled Terms. The Geographical codes (GC) and the corresponding Geographical Headings (GH) are used to index the countries or regions occurring in an article. In addition marine areas, intergovernmental organisations, physical geography are included in the Geographical Codes. The text versions (GH) and the code versions (GC) are available online and can be linked using the display command. The Subject Categories or Section Codes (SC) respectively Section Headings (SH), subdivide the whole AGRIS scope into sections of specific subject fields.

The text version (SH) and the code version (SC) are available online and can be linked using the display command. Descriptors (UT – Uncontrolled Term) were not assigned to documentary ARGIS records up to 1979, and only rarely since 1979. A vocabulary based on controlled descriptors is not available. Approximately five per cent of the records contain abstracts.

19:29. Online   DIMDI

File name	AG86
Alternative name(s)	Agricultural Information System; International Information System for the Agricultural Sciences and Technology
Start year	1986
Number of records	800,000
Update period	Monthly
SDI period	Monthly
Price/Charges	Connect time: UK£03.24–07.03
	Online print: UK£0.15–0.33
	Offline print: UK£0.07–0.14

Downloading is allowed
Thesaurus is online

Notes

The file has been subdivided into two files by date (1985/6). File AG75 contains records covering the period 1975–1985 and AG86 contains the post-1986 records. Suppliers of online documents: British Library Document Supply Centre, Boston Spa, England; Harkers Information Retrieval System, Sydney, Australia; Zentralbibliothek der Landbauwissenschaft, Bonn, Germany. 10% of the records contain abstracts. There is menu driven user guidance in German and English.

Record composition

Abstract AB; Author AU; Bibliographical Level BL; Conference Names KN; Controlled Terms CT; Corporate Source CS; Document Type DT; Entry Date ED; Geographical Heading GH; Language LA; Number of Document ND; Section Headings SH; Source SO; Subject Codes SC; Title TI and Uncontrolled Terms UT

AG86 (1986+) contains the following indexing data elements: Subject Categories, Controlled Terms of the *Agrovoc-Thesaurus*. Controlled Terms: from 1986 all AGRIS-documents are indexed with descriptors of the *Agrovoc-Thesaurus* which uses a polyhierarchically structured vocabulary and replaces in AG86 the Commodity Codes and the Geographical Codes which are used in AG75. The Subject Categories or Section Codes (SC) respectively Section Headings (SH), subdivide the whole AGRIS scope into sections of specific subject fields. The text version (SH) and the code version (SC) are available online and can be linked using the display command. Descriptors (UT – Uncontrolled Term) were not assigned to documentary ARGIS records up to 1979, and only rarely since 1979. A vocabulary based on controlled descriptors is not available.

19:30. Online   ESA-IRS

File name	File 29
Alternative name(s)	Agricultural Information System; International Information System for the Agricultural Sciences and Technology
Start year	1989 (October 1991)

Number of records	1,400,000
Update period	Monthly
Database aids	AGRIS/Stairs User Manual
	FAO-AGRIS–22 (Rev.3) 1987 in
	English
Price/Charges	Subscription: UK£70.29
	Database entry fee: UK£42.17
	Offline print: UK£0.10
	SDI charge: UK£2.11 (Profile) 0.10
	(Print)

Notes

ESA-IRS is a gateway to International Atomic Energy Agency (IAEA) in Vienna where the database is actually held which means changing the search language to the IAEA's STAIRS language. For training file see TGRIS (File 118). An SDI service is available.

From 1993 ESA-IRS are charging an annual fee of 100 Accounting Units (c.UK£ 70.29) to all users. This is equivalent to the fee for full documentation and will not be charged to customers already paying for documentation.

Record composition

Abstract in English AB; Abstract in French ABFR; Abstract in Spanish ABES; Author AU; Commodity/Geographic Code (From 1975/85) RP; Controlled Terms (English) CT; Controlled Terms (French) CTFR; Controlled Terms (Spanish) CTES; Controlled Terms (Local) FT; First or Primary Subject Category Number CAT; Language LA; Record number in Agrindex RN; Report/Patent Number RP; Serial Information JR; Subject Categories CC; Title TI; Volume and Issue Number of Agrindex VVSS and Publication Year YEAR

Retrieval is via the STAIRS retrieval language as described in FAO-AGRIS-22.

19:31. Online International Atomic Energy Agency (IAEA)

File name	AGRIS
Alternative name(s)	Agricultural Information System;
	International Information System for
	the Agricultural Sciences and
	Technology
Start year	
Number of records	
Update period	
	Gateway available to ESA-IRS

19:32. CD-ROM SilverPlatter

File name	AGRIS
Alternative name(s)	Agricultural Information System;
	International Information System for
	the Agricultural Sciences and
	Technology
Format notes	Mac, IBM
Software	SPIRS/MacSPIRS
Start year	1975
Number of records	2 million+
Update period	Quarterly
Price/Charges	Subscription: UK£490 – 1,825.50

Notes

Five discs. Current disc (1991-present) is £490 single user, £735 for 2–8 users on network; current disc and archival set (1975 to present) £1,215 single user, £,822.50 2–8 users on network; archival swt purchase £820 single user, £1,230 2–8 users on network.

19:33. Tape Food and Agriculture Organization of the United Nations (FAO)

File name	AGRIS
Alternative name(s)	Agricultural Information System;
	International Information System for
	the Agricultural Sciences and
	Technology
Format notes	IBM
Software	STAIRS
Start year	1990
Number of records	100,000
Update period	Monthly

19:34. Database subset
Online ESA-IRS

File name	File 118 – Training AGRIS
Alternative name(s)	Agricultural Information System;
	International Information System for
	the Agricultural Sciences and
	Technology
Start year	Fixed set
Number of records	1,688 (October 1991)
Update period	Not updated
Price/Charges	Subscription: UK£70.29
	Database entry fee: UK£6.99

Notes

AGRIS Training file; fixed subset of AGRIS; for full details refer to main file AGRIS File 29. Services such as offline printing are not available.

19:35. Database subset
Online ASAS

File name	ROMAGRIS
Alternative name(s)	Agricultural Information System;
	International Information System for
	the Agricultural Sciences and
	Technology
Start year	1990
Number of records	100,000
Update period	Monthly

Notes

Contains the Romanian segments to AGRIS.

Alimentarium Information System

Information and Research Center on Health Services

19:37. Master record

Alternative name(s)	ALIMIS
Database type	Bibliographic
Number of journals	
Sources	
Start year	1900
Language	English
Coverage	
Number of records	8,000
Update size	2,500
Update period	Monthly

Keywords

Human Digestion

Description

Main information system on substances in human environment.

19:38. Online   UVTEI-UTZ

File name	ALIMIS
Alternative name(s)	ALIMIS
Start year	1900
Number of records	8,000
Update period	Monthly

For more details of constituent databases, see:
DVJB

Animal Knowledge Base
Pacific Veterinary Services

19:40. Master record

Database type	Textual, Bibliographic, Directory
Number of journals	
Sources	Journals
Start year	Current information
Language	English
Coverage	USA
Number of records	
Update size	—
Update period	Weekly
Index unit	Articles

Description

Information for veterinarians and other animal care professionals. Includes texts of peer-reviewed veterinary medicine articles on topics such as quarantine recommendations, diagnostic and treatment protocols and drug dosages. Also includes citations, with abstracts, to current literature and a directory of animal care specialists.

19:41. Online   GE Information Services (GEIS)

File name	Animal Knowledge Base
Start year	Current information
Number of records	
Update period	Weekly

Automated System of Scientific and Technical Information
ZNIIinformazii

19:42. Master record

Database type	Bibliographic
Number of journals	
Sources	
Start year	1985
Language	English
Coverage	
Number of records	600,000
Update size	—
Update period	

Keywords

Physics; Optics

Description

Bibliographic database on optics and related subjects.

19: 43. Diskette   ZNIIinformazii

File name	
Start year	1985

Number of records	600,000
Update period	

Bakteriologiai adatbazis
Johan Bela Orszagos
KözegeszsegÜgyi

19:44. Master record

Database type	Bibliographic, Factual
Number of journals	
Sources	
Start year	
Language	English
Coverage	
Number of records	
Update size	—
Update period	

Keywords

Bacteria

Description

In-house database on micro-organisms.

19:45. Online   Johan Bela Orszagos Kozegeszsegugyi

File name	EUMIKRO
Start year	
Number of records	
Update period	

Banco de Información Sobre Medicina Veterinaria (BIVE)
Universidad Nacional Autonoma de Mexico, Facultad de Medicina Veterraria-y-Zootecnica

19:46. Master record

Database type	Bibliographic
Number of journals	
Sources	Journals, Monographs, Reports and Conference proceedings
Start year	1984
Language	Spanish
Coverage	Caribbean, Latin America, Mozambique, Portugal and Spain
Number of records	5,000
Update size	—
Update period	Varies

Description

Contains citations to Spanish-language literature on veterinary medicine. Covers basic animal medicine (for example, anatomy, biochemistry, epidemiology, genetics, microbiology, immunology, pharmacology, toxicology), hygiene and public health, and animal technology fields (for example, apiculture, aquaculture, animal husbandry).

Spanish-language literature.

19:47. Online   Universidad Nacional Autonoma de Mexico, Servicio de Consultie a Bancos de Informacion

File name	
Start year	1984

Number of records   5,000
Update period   Varies

Bancos Bibliográficos Mexicanos
Universidad de Colima, Dir Gen de Int Acad Des Bib

19:48. Master record

Alternative name(s)	Bancos Bibliograficos Mexicanos; Mexican Bibliographic Database
Database type	Library catalogue/cataloguing aids, Bibliographic
Number of journals	
Sources	Monographs and Journals
Start year	
Language	Spanish
Coverage	Mexico and Latin America
Number of records	
Update size	–
Update period	Twice a year

Keywords

Culture; Fishing; Economics

Description

Contains union catalogue of Mexico University Libraries. Covers: political campaigns of Mexican Presidents, Latin American economics, Mexican literature, education, health science, social sciences, fishery, veterinary medicine, research directory, Colima-Mexico – its culture, history, law and economics.

19:49. CD-ROM   Universidad de Colima

File name	Bancos Bibliográficos Mexicanos
Alternative name(s)	Bancos Bibliograficos Mexicanos; Mexican Bibliographic Database
Format notes	IBM
Software	SIABUC
Start year	
Number of records	
Update period	Twice a year
Price/Charges	

BGA-Pressedienst
Bundesgesundheitsamt – BGA

19:50. Master record

Database type	Textual
Number of journals	
Sources	Press releases
Start year	1980
Language	German
Coverage	Germany
Number of records	462 documents
Update size	50 documents
Update period	As needed

Keywords

Drugs; HIV; Infectious Diseases; Pollution

Description

This is a full-text database in the German language in the field of human and veterinary medicine and related fields. It corresponds to the printed press releases from the Bundesgesundheitsamt (BGA, that is, Federal Health Office) of the Federal Republic of Germany. The database contains the full text of the original documents. Subject coverage includes espe-cially: drugs (for example, express information on drugs), infectious diseases (for example, AIDS), social medicine and epidemiology, toxicology, water, soil, air pollution, environmental chemicals in food, radiation health.

19:51. Online   DIMDI

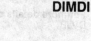

File name	BP80
Start year	1980
Number of records	418 documents
Update period	As needed
Price/Charges	Connect time: UK£0.16–0.34
	Online print: UK£03.88–08.62
	Offline print: UK£0.07–0.14

Downloading is allowed

Record composition

DIMDI Number ENR; Machine Date MD; Number of Document ND; Publication Year PY; Source SO and Title TI

Since January 29, 1992 the database can be searched using DIMDI's User guidance GRIPS-Menu. Freetext searches have to be carried out. There is neither controlled nor uncontrolled vocabulary in the database. Only the user guidance is in English, search terms have to be entered in German.

The press releases are continuously numbered per year by the BGA, for example the thirty first press release in 1991 has the number 31/91. In the field ND (Number of Document) this number is transformed to the format YYnn (YY=two digits for the year, nn=serial number), for example, 9131.

Bibliographia Medica Cechoslovaca
Vyzkumny ustav vnejsich ekonomickych

19:52. Master record

Database type	Bibliographic
Number of journals	
Sources	
Start year	1983
Language	English
Coverage	
Number of records	80,000
Update size	12,000
Update period	

Description

The database contains references on medical science serials.

19:53. Online   VTEI

File name	BMC
Start year	1983
Number of records	80,000
Update period	

BioBusiness
BIOSIS

19:54. Master record

Database type	Bibliographic
Number of journals	500
Sources	Conference proceedings, journals, monographs, newsletters, research reports and patents (US)
Start year	1985
Language	English
Coverage	International

Number of records	480,000
Update size	42,000
Update period	Monthly
Database aids	BioBusiness Search Guide, Philadelphia, BIOSIS, How to search BioBusiness,Philadelphia, BIOSIS and Newsletters: BioSearch, BioScene.

Keywords

Cosmetics; Fishing; Forestry; Genetic Engineering; Immunology

Description

BioBusiness is a bibliographic database which focuses specifically on the business applications of biomedical research. It contains citations, with abstracts, to the worldwide periodical literature on business applications of biological and biomedical research. Subjects covered include: agriculture and forestry, animal production, biomass conversion, crop production, diet and nutrition, fermentation, food technology, cosmetics, genetic engineering, health care, industrial microbiology, pharmaceutical products, medical technology, medical diagnostics, medical instrumentation, occupational health, pesticides, pharmaceuticals, protein production, toxicology, veterinary science, waste treatment, energy and the environment, and other industries affected by biotechnological developments. Also covers patents in such areas as immunological testing, food processes, and fishing. For each patent record, includes inventor's name and address, patent title and number, patent classes, date granted, and assignee. BioBusiness can be used to discover: the latest legislation and regulatory controls affecting implementation of biotechnology research; the impact of economic fluctuations on price and production forecasts for agricultural commodities; the financial effects of recycling programs on business; the increased use of natural ingredients in cosmetic and personal care products; the applications of bioengineering in pharmaceuticals; trends in the development and marketing of food products; etc.

A broad spectrum of life science, business and management journals are scanned. Abstracts are included for approximately 55–60% of the records.

Both controlled and uncontrolled terms are used for indexing. The concept codes used are different from the BIOSIS concept codes.

19:55. Online   BIOSIS Life Science Network

File name	
Start year	1985
Number of records	480,000
Update period	Monthly
Price/Charges	Connect time: US$9.00
	Online print: US$6.00 per 10; 2.25 per abstract; 3.50 per full text article

Downloading is allowed
Also available via the Internet by telnetting to LSN.COM.

Notes

On Life Science Network users can search this database or they can scan a group of subject-related databases. There is a charge of $2.00 per scan of subject-related databases. To search one database and display up to ten citations costs $6.00. Most charges are for information retrieved. There are no charges if there are no results and no charge to transfer results to a printer or diskette. Articles may also be ordered via an online document delivery request. A telecommunications software package is also avail-

able, costing $12.95, providing an automatic connection to Life Science Network for heavy users of the service, with capability to transfer to print or disk and customised colour options.

19:56. Online   BRS

File name	BBUS
Start year	1985
Number of records	480,000
Update period	Weekly
Price/Charges	Connect time: UK£88.00/98.00
	Online print: UK£0.46/0.54
	Offline print: UK£0.52

Downloading is allowed

19:57. Online   CISTI, Canadian Online Enquiry Service CAN/OLE

File name	
Start year	1985
Number of records	480,000
Update period	Monthly

Downloading is allowed

19:58. Online   Data-Star

File name	BBUS
Start year	1985
Number of records	277,972
Update period	Weekly
Database aids	Data-Star Business Manual and Online manual (search NEWS-BBUS in NEWS)
Price/Charges	Subscription: UK£32.00
	Connect time: UK£63.60
	Online print: UK£0.41
	Offline print: UK£0.36
	SDI charge: UK£3.94

Downloading is allowed

Notes

From June 1993 Data-Star have introduced an annual fee/subscription per contract (that is, not per password) of SFr 80.00 (c.UK£ 32.00) payable every June. For North American customers billed in dollars who also use DIALOG, the DIALOG fee also covers access to Data-Star. Academic customers, 'commitment' customers and customers currently billed in dollars are exempt.

Record composition

Abstract AB; Accession Number and Update Code AN; Author AU; Author Affiliation IN; Company Name CO; Concept Codes CC; Descriptors DE; Language of Article LG; Named Person(s) NA; Publication Details PU; Source SO; Title TI; Update Codes UP and Year of Publication YR

19:59. Online   DIALOG

File name	File 285
Start year	1985
Number of records	371,575
Update period	Weekly
Price/Charges	Connect time: US$126.00
	Online print: US$0.85
	Offline print: US$0.85
	SDI charge: US$10.50

Downloading is allowed

Notes

DIALINDEX Categories: AGRIBUS, BIOBUS, BIOTECH, PHARMINA.

19:60. Online   ESA-IRS

File name	File 137
Start year	1985
Number of records	372,000 (October 1991)
Update period	Weekly

Price/Charges — Subscription: UK£70.29
Database entry fee: UK£3.49
Online print: UK£0.74
Offline print: UK£0.79
SDI charge: UK£3.49

Downloading is allowed

Notes

The default supplier of original document is British Library Documentation Supply Centre.

From 1993 ESA-IRS are charging an annual fee of 100 Accounting Units (c.UK£ 70.29) to all users. This is equivalent to the fee for full documentation and will not be charged to customers already paying for documentation.

Record composition

Abstract /AB; Additional Source Information NT; Author AU; Concept Code CC; Concept Code Name CN; Corporate Source CS; ISBN BN; Journal Name JN; Language LA; Named Company NM; Named Person SP; Native Number NN; Patent Assignee PH; Patent Number PN; Publication Year PY; Subfile (1) SF; Title /TI; Uncontrolled Terms /UT and US Patent Classification PC

19:61. Online   STN

File name	BIOBUS
Start year	1985
Number of records	480,000
Update period	Weekly

Downloading is allowed

19: 62. Tape   BIOSIS

File name	
Format notes	9-track, 800, 1600 or 6250 bpi, variable length records, variable block size
Start year	1985
Number of records	480,000
Update period	Monthly

Notes

Corresponds to the BioBusiness online database. Annual lease price is $2,350 plus additional usage charges; contact BIOSIS for archival tape prices.

Biological and Agricultural Index
HW Wilson Company

19:63. Master record

Alternative name(s)	BAI; Wilson Biological and Agricultural Index
Database type	Bibliographic
Number of journals	200+
Sources	Journals
Start year	1983 (July)
Language	English
Coverage	International
Number of records	184,000
Update size	54,000
Update period	Twice per week
Index unit	Articles, Book reviews, Symposia, Conference papers and Letters to the editor (selected)

Keywords

Plant Sciences; Physiology; Horticulture; Forestry; Animal Sciences; Agricultural Economics; Agro-chemicals; Agricultural Engineering

Description

Indexing of 226 key periodicals in the life sciences; a separate index of current book reviews. The major areas covered include: Agriculture; Agricultural chemistry, economics, engineering and research; Animal husbandry; Biochemistry; Biology; Botany; Cytology; Ecology; Entomology; Environmental sciences; Food science; Forestry; Genetics; Horticulture; Marine biology and limnology; Microbiology; Nutrition; Physiology; Plant pathology; Soil science; Veterinary medicine; Zoology.

Corresponds to *Biological and Agricultural Index.*

English-language periodicals on biology and agriculture.

Articles indexed under specific, accessible subject headings in a single alphabet; extensive cross referencing; title enhancement for titles with ambiguous titles; complete bibliographic data on each article indexed.

19:64. Online   OCLC EPIC; OCLC FirstSearch

File name	
Alternative name(s)	BAI
Start year	
Number of records	
Update period	

19:65. Online   WilsonLine

File name	BAI
Alternative name(s)	BAI; Wilson Biological and Agricultural Index
Start year	1983 (July)
Number of records	
Update period	Twice per week

19:66. CD-ROM   Wilsondisc

File name	
Alternative name(s)	BAI; Wilson Biological and Agricultural Index
Format notes	IBM
Software	WilsonDisc
Start year	1983 (July)
Number of records	
Update period	Quarterly
Price/Charges	Subscription: US$1,495

Notes

Subscription fee includes unlimited online access to BAI file through WilsonLine.

Biotechnology
VNII Sistem Upr., ekon. Issl. i Informazii mikrobiol. Prom. ArmNIINTI

19:67. Master record

Database type	Bibliographic
Number of journals	
Sources	
Start year	1984
Language	English
Coverage	
Number of records	35,000
Update size	—
Update period	

Keywords

Biotechnology

Description

Bibliographic source on biotechnology.

19:68. Diskette · VNII Sistem Upr., ekon. Issl. i Informazii mikrobiol. Prom.

File name
Start year · 1984
Number of records · 35,000
Update period

BioWorld Online
BioWorld

19:69. Master record

Database type · Textual, Directory, Factual, Bibliographic
Number of journals
Sources
Start year · Current
Language · English
Coverage · International
Number of records
Update size · —
Update period · Daily

Description

Provides a variety of information on the biotechnology business. Includes news from *BioWorld Today*, Bioworld Online and *BioVenture View*, reports on relevant company stocks and financial data on publicly owned biotechnology companies, a record of forthcoming events, and citations to biotechnology literature. A directory of biotechnology companies gives name, contact person, address, commercial alliances, partnerships, investment data, management history, product development and sales. The directory covers 900 companies worldwide, specialising in medicine, veterinary science, agriculture, food and brewing and other disciplines. There is also an electronic mail service.

19:70. Online · NIFTY Corporation, NIFTY-Serve

File name
Start year · Current
Number of records
Update period · Daily

CAB Abstracts
CAB International

19:71. Master record

Database type · Bibliographic
Number of journals · 14,000
Sources · Books, company reports, conference proceedings, dissertations, grey literature, journals, monographs, patents, research reports, standards and theses
Start year · 1972
Language · English (original language titles)
Coverage · International

Number of records · 2,800,000
Update size · 150,000
Update period · Monthly
Abstract details · CAB's own indexers write detailed informative English-language summaries for each record.
Thesaurus · CAB Abstracts Thesaurus
Database aids · CAB Abstracts Online Manual, CAB Serials Checklist, CAB Section Code Lists, CAB International Database News. and IULAS (International Union List of Agricultural Serials)

Keywords

Agricultural Economics; Agrochemicals; Anatomy; Animal Breeding; Animal Diseases; Bioagriculture; Crop Protection; Diet; Entomology; Environmental Health; Forestry; Horticulture; Immunology; Medical Entomology; Medical Immunology; Medical Mycology; Medical Parasitology; Mycology; Nutrition; Paper
and Packaging; Pathology; Pest Management; Physiology; Plant Diseases; Plant Genetics; Pollution; Public Health; Rural Sociology; Soil Management; Sport; Tourism; Travel; Veterinary Entomology; Veterinary Mycology; Water Management

Description

Contains citations, with abstracts, to the worldwide literature in the agricultural sciences and related areas of applied biology. Subjects covered include agricultural engineering; agricultural entomology; animal breeding; biocontrol; biodeterioration and biodegradation; biotechnology; crop protection; dairy science and technology; economics; engineering; environment; forestry and forest products; genetics; herbicides; helminthology; horticulture; irrigation; leisure, recreation and tourism; medical and veterinary entomology; microbiology; mycology; nutrition (human and animal); parasitology (human and animal); plant breeding and pathology; protozoology; rural development and sociology; soil science and fertilizers and arid lands (1980 to 1982). Coverage of veterinary medicine begins in 1972. Also contains useful material on rural development in third world countries. Animal breeding and production, animal nutrition & dairy science and technology, covers: animals including farm mammals of economic or domestic importance; laboratory mammals; poultry, game and other birds of economic importance; fish, molluscs and crustacea; and certain invertebrates used in genetic studies. Subjects covered include performance traits and products; breeding and genetics; biotechnology; reproduction; nutrition; the dairy industry; housing and equipment for livestock and in aquaculture; and nongenetic effects on animals. Crop protection and pests covers: entomology; plant pathology; nematology and weed science for the full ranges of agricultural, horticultural, plantation and forestry crops. Covers areas of pest taxonomy; biology; ecology; management; and economic and social impact. Environmental health and toxicology covers: environmental agrochemicals (insecticides, fungicides, pesticides, fertilisers); groundwater contamination, runoff and leaching; heavy metals in soil, crops and animals; reclamation and re-vegetation of polluted sites; environmental impact of farming; waste management, treatment and disposal; toxicology (toxic plants, wastes, food poisoning, carcinogens); and steroids and hormones in animals. Forestry covers: silviculture and forestry management; tree biology; forest pests and their control; forest land use; wood properties; timber extraction, conversion and management; wood products; marketing and trade; agroforestry systems and related land use; plant and animal species for agroforestry; environmental and service aspects of agroforestry systems; and sociological, cultural and economic aspects of agroforestry systems. Horticulture covers: literature on temperate tree fruits and nuts; small fruits; viticulture; vegetables; temperate, tropical and greenhouse; ornamental plants; minor industrial crops; subtropical and tropical fruits and plantation crops. Leisure, recreation and tourism covers: leisure industries, travel and transport, marketing of services and products, natural resources and environmental issues, facility management and planning, sport, and leisure and tourism policies. Plant genetics covers: material on breeding; genetic resources; varieties; molecular and general genetics; in vitro culture; cytology and ploidy; reproductive behaviour; evolution and taxonomy; stress tolerance; disease and pest resistance; and quality and yield components. Soil science covers: soil management; crop management; fertilisers and amendments; agricultural meteorology; pollution; land reclamation; irrigation and drainage; plant nutrition and plant water relations. Veterinary science covers: animals including farm animals; pets; game animals; all animals of economic importance, including farmed fish and shellfish; commercially important wild fish; zoo animals and wild animals. Subjects include viral and bacterial diseases; protozoology; mycology; helminthology; arthropod parasites; toxicology; immunology; pharmacology and therapeutics; physiology; biochemistry and anatomy; zootechny, hygiene and food inspection, and related areas. About 85% of items are abstracted in English with each abstract containing 80–100 words. Sources are published in 74 languages.

Corresponds to the fifty main journals and specialised journals published by the Commonwealth Agricultural Bureaux (CAB) International, an international, intergovernmental organisation registered with the United Nations. Membership is open to all governments wishing to participate. *The International Union List of Agricultural Serials*, a compilation of the serials indexed in AGRICOLA, AGRIS and CAB lists which database indexes a given title. Several hosts have separate subfiles by subject. On all BRS services four subsets are available separately; on agricultural economics, rural development and sociology; on human nutrition; on leisure, recreation and tourism; and on medical and veterinary sciences. On Data-Star, three subsets are available separately: on human nutrition, on human parasitology and mycology; and on medical and veterinary sciences. On DIMDI there are eleven subsets available separately: Animal; Animal Production; Economics; Engineering; Forestry; Human; Nutrition; Plant; Plant Protection; Tourism; and Veterinary Science.

From 1972 to 1983 the Controlled Terms take the form of subject index entries and additional index entries. The number of controlled terms allocated varies from one item/abstract to another. Various collections of uncontrolled, semi-controlled and controlled terms and phrases (keyword units) were used. The Controlled Terms vary between abstract journals. The most strictly controlled list of terms are used in *Index Veterinarius*, which from 1972 to 1976 used *Veterinary Subject Headings* (CAB, 1972) and from 1977 the *Veterinary Multilingual Thesaurus* (there is about 60% agreement between them). The Controlled Terms are the subject index entries used to generate the printed subject indices of the abstract journals, while the additional index entries, where present are

used to facilitate retrieval. No hierarchical structure is available for controlled terms. The controlled terms comprise various categories of descriptors and names of organisms are in Latin or in English. Various systems of chemical notation and geographical terms are also used. From 1984 onwards controlled indexing terms are allocated from the *CAB Thesaurus*. A cumulative, alphabetic list of all Controlled Terms, including the descriptors from 1972/83 plus the descriptors of the *CAB Thesaurus* can be accessed by the DISPLAY-command. Almost every abstract is accompanied by a Section Code except the title-only items in *Index Veterinarius*. Usually the Section Codes are structured hierarchically corresponding to the sections and subsections of the CABI abstract journals. Two types of Section Codes are in use: Primary Sequencing Codes and Cross Reference Codes. Primary Sequencing Codes describe the main topic of an article and place an abstract within a given section of an abstract journal. These sections are often subdivided into several subsections; accordingly the assigned Primary Sequencing Codes are taken from the lower levels of the hierarchy. One to two Primary Sequencing Codes are allocated to each abstract.

Cross Reference Codes, which do not occur in every abstract, cover the secondary aspects of an article and refer to another relevant journal section. Where allocated, they are taken from the higher levels of the hierarchy. Four to five Cross Reference Codes may be assigned to an abstract. The Section Codes are up to ten characters long, prefixed by a two character abstract journal code. Different codes and headings are used in each abstract journal so two different codes may be allocated. Section Headings refer to chapter headings and are broader terms to the Section Codes which makes it possible to use them for coarse subdivisions of a subject. (See CAB Abstracts Online for further advice).

19:72. Online   BIS

File name	CABA
Start year	
Number of records	
Update period	

19:73. Online   BRS, Morning Search, BRS/Colleague

File name	
Start year	
Number of records	
Update period	Monthly
Price/Charges	Connect time: US$62.00/72.00
	Online print: US$0.47/0.55
	Offline print: US$0.55
	SDI charge: US$12.50

Downloading is allowed

Notes

Indexing is detailed and comprehensive using a controlled vocabulary.

19:74. Online   CISTI, Canadian Online Enquiry Service CAN/OLE

File name	CAB
Start year	
Number of records	
Update period	
Price/Charges	Connect time: Canadian $40.00
	Online print: Canadian $0.45
	Offline print: Canadian $0.45

Notes

CISTI accessible only in Canada.

19:75. Online — Data-Star

File name	CABI
Start year	1984
Number of records	1,000,000
Update period	Monthly
Database aids	Data-Star Biomedical, Business and Chemical Manuals. and Online manual (search NEWS-CABI in NEWS)
Price/Charges	Subscription: SFr80.00
	Connect time: SFr50.80
	Online print: SFr127.00
	Offline print: SFr1.01
	SDI charge: SFr12.40

Downloading is allowed
Thesaurus is online

Notes
From June 1993 Data-Star have introduced an annual fee/subscription per contract (that is, not per password) of SFr 80.00 (c.UK£ 32.00) payable every June. For North American customers billed in dollars who also use DIALOG, the DIALOG fee also covers access to Data-Star. Academic customers, 'commitment' customers and customers currently billed in dollars are exempt.

Record composition
Abstract AB; Accession Number and Update Code AN; Article Type AT; Author(s) AU; Author Affiliation IN; Descriptors DE; Foreign Title TT; Geographic Descriptor CN; ISBN Number IS; Language of summary in original LS; Original Language LG; Publication Year YR; References AV; Section heading(s) SC; Source SO; Title TI; Update Code UP and Updated Code UD

19:76. Online — DIALOG, Knowledge Index

File name	File 50
Start year	1972 – 1983
Number of records	13,000
Update period	Monthly
Price/Charges	Connect time: US$54.00
	Online print: US$0.90
	Offline print: US$0.90
	SDI charge: US$15.00

Downloading is allowed
Thesaurus is online

Notes
This database is also available to home users during evenings and weekends at a reduced rate on the Knowledge Index service of DIALOG – file name in this case is CAB ABSTRACTS, and searches are made with simplified commands or menus.

DIALINDEX Categories: AGRI, BIOTECH, CAB, ENVIRON, FOODSCI, LEISURE, NUTRIT, VETSCI. The One-Search facility enables the two files of AGRICOLA, the one file of AGRIS and the two files of CAB to be searched simultaneously.

19:77. Online — DIALOG, Knowledge Index

File name	File 53
Start year	1984
Number of records	2,500,000
Update period	Monthly
Price/Charges	Connect time: US$54.00
	Online print: US$0.90
	Offline print: US$0.90

Downloading is allowed

Notes
This database is also available to home users during evenings and weekends at a reduced rate on the Knowledge Index service of DIALOG – file name in this case is CAB ABSTRACTS, and searches are made with simplified commands or menus.

DIALINDEX Categories: AGRI, BIOTECH, CAB, ENVIRON, FOODSCI, LEISURE, NUTRIT, VETSCI.

19:78. Online — DIMDI

File name	CV72
Software	GRIPS
Start year	1972
Number of records	2,842,569
Update period	Monthly
SDI period	1 month
Database aids	Memocard CAB ABSTRACTS and User Manual CAB ABSTRACTS
Price/Charges	Connect time: UK£18.74–22.53
	Online print: UK£0.40–0.58
	Offline print: UK£0.33–0.40

Downloading is allowed
Thesaurus is online

Notes
Contains all citations included in the abstract journals of the CAB. Abstracted records are 82% of the total. The unit record contains information about author(s), title and other bibliographic data as well as institutions, keywords, subunit(s) and abstracts (eighty-four per cent). More complex subjects or clearly defined subject areas are represented in the following DIMDI subfiles consisting of one or several subunits which can be used like individual databases: CAB Ado; CAB Animal; CAB Animal Products; CAB Economics; CAB Engineering; CAB Forestry; CAB Human; CAB Nutrition; CAB Plant; CAB Plant Protection; CAB Leisure Recreation Tourism; CAB Veterinary Science. Suppliers of online documents: British Library Document Supply Centre, Boston Spa, England; Harkers Information Retrieval System, Sydney, Australia; Instituto de Informacion y Documentacion en Ciencia y Tecnologia, Madrid, Spain; Universitätsbibliothek und TIB, Hannover, Germany; Zentralbibliothek der Landbauwissenschaft, Bonn, Germany.

Record composition
Additional Author AA; Abstract AB; Abstractor's Initials AI; Abstract Language AL; Author AU; Author's Variants AV; Classification Code CC; Corporate Author CA; Corporate Source CS; Controlled Terms CT; Decimal Code DC; Document Type DT; Entry Date ED; Entry Month EM; Free Text FT; Geographical Codes GC; Geographical Heading GH; Journal Title JT; Language LA; Abstract Number NA; Document Number ND; Cross Reference Number NX; Original Field OF; Order Number OD; Publisher's Name PU; Preprocessed Searches PPS; Publication Year PY; ISBN SB; Section Code SC; Subfile SF; Section Headings SH; Source SO; Secondary Journal Source SSO; Subunit SU and Title TI

The Basic Index includes the data fields: Title, Abstract, Controlled Term, Section Heading, Geographical Heading. Controlled Terms from 1984 correspond to the polyhierarchic structured CAB thesaurus; prior to 1984: mixture of terms. Access points with Producer's equivalent name in brackets: Subunits (SU) (Abstract Journals); Section Codes (SC) (Sequencing Code Numbers); Section Headings (SH)

(Section Headings); Decimal Codes (DC) (Decimal Codes); Geographical Codes (GC) (Geographical Codes); Controlled Terms (CT) Subject Index Entries; Geographical Headings (GH) Countries.

19:79. Online — ESA-IRS

File name	File 124
Start year	1986+
Number of records	760,000
Update period	Monthly
Price/Charges	Subscription: UK£70.29
	Database entry fee: UK£3.51
	Online print: UK£0.07 – 0.60
	Offline print: UK£0.64
	SDI charge: UK£2.46

Downloading is allowed
Thesaurus is online

Notes

From 1993 ESA-IRS are charging an annual fee of 100 Accounting Units (c.UK£ 70.29) to all users. This is equivalent to the fee for full documentation and will not be charged to customers already paying for documentation.

Record composition

Abstract /AB; Abstract Journal AJ; Author AU; Bureau Bees Decimal Code (1) BD; CAB Record No. NR; Classification Code CC; Classification Name CN; Controlled Terms /CT; Corporate Source CS; Fertilizer Decimal Code (1) SD; Journal Announcement (Updates) UP; Journal Name JN; Language LA; Native Number NN; Publication Year PY; Publisher PB; Summary Language SL; Title /TI and UDC Number UC

19:80. Online — ESA-IRS

File name	File 132
Start year	1972+
Number of records	2,600,000
Update period	Monthly
Price/Charges	Subscription: UK£70.29
	Database entry fee: UK£3.51
	Online print: UK£0.07 – 0.60
	Offline print: UK£0.64
	SDI charge: UK£2.46

Downloading is allowed
Thesaurus is online

Notes

From 1993 ESA-IRS are charging an annual fee of 100 Accounting Units (c.UK£ 70.29) to all users. This is equivalent to the fee for full documentation and will not be charged to customers already paying for documentation.

Record composition

Abstract /AB; Abstract Journal AJ; Author AU; Bureau Bees Decimal Code (1) BD; CAB Record No. NR; Classification Code CC; Classification Name CN; Controlled Terms /CT; Corporate Source CS; Fertilizer Decimal Code (1) SD; Journal Announcement (Updates) UP; Journal Name JN; Language LA; Native Number NN; Publication Year PY; Publisher PB; Summary Language SL; Title /TI and UDC Number UC

19:81. Online — ESA-IRS

File name	File 16
Start year	1972–1985
Number of records	1,900,000
Update period	Closed File

Price/Charges	Subscription: UK£70.29
	Database entry fee: UK£3.51
	Online print: UK£0.07 – 0.60
	Offline print: UK£0.64
	SDI charge: UK£2.46

Downloading is allowed
Thesaurus is online

Notes

From 1993 ESA-IRS are charging an annual fee of 100 Accounting Units (c.UK£ 70.29) to all users. This is equivalent to the fee for full documentation and will not be charged to customers already paying for documentation.

Record composition

Abstract /AB; Abstract Journal AJ; Author AU; Bureau Bees Decimal Code (1) BD; CAB Record No. NR; Classification Code CC; Classification Name CN; Controlled Terms /CT; Corporate Source CS; Fertilizer Decimal Code (1) SD; Journal Announcement (Updates) UP; Journal Name JN; Language LA; Native Number NN; Publication Year PY; Publisher PB; Summary Language SL; Title /TI and UDC Number UC

19:82. Online — Japan Information Center of Science and Technology (JICST)

File name	CABA
Start year	1979
Number of records	1,590,000
Update period	Monthly
Price/Charges	Connect time: US$55.00
	Online print: US$0.20
	Offline print: US$0.20
	SDI charge: US$11.48

Downloading is allowed

Record composition

Abstract AB; Accession Number AN; Author AU; Broader Terms BT; Classification Codes CC; Controlled Terms CT; Corporate Source CS; Country of Publication CY; Document Type DT; Language LA; Source SO and Title TI

19:83. Online — STN

File name	CABA
Start year	1979
Number of records	1,900,000
Update period	Monthly
Price/Charges	Connect time: DM85.00
	Online print: DM1.34
	Offline print: DM1.42
	SDI charge: DM17.57

Also available on JICST.

19:84. Online — University of Tsukuba

File name	CAB Abstracts
Start year	
Number of records	
Update period	

Notes

Access through University of Tsukuba limited to affiliates of the University of Japan.

19:85. CD-ROM — SilverPlatter

File name	CABCD Vol.1 1984–86
Format notes	IBM, Mac, NEC
Software	SPIRS
Start year	1984–1986

Number of records
Update period — Annually
Database aids — Silverplatter CAB User Manual, Quick Reference Cards and SPIRS User Manual
Price/Charges — Subscription: UK£1,425–2,850
Thesaurus is online

Notes

Nearly sixty-five per cent of the records are drawn from English language sources, the remainder from articles in over 75 languages. Approximately ninety-five per cent of records have an English language abstract. CABCD has 930,000 records in total, with 130,000 records being added each year. It is available in separate discs as four volumes to date, dating from 1984 through to 1995. There are various price ranges depending on number of volumes purchased. Vol.1, 1984–1986, costs UK£ 1,425 for single users, £2,850 for 2–8 networked users.

Record composition

English language title; foreign language title (where appropriate); author; author's address; source title; citation details; publication year; publication type; language of original document; summary language; abstract; subject index terms; geographic index terms and subfile codes (CABI Abstract Journal code)

The Index command can be used to provide access to a list of all words, descriptors and hyphenated phrases which have been indexed in the free-text fields. The index excludes information present in the limit fields, such as language and date. The index is arranged alphabetically word by word, and can be browsed and terms selected which are then searched for automatically using the OR operator. Use of the Index shows up inevitable spelling mistakes.

19:86. CD-ROM SilverPlatter

File name — CABCD Vol.2 1987–89
Format notes — IBM, Mac, NEC
Software — SPIRS
Start year — 1987–1989
Number of records
Update period — Annually
Database aids — Silverplatter CAB User Manual, Quick Reference Cards and SPIRS User Manual
Price/Charges — Subscription: UK£2,850 5,700
Thesaurus is online

Notes

Nearly sixty-five per cent of the records are drawn from English language sources, the remainder from articles in over 75 languages. Approximately ninety-five per cent of records have an English language abstract. This is the second volume of CABCD. CABCD has 930,000 records in total, with 130,000 records being added each year. It is available in separate discs as four volumes to date, dating from 1984 through to 1995. There are various price ranges depending on number of volumes purchased: Vol.2, 1987–1989, £2,850 for single users, £5,700 for 2–8 networked users.

Record composition

English language title; foreign language title (where appropriate); author; author's address; source title; citation details; publication year; publication type; language of original document; summary language; abstract; subject index terms; geographic index terms and subfile codes (CABI Abstract Journal code)

The Index command can be used to provide access to

a list of all words, descriptors and hyphenated phrases which have been indexed in the free-text fields. The index excludes information present in the limit fields, such as language and date. The index is arranged alphabetically word by word, and can be browsed and terms selected which are then searched for automatically using the OR operator. Use of the Index shows up inevitable spelling mistakes.

19:87. CD-ROM SilverPlatter

File name — CABCD Vol.3 1990–92
Format notes — IBM, Mac, NEC
Software — SPIRS
Start year — 1990–92
Number of records
Update period — Annually
Database aids — Silverplatter CAB User Manual, Quick Reference Cards and SPIRS User Manual
Price/Charges — Subscription: UK£1,710–9,000
Thesaurus is online

Notes

Nearly sixty-five per cent of the records are drawn from English language sources, the remainder from articles in over 75 languages. Approximately ninety-five per cent of records have an English language abstract. CABCD has 930,000 records in total, with 130,000 records being added each year. This is the third volume of CABCD. It is available in separate discs as four volumes to date, dating from 1984 through to 1995. There are various price ranges depending on number of volumes purchased: Vol.3, 1990–1992, £3,845 for single users, £7,690 for 2–8 networked users; Vol.3 1992 renewal purchase £1,710 for single users, £3,420 for 2- 8 networked users.

Record composition

English language title; foreign language title (where appropriate); author; author's address; source title; citation details; publication year; publication type; language of original document; summary language; abstract; subject index terms; geographic index terms and subfile codes (CABI Abstract Journal code)

The Index command can be used to provide acces to a list of all words, descriptors and hyphenated phrases which have been indexed in the free-text fields. The index excludes information present in the limit fields, such as language and date. The index is arranged alphabetically word by word, and can be browsed and terms selected which are then searched for automatically using the OR operator. Use of the Index shows up inevitable spelling mistakes.

19:88. CD-ROM SilverPlatter

File name — CABCD Vol.4 1993–95
Format notes — IBM, Mac, NEC
Software — SPIRS
Start year — 1993–95
Number of records
Update period — Annually
Database aids — Silverplatter CAB User Manual, Quick Reference Cards and SPIRS User Manual
Price/Charges — Subscription: UK£4,500 – 9,000
Thesaurus is online

Notes

Nearly sixty-five per cent of the records are drawn from English language sources, the remainder from articles in over 75 languages. Approximately ninety-five per cent of records have an English language abstract. This is the prospective fourth volume of

CABCD. CABCD has 930,000 records in total, with 130,000 records being added each year. It is available in separate discs as four volumes to date, dating from 1984 through to 1995. There are various price ranges depending on number of volumes purchased: Vol.4 1993–1995 £4,500 for single users, £9,000 for 2–8 networked users. Prices on application for purchase of Vol.4 1993.

Record composition

English language title; foreign language title (where appropriate); author; author's address; source title; citation details; publication year; publication type; language of original document; summary language; abstract; subject index terms; geographic index terms and subfile codes (CABI Abstract Journal code)

The Index command can be used to provide access to a list of all words, descriptors and hyphenated phrases which have been indexed in the free-text fields. The index excludes information present in the limit fields, such as language and date. The index is arranged alphabetically word by word, and can be browsed and terms selected which are then searched for automatically using the OR operator. Use of the Index shows up inevitable spelling mistakes

19:89. Diskette CAB International

File name	CABI Abstract Journals on Floppy Disk
Format notes	IBM
Start year	
Number of records	
Update period	Same as for printed journal
Price/Charges	

Notes

Any one of the CAB International Abstract Journals may be received on floppy disk, according to the purchaser's requirements. Update frequency is the same as for the particular printed journal (monthly, bimonthly or quarterly). Price is double the cost of the equivalent printed journal. The diskettes are supplied without retrieval software, but the subscriber has the choice of three formats – comma delimited, CDS-ISIS or Pro-Cite – to enable use with most commercial database management software, with Micro CDS-ISIS or with Pro-Cite.

19:90. Database subset
Online BRS Online Service, Morning Search, BRS/Colleague

File name	CAB: Veterinary and Medical
Start year	1980–1990
Number of records	8,200
Update period	Monthly
Price/Charges	Connect time: US$62.00/72.00
	Online print: US$0.47/0.55
	Offline print: US$0.55
	SDI charge: US$12.50

Downloading is allowed

Notes

A subset of CAB Abstracts containing all documents from: *Index Veterinarius; Veterinary Bulletin; Reviews of Applied Entomology, Series B; Review of Medical and Veterinary Mycology; Nutrition Abstracts and Reviews, Series B; Helminthology Abstracts, Series A; Animal Disease Occurrence* (ceased publication 1989) and *Small Animal Abstracts* (ceased publication in 1989).

19:91. Database subset
Online Data-Star

File name	VETS
Start year	1984
Number of records	150,000
Update period	Monthly
Database aids	Data-Star Biomedical Manual
Price/Charges	Subscription: SFr80.00
	Connect time: SFr127.00
	Online print: SFr1.01
	Offline print: SFr1.04
	SDI charge: SFr12.40

Downloading is allowed
Thesaurus is online

Notes

A bibliographic source of information on all aspects of veterinary science and medicine. Documents comprising bibliographic details with or without an abstract are included for literature on all aspects of veterinary medicine. Subjects covered include: diseases of livestock, poultry, pets, laboratory animals, zoo animals, farmed fish and shellfish and certain wild animals; anatomy, physiology, biochemistry, pharmacology, surgery, radiography, toxicology, immunology and immunogenetics of domestic animals; bacteriology, virology, mycology, protozoology, helminthology and entomology related to animal diseases; zoonoses; meat inspection and economics of animal diseases. Abstracts sources include: *Veterinary Bulletin, Index Veterinarius and Small Animal Abstracts* and, in part, *Helminthological Abstracts, Review of Medical and Veterinary Entomology; Protozoological Abstracts, Review of Medical and Veterinary Mycology, Animal Breeding Abstracts, Diary Science Abstracts and Nutrition Abstracts and Reviews Series B, Livestock Feeds and Feeding.*

From June 1993 Data-Star have introduced an annual fee/subscription per contract (that is, not per password) of SFr 80.00 (c.UK£ 32.00) payable every June. For North American customers billed in dollars who also use DIALOG, the DIALOG fee also covers access to Data-Star. Academic customers, 'commitment' customers and customers currently billed in dollars are exempt.

Record composition

Abstract AB; Accession Number and Update Code AN; Article Type AT; Author AU; Author Affiliation IN; Description DE; Foreign Title TT; Geographic Descriptor CN; ISBN Number IS; Language of Original Summary; Original Language LG; Publication Year YR; Section code and heading SC; Source SO; Title TI and Update Code UP

19:92. Database subset
Online DIALOG, Knowledge Index

File name	File 250 – ONTAP CAB Abstracts Training File
Start year	January – March 1985
Number of records	34,388
Update period	Closed File
Price/Charges	Connect time: US$15.00

Notes

The low-cost training file containing records from the January to March 1985 updates to File 50, the main CAB Abstracts file on DIALOG. Offline prints are not available in ONTAP files.

19:93. Database subset
Online   DIMDI

File name	C473 – CAB NUTRITION
Start year	1973
Number of records	360,891
Update period	Monthly
SDI period	1 month
Price/Charges	Connect time: UK£18.74–22.53
	Online print: UK£0.40–0.58
	Offline print: UK£0.33–0.40

Downloading is allowed

Notes

Contains citations on human nutrition and animal feeding from CAB Abstracts. Searches are possible from January 1961. 95% of the records have abstracts.

CAB NUTRITION is defined as subfile to VCAB ABSTRACTS with: FIND SU=(0N;0U;1C;1N;2N).

19:94. Database subset
Online   DIMDI

File name	C773 – CAB ANIMAL PROD
Start year	1972
Number of records	541,364
Update period	Monthly
SDI period	1 month
Price/Charges	Connect time: UK£18.74–22.53
	Online print: UK£0.40–0.58
	Offline print: UK£0.33–0.40

Downloading is allowed

Notes

Contains the relevant citaions on animal breeding and production from CAB Abstracts. Journals referenced: *Animal Breeding Abstracts; Dairy Science Abstracts; Nutrition Abstracts and Reviews (B.Livestock Feeds and Feeding); Nutrition Abstracts* (1973–1976); *Poultry Abstracts; Pig News and Information.* Searches are possible from January 1973. 95% of the records have abstracts.

CAB ANIMAL PROD is defined as subfile to CAB ABASTRACTS with: FIND SU=(0A;0D;0N;1N;2N; 7A;7D).

19:95. Database subset
Online   DIMDI

File name	C872 – CAB VET SCIENCE
Start year	1972
Number of records	678,064
Update period	Monthly
SDI period	1 month
Price/Charges	Connect time: UK£18.74–22.53
	Online print: UK£0.40–0.58
	Offline print: UK£0.33–0.40

Downloading is allowed

Notes

Contains citations on veterinary science from CAB Abstracts. Journals referenced: *Helminothological Abstracts (A. Animal and Human); Index Veterinarius; Review of Applied Entomology (B. Medical and Veterinary); Review of Medical and Veterinary Mycology; Veterinary Bulletin; Protozoological Abstracts* (from 1977); *Animal Disease Occurrence* (from 1980); *Small Animal Abstracts* (from 1984). Searches are possible from January 1972. 95% of the records have abstracts.

CAB VET SCIENCE is defined as subfile to CAB ABSTRACTS with: FIND SU= (0H;0I;0L;0V;0Y; 2V;7V).

19:96. Database subset
Online   DIMDI

File name	C980 – CAB ADO
Alternative name(s)	Animal Disease Occurrence
Start year	1980
Number of records	
Update period	Twice a year
Price/Charges	Connect time: UK£18.74–22.53
	Online print: UK£0.40–0.58
	Offline print: UK£0.33–0.40

Downloading is allowed

Notes

Equivalent to the printed *Animal Disease Occurrence.* Covers epidemiology of animal diseases. Contains records on the incidence of animal diseases worldwide. Data include the country of occurrence, number of animals affected, duration of the disease, number of deaths, and economic effects. Each record includes a citation to the source publication. All documents have abstracts. Approximately ninety per cent of the ADO documents are also published in the Veterinary Bulletin but without additional factual data.

Record composition
Animal Species ANI

19:97. Database subset
Online   DIMDI

File name	CX72 – CAB ANIMAL
Start year	1972
Number of records	1,629,488
Update period	Monthly
SDI period	1 month
Price/Charges	Connect time: UK£18.74–22.53
	Online print: UK£0.40–0.58
	Offline print: UK£0.33–0.40

Downloading is allowed

Notes

Contains the animal relevant documents of CAB Abstracts. Journals referenced: *Animal Breeding Abstracts; Apicultural Abstracts; Dairy Science Abstracts; Helminthological Abstracts (A. Animal and Human); Index Veterinarius; Review of Applied Entomology (B. Medical and Veterinary); Review of Applied Entomology (B. Medical and Veterinary); Review of Medical and Veterianry Mycology; Nutrition Abstracts and Reviews (A. Human and Experimental)* (from 1977); *World Agricultural Economics and Rural Sociology Abstracts; Nutrition Abstracts and Reviews (A. Human and Experimental); Veterinary Bulletin; Protozoological Abstracts* (from 1977); *Nutrition Abstracts* (1973–1976); *Rural Extension, Education and Training Abstracts* (from 1978); *Rural Development Abstracts; Animal Disease Occurence; Leisure, Recreation and Tourism Abstracts; Poultry Abstracts; Pig News and Information; Biocontrol News and Information; Biodeterioration Abstracts; Small Animal Abstracts; Agricultural Engineering Abstracts.* Searches are possible from January 1972. 70% of the records have abstracts.

19:98. Database subset
Online   ESA-IRS

File name	File 112 – Training CAB Abstracts
Start year	1984/5
Number of records	28,000
Update period	None
Thesaurus is online	

Notes

Training file and subset of the full CAB Abstracts file which has the file numbers 16 (1972–1985), 124 (1986 to date) and 132 (1972 to date). It is available at a low access fee for user training. Services such as offline prints, automatic curent awareness and document ordering are not available with the traiing file.

Record composition

Abstract /AB; Abstract Journal AJ; Author AU; CAB Record Number NR; Classification Codes CC; Classification Names CN; Controlled Terms /CT; Corporate Source CS; Journal Announcement (Updates) UP; Journal Name JN; Language LA; Native Accession Number NN; Publication Year PY; Publisher PB; Summary Language SL; Title /TI and UDC Numbers UC

19:99. Database subset

CD-ROM   **SilverPlatter**

File name	BeastCD (CAB Spectrum series)
Alternative name(s)	CABBeastCD (CAB Spectrum series)
Format notes	IBM, Mac, NEC
Software	SPIRS/MacSPIRS
Start year	1973
Number of records	340,000
Update period	Annually
Price	UK£2,890 – 5,780
	Subscription: UK£910 – 1,820

Notes

Subset of CAB Abstracts database covering: animal breeding and production, animal nutrition, dairy science and technology; management and biotechnology of economically valuable animals and of laboratory species relevant to agriculture. Contains all records published in *Animal Breeding Abstracts* (1983-), *Nutrition Abstracts and Reviews-Series B: Livestock Feeds and Feeding* (1931-) and relevant records from *Dairy Science Abstracts* (1939-), *Pig News and Information*, *Poultry Abstracts* and *AgBiotech News and Information*. Animals covered include farm mammals of economic importance; laboratory mammals; poultry; game and other birds of economic importance; fish, molluscs, and crustaceans; and certain invertebrates used in genetic studies. Subjects covered include performance traits and products; breeding and genetics; biotechnology; reproduction; nutrition; the dairy industry; housing and equipment for livestock and in aquaculture; and non-genetic effects on animals and traits.

A full set of archival discs covering 1973–1991 is available for outright purchase at UK£ 2,890 for single user, £5,780 for 2–8 networked users (member country). Annual renewal costs are £910 for single users, £1,820 for 2–8 networked users (member country). There are various journals options and print/updates prices on application to CAB or SilverPLatter. There is also a VetCD/BeastCD combined set available: full set £5,495 for single users, £10,990 for 2–8 networked users; annual renewal £1,655 for single users, £3,310 for 2–8 networked users.

In-depth indexing, using controlled terms from the *CAB Thesaurus.*

19:100. Database subset

CD-ROM   **SilverPlatter**

File name	VetCD (CAB Spectrum series)
Alternative name(s)	CABVetCD (CAB Spectrum series)
Format notes	IBM, Mac, NEC
Software	SPIRS/MacSPIRS

Start year	1973
Number of records	300,000
Update period	Annually
Price	UK£3,980 – 7,960
	Subscription: UK£1,155 – 2,310

Notes

Covers veterinary science and relevant records from CAB Abstracts database in such areas as protozoology; mycology; helminthology; and applied entomology. Contains abstracts and citations published in the following CABI abstract journals: *Index Veterinarius* (1933–), *Veterinary Bulletin* (1931–), *Helminthological Abstracts, Protozoological Abstracts, Review of Medical and Veterinary Entomology* and *Review of Medical and Veterinary Mycology*. Animals covered include farm animals, pets and game animals; all animals of economic importance including farmed fish and shellfish; commercially important wild fish; zoo animals and wild animals. Other subjects covered include: viral and bacterial diseases, arthropod parasites, toxicology, immunology, pharmacology, biochemistry, food inspection and other related areas.

Archival disc covering 1973–1991 is available for outright purchase at UK£3,980 for single users, £7,960 for 2–8 networked users (member country). Annual renewals cost UK£1,155 for single users, £2,310 for 2–8 networked users. There are various journals options and print/updates prices on application to CAB or SilverPLatter. There is also a VetCD/BeastCD combined set available: full set £5,495 for single users, £10,990 for 2–8 networked users; annual renewal £1,655 for single users, £3,310 for 2–8 networked users.

In-depth indexing using controlled terms from the *CAB Thesaurus.*

This database can also be found on:
Human Nutrition on CD-ROM

Cambridge Scientific Abstracts Life Sciences

Cambridge Scientific Abstracts

19:102. Master record

Alternative name(s)	CSAL
Database type	Bibliographic
Number of journals	
Sources	Journals, Books, Conference papers, Technical reports, Patents, Theses and Dissertations
Start year	1978
Language	English
Coverage	International
Number of records	1,164,810
Update size	–
Update period	Monthly

Keywords

Acute Poisoning; Aging; Air Pollution; Algology; Amino-Acids; Anatomy; Antibiotics; Aquaculture; Atmospheric Science; Bacteriology; Behavioural Ecology; Bioengineering; Biological Membranes; Biotechnology; Bone Disease; Calcium Metabolism; Chemoreception; Chronic Poisoning; Clinical Medicine; Clinical Toxicology; DNA; Drugs; Ecology; Ecosystems; Endocrinology; Entomology – Agricultural; Entomology – Applied; Entomology – Human; Entomology – Veterinary; Environmental

Biology; Ethology; Genetic Engineering; Hazardous Substances; HIV; Histology; Human Ecology; Immune Disorders; Immunology; Infectious Diseases; Land Pollution; Marine Biotechnology; Marine Engineering; Microbiology; Molecular Biology; Molecular Neurobiology; Mycology; Naval Engineering; Noise Pollution; Oceanography; Neurology; Neuropharmacology; Neurophysiology – Animal; Neuroscience; Nucleic Acids; Nutrition; Oncology; Occupational Health and Safety; Osteoporosis; Osteomalacia; Pathology; Peptides; Pharmaceuticals; Pheromones; Physiology; Pollution; Proteins; Protozoology; Psychophysics; Public Health; Radiation; Rhinology; RNA; Sleep; Smoking; Substance Abuse; Taste Perception; Thermal Pollution; Viral Genetics; Water; Water Pollution

Description

A superfile providing access to the following abstracting services:

Life Sciences Collection;
Aquatic Sciences and Fisheries Abstracts;
Oceanic Abstracts; and
Pollution Abstracts.

Covers the worldwide technical literature on medical and biological disciplines from journals, books, conference papers, technical reports, patents, theses and dissertations.

19:103. Online   BRS

File name	Cambridge Scientific Abstracts Life Sciences
Alternative name(s)	CSAL
Start year	1978
Number of records	1,164,810
Update period	Monthly

Notes

A superfile providing access to the following abstracting services: the Life Science Collection, Aquatic Sciences and Fisheries Abstracts, Oceanic Abstracts and Pollution Abstracts.

For more details of constituent databases, see:
Life Sciences Collection
Aquatic Sciences and Fisheries Abstracts
Oceanic Abstracts
Pollution Abstracts

CompuKennel Online Information Network

CompuKennel Information Service Inc

19:105. Master record

Database type	Directory, Textual
Number of journals	
Sources	
Start year	Racing statistics, most recent 3 months
Language	English
Coverage	USA
Number of records	
Update size	–
Update period	Varies; Racing statistics, daily

Keywords

Animal Breeding; Animal Racing; Sport

Description

Contains information on greyhound racing and breeding. For each dog, includes the names of its owner and trainer, established racing weight, the racetrack at which it is currently running and its track performance, and evaluation of its racing history according to various performance criteria. Also provides bloodstock information containing an animal's certificate of registry data, including date whelped, names of sire and dam, litter number, and left and right ear tattoo numbers. Breeding information covers each animal's bloodline for five generations. Also contains articles dealing with issues in veterinary care, a medical question and answer forum, and online advertising for racing dogs, brood stock, and industry services and equipment.

Sources include materials supplied by the National Greyhound Association.

19:106. Online   CompuKennel Information Service Inc

File name	
Start year	Racing statistics, most recent 3 months
Number of records	
Update period	Racing statistics, daily

CRIS/USDA Current Research Information System

US Department of Agriculture, Cooperative State Research Service

19:107. Master record

Alternative name(s)	Current Research Information System
Database type	Directory
Number of journals	
Sources	Project descriptions
Start year	New, ongoing and recently completed projects; terminated projects retained for 2 years
Language	English
Coverage	USA
Number of records	37,326
Update size	5,400
Update period	Monthly

Keywords

Community Development; Conservation; Food and Drink; Forestry; Health and Safety; Nutrition

Description

Contains descriptions of ongoing and recently completed research projects in agriculture, forestry, biology, and related life sciences. Covers research sponsored or conducted USDA research agencies, state agricultural experiment stations, state forestry and veterinary medicine schools, and other cooperating state institutions in the biological, physical, social, and behavioural sciences. The database includes the HNRIMS subfile, which contains project information on human nutrition research of USDA, NIH and other federal agencies. CRIS records include summaries of the objectives and approach used in the research. Annual progress and publication reports are also included for most records. Covers natural resource conservation and management; crop and livestock production; plant and animal protection; product development; marketing and economics; food and nutrition; consumer health and safety; family life; housing; rural development; environmental protection; forestry; outdoor recreation; and community, area, and regional development.

19:108. Online — DIALOG

File name	File 60
Alternative name(s)	Current Research Information System
Start year	New, ongoing and recently completed projects; terminated projects retained for 2 years
Number of records	37,326
Update period	Monthly
Price/Charges	Connect time: US$45.00
	Offline print: US$0.15

19:109. CD-ROM — SilverPlatter

File name	
Alternative name(s)	Current Research Information System
Start year	New, ongoing and recently completed projects; terminated projects retained for 2 years
Number of records	35,115
Update period	Monthly

This database can also be found on:
Agrisearch

CRYINFO
Institut Problem Kriobiologii i Kriomedizinij

19:111. Master record

Database type	Bibliographic
Number of journals	
Sources	
Start year	1962
Language	English
Coverage	
Number of records	2,800
Update size	—
Update period	

Keywords

Cryobiology

Description

Cryobiology information system.

19:112. Diskette — Institut Problem Kriobiologii i Kriomedizinij

File name	
Start year	1962
Number of records	2,800
Update period	

CSIRO Research in Progress
Commonwealth Scientific Industrial Research Organization

19:113. Master record

Alternative name(s)	SIRO
Database type	Directory
Number of journals	
Sources	Project descriptions and Research communications
Start year	Current information
Language	English
Coverage	Australia

Number of records	265
Update size	—
Update period	Annually
Index unit	Research programmes and Project

Keywords

Information Science; Manufacturing; Nutrition

Description

Contains references to current CSIRO-sponsored research programmes and associated projects. Covers programmes in animal health, biotechnology, human nutrition, agriculture, water and land resource management, manufacturing, minerals processing, and information science. Includes programme name and description, division name, address, and telephone number, and programme leaders. For each research project, includes title and description, research organisation name and location, and associated research programme.

Data are obtained from surveys of CSIRO divisions. Corresponds to the *Directory of CSIRO Research Programs*.

19:114. Online — CSIRO Australis

File name	
Alternative name(s)	SIRO
Start year	Current information
Number of records	265
Update period	Annually

Current Contents Search Bibliographic Database
Institute for Scientific Information

19:115. Master record

Database type	Bibliographic
Number of journals	1,300
Sources	Journals
Start year	Most recent twelve months
Language	English
Coverage	International
Number of records	1,547,676
Update size	728,000
Update period	Weekly
Index unit	Articles, reviews, letters, notes and Editorials

Keywords

Applied Science; Atmospheric Science; Clinical Medicine; Immunology; Inorganic Chemistry; Molecular Biology; Neuroscience; Organic Chemistry; Polymers; Statistics; Astrophysics; Spectroscopy; Pathology; Physics; Water Supply

Description

Contains citations to articles listed in the tables of content of leading journals in the sciences, social sciences, and arts and humanities. There are seven subsets:

Clinical medicine (CLIN): Covers a broad range of disciplines including: allergy, anaesthesiology, biomethods, cardiology, clinical and medicinal chemistry, clinical psychiatry, dentistry, dermatology, epidemiology, family medicine, gastroenterology and hepatology, general and internal medicine, geriatrics and gerontology, hematology, infectious diseases, medical technology and laboratory medicine, neurology, oncology, ophthalmology, orthopedics, otorhinolaryngology, paediatrics, pharmacy, physical medicine and rehabilitation, radiology and nuclear medicine, reproductive systems, respiratory medicine, sports sciences, surgery, and urology.

Life sciences (LIFE): Covers: anatomy, biochemistry, biophysics, cytology, endocrinology, experimental medicine, experimental biology, genetics, gerontology, hematology, histology, immunology, microbiology, molecular biology, neuroscience, parasitology, pathology, pharmaceutical chemistry, pharmacology, physiology, radiology and nuclear medicine, toxicology and virology.

Arts and humanities (ARTS).

Engineering, technology, and applied sciences (ENG):

Social and behavioural sciences (BEHA): Covers business, economics, education, geography, history, law, library and information science, management, planning and development, political science, psychiatry, psychology, public health, rehabilitation, sociology.

Agriculture, biology, and environmental sciences (AGRI): Covers agricultural chemistry, economics, engineering, agronomy, animal behaviour, animal husbandry, applied microbiology, biotechnology, botany, conservation, crop science, dairy science, ecology, entomology, environmental sciences, fishery science and technology, forestry, horticulture, marine biology, mycology, nutrition, oceanology, orinthology, pest control, soil science, taxonomy, veterinary medicine and pathology, water research and engineering, wildlife management and zoology.

Physical, chemical, and earth sciences (PHYS): Covers analytical chemistry, applied physics, astronomy, astrophysics, atmospheric sciences, chemical physics, chemistry, condensed matter, crystallography, geology and geophysics, inorganic and nuclear chemistry, mathematics, meteorology, nuclear physics, organic chemistry, paleontology, physical chemistry, physics, polymer chemistry, spectroscopy, statistics and probability.

Includes title, authors, bibliographic data, abstracts and keywords, and, when available, reprint authors' addresses.

Current Contents Search is the online version of ISI's popular Current Contents series of publications. Current Contents is a weekly service that reproduces the tables of contents from current issues of leading journals in the sciences, social sciences, and arts and humanities. All ISI databases have a linked service known as The Genuine Article which can deliver the full text of located articles by mail, facsimile transmission or courier. Orders can be placed via the host service in use, mail, facsimile transmission, telephone or telex. Diskette products have a single-keystroke order information facility. The minimum charge is US$ 11.25 within USA and Canada and US$ 12.20 elsewhere.

Leading journals in the sciences, social sciences, and arts and humanities.

Keywords supplied by the author are included. In addition, ISI adds Keywords Plus which are generated by analysis of titles of articles that appear in the list of citations.

19:116. Online — BRS, Morning Search, BRS/Colleague

File name	CBIB
Start year	
Number of records	
Update period	
Price/Charges	Connect time: US$85.00/95.00
	Online print: US$0.57/0.65
	Offline print: US$0.65
	SDI charge: US$6.50

Notes

The database is a twelve month rolling file. A special print format, CONT, allows the user to print a Table of Contents format that closely mirrors the print product.

19:117. Online — BRS, Morning Search, BRS/Colleague

File name	CTOC
Alternative name(s)	Current Contents Search Tables of Contents Database
Start year	Most recent twelve months
Number of records	1,547,676
Update period	Weekly
Price/Charges	Connect time: US$85.00/95.00
	Online print: US$1.45/1.53
	Offline print: US$1.33
	SDI charge: US$6.50

Notes

A special print format, CONT, allows the user to print a Table of Contents format that closely mirrors the print product.

19:118. Online — Data-Star

File name	CCCC
Start year	1992 (March)
Number of records	
Update period	Weekly
Price/Charges	Subscription: SFr80.00
	Connect time: SFr150.00
	Online print: SFr1.27 – 3.30
	Offline print: SFr1.59 – 3.62
	SDI charge: SFr10.00

Notes

The database is a twelve month rolling file.

CCCC contains single bibliographic records; the contents page of a journal issue is attached to ONE of the documents from that issue. CCCC may be searched as a conventional bibliographic file and the results printed out in the normal way or by limiting the search with command CP=CP results will be limited to records containing the contents pages, these may then be printed out (.P CP 1). As the Genuine Article document ordering number is appended to each record, it is possible to search in that number (for example, JY699.GA.) – the result will show the number of articles in that issue and thus the length of the contents page. Some journals have extremely long contents pages and it is useful to know before printing. The SF field indicates in which other ISI databases the same record appears. Type DOCZ at any time to find the total number of records currently in the database.

From June 1993 Data-Star have introduced an annual fee/subscription per contract (that is, not per password) of SFr 80.00 (c.UK£ 32.00) payable every June. For North American customers billed in dollars who also use DIALOG, the DIALOG fee also covers access to Data-Star. Academic customers, 'commitment' customers and customers currently billed in dollars are exempt.

Record composition

Accession Number AN; Occurence Table OC; Author AU; Institution IN; Country Name CN; Title TI; Source SO; Page Numbers PP; ISSN IS; Publication Year YR; Language LG; Journal Category JC; Publication

Type PT; Genuine Article Number GA; Descriptors DE; Keywords Plus KP; Author Keywords KW; Current Contents Edition CC; Supplementary File SF; Number of Cited References NU (Display only); Abstract Availability AV; Abstract AB; Contents Page CP; Update yymmdd UD (Limit only) and Update yymm UP (Limit only)

19:119. Online   DIALOG

File name	File 440
Start year	Current six months to one year
Number of records	1,477,528
Update period	Weekly
Price/Charges	Connect time: US$102.00
	Online print: US$0.80 – 2.10
	Offline print: US$0.80 – 2.10
	SDI charge: US$7.00

19:120. Tape   Institute for Scientific Information

File name	Current Contents Search
Format notes	Tape reels: 6250 BPI (EBCDIC or ASCII), fixed 90-character records. Cartridges: 38,000 BPI (EBCDIC or ASCII), fixed 90-character records. Both tapes and cartridges have a block size of 9,000 records.
Start year	Most recent twelve months
Number of records	1,547,676
Update period	Weekly

Notes
The tape provides the same coverage as other Current Contents products and allows searching within and across as many of the individual editions as required.

Includes author keywords, Key Words Plus, author addresses and searchable English-language abstracts.

19:121. Database subset
Online   BRS, Morning Search, BRS/Colleague

File name	AGRI
Alternative name(s)	CBIB: Agriculture, Biology, and Environmental Sciences
Start year	
Number of records	
Update period	
Price/Charges	Connect time: US$85.00/95.00
	Online print: US$0.57/0.65
	Offline print: US$0.65

Notes
A special print format, CONT, allows the user to print a Table of Contents format that closely mirrors the print product.

19:122. Database subset

Online   DIMDI

File name	I183 – SCIAGRI
Software	GRIPS
Start year	1983
Number of records	889,860
Update period	Weekly
SDI period	1 week
Database aids	User Manual SCISEARCH/SOCIAL SCISEARCH and Memocard SCISEARCH
Price/Charges	Connect time: UK£14.41–20.32 (Group I); 15.57–23.24 (Group II); 18.50–43.71 (Group III) Online print: UK£0.39–0.57 Offline print: UK£0.31–0.37

Downloading is allowed

Notes
SCIAGRI corresponds to the Current Contents edition Agriculture, Biology and Environmental Sciences. Approximately eleven per cent of records contain abstracts. Searches are possible from January 1983. There are preferential costs for subscribers to the printed product. Groups shown for pricing refer to: 1. Users in the Federal Republic of Germany active in the field of biosciences, with the exception of private companies. Under temporary federal grant there is a rebate for this group of users; 2. Other users who are subscribers of the equivalent printed product. These users have to inform ISI that they wish this preferential rate; 3. Other users who are not subscribers of the equivalent printed product.

Record composition
Abstract AB; Abstract Indicators AI; Author AU; Author's Keywords IT; Cluster Code CC; Cluster Term CT; Cluster Weight /W; Corporate Country CCO; Corporate Source CS; Document Type DT; Entry Date ED; Free Text FT; Journal Title JT; Keywords Plus UT; Language LA; Number of Document ND; Number of References RN; Publication Year PY; Reference RF; Referenced Journal RJ; Referenced Patent No. RP; Subject Code SC; Subject Heading SH; Source SO; Subunit SU and Title TI

The basic index includes the following data fields: Title, Controlled Term, Index Term, Uncontrolled Term and Abstract.

19:123. Database subset
Online   DIMDI

File name	IL89 – Current Contents/SciSearch
Software	GRIPS
Start year	Latest 12 months
Number of records	729,304
Update period	Weekly
SDI period	1 week
Database aids	User Manual SCISEARCH/Social SCISEARCH and Memocard SCISEARCH
Price/Charges	Connect time: UK£14.41–20.32 (Group I); 15.57–23.24 (Group II); 18.50–43.71 (Group III) Online print: UK£0.39–0.57 Offline print: UK£0.31–0.37

Downloading is allowed

Notes
This is a separate database on DIMDI of Current Contents/ SciSearch. IL89 contains the documents of the last twelve months from Social SciSearch. It corresponds to the subject content of SciSearch, the only difference from the main file on DIMDI (IS74) is the output format. Suppliers of online documents: British Library Document Supply Centre, Boston Spa, England; Harkers Information Retrieval System, Sydney, Australia; The Information Store, San Francisco, USA; Institute for Scientific Information, Philadelphia, USA.

There are preferential costs for subscribers to the printed product. Groups shown for pricing refer to: 1. Users in the Federal Republic of Germany active in the field of biosciences, with the exception of private companies. Under temporary federal grant there is a rebate for this group of users; 2. Other users who are subscribers of the equivalent printed product. These users have to inform ISI that they wish this preferential rate; 3. Other users who are not subscribers of the equivalent printed product.

Record composition

Abstract Indicator AI; Abstract AB; Author AU; Author's Keywords IT; Cluster Code CC; Corporate Country CCO; Corporate Source CS; Document Type DT; Entry Date ED; Free Text FT; Index Term IT; Journal Title JT; Keywords Plus UT; Language LA; Number of Document ND; Number of References RN; Publication Year PY; Reference RF; Referenced Journal RJ; Referenced Patent No. RP; Source SO; Subject Code SC; Subject Heading SH; Subunit SU; Title TI and Uncontrolled Term (Keywords Plus) UT

After the SHOW-, PRINT or DLOAD- command the output of documents is displayed in the table of contents format. The basic index includes the data fields: Title, Index Term and Uncontrolled Term.

19:124. Database subset

Diskette	Institute for Scientific Information
File name	Current Contents on Diskette – Agriculture, Biology, Environmental Sciences
Format notes	IBM, NEC, Mac
Software	Proprietary Vn.3.0
Start year	
Number of records	
Update period	Weekly
Price/Charges	Subscription: US$427

Notes

Contains citations to articles listed in the tables of contents of about 1,000 journals and 300 book series in agriculture, environment and the life sciences. Equivalent to the print *Current Contents/Agriculture, Biology & Environmental Sciences*; and in part to the Current Contents Search online database.

Reduced subscription for print subscribers. The latest version of the software (August 1992) allows search profiles to be run against six issues at one time; better file compression to use less hard disk space; expanded online, context sensitive help; better truncation (including left-hand) facilities; and new output options. KeyWords Plus (tm) provides users with search terms taken from an article's bibliography: in this way users should identify many more articles. KeyWords Plus (tm) also allows users to determine on inspection how closely the article pertains to their area of interest. Users are now also able to transfer multiple search terms from the dictionaries to search statements.

Record composition

ISBN; ISSN and Publisher

19:125. Database subset

Diskette	Institute for Scientific Information
File name	Current Contents on Diskette with Abstracts – Agriculture, Biology, Environmental Sciences
Format notes	IBM, NEC, Mac
Software	Proprietary Vn.3.0
Start year	
Number of records	
Update period	Weekly
Price/Charges	Subscription: US$750

Notes

Contains citations with abstracts to articles listed in the tables of contents of about 1,000 journals and 300 book series in agriculture, environment and the life sciences. Equivalent to the print *Current Contents/*

Agriculture, Biology & Environmental Sciences; and in part to the Current Contents Search online database.

Reduced subscription for print subscribers. The latest version of the software (August 1992) allows search profiles to be run against six issues at one time; better file compression to use less hard disk space; expanded online, context sensitive help; better truncation (including left-hand) facilities; and new output options. KeyWords Plus (tm) provides users with search terms taken from an article's bibliography: in this way users should identify many more articles. KeyWords Plus (tm) also allows users to determine on inspection how closely the article pertains to their area of interest. Users are now also able to transfer multiple search terms from the dictionaries to search statements.

Record composition

ISBN; ISSN and Publisher

19:126. Database subset

Tape	Institute for Scientific Information
File name	CC Search/Agriculture, Biology & Environmental Sciences
Start year	Current
Number of records	
Update period	Weekly
Price/Charges	Subscription: US$15,000 – 18,750

Notes

Contains citations to articles listed in the tables of contents of about 1,000 journals and 300 book series in agriculture, environment and the life sciences. Equivalent to the print *Current Contents/Agriculture, Biology & Environmental Sciences*; and in part to the Current Contents Search online database.

Reduced subscription for print subscribers. The latest version of the software (August 1992) allows search profiles to be run against six issues at one time; better file compression to use less hard disk space; expanded online, context sensitive help; better truncation (including left-hand) facilities; and new output options. KeyWords Plus (tm) provides users with search terms taken from an article's bibliography: in this way users should identify many more articles. KeyWords Plus (tm) also allows users to determine on inspection how closely the article pertains to their area of interest. Users are now also able to transfer multiple search terms from the dictionaries to search statements.

Annual lease price is $15,000 (academic), $18,750 (corporate).

Record composition

ISBN; ISSN and Publisher

Danmarks Veterinaer-og Jordbrugsbase

Danmarks Veterinaer og Jordbrugsbibliotek (Danish Veterinary and Agricultural Library)

IS Datacentralen

19:127. Master record

Database type	Bibliographic, Library catalogue/cataloguing aids
Number of journals	
Sources	Monographs
Start year	1979
Language	Danish
Coverage	Denmark
Number of records	15,252
Update size	2,000
Update period	Every second year

Keywords
Animal Husbandry; Horticulture

Description
The database contains references to books in Danmarks Veterinar- og Jordbrugsbibliotek (Danish Veterinary and Agricultural Library) since 1979. Subjects covered: agriculture, forestry and horticulture, foodstuffs, biochemistry, veterinary medicine and animal husbandry. DVJB in included in both ALBVA and ALIS.

19:128. Online　　　　　　DC Host Centre

File name	DVJB
Start year	1979
Number of records	15,252
Update period	Every second year
Price/Charges	Connect time: Danish kroneFree

19:129. Online　　　　　　DTB

File name	DVJB
Start year	1979
Number of records	15,252
Update period	Every second year

19:130. Online　　Forskningsbibliotekernes EDB Kontor

File name	DVJB
Start year	1979
Number of records	15,252
Update period	Every second year

This database can also be found on:
ALBA
ALIS

Database of the Moscow Institute of Thermal Engineering
Moskowskii Institut Tjeplotechniki

19:132. Master record

Database type	Bibliographic
Number of journals	
Sources	
Start year	
Language	English
Coverage	
Number of records	6,000
Update size	—
Update period	

Keywords
Food Products; Beverages; Nutritive Engineering

Description
Database on food and nutritive engineering.

19:133. Diskette　　Moskowskii Institut Tjeplotechniki

File name	Database of the Moscow Institute of Thermal Engineering
Start year	
Number of records	6,000
Update period	

Database on Pesticide Control Systems
Institut eksperimentalnoj Meteorologie

19:134. Master record

Database type	Bibliographic, Factual
Number of journals	
Sources	
Start year	1985
Language	English
Coverage	
Number of records	
Update size	
Update period	

Keywords
Pesticides; Public Administration

Description
Contains factual data on pesticide control means.

19:135. Diskette　　Institut eksperimentalnoj Meteorologie

File name	
Start year	1985
Number of records	
Update period	

Database on Planned Publications
NPO 'Wjesojusnaja knishnaja Palata'

19:136. Master record

Database type	Bibliographic
Number of journals	
Sources	
Start year	
Language	English
Coverage	
Number of records	100,000
Update size	—
Update period	

Description
General future publications in the USSR.

19:137. Other media　　NPO 'Wjesojusnaja knishnaja Palata'

File name	
Start year	

Number of records   100,000
Update period

DHSS-MEDTEH
UK Departments of Health and Social Security Library

19:140. Master record

Alternative name(s)	Medical Toxicology and Environmental Health
Database type	Bibliographic, Textual
Number of journals	2,000
Sources	Administrative circulars, books, conference proceedings, government documents, government publications, journals, pamphlets, official publications and reports
Start year	1888
Language	English
Coverage	International
Number of records	26,600
Update size	—
Update period	Weekly
Index unit	Articles
Thesaurus	DHSS-Data Thesaurus, Dept of Health, London, 1985

Keywords

Air Pollution; Cancer; Cosmetics; Food Additives; Food Contaminants; Laboratory Practice; Mutation; Noise Pollution; Nutrition; Pesticides; Radiation Biology; Smoking; Veterinary Medicines; Water Pollution

Description

DHSS-MEDTECH offers specialised information covering medical toxicology and environmental health, using the resources of the Department of Health library in London. It includes more strictly scientific and medical information than the wider ranging DHSS-DAT database. It contains citations with abstracts to literature on environmental, chemical, toxicological, food and nutrition issues, and includes more strictly scientific and medical information in these subject areas than the wider ranging DHSS-DATA database. Subjects covered include: government and regulatory authorities, carcinogenicity and mutagenicity, chemicals in food (such as contaminants, preservatives and additives); consumer products; industrial chemicals; pesticides, radiation, air, water and noise pollution; radiation biology; veterinary medicines; laboratory practices; cosmetics; toxicology and the health consequences of smoking. An important feature of the database is the inclusion of full details, including sources of supply, of DOH publications.

Materials from 1888 to 1983 have recently been added to the database. Abstracts are available for documents added to the database from 1984.

The data field Note contains information such as: bibliography, annual, named individuals and additional publication details. DHMT covers a variety of multi-word sources, not all of which are hyphenated, for example details of monographs, reports, etc. These should be searched in freetext using adjacency operators to link terms and qualified by the use of .SO.

19:141. Online   Data-Star

File name	DHMT
Alternative name(s)	Medical Toxicology and Environmental Health
Start year	1888
Number of records	26,600
Update period	Weekly
Database aids	Data-Star Biomedical Manual and Online manual (search NEWS-DHMT in NEWS)
Price/Charges	Subscription: SFr80.00
	Connect time: SFr127.20
	Online print: SFr0.39
	Offline print: SFr0.80
	SDI charge: SFr6.80

Notes

To search DHSS-DATA and DHSS-MEDTEH simultaneously use the DHZZ-Superlabel.

From June 1993 Data-Star have introduced an annual fee/subscription per contract (that is, not per password) of SFr 80.00 (c.UK£ 32.00) payable every June. For North American customers billed in dollars who also use DIALOG, the DIALOG fee also covers access to Data-Star. Academic customers, 'commitment' customers and customers currently billed in dollars are exempt.

Record composition

Accession Number and Update Code AN; Author(s) AU; Corporate Author(s) CA; Descriptor(s) DE; Language LG; Notes NT; Publication Type PT; Publication Year PY; Publication Year (archive) YA; Source SO; Title TI and Update Code UP

Dissertations
Gosudarstwennaja Biblioteka SSSR im. W. I. Lenina

19:142. Master record

Database type	Reference
Number of journals	
Sources	
Start year	
Language	English
Coverage	
Number of records	
Update size	—
Update period	

Description

General referral to theses.

19:143. Other media   Gosudarstwennaja Biblioteka SSSR im. W. I. Lenina

File name	Dissertations
Start year	
Number of records	
Update period	

Easy Vet
IMS America Ltd, Hospital/Laboratory/Veterinary Database Division

19:144. Master record

Database type	Statistical, Textual
Number of journals	
Sources	Journal

Start year	1982
Language	English
Coverage	USA
Number of records	21,000
Update size	—
Update period	Quarterly

Keywords

Animal Health Care Products; Drugs; Pharmaceutical Industry; Pharmaceutical Products; Veterinary Science

Description

Contains time series on sales of animal health-care products. Includes pharmaceuticals, biologicals, and diagnostic aids purchased for therapy, diagnosis, and health maintenance. Provides estimated total national sales and breakdowns of sales by veterinarians, drug stores, livestock supply stores, farming cooperatives, poultry owners, feed lots, feed mills, and feed manufacturers.

Corresponds to *US Pharmaceutical Market: Animal and Poultry*.

19:145. Online   IMS America Ltd
File name
Start year	1982
Number of records	21,000
Update period	Quarterly

Notes

Subscription to *US Pharmaceutical Market: Animal and Poultry* required.

ELFIS
Zentralstelle für Agrardokumentation und Information (ZADI)

19:146. Master record
Alternative name(s)	Ernährungs-, Land- und Forstwirtschaftliches Informationssystem; Information System on Food Agriculture Forestry
Database type	Bibliographic
Number of journals	
Sources	Conference proceedings, journals, monographs, research communications and reports
Start year	1984
Language	German
Coverage	Germany
Number of records	149,462
Update size	18,000
Update period	Quarterly
Thesaurus	Agrovoc Thesaurus

Keywords

Food Science; Nutrition

Description

ELFIS contains citations to literature on agriculture, veterinary science, and food sciences and technology. It is produced by the Documentation Centres of FIS-ELF. The subjects covered include: microbiology; biotechnology; plant production; grasslands farming; forage growing; plant breeding; timber industry; viticulture; phytomedicine; sugar technology; horticulture; forestry; dairy science; agricultural engineering; soil science; vegetation science; home economics; human nutrition; cereal processing; the brewing industry;

economics; labour management; conservation and landscape management.

Approximately 26 per cent of the records contain abstracts.

German and German-language serials, books and reports since 1984.

ELFIS documents are indexed with the subject codes, commodity codes and geographical codes of the AGRIS Classification Scheme of the FAO, with the controlled terms of the German version of the *Agrovoc-thesaurus* and with uncontrolled terms. Subject codes describe the broader aspects of an article.

19:147. Online   DIMDI
File name	AN85
Alternative name(s)	Ernaehrungs-, Land- und Forstwirtschaftliches Informationssystem; Information System on Food Agriculture Forestry
Software	GRIPS
Start year	1984
Number of records	149,462
Update period	Quarterly
SDI period	Monthly
Database aids	DIMDI Memocard
Price/Charges	Connect time: UK£03.24–07.03
	Online print: UK£0.15–0.33
	Offline print: UK£0.07–0.14

Downloading is allowed
Thesaurus is online

Notes

Suppliers of online documents: British Library Document Supply Centre, Boston Spa, England; Harkers Information Retrieval System, Sydney, Australia; Zentralbibliothek der Landbauwissenschaft, Bonn, Germany.

Record composition

Abstract AB; Author AU; Commodity Codes CC; Conference Name KN; Controlled Terms CT; Geographic Codes GC; Language LA; Document Number ND; Source SO; Subject Codes SC; Title TI and Uncontrolled Terms UT

The unit record includes author(s), title and relevant bibliographic data, affiliation, descriptors, subject field(s) and abstracts (26%). All titles are in German language with an English translation. German and English title words can be searched via freetext.

Environmental Teratology
Oak Ridge National Laboratory, Environmental Teratology Information Centre

19:148. Master record
Alternative name(s)	ETIC; Environmental Teratology Information Center Files
Database type	Bibliographic, Directory
Number of journals	
Sources	Journals
Start year	1975 (earliest materials from 1912)
Language	English
Coverage	International

Number of records	45,000
Update size	–
Update period	Quarterly
Index unit	Articles

Description

Produced by the Environmental Mutagens, Carcinogen and Teratogen Information Program of the ORNL, this database contains citations to the worldwide literature on teratology – the science dealing with causes, mechanisms, and manifestations of structural or functional alterations in animal development. Covers the testing and evaluation for teratogenic activity of chemical, biological, and physical agents and of dietary deficiencies in warm-blooded animals, plus developmental and reproductive teratology. Primary emphasis is on literature that covers the administration of an agent to pregnant animals and examination of offspring at or near birth for structural or functional anomalies. Records also contain Chemical Abstracts Service Registry Numbers.

19:149. Online BLAISE-LINK
(as a part of TOXNET)

File name	ETICBACK
Alternative name(s)	ETIC
Start year	
Number of records	
Update period	

Notes

The backfile of Environmental Teratology giving citations to articles published between 1950 and 1988, providing full bibliographic details, keywords, chemical names and CAS Registry Numbers to articles dealing with teratology and developmental/reproductive toxicology.

19:150. Online CISTI MEDLARS
(as a part of TOXNET)

File name	ETICBACK
Alternative name(s)	ETIC
Start year	
Number of records	
Update period	

Notes

The backfile of Environmental Teratology giving citations to articles published between 1950 and 1988, providing full bibliographic details, keywords, chemical names and CAS Registry Numbers to articles dealing with teratology and developmental/reproductive toxicology.

19:151. Online National Library of
Medicine
(as a part of TOXNET)

File name	ETICBACK
Alternative name(s)	ETIC; Environmental Teratology Information Center Files
Start year	
Number of records	
Update period	

Notes

The backfile of Environmental Teratology giving citations to articles published between 1950 and 1988, providing full bibliographic details, keywords, chemical names and CAS Registry Numbers to articles dealing with teratology and developmental/reproductive toxicology.

This database can also be found on:

TOXLINE
TOXLINE Plus
PolTox I: NLM, CSA, IFIS
Developmental and Reproductive Toxicology – DART

Farmadisco
CD Systems
OEMF

19:153. Master record

Alternative name(s)	Informatore, L' Farmaceutico; Info-Farmadisco
Database type	Textual, Directory, Bibliographic, Factual
Number of journals	
Sources	Databases
Start year	1970
Language	Italian
Coverage	Italy
Number of records	
Update size	–
Update period	Semiannually

Keywords

Drugs; Pharmaceutical Products

Description

Pharmaceutical data on all medicinal products, with active ingredients and their anatomic, therapeutic, and chemical classification. Also includes cosmetic, dietary, and veterinary products; and names and addresses of manufacturers of drugs and borderline products. Contains:

useful telephone numbers;
List of ASS.INDE members;
Medicinal products only available on non-repeatable prescriptions;
Summary table of mandatory drugs to be stocked by pharmacies;
Alphabetical list of the pharmaceutical substances monographs with the relative type of confection;
Adverse reaction to drugs – Definition and Codes – WHO/OMS list;
Medicinal herbs, listed with the necessary instructions for preparing magistral galenic preparations;
Laboratories (full addresses, deposits and representatives, and relative level of production, plus a list of Italian wholesalers); and
Index Magnus, with over 60,000 references.

In addition, one section has medicinal products subdivided by ATC in order of active element. A description of the type of confection is given for each medicinal product and its *SSN Therapeutical Manual* (A-B-C) category and producing company is also given. Users can move from any of the archives to others, for example, from a substance card to all specialities in Informatore Farmaceutico containing that substance, or to all the firms producing that same substance.

Contains the contents of the two volumes of the print edition.

19:154. CD-ROM OEMF

File name	Farmadisco
Alternative name(s)	Informatore, L' Farmaceutico; Info-Farmadisco
Format notes	IBM
Software	CD-Hyper
Start year	1970

Number of records	
Update period	Semiannually
Price/Charges	Subscription: US$1,089

Fish and Fisheries Worldwide
National Information Services Corporation (NISC)

19:155. Master record
CD-ROM   **National Information Services Corporation (NISC)**

Database type	Bibliographic, Directory, Addresses/Telephone directory
Number of journals	
Sources	Journals, monographs, pamphlets, conference proceedings, reports, government publications, theses and grey literature
Start year	1971
Language	English
Coverage	International
Number of records	135,000
Update size	—
Update period	Twice per year
Index unit	Articles

Keywords
Ichthyology; Toxicology; Oceanography

Description
Citations of the world's literature on fisheries and fish-related topics. Drawn from several leading sources, including:

Fisheries Review from the US Fish and Wildlife Service (76,000 entries from 1971 onwards);

FISHLIT database from the JLB Smith Institute of Ichthyology, Rhodes University (30,000 records drawn from over 1,000 relevant journals – 1985 to present);

Fish Health News Abstracts (1978–1985, equivalent to the publication produced by the US Fish and Wildlife Service) fish health references up to 1985 when they were first included in the Fisheries Review database; and

Aquaculture which covers marine, freshwater and brackish organisms (over 10,000 citations from 1970 to 1984).

Covers such topics in Aquaculture as: fish culture and propagation; fish farming; hatcheries and propogation; aquarium fish; warmwater culture; growing requirements culture techniques and equipment; management of aquaria; farm ponds; small impoundments; dams; cage culture and marine ranching; intensive and extensive culture; and regulations and legislation. Ecology and the Environment covers marine, brackish, estuarine and freshwater environments; habitats; aquatic communities and fish assemblages; limnology and oceanography; species interactions and food webs; natural history; mathematical models; biogeography; and freshwater and marine fish. Physiology topics include biology and physiology; biochemistry; histochemistry; age and growth; nutrition; and reproduction. Fisheries subject areas cover fishery regulations and legislation; management topics; fishery stations; surveys, marking; tagging and returns, data analysis; stock assessment and identification; fishing

gear and techniques; management techniques and equipment; and mathematical modelling. Fish diseases are covered: parasitic, viral and bacterial diseases; nutritional and physiological diseases; fungal and protozoan diseases; diagnostic procedures; pathology; fish health studies; immunization; drug clearance; and disease treatment and control measures. Experimental research coverage includes research technologies and equipment; cell and tissue culture; genetics and behaviour; genetic engineering; genetics variation studies; electrophoretic studies; mathematical modelling; biochemistry; and hybridisation. Academic ichthyology covers taxonomy, phylogeny and evolution; morphological studies; meristics and morphometrics; and electron microscopy and histology. Also covered are distribution (biogeography; movement, seasonal and depth distributions; geographic distribution; and migration), economic aspects (aquatic plants and their control; fisheries management) and pollution studies (pesticides and industrial pollution; toxicology and bioassays). There is also a directory with the latest addresses of fish scientists with over 5,000 publishing ichthyologists and fishery scientists.

Notes
For related CD-ROMs see 'Fisheries Review/Wildlife Review' and 'Wildlife Worldwide'. The combination of these four databases means that gaps which may exist in one database have been greatly reduced or eliminated by the other files. Searches can be performed on all databases simultaneously, individually or in user-designated groups. Extensive keyword indexing as well as taxonomic and geographic identifiers mean that searches can be performed by species or by geographic areas from broad, regional basis to a narrow, specific locality.

For more details of constituent databases, see:
Fisheries Review/Wildlife Review
FISHLIT
Fish Health News Abstracts
Aquaculture

Food Products
VNIKTI cholodilnoj Promishlennosti

19:157. Master record

Database type	Factual
Number of journals	
Sources	
Start year	1980
Language	English
Coverage	
Number of records	
Update size	—
Update period	

Keywords
Food Products; Beverages

Description
Factographic information on chilling and freezing food.

19:158. Diskette   **VNIKTI cholodilnoj Promishlennosti**

File name	
Start year	1980

Number of records
Update period

Foreign Serials
GPNTB SSSR

19:159. Master record
Database type	Bibliographic
Number of journals	
Sources	Journals
Start year	1982
Language	English
Coverage	
Number of records	26,500
Update size	1,000
Update period	

Description
Foreign serials held by Soviet libraries. Equivalent to *The All-Union Summary Catalog Of Foreign Serials.*

19:160. Other media   GPNTB SSSR
File name	Foreign Serials
Start year	1982
Number of records	26,500
Update period	

Genek, feherjek es peptidek adatait elemzö programcsomag
Orszagos Sugarbiologiai es

19:161. Master record
Database type	Bibliographic, Factual
Number of journals	
Sources	
Start year	
Language	English
Coverage	
Number of records	
Update size	—
Update period	

Description
In-house DNA database, factographic.

19:162. Online   Orszagos Sugarbiologiai es
File name	BIOANAL
Start year	
Number of records	
Update period	

Institutbiblioteker ved Landbohoejskolen
Danmarks Veterinaer og Jordbrugsbibliotek

19:167. Master record
Database type	Library catalogue/cataloguing aids
Number of journals	
Sources	
Start year	
Language	Danish
Coverage	Denmark
Number of records	2,600
Update size	—
Update period	Every second year

Description
References to literature in seminar libraries at the Royal Veterinary and Agricultural High School. Is included in ALBA.

19:168. Online   Danmarks Veterinaer og Jordbrugsbibliotek
File name	LIBI
Start year	
Number of records	2,600
Update period	Every second year

19:169. Online
File name	LIBI
Start year	
Number of records	2,600
Update period	Every second year

This database can also be found on:
ALBA

Kardiologiai adatbazisok
Orszagos Kardiologiai Intezet

19:172. Master record
Database type	Bibliographic
Number of journals	
Sources	
Start year	
Language	English and French
Coverage	
Number of records	
Update size	—
Update period	

Keywords
Cardiology

Description
Main information system on cardiovascular treatment.

19:173. Online   Orszagos Kardiologiai Intezet
File name	SZIVTARS
Start year	
Number of records	
Update period	

Kardiologiai szakirodalmi adatbazis
Orszagos Kardiologiai Intezet

19:174. Master record
Database type	Bibliographic
Number of journals	
Sources	
Start year	
Language	English
Coverage	
Number of records	
Update size	—
Update period	

Keywords
Cardiology

Description
In-house cardiological treatment and diagnostics system.

19:175. Online　　Orszagos Kardiologiai Intezet

File name　　CBOOKS
Start year
Number of records
Update period

Könyvtari adatbazis
Orszagos Haematologiai es

19:176. Master record

Database type　　Bibliographic
Number of journals
Sources
Start year
Language　　English
Coverage
Number of records
Update size　　–
Update period

Keywords

Haematology

Description

In-house information on haematology.

19:177. Online　　　　　　OHVI

File name　　ASCA
Start year
Number of records
Update period

LANTDOK
Sveriges Lantbruksuniversitets Bibliotek (SLUB)

19:178. Master record

Alternative name(s)　　Swedish Agricultural Literature
Database type　　Bibliographic
Number of journals
Sources　　Statutes and Government documents (Swedish)
Start year　　1983
Language　　Swedish (keywords), English and Swedish
Coverage　　Sweden
Number of records　　35,000
Update size　　5,000
Update period　　Irregular

Keywords

Forestry; Food Science; Horticulture; Fisheries; Nutrition

Description

LANTDOK contains bibliographic information on all important Swedish documents (from 1983) on agricultural science. The main scope is the same as that of AGRIS. The LANTDOK database covers two additional types of records: documents written for others than researchers; documents published by Swedes outside Sweden (AGRIS covers these items via the regional centre for the country of publication). This means that such material as laws, statutes, statistics, parliamentary material, etc is covered. The following categories are excluded from the database: newspapers, material produced for the public (home gar-

dening, home ornamental plants, popular books on pets, etc), patents, minor documents, such as book reviews, letters to the editor etc, provided they give little or no real matter information. The input is produced by the library of the Swedish University of Agricultural Sciences. Most of the work is done at the Ultuna library, the specialised branch libraries at Alnarp (horticultural sciences, landscape planning) and Umeå (forestry) cover their fields respectively. LANTDOK is a part of the catalogue system LUKAS of the Swedish University of Agricultural Sciences Library and can be searched simultaneously with SLUBIB. Subjects covered include: agriculture, forestry, horticulture, fisheries, food science, environment, veterinary medicine.

Corresponds to *Svensk Lantbruksbibliografi.*

All records are given with descriptors, at present in English and using the AGRIS vocabulary *Agrovoc.* There are both narrower and broader terms.

19:179. Online　　　　　Sveriges Lantbruksuniversitet Bibliotek (SLUB)

File name　　LANTDOK
Alternative name(s)　　Swedish Agricultural Literature
Start year　　1983
Number of records　　35,000
Update period　　Irregular

Life Sciences Collection
Cambridge Scientific Abstracts

19:180. Master record

Alternative name(s)　　LSC; CSA Life Sciences Collection
Database type　　Bibliographic
Number of journals　　5,000
Sources　　Journals, books, serial monographs, conference proceedings, patents (US), patents (UK), patents (Japanese) and reports
Start year　　1978
Language　　English
Coverage　　International
Number of records　　1,500,000
Update size　　Monthly
Update period　　Monthly

Keywords

Acute Poisoning; Aging; Algology; Amino-Acids; Anatomy; Antibiotics; Aquaculture; Bacteriology; Behavioural Ecology; Bioengineering; Biological Membranes; Biotechnology; Bone Disease; Calcium Metabolism; Chemoreception; Chronic Poisoning; Clinical Medicine; Clinical Toxicology; DNA; Drugs; Ecology; Ecosystems; Endocrinology; Entomology – Agricultural; Entomology – Applied; Entomology – Human; Entomology – Veterinary; Environmental Biology; Ethology; Genetic Engineering; Hazardous Substances; HIV; Histology; Human Ecology; Immune Disorders; Immunology; Infectious Diseases; Marine Biotechnology; Microbiology; Molecular Biology; Molecular Neurobiology; Mycology; Neurology; Neuropharmacology; Neurophysiology – Animal; Neuroscience; Nucleic Acids; Nutrition; Oncology; Occupational Health and Safety; Osteoporosis; Osteomalacia; Pathology; Peptides; Pharmaceuticals; Pheromones;

Physiology; Pollution; Proteins; Protozoology; Psychophysics; Public Health; Radiation; Rhinology; RNA; Sleep; Smoking; Substance Abuse; Taste Perception; Viral Genetics

Description

Life Sciences Collection contains abstracts of information in the fields of (and corresponding to abstract journals from CSA): animal behaviour; biochemistry-amino-acid, peptide and protein; biochemistry – nucleic acids; biochemistry-biological membranes; biotechnology research (from 1984 to date); calcified tissue; chemoreception; ecology; endocrinology; entomology; genetics; human genomes; basic research and clinical applications; immunology, marine biotechnology, microbiology-algology, mycology and protozoology; microbiology-bacteriology; microbiology-industrial and applied microbiology; oncology-oncogenes and growth factors; neurosciences (from 1983 to date); toxicology; virology and AIDS. AIDS is covered in depth. The worldwide coverage is of journal articles, books, conference proceedings, report literature, patents, theses and dissertations.

Corresponds to the series of abstracting journals published by CSA: *Animal Behavior Abstracts; Biochemistry Abstracts-Amino-acid, Peptide and Protein; Biochemistry Abstracts-Biological Membranes; Biochemistry Abstracts-Nucleic Acids; Calcified Tissue Abstracts; Biotechnology Research Abstracts* (from 1984 to date); *Chemoreception Abstracts; Ecology Abstracts; Endocrinology Abstracts; Entomology Abstracts; Genetics Abstracts; Human Genome Abstracts; Basic Research and Clinical Applications; Immunology Abstracts; Marine Biotechnology Abstracts; Microbiology Abstracts-Algology, Mycology and Protozoology; Microbiology Abstracts-Bacteriology; Microbiology Abstracts-Industrial and Applied Microbiology; Neurosciences Abstracts* (from 1983 to date)*; Oncogenes and Growth Factors Abstracts; Toxicology Abstracts; Virology and AIDS Abstracts.* Most recently added were *Marine Biotechnology Abstracts* and *Oncogenes and Growth Factors Abstracts.* Also includes *Oncology Abstracts* and *Feeding, Weight and Obesity Abstracts* for the period they were published.

19:181. Online   BIOSIS Life Science Network

File name	Life Sciences Collection
Start year	1978
Number of records	1,500,000
Update period	Monthly
Price/Charges	Connect time: US$9.00
	Online print: US$6.00 per 10; 2.25
	per abstract; 3.50 per full text article

Also available via the Internet by telnetting to LSN.COM.

Notes

On Life Science Network users can search this database or they can scan a group of subject-related databases. There is a charge of $2.00 per scan of subject-related databases. To search one database and display up to ten citations costs $6.00. Most charges are for information retrieved. There are no charges if there are no results and no charge to transfer results to a printer or diskette. Articles may also be ordered via an online document delivery request. A telecommunications software package is also available, costing $12.95, providing an automatic connection to Life Science Network for heavy users of the service, with capability to transfer to print or disk and customised colour options.

19:182. Online   DIALOG

File name	File 76
Start year	1978
Number of records	1,392,381
Update period	Monthly
Price/Charges	Connect time: US$90.00
	Online print: US$0.75
	Offline print: US$0.75
	SDI charge: US$9.50

19:183. Online   STN

File name	LIFESCI
Start year	1978
Number of records	1,500,000
Update period	Monthly

19:184. CD-ROM   Compact Cambridge

File name	Life Sciences Collection
Alternative name(s)	LSC; CSA Life Sciences Collection
Format notes	NEC, 9800, IBM
Start year	1982
Number of records	
Update period	Quarterly
Price	UK£1,165 – 2,985 (Initial with backfiles)
	Subscription: UK£985

Notes

Contains eighteen subject orientated subfiles in the life and biosciences field, covering some 5,000 core journals, books, serial monographs, etc. Over 98,000 abstracts are added each year. Subscribers to CSA's life sciences print journals receive a £500 credit towards the first year's subscription to LSC CD-ROM 1982-present or 1985-present.

19:185. Tape   Cambridge Scientific Abstracts

File name	Life Sciences Collection on Magnetic Tape
Alternative name(s)	LSC; CSA Life Sciences Collection
Format notes	9-track, unlabelled, 1600 bpi, EBCDIC
Start year	1982
Number of records	
Update period	Monthly
Price/Charges	Subscription: US$13,950

Notes

The series of abstracting journals published by CSA are available on this tape as a collection. They are also available separately as tape subsets of the Life Sciences Collection, the online database to which this tape corresponds.

Price for the current year tape is $13,950; single-year archival file is $7,100.

19:186. Database subset Tape   Cambridge Scientific Abstracts

File name	Animal Behavior Abstracts on Magnetic Tape
Format notes	9-track, unlabelled, 1600 bpi, EBCDIC
Start year	1978
Number of records	
Update period	Quarterly

Notes

A subset of the Life Sciences Collection. Contains citations, with abstracts, to the worldwide literature on ethology, the study of animal behaviour. Covers neurophysiology, behavioural ecology, biochemical, anatomical and neurophysiological correlates, sleep, brain stimulation, drug studies, hormones, habituation, reinforcement, avoidance, discrimination, complex learning, memory, theoretical models, communication, aggression, social spacing and dominance in animals.

Corresponds to *Animal Behavior Abstracts* and in part to the Life Sciences Collection online database. Contact CSA for pricing information.

19:187. Database subset

Tape	Cambridge Scientific Abstracts
File name	Cambridge Microbiology Abstracts Series on Magnetic Tape
Format notes	9-track, unlabelled, 1600 bpi, EBCDIC
Start year	1978
Number of records	
Update period	Monthly

Notes

A subset of the Life Sciences Collection. Contains three databases of information on microbiology.

Industrial & Applied Microbiology contains citations, with abstracts, to the worldwide literature on practical applications of microbiology. Covers pharmaceutical, food and beverage, agricultural and environmental applications, and methodology and research. Includes antibiotics and antimicrobial agents; vaccines and serum production; food contamination, ripening and fermentation processes; soil microbiology; plant diseases caused by microorganisms; composting; hydrocarbons; methane production; pollution; and isolation, identification and characterization of microorganisms. Also incudes registered US patents. Corresponds to *Cambridge Microbiology Abstracts, Section A; Industrial and Applied Microbiology*, and in part to the Life Sciences Collection online database.

Bacteriology contains citations, with abstracts, to the worldwide literature on bacteriology. Covers immunology, taxonomy, methods, cell properties, genetics, antibiotics and antimicrobials, toxins, medical, veterinary and invertebrate bacteriology, plant diseases, and ecological aspects. Corresponds to *Cambridge Microbiology Abstracts, Section B: Bacteriology*, and in part to the Life Sciences Collection online database.

Algology, Mycology and Protozoology contains citations, with abstracts, to the worldwide literature on algae, fungi, protozoa and lichens. Includes reproduction, growth, life cycles, biochemistry, genetics, and infection and immunity in humans, other animals and plants. Covers taxonomy, structure and function, ecology and distribution, effects of physical and chemical factors, methodology, media and culture, nutrition, mycotoxins, parasitism and diseases, viruses and bacteria, soil microbiolgy and mycorrhiza, spoilage and biodegradation, and pollution. Corresponds to *Cambridge Microbiology Abstracts, Section C: Algology, Mycology and Protozoology*, and in part to the Life Sciences Collection online database. Pricing information may be obtained from Cambridge Scientific Abstracts.

19:188. Database subset

Tape	Cambridge Scientific Abstracts
File name	Entomology Abstracts on Magnetic Tape
Format notes	9-track, unlabelled, 1600 bpi, EBCDIC
Start year	1982

Number of records	
Update period	Monthly

Notes

A subset of the Life Sciences Collection. Contains citations, with abstracts, to the worldwide literature on insects, arachnids, myriapods, onychophorans and terrestrial isopods. Covers geographic distribution, nomenclature, new species, techniques and methodology, morphology of all life cycle stages, physiology, anatomy, histology, biochemistry, toxicology and resistance, ecology, behaviour, and medical, veterinary, agricultural and applied entomology. Corresponds to *Entomology Abstracts* and in part to the Life Sciences Collection online database. Contact CSA for pricing information.

This database can also be found on:
Cambridge Scientific Abstracts Life Sciences
Human Nutrition on CD-ROM

MAKSI1
Gosudarstwennaja Biblioteka SSSR im. W. I. Lenina

19:190. Master record

Database type	Bibliographic
Number of journals	
Sources	
Start year	1974
Language	English
Coverage	
Number of records	42,000
Update size	—
Update period	

Keywords

Public Administration

Description

Records of serials available in the CMEA libraries.

19:191. Other media

	Gosudarstwennaja Biblioteka SSSR im. W. I. Lenina
File name	
Start year	1974
Number of records	42,000
Update period	

Medical and Microbiological Industry
Zentr. bjuro ASU i TEI med. i mikrobiol. Prom.

19:192. Master record

Database type	Bibliographic
Number of journals	
Sources	
Start year	1980
Language	English
Coverage	

Number of records 140,000
Update size —
Update period

Description
Medical and microbiological database.

19:193. Diskette   Zentr. bjuro ASU i TEI med. i mikrobiol. Prom.
File name
Start year 1980
Number of records 140,000
Update period

Medicinal Herbs
ArmNIINTI

19:194. Master record
Database type Bibliographic
Number of journals
Sources
Start year 1989
Language English
Coverage
Number of records 1,000
Update size —
Update period

Keywords
Alternative Medicine; Homeopathy

Description
Bibliographic source on medicinal herbs, homeopathy.

19:195. Diskette   ArmNIINTI
File name
Start year 1989
Number of records 1,000
Update period

Merck Veterinary Manual
Merck Sharp & Dôhme Research Knowledge Access

19:196. Master record
Database type Textual, Image
Number of journals
Sources Monograph, Laws/regulations and Government documents (US)
Start year
Language English
Coverage USA
Number of records
Update size —
Update period Annually

Description
Contains the 6th edition of the *Merck Veterinary Manual*, with text, colour illustrations, and the text and images from Title 21 of the *Code of Federal Regulations*, Parts 500 – 599, the official compilation of drugs approved by the FDA for veterinary use.

19:197. CD-ROM   Knowledge Access
File name Merck Veterinary Manual
Format notes IBM
Software KAware 2
Start year

Number of records
Update period Annually

Ministerie WVC
Netherlands Ministry of Welfare, Health and Cultural Affairs

19:198. Master record
Database type Bibliographic
Number of journals
Sources Books, Reports, Government publications and Periodicals
Start year 1982
Language Dutch
Coverage Netherlands (primarily) and International (some)
Number of records 67,000
Update size 8,000
Update period Daily

Keywords
Elderly; Hospitals; Welfare; Social Services; Recreation; Libraries; Sport; Museums; Health Care; Emergency Services

Description
Citations, with abstracts, to the international literature on social services, health care, recreation and culture in the Netherlands, services to youth, the elderly, minority groups and handicapped people, veterinary and human medicine, hospitals, emergency services, sports, leisure, performing and fine arts, libraries and museums.

Corresponds to *WVC Documentatie*, with additional information online.

19:199. Online   Rijks Computer Centrum
File name
Start year 1982
Number of records 67,000
Update period Daily

MTA-SOTE Genek, feherjek es peptidek adatait szolgaltato adatbazis
MTA – SOTE Egyesitett Kutatasi

19:200. Master record
Database type
Number of journals
Sources
Start year
Language English
Coverage
Number of records
Update size —
Update period

Keywords
DNA

Description
DNA mapping database.

19:201. Online

MTA – SOTE Egyesitett Kutatasi

File name	BIOSEQ
Start year	
Number of records	
Update period	

Number of records	400
Update period	

Neurological Documentary Database

George Marinescu Hospital

19:202. Master record

Database type	Bibliographic
Number of journals	
Sources	
Start year	1987
Language	English
Coverage	
Number of records	7,000
Update size	1,000
Update period	Monthly

Keywords

Neurology; Surgery

Description

Bibliographic database system on neurology and surgery.

19:203. Other media

George Marinescu Hospital

File name	
Start year	1987
Number of records	7,000
Update period	Monthly

Orzsagos Munkavedelmi Tudomanyos Kutato Intezet Veszelyes vegyianyagok

Orszagos Munkavedelmi Tudomanyos

19:204. Master record

Database type	
Number of journals	
Sources	
Start year	
Language	English
Coverage	
Number of records	400
Update size	–
Update period	

Keywords

Hazardous Substances; Health and Safety; Public Administration

Description

Reference system on environmental data and toxicology

19:205. Online

IIF

File name	VESV
Start year	

PASCAL

Centre National de la Recherche Scientifique, Institut de l'Information Scientifique et Technique, Science Humaines et Sociales (CNRS/INIST)

19:206. Master record

Alternative name(s)	Programme Applique a la Selection et a la Compilation Automatique de la Litterature
Database type	Bibliographic
Number of journals	8,500
Sources	Books, conference proceedings, dissertations, journals, maps, monographs, patents (biotechnology), reports, technical reports and theses
Start year	1973
Language	English (titles and keywords), French and Spanish (keywords)
Coverage	International
Number of records	9 million
Update size	500,000
Update period	Monthly
Index unit	Articles
Thesaurus	Biomedical Thesaurus in 3 volumes
Database aids	PASCAL User Manual, PASCAL Classification Scheme and PASCAL Dictionary in 3 Volumes (French, English, Spanish): Exact Sciences, Technology, Medicine

Keywords

Bioagriculture; Biomedicine; Biotechnology; Cell Biology; Civil Engineering; Construction; Demography; Electrical Engineering; Epidemiology; Ergonomics; Immunology; Metallurgy; Microbiology; Mineralogy; Nutrition; Parasitology; Patents; Physics; Pollution; Public Health; Travel Medicine; Tropical Medicine

Description

PASCAL is a multidisciplinary and multilingual bibliographic database covering the core of scientific, technical and medical literature worldwide. Subjects covered include: Life sciences – biology, tropical medicine, biomedical engineering, biochemistry, biotechnology, pharmacology, microbiology, ophthalmology, dermatology, anaesthesia, human diseases, animal biology, reproduction, genetics, zoology, plant biology, agronomics, agricultural science, psychology; Earth sciences – mineralogy, mining economics, cristallography, stratigraphy, hydrology, paleontology; Physical sciences physics, information science, computer science, astronomy, electrical engineering, electronics, atoms and molecules, general, physical, analytical, inorganic and organic chemistry; Engineering sciences – energy, metallurgy, pollution, mechanical industries, construction, welding and brazing, civil engineering, building and public works, transportation.

In addition there are specialised subfiles in the following areas: information science, documentation, energy, metallurgy, civil engineering, earth sciences, biotechnology, zoology of invertebrates, agriculture and tropical medicine.

On ESA-IRS, DIALOG and QUESTEL searches can

be limited to one of the two subfiles PASCAL: Biotechnologies and PASCAL: Medécine Tropicale dating from 1982 on ESA-IRS and QUESTEL, but on DIALOG from 1986. Each subfile holds over 40,000 records.

Biotechnologies contains citations, with abstracts to the international biotechnology literature, covering biochemistry, cell biology, microbiology and applications of cultured microorganisms and cells in agriculture, energy, food processing, medicine, metallurgy and pollution control. Some patents are included in this area. Corresponds to *PASCAL THEMA 215: biotechnologies*.

Medécine Tropicale provides citations, with abstracts, to the international literature of tropical medicine, covering human and animal parasites and diseases, the biology and control of vectors, intermediate hosts and reservoirs, ergonomics, nutrition, physical and social demography, public health and medical issues relating to travellers. Corresponds to *PASCAL THEMA 235: Médecine Tropicale*.

These subfiles are available as part of PASCAL on DIALOG, QUESTEL and ESA-IRS.

PASCAL is the online version of the print publication *Bibliographie Internationale* (1984 onwards) and corresponds to the publication *Bulletin Signaletique* (1973–1983). The titles in the PASCAL file are in their original languages and are translated into French and/or English. Approximately fifty per cent of records have abstracts which are in French or English (from 1982 the titles and keywords are also given in English). Journal articles account for approximately ninety-three per cent of the file. 8,500 journals are regularly scanned. Source materials are published in various languages: English 63%, French 12%, Russian 10%, German 8% and other languages 7%.

The controlled terms are in French and also in English for records since 1982 and in Spanish for records since 1977. German controlled terms are also provided in the area of metallurgy.

19:207. Online CompuServe Information Service

File name	IQUEST File 1284
Alternative name(s)	Programme Applique a la Selection et a la Compilation Automatique de la Litterature
Start year	1973
Number of records	9 million
Update period	Monthly
Price/Charges	Subscription: US$8.95 per month Database entry fee: US$9/search; some databases carry a surcharge ($2–75) Online print: US$10 references free; then $9 per ten; abstracts $3 each

Downloading is allowed

Notes

Accessed via IQUEST or IQMEDICAL, this database is offered by a Questel gateway. IQUEST can either search across all databases, a database of the user's choice or selected multiple databases.

19:208. Online DIALOG

File name	File 144
Alternative name(s)	Programme Applique a la Selection et a la Compilation Automatique de la Litterature
Start year	1973

Number of records	3,866,245
Update period	Monthly
Price/Charges	Connect time: US$60.00 Online print: US$0.50 Offline print: US$0.50 SDI charge: US$12.00

Notes

DIALINDEX Categories: AGRI, BIOCHEM, BIOSCI, BIOTECH, CHEMLIT, EECOMP, ENERGY, ENERGYP, GEOLOGY, GEOLOGYP, GEOPHYS, MATERIAL, MEDICINE, METALS, PHYSICS, SCITECHB.

19:209. Online ESA-IRS

File name	File 14
Alternative name(s)	Programme Applique a la Selection et a la Compilation Automatique de la Litterature
Start year	1973
Number of records	8,263,000 (October 1991)
Update period	Monthly
Price/Charges	Subscription: UK£70.29 Database entry fee: UK£3.51 Online print: UK£0.07 – 0.56 Offline print: UK£0.50 SDI charge: UK£3.51

Notes

QUESTALERT and QUESTORDER are both available on this file. The LIMIT ALL command can be used to limit all subsequent sets. This can be cancelled by entering a new LALL or a BEGIN command.

From 1993 ESA-IRS are charging an annual fee of 100 Accounting Units (c.UK£ 70.29) to all users. This is equivalent to the fee for full documentation and will not be charged to customers already paying for documentation.

Record composition

Abstract /AB; Author AU; Classification Code CC; Classification Number CN; CODEN CO; Controlled Terms (Descriptors) /CT; Controlled Terms in English /KE; Controlled Terms in French /KF; Controlled Terms in Spanish or German /KO; Corporate Source CS; Country/Place of Publication CY; Document Type DT; Domain (Subfile) DO; Generic Controlled Terms (Broader Terms) /CT*; Geographical Coordinates GC; International Patent Classification PC; ISBN BN; ISSN SN; Journal Name JN; Language LA; Language of Summary LS; Location of Document LC; Major Controlled Terms /CT* or /MAJ; Map Type CA; Meeting Date MD; Meeting Location ML; Meeting Title MT; Native Number NN; Report Number RN; Patent Application Number PA; Patent Holder (Corporate) PH; Patent Number PN; Patent Priority PP; Publication Year PY; Publisher PB; Report Number RN; Single Controlled Terms /ST; Source SO; Titles (English) /ET; Titles (French) /FT; Titles (other) /0T and Titles (all) /TI

The titles are in their original language and are translated into French and/or English. The Controlled Terms are in French and also in English for records since 1982, and Spanish for records since 1984. German controlled terms are also provided in the area of metallurgy. Abstracts are in French or English (English especially from 1990 onwards). The EXPAND command can be used to display the PASCAL thesaurus. The basic index includes the following data fields: Abstract, Controlled Terms in any language, Controlled Terms in English, Controlled Terms in French, Controlled Terms in Spanish or German, Generic Controlled Terms, Single Controlled

Terms, Titles (English), Titles (French), Titles (Other). The Classification Name is the principal hierarchical category corresponding to the classification code of the record. Some fields are searchable in both French and English. The data field Source may include: monographic source, collective source or title of collection. The prefix 'SO=' corresponds to the information displayed immediately after the title. It does not correspond to the field labelled 'Source Information' in the displayed record. To search for journal names the prefix 'JN=' should be used. Role indicators which are used with substances to identify the role they play in a chemical reaction or process are placed after the name of the substance with the symbol | as separator in file 205 and the symbol ! as separator in file 204. Role indicators have been used in chemistry-and physics-related records since 1979 and in metallurgy related reocrds since 1980. They are as follows: ENT: Primary material, FIN: End product, ACT: Active product, SUB: Substrate, solvent, etc, ANA: Analytically determined compound, SEC: Secondary material.

19:210. Online   ESA-IRS

File name	File 204
Alternative name(s)	Programme Applique a la Selection et a la Compilation Automatique de la Litterature
Start year	1973 – 1983
Number of records	4,900,000
Update period	Closed File
Price/Charges	Subscription: UK£70.29
	Database entry fee: UK£3.51
	Online print: UK£0.07 – 0.56
	Offline print: UK£0.50
	SDI charge: UK£3.51

Downloading is allowed
Thesaurus is online

Notes

QUESTALERT and QUESTORDER are both available on this file. The LIMIT ALL command can be used to limit all subsequent sets. This can be cancelled by entering a new LALL or a BEGIN command.

From 1993 ESA-IRS are charging an annual fee of 100 Accounting Units (c.UK£ 70.29) to all users. This is equivalent to the fee for full documentation and will not be charged to customers already paying for documentation.

Record composition

Abstract /AB; Author AU; Classification Code CC; Controlled Terms (Descriptors) /CT; Corporate Source CS; Country/Place of Publication CY; Document Type DT; ISBN BN; ISSN SN; Journal Name JN; Language LA; Major Controlled Terms /CT* or /MAJ; Map Type CA; Native Number NN; Report Number RN; Single Controlled Terms /ST; Titles (English) /ET; Titles (French) /FT; Titles (other) /OT and Titles (all) /TI

The EXPAND command can be used to display the PASCAL thesaurus. The basic index includes the following data fields: Abstract, Controlled Terms (Descriptors), Major Controlled Terms, Single Controlled Terms, Titles (English), Titles (French), Titles (other), Titles (all). Examples of documents types in file 204 include: Journal Article (Code TP), Patent (TB), Conference (TC), Book (TL), Map (TM), Miscellaneous (TS), Monography (LM), Thesis (TT), Report (TR). Role indicators which are used with substances to identify the role they play in a chemical reaction or process are placed after the name of the substance with the symbol | as separator in file 205 and the symbol ! as separator in file 204. Role indi-

cators have been used in chemistry-and physics-related records since 1979 and in metallurgy related reocrds since 1980. They are as follows: ENT: Primary material, FIN: End product, ACT: Active product, SUB: Substrate, solvent, etc, ANA: Analytically determined compound, SEC: Secondary material.

19:211. Online   ESA-IRS

File name	File 205
Alternative name(s)	Programme Applique a la Selection et a la Compilation Automatique de la Litterature
Start year	1984
Number of records	
Update period	Monthly
Price/Charges	Subscription: UK£70.29
	Database entry fee: UK£3.51
	Online print: UK£0.07 – 0.56
	Offline print: UK£0.50
	SDI charge: UK£3.51

Downloading is allowed
Thesaurus is online

Notes

QUESTALERT and QUESTORDER are both available on this file. The LIMIT ALL command can be used to limit all subsequent sets. This can be cancelled by entering a new LALL or a BEGIN command.

From 1993 ESA-IRS are charging an annual fee of 100 Accounting Units (c.UK£ 70.29) to all users. This is equivalent to the fee for full documentation and will not be charged to customers already paying for documentation.

Record composition

Abstract /AB; Author AU; Classification Code CC; Classification Number CN; CODEN CO; Controlled Terms (Descriptors) in any language /CT; Controlled Terms in English /KE; Controlled Terms in French /KF; Controlled Terms in Spanish or German /KO; Corporate Source CS; Country of Publication CY; Document Type DT; Domain (Subfile) DO; Generic Controlled Terms (Broader Terms) /CT*; Geographical Coordinates GC; International Patent Classification PC; ISBN BN; ISSN SN; Journal Name JN; Language LA; Language of Summary LS; Location of Document LC; Map Type CA; Meeting Date MD; Meeting Location ML; Meeting Title MT; Native Number NN; Patent Application Number PA; Patent Holder (Corporate) PH; Patent Number PN; Patent Priority PP; Publication Year PY; Publisher PB; Report Number RN; Single Controlled Terms /ST; Source SO and Titles /TI

The basic index includes the following data fields: Abstract, Controlled Terms in any language, Controlled Terms in English, Controlled Terms in French, Controlled Terms in Spanish or German, Generic Controlled Terms, Single Controlled Terms, Titles. The Classification Name is the principal hierarchical category corresponding to the classification code of the record. Some fields are searchable in both French and English. The data field Source may include: monographic source, collective source or title of collection. The prefix 'SO=' corresponds to the information displayed immediately after the title. It does not correspond to the field labelled 'Source Information' in the displayed record. To search for journal names the prefix 'JN=' should be used. Role indicators which are used with substances to identify the role they play in a chemical reaction or process are placed after the name of the substance with the symbol | as separator in file 205 and the symbol ! as separator in file 204. Role indicators have been used in chemistry-and physics-related records since 1979 and in metallurgy related reocrds since 1980. They are as follows: ENT: Primary material, FIN: End product, ACT: Active product, SUB: Substrate, solvent, etc, ANA: Analytically determined compound, SEC: Secondary material.

19:212. Online   Questel

File name	PASC73
Alternative name(s)	Programme Applique a la Selection et a la Compilation Automatique de la Litterature
Start year	1973
Number of records	9 million
Update period	

19:213. CD-ROM   Centre National de la Recherche Scientifique, Institut de l'Information Scientifique et Technique, Science Humaines et Sociales (CNRS/INIST)

File name	PASCAL CD-ROM
Alternative name(s)	Programme Applique a la Selection et a la Compilation Automatique de la Litterature; CD-ROM PASCAL
Format notes	IBM
Software	GTI
Start year	1987
Number of records	450,000
Update period	Quarterly
Price/Charges	Subscription: FFr15,000 – 17,790

Notes

Each disc corresponds to one year update of the PASCAL database i.e. approximately 500,000 records. An annual subscription with quarterly updates. Costs 15,000 FFr for current year (1990, 1 disc); 7,500 Ffr for each backfile disc (1987, 1988, 1989, 1 disc each). The full collection with the current year subscription costs 35,000 – 41,150 FFr Can be used in a LAN network provided the network conforms to the standards required for the MSCDEX extension. Several commercial packages exist to make it possible to operate PASCAL CD-ROM in a suitable network environment.

19:214. Tape   Centre National de la Recherche Scientifique, Institut de l'Information Scientifique et Technique, Science Humaines et Sociales (CNRS/INIST)

File name	PASCAL
Alternative name(s)	Programme Applique a la Selection et a la Compilation Automatique de la Litterature
Format notes	9-track 1,600 or 6,250 BPI magnetic tapes, EBCDIC character set, with or without IBM-OS label
Start year	1987
Number of records	500,000
Update period	Annually
Price/Charges	

Notes

Each tape corresponds to one year update of the PASCAL database, that is, approximately 500,000 records.

19:215. Videotex   Minitel

File name	PASCAL 362936011
Alternative name(s)	Programme Applique a la Selection et a la Compilation Automatique de la Litterature
Start year	
Number of records	
Update period	

19:216. Database subset
Online   ESA-IRS

File name	File 37 – Training Pascal
Alternative name(s)	Programme Applique a la Selection et a la Compilation Automatique de la Litterature
Start year	1984–1985
Number of records	48,325(October 1991)
Update period	Not updated
Price/Charges	Connect time: UK£6.99 per hour
Downloading is allowed	
Thesaurus is online	

Notes

Training database (subfile of PASCAL main file, File 14). Neither QUESTALERT nor QUESTORDER are available. Services such as offline prints are also not available.

Record composition

Abstract /AB; Author AU; Classification Code CC; Classification Name CN; CODEN CO; Controlled terms in any language /CT; Controlled terms in English /KE; Controlled terms in French /KF; Controlled terms in Spanish or German /KO; Corporate Source CS; Country of Publication CY; Document Type DT; Domain DO; Generic controlled terms (broader terms) /CT*; Geographical Coordinates GC; ISBN BN; ISSN SN; Journal Name JN; Language LA; Language of Summary LS; Location of Document LC; Map Type CA; Meeting Title MT; Meeting Date MD; Meeting Location ML; Native Number NN; Patent Application Number PA; Patent Holder (Corporate) PH; Patent Number PN; Patent Priority PP; Publication Year PY; Publisher PB; Report Number RN; Single Controlled Terms /ST; Source SO and Titles /TI

The EXPAND command can be used to display the PASCAL thesaurus. The basic index includes the following data fields: Abstract, Controlled terms in any language, Controlled terms in English, Controlled terms in French, Controlled terms in Spanish or German, Generic controlled terms (broader terms), Single controlled terms, Titles. The classification name is the principal hierarchical category corresponding to the classification code of the record. Some fields are searchable in both French and English. Pascal can be divided into a number of subfiles (domains), a list of which can be obtained by entering the command E DO =. Source (SO=) may include: monographic source, collective source, or title of collection. The 'SO=' field is placed between title and author in the displayed record. To search for journal names the prefix 'JN=' should be used. Role indicators which are used with substances to identify the role they play in a chemical reaction or process are placed after the name of the substance with the symbol | as separator in file 205 and the symbol ! as separator in file 204. Role indicators have been used in chemistry-and physics-related records since 1979 and in metallurgy related reocrds since 1980. They are as follows: ENT: Primary material, FIN: End product, ACT: Active product, SUB: Substrate, solvent, etc, ANA: Analytically determined compound, SEC:

Secondary material. The LIMIT ALL command can be used to limit all subsequent sets. The limitation can be cancelled by entering a new LALL or a BEGIN command.

This database can also be found on:
Metropolitan
Medata-ROM

Pesticide Activity
VNII chimicheskich Sredstw Sachiti Rastjenii

19:218. Master record

Database type	Factual
Number of journals	
Sources	
Start year	
Language	English
Coverage	
Number of records	4,500
Update size	—
Update period	

Keywords

Hazardous Chemicals; Pesticides; Public Administration

Description

Factorgraphic information on pesticide properties.

19:219. Diskette   VNII chimicheskich Sredstw Sachiti Rastjenii

File name	
Start year	
Number of records	4,500
Update period	

Pharmaceutical and Healthcare Industry News Database
Pharmaprojects PJB Publications Ltd

19:220. Master record

Alternative name(s)	PHIND
Database type	Textual
Number of journals	4
Sources	Newsletters
Start year	1980
Language	English
Coverage	International
Number of records	113,270
Update size	—
Update period	Daily
Index unit	Newsletters, articles and reports
Database aids	User guide available from producer

Keywords

Applied Science; Herbicides; Marketing; Medical Diagnostics; Pesticides; Plant Protection; Product Liability

Description

This database contains information on product developments, markets, regulatory affairs of importance to the international pharmaceutical, medical device, veterinary and agrochemical industries. All publications have already been made available online in abstract form, but this is the only database which contains the full-text of every report and the only one which makes these reports available before publication. It includes all the text, pre-publication, current and archival material from four major international industry newsletters:

Scrip World Pharmaceutical News (1/82+, issue number 655) which contains world pharmaceutical news and is the most widely read international pharmaceutical industry newsletter, being used at all levels within pharmaceutical companies, regulatory authorities, financial instituions, service industries and others to gain an insight into significant events throughout the world, paying special attention to product developments, regulatory affairs, market intelligence, company results and personnel;
Clinica World Medical Device News (10/80+ issue number 1) which contains world medical device news and provides a similar service for the device and diagnostic industry;
Animal Pharm World Animal Health News (1/82+, issue number 1) which contains world animal health news; and
Agrow World Agrochemical News (10/85+, issue number 1) which contains world agrochemical news and is aimed at the herbicide, pesticide, rodenticide and plant growth regulator industries.

All four print publications follow a similar structure and contains sections on: Product & Research News, Company News, International News, People and Conferences, plus regular monitoring ofregulatiory bodies such as the US Food and Drug Administration, the US Environmental Protection Agency, the European Economic Community and the World Health Organisation. Reports are added to a daily and current file within three working days of writing, before publication. Items destined for publication in *Scrip* or *Clinica* are therefore available online days before the printed newsletters will reach users.

Each report has been written on the basis of news gathered from a wide variety of sources, and the range of information available is evaluated for relevance to the major industrial areas covered and is amplified by investigative reporting. They are subsequently moved into the archival file after approximately three weeks. Covers company activities (marketing, mergers, acquisitions, sales), product research and development (clinical trials, launches, approvals, etc), regulatory decisions (labelling changes, pesticide bans, product liability, etc) and notices of conferences, symposia and executive appointments.

The database corresponds to *Agrow World Crop Protection News, Animal Pharm World Animal Health News, Clinica World Medical Device and Diagnostic News and Scrip World Pharmaceutical News.*

19:221. Online   BRS

File name	PHIC
Alternative name(s)	PHIND
Start year	1980
Number of records	113,270
Update period	Daily
Price/Charges	Connect time: US$145.00/155.00
	Online print: US$3.52/3.60
	Offline print: US$3.60
	SDI charge: US$5.00

Notes

This is the current file Pharmaceutical and Healthcare Industry News Database.

19:222. Online   **BRS**

File name	PHID
Alternative name(s)	PHIND
Start year	1980
Number of records	113,270
Update period	Daily
Price/Charges	Connect time: US$145.00/155.00
	Online print: US$3.52/3.60
	Offline print: US$3.60
	SDI charge: US$5.00

Notes

Contains details of company activities and product development on a daily basis before publication of the printed version.

19:223. Online   **BRS**

File name	PHIN
Alternative name(s)	PHIND
Start year	1980
Number of records	113,270
Update period	Daily
Price/Charges	Connect time: US$145.00/155.00
	Online print: US$0.77/0.85
	Offline print: US$1.10

Notes

Pharmaceutical and Healthcare Industry News Database – Backfile: records are removed from the daily and current file into this archival file after approximately three weeks.

19:224. Online   **CompuServe Information Service**

File name	IQUEST File 2074: SCRIP – Daily News
Alternative name(s)	PHIND
Start year	1986
Number of records	
Update period	Daily
Price/Charges	Subscription: US$8.95 per month
	Database entry fee: US$9/search; some databases carry a surcharge ($2–75)
	Online print: US$10 references free; then $9 per ten; abstracts $3 each

Notes

Accessed via IQUEST, this database is offered by a Data-Star gateway. IQUEST can either search across all databases, a database of the user's choice or selected multiple databases.

This is the daily news file of pre-publication material used for daily scanning of reports on topics of particular interest and is included in the SCRIP CURRENT NEWS database. For all information on a particular topic it is necessary to search both SCRIP CURRENT NEWS and SCRIP RETROSPECTIVE.

19:225. Online   **CompuServe Information Service**

File name	IQUEST File 2075: SCRIP – Current News
Alternative name(s)	PHIND
Start year	1986
Number of records	
Update period	Daily
Price/Charges	Subscription: US$8.95 per month
	Database entry fee: US$9/search; some databases carry a surcharge ($2–75)
	Online print: US$10 references free; then $9 per ten; abstracts $3 each

Notes

Accessed via IQUEST, this database is offered by a Data-Star gateway. IQUEST can either search across all databases, a database of the user's choice or selected multiple databases.

This is the file containing current news, including SCRIP – DAILY NEWS, and is used for scanning for recently written reports.

19:226. Online   **CompuServe Information Service**

File name	IQUEST File 2076: SCRIP – Retrospective
Alternative name(s)	PHIND
Start year	1986
Number of records	
Update period	Daily
Price/Charges	Subscription: US$8.95 per month
	Database entry fee: US$9/search; some databases carry a surcharge ($2–75)
	Online print: US$10 references free; then $9 per ten; abstracts $3 each

Notes

Accessed via IQUEST or IQMEDICAL, this database is offered by a Data-Star gateway. IQUEST can either search across all databases, a database of the user's choice or selected multiple databases.

This is the archive file of information, removed from SCRIP – CURRENT NEWS and SCRIP – DAILY NEWS files.

19:227. Online   **Data-Star**

File name	PHIC
Alternative name(s)	PHIND
Start year	Latest four to five weeks
Number of records	113,270
Update period	Daily
Database aids	Data-Star Business and Biomedical Manuals, Berne, Data-Star, 1989 and Online manual (search NEWS-PHIN in NEWS)
Price/Charges	Subscription: SFr80.00
	Connect time: SFr263.00
	Online print: SFr5.48
	Offline print: SFr5.81

Notes

This is the file containing current news, including PHID (up to five weeks of data). PHIC is used for scanning for recently written reports. PHIC includes PHID but PHID and PHIC are not included in PHIN. For all information on a particular topic both PHIN and PHIC must be searched.

From June 1993 Data-Star have introduced an annual fee/subscription per contract (that is, not per password) of SFr 80.00 (c.UK£ 32.00) payable every June. For North American customers billed in dollars who also use DIALOG, the DIALOG fee also covers access to Data-Star. Academic customers, 'commitment' customers and customers currently billed in dollars are exempt.

Record composition

Accession Number and Update Code AN; Date of Entry of Report DT; Date of Publication YD; Month of Publication YM; Occurrence Table OC; Source SO; Title TI; Text of Report TX; Update Code UP and Year of Publiction YR

19:228. Online   **Data-Star**

File name	PHID
Alternative name(s)	PHIND

Start year	Today only
Number of records	113,270
Update period	Daily
Database aids	Data-Star Business and Biomedical Manuals, Berne, Data-Star, 1989 and Online manual (search NEWS-PHIN in NEWS)
Price/Charges	Subscription: SFr80.00
	Connect time: SFr263.00
	Online print: SFr5.48
	Offline print: SFr5.81

Notes

PHID is the daily news file of pre-publication material used for daily scanning of reports on topics of particular interest. PHID is included in the database PHIC. For all information on a particular topic it is necessary to search both PHIN and PHIC.

From June 1993 Data-Star have introduced an annual fee/subscription per contract (that is, not per password) of SFr 80.00 (c.UK£ 32.00) payable every June. For North American customers billed in dollars who also use DIALOG, the DIALOG fee also covers access to Data-Star. Academic customers, 'commitment' customers and customers currently billed in dollars are exempt.

Record composition

Accession Number and Update Code AN; Date of Entry of Report DT; Date of Publication YD; Month of Publication YM; Occurrence Table OC; Source SO; Title TI; Text of Report TX; Update Code UP and Year of Publiction YR

19:229. Online   Data-Star

File name	PHIN
Alternative name(s)	PHIND
Start year	1980 (to circa five weeks ago)
Number of records	113,270
Update period	Daily
Database aids	Data-Star Business and Biomedical Manuals, Berne, Data-Star, 1989 and Online manual (search NEWS-PHIN in NEWS)
Price/Charges	Subscription: SFr80.00
	Connect time: SFr263.00
	Online print: SFr5.48
	Offline print: SFr5.81

Notes

This is the archive file of information, removed from PHID and/or PHIC files. For all information on a particular topic it is necessary to search both PHIN and PHIC.

From June 1993 Data-Star have introduced an annual fee/subscription per contract (that is, not per password) of SFr 80.00 (c.UK£ 32.00) payable every June. For North American customers billed in dollars who also use DIALOG, the DIALOG fee also covers access to Data-Star. Academic customers, 'commitment' customers and customers currently billed in dollars are exempt.

Record composition

Accession Number and Update Code AN; Date of Entry of Report DT; Date of Publication YD; Month of Publication YM; Occurrence Table OC; Source SO; Title TI; Text of Report TX; Update Code UP and Year of Publiction YR

19:230. Online   DIALOG

File name	File 129
Alternative name(s)	PHIND

Start year	1980
Number of records	179,399
Update period	Weekly
Price/Charges	Connect time: US$150.00
	Online print: US$0.90
	Offline print: US$0.90
	SDI charge: US$5.00

Notes

The Pharmacuetical and Healthcare Industry News Database (PHIND) is divided into two files – daily (File 130) and current information (File 129), which includes some unpublished articles, and archival material dating back to 1980.

19:231. Online   DIALOG

File name	File 130
Alternative name(s)	PHIND
Start year	1980
Number of records	179,399
Update period	Daily
Price/Charges	Connect time: US$150.00
	Online print: US$4.00
	Offline print: US$4.00
	SDI charge: US$5.00 (weekly)/ 2.00 (daily)

Notes

The Pharmaceutical and Healthcare Industry News Database (PHIND) on Dialog is divided into two files – daily (File 130) and current information (File 129), which includes some unpublished articles, and archival material dating back to 1980.

DIALINDEX Categories: BIOBUS, BIOTECH, PHARM, PHARMINA, PHIND.

19:232. Database subset
Online   Data-Star

File name	TRPI – Pharmaceutical and Healthcare Industry News Training File
Alternative name(s)	PHIND
Start year	
Number of records	
Update period	
Database aids	Data-Star Business and Biomedical Manuals, Berne, Data-Star, 1989 and Online manual (search NEWS-PHIN in NEWS)
Price/Charges	Connect time: Free

Record composition

Accession Number and Update Code AN; Date of Entry of Report DT; Date of Publication YD; Month of Publication YM; Occurrence Table OC; Source SO; Title TI; Text of Report TX; Update Code UP and Year of Publiction YR

Pharmacontacts
Pharmaprojects PJB Publications Ltd

19:233. Master record

Alternative name(s)	Company Directory Database
Database type	Directory
Number of journals	
Sources	Directories
Start year	Current information
Language	German and English
Coverage	International

Number of records   20,000
Update size   –
Update period   Monthly

Keywords

Agrochemicals; Crop Protection; Education –
Veterinary Medicine; Regulatory Agencies – Pharma-
ceuticals; Regulatory Agencies – Agrochemicals;
Regulatory Agencies – Veterinary Medicine;
Research and Development – Agriculture

Description

Pharmacontacts contains the names and addresses
of over 7,000 pharmaceutical companies, agrochemi-
cal/crop protection companies and 2,400 animal-
related health companies worldwide. In addition, details of 56 pharmaceutical and agrochemical regulatory bodies, research agencies in agrochemicals and
veterinary science, 161 veterinary regulatory bodies
and 140 veterinary institutions in this area are
included. Wherever possible, telephone, telex, and
telefax numbers are included.

The database, from the producers of PHIND, has
been extensively researched, being based on the
Scrip directories of pharmaceutical companies, the
Animal Pharm directory of animal health companies
(the *Agrow* directory of Agrochemical companies)
and, in future, on the *Clinica* directories of device and
diagnostic companies.

19:234. Online   BRS

File name   PHCO
Alternative name(s)   Company Directory Database
Start year   Current information
Number of records   20,000
Update period   Weekly
Price/Charges   Connect time: US$145.00/155.00
                        Online print: US$1.25/1.35
                        Offline print: US$0.82

19:235. Online   Data-Star

File name   PHCO
Alternative name(s)   Company Directory Database
Start year   Current information
Number of records   20,000
Update period   Monthly
Price/Charges   Subscription: UK£32.00
                        Connect time: UK£105.20
                        Online print: UK£0.88
                        Offline print: UK£0.54

Notes

From June 1993 Data-Star have introduced an annual
fee/subscription per contract (that is, not per password) of SFr 80.00 (c.UK£ 32.00) payable every June.
For North American customers billed in dollars who
also use DIALOG, the DIALOG fee also covers
access to Data-Star. Academic customers, 'commitment' customers and customers currently billed in
dollars are exempt.

Protein
Institut obchej Genetiki

19:236. Master record

Database type   Bibliographic
Number of journals
Sources
Start year   1985
Language   English
Coverage

Number of records
Update size   –
Update period

Keywords

Biotechnology

Description

Bibliographic   information   in   genetics   and
biotechnology.

19:237. Diskette   Institut obchej Genetiki

File name
Start year   1985
Number of records
Update period

Research Centers and Services Directory
Gale Research

19:238. Master record

Database type   Directory, Organisations
Number of journals
Sources   Directories
Start year   Current information
Language   English
Coverage   International
Number of records   38,489 organizations
Update size   –
Update period   Two times per year reload

Keywords

Astronomy; Food Science; Aerospace; Space
Research; Regional Studies

Description

Descriptions of organisations conducting research
from all countries. Fields of research include agriculture, food, veterinary science, biological and environmental sciences, astronomy, space science,
computers, mathematics, engineering, technology,
physical and earth sciences, business and economics, government and public affairs, labour, industrial relations, law, behavioural and social sciences,
education, humanities, religion and regional and area
studies. Also includes multidisciplinary programmes,
research coordinating offices and research parks.
Entries give names, addresses and description of field
of interest for government, university, independent
non-profit, and commercial research devlopment
centres, institutes, laboratories, bureaus, test facilities, experiment stations, research parks, foundations,
councils and any other research supporting organizations. The director or chief officer is listed with
address, telephone and FAX numbers, affiliated institutions, publications and services. Combines the contents of four printed directories.

Corresponds to *Research Centers Directory*, which
covers over 12,300 university-based and other non-
profit research facilities in the U.S. and Canada;
International Research Centers Directory, which
covers over 6,600 non-U.S. research organisations in
approximately 145 countries; *Government Research
Directory*, which covers more than 3,700 research
units of the U.S. federal government; and *Research
Services Directory*, which covers more than 3,400
private sector firms an individuals involved in for-profit
research activities.

19:239. Online DIALOG

File name	File 115
Start year	Current information
Number of records	27,500
Update period	Two times per year
Price/Charges	Connect time: US$96.00
	Online print: US$0.85
	Offline print: US$0.85

Ritka vercsoport tulajdonsagu donorok nyvilvantartasa

Orszagos Haematologiai es

19:240. Master record

Database type	Bibliographic, Factual
Number of journals	
Sources	
Start year	
Language	English
Coverage	
Number of records	3,100
Update size	—
Update period	

Keywords

Haematology

Description

Medical treatment and haematology database.

19:241. Online OHVI

File name	RARE
Start year	
Number of records	3,100
Update period	

SLUBIB

Sveriges Lantbruksuniversitets Bibliotek (SLUB)

19:242. Master record

Alternative name(s)	Sveriges Lantbruksuniversitets Bibliotek (SLUB)
Database type	Library catalogue/cataloguing aids, Bibliographic
Number of journals	
Sources	Books, journals and research reports
Start year	1968; foreign material, 1976 to date
Language	English and Swedish
Coverage	International
Number of records	75,000
Update size	9,000
Update period	Weekly
Index unit	Articles

Keywords

Forestry; Food Science; Horticulture; Fisheries; Nutrition

Description

SLUBIB contains references to the holdings of the libraries of the Swedish University of Agricultural Sciences (Sveriges lantbruksuniversitets bibliotek); Foreign books and research reports published 1968 and later, Swedish books and research reports published 1976 and later. Holdings of periodicals are included. SLUBIB is a part of the catalogue system

LUKAS of the Swedish University of Agricultural Sciences Library and can be searched simultaneously with LANTDOK. Subjects covered include: agriculture, forestry, horticulture, fisheries, food science, environment, veterinary medicine, library catalogues.

19:243. Online Sveriges Lantbruksuniversitet Bibliotek (SLUB)

File name	SLUBIB
Alternative name(s)	Sveriges Lantbruksuniversitets Bibliotek (SLUB)
Start year	1968; foreign material, 1976 to date
Number of records	75,000
Update period	Weekly

ST HU

Statens Husdyrbrugsforsoeg Biblioteket

19:244. Master record

Alternative name(s)	Statens Husdyrbrugforsoeg katalog
Database type	Library catalogue/cataloguing aids, Bibliographic
Number of journals	
Sources	Books and Journals
Start year	1960
Language	Multilingual, English (index terms) and Danish
Coverage	Denmark
Number of records	1,180
Update size	250
Update period	Daily

Description

The database contains literature references to the stock of books and periodicals held by the animal husbandry experiments department.

19:245. Online Statens Husdyrbrugsforsoeg Biblioteket

File name	ST HU
Alternative name(s)	Statens Husdyrbrugforsoeg Katalog
Start year	1960
Number of records	1,180
Update period	Daily

Notes

Subscription to UNI-C required.

Termeszettudomanyi Muzeum Allattar, Hazai gerincesek adatbazisa

Müszi Rt., Budapest

19:246. Master record

Database type	Reference
Number of journals	
Sources	
Start year	
Language	English
Coverage	

Number of records 12,557
Update size —
Update period

Description
Biological referral database on species.

19:247. Online
IIF
File name GERI
Start year
Number of records 12,557
Update period

TOXALL
National Library of Medicine

19:248. Master record

Alternative name(s)	Toxicology Information Online
Database type	Bibliographic
Number of journals	
Sources	Government documents (US), journals, monographs, research projects, Patents, Conference proceedings, Research communications and Symposia
Start year	1940, partly
Language	English
Coverage	International
Number of records	2,500,000
Update size	120,000
Update period	Monthly

Keywords
Aneuploidy; Accident Prevention; Biological Hazards; Chemical Substances; Chromosome Abnormalities; Drugs; Environmental Health; Epidemiology; Ergonomics; Hazardous Substances; Hazardous Waste; Health Physics; Industrial Materials; Industrial Processes; Metabolism; Occupational Health and Safety; Occupational Psychology; Pathology; Pesticides; Pollution; Safety Education; Standards; Vocational Training; Waste Management; Water Treatment

Description
TOXALL/TOXLINE (Toxicology Information Online) is the National Library of Medicine's extensive collection of online bibliographic information covering the toxicological effects of drugs, pesticides and other chemicals. The database contains references to published material and research in progress in areas such as adverse drug reactions, carcinogenesis, mutagenesis, teratogenesis, environmental pollution and food contamination, toxicology, pharmacology, analytical chemistry and occupational safety. Most of the citations include, in addition to the bibliographic information, abstracts and/or indexing term and/or indexing terms and/or CAS Registry numbers.

TOXALL is composed of several database segments of toxicological interest (from CA, BIOSIS Previews and MEDLINE) and of total contents of specialised toxicological data collections. As the data in the different subunits is provided by different producers, there is a relatively great number of duplicates in the database. In addition the structure of the records also varies, for example some include abstracts and some use *MeSH* Indexing, others do not.

The subfiles are, with starting date of coverage being the publication year shown:

ANEUPL (Aneuploidy file of the Environmental Mutagen Information Center) pre 1950 to the present;
Chemical-Biological Activities – CA (Chemical Abstracts);
CISDOC (International Labour Office) (ILO) Abstracts 1981 to the present;
CRISP (Toxicology Research Projects (RPROJ) 1988 to the present;
EMIC (Environmental Mutagen Information Center File of the Oak Ridge National Laboratory (ORNL) 1950 to the present;
EPIDEM (Epidemiology Information System File of the FDA) 1940 to the present;
ETIC (Environmental Teratology Information Center File of ORNL) 1950 to the present;
Federal Research in Progress (FEDRIP) 1982;
HAPAB (Health Aspects of Pesticides Abstract Bulletin of the Environmental Protection Agency (EPA) (see PESTAB));
HAYES (Hayes File on Pesticides);
HMTC (Abstract Bulletin of the US Army's Hazardous Materials Technical Center) 1982 to the present;
International Pharmaceutical Abstracts (IPA) 1969 to the present;
HEEP – see Toxicological Aspects of Environmental Health;
NIOSH (References of the National Institute for Occupational Safety and Health Technical Information Center (NIOSHTIC) database) 1984 to the present;
NTIS (Toxicology Document and Data Depository (TD3) of the National Technical Information Service (NTIS) 1979 to the present;
PESTAB (Pesticides Abstracts of the EPA (Formerly HAPAB) 1968–1981;
PPBIB (Poisonous Plants Bibliography) pre-1976;
RPROJ (Research Projects Directory);
Toxicological Aspects of Environmental Health (BIOSIS) (formerly BIOSIS/HEEP, Health Effects of Environmental Pollutants) 1970 to the present;
TMIC (Toxic Materials Information Center File);
TOXBIB (Toxicity Bibliography from the MEDLINE file) 1965 to the present;
TSCATS (Toxic Substances Control Act Test Submissions File of the EPA) (all relevant submissions).

References in TOXLINE are from producers that do not require royalty charges; references on toxicology from producers that do require royalty charges are placed in TOXLIT.

The database contains approximately 20,000 citations from between 1940 and 1965, 640,000 from 1965 to 1976, EMIC since 1960 and ETIC since 1965. About 45% of the records added per year are from the TOXBIB subfile, which is derived from MEDLINE. Approximately eighty-two per cent of documents contain abstracts. Some hosts only carry TOXLINE. TOXLIT comprises IPA (International Pharmaceutical Abstracts), CA (Chemical Abstracts) and Toxicological Aspects of Environmental Health (BIOSIS) (formerly BIOSIS/HEEP).

The datafield Controlled Terms contains vocabulary from all of the subunits. The datafields CAS Registry Number, Chemical Abstracts Classification Codes and ILO Classification Codes can only be searched directly. The datafield Controlled Terms can be searched directly as well as through freetext and the data fields Title and Abstract can only be searched through freetext. The following points are recommended for drugs and chemicals: always use Registry

1333

numbers when available; for a broad concept search use as many synonyms as possible in title, keywords and abstract; for TOXBIB only use controlled terms from MeSH.

19:249. Online

DIMDI

File name	TX65 – TOXALL
Start year	1940, partly
Number of records	3,466,353
Update period	Monthly
SDI period	1 month
Price/Charges	Connect time: UK£35.99–39.78
	Online print: UK£0.52–0.70
	Offline p;rint: UK£0.48–0.55

Downloading is allowed

Notes

As TOXALL is composed of several database segments of toxicological interest (from Chemical Abstracts Service, MEDLINE, BIOSIS Previews) and total contents of specialised toxicological data collections, single citations may occur more than once. DIMDI recommends using CHEMLINE for the retrieval of synonyms and CAS Registry Numbers of chemical substances before starting a TOXALL search. It also advises that a search for chemical substances should not be restricted to the CAS Registry Number field because several TOXALL subunits do not contain this field. The TOXALL subunits are pooled to create the subfiles TOXLINE and TOXLIT which can be accessed separately by using their poolkeys. TOXLIT contains the subunits CA, BIOSIS/HEEP (up to July 1985: HEEP) and IPA. TOXLINE contains the other subunits ANEUPL, DART, EMIC, ETIC, FEDRIP, HAYES, HMTC, ILO, NIOSH, PESTAB/HAPAB, PPBIB, RPROJ, TD3, TMIC, TOXBIB, TSCATS. Documents total over 3 million since 1965 (about 20,000 citations from 1940 to 1965, 640,000 from 1965 to 1876, EMIC since 1960, ETIC since 1950).

Suppliers of online documents: British Library Document Supply Centre, Boston Spa, England; Harkers Information Retrieval System, Sydney, Australia; Instituto de Informacion y Documentacion en Ciencia y Tecnologica, Madrid, Spain; State Central Scientific Medical Library Supplier Center, Moscow, USSR. 82% of records contain abstracts. Searches are available from January 1965.

Record composition

Abstract AB; Author AU; BIOSIS Section Heading BISH; Chemical Abstracts Section Code CASC; Chemical Abstracts Section Heading CASH; CAS Reg. No CR; Corporate Source CS; Controlled Term CT; Country CY; Document Date DT; Date Received REC; Entry Month EM; Free Text FT; Gene Symbol GE; International Labour Office Classification Code ILCC; International Labour Organisation Section Heading ILSC; International Pharmaceutical Abstracts Section Code IPSC; International Pharmaceutical Association Section Heading IPSH; ISSN SS; Journal Code JC; Journal Title JT; Language LA; Machine Date MD; Number of Document ND; Number of Supporting Agency NS; Number of Unit Record (DIMDI) NU; Order Number OD; Preprocessed Search PPS; Price PR; Publication Year PY; Qualifier AF; Secondary Source SEC; Source SO; Subunit SU; Supporting Agency SA; Title TI; Toxic Substances Control Act Section Code TSCC; Type of Award TA and ZIP Code ZP.

CALL TOXDUP provides the user with a means to define their own hitlist of subunits from TOXALL and its subfiles TOXLINE and TOXLIT and thereby identify duplicate records.

19:250. Database subset
Online

BLAISE-LINK

File name	TOXLINE
Start year	
Number of records	
Update period	

19:251. Database subset
Online

BLAISE-LINK

File name	TOXLIT
Start year	
Number of records	
Update period	

19:252. Database subset
Online

BRS

File name	TOXL
Start year	1965
Number of records	
Update period	Monthly
Price/Charges	Connect time: US$26.00/36.00
	Online print: US$0.07/0.15

Notes

Records from the IPA and BIOSIS subfiles are excluded from this database.

19:253. Database subset
Online

BRS

File name	XTOL
Start year	1965
Number of records	
Update period	Monthly
Price/Charges	Connect time: US$26.00/36.00
	Online print: US$0.07/0.15

Notes

This is a subtitle of BRS's TOXL database and contains documents from all TOXLINE subfiles except the MEDLINE-derived subfile TOXBIB. It contains approximately thirty per cent of the documents in TOXLINE covering the pharmacological, biomedical, physiological and toxicological effects of drugs and other chemicals. Data from proprietary sources is excluded.

19:254. Database subset
Online CompuServe Information Service

File name	IQUEST File 2576 – TOXLINE
Start year	1965
Number of records	
Update period	Monthly
Price/Charges	Subscription: US$8.95 per month
	Database entry fee: US$9/search; some databases carry a surcharge ($2–75)
	Online print: US$10 references free; then $9 per ten; abstracts $3 each

Downloading is allowed

Notes

Coverage dates vary depending on subfile. Accessed via IQUEST or IQMEDICAL, this database is offered by a DIALOG gateway. IQUEST can either search across all databases, a database of the user's choice or selected multiple databases.

19:255. Database subset
Online **Data-Star**

File name	TOXX (TOXLINE)
Start year	Current month
Number of records	1,152,262
Update period	Monthly
Database aids	Data-Star Biomedical Manual and Online Guide (search NEWS-TOXL in NEWS)
Price/Charges	Connect time: SFr78.00
	Online print: SFr0.21–0.24
	Offline print: SFr6.80
	SDI charge: SFr0.24

Notes
The current month file does not include references from Toxicology Research Projects (CRISP); Epidemiology Information System File of the FDA (EPIDEM); the Federal Research in Progress Database (FEDRIP); the Abstracts Bulletin of the US Army's Hazardous Materials Technical Centre (HMTC); or the Toxic Substances Control Act Test Submissions File of the EPA (TSCATS). For TOXBIB use also *Medical Subject Headings Annotated Alphabetic List (MeSH)* and Tree Structures (TREE) published annually.

From June 1993 Data-Star have introduced an annual fee/subscription per contract (that is, not per password) of SFr 80.00 (c.UK£32.00) payable every June. For North American customers billed in dollars who also use DIALOG, the DIALOG fee also covers access to Data-Star. Academic customers, 'commitment' customers and customers currently billed in dollars are exempt.

Record composition
Abstract AB; Accession number and secondary source ID or by code for faster retrieval AN; Author(s) AU; Availability, Order-ID-number, Prices AV; Award type AW; CAS Registry number(s) RN; Classification code CC; Comment CM; Corporate name CA; Entry month EM; Gene symbol GS; Institution, address IN; Keywords KW; Journal coden CD; Language of original LG; MESH-Descriptors in TOXBIB DE; Publication type PT; Source and ISSN-number in TOXBIBSO; Supporting agency SA; Title TI and Year of publication YR

19:256. Database subset
Online **Data-Star**

File name	TOXL (TOXLINE)
Start year	1981 to date
Number of records	1,152,262
Update period	Monthly
Database aids	Data-Star Biomedical Manual and Online guide (search NEWS-TOXL in NEWS)
Price/Charges	Subscription: SFr80.00
	Connect time: SFr78.00
	Online print: SFr0.21–0.24
	Offline print: SFr6.80
	SDI charge: SFr0.24

Notes
For TOXBIB users should also consult *Medical Subject Headings Annotated Alphabet List (MeSH)* and Tree Structures (TREE) published annually.

From June 1993 Data-Star have introduced an annual fee/subscription per contract (that is, not per password) of SFr80.00 (c.UK£32.00) payable every June. For North American customers billed in dollars who

also use DIALOG, the DIALOG fee also covers access to Data-Star. Academic customers, 'commitment' customers and customers currently billed in dollars are exempt.

Record composition
Abstract AB; Accession number and secondary source ID or by code for faster retrieval AN; Author(s) AU; Availability, Order-ID-number, Prices AV; Award type AW; CAS Registry number(s) RN; Classification code CC; Comment CM; Corporate name CA; Entry month EM; Gene symbol GS; Institution, address IN; Keywords KW; Journal coden CD; Language of original LG; MESH-Descriptors in TOXBIB DE; Publication type PT; Source and ISSN-number in TOXBIBSO; Supporting agency SA; Title TI and Year of publication YR

19:257. Database subset
Online **Data-Star**

File name	TO80 (TOXLINE)
Start year	Pre 1965–1980
Number of records	
Update period	Monthly
Database aids	Data-Star Biomedical Manual and Online guide (search NEWS-TOXL in NEWS)
Price/Charges	Subscription: SFr80.00
	Connect time: SFr78.00
	Online print: SFr0.21–0.24
	Offline print: SFr6.80
	SDI charge: SFr0.24

Notes
The Health Aspects of Pesticides Abstracts Bulletin of the Environmental Protection Agency (HAPAB) is only available in the two files which extend back further than 1965 – TO80 and TOZZ – that is before it was renamed Pesticides Abstracts.

This file does not include references from Toxicology Research Projects (CRISP); Epidemiology Information System File of the FDA (EPIDEM); the Federal Research in Progress Database (FEDRIP); the Abstracts Bulletin of the US Army's Hazardous Materials Technical Centre (HMTC); or the Toxic Substances Control Act Test Submissions File of the EPA (TSCATS). For TOXBIB users should also consult *Medical Subject Headings Annotated Alphabet List (MeSH)* and Tree Structures (TREE) published annually.

From June 1993 Data-Star have introduced an annual fee/subscription per contract (that is, not per password) of SFr80.00 (c.UK£32.00) payable every June. For North American customers billed in dollars who also use DIALOG, the DIALOG fee also covers access to Data-Star. Academic customers, 'commitment' customers and customers currently billed in dollars are exempt.

Record composition
Abstract AB; Accession number and secondary source ID or by code for faster retrieval AN; Author(s) AU; Availability, Order-ID-number, Prices AV; Award type AW; CAS Registry number(s) RN; Classification code CC; Comment CM; Corporate name CA; Entry month EM; Gene symbol GS; Institution, address IN; Keywords KW; Journal coden CD; Language of original LG; MESH-Descriptors in TOXBIB DE; Publication type PT; Source and ISSN-number in TOXBIBSO; Supporting agency SA; Title TI and Year of publication YR

19:258. Database subset

Online **Data-Star**

File name	TOZZ (TOXLINE)
Start year	Pre 1965
Number of records	1,152,262
Update periods	Monthly
Database aids	Data-Star Biomedical Manual and Online guide (search NEWS-TOXL in NEWS)
Price/Charges	Subscription: UK£32.00
	Connect time: UK£31.20
	Online print: UK0.00–0.71
	Offline print: UK£0.08–0.10
	SDI charge: UK£2.72

Notes

Data-Star recommends the following search tactics in relation to drugs and chemicals: always use Registry numbers when available; for a broad concept search use as many synonyms as possible in title, keyword and abstract, for multi-word names use ADJ or WITH and for TOXBIB only use specific DE-searching using online MeSH and Tree. The Health Aspects of Pesticides Abstracts Bulletin of the Environmental Protection Agency (HAPAB) is only available in the two files which extend further back than 1965 – TO80 and TOZZ – that is before it was renamed Pesticides Abstracts. For TOXBIB users should also consult *Medical Subject Headings Annotated Alphabet List (MeSH)* and Tree Structures (tree) published annually.

From June 1993 Data-Star have introduced an annual fee/subscription per contract (that is, not per password) of SFr80.00 (c.UK£32.00) payable every June. For North American customers billed in dollars who also use DIALOG, the DIALOG fee also covers access to Data-Star. Academic customers, 'commitment' customers and customers currently billed in dollars are exempt.

Record composition

Abstract AB; Accession number and secondary source ID or by code for faster retrieval AN; Author(s) AU; Availability, Order-ID-number, Prices AV; Award type AW; CAS Registry number(s) RN; Classification code CC; Comment CM; Corporate name CA; Entry month EM; Gene symbol GS; Institution, address IN; Keywords KW; Journal coden CD; Language of original LG; MESH-Descriptors in TOXBIB DE; Publication type PT; Source and ISSN-number in TOXBIBSO; Supporting agency SA; Title TI and Year of publication YR

19:259. Database subset

Online **Data-Star**

File name	TRTO – Training file (TOXLINE)
Start year	
Number of records	
Update period	Monthly
Price/Charges	Connect time: Free
	Online print: Free

Notes

Data-Star recommends the following search tactics in relation to drugs and chemicals: always use Registry numbers when available; for a broad concept search use as many synonyms as possible in title, keyword and abstract, for multi-word names use ADJ or WITH and for TOXBIB only use specific DE-searching. For TOXBIB users should also consult *Medical Subject Headings Annotated Alphabet List (MeSH)* and Tree Structures (tree) published annually.

Record composition

Abstract AB; Accession number and secondary source ID or by code for faster retrieval AN; Author(s) AU; Availability, Order-ID-number, Prices AV; Award type AW; CAS Registry number(s) RN; Classification code CC; Comment CM; Corporate name CA; Entry month EM; Gene symbol GS; Institution, address IN; Keywords KW; Journal coden CD; Language of original LG; MESH-Descriptors in TOXBIB DE; Publication type PT; Source and ISSN-number in TOXBIBSO; Supporting agency SA; Title TI and Year of publication YR

19:260. Database subset

Online **DIALOG**

File name	File 156
Start year	
Number of records	1,647,025
Update period	Monthly
Price/Charges	Connect time: US$66.00
	Online print: US$0.25
	Offline print: US$0.25
	SDI charge: US$7.50

Notes

Coverage dates vary depending on subfile.

19:261. Database subset

Online **DIMDI**

File name	TX165 – TOXLINE
Start year	1940, partly
Number of records	1,196,643
Update period	Monthly
SDI pweios	1 month
Price'Charges	Connect time: UK£05.20–8.99
	Online print: UK£0.16–0.34
	Offline print: UK£0.09–0.15

Downloading is allowed

Notes

TOXLINE is a TOXALL-subfile containing the following subunits ANEUPL, EMIC EPIDEM, ETIC, FEDRIP, HAYES, HMTC, ILO, NIOSH, PESTAB/HAPAB, PPBIBB, RPROJ, TD3, TMIC, TOXBIB, TSCATS. Public Health Services (USA)-supported research from FEDRIP is not included in TOXLINE because that information is already available in the RPROJ subunit.

Suppliers of online documents: British Library Document Centre, Boston Spa, England; Harkers Information Retrieval System, Sydney, Australia; Instituto de Informacion y Documentacion en Ciencia y Tecnologica, Madrid, Spain; State Central Scientific Medical Library Supplier Center, Moscow, USSR. 82% of records have abstracts.

Record composition

Abstract AB; Author AU; BIOSIS Section Heading BISH; Chemical Abstracts Section Code CASC; Chemical Abstracts Section Heading BISH; CAS Reg. No CR; Corporate Source CS; Controlled Term CT; Country CY; Date Project Begins DB; Date Project Ends DE; Date Received REC; Document Date DT; Entry Month EM; Free Text FT; Gene Symbol GE; International Labour Office Section Code ILSC; International Labour Office Section Code ILSC; International Labour Organisation Section Heading ILSC; International Pharmaceutical Abstracts Section Code IPSC; International Pharmaceutical Association Section Heading Heading IPSH; ISSN SS; Journal Code CJ; Journal Title JT; Language LA; Machine Date MD; Number of Document ND; Number of Supporting Agency NS; Number of Unit Record

(DIMDI) NU; Order Number OD; Preprocessed Search PPS; Price PR; Publication Year PY; Qualifier AF; Secondary Source SEC; Source SO; Subunit SU; Supporting Agency SA; Title TI; Toxic Substances Control Act Section Code TSCC; Type of Award TA and ZIP Code ZP

19:262. Database subset

Online   **DIMDI**

File name	T265 – TOXLIT
Start year	1965
Number of records	2,269,710
Update period	Monthly
SDI period	1 month
Database aids	Online User Manual/TOXALL
Price/Charges	Connect time: UK£33.36–37.15
	Online print: UK£0.53–0.71
	Offline print: UK£0.50–0.56

Downloading is allowed

Notes

TOXLIT is a TOXALL-subfile containing the following subunits BIOSIS/HEEP,CA and IPA. From Chemical Abstracts the following segments are taken: CABAC Chemical/Biological Activities, plus other parts of CA referring to toxicology, pharmacology and biochemistry.

Suppliers of online documents: British Library Document Supply Centre, Boston Spa, England; Harkers Information Retrieval System, Sydney, Australia; Instituto de Informacion y Documentacion en Ciencia y Technologica, Madrid, Spain; State Central Scientific Medical Library Supplier Center, Moscow, USSR. Searches are possible from January 1965. 82% of records have abstracts.

Record composition

Abstract AB; Author AU; BIOSIS Section Heading BISH; Chemical Abstracts Section Code CASC; Chemical Abstracts Section Heading CASH; CAS Reg. No CR; Controlled Term CT; Corporate Source CS; Country CY; Date Received REC; Document Date DT; Entry Month EM; Free Text FT; International Labour Office Section Code ILSC; International Labour Office Section Heading ILSH; International Pharmaceutical Abstracts Section Code IPSC; International Pharmaceutical Association Section Heading IPSH; ISSN SS; Journal Code JC; Journal Title JT; Language LA; Machine Date MD; Number of Document ND; Number of Supporting Agency NS; Number of Unit Record (DIMDI) NU; Order Number OD; Preprocessed Search PPS; Price PR; Publication Year; Qualifier AF; Source SO; Subunit SU; Supporting Agency SA; Title TI; Toxic Substances Control Act Section code TSCC; Type of Award TA and ZIP Code ZP

19:263. Database subset

Online   **Japan Information Center of Science and Technology (JICST)**

File name	TOXLINE
Alternative name(s)	Toxicology Information Online
Start year	
Number of records	
Update period	

19:264. Database subset

Online   **Japan Information Center of Science and Technology (JICST)**

File name	TOXLIT
Alternative name(s)	Toxicology Information Online
Start year	
Number of records	
Update period	

19:265. Database subset

Online   **National Library of Medicine**

File name	TOXLINE
Start year	Varies by file
Number of records	
Update period	Monthly

19:266 Database subset

Online   **National Library of Medicine**

File name	TOXLIT
Start year	1965
Number of records	
Update period	Monthly

19:267. Database subset

Tape   **National Library of Medicine**

File name	TOXLINE
Format notes	IBM
Start year	Varies by file
Number of records	
Update period	Monthly

Notes

Corresponds to the TOXLINE online database. Contact NLM for pricing information.

19:268. Database subset

Tape   **National Library of Medicine**

File name	TOXLIT
Format notes	IBM
Start year	1965
Number of records	
Update period	Monthly

Notes

Corresponds to the TOXLIT online database. Contact NLM for pricing information.

This database can also be found on:
PolTox I: NLM, CSA, IFIS
Toxline on SilverPlatter
Toxline Plus

For more details of constituent databases, see:
TOXLIT
TOXLINE

TOXLINE
National Library of Medicine

19:269. Master record

Database type	Bibliographic, Factual
Number of journals	17,400
Sources	Journals
Start year	1945
Language	English
Coverage	International
Number of records	660,000
Update size	–
Update period	Monthly

Keywords

Aneuploidy; Chromosome Abnormalities; Drugs; Occupational Health and Safety; Pesticides; Pollution; Water Treatment

Description

TOXLINE is a part of TOXALL with references from producers that do not require royalty charges; references on toxicology from producers that do require royalty charges are placed in TOXLIT. The database contains approximately 20,000 citations from between 1940 and 1965, 640,000 from 1965 to 1976, EMIC since 1960 and ETIC since 1965. Approximately eighty-two per cent of documents contain abstracts. Some hosts only carry TOXLINE.

For more details of constituent databases, see:
Aneuploidy
CISDOC
Environmental Mutagens – EMIC
Environmental Teratology – ETIC
Epidemiology Information System – EPIDEM
Federal Research in Progress – FEDRIP
Hayes File on Pesticides – HAYES
Hazardous Materials Technical Center – HMTC
International Pharmaceutical Abstracts – IPA
NIOSHTIC, subset
Pesticides Abstracts – PESTAB (post-1965)
Pesticides Abstracts – HAPAB (pre-1965)
Poisonous Plants Bibliography – PPBIB
Toxic Substances Control Act Test Submissions – TSCATS
MEDLINE, subset – Toxicity Bibliography – TOXBIB
Toxicological Aspects of Environmental Health – BIOSIS (formerly HEEP)
Toxicology/Epidemiology Research Projects – RPROJ – CRISP
Toxicology Document and Data Depository – NTIS, subset
Toxic Materials Information Center File – TMIC

This database can be found on:
TOXALL
PolTox I: NLM, CSA, IFIS
Toxline on SilverPlatter
Toxline Plus

TOXLIT
National Library of Medicine

19:270. Master record

Database type	Bibliographic
Number of journals	
Sources	
Start year	
Language	
Coverage	
Number of records	
Update size	–
Update period	

Keywords
Aneuploidy; Chromosome Abnormalities; Drugs; Occupational Health and Safety; Pesticides; Pollution; Water Treatment

Description
TOXLIT is a part of TOXALL with references from producers that require royalty charges; references on toxicology from producers that do not require royalty charges are placed in TOXLINE. The database contains approximately 20,000 citations from between 1940 and 1965, 640,000 from 1965 to 1976, EMIC since 1960 and ETIC since 1965. Approximately eighty- two per cent of documents contain abstracts. Some hosts only carry TOXLINE.

For more details of constituent databases, see:
Chemical Abstracts – CA
Biological Abstracts – BIOSIS
International Pharmaceutical Abstracts – IPA

This database can be found on:
TOXALL
PolTox I: NLM, CSA, IFIS
Toxline on SilverPlatter
Toxline Plus

Toxikologiai adatbazis
Johan Bela Orszagos KözegeszsegÜgyi

19:271. Master record

Database type	Reference
Number of journals	
Sources	
Start year	
Language	English
Coverage	
Number of records	
Update size	–
Update period	

Description
Referral database system on micro-organisms.

19:272. Online
Johan Bela Orszagos Kozegeszsegugyi

File name	EUTOX
Start year	
Number of records	
Update period	

VETDOC
Derwent Publications Ltd

19:273. Master record

Alternative name(s)	Veterinary Literature Documentation
Database type	Bibliographic
Number of journals	
Sources	Journals
Start year	1968
Language	English
Coverage	International
Number of records	96,000
Update size	4,800
Update period	Quarterly
Index unit	Articles

Keywords
Veterinary Drugs

Description
VETDOC contains citations, with abstracts, to the worldwide journal literature on veterinary drugs, vaccines, growth promotants, toxicology and hormonal control of breeding for domestic and farm animals. Subject areas covered include analysis, biochemistry, chemistry, endorinology, microbiology, pathology, pharmacoloyg, zoology and management.

The database corresponds to the biweekly *Vetdoc Abstract Journal and Associated Classified Editions*. Each record contains indepth keywording and fragmentation codes.

19:274. Online
ORBIT

File name	UDBV
Start year	1983
Number of records	96,000
Update period	Quarterly
SDI period	Monthly
Price/Charges	Connect time: US$60.00
	Online print: US$0.25/0.25
	Offline print: US$0.25/0.25
	SDI charge: US$8.50

Downloading is allowed

Notes
The corresponding file VETD contains records for the years 1968–1982. Electronic SDI service is now available within two hours on ORBIT. They can be downloaded and reformatted on a word processor. Results are retrieved in the low cost PRINTS file, $15 per connect hour. Online access is restricted to VETDOC subscribers.

19:275. Online   ORBIT

File name	VETD
Start year	1968–1982
Number of records	
Update period	Quarterly
SDI period	Monthly
Price/Charges	Connect time: US$60.00
	Online print: US$0.25/0.25
	Offline print: US$0.25/0.25
	SDI charge: US$8.50

Downloading is allowed

Notes
See corresponding file UDBV for records from 1983 onwards. Electronic SDI service is now available within two hours on ORBIT. They can be downloaded and reformatted on a word processor. Results are retrieved in the low cost PRINTS file, $15 per connect hour. Online access is restricted to VETDOC subscribers.

Veterinary Science
Wsesojusnyj institut nauchnoj technicheskoj informazii

19:276. Master record

Database type	Bibliographic
Number of journals	
Sources	
Start year	1984
Language	English
Coverage	
Number of records	47,000
Update size	4,800
Update period	

Description
Scientific database on veterinary medicine. Viniti's Separate Publication *Veterinary Science*

19:277. Online   **Wsesojusnyj institut nauchnoj technicheskoj informazii**

File name	
Start year	1984
Number of records	47,000
Update period	

Virginia Disc: VADISC 1
Nimbus Records Ltd
Virginia Polytechnic Institute and State University

19:278. Master record

Database type	Computer software, Bibliographic, Textual, Factual, Statistical, Image, Cartographic, Multimedia
Number of journals	
Sources	
Start year	
Language	English
Coverage	
Number of records	
Update size	—
Update period	
Database aids	Twelve-page description of software and data and User Agreement

Keywords
Nutrition

Description
The Virginia Disc series was conceived to demonstrate the feasibility of local publishing of CD-ROMs, especially by universities, and to stimulate interest in both CD-ROM and innovative approaches to information storage and retrieval. Manifold data, images, computer science, consumer information and software included in 35 searchable collections.

VADISC 1 contains about 6,000 files totalling about 600 Mbytes and includes over thirty searchable databases and a 30-minute slide demonstration of the contents. Some data may be downloaded, some may be searched with the software packages included. Major software packages include FoxBASE+ (compiled dBASE III Plus programs); HyperLink (hypertext package); PC-Write (shareware editor/word processor) Personal Librarian (full-text retrieval software with Boolean logic, truncation, wild cards, proximity operators and ranking of search results); Perfect Hash Functions (Software routines which demonstrate the applicability of perfect hashing as a method of accessing data on CD-ROMs); TOPIC (full-text retrieval software incorporating artificial intelligence and fuzzy set concepts supporting reusable topic specifications that can form the kernel of more complex queries); and Window Book Technology (hypertext system).

The data collections included are:

Four collections from the Association for Computing Machinery (use Personal Librarian);
Computer World – a collection of 2351 computer articles (TOPIC);
Electronic Mail Digest Archives (TOPIC);
Inter-American Compendium of Registered Veterinary Drug products (FoxBASE+);
IPIS-Hypertext – the Integrated Preservation Information System (HyperLink);
King James Bible (Personal Librarian);
Rutgers' Information Retrieval Database (Dr Tefko Saracevic) on the elements involved in information seeking, searching and retrieving, particularly relating to the cognitive context and human decisions and interactions involved (Personal Librarian);
University of Melbourne Computer Science Bibliography (Personal Librarian);
University Self Study – survey of last ten years at VPI&SU providing variable information in full-text form (Personal Librarian);
US Department of Agriculture Extension Information – possibly the single most important collection on the disc, including a list of Virginia publication titles (Personal Librarian); general information fact sheets on agriculture, clothing and textiles, gardening, health and nutrition, home and financial management, home economics, pests, rural community development and youth leadership (Personal Librarian); Florida Agricultural Information Retrieval System (FAIRS) with data; Florida Pest Control Guides; Virginia Master Gardener Handbook (Window Book or Personal Librarian); Recipe Nutrition Analysis; Pesticide Spray Bulletin (Personal Librarian);
US Geographical and Population Data (FoxBASE+);
Virginia Genealogical Database (Personal Librarian);
Virginia Tech Faculty Expertise Database (Personal Librarian).

Public Domain data collections include:

Artificial Intelligence List (eMail messages);
Architectural Images (AUTOCAD files requiring VGA or Targa board);
Dual Independent Map Format file of US state boundaries;

Florida Extension Images of flora and fuana native to Florida (require VGA or Targa board);

Information Retrieval List (eMail messages);

Information Retrieval Test Collections including ADI, CACM, CISI, Cranfield, MEDLINE, NPL, TIME and LISA (Sheffield);

Survey Points in Virginia, Washington DC and Baltimore;

University of Maryland CVL Images – a collection of 200 varied images;

US Geological data of digital elevation models, digital line graph data, land use/land cover data and population/place data.

In addition a DVI directory has files that are usable with Pro750 trademark symbol Application Development Platform from Intel or other compatible DVI systems – full motion video sequences, photographic stills and images.

19:279. CD-ROM   Virginia Polytechnic Institute and State University

File name	
Software	Needs MS-DOS V3.3 or above and Microsoft Extensions V2.0 or above.
Start year	
Number of records	
Update period	
Database aids	Twelve-page description of software and data and User Agreement

OTHER TOPICS

1st Medical Response
Micromedex Inc

20:1. Master record

Database type	Factual, Directory, Textual, Bibliographic
Number of journals	
Sources	
Start year	
Language	English
Coverage	USA (primarily) and International (some)
Number of records	
Update size	—
Update period	Quarterly

Keywords
First Aid; Hazardous Chemicals; Occupational Health and Safety

Description
Protocols for developing training programmes or establishing protocols for first aid or initial response to accidents, injuries or illnesses occurring in the workplace.

This database can be found on:
TOMES Plus

Ärzte Zeitung Datenbank
Ärzte Zeitung Verlagsgesellschaft mbH

20:3. Master record

Alternative name(s)	Ärzte Zeitung Datenbank; Arzte Zeitung Datenbank
Database type	Textual
Number of journals	450
Sources	Journals, newspapers, press releases, research reports and surveys
Start year	1984
Language	German
Coverage	Germany (primarily) and International (some)
Number of records	100,000
Update size	—
Update period	Weekly

Keywords
Clinical Research; Diagnosis; Therapy

Description
This database covers medical trends, management of health services and the pharmaceutical industry. The main subjects covered include: developments in current medical and clinical research, diagnosis, therapy and treatment, health-care planning and social issues, national and international health policies, health management, office management and relevant company and industry news, market data and trends in the pharmaceutical industry.

This is the online equivalent to the printed *Ärzte-Zeitung* (daily) and selected articles from *Arzneimittel Zeitung* (bi-weekly). Approximately seventy per cent of the news is devoted to West Germany and the database is also strong on developments in Eastern Europe; other countries (including Western Europe and North American) are covered to a lesser extent. Information is taken from 450 national and international newspapers and journals and from press releases of companies, government agencies, and national and international organisations. Original research and statistical surveys on specific topics is also provided from *Aerzte Zeitung*'s editorial staff in Munich, Frankfurt, Bonn, Hamburg, Berlin and New York.

There are seven broad groups of subject categories: Forschung-und-Prazis, Gesundheitspolitik, Kultur, Medizin, Panorama, WIrtachaft-Politik and Undefined.

20:4. Online — Bertelsmann InformationsService GmbH (BIS)

File name	AEZT
Alternative name(s)	Ärzte Zeitung Datenbank; Arzte Zeitung Datenbank
Start year	
Number of records	
Update period	

20:5. Online — Data-Star

File name	AEZT
Alternative name(s)	Ärzte Zeitung Datenbank; Arzte Zeitung Datenbank
Start year	1984
Number of records	100,000
Update period	Weekly
Database aids	Data-Star Business Manual and Online manual (search NEWS-AEZT in NEWS)
Price/Charges	Subscription: SFr80.00
	Connect time: SFr115.00
	Online print: SFr0.45
	Offline print: SFr0.73
	SDI charge: SFr7.80

Thesaurus is online

Notes
From June 1993 Data-Star have introduced an annual fee/subscription per contract (that is, not per password) of SFr 80.00 (c.UK£ 32.00) payable every June. For North American customers billed in dollars who also use DIALOG, the DIALOG fee also covers access to Data-Star. Academic customers, 'commitment' customers and customers currently billed in dollars are exempt.

AfterCare Instructions: Injury and Illness

Micromedex Inc

20:6. Master record

Alternative name(s)	Computerized Clinical Information System: AfterCare Instructions: Injury and Illness; CCIS: AfterCare Instructions: Injury and Illness; Injury and Illness: AfterCare Instructions; AfterCare Instructions
Database type	Factual, Textual, Numeric, Directory
Number of journals	
Sources	
Start year	1988
Language	English and Spanish
Coverage	International
Number of records	
Update size	—
Update period	Quarterly

Keywords

Clinical Medicine; Drugs

Description

The AfterCare database consists of two individual modules, available separately or as a combination. Injury and Illness contains instructions for injury and illness, which can be personalised for each patient, can be accessed by more than 500 titles in 22 subject categories. The other module is USP DI Volume 2. Injury and Illness provides printed instructions for health care professionals to give to patients who have been discharged from the emergency department or clinic or who have received medication from a pharmacy. Each instruction sheet can be located by the medical or common name of the sign, symptom or diagnosis. Brief information regarding thirty generic drugs specific to the emergency department or clinic setting is included. All instructions are researched, prepared and reviewed by members of the Micromedex editorial staff and board, comprising over 350 physicians and pharmacists. Information is available in both English and Spanish.

20:7. CD-ROM   Micromedex Inc

File name	AfterCare Instructions: Injury and Illness
Alternative name(s)	Computerized Clinical Information System: AfterCare Instructions: Injury and Illness; CCIS: AfterCare Instructions: Injury and Illness; Injury and Illness: AfterCare Instructions; AfterCare Instructions
Start year	1988
Number of records	
Update period	Quarterly

Notes

This database is available as a standalone product, as well as being a part of CCIS, Computerized Clinical Information System.

This database can also be found on:
CCIS

Alcohol Information for Clinicians and Educators Database

Project CORK Institute, Dartmouth Medical School

20:8. Master record

Database type	Bibliographic, Library catalogue/cataloguing aids
Number of journals	
Sources	Conference papers, government documents, journals, monographs and reports
Start year	1978
Language	English
Coverage	International
Number of records	9,000+
Update size	1,200
Update period	Quarterly
Hosts have included	BRS (until 31.12.92.)

Keywords

Alcohol Abuse; Drug Abuse

Description

This database provides an index to the collection of information about alcohol and alcoholism and other drugs in the Project Cork Resource Center which was started in 1978 to provide information services to physicians and medical educators as they worked to integrate alcohol education into the medical school curriculum. It also includes biomedical, social science and social policy literature. The scope of the collection was expanded throughout 1990 to include drugs other than alcohol. The multidisciplinary collection is used by health care providers, administrators, policy makers and educators. Materials selected for the collection include journals, books, government reports, and documents and presentations.

The database corresponds in part to *Alcohol Clinical Update*, a newsletter that contains selected material from the database.

Controlled vocabulary developed by the Project Cork Resource Center.

BRS discontinued this database at the end of 1992.

Alzheimer's Disease

Alzheimer's Disease Education and Referral Center

20:9. Master record

Database type	Bibliographic, Textual
Number of journals	
Sources	Journals, Monographs, Pamphlets and A-V material
Start year	1987
Language	English
Coverage	USA (primarily) and International (some)
Number of records	
Update size	—
Update period	Quarterly
Index unit	Articles

Description

Contains citations, with abstracts, to journal articles, books, pamphlets, and audiovisual materials related to Alzheimer's disease.

Language is primarily English, with some coverage of materials in other languages.

This database can be found on:
Combined Health Information Database

American Type Culture Collection

American Type Culture Collection Institute for Fermentation

20:10. Master record

Database type	Textual, Directory
Number of journals	
Sources	
Start year	
Language	English
Coverage	International
Number of records	
Update size	—
Update period	Annually
Index unit	Microorganism

Description

Contains microorganism reference catalogues which can be searched by name, culture collection designation, growth temperature, or GC content, depending on catalogue searched. Catalogues include Animal Viruses and Antisera; Bacteria and Bacteriophages; Cell Lines and Hybridomas; Clones, Vectors, Libraries and Hosts; Plant Viruses and Hosts; Protozoa and Algae; and Yeasts and Filamentous Fungi.

Users may search all the catalogues simultaneously or limit their search to one catalogue.

20:11. Online — BIOSIS Life Science Network

File name	ATCC
Start year	
Number of records	
Update period	
Price/Charges	Connect time: US$9.00
	Online print: US$6.00 per 10; 2.25 per abstract; 3.50 per full text article

Also available via the Internet by telnetting to LSN.COM.

Notes

On Life Science Network users can search this database or they can scan a group of subject-related databases. There is a charge of $2.00 per scan of subject-related databases. To search one database and display up to ten citations costs $6.00. Most charges are for information retrieved. There are no charges if there are no results and no charge to transfer results to a printer or diskette. Articles may also be ordered via an online document delivery request. A telecommunications software package is also available, costing $12.95, providing an automatic connection to Life Science Network for heavy users of the service, with capability to transfer to print or disk and customised colour options.

20:12. CD-ROM — Hitachi Software Engineering

File name	CD-Strains
Format notes	IBM
Software	CD-Strains

Start year	
Number of records	
Update period	Annually

AMIA Communications Network

American Medical Informatics Association (AMIA)

20:13. Master record

Alternative name(s)	AAMSI Communications
Database type	Bibliographic, Textual, Textual (book reviews), Directory
Number of journals	8+
Sources	Journals, Book reviews, Suppliers, Own publications and Newsletter
Start year	Current
Language	English
Coverage	International
Number of records	
Update size	—
Update period	Quarterly
Index unit	Articles, Book reviews and Companies

Description

Contains information on the use of computer and information systems in medicine. Includes citations to articles in the current quarter's issues of *Computers in Health Care*, *Computers in Biology and Medicine*, *Medical Informatics*, *Computer Programs in Biomedicine*, and *Journal of Medical Systems*, as well as selected other journals (for example, *New England Journal of Medicine* and *American Journal of Public Health*). Also includes book reviews; information on vendors of computerised medical systems (including name, address and product descriptions); a message from the AAMSI President; an editorial; full text of a feature article from the AAMSI News newsletter; AAMSI organizational news; a list of such professional activities as workshops and seminars; and a calendar of professional meetings for the coming two years.

An electronic bulletin board, the AAMSI Medical Forum, is also available.

20:14. Online — CompuServe Information Service

File name	
Alternative name(s)	AAMSI Communications
Start year	
Number of records	
Update period	
Price/Charges	Subscription: US$8.95 per month
Downloading is allowed	

Annals of Neurology

Little, Brown and Company

20:15. Master record

Database type	Textual, Factual
Number of journals	
Sources	Newsletter
Start year	1984
Language	English
Coverage	International

Number of records
Update size   –
Update period
Index unit   Articles, Letters and Reviews

Keywords
Neurology

Description
Chronicles current research developments and clinical topics relevant to the practice of neurology. Regular sections include: brief communications, editorial, letters to the editor, neurological progress, neurological review, neurological issues and notes and letters.

Annals of Neurology is the official journal of the American Neurological Association and the Child Neurology Association.

20:16. Online   Mead Data Central
(as a NEXIS database)

File name   ANN – NEXIS
Start year   1984–1987
Number of records
Update period
Price/Charges   Subscription: US$1,000 – 3,000
                    (Depending on needs)
                    Connect time: US$49.00
                    (Telecomms + connect time)
                    Database entry fee: US$24.00
                    (Search charge)
                    Online print: US$0.04 per line

Notes
Library: GENMED; Group file: ARCJNL.

A subscription charge which covers all transactional charges, connect time, telecommunications and the small administration charge can take the place of the individual charges. Subscriptions are negotiated with customers and vary according to the number of menus (thus, files) that are to be used – typically a minimum subscription would be about US$ 1,000. All charges include training and a 24-hour help line.

Record composition
Publication; Cite; Date; Section; Length; Title; Source; Author; Abstract (SUM-ABS); Text; Additional information (SUPP-INFO); Reference (BIBLIO-REF); Graphic; Correction; Correction Date; Discussion and Editor's Note

This database can also be found on:
NEXIS
Comprehensive Core Medical Library
IQUEST File 1189

Annals of Plastic Surgery
Little, Brown and Company

20:18. Master record
Database type   Bibliographic, Factual, Textual
Number of journals
Sources   Newsletter
Start year   1984
Language   English
Coverage   International
Number of records
Update size   –
Update period
Index unit   Articles, Letters and Reviews

Keywords
Surgery; Plastic Surgery

Description
Covers current research and developments and clinical topics relevant to the practice of plastic surgery. Regular sections include: case reports, gadgetry, 'How I do it', letters to the editor, original articles and overviews.

20:19. Online   Mead Data Central
(as a NEXIS database)

File name   ANPS – NEXIS
Start year   1984–1987
Number of records
Update period
Price/Charges   Subscription: US$1,000 – 3,000
                    (Depending on needs)
                    Connect time: US$49.00
                    (Telecomms + connect time)
                    Database entry fee: US$24.00
                    (Search charge)
                    Online print: US$0.04 per line

Notes
Library: GENMED; Group file: ARCJNL.

A subscription charge which covers all transactional charges, connect time, telecommunications and the small administration charge can take the place of the individual charges. Subscriptions are negotiated with customers and vary according to the number of menus (thus, files) that are to be used – typically a minimum subscription would be about US$ 1,000. All charges include training and a 24-hour help line.

Record composition
Publication; Cite; Date; Section; Length; Title; Source; Author; Abstract (SUM-ABS); Text; Additional information (SUPP-INFO); Reference (BIBLIO-REF); Graphic; Correction; Correction Date; Discussion and Editor's Note

This database can also be found on:
NEXIS

APINMAP Database
UNESCO Asian and Pacific Information Network on Medicinal and Aromatic Plants (APINMAP)

20:21. Master record
Alternative name(s)   Asian and Pacific Information
                        Network on Medicinal and Aromatic
                        Plants
Database type   Bibliographic
Number of journals
Sources
Start year   Current
Language   English
Coverage   Asia and Pacific
Number of records
Update size   –
Update period   Daily

Keywords
Alternative Medicine; Medicinal Plants

Description
A database of information on the medicinal and aromatic plants and spices of Asia and the Pacific region. Available to network members and to external users with restrictions. Also available as a printout.

Indexing terms are drawn from the *Medical Subject Headings* of the US National Library of Medicine (*MeSH*), *Index Kiwensis* and *PIDVOC*. The Chemical Abstracts Registry Number is also indexed.

20:22. Diskette — UNESCO Asian and Pacific Information Network on Medicinal and Aromatic Plants (APINMAP)

File name	APINMAP Database
Alternative name(s)	Asian and Pacific Information Network on Medicinal and Aromatic Plants
Format notes	IBM
Software	CDS/ISIS (Mini-micro version)
Start year	Current
Number of records	
Update period	Daily

Archives of Dermatology
American Medical Association

20:23. Master record

Database type	Bibliographic, Factual, Textual
Number of journals	1
Sources	Newsletter
Start year	1982
Language	English
Coverage	International
Number of records	
Update size	–
Update period	Annually

Keywords
Dermatology; Surgery

Description
Covers current research developments and clinical topics relevant to the practice of dermatology including dermatopathology, dermatologic surgery and immunodermatology. Sections include: Full text and images of original contributions; Editorials; Book reviews; Clinical notes; Letters to the editor; Photograph essays; Commentaries; Review articles; Case reports.

20:24. Online — Mead Data Central (as a NEXIS database)

File name	ARD – NEXIS
Alternative name(s)	NEXIS – Archives of Dermatology
Start year	1982
Number of records	
Update period	Monthly
Price/Charges	Subscription: US$1,000 – 3,000 (Depending on needs) Connect time: US$49.00 (Telecomms + connect time) Database entry fee: US$14.00 (Search charge) Online print: US$0.04 per line

Notes
Library: GENMED; Group file: JNLS.

A subscription charge which covers all transactional charges, connect time, telecommunications and the small administration charge can take the place of the individual charges. Subscriptions are negotiated with customers and vary according to the number of menus (thus, files) that are to be used – typically a minimum subscription would be about US$ 1,000. All charges include training and a 24-hour help line.

Record composition
Publication; Cite; Date; Section; Series; Length; Title; Source; Author; Abstract (SUM-ABS); Text; Additional information (SUPP-INFO); Reference (BIBLIO-REF); Graphic; Correction; Correction Date; Discussion; Editor's Section (ED/SECT) and Editor's Note

20:25. CD-ROM — CMC ReSearch

File name	Archives of Dermatology
Format notes	IBM
Start year	1985
Number of records	
Update period	Annually
Price/Charges	Subscription: UK£265

Notes
Contains five years of the *Archives of Dermatology*.

This database can also be found on:
NEXIS
American Medical Association Journals Online
Medtext

Archives of Internal Medicine
American Medical Association

20:27. Master record

Database type	Bibliographic, Factual, Textual
Number of journals	1
Sources	Newsletter
Start year	1982
Language	
Coverage	
Number of records	
Update size	–
Update period	Monthly
Index unit	Articles, letters and reviews

Keywords
Internal Medicine

Description
Archives of Internal Medicine covers current research developments and clinical topics including the diagnosis and other practical management of various diseases identified in the field of internal medicine. Coverage includes cardiovascular diagnosis; clinical epidemiology; clinical ethics; critical care medicine; pathophysiology; primary care medicine; and Rankin Clinical Research. Sections include: Full text of original contributions; Editorials; Book reviews; Clinical notes; Letters to the editor; Photograph essays; Commentaries; Review articles; and Case reports.

20:28. Online — Mead Data Central (as a NEXIS database)

File name	ARIM – NEXIS
Alternative name(s)	NEXIS – Archives of Internal Medicine
Start year	1982
Number of records	
Update period	Monthly
Price/Charges	Subscription: US$1,000 – 3,000 (Depending on needs) Connect time: US$49.00 (Telecomms + connect time) Database entry fee: US$14.00 (Search charge) Online print: US$0.04 per line

Notes

Library: GENMED; Group File: JNLS.

A subscription charge which covers all transactional charges, connect time, telecommunications and the small administration charge can take the place of the individual charges. Subscriptions are negotiated with customers and vary according to the number of menus (thus, files) that are to be used – typically a minimum subscription would be about US$ 1,000. All charges include training and a 24-hour help line.

Record composition

Publication; Cite; Date; Section; Length; Title; Source; Author; Abstract (SUM-ABS); Text; Additional information (SUPP-INFO); Reference (BIBLIO-REF); Graphic; Correction; Correction Date; Discussion and Editor's Note

20:29. CD-ROM   CMC ReSearch

File name	Archives of Internal Medicine on CD-ROM
Format notes	IBM
Software	DiscPassage
Start year	Most recent five years
Number of records	
Update period	Annually
Price/Charges	Subscription: UK£265

Notes

Contains five years of the *Archives of Internal Medicine*. Images from the text are included.

This database can also be found on:
NEXIS
American Medical Association Journals Online
Medtext

Archives of Neurology
American Medical Association

20:31. Master record

Database type	Bibliographic, Factual, Textual
Number of journals	
Sources	Newsletter
Start year	1982
Language	English
Coverage	International
Number of records	
Update size	—
Update period	Monthly
Index unit	Articles, letters and reviews

Keywords

Neurology

Description

Archives of Neurology chronicles current research developments and clinical topics relevant to the practice of neurology: child neurology; controversies in neurology; history of neurology; etc. Sections include full text of original contributions; Editorials; Book reviews; Clinical notes; Letters to the editor; Photograph essays; Commentaries; Review articles; and Case reports.

20:32. Online   Mead Data Central
(as a NEXIS database)

File name	ARN – NEXIS
Start year	
Number of records	
Update period	Monthly

Price/Charges	Subscription: US$1,000 – 3,000 (Depending on needs)
	Connect time: US$49.00 (Telecomms + connect time)
	Database entry fee: US$14.00 (Search charge)
	Online print: US$0.04 per line

Notes

Library: GENMED; Group File: JNLS.

A subscription charge which covers all transactional charges, connect time, telecommunications and the small administration charge can take the place of the individual charges. Subscriptions are negotiated with customers and vary according to the number of menus (thus, files) that are to be used – typically a minimum subscription would be about US$ 1,000. All charges include training and a 24-hour help line.

Record composition

Publication; Cite; Date; Section; Length; Title; Source; Author; Abstract (SUM-ABS); Text; Additional information (SUPP-INFO); Reference (BIBLIO-REF); Graphic; Correction; Correction Date; Discussion and Editor's Note

20:33. CD-ROM   CMC ReSearch

File name	Archives of Neurology
Format notes	IBM
Software	DiscPassage
Start year	
Number of records	
Update period	Annually
Price/Charges	Subscription: UK£265

Notes

Includes five years of the *Archives of Neurology*. Images from the text are included.

This database can also be found on:
NEXIS
American Medical Association Journals Online
Medtext

Archives of Ophthalmology
American Medical Association

20:35. Master record

Database type	Bibliographic, Textual, Factual
Number of journals	
Sources	Newsletter
Start year	1982
Language	English
Coverage	International
Number of records	
Update size	—
Update period	Monthly
Index unit	Articles, letters and reviews

Keywords

Ophthalmology

Description

Archives of Ophthalmology chronicles current research developments and clinical topics relevant to the practice of ophthalmology. Sections include: Full text of original contributions; Editorials; Book reviews; Clinical notes; Letters to the editor; Photograph essays; Commentaries; Review articles; Case reports.

20:36. Online — Mead Data Central (as a NEXIS database)

File name	AROP – NEXIS
Alternative name(s)	NEXIS – Archives of Ophthalmology
Start year	1982
Number of records	
Update period	Monthly
Price/Charges	Subscription: US$1,000 – 3,000 (Depending on needs) Connect time: US$49.00 (Telecomms + connect time) Database entry fee: US$24.00 (Search charge) Online print: US$0.04 per line

Notes

Library: GENMED; Group file: JNLS.

A subscription charge which covers all transactional charges, connect time, telecommunications and the small administration charge can take the place of the individual charges. Subscriptions are negotiated with customers and vary according to the number of menus (thus, files) that are to be used – typically a minimum subscription would be about US$ 1,000. All charges include training and a 24-hour help line.

Record composition

Publication; Cite; Date; Section; Length; Title; Source; Author; Abstract (SUM-ABS); Text; Additional information (SUPP-INFO); Reference (BIBLIO-REF); Graphic; Correction; Correction Date; Discussion and Editor's Note

20:37. CD-ROM — CMC ReSearch

File name	Archives of Ophthalmology on CD-ROM
Format notes	IBM
Software	DiscPassage
Start year	
Number of records	
Update period	Annually
Price/Charges	Subscription: UK£265

Notes

Contains five years of the *Archives of Ophthalmology*. This includes: Full text and images of original contributions; Editorials; Book reviews; Clinical notes; Letters to the editor; Photograph essays; Commentaries; Review articles; Case reports.

This database can also be found on:
NEXIS
American Medical Association Journals Online
Medtext

Archives of Otolaryngology, Head and Neck Surgery
American Medical Association

20:39. Master record

Database type	Bibliographic, Textual, Factual
Number of journals	
Sources	Newsletter
Start year	1982
Language	English
Coverage	International
Number of records	
Update size	–
Update period	Monthly
Index unit	Articles, letters and reviews

Keywords

Otolaryngology; Plastic Surgery; Surgery

Description

Archives of Otolaryngology, Head and Neck Surgery chronicles current research developments and clinical topics relevant to the practice of otolaryngology, including head and neck surgery, facial plastic and reconstructive surgery as well as communicative disorders. Sections include: Full text and images of original contributions; Editorials; Book reviews; Clinical notes; Letters to the editor; Photograph essays; Commentaries; Review articles; and Case reports.

20:40. Online — Mead Data Central (as a NEXIS database)

File name	AROT – NEXIS
Alternative name(s)	NEXIS – Archives of Otolaryngology, Head and Neck Surgery
Start year	1982
Number of records	
Update period	Monthly
Price/Charges	Subscription: US$1,000 – 3,000 (Depending on needs) Connect time: US$49.00 (Telecomms + connect time) Database entry fee: US$24.00 (Search charge) Online print: US$0.04 per line

Notes

Library: GENMED; Group File: JNLS.

A subscription charge which covers all transactional charges, connect time, telecommunications and the small administration charge can take the place of the individual charges. Subscriptions are negotiated with customers and vary according to the number of menus (thus, files) that are to be used – typically a minimum subscription would be about US$ 1,000. All charges include training and a 24-hour help line.

20:41. CD-ROM — CMC ReSearch

File name	Archives of Otolaryngology, Head and Neck Surgery on CD-ROM
Format notes	IBM
Software	DiscPassage
Start year	Most recent five years.
Number of records	
Update period	Annually
Price/Charges	Subscription: UK£265

Notes

This disc includes five years of the *Archives of Otolaryngology, Head, and Neck Surgery*. Images from the text are included.

This database can also be found on:
NEXIS
American Medical Association Journals Online
Medtext

Archives of Pathology and Laboratory Medicine
American Medical Association

20:42. Master record

Database type	Bibliographic, Textual, Factual
Number of journals	
Sources	Newsletter
Start year	1982
Language	English
Coverage	International

Number of records
Update size —
Update period Monthly
Index unit Articles, letters and reviews

Keywords
Laboratory Medicine; Pathology

Description
Archives of Pathology and Laboratory Medicine chronicles current research developments and clinical topics relevant to the practice of pathology, including clinical applications to diagnosis and laboratory monitoring of therapy. Sections include: Full text of original contributions; Editorials; Book reviews; Clinical notes; Letters to the editor; Photograph essays; Commentaries; Review articles; Case reports.

20:43. Online
**Mead Data Central
(as a NEXIS database)**

File name ARP – NEXIS
Alternative name(s) NEXIS – Archives of Pathology and Laboratory Medicine
Start year 1982
Number of records
Update period Monthly
Price/Charges Subscription: US$1,000 – 3,000 (Depending on needs)
Connect time: US$49.00 (Telecomms + connect time)
Database entry fee: US$24.00 (Search charge)
Online print: US$0.04 per line

Notes
Library: GENMED; Group file: JNLS.

A subscription charge which covers all transactional charges, connect time, telecommunications and the small administration charge can take the place of the individual charges. Subscriptions are negotiated with customers and vary according to the number of menus (thus, files) that are to be used – typically a minimum subscription would be about US$ 1,000. All charges include training and a 24-hour help line.

Record composition
Publication; Cite; Date; Section; Length; Title; Source; Author; Abstract (SUM-ABS); Text; Additional information (SUPP-INFO); Reference (BIBLIO-REF); Graphic; Correction; Correction Date; Discussion and Editor's Note

20:44. CD-ROM
CMC ReSearch

File name Archives of Pathology and Laboratory Medicine on CD-ROM
Format notes IBM
Software DiscPassage
Start year Most recent five years
Number of records
Update period Annually
Price/Charges Subscription: UK£265

Notes
This disc contains five years of the *Archives of Pathology and Laboratory Medicine*. Images from text are included.

This database can also be found on:
NEXIS
American Medical Association Journals Online
Medtext

Archives of Surgery
American Medical Association

20:45. Master record
Database type Bibliographic, Textual, Factual
Number of journals
Sources newsletter
Start year 1982
Language English
Coverage International
Number of records
Update size —
Update period Monthly
Index unit articles, letters and reviews

Keywords
Surgery

Description
Archives of Surgery chronicles current research developments and clinical topics relevant to the practice of surgical medicine. Sections include: Full text of original contributions; Editorials; Book reviews; Clinical notes; Letters to the editor; Photograph essays; Commentaries; Review articles; Case reports.

20:46. Online
**Mead Data Central
(as a NEXIS database)**

File name ARS – NEXIS
Alternative name(s) NEXIS – Archives of Surgery
Start year 1982
Number of records
Update period Monthly
Price/Charges Subscription: US$1,000 – 3,000 (Depending on needs)
Connect time: US$49.00 (Telecomms + connect time)
Database entry fee: US$24.00 (Search charge)
Online print: US$0.04 per line

Notes
Library: GENMED; Group File: JNLS.

A subscription charge which covers all transactional charges, connect time, telecommunications and the small administration charge can take the place of the individual charges. Subscriptions are negotiated with customers and vary according to the number of menus (thus, files) that are to be used – typically a minimum subscription would be about US$ 1,000. All charges include training and a 24-hour help line.

Record composition
Publication; Cite; Date; Section; Length; Title; Source; Author; Abstract (SUM-ABS); Text; Additional information (SUPP-INFO); Reference (BIBLIO-REF); Graphic; Correction; Correction Date; Discussion and Editor's Note

20:47. CD-ROM   CMC ReSearch

File name	Archives of Surgery on CD-ROM
Format notes	IBM
Software	DiscPassage
Start year	1985
Number of records	
Update period	Annually
Price/Charges	Subscription: UK£265

Notes

This disc contains five years of the *Archives of Surgery*. Includes images from the text.

This database can also be found on:
NEXIS
American Medical Association Journals Online
Medtext

Arthritis and Musculoskeletal and Skin Diseases

National Arthritis and Musculoskeletal and Skin Diseases Information Clearinghouse (NAMSIC)

20:48. Master record

Database type	Bibliographic
Number of journals	
Sources	Journals, Monographs, Pamphlets and A-V material
Start year	1978
Language	English
Coverage	USA (primarily) and International (some)
Number of records	
Update size	—
Update period	Quarterly

Description

Contains citations, with abstracts, to journal articles, books, pamphlets, and audiovisual materials on arthritis and related musculoskeletal and skin diseases.

Language is primarily English, with some coverage of materials in other languages.

This database can be found on:
Combined Health Information Database

Arzneimittel-Interaktionen des SAV

Schweizerischer Apothekerverein

20:50. Master record

Database type	Textual, Factual
Number of journals	
Sources	
Start year	
Language	German
Coverage	Switzerland
Number of records	
Update size	—
Update period	
Hosts have included	AEK (AerzteKasse)

Keywords

Drugs; Pharmaceuticals; Surgery

Description

This is one of ten databases in the medical and pharmaceutical fields on the MediROM database. It is possible to establish logical links between the data of some of the databases.

This database can be found on:
MediROM

Asbestos Control Report

Business Publishers Inc

20:54. Master record

Database type	Textual
Number of journals	1
Sources	Newsletter
Start year	1987
Language	English
Coverage	USA
Number of records	
Update size	—
Update period	Monthly

Keywords

Asbestos; Asbestosis; Hazardous Waste; Liability Insurance; Occupational Health and Safety; Standards; Waste Disposal

Description

Contains the full text of *Asbestos Control Report*, a newsletter covering state and federal activities in asbestos control techniques and regulation. Includes company activities, worksite health and safety, federal asbestos standards, medical research efforts and findings, asbestos-contaminated waste disposal, liability insurance, bidding, contract management, pending litigation and court decisions.

Corresponds to *Asbestos Control Report* newsletter. On DIALOG and Data-Star this database is available as part of the PTS Newsletter Database, supplied by Predicast.

20:55. Online   NewsNet Inc

File name	
Start year	1987
Number of records	
Update period	Monthly

This database can also be found on:
PTS Newsletter Database

Asbestos

University of Sherbrooke

20:57. Master record

Database type	Bibliographic
Number of journals	
Sources	Journals, Monographs, Government documents, Research communications, Reports, Trade journals, Bibliographies and Databases
Start year	Technological documents, 1970; medical documents, 1890
Language	English
Coverage	International

Number of records
Update size   –
Update period   Quarterly

Keywords
Asbestos; Hazardous Substances; Occupational
Health and Safety; Mineralogy; Patents

Description
Contains citations, with abstracts, to the worldwide
literature on all aspects of asbestos, including technology, chemistry, geology, mineralogy, construction,
economics, biology, mining, patents, production, products, pollution, control, laws and regulations, health
and safety, statistics, and medical research concerning asbestos-related diseases.

20:58. Online   University of Sherbrooke
File name
Start year   Technological documents, 1970;
                     medical documents, 1890
Number of records
Update period   Quarterly

Aviation Compendium
Avantext Inc

20:59. Master record
Database type   Factual, Directory
Number of journals
Sources
Start year
Language
Coverage   USA and Canada
Number of records
Update size   –
Update period
Index unit   aircraft

Keywords
Aviation

Description
Contains a complete list of every registered aircraft in
the United States and Canada with owner's name and
address plus details of engine manufacturer, fuel burn
rate, number of seats, year built, etc. Also lists every
pilot and mechanic with data on certificates and ratings, type and date of last medical, etc. Also contains
detailed information on airports, medical examiners,
flight schools, air taxi operators, FAA certified maintenance facilities, and so on.

20:60. CD-ROM   Avantext Inc
File name   Aviation Compendium
Format notes   Mac, IBM
Start year
Number of records
Update period

Badekurorte
20:61. Master record
Database type   Textual, Factual
Number of journals
Sources
Start year
Language   German
Coverage   Switzerland

Number of records
Update size   –
Update period
Hosts have included   AEK (AerzteKasse)

Keywords
Drugs; Pharmaceuticals; Surgery

Description
This is one of ten databases in the medical and pharmaceutical fields on the MediROM database. It is
possible to establish logical links between the data of
some of the databases.

This database can be found on:
MediROM

BiblioMed Infectious Diseases
National Library of Medicine

20:63. Master record
CD-ROM   Healthcare Information
                                  Services Inc
Database type   Bibliographic, Textual
Number of journals   200
Sources   Monographs and journals
Start year   Most recent ten years
Language   English
Coverage   International
Number of records   400,000
Update size   –
Update period   Quarterly

Keywords
Infectious Diseases

Description
Selected subset of MEDLINE, for last ten years, with
full abstracts. Also contains full text of the *Yearbook of
Infectious Diseases* as well as *H&H's Drug
Interactions and Updates*.

For more details of constituent databases, see:
MEDLINE
Yearbook of Infectious Diseases
H&H's Drug Interactions and Updates

BIFOS
Federal Ministry for Youth, Family Affairs, Women and Health

20:65. Master record
Alternative name(s)   Betaeubungsmittelrecht-
                           Informationssystem
Database type   Factual, Textual
Number of journals
Sources   Law reports
Start year   1984–1987
Language   German
Coverage   Germany
Number of records   99,000
Update size   30,000
Update period   Annually

Keywords
Drug Abuse

Description

BIFOS is a non-bibliographic German Language database containing references to Federal Republic of Germany and West Berlin court decisions for cases involving the law on dangerous drugs (Beteaubungsmittelgesetz – BtMG). Records include defendant's age, sex, and nationality, charge, relevant statutes applied, sentence, and location and type of court, names of the drugs and sanctions.

For the year 1984 only approximately 50% of all decisions were stored. From 1985 onwards all annual decisions are available. The annual data can only be released after the report to parliament on drugs of the Federal Minister for Youth, Family Affairs, Women and Health has been published.

20:66. Online — DIMDI

File name	BT84
Alternative name(s)	Betaeubungsmittelrecht-Informationssystem
Start year	1984
Number of records	17,162
Update period	Not updated
Price/Charges	Connect time: UK£03.88–08.62
	Online print: UK£0.16–0.34
	Offline print: UK£0.07–0.14

Downloading is allowed

Notes

For 1984 only 50% of all decisions have been stored.

20:67. Online — DIMDI

File name	BT85
Alternative name(s)	Betaeubungsmittelrecht-Informationssystem
Start year	1985
Number of records	25,364
Update period	Not updated
Price/Charges	Connect time: UK£03.88–08.62
	Online print: UK£0.16–0.34
	Offline print: UK£0.07–0.14

Downloading is allowed

20:68. Online — DIMDI

File name	BT86
Alternative name(s)	Betaeubungsmittelrecht-Informationssystem
Start year	1986
Number of records	26,638
Update period	Not updated
Price/Charges	Connect time: UK£03.88–08.62
	Online print: UK£0.16–0.34
	Offline print: UK£0.07–0.14

20:69. Online — DIMDI

File name	BT87
Alternative name(s)	Betaeubungsmittelrecht-Informationssystem
Start year	1987
Number of records	29,856
Update period	Not updated
Price/Charges	Connect time: UK£03.88–08.62
	Online print: UK£0.16–0.34
	Offline print: UK£0.07–0.14

Biomedical Polymers
Elsevier Advanced Technology Publications

20:72. Master record

Database type	Textual
Number of journals	1
Sources	Newsletter

Start year	Jan 1988 to Aug 1988
Language	English
Coverage	International
Number of records	—
Update size	—
Update period	Closed File

Keywords

Polymers

Description

Contains full text of *Biomedical Polymers*, a monthly newsletter on research, development, and applications in polymers for medical uses.

Corresponds to the monthly *Biomedical Polymers* newsletter, now incorporated into Biomedical Materials. Supplied to Data-Star and DIALOG by Predicasts.

This database can be found on:
PTS Newsletter Database (as Biomedical Materials)

BioPatents
BIOSIS

20:74. Master record

Database type	Bibliographic
Number of journals	
Sources	Patents
Start year	Current 18 months
Language	English
Coverage	USA
Number of records	9,000
Update size	—
Update period	Every two weeks
Index unit	Patents

Keywords

Biomedicine; Bioagriculture

Description

Contains citations to patents granted in the USA in specialized life science fields. Covers biotechnology, biomedicine, agriculture, and food technology. Includes patent number, inventor, date patent was granted, assignee, and bibliographic information.

20:75. Online — BIOSIS Life Science Network

File name	
Start year	Current 18 months
Number of records	9,000
Update period	Every two weeks
Price/Charges	Connect time: US$9.00
	Online print: US$6.00 per 10; 2.25
	per abstract; 3.50 per full text article

Also available via the Internet by telnetting to LSN.COM.

Notes

Initiation fee of $50 to BIOSIS required. On Life Science Network users can search this database or they can scan a group of subject-related databases. There is a charge of $2.00 per scan of subject-related databases. To search one database and display up to ten citations costs $6.00. Most charges are for information retrieved. There are no charges if there are no results and no charge to transfer results to a printer or diskette. Articles may also be ordered via an online document delivery request. A telecommunications software package is also available, costing $12.95, providing an automatic connection to Life Science Network for heavy users of the service, with capability to transfer to print or disk and customised colour options.

Biotechnologies La Cellule

Centre National d'Enseignement à Distance

20:76. Master record

Database type	Multimedia
Number of journals	
Sources	
Start year	
Language	French
Coverage	
Number of records	
Update size	–
Update period	Not updated

Description

Contains five modules in French, each lasting one hour, covering biotechnology, cell use and enzymes.

20:77. CD-ROM   Centre National d'Enseignement à Distance

File name	Biotechnologies La Cellule
Format notes	IBM
Start year	
Number of records	
Update period	Not updated

Boirondoc

Institut Boiron

20:78. Master record

Database type	Bibliographic
Number of journals	
Sources	Journals and Theses
Start year	
Language	French
Coverage	France
Number of records	3,200
Update size	–
Update period	Every two weeks
Index unit	Articles and Theses

Keywords

Homeopathy

Description

Citations to articles and theses on homeopathy. Documents can be ordered online.

20:79. Online   SUNIST

File name	
Start year	

Number of records	3,200
Update period	Every two weeks

British Journal of Surgery

Butterworth Scientific Ltd

20:80. Master record

Database type	Textual, Factual
Number of journals	1
Sources	Newsletter
Start year	1985
Language	English
Coverage	International
Number of records	
Update size	
Update period	
Index unit	Articles

Keywords

Surgery

Description

The British Journal of Surgery is a well-organised reference tool which chronicles current research developments and clinical topics relevant to surgical practice and also contains information addressing scientific, educational, ethical and humanistic issues. The journal contains standard topical sections reporting on a wide variety of topics; these include: Abstracts, Association of Surgeons of Great Britain and Ireland, Book Reviews, British Association of Endocrine Surgeons Abstract, British Association of Endocrine Surgeons, Case Reports, Correspondence, Frontiers in Colorectal Disease, Reviews, short notes, case reports, surgical practice, Surgical Research Society Abstracts, Surgical Workshop, Vascular Surgical Society Abstracts, and the editorial.

20:81. Online   Mead Data Central (as a NEXIS database)

File name	BJS – NEXIS
Alternative name(s)	NEXIS – British Journal of Surgery
Start year	1985–1987
Number of records	
Update period	
Price/Charges	Subscription: US$1,000 – 3,000 (Depending on needs)
	Connect time: US$49.00 (Telecomms + connect time)
	Database entry fee: US$24.00 (Search charge)
	Online print: US$0.04 per line

Notes

Library: GENMED; Group files: ARCJNL.

A subscription charge which covers all transactional charges, connect time, telecommunications and the small administration charge can take the place of the individual charges. Subscriptions are negotiated with customers and vary according to the number of menus (thus, files) that are to be used – typically a minimum subscription would be about US$ 1,000. All charges include training and a 24-hour help line.

Record composition

Publication; Cite; Date; Section; Length; Title; Source; Author; Abstract (SUM-ABS); Text; Additional information (SUPP-INFO); Reference (BIBLIO-REF); Graphic; Correction; Correction Date and Discussion

This database can also be found on:
NEXIS
IQUEST File 1189
Comprehensive Core Medical Library

Canadiana
Canadian Centre for Occupational Health and Safety (CCOHS)

20:83. Master record

Database type	Bibliographic, Textual
Number of journals	
Sources	Journals, Grey literature, Books, Monographs, Periodicals and Conference proceedings
Start year	1980
Language	English and French
Coverage	Canada (primarily) and International (some)
Number of records	14,300 (October 1991)
Update size	–
Update period	Quarterly

Keywords
Hazardous Substances; Occupational Health and Safety; Occupational Medicine; Radiation

Description
Bibliographic references, with in-depth abstracts, covering the whole field of occupational health and safety, hazardous substances, radiation protection, legislation, occupational medicine and respiratory disorders.

Documents published in Canada, about Canadian subjects, or by Canadian authors.

20:84. Online   CCINFOline

File name	Canadiana
Start year	
Number of records	
Update period	Monthly

20:85. Online   ESA-IRS

File name	File 226
Start year	1980
Number of records	14,300 (October 1991)
Update period	Quarterly

Notes
From 1993 ESA-IRS are charging an annual fee of 100 Accounting Units (c.UK£ 70.29) to all users. This is equivalent to the fee for full documentation and will not be charged to customers already paying for documentation.

This database can also be found on:
CCINFOdisc Series B1 – OHS CanData

Cataloghi Impossibili – Vol 10 Medicine and Pharmacology
Fototeca Storica Nazionale

20:87. Master record

Database type	Bibliographic, Library catalogue/cataloguing aids, Image, Textual
Number of journals	
Sources	

Start year	Prehistory
Language	Italian
Coverage	International
Number of records	200
Update size	–
Update period	Varies

Keywords
Medical History

Description
A selection of 200 images drawn from the 6,000 images of the FSN medical collection, which is the largest private collection of art work on the subject in the world. From prehistory to modern times, includes rock paintings, renaissance frescos, 700 illustrated miniatures from ancient parchments, and the rarest incunabulae. Depicts the doctor and his practice throughout history; the sorcerer and the clinician, and the general history of the profession.

One of the twelve volumes of An Impossible Catalogue.

20:88. CD-ROM   Fototeca Storica Nazionale

File name	Cataloghi Impossibili – Vol 10 Medicine and Pharmacology
Format notes	IBM
Software	Volare
Start year	Prehistory
Number of records	200
Update period	Varies
Price	Lire150,000

CCINFOdisc Series A1 – MSDS
Canadian Centre for Occupational Health and Safety (CCOHS)

20:89. Master record

CD-ROM   Canadian Centre for Occupational Health and Safety (CCOHS)

Alternative name(s)	MSDS
Database type	Textual, Factual, Directory, Numeric
Number of journals	
Sources	Chemical manufacturers, Chemical distributors, data sheets, Government documents, Journals, Monographs and Suppliers
Start year	Current information
Language	English and French
Coverage	Canada (primarily), International (some) and USA (some)
Number of records	
Update size	–
Update period	Quarterly

Keywords
Dangerous Chemicals; First Aid; Hazardous Substances; Occupational Health and Safety; Waste Management

Description
Contains full text of two databases, in both French and English, containing trade names, chemical information, regulatory information on pesticide products and pest management research information systems:

MSDS/FTSS includes over 72,500 Material Safety

Data Sheets on chemical trade name products, as supplied by the manufacturers.

Cheminfo/Infochim, produced by the CCOHS, covers the properties, uses, occurrences, health effects and hazards of pure chemicals, natural substances, and mixtures resulting from industrial processes – for each chemical, provides name, synonyms, CAS number, molecular and structural formula, as well as information about its uses and occurrences, physical properties, appearance, reactivity, warning properties (odours, irritation), animal toxicity data; information is gathered from journals, monographs, government documents, and from MSDS from chemical manufacturers.

Equivalent to the online databases: MSDS/FTSS; Cheminfo/Infochim. FTSS is the French-language equivalent of MSDS, Infochim is the French-language equivalent of Cheminfo, MSDS is also known as Trade Names, the French-language equivalent being Noms de Marque.

For more details of constituent databases, see:
MSDS/FTSS
Cheminfo/Infochim

CCINFOdisc Series A2 – CHEM Data

Canadian Centre for Occupational Health and Safety (CCOHS)

20:91. Master record

CD-ROM	Canadian Centre for Occupational Health and Safety (CCOHS)
Alternative name(s)	CHEM Data; Chemical Information
Database type	Bibliographic, Textual, Numeric, Factual, Directory, Computer software
Number of journals	
Sources	Chemical manufacturers, Databases, data sheets, Journals, Government departments, Government documents, Monographs, Producers documents, Research communications, Research reports, Suppliers, Thesaurus and Laws/regulations
Start year	Current information
Language	English and French
Coverage	Canada (primarily), USA (some) and International (some)
Number of records	
Update size	–
Update period	Quarterly

Keywords

Biological Control; Chemical Hazards; Chemicals; Chemical Toxicology; Dangerous Chemicals; Environmental Health; Hazardous Materials; First Aid; Herbicides; Mineralogy; Nickel; Occupational Health and Safety; Occupational Medicine; Pest Control; Pesticide Residues; Pesticides; Pharmaceuticals; Teratology; Transport; Weed Control

Description

Contains both full-text and bibliographic information in several files of descriptive, toxicological and transportation data for chemical substances, and educational meterials on a variety of occupational safety and health topics.

Cheminfo/Infochim (English and French), which is produced by the CCOHS, on the properties, uses, occurrences, health effects and hazards of pure chemicals, natural substances, and mixtures resulting from industrial processes – for each chemical, provides name, synonyms, CAS number, molecular and structural formula, as well as information about its uses and occurrences, physical properties, appearance, reactivity, warning properties (odours, irritation), animal toxicity data; information is gathered from journals, monographs, government documents, and from MSDS from chemical manufacturers;

RIPP/RIPA (English and French), which is Agriculture Canada's Regulatory Information on Pesticide Products.

PRIS/SILD (English and French), six of Agriculture Canada's databases on pesticide research.

TDG/Hazardous Materials, giving US and Canadian regulations on the transportation of dangerous goods.

New Jersey Hazardous Substance Fact Sheets, information sheets from the NJ Department of Health.

DSL/NDSL, LI/EDS (English and French), Environment Canada's listing of chemicals in use in Canada.

NiPERA CAB, Nickel Producer's ERA bibliographic database of nickel-related health documents.

CESARS, contains toxicological data on approximately 195 chemicals, covering their physical and chemical properties and toxicity.

OH&S Software database, the equivalent of the hard copy publication Occupational Health & Safety Software Packages, offers descriptions of commercial computer software programs. The database currently contains some 186 Canadian and US programs.

Contains full text of Chemical Hazard Summaries, covering chemicals in common use in Canadian workplaces, Fiches Toxologiques (French-language equivalent of Chemical Hazard summaries) and New Jersey Hazardous Substance Fact sheets.

For more details of constituent databases, see:
Cheminfo/Infochim
RIPP/RIPA
PRIS/SILD
TDG/Hazardous Materials
New Jersey Hazardous Substance Fact Sheets
DSL/NDSL, LI/EDS
NiPERA CAB
CESARS
OH&S Software database

CCINFOdisc Series C1 – NIOSHTIC

National Institute of Occupational Safety and Health (NIOSH)

20:93. Master record

CD-ROM	Canadian Centre for Occupational Health and Safety (CCOHS)
Alternative name(s)	NIOSHTIC; NIOSHTIC and DIDS Databases
Database type	Bibliographic, Factual, Directory
Number of journals	
Sources	journals, monographs and reports

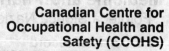

Start year
Language English
Coverage International
Number of records
Update size —
Update period Quarterly

Keywords

Accident Prevention; Biological Hazards; Epidemi-
ology; Ergonomics; Hazardous Waste; Health
Physics; Industrial Materials; Industrial Processes;
Metabolism; Occupational Health and Safety;
Pathology; Safety Education; Vocational Training;
Waste Management

Description

Contains two databases:

NIOSHTIC, database of bibliographic references prepared by the US National Institute for Occupational
Safety and Health (NIOSH), covering international
health and safety documents.
DIDS (Document Information Directory System), a listing of NIOSH documents and reports, with ordering
information.

Notes

10% discount on set of MSDS, CHEM Source, OSH
CanData, OSH InterData, NIOSHTIC and RTECS
with Microinfo.

For more details of constituent databases, see:
NIOSHTIC
DIDS

CCIS
Micromedex Inc

20:95. Master record
CD-ROM **Micromedex Inc**

Alternative name(s) Computerized Clinical Information
System
Database type Bibliographic, Factual, Textual,
Directory, Numeric
Number of journals
Sources
Start year 1974
Language English and Spanish (some)
Coverage International
Number of records
Update size —
Update period Quarterly

Keywords

Acute Medicine; Clinical Medicine; Dangerous
Chemicals; Diagnosis; Drugs; Drug Therapy;
Emergency Medicine; Epidemiology; Hazardous
Substances; Occupational Health and Safety;
Pharmaceutical Products; Pharmaceuticals;
Pharmacokinetics; Poisons; Radiography

Description

The Computerized Clinical Information System (CCIS)
is a compilation of the Micromedex databases: the
Poisindex, Drugdex and Emergindex databases are
referred to as primary databases; all other databases
are referred to as supplementary databases:
Martindale, AfterCare Instructions (in two modules,
Injury and Illness and USP DI Drug Information
Leaflets), TOMES system (including TOMES Plus),
Identidex, Dosing & Therapeutic Tools, USP DI
Volume I, Reprorisk and P&T Quik.

The primary databases (Poisindex, Drugdex and
Emergindex) are offered on annual subscription with a
choice of – System I: any one of the primary titles,
System II: any two of the primary titles, System III: all
three of the primary titles. Any of the primary databases can be purchased separately for a cost plus a
first year software licence fee of £280. There are
optional and variable subscriptions for the supplementary databases. The price is determined by the
primary system type purchased and the price is added
to the cost for the primary system selected. They are
also available on a standalone basis, for which a £65
licence fee per standalone product at list price applies.
Prices are as follows (first price is standalone cost,
price in brackets is cost when combined with a primary
system) : AfterCare Instructions: Injury/Illness £425
(£215); AfterCare Instructions: AfterCare USP DI
£360 (£180); AfterCare Combo (a combination of the
latter two databases) £620 (£310); Drug Interactions
£230 (£115); Identidex £520 (the supplementary
Identidex system is included with Poisindex free of
charge); Martindale £250 (£125); P&T Quik £195
(available only as diskette); Reprorisk £455 (£230);
TOMES £1,300 (£650); Know Abuse £100; Identidex
and Dosing & Therapeutic Tools are included with the
primary systems at no extra cost; Martindale,
Reprorisk, P&T Quik (diskette version), Know Abuse,
USP DI Volume 1, Identidex and AfterCare may be
purchased as standalone products. Reprorisk may
also be purchased as a part of TOMES Plus, but is not
included in the standard subscription.

TOMES and TOMES Plus are important standalone
products, they are not designated as 'primary' for the
purpose of pricing to facilitate the system's concept of
pricing. TOMES Plus is a separate disc and product,
not part of the CCIS system. Licence fees are not
charged for these two products. Additional disc pricing
is available for customers wanting to add additional
systems to the same physical facility – price for this
additional disc is £685 plus the licence fee (which is
required for each new installation). Contact
Micromedex for details.

For more details of constituent databases, see:
CCIS: AfterCare Instructions: Injury and Illness
CCIS: AfterCare Instructions: Drug Information for the Health
Professional: USP DI Volume 1
CCIS: AfterCare Instructions: USP DI Drug Information Leaflets
– USP DI Volume 2
CCIS: Dosing & Therapeutic Tools
CCIS: Drugdex
CCIS: Emergindex
CCIS: Identidex
CCIS: Martindale: The Extra Pharmacopoeia
CCIS: P&T Quik
CCIS: Poisindex
CCIS: Reprorisk
CCIS: TOMES

CCOHS Publications Disc
Canadian Centre for Occupational
Health and Safety (CCOHS)

20:97. Master record
Database type Factual
Number of journals
Sources
Start year
Language
Coverage Canada

Number of records
Update size   —
Update period   Twice a year

Keywords
Chemical Substances; Environmental Health; Hazardous Substances; Infectious Diseases; Lung Disease; Occupational Health and Safety; Radiation

Description
Contains International Chemical Safety Cards and Environmental Health Criteria Documents from the International Programme on Chemical safety; Hazardous Substance Fact Sheets from the New Jersey Department of Health Right to Know Program; publications on chemicals and health, understanding MSDSs, working environments, video display terminals, infectious diseases, radiation, noise and vibration, lung disease, farming and outdoor work, guides to safe use of hazardous materials, from the Canadian Centre for Occupational Health and Safety; plus an international collection of case histories of actual control measures implemented to reduce health and safety hazards in the workplace.

20:98. CD-ROM   CCOHS
File name   OSH Publications
Format notes   IBM
Start year
Number of records
Update period   Twice a year
Price/Charges   Subscription: UK£800

Chemdata
Harwell Laboratories
UK Fire Brigade

20:99. Master record
Database type   Factual
Number of journals
Sources
Start year   1975
Language   English and German
Coverage   Europe
Number of records   18,000
Update size   —
Update period

Keywords
Dangerous Chemicals; First Aid; Hazardous Substances

Description
Harwell Laboratories' and the UK Fire Brigades' collection (fifteen years' worth) of data on dangerous goods. Safety measures for 18,000 substances are included, explained, for the first time, in English and German.

20:100. CD-ROM   Springer-Verlag
File name   Dangerous Goods – Chemdata
Format notes   IBM
Software   OptiSearch
Start year
Number of records
Update period
Price/Charges   Subscription: DM6,500

Notes
Harwell Laboratories' and the UK Fire Brigades' collection of data on dangerous goods. Safety measures for 18,000 substances are included. One database including information on: Names; Substance infor-

mation; Carriage classification; Appearance; Health risks; controlling the results of the accident; Safety measures; Water pollution; Equipment; First aid; Medical advice; manufacturers names and addresses. Searchable by: Pictogram, name, UN number, colour, consistency, smell and numerical searches.

ISSN 0934–3520

This database can also be found on:
Dangerous Goods
Dangerous Goods – Hommel, VCI, Merck, Chemdata
Dangerous Goods – Chemdata, Operation Files, BAG Toxic Substances Lists, SUVA

Chemical Safety NewsBase
Royal Society of Chemistry

20:102. Master record
Alternative name(s)   CSNB
Database type   Bibliographic
Number of journals   250
Sources   A-V material, books, conference
                           proceedings, films, journals,
                           laws/regulations, monographs,
                           press releases, technical reports
                           and standards
Start year   1981
Language   English
Coverage   International
Number of records   29,000+
Update size   3,600
Update period   Monthly
Index unit   Articles
Database aids   User-Aid Manual, Cambridge, Royal
                           Scoiety of Chemistry, 1990 UK £18
                           (US$ 15)

Keywords
Allergens; Animal Hazards; Chemical Substances; Dangerous Chemicals; Dermatology; Epidemiology; Explosion; Fire; Genetic Risks; Hazardous Chemicals; Microbiological Hazards; Occupational Health and Safety; Radiation; Reproductive Hazards; Standards; Toxic Substances; Waste Management

Description
Produced by the Royal Society of Chemistry the Chemical Safety NewsBase is a merger of the databases Laboratory Hazards Bulletin and Chemical Hazards in Industry. As of 1993, coverage has been extended to include health and safety matters in the office environment. It contains citations, with abstracts, to the worldwide literature on health and safety effects of chemicals in the chemical industry, and to animal and microbiological hazards encountered by employees in chemical, biochemical, medical, and other types of laboratories. Items are taken from over 200 major primary sources including both specialist occupational health publications and chemical, biochemical, toxicological and medical research journals. Subject scope spans medicine, biochemistry, toxicology, epidemiology, occupational health and safety and legislation. Subjects covered include: chemical reactions; fires and explosions; biological effects of chemicals, animals and microorganisms; transportation and storage of chemicals; hazardous waste management; safe practices and equipment; legislation and standards for industrial chemical usage; laboratory design and management; emergency planning; toxic chemicals; carcinogens and mutagens; research on laboratory animals; radiation;

harmful biological effects of chemicals, including genetic risks; allergens, irritants and dermatitis; labelling; waste disposal; fumes; leaks, spills and unplanned release; animal and microbiological hazards; reproductive hazards; general and miscellaneous biological effects; occupational health, hygiene and monitoring; precautions; forthcoming events; publications and organisations, and feedback. It also includes Chemical Abstracts Service (CAS) Registry Numbers for cited substances. Items on well-known hazards are not included unless new information is given and items on full production plant hazards are also excluded. The database is of interest of safety inspectors and all those involved in occupational medicine and safety at work. Risks which are already widely known are only covered in connection with new publications, although the database does contain various works on general aspects of health and safety. The excerpts and abstracts are in English.

The database corresponds to the printed publications: *Chemical Hazards in Industry, Laboratory Hazards Bulletin* and *Hazards in the Office* (the latter from the beginning of 1993, when a bimonthly publication is available).

Sources include specialist occupational health publications, and chemical, biochemical, toxicological, and medical journals, books, reports, references to conferences, courses and forthcoming events, non- print materials (for example, films, posters), and organizations that provide information on hazards.

Bibliographic information, indexing terms, abstracts and CAS Registry numbers are all searchable.

20:103. Online　　　　　　　　Data-Star

File name	CSNB
Alternative name(s)	CSNB
Start year	1981
Number of records	25,000+
Update period	Monthly
Database aids	Data-Star Chemical Manual and Online manual (search for NEWS-CSNB in NEWS)
Price/Charges	Subscription: SFr80.00
	Connect time: SFr175.00
	Online print: SFr1.88
	Offline print: SFr1.34
	SDI charge: SFr13.30

Downloading is allowed
Thesaurus is online

Notes

From June 1993 Data-Star have introduced an annual fee/subscription per contract (that is, not per password) of SFr 80.00 (c.UK£ 32.00) payable every June. For North American customers billed in dollars who also use DIALOG, the DIALOG fee also covers access to Data-Star. Academic customers, 'commitment' customers and customers currently billed in dollars are exempt.

Record composition

Abstract AB; Accession Number and Update Code AN; Author AU; Author Affiliation IN; CAS Registry Numbers RN; Company Source CO; Descriptors DE; Journal Coden CD; Language LG; Publication Type PT; Publisher PB; Section Number SC; Source SO; Subject Identifiers ID; Title TI; Update Code UP and Year YR

20:104. Online　　　　　　　　DIALOG

File name	File 317
Alternative name(s)	CSNB
Start year	1981 (January)
Number of records	27,160
Update period	Monthly
Price/Charges	Connect time: US$150.00
	Online print: US$1.40
	Offline print: US$1.40
	SDI charge: US$15.00

Notes

DIALINDEX Categories: CHEMLIT, RNCHEM, SAFETY, TOXICOL.

20:105. Online　　　　　　　　ESA-IRS

File name	File 90
Alternative name(s)	CSNB
Start year	1981
Number of records	24,700 (October 1991)
Update period	Monthly
Price/Charges	Subscription: UK£70.29
	Database entry fee: UK£3.49
	Online print: UK£0.56
	Offline print: UK£0.53
	SDI charge: UK£2.80

Notes

From 1993 ESA-IRS are charging an annual fee of 100 Accounting Units (c.UK£ 70.29) to all users. This is equivalent to the fee for full documentation and will not be charged to customers already paying for documentation.

Record composition

Abstract /AB; Author AU; Class Code CC; Class Name CC; CODEN CO; Controlled Terms /CT /TERMS; Corporate Source CS; Document TYpe DT; ISBN BN; ISSN SN; Journal Name JN; Language LA; Meeting Information MI; Native Number NN; Publication Date PD; Publisher PB; Registry Number RN and Title /TI

20:106. Online　　　　　　　　ORBIT

File name	CSNB
Alternative name(s)	CSNB
Start year	1981
Number of records	27,000+
Update period	Monthly
Database aids	Quick Reference Guide (10/88) Free (single copy) and Database Manual (1990) US$15
Price/Charges	Connect time: US$110.00
	Online print: US$0.90
	Offline print: US$0.60
	SDI charge: US$6.25

Notes

Electronic SDI service is now available within two hours on ORBIT. They can be downloaded and reformatted on a word processor. Results are retrieved in the low cost PRINTS file, $15 per connect hour.

Unique features: subject/substance/CAS Registry Number indexing.

20:107. Online　　　　　　　　STN

File name	CSNB
Alternative name(s)	CSNB
Start year	1984
Number of records	30,281
Update period	Monthly

Price/Charges	Connect time: DM210.00
	Online print: DM2.10
	Offline print: DM1.40
	SDI charge: DM14.00

Notes

Supplied to STN International by FIZ Chemie GmbH.

Cheminfo
Canadian Centre for Occupational Health and Safety (CCOHS)

20:108. Master record

Alternative name(s)	Infochim
Database type	Factual, Textual, Numeric
Number of journals	
Sources	Data sheets, Suppliers, Journals, Monographs and Government documents
Start year	Current information
Language	English
Coverage	Canada (primarily), International (some) and USA (some)
Number of records	
Update size	–
Update period	Varies

Keywords

First Aid; Occupational Health and Safety

Description

Produced by the CCOHS, Cheminfo contains descriptive, health, and precautionary data on pure chemicals, natural substances, and chemical mixtures resulting from or used in industrial processes. For each chemical, provides substance identification, including name, synonyms, Chemical Abstracts Service (CAS) Registry Number, and molecular and structural formula, as well as information about its uses and occurrences, physical properties, appearance, reactivity, warning properties (for example, odours, irritation), animal toxicity data, proposed Workplace Hazardous Materials Information System (WHMIS) classification, fire and explosion hazards, and human health effects from short-term acute or chronic exposure. Also provides information on occupational control measures, including airborne exposure limits, ventilation, personnel protective equipment and clothing, respiratory protection guidelines, and recommendations on storage and handling, spill and leak procedures, cleanup, disposal, and emergency first aid.

Sources include Material Safety Data Sheets from chemical manufacturers. During the late 1980s/early 1990s, the American National Standards Institute (ANSI) developed a standard for the presentation of MSDS which has been endorsed by the International Council of Chemical Associations; the ANSI recommendations for format and content have been incorporated into Cheminfo. CCOHS is also adding information required under the ISHA Hazard Communications Standard to each record. Corresponds to the Cheminfo online database. French-language equivalent is Infochim.

20:109. Online   CCINFOline

File name	
Alternative name(s)	Infochim
Start year	Current information

Number of records	
Update period	Varies

This database can also be found on:
CCINFOdisc Series A1 – MSDS
CCINFOdisc Series A2 – CHEM Data

Chemtox Database
Resource Consultants Inc

20:111. Master record

Database type	Textual, Directory, Factual
Number of journals	
Sources	Laws/regulations and Government documents
Start year	Current information
Language	English
Coverage	USA (primarily) and International (some)
Number of records	5,400
Update size	–
Update period	Quarterly
Index unit	Chemicals

Keywords

Carcinogens; Dangerous Chemicals; First Aid; Hazardous Substances; Occupational Health and Safety

Description

Contains information on 5,400 common hazardous chemicals. Includes chemicals regulated by the Occupational Health and Safety Act (OSHA); Clean Water Act; Safe Drinking Water Act; Clean Air Act; Resource Conservation Recovery Act (RCRA); Comprehensive Environmental Response, Compensation and Liability Act (CERCLA or Superfund); Superfund Amendments and Reauthorization act (SARA); and the US Department of Transportation's (DOT) Hazardous Materials Transportation Act, Ports and Waterways Act and Pipeline Safety Act. Also covers chemicals reviewed by the American Conference of Governmental Industrial Hygienists (ACGIH); Deutsche Forschungsgeminschaft; National Institute for Occupational Safety and Health (NIOSH); US Toxicology Program (NTP); EPA Carcinogen Assessment Group; International Agency for Research on Cancer (IARC); Federal Insecticide, Fungicide and Rodenticide Act (FIFRA); Nuclear Regulatory Commission (NRC); Extraordinarily Hazardous Substances by the New Jersey Department of Environmental Protection; Workplace Hazardous Materials Information System (WHMIS); and Science Advisory Panel to the California Governor's List (Proposition 65). For each chemical includes: identifiers (name, CAS number, synonyms, formula, chemical class, Registry of Toxic Effects of Chemical Substances (RTECS) number, DOT ID number, STCC number, EPA ID number); physical and chemical properties; toxicological data; regulatory data; data related to transport, including emergency response; spill and disposal data; personal protection data; symptoms of chemical exposure; analytical methods. Users can generate Material Safety Data Sheets (MSDS) for each chemical.

20:112. Diskette   Resource Consultants Inc

File name	Chemtox Database
Format notes	IBM
Software	Revelation DBMS
Start year	Current information

Number of records 5,400
Update period Quarterly
Price/Charges Subscription: US$700

Chest
CMC ReSearch

20:113. Master record

Database type Textual
Number of journals 1
Sources journal
Start year
Language English
Coverage USA
Number of records
Update size —
Update period Annually
Index unit Articles

Keywords
Physiology

Description
Full text with illustrations from the journal *Chest* from the American Academy of Chest Physicians. Contains reviewed original investigations as well as special features such as: Clinical Investigations in Critical Care, Roentgenogram of the Month, case reports, and book reviews. Covers 1985 – 1990.

20:114. CD-ROM   CMC ReSearch

File name Chest
Format notes IBM
Software DiscPassage
Start year
Number of records
Update period Annually
Price US$395
  Subscription: US$150

Chinese Medical Plant Database
Computing Institute, Chinese Academy of Sciences

20:115. Master record

Alternative name(s) CMP
Database type Factual, Directory, Bibliographic
Number of journals
Sources Dictionaries
Start year 1989
Language English and Chinese
Coverage China
Number of records 27,000
Update size —
Update period Continuously

Keywords
Alternative Medicine; Herbal Remedies; Plant Sciences

Description
Contains both bibliographic and factual data covering Chinese native medical plants used in traditional Chinese medicine and western medicine and plants transplanted into China from abroad. Data sources are dictionaries of traditional Chinese medicines and Chinese herb books of medicinal plants. All data has been evaluated by Chinese specialists before being incorporated into the database.

Botanical data covers plant family, medicinal components, medicinal features, name, region where found, preservation instructions and curative properties.

As of 1993, the database contains details of 2,000 medicinal plants, 5,000 traditional Chinese medicines and 20,000 bibliographic references.

20:116. Online   Scientific Database System

File name Chinese Medical Plant Database
Alternative name(s) CMP
Start year 1989
Number of records 27,000
Update period Continuously

Notes
Retrieval is by key word, CAS Registry Number, chemical name, chemical structures, molecular formula and molecular weight.

Record composition
Index terms; CAS Registry Number; Chemical Name; Chemical Structure; Molecular Formula and Molecular Weight

Chinese Optical Abstracts
Changchun Optical and Mechanical Institute

20:117. Master record

Alternative name(s) COA
Database type Bibliographic
Number of journals
Sources Journals
Start year 1985
Language Chinese
Coverage China
Number of records 35,000
Update size 4,800
Update period Twice per month
Index unit Articles

Keywords
Ophthalmology; Optics; Optical Engineering; Optical Science; Spectroscopy; Fibre Optics; Lasers

Description
Covers publications and documents in Chinese dealing with optics, photoelectronics and optical applications. Subjects covered include photometry, colorimetry, radiation, luminescence, mgeometric optics, physical optics, thin film optics, fibre optics, spectroscopy, lasers, optical communications, optical testing and measurement, optical technology and instruments, etc.

20:118. Online   Changchun Optical and Mechanical Institute

File name Chinese Optical Abstracts
Alternative name(s) COA
Start year 1985
Number of records 35,000
Update period Twice per month
Price/Charges Database entry fee: US$7.00 per search
  Online print: US$0.15

Cholesterol, High Blood Pressure, and Smoking Education

National Heart, Lung, and Blood Institute

20:119. Master record

Database type	Bibliographic
Number of journals	
Sources	Journals, Monographs, Pamphlets, Reports and Educational materials
Start year	1981
Language	English
Coverage	USA (primarily) and International (some)
Number of records	
Update size	–
Update period	Quarterly

Description

Contains citations, with abstracts, to books, journal articles, pamphlets, reports, and educational materials on cholesterol, high blood pressure, and smoking.

Language is primarily English, with some coverage of materials in other languages.

This database can be found on:
Combined Health Information Database

Citizens Emergency Travel Advisory Service

US Department of State, Citizens Emergency Center

20:121. Master record

Alternative name(s)	Department of State Travel Advisory Service
Database type	Factual, Textual
Number of journals	
Sources	Government departments (US)
Start year	Current information
Language	English
Coverage	International
Number of records	
Update size	–
Update period	Continuously

Keywords

Crime; Epidemiology; Political Unrest; Travel; Travel Medicine; Warfare

Description

Contains information for travellers outside the United States on possible hazardous travel conditions in foreign countries, including information on warfare, crime, political and civil unrest, outbreaks of communicable diseases and other conditions.

20:122. Online — CompuServe Information Service

File name	Citizens Emergency Travel Advisory Service
Alternative name(s)	Department of State Travel Advisory Service
Start year	Current information

Number of records	
Update period	Continuously
Price/Charges	Subscription: US$8.95 per month
Downloading is allowed	

Communicable Disease Data Base

World Health Organisation – Pan American Health Organization. Caribbean Epidemiology Centre.

20:123. Master record

Database type	Numeric
Number of journals	
Sources	
Start year	1976
Language	English
Coverage	
Number of records	13,000
Update size	–
Update period	Weekly

Keywords

Epidemiology; Infectious Diseases

Description

A database of communicable diseases information. Subject scope is disease transmission, epidemiology and infectious diseases.

Available to UN system organisations; external users; data is made available on demand to health workers, especially for research and planning. Available only as a printout. Printed products – *Annual review of communicable diseases; CAREC surveillance report*.

20:124. Printout — World Health Organisation – Pan American Health Organization. Caribbean Epidemiology Centre

File name	Communicable Disease Data Base
Format notes	IBM
Software	dBASE III
Start year	1975
Number of records	
Update period	

Notes

Available only as a printout.

Comprehensive Core Medical Library

BRS

20:125. Master record

Database type	Textual
Number of journals	
Sources	Journals and monographs

Start year | Textbooks, current editions; journals, see Description
Language | English
Coverage | English-speaking countries (primarily)
Number of records | —
Update size | —
Update period | Weekly
Index unit | Articles, book chapters, book reviews, editorials and letters to the editor

Keywords

HIV; Anatomy

Description

CCML contains full text of major medical textbooks and over seventy medical journals. The database is designed to help both information and medical professionals obtain the full text of authoritative medical information quickly and efficiently. It can be used to locate contextual references, additional references from bibliographies and footnotes, and access the full text of articles, chapters, letters to the editor, editorials and book reviews. Retrospective coverage and updating varies by source. It includes the American College of Obstetricians and Gynecologists' *Precis III* and *Standards for Obstetric-Gynecologic Services* (6th edition); Berkow's *The Merck Manual*; Blacklow's *MacBryde's Signs and Symptoms*; Boucek's *Coronary Artery Disease, Pathological and Clinical Assessment*; Cohen's *Emergencies in Obstetrics and Gynecology*; Griffith's *Instructions for Patients*; Hollingworth's *Pregnancy, Diabetes, and Birth*; Kaplan's *Comprehensive Textbook of Psychiatry*; Karliner's *Coronary Care*; Mandell, Douglas, and Bennett's *Principles and Practice of Infectious Diseases* (2nd edition); Margulies and Thaler's *The Physician's Book of Lists*; Ogilvie's *Birch's Emergencies in Medical Practice*; Parillo's *Major Issues in Critical Care Medicine*; Percival's *Holland and Brews Manual of Obstetrics*; Rakel's *Conn's Current Therapy* (1985, 1986, 1987, 1988); Rowland's *Merritt's Textbook of Neurology*; Sabiston's *Texbook of Surgery* (12th edition); Schiff's *Diseases of the Liver*; Schwartz's *Principles and Practice of Emergency Medicine* (2nd edition); Williams' *Gray's Anatomy*; and Wyngaarden's *Cecil Textbook of Medicine*. Publishers include Churchill Livingstone, J.B. Lippincott, and W.B. Saunders. Also includes the serials *Cardiology Clinics, Emergency Medicine Clinics of North America*, and *Medical Clinics of North America*, published by W.B. Saunders. The complete list of journals and yearbooks covered as at 12/92 follows:

Journals:

ACOG Technical Bulletin (3/73–)
Age and Ageing (7/86–)
AIDS: Papers from Science (1/82–12/85)
American Family Physician (7/91–)
American Heart Journal (1/86–)
American Journal of Cardiology (1/86–)
American Journal of Medicine (5/86–)
American Journal of Obstetrics and Gynaecology (1/86–)
American Journal of Physical Medicine and Rehabilitation (4/91–)
American Journal of Psychiatry (8/85–)
American Journal of Public Health (7/85–)
American Journal of Roentgenology (11/90–)
American Journal of Surgery (2/86–)
Anesthesia and Analgesia (1/88–)
Anesthesiology (8/86–)

Annals of Internal Medicine (8/84–)
Annals of Neurology (9/86–)
Annals of Rheumatic Diseases (1/87–11/88)
Annals of Surgery (2/85–)
Annals of Thoracic Surgery (1/91–)
Archives of Disease in Childhood (7/85–)
Arteriosclerosis (1/86–)
Arthritis and Rheumatism (1/86–)
British Heart Journal (1/86–)
British Journal of Diseases of the Chest (1/87–7/88)
British Journal of Obstetrics and Gynaecology (1/87–)
British Journal of Rheumatology (2/86–)
British Journal of Surgery (5/86–)
British Journal of Urology (7/87–)
British Medical Journal (7/83–)
Canadian Medical Association Journal (11/86–)
Cancer Treatment Reports (1/85–12/87)
Circulation (7/87–)
Circulation Research (7/88–)
Clinical Chemistry (6/92–)
Clinical Diabetes (1/86–)
Clinical Orthopaedics (5/85–)
Clinical Pediatrics (6/85–5/90)
Clinical Pharmacology and Therapeutics (7/85–)
Critical Care Medicine (11/90–)
Diabetes (1/86–)
Diabetes Care (1/86–)
Emergency Medicine Reports (11/85–10/86)
Fertility and Sterility (3/86–4/89)
Gastroenterology (7/91–)
Genitourinary Medicine (4/88–)
Gut (4/86–)
Harvard Medical School Health Letter (11/85–)
Heart and Lung (1/86–1/89)
Hypertension and Arteriosclerosis (7/88–)
Journal of Allergy and Clinical Immunology (1/86–)
Journal of American Board of Family Practice (1/88–)
Journal of the American College of Cardiology (1/89–)
Journal of American Medical Association (1/92–)
Journal of Bone and Joint Surgery (7/85–)
Journal of Clinical Chemistry (6/92–)
Journal of Clinical Investigation (7/86–)
Journal of Clinical Pathology (1/86–)
Journal of Laboratory and Clinical Medicine (1/86–)
Journal of Neurology, Neurosurgery and Psychiatry (2/86–)
Journal of Pediatrics (1/86–)
Journal of Reconstructive Surgery (11/90–)
Journal of the National Cancer Institute (1/85–3/88)
Journal of Trauma (11/90–)
Journal of Urology (10/90–)
Lancet (7/83–)
Medical Letter (8/82–)
Medical Science Research (1/87–5/88)
Medicine (11/85–)
Morbidity and Mortality Weekly Report (6/85–9/90)
Nature (10/85–9/89)
Neurology (1/87–)
New England Journal of Medicine (1/83–)
Obstetrical and Gynecological Survey (1/86–)
Obstetrics and Gynaecology (1/88–)
Pediatrics (7/85–)
Physical Therapy (3/86–)
Quarterly Journal of Medicine (5/86–8/88)
Seminars in Liver Disease (2/86–8/87)
Seminars in Neurology (3/86–3/88)
Seminars in Respiratory Medicine (7/85–10/88)
Sexually Transmitted Diseases (4/85–)
Stroke (7/88–)
Thorax (1/86–1/89)

Year Books:

Year Book of Anesthesia
Year Book of Cancer

Year Book of Cardiology
Year Book of Critical Care Medicine
Year Book of Dentistry
Year Book of Dematology
Year Book of Diagnostic Radiology
Year Book of Digestive Diseases
Year Book of Drug Therapy
Year Book of Emergency Medicine
Year Book of Endocrinology
Year Book of Family Practice
Year Book of Hand Surgery
Year Book of Hematology
Year Book of Infectious Diseases
Year Book of Medicine
Year Book of Neurology and Neurosurgery
Year Book of Nuclear Medicine
Year Book of Obstetrics and Gynaecology
Year Book of Ophtalmolgy
Year Book of Orthapaedics
Year Book of Otolaryngology
Year Book of Patology
Year Book of Pediatrics
Year Book of Plastic Surgery
Year Book of Podiatric Medicine
Year Book of Perinatal/Neonatal Medicine
Year Book of Psychiatry
Year Book of Pulmonary Disease
Year Book of Rehabilitation
Year Book of Sports Medicine
Year Book of Surgery
Year Book of Urology
Year Book of Vascular Surgery.

20:126. Online   BRS

File name	CCML
Alternative name(s)	CCML
Start year	
Number of records	
Update period	Weekly
Price/Charges	Connect time: US$41.00/51.00
	Online print: US$0.91/0.99
	Offline print: US$0.99
	SDI charge: US$10.30

20:127. Online   CompuServe Information Service

File name	IQUEST File 1189
Start year	1982
Number of records	
Update period	Every two weeks
Price/Charges	Subscription: US$8.95 per month
	Database entry fee: US$9/search; some databases carry a surcharge ($2–75)
	Online print: US$10 references free; then $9 per ten; abstracts $3 each

Downloading is allowed

Notes
Accessed via IQUEST or IQMEDICAL, this database is offered by a BRS gateway. IQUEST can either search across all databases, a database of the user's choice or selected multiple databases.

20:128. Database subset
Online   BRS

File name	PCTJ – Comprehensive Core Medical Library Practice File
Alternative name(s)	CCML
Start year	
Number of records	
Update period	

Price/Charges	Connect time: US$Free/10.00
	Online print: US$Free

Notes
The training file for CCML.

20:129. Database subset
Online   BRS

File name	AACC
Start year	1986 (October)
Number of records	
Update period	Weekly
Price/Charges	Connect time: US$41.00/51.00
	Online print: US$0.91/0.99
	Offline print: US$0.99

Notes
AACC contains full text of articles, editorials, letters and other materials identified as pertaining to Acquired Immune Deficiency Syndrome (AIDS) and AIDS related subjects from medical journals included in the Comprehensive Core Medical Library.

AACC simplifies full-text searching for AIDS-related topics.

20:130. Database subset
Online   BRS

File name	JOUR
Start year	
Number of records	
Update period	Weekly
Price/Charges	Connect time: US$41.00/51.00
	Online print: US$0.91/0.99
	Offline print: US$0.99

Notes
This database contains the full text of all the medical journals included in the Comprehensive Core Medical Library.

20:131. Database subset
Online   BRS

File name	MEDB
Start year	Concurrent with publication of new editions
Number of records	
Update period	Varies
Price/Charges	Connect time: US$41.00/51.00
	Online print: US$0.91/0.99
	Offline print: US$0.99

Notes
This database contains the full text of the medical textbooks and reference works included in the Comprehensive Core Medical Library.

20:132. Database subset
Online   CompuServe Information Service

File name	CCMLAIDS
Start year	1982
Number of records	
Update period	Weekly
Price/Charges	Subscription: US$8.95 per month

Downloading is allowed

Notes
CCMLAIDS contains full text of articles, editorials, letters and other materials identified as pertaining to Acquired Immune Deficiency Syndrome (AIDS) and AIDS related subjects from medical journals included in the Comprehensive Core Medical Library.

AACC simplifies full-text searching for AIDS-related topics.

20:133. Database subset
Online   CompuServe Information Service

File name	IQUEST File 2543 – AIDS Articles
Start year	1983
Number of records	
Update period	Weekly
Price/Charges	Subscription: US$8.95 per month Database entry fee: US$9/search; some databases carry a surcharge ($2–75) Online print: US$10 references free; then $9 per ten; abstracts $3 each

Downloading is allowed

Notes

The file contains full text of articles, editorials, letters and other materials identified as pertaining to Acquired Immune Deficiency Syndrome (AIDS) and AIDS related subjects from medical journals included in the Comprehensive Core Medical Library.

Accessed via IQUEST or IQMEDICAL, this database is offered by a BRS gateway. IQUEST can either search across all databases, a database of the user's choice or selected multiple databases.

20:134. Database subset
Online   CompuServe Information Service

File name	IQUEST File 7031 – Lancet
Start year	1983
Number of records	
Update period	Weekly
Price/Charges	Subscription: US$8.95 per month Database entry fee: US$9/search; some databases carry a surcharge ($2–75) Online print: US$10 references free; then $9 per ten; abstracts $3 each

Downloading is allowed

Notes

Full text of the articles, book reviews, notes and news in Lancet. Accessed via IQUEST or IQMEDICAL, this database is offered by a BRS gateway. IQUEST can either search across all databases, a database of the user's choice or selected multiple databases.

For more details of constituent databases, see:
American Family Physician
American Journal of Psychiatry
American Journal of Public Health
Annals of Internal Medicine
Annals of Neurology
British Journal of Surgery
British Medical Journal
Canadian Medical Association Journal
Cancer Treatment Reports
Clinical Pediatrics
Critical Care Medicine
Journal of American Medical Association
Morbidity and Mortality Weekly Report
New England Journal of Medicine
Obstetrics and Gynaecology
Pediatrics
Sexually Transmitted Diseases

Conquest Marketing Information System
Donnelley Marketing Information Services

20:135. Master record

Database type	Factual, Statistical, Textual, Numeric, Cartographic, Directory, Mapped statistical, Computer software, Organisational/Biographical
Number of journals	
Sources	
Start year	1970
Language	English
Coverage	USA and Canada
Number of records	
Update size	–
Update period	Annually

Keywords

Demography; Health Care Market; Hospital Facilities; Physicians; Product Catalogues; Shopping Centres (US); Television

Description

A US consumer information database with more than 25 files offering access to current year demographic estimates and five years of data on key demographic variables. Includes details of 1980 and 1970 US Census data; 30,000 shopping centres; more than 7.5 million commercial businesses; sales potentials for 21 types of retail stores; retail sales estimates; consumer lifestyles; product usage and median data; business statistics and listings; financial deposit and location data; shopping centres; grocery stores; geographic boundaries and streets.

There is also access to ClusterPLUS, the only updated life style segmentation system. Industry packages include Conquest/Financial, Conquest/Advertising, Conquest/Canada, TV Conquest, Conquest/Health Care, and Cable Conquest.

20:136. Database subset
CD-ROM   Donnelley Marketing Information Services

File name	Conquest DRG Forecasting Models
Start year	
Number of records	
Update period	Annually
Price/Charges	Subscription: US$4,000

Notes

Contains current year estimates and five year projections of physician caseloads for Diagnosis Related Groups (DRGs) and Major Diagnostic Changes (MDCs). Part of Conquest Marketing information System

20:137. Database subset
CD-ROM   Donnelley Marketing Information Services

File name	Conquest Physician Specialty Counts
Software	TargetScan 2.3
Start year	
Number of records	500,000
Update period	Annually
Price/Charges	Subscription: US$3,000

Notes

Contains summary data on the number of physicians in each ZIP code area. Covers over 500,000 physicians in thirty-six specialties. Part of Conquest Marketing Information System

20:138. Database subset
CD-ROM   **Donnelley Marketing Information Services**

File name	Conquest Physician's Reference Files
Software	TargetScan 2.3
Start year	
Number of records	
Update period	Annually

Notes

Contains physician's names, speciality code and office location by latitude and longitude. Part of Conquest Marketing Information System.

Critical Care Medicine
CMC ReSearch

20:139. Master record

Database type	Textual, Factual
Number of journals	1
Sources	Journal
Start year	
Language	
Coverage	
Number of records	290,000
Update size	–
Update period	Annually

Keywords

Critical Care Medicine

Description

Full text, tables and images, covering each issue from 1985–1989 of *Critical Care Medicine*, the much-respected Williams and Wilkins publication. Provides the latest news about advances in equipment, diagnosis and treatment, research and reports on clinical breakthroughs, and original articles.

20:140. CD-ROM   CMC ReSearch

File name	Critical Care Medicine: 1985–1990
Format notes	IBM
Software	DiscPassage
Start year	
Number of records	
Update period	Annually
Price	US$395
	Subscription: US$150

This database can also be found on:
Critical Care Medicine – Personal MEDLINE
Comprehensive Core Medical Library
IQUEST File 1189

Cumulative Trauma Disorders News

20:141. Master record

Alternative name(s)	CTD News
Database type	Factual, Textual
Number of journals	1
Sources	Newsletter

Start year	Current year
Language	English
Coverage	International
Number of records	
Update size	–
Update period	Monthly

Keywords

Cumulative Trauma Disorders

Description

Provides news on CTD such as carpal tunnel syndrome, stress and back pain. Includes news of litigation and regulations as well as prevention and treatment.

20:142. Online   CompuServe Information Service

File name	IQUEST File 3130
Alternative name(s)	CTD News
Start year	Current year
Number of records	
Update period	Monthly
Price/Charges	Subscription: US$8.95 per month
	Database entry fee: US$9/search; some databases carry a surcharge ($2–75)
	Online print: US$10 references free; then $9 per ten; abstracts $3 each

Downloading is allowed

Notes

Accessed via IQUEST or IQMEDICAL, this database is offered by a NewsNet gateway. IQUEST can either search across all databases, a database of the user's choice or selected multiple databases.

20:143. Online   NewsNet Inc

File name	
Alternative name(s)	CTD News
Start year	Current year
Number of records	
Update period	Monthly

Dalctraf
Dalctraf HB

20:144. Master record

Database type	Bibliographic
Number of journals	
Sources	
Start year	1980
Language	English
Coverage	International
Number of records	3,000
Update size	450
Update period	Monthly

Keywords

Alcohol Abuse; Drug Abuse; Road Safety

Description

Dalctraf registers international literature in the biomedical and social sciences related to the incidence and effects of alcohol and drugs on traffic safety. It is one of the files in the DRUGAB information system. See also Alconarc and Nordrug.

Equivalent to *Alcohol, Drugs and Traffic Safety. Current Research Literature.*

20:145. Online   DAFA Data AB

File name	Dalctraf
Start year	1980
Number of records	3,000
Update period	Monthly

This database can also be found on:
Drugab

Dangerous Goods – Chemdata, Operation Files, BAG Toxic Substances Lists, SUVA

Springer-Verlag

20:146. Master record

CD-ROM   Springer-Verlag

Alternative name(s)	Gefahrgut – Chemdata, Operation Files, BAG Toxic Substances Lists, SUVA; Chemdata, Operation Files, BAG Toxic Substances List, SUVA
Database type	Factual
Number of journals	
Sources	
Start year	
Language	English, German and French (some)
Coverage	
Number of records	
Update size	–
Update period	

Keywords

Chemical Substances; Dangerous Chemicals; First Aid; Hazardous Substances; Industrial Health and Safety; Toxic Substances

Description

Four databases from the Springer-Verlag collection of Dangerous Goods databases including information on: Names; Substance information; Carriage classification; Appearance; Health risks; controlling the results of the accident; Safety measures; Water pollution; Equipment; First aid; Medical advice; manufacturers names and addresses. Searchable by: Pictogram, name, UN number, colour, consistency, smell and numerical searches.

Chemdata: Harwell Laboratories' and the UK Fire Brigades' collection of data on dangerous goods. Safety measures for 18,000 substances are included.

Operation Files: The operation files for chemical incidents of the Swiss Fire Brigades Association; Illustrations and clear presentation give instructions on the correct procedures in accidents. dangerous goods classes including many substances and preparations are summarised on separate pages in German and French.

BAG Toxic Substances List: The Swiss Toxic Substances List contains poison classes and the addresses of registered companies. 76,000 substances and products are included with their trade name and all available synonyms.

SUVA: The Swiss Accident Insurance Institution, is the editor of the safety codes of liquids and gases. The physical values in this list are of importance when judging the safety of substances.

ISSN 0934–3563

For more details of constituent databases, see:
Chemdata
Operations File/Einsatzakten SFA
BAG Toxic Substances List/BAG-Giftlisten
SUVA

Dangerous Goods – Hommel, VCI, Merck Catalogue, Chemdata

Springer-Verlag

20:147. Master record

CD-ROM   Springer-Verlag

Alternative name(s)	Gefahrgut – Hommel, VCI, Merck Catalogue, Chemdata; Hommel, VCI, Merck Catalogue, Chemdata
Database type	Factual
Number of journals	
Sources	
Start year	
Language	English and German
Coverage	Europe
Number of records	
Update size	–
Update period	

Keywords

Dangerous Chemicals; First Aid; Hazardous Substances; Industrial Health and Safety; Toxic Substances

Description

Four databases from the Springer-Verlag collection on Dangerous Goods, including information on: Names; Substance information; Carriage classification; Appearance; Health risks; controlling the results of the accident; Safety measures; Water pollution; Equipment; First aid; Medical advice; manufacturers names and addresses. Searchable by: Pictogram, name, UN number, colour, consistency, smell and numerical searches.

Hommel: *Handbook of Dangerous Goods*, 1,500 substances: Technical and Physical data, reactions, environmental data and instructions concerning intervention, first aid, and medical treatment are given.

VCI: *The Handbook of Firms* in the chemical industry, published by Econ-Verlag, lists the addresses and products of chemical manufacturers and wholesalers in Germany.

Merck Catalogue (formerly Fluka): *The Merck Catalogue* contains the entire program of chemicals and biochemicals supplied by this company. Included are: Names; Trade names; Synonyms; Industrial health and safety standards. Information on 13,000 substances is given.

Chemdata: Harwell Laboratories' and the UK Fire Brigades' collection of data on dangerous goods. Safety measures for 18,000 substances are included.

ISSN 0934–3547

For more details of constituent databases, see:
Hommel
VCI
Merck Catalogue
Chemdata

Dangerous Goods – Hommel, VCI, Merck Catalogue, Operation Files, BAG Toxic Substances Lists, SUVA

Springer-Verlag

20:148. Master record
CD-ROM **Springer-Verlag**

Alternative name(s)	Gefahrgut – Hommel, VCI, Merck Catalogue, Operation Files, BAG Toxic Substances Lists, SUVA; Hommel, VCI, Merck Catalogue, Operation Files, BAG Toxic Substances Lists, SUVA
Database type	Factual
Number of journals	
Sources	
Start year	
Language	English and German
Coverage	Europe
Number of records	
Update size	–
Update period	

Keywords
Chemical Substances; Dangerous Chemicals; First Aid; Hazardous Substances; Industrial Health and Safety; Toxic Substances

Description
Six databases from the Dangerous Goods collection from Springer-Verlag, including information on: Names; Substance information; Carriage classification; Appearance; Health risks; controlling the results of the accident; Safety measures; Water pollution; Equipment; First aid; Medical advice; manufacturers names and addresses. Searchable by: Pictogram, name, UN number, colour, consistency, smell and numerical searches.

Hommel: *Handbook of Dangerous Goods*, 1,500 substances: Technical and Physical data, reactions, environmental data and instructions concerning intervention, first aid, and medical treatment are given.

VCI: *The Handbook of Firms* in the chemical industry, published by Econ- Verlag, lists the addresses and products of chemical manufacturers and wholesalers in Germany.

Merck Catalogue (formerly Fluka): *The Merck Catalogue* contains the entire program of chemicals and biochemicals supplied by this company. Included are: Names; Trade names; Synonyms; Industrial health and safety standards. Information on 13,000 substances is given.

Operation Files: The operation files for chemical incidents of the Swiss Fire Brigades Association; Illustrations and clear presentation give instructions on the correct procedures in accidents. dangerous goods classes including many substances and preparations are summarised on separate pages in German and French.

BAG Toxic Substances List: The Swiss Toxic Substances List contains poison classes and the addresses of registered companies. 76,000 substances and products are included with their trade name and all available synonyms.

SUVA: The Swiss Accident Insurance Institution, is the editor of the safety codes of liquids and gases. The physical values in this list are of importance when judging the safety of substances.

ISSN 0934–3555

For more details of constituent databases, see:
Hommel
VCI
Merck Catalogue
Operation Files/Einsatzakten SFA
BAG Toxic Substances List/BAG-Giftlisten
SUVA

Dangerous Goods – Hommel, VCI, Merck Catalogue

Springer-Verlag

20:149. Master record
CD-ROM **Springer-Verlag**

Alternative name(s)	Gefahrgut – Hommel, VCI, Merck Catalogue; Hommel, VCI, Merck Catalogue
Database type	Factual
Number of journals	
Sources	
Start year	
Language	English and German
Coverage	Europe
Number of records	
Update size	–
Update period	

Keywords
Dangerous Chemicals; First Aid; Hazardous Substances; Industrial Health and Safety; Toxic Substances

Description
Three databases from the Springer-Verlag collection on Dangerous Goods, including information on: Names; Substance information; Carriage classification; Appearance; Health risks; Controlling the results of the accident; Safety measures; Water pollution; Equipment; First aid; Medical advice; manufacturers names and addresses. Searchable by: Pictogram, name, UN number, colour, consistency, smell and numerical searches.

Hommel: *Handbook of Dangerous Goods*, 1,500 substances: Technical and Physical data, reactions, environmental data and instructions concerning intervention, first aid, and medical treatment are given.

VCI: *The Handbook of Firms* in the chemical industry, published by Econ-Verlag, lists the addresses and products of chemical manufacturers and wholesalers in Germany.

Merck Catalogue (formerly Fluka): *The Merck Catalogue* contains the entire program of chemicals and biochemicals supplied by this company. Included are: Names; Trade names; Synonyms; Industrial health and safety standards. Information on 13,000 substances is given.

ISSN 0934–3512

For more details of constituent databases, see:
Hommel
VCI
Merck Catalogue

Dangerous Goods – Operation Files, BAG Toxic Substances Lists, SUVA

Springer-Verlag

20:150. Master record

CD-ROM   **Springer-Verlag**

Alternative name(s)	Gefahrgut – Operation Files, BAG Toxic Substances Lists, SUVA; Operation Files, BAG Toxic Substances Lists, SUVA
Database type	Factual
Number of journals	
Sources	
Start year	
Language	English and German
Coverage	Europe
Number of records	
Update size	–
Update period	

Keywords
Chemical Substances; Dangerous Chemicals; First Aid; Industrial Health and Safety; Toxic Substances

Description
Three databases from the Springer-Verlag collection of Dangerous Goods databases, including information on: Names; Substance information; Carriage classification; Appearance; Health risks; controlling the results of the accident; Safety measures; Water pollution; Equipment; First aid; Medical advice; manufacturers names and addresses. Searchable by: Pictogram, name, UN number, colour, consistency, smell and numerical searches.

Operation Files: The operation files for chemical incidents of the Swiss Fire Brigades Association; Illustrations and clear presentation give instructions on the correct procedures in accidents. dangerous goods classes including many substances and preparations are summarised on separate pages in German and French.

BAG Toxic Substances Lists: The Swiss Toxic Substances List contains poison classes and the addresses of registered companies. 76,000 substances and products are included with their trade name and all available synonyms.

SUVA: The Swiss Accident Insurance Institution, is the editor of the safety codes of liquids and gases. The physical values in this list are of importance when judging the safety of substances.

ISSN 0934–3539

For more details of constituent databases, see:
Operation Files/Einsatzakten SFA
BAG Toxic Substances Lists/BAG-Giftlisten
SUVA

Dangerous Goods

Springer-Verlag

20:151. Master record

CD-ROM   **Springer-Verlag**

Alternative name(s)	Gefahrgut
Database type	Factual
Number of journals	
Sources	

Start year	
Language	English, German and French (some)
Coverage	Europe
Number of records	526,000
Update size	–
Update period	

Keywords
Chemical Substances; Dangerous Chemicals; First Aid; Hazardous Substances; Industrial Health and Safety; Toxic Substances

Description
Contains seven databases on potentially hazardous chemicals, with a common index and searching interface, containing over 400,000 names, synonyms and product names, plus 126,000 environmentally risky substances, with individual profiles for fire brigades, police, rescue services and so on. It is restricted to those carried in bulk in Europe and provides 'first response' data, of the type likely to be useful to the emergency services and to transport authorities.

Information included: Names; Substance information; Carriage classification; Appearance; Health risks; Controlling the results of the accident; Safety measures; Water pollution; Equipment; First aid; Medical advice; manufacturers' and wholesalers' names and addresses. Searchable by: Pictogram, name, UN number, colour, consistency, smell and numerical searches.

Hommel: *Handbook of Dangerous Goods*, 1,500 substances: Technical and Physical data, reactions, environmental data and instructions concerning intervention, first aid, and medical treatment are given.

Chemdata: Harwell Laboratories' and the UK Fire Brigades' collection (fifteen years' worth) of data on dangerous goods. Safety measures for 18,000 substances are included, explained, for the first time, in English and German.

Operation files: The operation files for chemical incidents of the Swiss Fire Brigades Association; Illustrations and clear presentation give instructions on the correct procedures in accidents. Dangerous goods classes including many substances and preparations are summarized on separate pages in German and French.

Merck (formerly Fluka): *The Merck Catalogue* contains the entire program of chemicals and bio chemicals supplied by this company. Included are: names; trade names; synonyms; industrial health and safety standards; MAK-values; and packaging and storage categories. Information on 13,000 substances is given.

BAG Toxic Substances List: The Swiss Toxic Substances List contains poison classes and the addresses of registered companies. 76,000 substances and products are included with their trade name and all available synonyms.

SUVA: The Swiss Accident Insurance Institution, is the editor of the safety codes of liquids and gases. The physical values in this list are of importance when judging the safety of substances.

VCI: *The Handbook of Firms* in the chemical industry, published by Econ-Verlag, lists the addresses and products of chemical manufacturers and wholesalers in the Federal Republic of Germany. This is a multilingual database – all printed documentation is in German only. Prompts and messages during searching may be selected from a choice of German, English and French. The data is in a variety of languages depending on the database being searched. Most are mainly German, but Chemdata is also in English; Merck provides English hazard phrases; BAG is mixed German/English and the Swiss Fire Brigade is in French and German; Hommel has German text with English headings and mixed German/English phraseology for technical data.

ISSN 0934–3571.

The Dangerous Goods collection of databases is available in various combinations on CD-ROM through Springer-Verlag:

a complete collection of seven databases (DM 15,300);
Hommel, VCI, Merck Catalogue, Chemdata (DM 12,350);
Hommel, VCI, Merck Catalogue, Operation Files, BAG Toxic Substances Lists, SUVA (DM 9,975);
Chemdata, Operation Files, BAG Toxic Substances Lists, SUVA (DM 9,975);
Hommel, VCI, Merck Catalogue (DM 6,500);
Chemdata (DM 6,500);
Operation Files, BAG Toxic Substances Lists, SUVA (DM 4,500).

For more details of constituent databases, see:
Chemdata
Operation Files/Einsazakten SFA
Merck Catalogue
BAG Toxic Substances List/BAG-Giftlisten
SUVA
VCI
Hommel

Database on Medicine and Health Care
VNII Medzinskoj i Mediko-technicheskoj Informazij

20:152 Master record

Database type	Bibliographic
Number of journals	
Sources	
Start year	1988
Language	English
Coverage	International
Number of records	120,000
Update size	—
Update period	

Description
Bibliographic source on international biomedicine.

20:153 Diskette — VNII Medzinskoj i Mediko-technicheskoj Informazij

File name	
Start year	1988
Number of records	120,000
Update period	

Diabetes (DM)
National Diabetes Information Clearinghouse

20:154 Master record

Database type	Bibliographic
Number of journals	
Sources	Journals, Monographs, Pamphlets and A-V material
Start year	1973
Language	English
Coverage	USA (primarily) and International (some)
Number of records	
Update size	—
Update period	Quarterly

Description
Contains citations, with abstracts, to journal articles, brochures, books, and audiovisual materials on diabetes.

Language is primarily English, with some coverage of materials in other languages.

This database can also be found on:
Combined Health Information Database

Dictionnaire Vidal
Bureau van Dijk
OVP – Editions du Vidal

20:155 Master record

Alternative name(s)	Vidal 1992; CD-ROM Vidal
Database type	Directory, Textual
Number of journals	
Sources	Book
Start year	
Language	French
Coverage	France
Number of records	9,000
Update size	—
Update period	Annually
Index unit	Drug

Keywords
Drugs; Pharmaceuticals; Surgery

Description
The *Dictionnaire Vidal*: the reference book in France for physicians and pharmacists. It contains fully detailed prescribing information on more than 9,000 pharmaceuticals, plus information on drug interaction and side effects. Features include automatic interaction checking and split screen comparisons. Covers 31st May 1990 to 31st May 1991.

Equivalent to the *Dictionnaire Vidal* or *Vidal Directory*, the drug reference book of France.

Free-text searching on every word. Can be searched by product name, active ingredient, therapeutic category, company name, or word.

20:156 CD-ROM   OVP – Editions du Vidal

File name	CD-ROM Vidal
Alternative name(s)	Vidal 1992; CD-ROM Vidal
Format notes	IBM
Software	Proprietary
Start year	
Number of records	9,000
Update period	Annually
Price/Charges	Subscription: US$710

Notes

Extra subscription options include: 'Rote Liste' (Bundesverband der Pharazeutischen Industrie eV) in German (US$155); 'Physician's Desk Reference' (Medical Economics Company) in English (US$710); 'Index Nominum' (Société Suisse de Pharmacie) in English (US$460); 'Breviaire Des Medicaments' (Documed) in French and German (US$460).

This database can also be found on:
MediROM
PharmaROM

DIDS
National Institute of Occupational Safety and Health (NIOSH)

20:158 Master record

Alternative name(s)	Document Information Directory System
Database type	Factual, Directory
Number of journals	
Sources	Journals, Monographs and Technical reports
Start year	
Language	English
Coverage	International
Number of records	
Update size	–
Update period	

Keywords

Accident Prevention; Biological Hazards; Epidemiology; Ergonomics; Hazardous Waste; Health Physics; Industrial Materials; Industrial Processes; Metabolism; Occupational Health and Safety; Pathology; Safety Education; Vocational Training; Waste Management

Description

Contains a listing of all of the NIOSH publications and reports, with ordering information.

20:159 Online   CCINFOline

File name	
Alternative name(s)	Document Information Directory System
Start year	
Number of records	
Update period	

This database can also be found on:
CCINFOdisc Series C1 – NIOSHTIC

Digestive Diseases (DD)
National Digestive Diseases Information Clearinghouse

20:161 Master record

Database type	Bibliographic
Number of journals	
Sources	Monographs

Start year	1980
Language	English
Coverage	USA (primarily) and International (some)
Number of records	
Update size	–
Update period	Quarterly

Description

Contains citations, with abstracts, to professional and patient education literature on digestive diseases.

Language is primarily English, with some coverage of materials in other languages.

This database can be found on:
Combined Health Information Database

Diseases of the Colon and Rectum
JB Lippincott Company

20:163 Master record

Database type	Textual, Factual
Number of journals	1
Sources	Journal
Start year	1984
Language	English
Coverage	International
Number of records	
Update size	–
Update period	
Index unit	Articles, Letters and Reviews

Keywords

Surgery

Description

Chronicles current research developments and clinical research topics relevant to the practice of colon and rectal surgery. The print product is the official journal of the American Society of Colon and Rectal Surgeons.

20:164 Online   Mead Data Central (as a NEXIS database)

File name	DCR – NEXIS
Start year	1984–1990
Number of records	
Update period	
Price/Charges	Subscription: US$1,000 – 3,000 (Depending on needs)
	Connect time: US$49.00 (Telecomms + connect time)
	Database entry fee: US$24.00 (Search charge)
	Online print: US$0.04 per line

Notes

Library: GENMED; Group File: ARCJNL.

A subscription charge which covers all transactional charges, connect time, telecommunications and the small administration charge can take the place of the individual charges. Subscriptions are negotiated with customers and vary according to the number of menus (thus, files) that are to be used – typically a minimum subscription would be about US$ 1,000. All charges include training and a 24-hour help line.

Record composition

Publication; Cite; Date; Section; Length; Title; Source; Author; Abstract (SUM-ABS); Text; Additional information (SUPP-INFO); Reference (BIBLIO-REF); Graphic; Correction; Correction Date; Discussion and Editor's Note

This database can also be found on:
NEXIS

Dosing & Therapeutic Tools

Micromedex Inc

20:166 Master record

Alternative name(s)	Computerized Clinical Information System: Dosing & Therapeutic Tools; CCIS: Dosing & Therapeutic Tools
Database type	Bibliographic, Factual, Textual, Directory, Numeric
Number of journals	
Sources	
Start year	1985
Language	English
Coverage	International
Number of records	
Update size	–
Update period	Quarterly

Keywords

Clinical Medicine; Diagnosis; Drug Therapy; Drugs; Pharmaceuticals

Description

Contains a library of resources related to medical dosages and therapeutic tools.

Diagnostic and Therapeutic Pearls contains brief charts or tables of significant medical, pharmaceutical or toxicological information not readily available separately. Covers medical terms and jargon, abbreviations and statistics.

Differential Diagnostic Lists contains lists of possible causes (for example, disease, drug, toxic agent) of clinical signs or symptoms, or laboratory findings that enable health care officials to narrow the possible causes of a specific finding.

EKG Rhythm Strips contains EKG rhythm strips that represent one-lead electrocardiogram of various cardiac rhythms and their descriptions. EKG rhythm strips are used as a teaching tool for medical personnel to recognise irregularities in heartbeats. Users can compare any two EKG strips in the database.

Nomograms contains nomograms (charts and graphs) that show correlation of potential clinical outcome with plasma or serum drug levels in an overdose situation. Users can compare serum drug level obtained at a known time after ingestion with the nomogram to predict ther potential for development of toxicity. Nomograms are available for acetaminophen, ibuprofen and salicylates.

Drug Dosing contains software that can be used to calculate the dosage and administration of medication for a specific patient. Users can calculate adult or paediatric dosages for emergency drugs and for selected other drugs (Dobutamine, Dopamine, Ethanol, Epinephrine, Lidocaine, N-Acetylcysteine, Nitroglycerin, Nitroprusside and Norephinephrine).

Calculators contains software that can be used to perform these calculations: alveolar-arterial oxygen gradient, anion gap, body weight and surface area, creatinine clearance, alcohols/ethylene glycol blodod level and SIU.

This database can be found on:
CCIS

DOT Emergency Response Guides

Micromedex Inc

20:168 Master record

Alternative name(s)	Emergency Respones Guides
Database type	Factual, Directory, Bibliographic
Number of journals	
Sources	
Start year	
Language	English
Coverage	International
Number of records	2,000
Update size	–
Update period	Quarterly

Keywords

Explosion; Fire; Hazardous Chemicals; Occupational Health and Safety

Description

DOT Emergency Response Guides prepared by the Department of Transportation – a reference source for initial response to releases, fires or explosions involving over 2,000 frequently transported chemicals.

This database can be found on:
TOMES Plus

Drugline

Läkemedelsinformationscentralen, Huddinge sjukhus

20:170 Master record

Database type	Factual, Textual
Number of journals	
Sources	Request forms
Start year	1982
Language	Swedish, English (some) and English (indexing)
Coverage	International
Number of records	3,500
Update size	400
Update period	Quarterly
Index unit	Drug

Keywords

Clinical Pharmacology; Drugs; Drug Therapy

Description

A problem-oriented drug information data bank. The information is based on questions received and answers prepared by clinical pharmacologists and pharmacists at the Drug Information Center (DIC), a subunit of the Institution for Clinical Pharmacology, Karolinska Institute at Huddinge Hospital, Sweden. Clinical pharmacologists and pharmacists help by reviewing information from the medical literature and databases not readily available to community physicians. Clinical questions are personally answered by referenced reviews after a literature search. Most requests deal with adverse drug reactions, including safety of drug treatment during pregnancy or breast feeding. There are also questions concerning choice of drug, pharmacokinetics and drug interactions. Drugline was created in cooperation with the Medical Information Centre (MIC). The records include all data and text from the rquest forms, except names of requester and patient.

Previously produced by MIC/Karolinska Institute Library and Information Center.

Topics are indexed by *Medical Subject Headings* (*MeSH*)

20:171 Online   MIC/Karolinska Institute Library and Information Center (MIC KIBIC)

File name	DRUGLINE
Start year	1982
Number of records	3,500
Update period	Quarterly

Notes

Special conditions for use apply.

DXplain

Massachusetts General Hospital
American Medical Association

20:172 Master record

Database type	Factual, Textual
Number of journals	
Sources	
Start year	Current information
Language	English
Coverage	USA
Number of records	2,000
Update size	As new data becomes available
Update period	Varies

Keywords

Biomedicine

Description

Contains descriptions of diseases, including related clinical and laboratory data. Provides diagnostic assistance by presenting plausible explanations for clinical data entered by the user. Users can also enter new information to update the database.

20:173 Online   AMA/NET

File name	
Start year	Current information
Number of records	2,000
Update period	Varies

Notes

Initiation fee of $30 for AMA members or $50 for non-members to AMA/NET required.

Ei/SPIE Critical Papers

Engineering Information Inc
International Society for Optical Engineers

20:174 Master record

Database type	Bibliographic
Number of journals	
Sources	Journals

Start year	1993
Language	English
Coverage	International
Number of records	
Update size	—
Update period	Twice per month
Index unit	Journals

Keywords

Ophthalmology; Optics

Description

Compiles the latest citations and abstracts from various journals and proceedings into five biweekly newsletters on aspects of optics.

20:175 Diskette   Engineering Information Inc

File name	Ei/SPIE Critical Papers
Format notes	IBM
Software	Ei Order
Start year	1993
Number of records	
Update period	Twice per month

Ei/SPIE Page One

Engineering Information Inc
International Society for Optical Engineers

20:176 Master record

Database type	Bibliographic
Number of journals	120
Sources	Journals and Conference proceedings
Start year	1993
Language	English
Coverage	International
Number of records	
Update size	—
Update period	Twice per month
Index unit	Journals and Conference proceedings

Keywords

Ophthalmology; Optics

Description

Provides the tables of contents for over 120 journals and 200 proceedings as an ASCII file.

20:177 Diskette   Engineering Information Inc

File name	
Format notes	IBM
Software	Ei Order
Start year	1993
Number of records	
Update period	Twice per month

Electronic Library of Medicine

Little, Brown and Company

20:178 Master record

Database type	Factual
Number of journals	
Sources	Books

Start year
Language
Coverage
Number of records
Update size   –
Update period   Quarterly

Keywords

Drugs; Pharmaceuticals

Description

Contains diagnostic and therapeutic information for some thirteen medical disciplines. Also includes volume one of the *US Pharmacopoetal Drug Information.*

20:179 CD-ROM   Little, Brown and Company

File name   Electronic Library of Medicine
Format notes   IBM
Software   Proprietary
Start year
Number of records
Update period   Quarterly

EMBASE
Elsevier Science Publishers

20:180 Master record

Alternative name(s)   Excerpta Medica
Database type   Bibliographic
Number of journals   4,700
Sources   Case studies, clinicians, journals, monographs, research communications, reviews, surveys and symposia
Start year   1974
Language   English
Coverage   International
Number of records   4,950,000+
Update size   350,000
Update period   Weekly
Index unit   Articles
Abstract details   Adaptations of the authors' summaries and selected on the basis of content and length by an international group of practicing medical and other qualified specialists and when necessary modified, shortened or extended to obtain the optimal information value. A group of over 2,000 biomedical specialists assists with the preparation of abstracts in particular subject areas and articles in non-Western European languages
Thesaurus   EMTREE Thesaurus METAGS
Database aids   Guide to the Classification and Indexing System, MALIMET (available online and on microfiche), Mini-Malimet, MECLASE Drug Trade Names (DN) and EMBASE List of Journals Abstracted

Keywords

HIV; Anaesthesia; Anatomy; Anthropology; Bio-engineering; Biotechnology; Cancer; Cardiology; Clinical Medicine; Clinical Neurology; Cosmetics; Drugs; Environmental Health; Environmental Pollution; Environmental Toxicology; Epilepsy; Food Additives; Food Contaminants; Forensic Medicine; Forensic Science; Gastroenterology; Gynaecology; Immunology; Industrial Medicine; Nephrology; Neuroscience; Neuromuscular Disorders; Nuclear Medicine; Obstetrics; Occupational Health and Safety; Patents; Pathology; Pharmaceuticals; Pollution; Public Health; Radiology; Toxic Substances; Waste Management

Description

EMBASE is the trademark for the English language Excerpta Medica database. Excerpta Medica was founded as a non-profit making organisation in 1946 with the goal of improving the availability and dissemination of medical knowledge through the publication of a series of abstract journals. The database contains citations, with abstracts, to the worldwide biomedical literature on human medicine and areas of biological sciences related to human medicine with an emphasis on the pharmacological effects of drugs and chemicals. The four main categories of primary literature sources are: specialist medical publications; general biomedicine publications; specialist non-medical publications and general scientific publications. Subjects covered include: anatomy; anesthesiology (including resuscitation and intensive care medicine); anthropology; pharmacology of anesthetic agents, spinal, epidural and caudal anesthesia and acupuncture (as anesthetic); autoimmunity; biochemistry; bioengineering; cancer; dangerous goods; dermatology; developmental biology; drug adverse reactions; drug dependence; drug effects; endocrinology; environmental health and pollution control (covering chemical pollution and its effect on man, animals, plants and microorganisms; measurement, treatment, prevention and control); exocrine pancreas; forensic science; gastroenterology (including diseases and disorders of: digestive systems; mouth; pharynx and more); genetics; gerontology and geriatrics; health economics; hematology; hepatobiliary system; hospital management; immunology (including immunity; hypersensitivity; histocompatibility and all aspects of the immune system); internal medicine; legal and socioeconomic aspects; mesentary; meteorological aspects; microbiology; nephrology (covering diagnosis; treatment; epidemiology; prevention; infections; glomerular and tubular disorders; blood purification; dialysis; kidney transplantation; toxic nephropathy and including important clinical abstracts with epidemiological studies and major clinical trials, with particular emphasis on hypertension and diabetes); neurosciences (especially clinical neurology and neurosurgery, epilepsy and neuromuscular disorders but also covering non-clinical articles on neurophysiology and animal models for human neuropharmacology); noise and vibration; nuclear medicine; obstetrics and gynaecology (including endocrinology and menstrual cycle, infertility, prenatal diagnosis and fetal monitoring, anti-conceptions, breast cancer diagnosis, sterilisation and psychosexual problems and neonatal care of normal children); occupational health and industrial medicine; opthalmology; otorhinolaryngology; paediatrics; pathology (including general pathology and organ pathology, pathological physiology and pathological anatomy, as well as laboratory methods and techniques used in pathology. General pathology topics range from cellular pathology, fetal and neonatal pathology, including congenital disorders, injury (both chemical and physical), inflammation and infection, immuno-pathology, collagen diseases and cancer pathology); peritoneum; pharmacology (including the effects and use of all drugs; experimental aspects of pharmacokinetics and pharmacodynamics; drug information); physiology; psychiatry and psychology (including addiction; alcoholism; sexual behaviour; suicide; mental deficiency and the clinical use or abuse of psychotropic and psychomimetic agents);

public health; radiation and thermal pollution; radiology (including radiodiagnosis, radiotherapy and radiobiology, ultrasound diagnosis, thermography, adverse reactions to radiotherapy and techniques and apparatus, radiobiology of radioisotopes, aspects of radiohygiene, new labelling techniques and tracer applications); rehabilitation; surgery; toxicology (including pharmaceutical toxicology; foods, food additives, and contaminants; cosmetics, toiletries, and household products; occupational toxicology; waste material in air, soil and water; toxins and venoms; chemical teratogens, mutagens, and carcinogens; phototoxicity; regulatory toxicology; laboratory methods and techniques; and antidotes and symptomatic treatment); urology; wastewater treatment and measurement. The database is particularly strong in drug-related literature, where records include manufacturers and drug trade names and generic names. Information on veterinary medicine, nursing and dentistry is generally excluded.

Excerpta Medica is extremely current as articles are indexed within 30 days of receipt and are online very soon after that. Approximately 900 journals (the Rapid Input Processing (RIP)) are processed with priority which means that within eleven weeks of the receipt of the original document, the completely-indexed records are available. More than 100,000 records are given this priority treatment. Some hosts have companion databases giving training or details of the indexing vocabularies and thesauri.

EMBASE concentrates on journal articles although about 1,000 books per annum were indexed between 1975 and 1980. The source journals include all forty-six sections of *Excerpta Medica*, the *Drug Literature Index* and *Adverse Reactions Titles*. New titles are added and old titles deleted at a rate of about 200–300 per year. The database covers sources from 110 countries with the following geographical scope: North America 36%, Western Europe 35%, United Kingdom 14%, USSR and Eastern Europe 7%, Asia 6%, Central and South America 1%, Austalia & South Pacific 1%, Africa and Middle East 1%. Approximately 50% of the citations are from drug and pharmaceutical literature and approximately 40% of citations added to the database each year do not appear in the corresponding printed abstract journals and indexes. Approximately 65% of the citations contain abstracts of on average 200 words with a maximum of 800 words which indicate the content of the articles and are not intended to summarise the results or express opinions. This makes free-text searching of the abstracts, titles and other searchable elements of the citation valuable. This compares with approximately sixty-five per cent of the records in MEDLINE and fifty-four per cent in BIOSIS. The records of the other leading bioscience database, SciSearch, now do contain abstracts. Approximately 75% of the articles are in the English language. Of the other leading bioscience databases, approximately eighty-eight per cent of articles on SciSearch are in English, eighty-six per cent of articles on BIOSIS and seventy-four per cent on MEDLINE. In addition approximately thirty-seven per cent of records with non-English sources contain English-language abstracts online. This compares with sixty-seven per cent on BIOSIS and twenty-six per cent on MEDLINE. SciSearch does now contain abstracts. Important publications NOT indexed in EMBASE include Meyler's *Side Effects of Drugs*, 1972–1980 published by Excerpta Medica and *Side Effects of Drugs Annual*, 1981 to the present, published by Elsevier.

A core collection of 3,500 biomedical journals supplemented by journals in the areas of agriculture, technology, economics, chemistry, environmental protection and sociology. General criteria used for selection are first that the document should be of potential relevance to medicine and secondly the information should be of lasting value for which reasons news items and comments are generally excluded.

EMBASE section headings are based on medical specialities; a total of forty-seven subfiles group together citations on topics such as anatomy, paediatrics, opthalmology, gastroenterelogy, cancer, plastic surgery, occupational health. Each subfile or section has its own hierarchical scheme. The thesaurus *MALIMET* (*Master List of Medical Terms*) is used which contains more than 250,000 preferred terms and 255,000 synonyms which are mapped to the preferred terms when used. It is used for indexing highly specific concepts such as names of drugs and chemicals; diseases and syndromes; anatomical and physiological aspects and diagnostic and therapeutic methods. *MALIMET* is growing at a rate of over 12,000 descriptors per annum, mainly through drug names and names of chemical compounds. The size of the complete *MALIMET* thesaurus for EMBASE (more than 250,000 preferred terms compared to 15,000 in *MeSH*) may indicate its tendency to provide a greater variety of possible terms and therefore, less consistent application in indexing. In 1993, all non-drug *MeSH* terms were included in the thesaurus mapped to *MALIMET* terms so that a search strategy can be transferred from MEDLINE.

Indexing incorporates the following rules: natural word order (acute leukemia, not leukemia acute); American spelling (tumor, not tumour), singular noun forms and not plural or adjectival forms (stomach tumor, not gastric tumors, but optic nerve, not eye nerve); the most specific term must be used. Since 1979, *MALIMET* terms have been weighted. Class A terms (weighted) indicate the main concepts while Class B terms (not weighted) indicate the less important concepts of a document. In addition to *MALIMET* broad concepts are indexed with EMCLAS and EMTAGS. EMCLAS is a poly-hierarchical decimal classification scheme of the forty-six subject subfiles which make up the sections of the printed *Excerpta Medica* containing approximately 6,500 entries. It is then further subdivided into a five level hierarchy of sub-categories. Indexing is performed by medical specialists and scientists whose specialism corresponds to the subject areas forming the major subdivisions of EMCLAS. The indexing builds up sequentially as the article is indexed by each of the sections for which it is relevant. On average each document is indexed for 3.5 different sections.

EMTAGS is a group of approximately 220 codes which represent general concepts such as groups, gender, organ systems, experimental animals and article type. In January 1991 about 10% of the terms were changed including important descriptors such as CANCER or BENIGN NEOPLASM.

EMBASE editors also add 'uncontrolled' drug terms to augment *MALIMET* descriptors in selected records. EMBASE provides a hierarchical classification system (EMTREES) reflecting fifteen broad facets of biomedicine. From January 1991 a new version of EMTREE went online comprising 35,000 terms. New descriptors and changes in the hierarchy were made in the following areas: anatomy of the eye; diseases; drugs; techniques; biological phenomea and document types. Prior to 1988 Section Headings based on medical speciality areas were used instead of EMTREES to index EMBASE citations. In both classification schemes, codes are constructed to facilitate broad concept retrieval through truncation. In addition three uncontrolled vocabularies are used: Medical Secondary Text; Drug (Trade Names) and Manufacturers' Names are used. Medical Secondary Text consists of free-text words, numbers and phrases, describing concepts which are not fully covered by the controlled terms, for example quantiative information such as the number of patients or experimental animals. Drug (Trade) Names consists of trade names of drugs referred to in an original document with the main aspect of biological effects of compounds listed. Manufacturers' Names lists the names of drug manufacturers. The value of controlled indexing is important when searching for topics where a subject population has been specified.

Relatively few bioscience databases provide consistent indexing for subject populations (that is, humans or specific test animals) and related characteristics commonly requested such as age groups, gender, occupation and racial or ethnic groups. EMBASE provides extensive consistent indexing for the identification of test animals and age groups with a less consistent approach for the indexing of humans, occupational groups, racial/ethnic groups and gender. In addition, in most bioscience files a form of pharmaceutical nomenclature exists. For EMBASE the preferred search terms are generic name, classification by action/use and CAS Reigstry Number although restrictions by date, subfile and vendor may apply to the latter and vendor documentation should be consulted for guidelines. The search terms Enzyme Commission Number, investigational code, chemical name and trade name should be cross-referenced to the preferred terminology in the thesaurus. In 1993, improved CAS Registry Numbers mean that there is a single Number assigned for every substance.

20:181 Database subset
Online   AMA/NET

File name	AMA/NET Empires
Alternative name(s)	Excerpta Medica
Start year	1984
Number of records	
Update period	Weekly

Notes

AMA/NET Empires contains citations, with some abstracts, to articles in key clinical journals. Articles are coded by medical specialty. Citations include full bibliographic information, subject indexing, drug terminology and drug manufacturers. The source of the database is EMBASE. A subscription fee of $30 for members or $50 for non-members of AMA/NET required.

20:182 Database subset
CD-ROM   SilverPlatter

File name	Excerpta Medica – Anesthesiology
Alternative name(s)	Excerpta Medica
Format notes	Mac, IBM
Software	SPIRS/MacSPIRS
Start year	1980
Number of records	116,000
Update period	Quarterly
Price/Charges	Subscription: UK£755 – 1,132

Notes

One of the Elsevier speciality Excerpta Medica range, this CD-ROM includes all of the abstracts and citations relating to anaesthesiology selected and indexed by Excerpta Medica from 1980 to the present.

Includes relevant information from the 3,500 biomedical journals scanned plus every record from the top anaesthesiology journals. The database covers both clinical and experimental aspects of the subject and includes resuscitation and intensive care medicine, pharmacology of anaesthetic agents, spinal, epidural and caudal anaesthesia and acupuncture (when used as an anaestheic procedure). In addition, relevant abstracts from other clinical and basic disciplines are included.

Prices are: for single users UK£755, for 2–8 networked users £1,132.

20:183 Database subset
CD-ROM   SilverPlatter

File name	Excerpta Medica – Neurosciences
Alternative name(s)	Excerpta Medica
Format notes	IBM, Mac
Software	SPIRS/MacSPIRS
Start year	1980
Number of records	510,000
Update period	Quarterly
Price/Charges	Subscription: UK£755 – 1,132

Notes

One of the Elsevier speciality Excerpta Medica range, this database, consisting of two CD-ROM discs, is a subset of EMBASE and covers a wide range of neurosciences. It is especially strong in clinical neurology, epilepsy and neuromuscular disorders. Non-clinical articles on neurophysiology and animal models for human neuropharmacology are also covered but animal studies without relevance to human neuropathology are less extensively covered in the early 1980s. Relevant abstracts from other clinical and basic disciplines are also included.

Prices are: for single users UK£755, for 2–8 networked users £1,132.

Emergindex
Micromedex Inc

20:184 Master record

Alternative name(s)	Computerized Clinical Information System: Emergindex; CCIS: Emergindex
Database type	Bibliographic, Factual, Textual, Directory
Number of journals	50
Sources	
Start year	
Language	English
Coverage	USA and International
Number of records	
Update size	—
Update period	Quarterly
Thesaurus	MeSH-based

Keywords

Acute Medicine; Diagnosis; Emergency Medicine; Epidemiology; Pharmaceuticals; Radiography

Description

A clinical support tool for the diagnosis and treatment of diseases and trauma seen in acute care settings. A referenced clinical information system that presents pertinent data for the practice of acute care medicine. It is designed to help those who deal with acute medical/surgical disease and traumatic injuries to more quickly and efficiently diagnose and treat the multitude of problems encountered daily. The system comprises three files of information on emergency, traumatic injury and acute care medicine, diagnosis and treatment.

Clinical Reviews contains over 285 reviews of emergency and acute care treatment protocols. Covers clinical presentation, including etiology and epidemiology, laboratory and radiographic studies, diagnostic aids, differential diagnoses, non-pharmacologic and pharmacologic therapeutics and disposition.

Clinical Abstracts contains about 17,000 citations, with abstracts, to about fifty journals on emergency and critical care medicine worldwide. Includes clinical and experimental studies on nearly 300 diseases and injuries. Each record includes study problem or purpose, study type, population data, study design, methodology, results, conclusions, and references.

Prehospital Care Protocols contains over thirty protocols for emergency medical service (EMS) personnel for diagnosis and treatment of the injured or ill patient in the prehospital environment. Each protocol includes presentation, stabilisation, base contact, special concerns and references.

A primary product of the Computerized Clinical Information System from Micromedex. The primary databases are offered on annual subscription with a choice of – System I: any one of the primary titles, System II: any two of the primary titles, System III: all three of the primary titles. Any of the primary databases can be purchased separately. Any combination of these systems attracts a first year software licence fee of £280.

Users can search by subjects in a 40,000 term medical thesaurus based on the National Library of Medicine *Medical Subject Headings (MeSH)*.

20:185 Tape   Micromedex Inc

File name	Emergindex
Alternative name(s)	Computerized Clinical Information System: Emergindex; CCIS: Emergindex
Start year	1973
Number of records	
Update period	Quarterly

Notes

Annual subscription to CCIS required. AfterCare Instructions, also on CCIS, is available to subcribers of this database for an additional fee.

20:186 Database subset
Online   Mead Data Central
(as a NEXIS database)

File name	ABSTR – NEXIS
Start year	1980
Number of records	285 in Clinical Reviews; 17,000 in Clinical Abstracts
Update period	Quarterly
Price/Charges	Subscription: US$1,000 – 3,000 (Depending on needs) Connect time: US$49.00 (Telecomms + connect time) Database entry fee: US$24.00 (Search charge) Online print: US$0.04 per line

Notes

Library: GENMED; Group files: EMERDX and MEDEX.

On NEXIS, Emergindex is divided into two files: Clinical Abstracts (ABSTR) and Clinical Reviews

(DISEAS). ABSTR is designed as authoritative information to assist in the diagnosis and treatment of acute diseases and injuries. The clinical abstracts are an ongoing cumulative review of the world's medical literature specifically related to emergency and critical care medicine. When the file is selected, an introductory note about searching the file and a list of topics is automatically displayed.

A subscription charge which covers all transactional charges, connect time, telecommunications and the small administration charge can take the place of the individual charges. Subscriptions are negotiated with customers and vary according to the number of menus (thus, files) that are to be used – typically a minimum subscription would be about US$ 1,000. All charges include training and a 24-hour help line.

Record composition

Copyright Information PUBLICATION; Citation SOURCE; Descriptive Phrase TOPIC; Statement of Purpose/Problem PURPOSE; Population (Study Subjects) POPULATION; Number in Study TOTAL; Number of Males in Study MALE; Number of Females in Study FEMALE; Methodology METHODOLOGY; Results RESULTS; Descriptive Terms TERMS; Study Design DESIGN and Study Definition STUDY-TYPE Each abstract is indexed by key terms for easy reference to any topic relevant to acute care medicine.

20:187 Database subset
Online   Mead Data Central
(as a NEXIS database)

File name	DISEAS – NEXIS
Start year	1980
Number of records	285 in Clinical Reviews; 17,000 in Clinical Abstracts
Update period	Quarterly
Price/Charges	Subscription: US$1,000 – 3,000 (Depending on needs) Connect time: US$49.00 (Telecomms + connect time) Database entry fee: US$24.00 (Search charge) Online print: US$0.04 per line

Notes

Library: GENMED; Group files: EMERDX and MEDEX.

On NEXIS, Emergindex is divided into two files: Clinical Abstracts (ABSTR) and Clinical Reviews (DISEAS). DISEAS is an information system which includes reviews of acute medical/surgical diseases and traumatic injuries. The reviews are written primarily by physicians who are involved in the practice, research and teaching of emergency and critical medicine. The system includes a comprehensive dictionary of over 40,000 index terms and synonyms based on the National Library of Medicine's subject headings (*MeSH*) and special headings devised by a panel of emergency and critical care physicians.

A document in DISEAS consists of a single Clinical Review and accompanying index terms. Most of the documents are several screens long.

A subscription charge which covers all transactional charges, connect time, telecommunications and the small administration charge can take the place of the individual charges. Subscriptions are negotiated with customers and vary according to the number of menus (thus, files) that are to be used – typically a minimum subscription would be about US$ 1,000. All charges include training and a 24-hour help line.

Record composition

Topic TOPIC; Summary Information SUMM; Critical Focus CRIT; Clinical Presentation CLNP; Diagnosis DGNS; Differential Diagnosis DDGN; Clinical Information CLPR; Clinical Information Introduction INTRO; Clinical Information Associated Conditions ASSOC; Clinical Information Vital Signs VITS; Clinical Information Dermatologic Presentation; Clinical Information HEENT Presentation HENT; Clinical Information Neck Presentation NECK; Clinical Information Respiratory Presentation RESP; Clinical Information Cardiovascular Presentation CARD; Clinical Information Gastrointestinal Presentation GAST; Clinical Information Genitourinary Presentation GENT; Clinical Information Musculoskeletal Presentation MUSC; Clinical Information Neurologic Presentation NEUR; Clinical Information Endocrine Presentation ENDO; Clinical Information Infectious Presentation INFT; Clinical Information Hematologic Presentation HEMP; Clinical Information Psychiatric Presntation PSYCH; Clinical Information Miscellaneous Presentation MSYMP; Clinical Information Complications COMP; Laboratory Studies LAB; Laboratory Studies General Discussion LAB-DCSSN; Laboratory Studies Hematologic Data HEME; Laboratory Studies Electrolytes ELEC; Laboratory Studies Chemical Survey CHEM; Laboratory Studies Urinalysis URNL; Laboratory Studies Arterial Blood Gases ABGS; Laboratory Studies Bacteriology BACT; Laboratory Studies Serology SEROL; Laboratory Studies Electrocardiogram EKG; Laboratory Studies Miscellaneous MISC; Radiographic Studies XRAY; Radiographic Studies Plain Films FILM; Radiographic Studies Contrast Studies CONT; Radiographic Studies Nuclear Scans NUCL; Radiographic Studies CT Scans CT; Radiographic Studies Ultrasound SONO; Radiographic Studies Magnetic Resonance Imaging MRI; Diagnostic Aids DIAG; Diagnostic Aids Invasive Procedures INVS; Diagnostic Aids Noninvasive Procedures NINV; Differential Diagnosis DIFF; Differential Diagnosis General Discussion DIFF-DCSSN; Differential Diagnosis Trauma TRMA; Differential Diagnosis Infectious INFC; Differential Diagnosis Inflammatory INFL; Differential Diagnosis Metabolic META; Differential Diagnosis Vascular VASC; Differential Diagnosis Neoplastic NEOP; Differential Diagnosis Toxicologic TOXC; Differential Diagnosis Physical Agents PHYS; Differential Diagnosis Miscellaneous MDGN; Treatment TRMT; Treatment Management Overview MGMT; Treatment Therapy, Non-Pharmacologic THNP; Treatment THerapy, Pharmacologic THPH; Criteria DISP; Admission Criteria ADMIT; Home Criteria HOME; Consult Criteria CONS; Transfer Criteria TRNS and References REFS

Synonyms for Clinical Review document titles are built into the TOPIC segment to retrieve valuable equivalents for document titles which are acronyms or variations of disease names (for example, CARDIO-VASCULAR will retrieve several documents, each covering a specific symptom or type of cardiovascular disease). The standard form of author's name in the REFS segment is LAST NAME-COMMA-SPACE-INITIAL(S). Depending on the information available

from the publisher, there may be one initial or two initials without spaces between them.

This database can also be found on:
CCIS
NEXIS

Ergodata
Universite de Paris V

20:188 Master record

Alternative name(s)	Banque de Données Internationales de Biometrie Humaine et d'Ergonomie
Database type	Bibliographic, Factual, Numeric
Number of journals	
Sources	Standards, Monographs, Government documents, Patents and Journals
Start year	Ergonomic Bibliographic Database, 1972; other files, last 30 years
Language	French
Coverage	International
Number of records	9 million +
Update size	—
Update period	Ergonomic Bibliographic Database twice per month; other files, as new data is available

Keywords

Anthropology; Biomechanics; Ergonomics; Physiology

Description

Consists of three files of information on human factors and ergonomics.

Human Biometrics and Biomechanics Database. Contains about 8.8 million individual anthropometric measurements gathered over the last thirty years on a large number of world populations. Data cover age, sex, nationality, human body measurements and space requirements, measurements for access and motion, human body dynamics, and such physiological data as visual and auditory acuity. The database is designed to help researchers, designers, manufacturers and ergonomists deal with problems involving morphological measurements and the variability of populations. Also has applications in the fields of anthropology, biomechanics, man-machine interfaces, human factors analysis, and human physiology. Updated as new data become available.

Ergonomic Bibliographic Database. Contains citations, with abstracts, to literature on ergonomy from Fiesta, a database containing citations of interest to the defence industry.

Summary Files in Ergonomics. Contains about 500 citations, with abstracts, to summaries of current or recommended ergonomic standards for environments where humans and machines work together. Documents can be ordered online. Updated as new data become available.

Annual subscription fee of 1200 French francs required.

20:189 Online   Ergodata

File name	Ergodata
Start year	1950
Number of records	
Update period	

For more details of constituent databases, see:
Human Biometrics and Biomechanics Database
Ergonomic Bibliographic Database
Summary Files in Ergonomics
Fiesta

Ergonomic Bibliographic Database
Universite de Paris V

20:191 Master record

Database type	Bibliographic, Factual
Number of journals	
Sources	Monographs and Journals
Start year	1972
Language	French
Coverage	International
Number of records	
Update size	–
Update period	Twice per month

Keywords
Anthropology; Biomechanics; Ergonomics

Description
Contains citations, with abstracts, to literature on ergonomy from Fiesta, a database containing citations of interest to the defence industry.

Annual subscription fee of 1200 French francs required.

This database can be found on:
Ergodata

ERICA
Sweden Statens Naturvårdsverk (SNV)

20:193 Master record

Database type	Bibliographic, Library catalogue/cataloguing aids
Number of journals	
Sources	Libraries, Grey literature and Research reports
Start year	1970
Language	Swedish and English (keywords/abstracts)
Coverage	Sweden
Number of records	
Update size	–
Update period	

Keywords
Air Pollution; Civil Engineering; Conservation; Environmental Hygiene; Epidemiology; Ergonomics; Hazardous Waste; Environmental Hygiene; Natural Resources; Noise Pollution; Occupational Health and Safety; Soil Pollution; Toxic Waste; Water Pollution; Wildlife

Description
A database of citations on environmental research topics, ERICA refers to the holdings of the library, books from 1970 and onwards. This is also part of the NATUR database.

This database can be found on:
NATUR

Family Practice – Personal MEDLINE
Information providers: National Library of Medicine

20:195 Master record

CD-ROM	Macmillan New Media
Database type	Bibliographic
Number of journals	
Sources	
Start year	Most recent five years.
Language	
Coverage	
Number of records	
Update size	–
Update period	Annually/Quarterly

Keywords
Family Medicine

Description
References and abstracts from essential journals chosen by a specialist. Covers: etiology, diagnosis, therapy, pharmacology and administration as they relate to family practice, community medicine, preventive medicine, ambulatory care, internal medicine, referral and consultation, delivery of health care, clinical medicine, primary prevention.

A subset of MEDLINE, plus all abstracts from major journals in the field of family medicine.

Notes
Product no longer available as of December 1992.

Femoral Neck Fractures Treatment
Hodos

20:196 Master record

Database type	Multimedia, Courseware
Number of journals	
Sources	
Start year	
Language	English
Coverage	
Number of records	
Update size	–
Update period	

Keywords
Vocational Training; Clinical Medicine

Description
Training module to be used as a part of a teaching module for medical staff associated with the treatment of broken hips. The objectives are to substantially reduce costs and achieve greater success rates.

20:197 DVI · Hodos

File name	Femoral Neck Fractures Treatment
Format notes	IBM
Start year	

Number of records
Update period

Notes

Runs on standard IBM with ActionMedia card and incorporates still and motion video image graphics, audio and text.

Fiesta
Centre de Documentation de l'Armement

20:198 Master record

Database type	Bibliographic
Number of journals	200+
Sources	Monographs, Standards, Patents, Government documents and Journals
Start year	1972
Language	French
Coverage	International
Number of records	400,000+
Update size	24,000
Update period	Twice per month

Keywords

Atmospheric Science; Bioengineering; Fuels; Oceanography; Physics

Description

Contains citations, with abstracts, to literature on a wide variety of topics of interest to the defense community. Covers aeronautics and aerodynamics; astronomy and astrophysics; atmospheric sciences; behavioural and social sciences; biological and medical sciences; bioengineering; chemistry; earth sciences; oceanography; electronics and electrical engineering; non-propulsive energy conversion; materials; mathematical sciences; mechanical, industrial, civil, and marine engineering; military sciences; missile technology; navigations; communications; detection and countermeasures; nuclear science and technology; physics; propulsion; fuels; and space technology.

20:199 Online   Centre de Documentation de l'Armement

File name	Fiesta
Start year	1972
Number of records	400,000+
Update period	Twice per month

This database can also be found on:
Ergodata

Finlandiana
Institute for Occupational Health (Finland)

20:200 Master record

Database type	Bibliographic
Number of journals	220
Sources	Books, conference proceedings, dissertations, grey literature, journals, laws/regulations, research reports and standards
Start year	1980
Language	Finnish (titles) and English
Coverage	Finland (primarily) and International (some)
Number of records	21,000
Update size	2,000
Update period	Quarterly

Keywords

Occupational Health and Safety

Description

Finlandiana is the principal source of Finnish literature on occupational heath and safety. It contains bibliographic references covering the whole field of work-related aspects of health and safety. Subjects covered include: occupational safety, safety engineering, medicine and diseases, rehabilitation, respiratory disorders, industrial hygiene, environmental protection and occupational accidents. Titles of Finnish records are in the original language, but the detailed classification system as well as the controlled terms give easy access to these sources for the first time.

Finlandiana is produced by the Institute for Occupational Health, Helsinki, Finland, an Institute of the International Labour Organisation.

20:201 Online   ESA-IRS

File name	File 227
Start year	1980
Number of records	21,000
Update period	Quarterly
Database aids	Output Formats on ESA-IRS Infosheet, ESA-QUEST Mini Manual and ESA-QUEST Pocket Guide/Technical Notes

Downloading is allowed

Notes

The LIMIT ALL command can be used to limit all subsequent sets. The limitation is cancelled by entering a new LIMIT ALL or a BEGIN command. QUESTORDER can be used for the online ordering of original documents. From 1993 ESA-IRS are charging an annual fee of 100 Accounting Units (c.UK£ 70.29) to all users. This is equivalent to the fee for full documentation and will not be charged to customers already paying for documentation.

Record composition

Author AU; Classification Code CC; Classification Names CN; Controlled Terms /CT; Journal Name JN; Language LA; Native Accession Number NN; Publication Year PY and Title /TI

The basic index includes the controlled terms and title data fields.

First Aid
Infotouch

20:202 Master record

Database type	Multimedia
Number of journals	
Sources	
Start year	
Language	Dutch, English, French and German
Coverage	International
Number of records	
Update size	—
Update period	Not updated

Keywords

First Aid; Home Health Care

Description

Multimedia instruction on first aid.

20:203 CDTV   Infotouch

File name	First Aid
Format notes	Commodore
Software	Proprietary
Start year	
Number of records	
Update period	Not updated
Price	US$79

FOCUS ON: Global Change
Institute for Scientific Information

20:204 Master record

Alternative name(s)	Global Change
Database type	Bibliographic
Number of journals	
Sources	Journals, Books, Conference proceedings and Newspapers
Start year	
Language	English
Coverage	International
Number of records	
Update size	1,200
Update period	Every two weeks
Index unit	Articles
Abstract details	English-language author abstracts are included for approximately 70% of all articles and books indexed

Keywords

Demography; Epidemiology; Forestry; Fuels; Industrial Hygiene

Description

Abstracted citations and multidisciplinary guide to current research on environmental change and human interaction with the environment. Covers agriculture, aquatic sciences, atmospheric sciences, business, demography, earth sciences, ecology, economics, energy and fuels, environmental sciences, epidemiology, forestry, geography, humanities, industrial hygiene, law, medicine, meteorology and atmospheric sciences, natural resources, planning and development, politics and policy, social sciences, toxicology, transportation, waste and water treatments, and wildlife management.

Covers the science and social science journals as well as business and popular press.

ISI claim to acquire data as much as three months earlier than any other secondary sources, thus making this with both fast and targeted research. All ISI databases have a linked service known as The Genuine Article which can deliver the full text of located articles by mail, facsimile transmission or courier. Orders can be placed via the host service in use, mail, facsimile transmission, telephone or telex. Diskette products have a single-keystroke order information facility. The minimum charge is US$ 11.25 within USA and Canada and US$ 12.20 elsewhere.

Includes Keywords Plus.

20:205 Diskette   Institute for Scientific Information

File name	FOCUS ON: Global Change
Alternative name(s)	Global Change
Format notes	IBM, Mac, NEC
Start year	

Number of records	
Update period	Every two weeks
Price/Charges	Subscription: US$395

Notes

Includes abstracts, author keywords and Key Words Plus.

Foresight
Opthalmic Information Systems

20:206 Master record

Database type	Textual, Factual
Number of journals	
Sources	
Start year	1986
Language	English
Coverage	International
Number of records	
Update size	–
Update period	Quarterly

Keywords

Ophthalmology

Description

Contains information written and edited by leading opthalmologists on the diagnosis and treatment of eye diseases. Covers problems of the anterior segment, external and inflammatory diseases, glaucoma, intra-ocular tumours, medical and surgical retina, and neuro- and paediatric opthalmology. Also provides electronic services, including mail, conferencing, continuing medical education (CME) courses, and access to other Source databases.

Monthly subscription of $20 to Opthalmic Information Systems and monthly minimum of $10 to The Source required.

20:207 Online   SOURCE, The

File name	
Start year	1986
Number of records	
Update period	Quarterly

Notes

Available as a Private Network Service database only.

FTSS
Canadian Centre for Occupational Health and Safety (CCOHS)

20:208 Master record

Alternative name(s)	MSDS; Trade Names; Noms de Marque
Database type	Textual, Factual, Numeric
Number of journals	
Sources	Data sheets
Start year	Current information
Language	French
Coverage	Canada (primarily), International (some) and USA (some)
Number of records	72,500
Update size	–
Update period	Periodically, as new data become available

Keywords

First Aid; Hazardous Substances; Occupational Health and Safety; Waste Management

Description

Contains over 72,500 Material Safety Data Sheets for chemical trade name products used in the workplace. Each entry includes trade names, manufacturer and distributor names, addresses and phone numbers, description and physical properties, reactivity, health hazards, storage and handling, spill and leak procedures, cleanup and disposal, personal protection and first aid.

English-language equivalent data base is MSDS (Material Safety Data Sheets)

20:209 Online — CCINFOline

File name	
Alternative name(s)	MSDS; Trade Names; Noms de Marque
Start year	Current information
Number of records	72,500
Update period	Periodically, as new data become available

This database can also be found on:
CCINFOdisc Series A1 – MSDS

Grants Database
Oryx Press
DIALOG

20:210 Master record

Database type	Directory, Reference
Number of journals	
Sources	
Start year	Current information
Language	English
Coverage	International
Number of records	8,900
Update size	—
Update period	Monthly

Keywords

Grants

Description

Contains listings of c.9,000 available academic grants offered by federal, state and local governments; commercial organisations; associations; and private foundations. All grants included in the database carry application deadlines up to six months ahead. Each record contains grant programme description, requirements, restrictions, full name, address, and telephone number when available for each contact person and sponsoring organisation, funding amounts, and deadline and renewal information. Subject areas encompass over 90 academic disciplines and topics including: the arts, education, health, humanities, physical and life sciences, building grants, grants for women only, study abroad, writing, and more. Emphasis is in the area of medicine and health.

Information is compiled by the editorial staff of the Oryx Press. Corresponds to the annual printed *Directory of Research Grants, Directory of Biomedical and Health Care Grants, Directory of Grants in the Humanities,* and *Directory of Grants in the Physical Sciences.*

20:211 Online — DIALOG

File name	File 85
Start year	Current information
Number of records	8,900
Update period	Monthly

Price/Charges	Subscription: US$72.00
	Online print: US$0.50
	Offline print: US$0.50

20:212 CD-ROM — DIALOG

File name	File 85
Format notes	Mac, IBM
Software	DIALOG OnDisc Manager
Start year	Current information
Number of records	8,900
Update period	Quarterly
Price/Charges	Subscription: US$850
	Connect time: US$72.00
	Online print: US$0.50
	Offline print: US$0.50

Hälso- och sjukvårdens ansvarsnämnd
Hälso- och sjukvårdens ansvarsnämnd (Swedish Medical Responsibility Board)

20:213 Master record

Alternative name(s)	Hälso- och sjukvårdens ansvarsnämnds publicerade beslut; HSAN; Swedish Medical Responsibility Board
Database type	Textual
Number of journals	
Sources	
Start year	1986
Language	Swedish
Coverage	Sweden
Number of records	304
Update size	—
Update period	Irregular

Description

Contains summaries of decisions from the Swedish Medical Responsibility Board.

Corresponds to: *Ansvarsnämndens Referatsamling/ Aarsbok*

20:214 Online — DAFA Data AB

File name	Rättsbanken
Alternative name(s)	Hälso- och sjukvårdens ansvarsnämnds publicerade beslut; HSAN; Swedish Medical Responsibility Board
Start year	1986
Number of records	304
Update period	Irregular

Notes

DAFA require payment of an initiation fee of approximately $500.

Hazardline
Occupational Health Services Inc (OHS)

20:215 Master record

Database type	Factual
Number of journals	
Sources	Standards and Journals
Start year	Current information
Language	English
Coverage	USA
Number of records	78,000+
Update size	—
Update period	Daily

Keywords

Chemical Substances; First Aid; Hazardous Chemicals; Hazardous Substances; Occupational Health and Safety; Waste Management

Description

Contains regulatory, health, and precautionary data on 3,000 hazardous chemicals. Includes chemical name; chemical formula; synonyms, including brand and trade names; Chemical Abstracts Service (CAS) Registry Number; identification number from the Registry of Toxic Effects of Chemical Substances (see RTECS); United States Department of Transportation (DOT) UN/PLACARD number; United States Environmental Protection Agency (EPA) hazardous waste number; a physical description of the substance; chemical and physical properties; incompatibility with other chemical substances; standards and recommendations for personal protective clothing and goggles (including information from the American Conference of Governmental Industrial Hygienists (ACGIH) Guidelines for the Selection of Chemical Protective Clothing, Vol. 1); emergency procedures in the event of personal contact; respirator requirements; route of entry of the substance into the body; permissable exposure levels, including carcinogenic, mutagenic, and teratogenic data, CERCLA Hazard Ratings, EPA reportable quantities, Food and Drug Administration (FDA) acceptable daily intake and food tolerances; level of danger to life or health (NIOSH-OSHA Immediately Dangerous to Life or Health (IDLH) value or RTECS toxicity value); symptoms upon exposure; first aid, including antidotes and post-antidote regimens; relevant federal regulations and abstracts of state laws on hazardous materials, transportation, storage, recycling, treatment, radioactive materials, and state right-to-know laws; medical examinations and specific tests required by the Occupational Safety and Health Administration (OSHA); fire-fighting recommendations from the Bureau of Explosives; and guidelines and procedures for dealing with hazardous leaks, spills, and waste disposal. Users can retrieve data on specific chemical substances by searching on various criteria, including chemical name, synonym, keyword, chemical formula, CAS Registry Number, RTECS number, DOT UN/PLACARD number, or symptoms of exposure. Of use to industrial managers, occupational health specialists, safety managers, researchers and technical librarians.

Sources of data include OSHA and EPA standards and regulations, National Institute of Occupational Safety and Health (NIOSH) criteria documents, important and relevant court decisions, and selected relevant standards and guidelines from such other organizations as the American National Standards Institute.

20:216 Online　　　　BRS, BRS/Colleague

File name	HZBD
Start year	Current information
Number of records	78,000+
Update period	Monthly
Price/Charges	Connect time: US$122.00/132.00
	Online print: US$0.35/0.43
	Offline print: US$0.43

20:217 Online　　　CompuServe Information Service

File name	IQUEST File 1237
Start year	Current information
Number of records	78,000+
Update period	Monthly

Price/Charges	Subscription: US$8.95 per month
	Database entry fee: US$9/search; some databases carry a surcharge ($2–75)
	Online print: US$10 references free; then $9 per ten; abstracts $3 each

Downloading is allowed

Notes

Accessed via IQUEST or IQMEDICAL, this database is offered by a BRS gateway. IQUEST can either search across all databases, a database of the user's choice or selected multiple databases.

20:218 Online　　Executive Telecom System International, Human Resource Information Network (ETSI/HRIN)

File name	
Start year	Current information
Number of records	78,000+
Update period	Daily

Notes

Annual subscription to ETSI/HRIN required.

20:219 Online　　Occupational Health Services Inc (OHS)

File name	
Start year	Current information
Number of records	78,000+
Update period	Daily

Hazardtext

Micromedex Inc

20:220 Master record

Database type	Factual, Directory, Textual, Bibliographic
Number of journals	
Sources	
Start year	
Language	English
Coverage	USA (primarily) and International (some)
Number of records	
Update size	–
Update period	Quarterly

Keywords

Emergency Medicine; Hazardous Chemicals; Occupational Health and Safety

Description

Combines a summary of chemical toxicity, an overview of emergency medical treatment and reviews of the range and physicochemical parameters with a review of initial hazard response to incidents (fires, spills, leaks) from hazardous materials.

This database can be found on:
TOMES
TOMES Plus

Health and Disease

Infotouch

20:222 Master record

Database type	Multimedia, Encyclopedia
Number of journals	
Sources	

Start year	
Language	Dutch, English, French and German
Coverage	International
Number of records	
Update size	–
Update period	Not updated

Description

A medical encyclopedia including anatomy, physiology, diseases and methods of treatment.

20:223 CDTV   Infotouch

File name	Health & Disease
Format notes	Commodore
Start year	
Number of records	
Update period	Not updated
Price	US$80

Health Education

Centers for Disease Control, Center for Chronic Disease Prevention and Health Promotion

20:224 Master record

Database type	Bibliographic
Number of journals	
Sources	Journals, Monographs, Conference proceedings, Reports and Grey literature
Start year	1977
Language	English
Coverage	USA (primarily) and International (some)
Number of records	
Update size	–
Update period	Quarterly

Description

Contains citations, with abstracts, to curricular materials, reports, monographs, journal articles, conference proceedings, unpublished documents, and programme descriptions on health education and health promotion methods and activities. Covers such topics as patient education, school and community health education, occupational health education, risk reduction education, professional training, and research and evaluation. Corresponds to *Current Awareness in Health Education*.

Language is primarily English, with some coverage of materials in other languages.

This database can be found on:
Combined Health Information Database
CDP file
Health Education Bibliography

Health for All – Primary Care and Consumer Information

CD Resources

20:226 Master record

Database type	Factual, Textual
Number of journals	
Sources	

Start year	
Language	English
Coverage	International
Number of records	
Update size	–
Update period	Annually

Description

International and country-based full text documents, case studies, overviews and training materials from over 140 publications from the following sources – WHO, Pan American Health Organization, US Agency for International Development, US Centers for Disease Control, International Planned Parenthood Federation, and World Federation of Public Health Organizations. Coverage includes: Legislation; Health planning and management; Primary health care; Environmental and occupational health; Maternal and child care, etc.

20:227 CD-ROM   CD Resources

File name	Health for All – Primary Care and Consumer Information
Format notes	IBM
Software	Proprietary
Start year	
Number of records	
Update period	Annually
Price/Charges	Subscription: US$895

Notes

Aids Information and Education is included free of charge.

Health Indicators in AFRO

World Health Organisation – Regional Office for Africa

20:228 Master record

Alternative name(s)	AFRO/PHS
Database type	Factual, Numeric
Number of journals	
Sources	
Start year	1970–1988
Language	French
Coverage	Africa
Number of records	6,615
Update size	–
Update period	Daily

Keywords

Public Health

Description

A database of information on health indicators in Africa, produced by the World Health Organization in Africa.

Available to UN system organisations, and to external users with restrictions. Available also as printout.

20:229 Diskette   World Health Organisation – Regional Office for Africa

File name	Health Indicators in AFRO
Alternative name(s)	AFRO/PHS
Format notes	IBM
Software	Proprietary
Start year	1974–1987

Number of records
Update period   Daily

Health Promotion
National Health Information Clearinghouse

20:230 Master record
Database type   Bibliographic, Textual
Number of journals
Sources   Journals, Monographs, Pamphlets
                       and A-V material
Start year   1987
Language   English
Coverage   USA (primarily) and International
                       (some)
Number of records
Update size   —
Update period   Quarterly
Index unit   Articles

Description
Contains full text and citations, with abstracts, to Department of Health and Human Service Office of Disease Prevention and Health Promotion Healthfinder Publications. Covers 1986 to date. Produced by the National Health Information Clearinghouse.

Language is primarily English, with some coverage of materials in other languages.

This database can be found on:
Combined Health Information Database
Health Education Bibliography

Heracles
Sportdoc

20:231 Master record
Database type   Bibliographic
Number of journals
Sources   Journals, Monographs, Theses,
                       Conference proceedings and Films
Start year   1973
Language   French
Coverage   France (primarily) and International
                       (some)
Number of records   30,000
Update size   5,000
Update period   Every two months

Keywords
Sport

Description
Contains references, with abstracts, to the science and techniques of physical and sporting activities. Provides scientific and practical source materials on sports, recreation, sports medicine, and physical education.

20:232 Online   Européenne de Données
File name   Hera
Start year   1973

Number of records   30,000
Update period   Monthly

Herbalist CD-ROM
Hopkins Technology

20:233 Master record
Database type   Textual, Factual
Number of journals
Sources
Start year
Language   English
Coverage
Number of records   180
Update size   —
Update period

Keywords
Alternative Medicine; Herbal Remedies

Description
The Herbalist CD-ROM covers the use of herbal medicines within a holistic perspective and includes information on basic principles of herbalism, human systems, herbal actions and their activity, and Materia Medica covering over 180 herbs. Medical and scientific citations and illustrations are included. The text is written by David L Hoffmann.

20:234 CD-ROM   Hopkins Technology
File name
Format notes   IBM
Start year
Number of records   180
Update period
Price   US$99.95

Notes
It is possible to search by herb, ailment, body area or generic topic. Software runs under DOS or Windows.

Home Clinic
Shufunotomo Co Ltd
Dorling Kindersley Publishers Ltd

20:235 Master record
Database type   Textual
Number of journals
Sources
Start year
Language   Japanese
Coverage   International
Number of records
Update size   —
Update period   Varies

Keywords
Diagnosis

Description
Links 206 symptoms to disease to help the user in diagnosis of illnesses. Contains a 'Home Clinic' section and a 'Cyclopedia of Knowledge of Illness' section. In the Home Clinic section, selecting Yes or No according to the chart, produces the diagnosis of the symptoms and the cure.

Corresponds to *How to Understand Symptoms*.

20:236 CD-ROM 8cm — Shufunotomo Co Ltd

File name	Home Clinic
Format notes	Sony, Data, Discman
Software	Electronic Book
Start year	
Number of records	
Update period	Varies
Price	Yen3,500

Hommel
Springer-Verlag

20:237 Master record

Database type	Factual
Number of journals	
Sources	
Start year	
Language	English (headings) and German
Coverage	
Number of records	1,500
Update size	—
Update period	

Keywords

Dangerous Chemicals; Toxic Substances; Industrial Health and Safety

Description

Handbook of Dangerous Goods, 1,500 substances: Technical and Physical data, reactions, environmental data and instructions concerning intervention, first aid, and medical treatment are given. The text is in German with English headings and mixed German/English phraseology for technical data.

This database can be found on:
Dangerous Goods
Dangerous Goods – Hommel, VCI, Merck Catalogue
Dangerous Goods – Hommel, VCI, Merck Catalogue, Chemdata
Dangerous Goods – Hommel, VCI, Merck Catalogue, Operation Files, BAG Toxic Substances Lists, SUVA

Human Biometrics and Biomechanics Database
Universite de Paris V

20:239 Master record

Database type	Bibliographic, Factual, Numeric
Number of journals	
Sources	Standards, Monographs, Government documents, Patents and Journals
Start year	Last 30 years
Language	French
Coverage	International
Number of records	8,800,000
Update size	—
Update period	As new data becomes available

Keywords

Anthropology; Biomechanics; Ergonomics; Physiology

Description

Contains about 8.8 million individual anthropometric measurements gathered over the last thirty years on a large number of world populations. Data cover age, sex, nationality, human body measurements and space requirements, measurements for access and motion, human body dynamics, and such physiological data as visual and auditory acuity. The database is designed to help researchers, designers, manufacturers, and ergonomists deal with problems involving morphological measurements and the variability of populations. Also has applications in the fields of anthropology, biomechanics, man-machine interfaces, human factors analysis, and human physiology. Updated as new data become available.

Annual subscription fee of 1200 French francs required.

This database can be found on:
Ergodata

Igaku Chuo Zasshi, Title Guide
Igaku Chuo Zasshi Kanko-kai

20:241 Master record

Database type	Bibliographic
Number of journals	1,800
Sources	Journals
Start year	1985
Language	Japanese, and English, some titles
Coverage	Japan
Number of records	130,000
Update size	60,000
Update period	Monthly
Index unit	Articles

Keywords

Clinical Medicine

Description

Citations to articles on clinical medicine, excluding dentistry and pharmacology, in Japanese journals.

Corresponds in part to *Igaku Chuo Zasshi*.

Covers Japanese journals only.

20:242 Online — Maruzen Company Ltd, Maruzen Scientific Information Service (MASIS) Center

File name	
Start year	1985
Number of records	130,000
Update period	Monthly

Immunization AFRO
World Health Organisation – Regional Office for Africa

20:243 Master record

Alternative name(s)	AFRO/CEIS
Database type	Numeric
Number of journals	
Sources	

Start year	1974–1987
Language	English
Coverage	Africa
Number of records	
Update size	–
Update period	Twice a year

Keywords

Immunology

Description

A database of information on immunization in Africa by the World Health Organization.

Available to UN system organisations, and to external users with restrictions. Printed products – *Information system; summary for WHO/AFRO*.

In-house indexing – country, year.

20:244 Diskette World Health Organisation – Regional Office for Africa

File name	Immunization AFRO
Alternative name(s)	AFRO/CEIS
Format notes	IBM
Software	dBASE III; Lotus 1–2–3
Start year	1974–1987
Number of records	
Update period	Twice a year

Immunization Articles
World Health Organisation – Expanded Programme on Immunization

20:245 Master record

Database type	Bibliographic
Number of journals	
Sources	Articles
Start year	1940
Language	English and French
Coverage	International
Number of records	12,000
Update size	–
Update period	Daily
Index unit	Articles

Keywords

Immunisation; Public Health

Description

A bibliographical database of articles from the EPI, the Expanded Programme on Immunization from the World Health Organization.

Available to UN system organisations; also to external users. Printed product: Listing of EPI articles by subject/author. Also available as a printout.

In-house system of keywords.

20:246 Diskette World Health Organisation – Expanded Programme on Immunization

File name	Immunization Articles
Format notes	IBM
Software	CARDBOX-PLUS
Start year	1940

Number of records	12,000
Update period	Daily

Immunization Coverage Surveys
World Health Organisation – Expanded Programme on Immunization

20:247 Master record

Database type	Numeric
Number of journals	
Sources	
Start year	1978–1984
Language	English
Coverage	International
Number of records	
Update size	–
Update period	Daily

Keywords

Immunisation; Public Health

Description

A statistical database of surveys on immunization from the Expanded Programme on Immunization (EPI) information system.

Available to UN system organisations; also to external users. Printed product: *EPI information system*. The database is also available as a printout.

In-house indexing system of file names.

20:248 Diskette World Health Organisation – Expanded Programme on Immunization

File name	Immunization Coverage Surveys
Format notes	IBM
Software	Lotus 1–2–3
Start year	1978–1984
Number of records	
Update period	Daily

Immunization Demographic Data
World Health Organisation – Expanded Programme on Immunization

20:249 Master record

Database type	Numeric
Number of journals	
Sources	
Start year	1974
Language	English
Coverage	International
Number of records	
Update size	–
Update period	Daily

Keywords

Demography; Immunisation; Public Health; Regional Studies

Description

A statistical database of demographic data on immunisation worldwide from the EPI information system.

Available to UN system organisations; also to external users. Printed product: *EPI information system*. The database is also available as a printout.

In-house indexing system of file names.

20:250 Diskette World Health Organisation – Expanded Programme on Immunization

File name	Immunization Demographic Data
Format notes	IBM
Software	Lotus 1–2-3
Start year	1974
Number of records	
Update period	Daily

Immunization Morbidity

World Health Organisation – Expanded Programme on Immunization

20:251 Master record

Database type	Numeric
Number of journals	
Sources	
Start year	Current information
Language	English
Coverage	International
Number of records	
Update size	–
Update period	Twice a year

Keywords

Immunisation; Mortality

Description

A statistical database on morbidity in immunisation from the EPI information system.

Available to UN system organisations; also to external users. Printed product: *EPI information system*. Also the database is available as a printout.

In-house indexing system of file names.

20:252 Diskette World Health Organisation – Expanded Programme on Immunization

File name	Immunization Morbidity
Format notes	IBM
Software	Lotus 1–2-3
Start year	Current information
Number of records	
Update period	Twice a year

Immunization Programme Reviews

World Health Organisation – Expanded Programme on Immunization

20:253 Master record

Database type	Factual
Number of journals	
Sources	
Start year	1978
Language	English
Coverage	International
Number of records	
Update size	–
Update period	Daily

Keywords

Immunisation; Public Health

Description

A factual database of reviews from the EPI information system.

Available to UN system organisations; alsot ot external users. Printed product: *EPI information system*.

The database is also available as a printout.

20:254 Diskette World Health Organisation – Expanded Programme on Immunization

File name	Immunization Programme Reviews
Format notes	IBM
Software	Lotus 1–2-3
Start year	1978
Number of records	
Update period	Daily

Immunoclone Database, The

Centre Europeen de Recherches Documentaires sur les Immunoclones – CERDIC

20:255 Master record

Database type	Bibliographic, Directory, Factual, Textual
Number of journals	
Sources	Conference proceedings, databases, databases (NLM), journals, laboratories, monographs, patents, producers catalogues and research reports
Start year	1986
Language	English
Coverage	International
Number of records	36,000
Update size	–
Update period	Monthly
Database aids	Coder's Manual and ICDB Vocabulary List and ICDB Format, Villeneuve-Loubet, CERDIC

Keywords

Biotechnology; Immunology; Patents

Description

The Immunoclone Database contains information on cells of immunological interest such as hybridomas, transfectomas and T-cell clones and their products and monoclonal antibodies. Descriptions provide cell information including cell types, immunogen, immunocyte donors, immortal partners and such product information as type and designation of the product and reactivities. Full bibliographical details are provided for each entry. Particular information includes production, properties and availability of immunoreactive substances. The database does not include information on polyclonal antibodies (for example, serums) and kits.

The database is partially derived from EMBASE, MEDLINE and PASCAL. Approximately 70% of records are from literature sources, 20–25% from catalogues and 5% from patents. The descriptions are taken mainly from scientific literature, pharmceutical companies and research laboratories. A reloading update is produced monthly.

20:256 Online Data-Star

File name	IMMU
Start year	1986

Number of records	25,000
Update period	Monthly
Database aids	Data-Star Biomedical Manual and Online manual (search NEWS-IMMU in NEWS)
Price/Charges	Subscription: SFr80.00 Connect time: SFr101.25 Online print: SFr1.26 – 2.52 Offline print: SFr2.17

Notes

From June 1993 Data-Star have introduced an annual fee/subscription per contract (that is, not per password) of SFr 80.00 (c.UK£ 32.00) payable every June. For North American customers billed in dollars who also use DIALOG, the DIALOG fee also covers access to Data-Star. Academic customers, 'commitment' customers and customers currently billed in dollars are exempt.

Record composition

Authors AU; Accession Number and Update Code AN; Cell Information CL; Coding Identification and Date ED; Descriptors DE; Institution IN; Literature Type AT; Notes NT; Patents PA; Product Information PN; Reactivity RE; Source SO; Short Cell Designation SD; Update (YYMM) UP; Update (YYMMDD) UD and Year YR

Descriptors are keywords taken exclusively from Excerpta Medica's *Emtree*.

20:257 Online   DIMDI

File name	HD00 Database
Start year	1992
Number of records	36,000
Update period	Monthly reloads
Database aids	User Manual ICDB-Immunoclone Database and Memocard ICDB-Immunoclone Database
Price/Charges	Connect time: UK£15.80–20.55 Online print: UK£0.79–0.97 Offline print: UK£0.39–0.46

Downloading is allowed

Notes

This file was issued as a revised form of Hybridoma in February 1991. The whole file is reloaded monthly which means that a current awareness service is not available with this database. Approximately 90% of the records contain abstracts. The unit record contains informaton on the production, the properties and the commercial availability of the immunoclones and their products.

Record composition

Author AU; Application of Product AP; Cell Type CELL; Cell Typing TY; Corporate Source CS; Controlled Term CT; Cross Reference NX; Distributor DI; Donor DO; Document Type DT; Entry Month EM; Immunogen IM; Immortal Partner IP; Last Revision Date LR; Locator LO; Name of Cell NAMEC; Name of Product NAMEP; Number of Document ND; Notes NOTE; Non-Reactivity NREAC; Patents PAT; Reactivity REAC; Source; Storage Information STOR; Transfected DNA TD and Type of Product PROD

Each document consists of four parts: Part 1 – Technical Data; Part 2 – Description and availability of cell culture; Part 3 – Description and availability of the product; Part 4 – Source of information. The basic index includes: Cell Type, Name of Cell, Immunogen, Donor, Immortal Partner, Transfected DNA, Cell Typing, Type of Product, Name of Product Reactivity,

Non- Reactivity, Application of Product, Locator, Notes and Controlled Term.

For more details of constituent databases, see:
MEDLINE
EMBASE
PASCAL

Index Nominum
Société Suisse de Pharmacie

20:259 Master record

Database type	
Number of journals	
Sources	
Start year	
Language	English
Coverage	Switzerland
Number of records	
Update size	–
Update period	
Index unit	drug

Keywords

Drugs; Pharmaceuticals; Surgery

Description

One of the databases contained on the CD-ROMs MediROM and PharmaROM in the medical and health care fields, produced for Swiss physicians and pharmacists. Also included as an option with the CD-ROM Vidal.

This database can be found on:
MediROM
PharmaROM

Index to Scientific and Technical Proceedings
Institute for Scientific Information

20:260 Master record

Alternative name(s)	ISTP; ISTP&B; ISTP Search
Database type	Bibliographic
Number of journals	
Sources	Conference proceedings, journals, monographs and reports
Start year	1978
Language	English
Coverage	International
Number of records	2,300,000
Update size	96,000
Update period	Monthly
Index unit	Articles, Conference papers, discussions, Editorials, letters, meeting abstracts, notes, reviews and proceedings papers
Database aids	List of the Section Codes with the corresponding Section Headings, List of the Unified Variant Spellings and Excerpt from the Variant Spelling Dictionary

Keywords

Clinical Medicine

Description

ISTB database indexes unabstracted conference proceedings literature. Subjects covered include: agriculture and agricultural sciences; applied sciences; biology; chemical sciences; clinical medicine; engineering; environmental sciences; life sciences; mathematics; physical sciences; technology; and other scientific and technical areas.

The database corresponds to the printed Index to Scientific and Technical Proceedings. ISTP contains only published proceedings. The form of the publication is unimportant so that books by publishers or societies as well as reports, sets of preprints (if no other form of publication is available) and journals can be used. ISTP only contains those publications and proceedings whose main portion has been published for the first time and also includes complete papers and not just abstracts. If however complete individual papers are presented with abstracts, the abstracts are utilised. Approximately 3,000 published worldwide conference proceedings are included annually which corresponds to about 90,000 publications. The database also encompasses approximately 1,650 books including the Annual Review Series.

The approximate percentage contribution of each individual discipline is as follows: Life Sciences 35% (including Clinical Medicine 8%); Engineering Sciences and Applied Sciences 35%; Physics and Chemistry 20% and Agriculture and Biology 10%.

All ISI databases have a linked service known as The Genuine Article which can deliver the full text of located articles by mail, facsimile transmission or courier. Orders can be placed via the host service in use, mail, facsimile transmission, telephone or telex. Diskette products have a single-keystroke order information facility. The minimum charge is US$ 11.25 within USA and Canada and US$ 12.20 elsewhere.

The indexing of the publications follows its assignment to speciic categories and there are approximately 200 broad subjects.

20:261 Online   BIDS

File name	ISTP
Alternative name(s)	ISTP; ISTP&B; ISTP Search
Start year	
Number of records	
Update period	Monthly

20:262 Online   ORBIT

File name	ISTP
Alternative name(s)	ISTP; ISTP&B; ISTP Search
Start year	1982
Number of records	1 million+
Update period	Monthly
Database aids	Quick Reference Guide (7/90) Free (single copy)
Price/Charges	Connect time: US$95.00
	Online print: US$1.30/1.75
	Offline print: US$1.30/1.75
	SDI charge: US$8.00

Notes

Electronic SDI service is now available within two hours on ORBIT. They can be downloaded and reformatted on a word processor. Results are retrieved in the low cost PRINTS file, $15 per connect hour.

20:263 Online   Institute for Scientific Information

File name	ISTP Search
Alternative name(s)	ISTP; ISTP&B; ISTP Search
Start year	1978
Number of records	2,300,000
Update period	Monthly

20:264 Tape   Institute for Scientific Information

File name	ISTP Search
Alternative name(s)	ISTP; ISTP&B; ISTP Search
Format notes	9-track, labels or unlabelled, 1600 or 6250 bpi, ASCII or EBCDIC, 90 character fixed-length, records, block size 1620 or 9000.
Start year	1978
Number of records	2,300,000
Update period	Monthly
Price/Charges	Subscription: US$10,000

Notes

Corresponds in part to the printed Index to Scientific and Technical Proceedings and to the ISTP online database. All ISI databases have a linked service known as The Genuine Article which can deliver the full text of located articles by mail, facsimile transmission or courier. Orders can be placed via the host service in use, mail, facsimile transmission, telephone or telex.

The minimum charge is US$ 11.25 within USA and Canada and US$ 12.20 elsewhere. Prices for magnetic tape: annual lease $10,000 (academic); 12,500 (corporate).

Industrial Health and Hazards Update
Merton Allen Associates

20:267 Master record

Database type	Bibliographic, Textual
Number of journals	1
Sources	Newsletter, Government documents (US), Reports and Journals
Start year	1984
Language	English
Coverage	USA (primarily) and International (some)
Number of records	—
Update size	—
Update period	Monthly
Index unit	Articles

Keywords

Explosion; Fire; Hazardous Waste; Legislation; Industrial Health and Safety; Occupational Health and Safety; Product Liability; Standards

Description

Contains the full text of Industrial Health and Hazards Update, a newsletter providing abstracts of reports and brief news items on legal and technical aspects of industrial safety. Covers regulations and standards, current litigation, product liability, industry surveys, hazard evaluations for particular workplaces and toxicology research, occupational safety, health, illness, hazards and disease, fire and explosion, mitigation and control of hazardous situations, hazardous wastes, recycling and treatment, environmental emissions and more related topics. Sources include government reports, journals and news items.

Corresponds to the monthly Industrial Health and

Hazards Update newsletter. Reprints of most reviewed reports are available at nominal cost. DIALOG and Data-Star are available on PTS Newsletter Database, supplied by Predicasts.

20:268 Online — Executive Telecom System International, Human Resource Information Network (ETSI/HRIN)

File name
Start year   1984
Number of records
Update period   Daily

Notes

Annual subscription to ETSI/HRIN required.

20:269 Online — NewsNet Inc

File name
Start year   1984
Number of records
Update period   Daily

Notes

Monthly subscription to NewsNet required.

This database can also be found on:
PTS Newsletter Database

Infectious Diseases – Personal MEDLINE

Information providers: National Library of Medicine

20:273 Master record

CD-ROM — Macmillan New Media

Database type   Bibliographic
Number of journals
Sources
Start year   Most recent five years.
Language
Coverage
Number of records   270,000
Update size   –
Update period   Annually/Quarterly

Keywords

Infectious Diseases; Tropical Medicine

Description

References and abstracts on bacterial, fungal, viral and parasitic infections across a variety of specialities, including tropical medicine. Covers symptoms, general pathology, treatment, procedures and techniques, epidemiology and public health issues, bacterial and fungal diseases, viral diseases, parasitic diseases, animal diseases, neoplasms, stomatognathic diseases, otorhinlaryngologic diseases, ocular diseases, hemic and lymphatic diseases, immunologic diseases, neonatal diseases and abnormalities, dermatologic diseases, urologic and genital diseases, nutritional and metabolic disorders, and diseases of the musculoskeletal, digestive, respiratory, endocrine, cardiovascular, and nervous systems, and their causative organisms.

A subset of MEDLINE, plus all abstracts from major medical journals on infectious diseases.

Notes

Product no longer available as of December 1992.
For more details of constituent databases, see:
MEDLINE

Infochim
Canadian Centre for Occupational Health and Safety (CCOHS)

20:275 Master record

Alternative name(s)   Cheminfo
Database type   Factual, Textual, Numeric
Number of journals
Sources   Data sheets, Suppliers, Journals, Monographs and Government documents
Start year   Current information
Language   French
Coverage   Canada (primarily), International (some) and USA (some)
Number of records
Update size   –
Update period   Varies

Keywords

First Aid; Occupational Health and Safety

Description

Contains the French-language equivalent of Cheminfo database, produced by the CCOHS. Covers descriptive, health, and precautionary data on pure chemicals, natural substances, and chemical mixtures resulting from or used in industrial processes. For each chemical, provides substance identification, including name, synonyms, Chemical Abstracts Service (CAS) Registry Number, and molecular and structural formula, as well as information about its uses and occurrences, physical properties, appearance, reactivity, warning properties (for example, odours, irritation), animal toxicity data, proposed Workplace Hazardous Materials Information System (WHMIS) classification, fire and explosion hazards, and human health effects from short-term acute or chronic exposure. Also provides information on occupational control measures, including airborne exposure limits, ventilation, personnel protective equipment and clothing, respiratory protection guidelines, and recommendations on storage and handling, spill and leak procedures, cleanup, disposal, and emergency first aid.

Sources include Material Safety Data Sheets from chemical manufacturers. English-language equivalent is Cheminfo.

20:276 Online — CCINFOline

File name   Infochim
Alternative name(s)   Cheminfo
Start year   Current information
Number of records
Update period   Varies
This database can also be found on:
CCINFOdisc Series A1 – MSDS
CCINFOdisc Series A2 – CHEM Data

INFOGRIPPE
VNII Gruppa MS SSSR

20:277 Master record

Database type   Bibliographic
Number of journals
Sources

Start year	1973
Language	English
Coverage	
Number of records	1,100
Update size	—
Update period	

Keywords

Patents

Description

Database on medical patents.

20:278 Diskette   VNII Gruppa MS SSSR

File name	
Start year	1973
Number of records	1,100
Update period	

Information per le Industrie
Assolombarda

20:279 Master record

Database type	Bibliographic
Number of journals	
Sources	Journals
Start year	1974
Language	Italian
Coverage	Italy
Number of records	8,000
Update size	—
Update period	Annually
Index unit	Articles

Keywords

Pollution; Occupational Diseases; Occupational Health and Safety

Description

Citations, with abstracts, to articles on industrial accident prevention, occupational diseases and industrial pollution in Italy.

Corresponds to *Informazioni per le Industrie*.

20:280 Online   SIRIO

File name	
Start year	1974
Number of records	8,000
Update period	Annually

INFOTOX
Commission de la Santé et de la Securité du Travail (CSST)
Toxicological Index

20:281 Master record

Database type	Textual, Factual
Number of journals	
Sources	Data sheets
Start year	Current Information
Language	French
Coverage	Canada (Quebec)
Number of records	6,000
Update size	2,000
Update period	Quarterly

Keywords

Hazardous Chemicals; Legislation; First Aid; Chemicals; Biological Hazards; Occupational Health and Safety

Description

Contains safety data sheets for about 6,000 pure and compound chemical and biological products used in industry and commercial applications in Quebec, giving information on physico-chemical and toxicological properties, product regulations, hazard prevention and first aid.

Corresponds to *Repertoire Toxicologique*.

20:282 Online   Commission de la Santé et de la Securité du Travail (CSST)

File name	
Start year	Current Information
Number of records	6,000
Update period	Quarterly

Ingenieur-Edition
Fachinformationszentrum Technik (FIZ Technik)

20:283 Master record

Database type	Bibliographic
Number of journals	
Sources	
Start year	1989
Language	German
Coverage	Germany
Number of records	
Update size	—
Update period	Three times per year

Keywords

Biomedicine; Textiles; Materials; Information Technology; Mechanical Engineering; Textile Engineering; Electrical Engineering

Description

Targetted at the engineering departments of universities, this product brings together seven databases on mechanical engineering, materials, textile engineering, electrical engineering and electronics, information technology, biomedicine and management. Bibliographic references date back three years.

20:284 CD-ROM   Fachinformationszentrum Technik (FIZ Technik)

File name	Ingenieur-Edition
Format notes	IBM
Start year	1989
Number of records	
Update period	Three times per year
Price/Charges	Subscription: DM1,850 – 4,000

INIS
International Atomic Energy Agency (IAEA, INIS Section)

20:285 Master record

Alternative name(s)	International Nuclear Information System
Database type	Bibliographic, Textual
Number of journals	10,000
Sources	Grey literature, journals, theses, patents, journals, conference proceedings, dissertations, reports and monographs
Start year	1970
Language	English, with some titles and abstracts also in original languages
Coverage	International

Number of records	1,515,800
Update size	108,000
Update period	Twice per month
Index unit	Conference papers, articles and reports

Keywords

Applied Science; Physics; Nuclear Physics; Nuclear Technology

Description

Compiled by contributions from over ninety national and international centres, INIS gives worldwide coverage, with long and detailed abstracts, of literature on peaceful uses of nuclear science and technology, non-military applications and related areas, with an emphasis on neutron and nuclear physics; atomic and molecular physics; general physics; high energy physics; chemistry, materials and earth sciences; external radiation biology; radioisotope effects and kinetics; applied life sciences; health and safety; radiation protection and environment; radiology and nuclear medicine; isotopes, radiation sources and radiation applications; engineering; fission reactors; instrumentation; waste management; economics and sociology; nuclear law; nuclear documentation; nuclear safeguards and inspection; mathematical methods and computer codes; and legal aspects. References are contributed by 75 national centres and fourteen international organisations. Journal articles, books, conference proceedings, patents, theses, reports and unconventional literature not available elsewhere are included.

Equivalent to the printed abstract journal *INIS ATOMINDEX* (24 issues a year). The database references over 10,000 journal sources, of which about 5,000 are scanned on a regular basis. While the online version is not available on a US-based host, but is available in Canada, the information is included in the DOE ENERGY files on both DIALOG and STN. The INIS (International Nuclear Information System) database is produced by the International Atomic Energy Agency in collaboration with 79 Member States and fourteen Member Organisations. Each member is represented by an INIS Liaison Officer who is responsible for provision to the system. Conditions for access – approval of Liaison Office in user's country may be required. Contact IAEA for complete list of participating countries and addresses of Liaison Offices or consult current issue of *INIS ATOMINDEX*. The database is also available on microfiche.

Indexing/Classification tools are from the INIS Reference Series including: INIS Manual for Indexing; INIS Subject Categories and Scope Description; INIS Thesaurus.

20:286 Online — Australian Nuclear Science & Technology Organization (ANSTO-INIS)

File name	INIS
Alternative name(s)	International Nuclear Information System
Start year	1970
Number of records	1,515,800
Update period	Twice per month

20:287 Online — BELINDIS

File name	File 28
Alternative name(s)	International Nuclear Information System
Start year	1970
Number of records	1,515,800
Update period	Twice per month

20:288 Online — CISTI, Canadian Online Enquiry Service CAN/OLE

File name	INIS
Alternative name(s)	International Nuclear Information System
Start year	1970
Number of records	1,515,800
Update period	Twice per month
Price/Charges	Connect time: US$40.00
	Online print: US$0.20
	Offline print: US$0.20

Notes

An SDI service is available on CAN/SDI from the AECL Centre, twelve issues annually; also CAN/DOC – major supplier is OON, alternate suppliers, OCKA, OGU, OONTR, URGENT. Conditions for use of CAN/OLE: pay as you go. There are no initiation fees and no minimum charge. Users are charged only for the time spent on the computer, with online cost summaries and a monthly invoice. Abstracts are available.

20:289 Online — ESA-IRS

File name	File 28
Alternative name(s)	International Nuclear Information System
Start year	1976
Number of records	1,313,000 (October 1991)
Update period	Every two weeks
Database aids	Thesaurus IAEA-INIS-13 (rev. 23), Classification scheme IAEA-INIS-3 (rev.6), Serials list IAEA-INIS-11 (rev.12) and Applications list IAEA-INIS-6 (rev. 16)
Price/Charges	Connect time: UK£42.17
	Offline print: UK£0.19
	SDI charge: UK£2.11

Notes

Any element of the references can be interrogated using the STAIRS Retrieval Language. There is an SDI service. Online tutorials are available.

From 1993 ESA-IRS are charging an annual fee of 100 Accounting Units (c.UK£ 70.29) to all users. This is equivalent to the fee for full documentation and will not be charged to customers already paying for documentation.

20:290 Online — ICSTI

File name	INIS
Alternative name(s)	International Nuclear Information System
Start year	1970
Number of records	1,515,800
Update period	Twice per month

20:291 Online — International Atomic Energy Agency (IAEA)

File name	INIS
Alternative name(s)	International Nuclear Information System
Start year	1970
Number of records	1,515,800
Update period	Twice per month

20:292 Online — STN

File name	INIS
Alternative name(s)	International Nuclear Information System
Start year	1970

Number of records 1,623,876
Update period Twice a month
Price/Charges Connect time: DM160.00
Online print: DM1.00
Offline print: DM1.00
SDI charge: DM10.95

Notes
INIS is available in Canada, but not in the USA.

Bibliographic information, abstracts, indexing terms and element terms are searchable.

20:293 CD-ROM   SilverPlatter

File name INIS
Alternative name(s) International Nuclear Information System
Format notes IBM
Software SPIRS
Start year 1976
Number of records 1.2m
Update period Quarterly
Price/Charges Subscription: UK£625 – 2,460

Notes
The database provides the deepest and broadest coverage of nuclear power-related literature. Chuck Huber (*CD-ROM Professional* 5(6) p129) demonstrated the breadth of INIS's coverage comparing it with Compendex Plus, INSPEC and Enviro/Energyline Abstracts Plus where it won hands down in searches on both 'Chernobyl' and 'muon catalyzed fusion'. However, he pointed out that potential buyers should realise that INIS's very breadth of coverage could mean some of the material will be hard to obtain (Over 10,000 records were annotated on his review disc as being unavailable through INIS). 'There is no doubt that the INIS CD-ROM, especially at its relatively moderate price for a large technical database, should be strongly considered by libraries supporting nuclear energy and engineering programs.'
The complete database is published on five CD-ROMs. The current disc, by annual subscription, covers 1989 to date with archival discs covering 1976 to 1988. Requires a signed subscription and licence agreement. A fifty per cent discount is available to developing countries. One time purchase of the archival set costs UK£ 1,250 for single users and £1,875 for 2–8 networked users; annual subscription for the current disc costs £625 for single users and £938 for 2–8 networked users; subscription for the current and archival disc together costs £1,640 for single users and £2,460 for 2–8 networked users.

20:294 Tape   International Atomic Energy Agency (IAEA)

File name INIS
Alternative name(s) International Nuclear Information System
Format notes IBM
Software STAIRS
Start year 1970
Number of records 1,515,800
Update period Twice per month

20:295 Database subset
Online   ESA-IRS

File name File 26 – Training INIS
Alternative name(s) International Nuclear Information System
Start year Fixed set

Number of records 6,037
Update period Not updated

Notes
This is a training file of the INIS Database, File 28. Services such as offline printing are not available.

INRS-Bibliographique
Institut National de Recherche et de Securité, Service de Documentation

20:296 Master record

Database type Bibliographic, Textual
Number of journals
Sources
Start year 1981
Language French
Coverage International
Number of records 16,000
Update size 3,000
Update period Monthly

Keywords
Ergonomics; Explosion; Fire; Industrial Medicine; Noise Pollution; Occupational Health and Safety; Working Conditions

Description
A bibliographic database containing citations, with abstracts, to the international literature on every aspect of professional job risk prevention and the improvement of working conditions, hygiene and safety at work, including chemical, physical, mechanical and noise risks, explosion and fire hazards, protection materials and techniques, job-related diseases and industrial medicine and ergonomics.

20:297 Online   Européenne de Données

File name INRS
Start year 1982
Number of records 21,500
Update period Monthly

20:298 Online   G.CAM Serveur

File name
Start year 1981
Number of records 16,000
Update period Monthly

This database can also be found on:
CCINFOdisc Series B2 – InterData

Insurance Abstracts
University Microfilms International

20:299 Master record

Database type Bibliographic
Number of journals 120
Sources Journals
Start year 1979–1984
Language English
Coverage USA and Canada
Number of records 68,912
Update size —
Update period Closed File
Index unit Articles

Keywords
Insurance; Risk Management; Employee Benefits; Health Care Costs; Occupational Health and Safety; Pensions; Taxation

Description

Citations, with brief abstracts, to articles from journals and magazines in insurance and risk management. Topics include accident, health, automobile, fire, property and life insurance, employee benefit plans, pensions, workers' compensation, risk management, taxation and medical costs.

Corresponds to *Life Insurance Index* (1979–1984) and *Property and Liability Insurance Index* (1980–1981).

Indexed with a controlled vocabulary

20:300 Online   DIALOG

File name	File 168
Start year	1979 – 1984
Number of records	68,912
Update period	Closed File
Price/Charges	Connect time: US$54.00
	Online print: US$0.15
	Offline print: US$0.15

Interacciones con Analisis Clinicos

Consejo General de Colegios Oficiales de Farmaceuticos de España

20:301 Master record

Database type	Factual, Textual
Number of journals	
Sources	Databases, Journals and Monographs
Start year	Current Information
Language	Spanish
Coverage	Spain
Number of records	200
Update size	–
Update period	Periodically, as new data become available

Keywords

Drugs; Haematology; Pharmaceuticals; Urology

Description

Descriptions of the effects of about 200 drugs or their active ingredients on chemicals in the human body, as determined by blood and urine tests for such substances as bilirubin, calcium, cholesterol, corticosteroids, glucose, lactic acid, magnesium, potassium, prolactin, proteins, triglycerides, urea and uric acid.

20:302 Online   Consejo General de Colegios Oficiales de Farmaceuticos de España

File name	
Start year	Current Information
Number of records	200
Update period	Periodically, as new data become available

Interactions de la Société Suisse de Pharmacie

Société Suisse de Pharmacie

20:303 Master record

Database type	
Number of journals	
Sources	

Start year	
Language	French
Coverage	Switzerland
Number of records	
Update size	–
Update period	
Index unit	drug

Keywords

Drugs; Pharmaceuticals; Surgery

Description

One of the databases on both PharmaROM and MediROM.

This database can be found on:
MediROM
PharmaROM

Interactions of the Medical Letter

20:305 Master record

Alternative name(s)	Medical Letter's Interactions
Database type	
Number of journals	
Sources	
Start year	
Language	English
Coverage	Switzerland
Number of records	
Update size	–
Update period	

Keywords

Drugs; Pharmaceuticals; Surgery

Description

This database in the medical and pharmaceutical field forms part of the MediROM and PharmaROM CD-ROMs, originally intended for Swiss pharmacists.

This database can also be found on:
MediROM
PharmaROM

Internal Medicine '92

Macmillan New Media

20:307 Master record

Database type	Textual, Factual
Number of journals	
Sources	Journals
Start year	1992 (January – December)
Language	English
Coverage	International
Number of records	
Update size	–
Update period	Quarterly

Keywords

Internal Medicine

Description

Contains the full text of *The New England Journal of Medicine; Journal of the American Medical Association; The Lancet; British Medical Journal;* and *Annals of Internal Medicine.*

20:308 CD-ROM   Macmillan New Media

File name	Internal Medicine '92
Format notes	IBM
Software	BRS/Search

Start year	1992 (January – December)
Number of records	
Update period	Quarterly
Price	UK£280 – 420

Notes

One time purchase price for individuals £280; and for institutions is £420.

IRE-ITTD
International Research and Evaluation (IRE)

20:309 Master record

Alternative name(s)	International Research and Evaluation-Information and Technology Transfer Database
Database type	Bibliographic
Number of journals	
Sources	Annual reports, Bibliographies, Conference papers, Company filings, Dissertations, Essays, Evaluation studies, Data sheets, Feasibility studies, Handbooks, Journals, Laws/regulations, Manuals, Newsletters, Patents, Research reports, Speeches, Standards, Statistical compilations, Syllabi, Taxonomies, Technical reports, Theses, Monographs and Databases
Start year	1892
Language	English
Coverage	International
Number of records	3,000,000
Update size	400,000
Update period	Every two weeks

Keywords

Law Enforcement; Waste Management; Fibre Optics; Lasers; Earth Sciences; Construction; Civil Engineering; Patents; Standards; Criminal Justice

Description

Citations, some with abstracts, to materials across a wide subject spectrum, including energy, law enforcement, justice, waste management, fibre optics, lasers, transportation, medicine, health, earth sciences, construction, civil engineering and agriculture.

Corresponds in part to Energy Information Database, Law Enforcement and Criminal Justice Information Database and Waste Management and Resource Recovery.

20:310 Online — International Research and Evaluation (IRE)

File name	
Start year	1892
Number of records	3,000,000
Update period	Every two weeks

IRIS
Merck Sharp & Dôhme/Chibret Bureau van Dijk

20:311 Master record

Database type	Bibliographic
Number of journals	
Sources	

Start year	
Language	French (search keywords and menus), English (search keywords and menus) and Italian (search menus)
Coverage	International
Number of records	120,000
Update size	–
Update period	Quarterly

Keywords

Ophthalmology

Description

Contains about 120,000 bibliographical references on ophthalmology. The references are selected and processed by a team of the internal Centre de Documentation of MSD/Chibret in Clermont-Ferrand.

Not publicly available.

The references can be accessed by keywords taken from a bilingual (French/English) thesaurus, made up of 1,600 terms. Apart from the subject, access is possible by the words of the title, words of the abstract and author's name. Access menus are in French, English and Italian.

20:312 CD-ROM — Chibret International Documentation Centre

File name	IRIS
Format notes	IBM
Software	Proprietary
Start year	
Number of records	120,000
Update period	Quarterly

JICMARS
Joint Industry Committee of Medical Advertisers for Readership Surveys
Joint Industry Committee for National Readership Surveys

20:313 Master record

Database type	Factual
Number of journals	
Sources	Market research surveys
Start year	1977
Language	English
Coverage	UK
Number of records	1,000
Update size	–
Update period	Quarterly

Keywords

Marketing

Description

Results of market research surveys providing data on general practitioner readership of medical publications in the UK.

National Medical Readership Survey is published quarterly and sent to all subscribers

20:314 Online — IMS

File name	JICMARS
Start year	1977
Number of records	1,000
Update period	Quarterly

20:315 Online TELMAR (UK)

File name	JICMARS
Start year	1977
Number of records	1,000
Update period	Quarterly

Journal of Trauma: 1985–1989
CMC ReSearch

20:316 Master record

Database type	Factual
Number of journals	
Sources	
Start year	
Language	
Coverage	
Number of records	
Update size	–
Update period	Annually

Description

Contains five years of the full text, tables & images from Williams & Wilkins *Journal of Trauma*. The information focuses on traumatic injury and emphasizes clinical applications, techniques, and new developments in care. Covers 1985 – 1989.

20:317 CD-ROM CMC ReSearch

File name	Journal of Trauma: 1985–1989
Format notes	IBM
Software	DiscPassage
Start year	
Number of records	
Update period	Annually
Price	UK£265

Kidney and Urologic Diseases
National Kidney and Urologic Diseases Information Clearinghouse

20:318 Master record

Database type	Bibliographic
Number of journals	
Sources	Journals, Monographs, Pamphlets and A-V material
Start year	1987
Language	English
Coverage	USA (primarily) and International (some)
Number of records	
Update size	–
Update period	Quarterly

Description

Contains citations, with abstracts, to journal articles, brochures, books, documents, and audiovisual materials relating to kidney and urologic diseases.

Language is primarily English, with some coverage of materials in other languages.

This database can be found on:
Combined Health Information Database

Kosmet
International Federation of the Societies of Cosmetics Chemists (IFSCC)

20:320 Master record

Database type	Bibliographic
Number of journals	
Sources	

Start year	1968
Language	German and English
Coverage	International
Number of records	4,000
Update size	1,200
Update period	

Keywords

Dermatology; Physics; Applied Science

Description

Contains citations, with some abstracts, on cosmetic and perfume science and technology, specifically dealing with raw materials, manufacture, analysis, control and use. KOSMET covers articles from periodicals, congresses and seminars on all matters related to cosmetics and perfumes, in particular the scientific, technical and biomedical areas. It covers different aspects of product development, the knowledge of healthy skin and its adnexa (hair, nails, teeth, glands), the trading of perfumes and cosmetics, the research and development of raw materials, active ingredients, formulations, manufacture, analysis, safety, physico-chemical properties, biological properties, stability, packaging and clinical studies.

20:321 Online Data-Star

File name	KOSM
Start year	January 1985 periodicals and meetings; 1968 for IFSCC Congresses
Number of records	6,152
Update period	Monthly
Database aids	Data-Star Biomedical Manual, Berne, Data-Star 1989 and Online Manual (search NEWS-KOSM in NEWS)
Price/Charges	Subscription: UK£32.00 Connect time: UK£51.60 Online print: UK£0.50 Offline print: UK£0.60 SDI charge: UK£4.32

Notes

From June 1993 Data-Star have introduced an annual fee/subscription per contract (that is, not per password) of SFr 80.00 (c.UK£ 32.00) payable every June. For North American customers billed in dollars who also use DIALOG, the DIALOG fee also covers access to Data-Star. Academic customers, 'commitment' customers and customers currently billed in dollars are exempt.

Lab-Link II
Mallinckrodt Inc, Science Products Division

20:322 Master record

Database type	Textual
Number of journals	
Sources	Data sheets
Start year	Current information
Language	English
Coverage	USA
Number of records	1,400
Update size	–
Update period	Four times per year

Keywords
Hazardous Chemicals; Occupational Health and Safety; Laboratories; Manufacturing; First Aid; Fire; Explosion

Description
Contains Material Safety Data Sheets for over 1,400 chemical substances used in laboratories in the electronics and other industries. Each MSDS provides the following information: product identification information (chemical name, CAS Registry number, synonyms, molecular weight, chemical formula and hazardous ingredients), label information (precautionary measures and first aid guidelines), US Department of Transport Hazard Classification, physical properties (appearance, solubility, boiling and melting points, specific gravity, vapour density and pressure, evaporation point), fire and explosion capacity and extinguishing media, toxicity data and occupational control measures (airborne exposure limits, ventilation, need for personal respirators, skin and eye contact protection and special storage requirements).

20:323 Online — Chemical Information Systems Inc (CIS)

File name	
Start year	Current information
Number of records	1,400
Update period	Four times per year

Notes
Annual subscription of $300 to CIS required.

20:324 Online — Mallinckrodt Inc, Science Products Division

File name	
Start year	Current information
Number of records	1,400
Update period	Four times per year

Lasion CD-Derma General Dermatology
Lasion Europe NV

20:325 Master record

Database type	Textual, Image
Number of journals	
Sources	
Start year	
Language	Dutch, French and English
Coverage	
Number of records	
Update size	—
Update period	Varies

Keywords
Dermatology

Description
Provides high-quality images to visualise skin pathologies, with sophisticated browsing methods to assist in differential diagnosis and the retrieval of other information.

20:326 CD-ROM — Lasion Europe NV

File name	Lasion CD-Derma General Dermatology
Format notes	IBM
Start year	

Number of records	
Update period	Varies

Leucocyte Typing Database III
Oxford University Press

20:327 Master record

Database type	Numeric
Number of journals	
Sources	
Start year	1987
Language	English
Coverage	International
Number of records	
Update size	—
Update period	Periodically

Keywords
Immunology

Description
Contains data on human white blood cell (leucocyte) differentiation antigens. Data were collected in 1986 at the Third International Workshop on Human Leucocyte Differentiation Antigens where reactivity patterns for some 500 monoclonal antibodies were compared against nearly 100 leucocyte types. Software allows users to compare antibodies and reactivity patterns using Third Workshop data or other data sources.

Corresponds to *Leucocyte Typing III*.

20:328 Diskette — Oxford University Press

File name	Leucocyte Typing Database III
Format notes	IBM
Start year	1987
Number of records	
Update period	Periodically
Price	UK£200

Notes
Educational and research institutions receive 50% discount. Price qouted is for EEC countries – US$400 elsewhere.

Leuven Medical Informatics
Orda-B

20:329 Master record

Database type	Factual
Number of journals	
Sources	
Start year	1991
Language	
Coverage	
Number of records	
Update size	—
Update period	

Keywords
Electrocardiography

Description
Three databanks relating to measurements and diagnostic data.

Over 300 Mbytes of data in toto.

20:330 CD-ROM — Orda-B

File name
Format notes — IBM
Start year — 1991
Number of records
Update period

Library of the Future – Data Discman Edition – Volume 3
World Library

20:331 Master record

Database type — Textual
Number of journals
Sources
Start year
Language
Coverage
Number of records
Update size — –
Update period

Keywords

Drama; Medical History; Philosophy

Description

Contains the complete text of 125 classic works of literature, philosophy, drama, poetry, biology and medicine. Includes works by the Greek philosophers Plato and Aristotle, plays by Aeschylus, Euripides, Aristophanes, Shakespeare, the writings of Galen and Hippocrates on biology and medicine, Virgil's *Aeneid, Eclogues* and *Georgics, Discourses* of Epictetus and *On the Nature of Things* by Lucretius.

20:332 CD-ROM 8cm — World Library

File name — Library of the Future – Data Discman Edition – Volume 3
Format notes — Sony Data Discman
Start year
Number of records
Update period
Price — US$39.95

Life Sciences Collection
Cambridge Scientific Abstracts

20:333 Master record

Alternative name(s) — LSC; CSA Life Sciences Collection
Database type — Bibliographic
Number of journals — 5,000
Sources — Journals, books, serial monographs, conference proceedings, patents (US), patents (UK), patents (Japanese) and reports
Start year — 1978
Language — English
Coverage — International
Number of records — 1,500,000
Update size
Update period — Monthly

Keywords

Acute Poisoning; Aging; Algology; Amino-Acids; Anatomy; Antibiotics; Aquaculture; Bacteriology; Behavioural Ecology; Bioengineering; Biological Membranes; Biotechnology; Bone Disease; Calcium Metabolism; Chemoreception; Chronic Poisoning; Clinical Medicine; Clinical Toxicology; DNA; Drugs; Ecology; Ecosystems; Endocrinology; Entomology – Agricultural; Entomology – Applied; Entomology – Human; Entomology – Veterinary; Environmental Biology; Ethology; Genetic Engineering; Hazardous Substances; HIV; Histology; Human Ecology; Immune Disorders; Immunology; Infectious Diseases; Marine Biotechnology; Microbiology; Molecular Biology; Molecular Neurobiology; Mycology; Neurology; Neuropharmacology; Neurophysiology – Animal; Neuroscience; Nucleic Acids; Nutrition; Oncology; Occupational Health and Safety; Osteoporosis; Osteomalacia; Pathology; Peptides; Pharmaceuticals; Pheromones; Physiology; Pollution; Proteins; Protozoology; Psychophysics; Public Health; Radiation; Rhinology; RNA; Sleep; Smoking; Substance Abuse; Taste Perception; Viral Genetics

Description

Life Sciences Collection contains abstracts of information in the fields of (and corresponding to abstract journals from CSA): animal behaviour; biochemistry-amino-acid, peptide and protein; biochemistry – nucleic acids; biochemistry-biological membranes; biotechnology research (from 1984 to date); calcified tissue; chemoreception; ecology; endocrinology; entomology; genetics; human genomes; basic research and clinical applications; immunology, marine biotechnology, microbiology- algology, mycology and protozoology; microbiology-bacteriology; microbiology-industrial and applied microbiology; oncology-oncogenes and growth factors; neurosciences (from 1983 to date); toxicology; virology and AIDS. AIDS is covered in depth. The worldwide coverage is of journal articles, books, conference proceedings, report literature, patents, theses and dissertations.

Corresponds to the series of abstracting journals published by CSA: *Animal Behavior Abstracts; Biochemistry Abstracts-Amino-acid, Peptide and Protein; Biochemistry Abstracts-Biological Membranes; Biochemistry Abstracts-Nucleic Acids; Calcified Tissue Abstracts; Biotechnology Research Abstracts* (from 1984 to date); *Chemoreception Abstracts; Ecology Abstracts; Endocrinology Abstracts; Entomology Abstracts; Genetics Abstracts; Human Genome Abstracts; Basic Research and Clinical Applications; Immunology Abstracts; Marine Biotechnology Abstracts; Microbiology Abstracts-Algology, Mycology and Protozoology; Microbiology Abstracts-Bacteriology; Microbiology Abstracts-Industrial and Applied Microbiology; Neurosciences Abstracts* (from 1983 to date); *Oncogenes and Growth Factors Abstracts; Toxicology Abstracts; Virology and AIDS Abstracts.* Most recently added were *Marine Biotechnology Abstracts* and *Oncogenes and Growth Factors Abstracts.* Also includes *Oncology Abstracts and Feeding, Weight and Obesity Abstracts* for the period they were published.

20:334 Database subset
Online — Cambridge Scientific Abstracts

File name — CSA Neurosciences Abstracts
Alternative name(s) — Neuroscience Abstracts; Endocrinology Abstracts (former name)
Start year — 1983
Number of records
Update period — Monthly

Notes

A subset of the Life Sciences Collection online database. Corresponds to *Neuroscience Abstracts.*

20:335 Database subset
Online   Cambridge Scientific Abstracts

File name	Toxicology Abstracts
Start year	1974
Number of records	14,000
Update period	Monthly

Notes

A subset of the Life Sciences Collection online database. Corresponds to Toxicology Abstracts. Contains citations to the worldwide literature on toxicology. Covers clinical toxicology, including acute or chronic poisoning from drugs, medicines and chemicals; toxic risks in the workplace; and environmental toxicology. Sources include about 2,500 journals.

20:336 Database subset
Tape   Cambridge Scientific Abstracts

File name	CSA Neurosciences Abstracts on Magnetic Tape
Alternative name(s)	Neurosciences Abstracts; Endocrinology Abstracts (former name)
Format notes	9-track, unlabelled, 1600 bpi, EBCDIC.
Start year	1983
Number of records	
Update period	Monthly

Notes

A subset of the Life Sciences Collection. Contains citations, with abstracts, to the worldwide literature on the neurosciences. Covers vertebrate and invertebrate neurosciences, endocrinology, aging, degeneration and repair, neuropharmacology, molecular neurobiology, genetics, sleep, neural correlates of behaviour, and immunology. Gives author's name, affiliation and address, journal title, volume, issue, date, pagination, CODEN, abstract, language, document type, treatment code and descriptors. Corresponds to Neurosciences Abstracts (formerly Endocrinology Abstracts), and in part to the Life Sciences Collection online database. It is also available online through Cambridge Scientific Abstracts.

Pricing information may be obtained from Cambridge Scientific Abstracts.

20:337 Database subset
Tape   Cambridge Scientific Abstracts

File name	Ecology Abstracts on Magnetic Tape
Format notes	9-track, unlabelled, 1600 bp, EBCDIC.
Start year	1974
Number of records	
Update period	Monthly

Notes

A subset of the Life Sciences Collection. Contains citations, with abstracts, to the worldwide literature on ecology and the environment. Focus is on how microbes, plants and animals interact with each other and with the environment. Coverage includes evolutionary biology; economics and systems analysis as they relate to ecosystems; human ecology; habitats and food chains; erosion, climate, water resources and pollution; and resource and ecosystems management. Corresponds to Ecology Abstracts, and in part to the Life Sciences Collection online database.

Pricing information may be obtained from Cambridge Scientific Abstracts.

20:338 Database subset
Tape   Cambridge Scientific Abstracts

File name	Toxicology Abstracts on Magnetic Tape
Format notes	9-track, unlabelled, 1600 bpi, EBCDIC.
Start year	1978
Number of records	
Update period	Monthly

Notes

A subset of the Life Sciences Collection. Contains citations to the international literature on toxicology, covering clinical toxicology (including acute and chronic poisoning from drugs, medicines and chemicals), toxic risks in the workplace and environmental toxicology. Includes social poisons and substance abuse; natural toxins; legislation and recommended standards; studies of industrial and agricultural chemicals; household products, pharmaceuticals and other substances; effects of alcohol and smoking; radiation and radioactive materials; and toxicology methodology and analytical procedures. Corresponds to Toxicology Abstracts and in part to the Life Sciences Collection online database. Contact Cambridge Scientific Abstracts for pricing information.

This database can also be found on:
Cambridge Scientific Abstracts Life Sciences
Human Nutrition on CD-ROM

LifeSaver
Media Design Interactive

20:339 Master record

Database type	Courseware, Multimedia, Factual, Textual
Number of journals	
Sources	
Start year	
Language	English
Coverage	
Number of records	
Update size	—
Update period	Varies

Keywords
First Aid

Description

A complete paramedics first aid course on CD-ROM. Designed as an adjunct to first aid courses, LifeSaver uses a pop-up interface and animated contents pages to navigate around the program. Divided into twenty-four chapters in multimedia format including narration, colour pictures and 'hot text' with links to different areas of the course, over twenty video clips are used which can be stepped through frame by frame so that important techniques can be properly assimilated. LifeSaver has been prepared by a team of physicians working in US hospitals and some of the video material was obtained during 'real-life' emergencies.

20:340 CD-ROM — Media Design Interactive

File name	LifeSaver
Format notes	IBM, Mac
Start year	
Number of records	
Update period	Varies
Price	UK£99

Lithium Index

University of Wisconsin-Madison, Department of Psychiatry, Lithium Information Center

20:341 Master record

Database type	Bibliographic, Textual (reviews)
Number of journals	
Sources	
Start year	Current information
Language	English
Coverage	International
Number of records	125
Update size	—
Update period	Periodically, as new data become available

Keywords

Biochemistry; Clinical Medicine; Lithium – Clinical Uses

Description

Contains analyses of the international literature on medical uses of lithium, including interactions with other drugs, side effects, medical conditions and treatment guidelines. Summaries can be retrieved by clinical topics (pregnancy, teratogenesis, neurological side effects, kidney damage, sexual function, fertility, cardiovascular system, cutaneous side effects, etc).

20:342 Online — University of Wisconsin-Madison, Department of Psychiatry, Lithium Information Center

File name	
Start year	Current information
Number of records	125
Update period	Periodically, as new data become available

Martindale

Royal Pharmaceutical Society of Great Britain

20:343 Master record

Alternative name(s)	CCIS: Martindale: The Extra Pharmacopoeia; Martindale – The Extra Pharmacopoeia on CCIS
Database type	Bibliographic, Factual, Textual
Number of journals	
Sources	Government reports, journals, laws/regulations, official publications and WHO publications
Start year	Current
Language	English
Coverage	International

Number of records	60,000
Update size	—
Update period	Annually
Index unit	Articles
Thesaurus	Martindale Online: Drug Information Thesaurus. London: Pharmaceutical Society of Great Britain, 2nd ed., 1990
Database aids	Martindale Online help-desk (9 am. to 5pm. UK time) Tel. +44 1 582 8455 and Martindale Online User's Guide (Data-Star), London, Pharmaceutical Society of Great Britain, 1985

Keywords

Clinical Medicine; Hazardous Substances; Drugs; Drug Therapy; Pharmacokinetics

Description

Martindale is a full text database based on the textbook, *Martindale, The Extra Pharmacopoeia* published by the Royal Pharmaceutical Society of Great Britain. It offers an extensive resource of evaluated information on drugs and medicines in clinical and therapeutic use throughout the world, and on investigational drugs, compounds liable to abuse and ancillary substances including diagnostic agents, pharmaceutical adjuvants and toxic substances. The database contains information on more than 25,000 compounds that are used in the many thousands of preparations also included. The compounds cover most drugs and medicines used to treat diseases as well as many investigational drugs. It also covers ancilliary substances such as asbestos. The database supplies information on groups of compounds as well as on individual substances and is supported by selected abstracts.

The information available for each compound will usually include: nomenclature (synonyms, generic names, chemical names), CAS Registry numbers, physical and pharmaceutical properties such as appearance, pharmacopoeial status, units adverse effects and their treatment, precautions, standards, contra-indications and interactions, pharmacokinetics, actions, uses, dosage and administration, proprietary names and preparations.

The database corresponds to the printed *Martindale: The Extra Pharmacopoeia* (30th edition). It is updated annually over a five-year cycle, so that at the end of the cycle the whole database has been reassessed. Conditions for use note that all the information provided through Martindale Online and is copyright of the Royal Pharmaceutical Society of Great Britain. Payment for information obtained through Martindale Online includes the right to store the information in memory and to print and display it for private use only. Martindale Online has been prepared assuming that the user has the necessary training to interpret the information it provides.

Martindale Online developed a hierarchical thesaurus of more than 9,600 descriptors to facilitate searching on classes of drugs (a feature omitted from printed editions. The database can be searched by: old English terms or their modern synonyms; international trade name; generic name; chemical name; disease state.

20:344 Online — Data-Star

File name	MART
Start year	Current

Number of records	46,000
Update period	Annually on a 5 year cycle
Database aids	Data-Star Biomedical Manual and Data-Star Online Manual (search NEWS-MART in NEWS)
Price/Charges	Subscription: SFr80.00
	Connect time: SFr107.00
	Online print: SFr1.19
	Offline print: SFr0.92

Downloading is allowed

Notes

From June 1993 Data-Star have introduced an annual fee/subscription per contract (that is, not per password) of SFr 80.00 (c.UK£ 32.00) payable every June. For North American customers billed in dollars who also use DIALOG, the DIALOG fee also covers access to Data-Star. Academic customers, 'commitment' customers and customers currently billed in dollars are exempt.

Record composition

Abstract AB; Accession Number AN; Author(s) AU; CAS Registry Number RN; Cross reference(s) XR; Descriptors DE; Document Length LE; Document Type RF; Entry Date ED; Headings HE; Molecular formula and Molecula Weight MO; Notes and Warnings NT; Pharmacopoeia(s) PC; Preparations PR; Preparation Licence Holder and Number PL; Publication Year PY; Radiopharmaceutical Data RP; Source(s) SO; Synonym(s) SY; Text TX; Title TI; Update Code UP and Warning WA

20:345 Online   DIALOG

File name	File 141
Start year	Current edition
Number of records	43,393 describing 25,000 preparations or compunds
Update period	Annually
Price/Charges	Connect time: US$63.00
	Online print: US$0.50
	Offline print: US$0.50

Notes

DIALINDEX Categories: DRUGDIR, PHARM, PHARMR, RNMED, TOXICOL, TRADENMS.

20:346 CD-ROM   Micromedex Inc

File name	Martindale – The Extra Pharmacopoeia on CCIS
Alternative name(s)	CCIS: Martindale: The Extra Pharmacopoeia; Martindale – The Extra Pharmacopoeia on CCIS
Format notes	IBM
Software	Proprietary
Start year	Current
Number of records	60,000
Update period	Quarterly

Notes

This database is available as a standalone product, as well as being a part of CCIS, Computerized Clinical Information System. The 30th edition of Martindale is now available both in print and on this CD-ROM.

20:347 Tape   Micromedex Inc

File name	Martindale – The Extra Pharmacopeia on CCIS
Alternative name(s)	CCIS: Martindale: The Extra Pharmacopoeia; Martindale – The Extra Pharmacopoeia on CCIS
Software	Proprietary
Start year	1987
Number of records	
Update period	Quarterly

Notes

Annual subsription to CCIS required. This database is also available as a standalone CD product, as well as being a part of CCIS, Computerized Clinical Information System.

This database can also be found on:
CCIS

Material Safety Data Sheets

Occupational Health Services Inc (OHS)
National Safety Data Corporation

20:348 Master record

Database type	Textual, Factual, Courseware
Number of journals	
Sources	Monograph, Government departments, Institutions and Data sheets
Start year	Current information
Language	English
Coverage	USA (primarily)
Number of records	85,000
Update size	—
Update period	Daily

Keywords

Fire; Explosion; Hazardous Chemicals; First Aid; Occupational Health and Safety; Waste Management

Description

Identification, handling and hazard disclosure information on chemical substances that require documentation by chemical manufacturers under the Hazard Communication and Labeling Standard of the Occupational Safety and Health Administration. For each of the 85,000 chemicals covered the following data are given: substance indentification (chemical name, trade names and molecular formula), manufacturer's or importer's name, address and phone number, physical data (description, boiling and melting points, specific gravity, evaporation rate, exposure limits and water solubility), fire and explosion data (flash point, upper and lower ignition limits and fire-fighting techniques), toxicity and health effects, including first aid and antidotes, reactivity, including incompatibilities (for example, explosive reaction with hydrogen peroxide), decomposition and polymerisation, handling, storage transportation or disposal conditions to avoid and spill and leak procedures. Sources include the OSHA, National Institute for Occupational Safety and Health, US Environmental Protection Agency and Dreisbach's *Handbook of Poisoning*.

20:349 Database subset
Online   Executive Telecom
System International,
Human Resource
Information Network (ETSI/HRIN)

File name	OHS MSDS Summary Sheet
Start year	Current information
Number of records	10,000
Update period	Daily

Notes

Summaries of Material Safety Data Sheets for about 10,000 chemical giving for each substance chemical name, CAS Registry number, chemical formula, physical description, fire and explosion hazards, reactivity, protective equipment, emergency response procedures, health effects and first aid. This is intended as a supplement or training aid for the fuller information in the database Material Safety Data Sheets. Annual subscription to ETSI/HRIN required.

20:350 Database subset
Online   Occupational Health Services Inc (OHS)

File name	OHS MSDS Summary Sheet
Start year	Current information
Number of records	10,000
Update period	Daily

Notes

Summaries of Material Safety Data Sheets for about 10,000 chemical substances, giving for each substance chemical name, CAS Registry number, chemical formula, physical description, fire and explosion hazards, reactivity, protective equipment, emergency response procedures, health effects and first aid. This is intended as a supplement or training aid for the fuller information in the database Material Safety Data Sheets. Monthly subscription to OHS required

20:351 Database subset
CD-ROM   National Safety Data Corporation

File name	Material Safety Data Sheets (I)
Format notes	IBM
Software	Quantum Access
Start year	
Number of records	35,000
Update period	
Price	US$750

20:352 Database subset
CD-ROM   National Safety Data Corporation

File name	Material Safety Data Sheets (II)
Format notes	IBM
Software	Quantum Access
Start year	
Number of records	35,000
Update period	
Price	US$750

Mediasource – Natural Sciences Library

Applied Optical Media Corporation
Grant Heilman Photography Inc

20:353 Master record

Database type	Multimedia
Number of journals	
Sources	
Start year	
Language	English
Coverage	International
Number of records	
Update size	–
Update period	Varies

Description

Contains 1,500 images and ninety minutes of music and sound effects, with reuse rights for most desktop multimedia PC applications. Covers agriculture, astronomy, botany, chemistry, environmental science, geology, human biology, physics, weather and climate, and zoology.

20:354 CD-ROM   Applied Optical Media Corporation

File name	Mediasource – Natural Sciences Library
Format notes	IBM, Mac
Start year	
Number of records	
Update period	Varies
Price	US$395

20:355 DVI   Applied Optical Media Corporation

File name	Mediasource – Natural Sciences Library
Format notes	IBM, Mac
Start year	
Number of records	
Update period	Varies
Price	US$395

Medical Waste News

Business Publishers Inc

20:356 Master record

Database type	Textual
Number of journals	1
Sources	Newsletter
Start year	1988
Language	English
Coverage	USA
Number of records	
Update size	–
Update period	Twice per month

Keywords

Hazardous Substances; Medical Waste Management; Waste Management

Description

A newsletter on the medical waste disposal industry, including reports on the disposal of infectious waste resulting from medical procedures and treatments in hospitals and clinics. Includes Congressional and state actions and regulations relevant to medical waste.

Corresponds to *Medical Waste News* newsletter. Available on DIALOG and Data-Star as part of the PTS Newsletter Database.

20:357 Online   CompuServe Information Service

File name	IQUEST File 2782
Start year	Current year
Number of records	
Update period	Twice per month
Price/Charges	Subscription: US$8.95 per month Database entry fee: US$9/search; some databases carry a surcharge ($2–75) Online print: US$10 references free; then $9 per ten; abstracts $3 each

Downloading is allowed

Notes

Accessed via IQUEST or IQMEDICAL, this database is offered by a NewsNet gateway. IQUEST can either search across all databases, a database of the user's choice or selected multiple databases.

20:358 Online   NewsNet Inc

File name	
Start year	1988

Number of records
Update period   Twice per month
This database can also be found on:
PTS Newsletter Database

MEDIC
Lääketieteellinen keskuskirjasto (LKK)

20:360 Master record
Database type	Bibliographic
Number of journals	
Sources	Conference proceedings, Dissertations, Journals, Meeting abstracts and Monographs
Start year	1978
Language	Finnish (mainly), English (descriptors) and Multilingual
Coverage	Finland
Number of records	26,200
Update size	2,500
Update period	Monthly
Index unit	Articles

Keywords
Biomedicine

Description
References to articles from about sixty medical journals published in Finland, and monographs and series, for example, reports from research institutions and universities, meetings abstracts and academic dissertations. Subjects covered include: medicine; biomedicine and health care.

This is the online equivalent of the printed publication *Finmed*.

20:361 Online   Lääketieteellinen keskuskirjasto (LKK)
File name	MEDIC
Start year	1978
Number of records	26,200
Update period	Monthly

Notes
Charges based on a subscription fee.

Medicorom
Inter CD

20:362 Master record
Database type	Encyclopedia, Directory, Dictionary, Factual
Number of journals	
Sources	Books
Start year	
Language	French
Coverage	France
Number of records	
Update size	—
Update period	Twice a year
Index unit	Drugs, doctors, hospitals, clinics and trade shows

Description
Contains: a drug dictionary with 3,400 entries; drug interactions; professional encyclopedia; directory of doctors in France; directories of hospitals and clinics; diary of medical trade shows; six-language medical glossary, and other encyclopaedic and directory information of use to the medical community.

20:363 CD-ROM   Inter CD
File name	Medicorom
Format notes	IBM
Start year	
Number of records	
Update period	Semiannually
Price/Charges	Subscription: FFr14,600

Meditext
Micromedex Inc

20:364 Master record
Database type	Factual, Directory, Textual, Bibliographic
Number of journals	
Sources	
Start year	
Language	English
Coverage	International
Number of records	
Update size	—
Update period	Quarterly

Keywords
Clinical Medicine; Hazardous Chemicals; Occupational Health and Safety

Description
Detailed, comprehensive, and referenced protocols for the medical evaluation and treatment of individuals exposed to industrial chemical agents.

This database can be found on:
TOMES
TOMES Plus

MEDLINE
National Library of Medicine

20:365 Master record
Database type	Bibliographic
Number of journals	3,500
Sources	Conference proceedings, journals, monographs and reviews
Start year	1964
Language	English
Coverage	International
Number of records	7,500,000
Update size	370,000
Update period	Weekly except January and February which are updated monthly.
Index unit	Biographies, case studies, comparative studies, editorials, letters, news releases, obituaries, reviews, articles, book chapters and interview
Abstract details	Author abstracts (since 1975) are available for approximately 70% of the citations
Thesaurus	Medical Subject Headings (MeSH)
Database aids	MeSH Tree Structures, Permuted MeSH, MeSH Supplementary Chemical Records with CAS Registration Numbers or Enzyme Codes (from June 1980), Gene Symbols from January 1991), List of Serials Indexed for Online Users, includes NLM Journal codens, List of Journals Indexed in Index Medicus includes subject order serials index and Indexing Manual

Keywords

HIV; Anaesthesia; Anatomy; Applied Science; Biochemistry; Biotechnology; Cancer; Cardiology; Cardiovascular Diseases; Chemical Substances; Clinical Medicine; Forensic Science; Geriatrics; Gynaecology; Handicapped; Health and Safety; Immunology; Infectious Diseases; Medical History; Mental Health; Microbiology; Obstetrics; Occupational Health and Safety; Orthopaedics; Paediatrics; Patents; Pathology; Physiology; Pollution; Public Health; Radiology; Social Services; Toxicology

Description

MEDLINE (MEDlars (MEDical Literature ANalysis and Retrieval System) onLINE) is a vast source of medical information covering the whole field of medicine and health science information. It is the most current file and includes the current year and at least two additional years depending on the host utilised. MEDLINE backfiles are segmented and are available back to 1966. Subjects covered include (1) basic sciences/research in medicine such as bacteriology, biochemistry, environmental research, genetics, immunology, microbiology, parasitology, physiology and virology; and (2) applied sciences/clinical medicine such as anatomy, biomedical technology, clincial medicine, communication disorders, dental medicine, dermatology, environmental medicine, experimental medicine, forensic medicine, gerontology, gynaecology, health care services, hospital administration, immunology, medical education, medical psychology, medical technology, neurology, nutrition, occupational medicine, nursing oncology, opthalmology, orthopedics, parasitology, paramedical professions, pathology, pharmacy, pharmacology, physiology, policy issues, population, psychiatry, psychology, rehabilitation, research, social science medicine; social medicine, sport medicine, toxicology and veterinary medicine.

MEDLINE corresponds to the printed publications: *Index Medicus, Index to Dental Literature, International Nursing Index* and various other bibliographies. Author abstracts are provided for approximately seventy per cent of items in the database. The database also covers chapters and articles from selected monographs from 1976 to 1981. About 74% of citations are to English-language sources and the remaining citations represent over forty other languages. This compares with 88% English-language sources on SciSearch, 86% on BIOSIS and 75% in EMBASE, the other leading bioscience databases. 50% of records were added after January 1975. More than 90% of journals are evaluated cover to cover. The database contains 304,354 citations for the years 1964/5 but as the controlled vocabulary and retrieval is different from the later years, these years are often offered as a separate file. Citations are automatically transferred from MEDLINE to other NLM-databases, therefore many of the journals indexed are also found in CANCERLIT (approximately 85% overlap with MEDLINE), HEALTH (approximately 80% overlap with MEDLINE) and AIDSLINE (approximately 75% overlap with MEDLINE). For BIOETHICSLINE no automatic transfer takes place but many MEDLINE-journals related to biomedical ethics are also evaluated for BIOETHICSLINE. Journals are categorised on three different levels of priority. Those on the third level are indexed in less depth than journals on levels one and two. The time lag between the appearance of the publication and availability on magnetic tape is usually shorter for priority one and two than for priority three journals. Journals to be considered for MEDLINE are selected by an advisory committee of physicians, scientists, librarians and publishers of medical journals appointed by the NLM. Journal information which is not indexed includes abstracts on congresses, book reviews, hospital reports, communications from medical associations, announcements of new drugs by pharmaceutical companies. Regarding the length of abstracts, between 1975 and 1977 there was no limitation regarding the length of abstracts. Between 1977 and 1980 no abstract longer than 200 words and between 1981 and 1983 no abstract longer than 250 words was stored. Due to these limitations only 45% of the citations contain abstracts for this period of input. From 1984 onwards, abstracts exceeding 250 words or 400 words for abstracts of articles ten pages or more in length are included but truncated and these abstracts have the message 'ABSTRACTS TRUNCATED AT 250/400 WORDS' at their end. From 1984, 65% of the citations contain an abstract. This compares with 60% in EMBASE and 54% in BIOSIS. Records of the other leading bioscience database, SciSearch, now also contains abstracts. Since 1980, 26% of MEDLINE records with non-English sources contain English-language abstracts online. This compares with 67% on BIOSIS and 37% on EMBASE. Abstracts from articles from journal titles of priority 3 have only been stored since Spring 1989.

MEDLINE's Tree Structures classification is the most detailed alphanumeric scheme developed for online searching. It is directly related to the controlled vocabulary in the database. It is necessary to use the hardcopy search aids produced – *MeSH* annotated alphabetic list, TREE structures, Permuted terms etc. to obtain successful search results, and, as they are re-edited and published by NLM each year, to use the latest edition only, as new terminology is included annually. Generally, new sets become available in December for use in the following year. The MeSH descriptors have check tags for gender, age groups, human, animal, article type and can also be subdivided using standard subheadings. A two tier level of indexing is used with an average of twelve descriptors assigned, of which three to five descriptors are major or primary headings which appear in *Index Medicus* or other print sources. In addition to the controlled vocabulary terms, textwords or free-text terms may be used for retrieval from the title, abstract, authors address and other parts of the citation. Exploded treewords, which are the hierarchical arrangement of *Medical Subject Headings* can also be used for retrieval of broad categories of information.

Every Medical Subject Heading has at least one corresponding alpha-numeric code or tree number which determines its location in the hierarchically arranged Tree Structures. Some headings have more than one tree number because they are located in more than one tree. There are a total of fifteen broad subject categories or trees as follows: A. Anatomical Terms; B. Organisms; C. Diseases; D. Chemicals and Drugs; E. Analytical, Diagnostic and Therapeutic Technics and Equipment; F. Psychiatry and Psychology; G. Biological Sciences; H. Physical Sciences; I. Anthropology, Education, Sociology and Social Phenomena; J. Technology, Industry, Agriculture, Food; K. Humanities; L. Information Science and Communications; M. Named Groups of Persons; N. Health Care; and Z. Geographicals. These broad categories are then broken down into narrower subcategories. The hardcopy thesaurus indicates when narrower terms are available under a code.

In addition to numerous cross-references *MeSH* precoordinates frequently searched concepts for example PREGNANCY IN DIABETES. It also contains history notes indicating starting dates for consistent usage of indexer- added terms online and hints for retrospective searching on topics where preferred terminology has changed over time, for example ROBOTICS (87) search AUTOMATION 1966–86. MEDLINE also permits indexers to identify concepts lacking adequate descriptors in MeSH. Since June 1980 its identifier field has been used to index chemicals discussed in the full text of source documents ensuring access to names or numbers of compounds whether or not they are included among MeSH descriptors. Registry Numbers have been assigned in MEDLINE records since June 1980. MEDLINE also consistently adds Enzyme Commission (EC) numbers to records for sources which discuss enzymes).

The datafield Document Type was introduced to MEDLINE in 1991, Prior to this some of the Document Types had been MeSH-Terms for example historial article, review. Most of these *MeSH* terms have been deleted and replaced by a corresponding Document Type retrospectively. Indexing with *MeSH* is performed by specially trained staff in indexing institutes in the USA. The value of controlled vocabulary is important when searching for topics where a subject population has been specified. Relatively few bioscience databases provide consistent indexing for subject populations (that is, humans or specific test animals) and related characteristics commonly requested such as age groups, gender, occupation and racial or ethnic groups. In comparison with BIOSIS, EMBASE and SciSearch MEDLINE provides the most extensive consistent indexing for the subject population groups, humans, test animals, racial/ethnic groups, gender and age groups but provides less consistent indexing of occupational gropus, where fewer controlled terms are augmented with natural language keywords in strategies. A study on indexing consistency in MEDLINE has shown an average consistency for central concept main heading (equivalent to MeSH term/MAJOR; that is, *Toxicology in records) identification of 61.1% for central concept subheadings (for example, *MeSH term-TOXICITY), of 54.9% and for central main heading/subheading combinations (for example, *Skin Drug Effects) of 43.1%. In most bioscience files a form of pharmaceutical nomenclature exists. For MEDLINE the preferred search terms are generic name, classification by action/use and CAS Registry Number although restrictions by date, subfile and vendor may apply to the latter and vendor documentation should be consulted for guidelines. Restrictions also apply for the search term Enzyme Commission Number and vendor documentations should again be consulted for guidelines. For the search terms investigational code, chemical name and trade name, the terminology is inconsistent and alternative names should be used in search strategies. Retrospective searching however may require the entry of other names used for the same substance at earlier stages in its development life cycle. The use of synonyms is advisable when searching compounds yet to be added as controlled *MeSH* descriptors.

In 1993, after the annual reload, there are some new features available: new file labels; page, issue and volume numbers in the source paragraph are now searchable, it is now possible to retrieve articles where the user has incomplete information eg. an article written by Schellenberg., published in a journal on Page 668; review articles are now searchable with a .LIMIT-command; 94 descriptors have been replaced by more up-to-date terminology; 421 new and updated *MeSH* terms and new publication types in the PT field.

20:366 Database subset

CD-ROM   **Aries Systems Corporation**

File name	Core Journals MEDLINE
Format notes	Mac, IBM
Software	Knowledge Finder
Start year	Most recent five years.
Number of records	
Update period	Quarterly
Price/Charges	Subscription: US$895 – 1,495

Notes

MEDLINE subset covering 270 primary clinical journals, including abridged *Index Medicus*, and Brandon Hill lists.

20:367 Database subset
CD-ROM   **Aries Systems Corporation**

File name	NeuroLine
Format notes	IBM, Mac
Software	Knowledge Finder 2.0
Start year	
Number of records	
Update period	Quarterly
Price/Charges	Subscription: US$395

Notes

Archive subset of MEDLINE for Neurology-related journals covering the previous ten years, plus the current year's MEDLINE.

20:368 Database subset
CD-ROM   **Aries Systems Corporation**

File name	OpthaLine
Format notes	IBM, Mac
Software	Knowledge Finder 2.0
Start year	
Number of records	
Update period	Quarterly
Price/Charges	Subscription: US$395

Notes

Archival subset of MEDLINE for opthalmology covering the previous ten years, plus the current year's MEDLINE.

20:369 Database subset
CD-ROM   **Aries Systems Corporation**

File name	OrthoLine Biomedical Literature Reference Volume 2
Format notes	IBM, Mac
Software	Knowledge Finder
Start year	Most recent ten years
Number of records	
Update period	Annually/Quarterly/Monthly
Price/Charges	Subscription: US$595 – 2,595

Notes

Archival MEDLINE subset, containing the most recent ten full years of the orthopaedics literature from MEDLINE.

Price varies depending on frequency of updates: Monthly, Quarterly, or Annually.

20:370 Database subset
CD-ROM   **Aries Systems Corporation**

File name	RadLine
Format notes	IBM, Mac
Software	Knowledge Finder 2.0
Start year	
Number of records	
Update period	Quarterly
Price/Charges	Subscription: US$395

Notes

Archival subset of MEDLINE for Radiology covering about one hundred journals and the previous ten years.

Radiology citations based on some two hundred *MeSH* terms.

20:371 Database subset
CD-ROM   **Aries Systems Corporation**

File name	SurgAnLine
Format notes	IBM, Mac
Software	Knowledge Finder 2.0
Start year	
Number of records	
Update period	Quarterly
Price/Charges	Subscription: US$395

Notes

Archival subset of MEDLINE for surgery and anaesthesia covering the previous ten years, plus the current year's MEDLINE.

20:372 Database subset
CD-ROM   **DIALOG OnDisc**

File name	MEDLINE Clinical Collection
Format notes	Mac, IBM
Software	DIALOG OnDisc Manager
Start year	Most recent five years.
Number of records	
Update period	Quarterly
Price/Charges	Subscription: US$725

Notes

Subset of MEDLINE focusing on clinical medicine and including the *Abridged Index Medicus*. Contains five years of references and abstracts from approximately 150 journals in clinical medicine. Also includes citations from: *A Library for Internists V Recommended by the American College of Physicians*; Brandon and Hill's *Selected List of Books and Journals for the Small Medical Library*.

20:373 Database subset
CD-ROM   **Healthcare Information Services Inc**

File name	BiblioMed
Format notes	IBM
Software	Proprietary
Start year	Most recent three years
Number of records	300,000
Update period	Quarterly
Price/Charges	Subscription: US$950

Notes

Selected subset of MEDLINE covering general medicine, with 300,000 abstracts and citations from 550 top clinical and medical journals. Aimed at a clinical medical practice.

20:374 Database subset
CD-ROM   **INSERM Questel**

File name	CD-MED – Anaesthesia and Resuscitation
Format notes	IBM
Software	CD-Answer
Start year	Most recent four to five years
Number of records	150,000
Update period	Quarterly
Price/Charges	Subscription: FFr6,000

Notes

A specialist subset of MEDLINE covering all aspects of local, regional and general anaesthesia and resuscitation. All aspects are taken into account: epidemiology, etiology, diagnosis, treatment and prevention. Includes a directory of research laboratories.

A bilingual medical dictionary allows searching in English or French.

20:375 Database subset
CD-ROM   **SilverPlatter**

File name	MEDLINE Professional
Format notes	IBM, Mac
Software	SPIRS/MacSPIRS
Start year	1966
Number of records	630,000
Update period	Six times per year
Price/Charges	Subscription: UK£285 – 863

Notes

Contains a subset of MEDLINE for clinical medicine on one disc. An archival disc is also available extending coverage back to 1981. Subscription costs are: regular subscription £575 for single users, £863 for 2–8 networked users; special price for individual users £325; archival subscription £358 for single users, £537 for 2–8 networked users; archival subscription for individual users £285.

20:376 Database subset
CD-ROM   **SilverPlatter**

File name	MEDLINE Professional Archival Disc
Format notes	IBM, Mac
Software	SPIRS
Start year	1981
Number of records	
Update period	Annually
Price/Charges	Subscription: UK£285 – 537

Notes

Contains an archival subset of MEDLINE for clinical medicine on one disc covering from 1985 back to 1981. Prices are: archival subscription £358 for single users, £537 for 2–8 networked users; archival subscription for individual users £285.

Microbial Resources Database of China
Institute of Microbiology

20:377 Master record

Alternative name(s)	MRDC
Database type	Factual, Statistical
Number of journals	
Sources	

Start year	1986
Language	Chinese and English
Coverage	China
Number of records	
Update size	—
Update period	

Keywords

Microbe Collections; Microbiology

Description

The database contains information as follows:

Microbial character data on microbes;
Microbial product market information;
Microbial nomenclature data;
Microbial terminology data; and
10452 RKC codes in both Chinese and English for international exchange.

Microbial characteristics of 3,000 strains, including about 49 genera of bacteria, ten genera for yeast and thirteen genera for actinomycetes are included. The database includes genera number, name, properties and has a statistical function.

Equivalent to the print, *Chinese Catalogue of Strains*.

20:378 Online — Scientific Database System

File name	Microbial Resources Database of China
Alternative name(s)	MRDC
Start year	1986
Number of records	
Update period	

MSDS

Canadian Centre for Occupational Health and Safety (CCOHS) Occupational Health Services Inc (OHS)

20:379 Master record

Alternative name(s)	FTSS; Trade Names; Noms de Marque
Database type	Textual, Factual, Numeric, Directory
Number of journals	
Sources	Data sheets, Chemical manufacturers and Chemical distributors
Start year	Current information
Language	English
Coverage	Canada (primarily), International (some) and USA (some)
Number of records	75,000+
Update size	—
Update period	Periodically, as new data become available

Keywords

Dangerous Chemicals; First Aid; Hazardous Substances; Occupational Health and Safety; Waste Management

Description

Produced by the Canadian Centre for Occupational Health and Safety, MSDS contains the complete text, in French and English, of over 75,000 Material Safety Data Sheets for chemical trade name products used in the workplace. Each entry includes trade names, manufacturer and distributor names, addresses and phone numbers, description and physical properties,

reactivity, health hazards, storage and handling, spill and leak procedures, cleanup and disposal, personal protection and first aid.

French-language equivalent data base is FTSS Data Base.

20:380 Online — CCINFOline

File name	MSDS/FTSS
Alternative name(s)	FTSS; Material Safety Data Sheets; Trade Names; Noms de Marque
Start year	Current information
Number of records	72,500
Update period	Periodically, as new data become available

20:381 Online — STN

File name	MSDS-CCOHS
Alternative name(s)	FTSS; Trade Names; Noms de Marque
Start year	1991
Number of records	75,815
Update period	Quarterly
Price/Charges	Connect time: DM83.00
	Online print: DM13.50
	Offline print: DM14.35

Notes

Trade names, company names, issue or re-issue date and the full text of the MSDS are searchable.

This database can also be found on:
CCINFOdisc Series A1 – MSDS

Multiple Sclerosis Research Projects

International Federation of Multiple Sclerosis Societies (IFMSS)

20:383 Master record

Database type	Directory
Number of journals	
Sources	
Start year	Current information
Language	English
Coverage	International
Number of records	
Update size	—
Update period	Twice per year

Keywords

Multiple Sclerosis

Description

Descriptions of funded multiple sclerosis research worldwide. Each project entry includes title, names of researchers, name and address of the research institution, funding details, start and end date, duration and project summary.

20:384 Online — BIOSIS Life Science Network

File name	
Start year	Current information
Number of records	
Update period	Twice per year
Price/Charges	Connect time: US$9.00
	Online print: US$6.00 per 10; 2.25 per abstract; 3.50 per full text article

Also available via the Internet by telnetting to LSN.COM.

Notes

On Life Science Network users can search this database or they can scan a group of subject-related databases. There is a charge of $2.00 per scan of subject-related databases. To search one database and display up to ten citations costs $6.00. Most charges are for information retrieved. There are no charges if there are no results and no charge to transfer results to a printer or diskette. Articles may also be ordered via an online document delivery request. A telecommunications software package is also available, costing $12.95, providing an automatic connection to Life Science Network for heavy users of the service, with capability to transfer to print or disk and customised colour options.

NATUR
Sweden Statens Naturvårdsverk (SNV)

20:385 Master record

Database type	Bibliographic, Library catalogue/cataloguing aids, Textual
Number of journals	
Sources	Libraries, Grey literature and Research reports
Start year	1970
Language	Original language (titles), Swedish and English (keywords/abstracts)
Coverage	Sweden
Number of records	30,000
Update size	2,000
Update period	Daily

Keywords

Air Pollution; Civil Engineering; Conservation; Environmental Hygiene; Epidemiology; Ergonomics; Hazardous Waste; Natural Resources; Noise Pollution; Occupational Health and Safety; Occupational Medicine; Soil Pollution; Toxic Waste; Water Pollution; Wildlife

Description

NATUR contains references to the literature at the Swedish Environmental Protection Agency. It consists of four subdatabases: 1) ERICA refers to the holdings of the library, books from 1970 and onwards, 2) SERIX contains references to environmental research reports, most of which are so called 'grey literature', that is, it is not formally published and therefore hard to retrieve, 3) SERIXX older part of SERIX, publishing years 1975 to 1989 and 4) descriptions of environmental research projects PROJEKT. Topics covered include: air, noise, water and soil pollution; toxic wastes; natural resources and wildlife; environmental monitoring and technology; environmental hygiene, epidemiology, ergonomics, occupational health and safety and hygiene. Each record includes title of document, project leader or report author, editor, corporate body, sponsor, research organisation abstract (when available), controlled terms (keywords), subject classification, codes for geographic region, lakes, rivers and chemical compounds (CAS numbers).

Corresponds to *Swedish Environmental Research*. Titles are in the original language; abstracts are in the original language or English; keywords are in English and Swedish.

20:386 Online   DAFA Data AB

File name	NATUR
Start year	1970

Number of records	30,000
Update period	Daily

For more details of constituent databases, see:
ERICA
PROJEKT
SERIX

NIOSHTIC
National Institute of Occupational Safety and Health (NIOSH)

20:388 Master record

Database type	Bibliographic, Textual
Number of journals	400; 70,000 monographs/reports
Sources	Journals, monographs and technical reports
Start year	1800
Language	English
Coverage	International
Number of records	170,000
Update size	12,000
Update period	Quarterly
Index unit	Articles
Thesaurus	NIOSH Controlled Vocabulary

Keywords

Accident Prevention; Biological Hazards; Epidemiology; Ergonomics; Hazardous Waste; Health Physics; Industrial Materials; Industrial Processes; Metabolism; Occupational Health and Safety; Occupational Medicine; Pathology; Safety Education; Vocational Training; Waste Management

Description

NIOSHTIC includes citations with abstracts relating to industrial hygiene, materials and processes in the workplace – occupational health and safety, occupational medicine, injury prevention and ergonomics. Coverage is of literature on, or relating to, the effects of working environment and conditions and work processes and materials on the safety and health of the worker; methods and instrumentation for the determination of such effects; measures for elimination of work hazards; and protective equipment for prevention of injuries to the worker. Subject areas of the documents are generally interdisciplinary and coverage includes occupational medicine, legislation, toxicology, epidemiology, pathology, histology, health physics, injury prevention, industrial hygiene, safety processes and materials, behavioural sciences, education and training, control technology, ergonomics, biochemistry, hazardous agents. Entries include CAS Registry numbers where relevant.

NIOSHTIC is the product of the Technical Information Branch, a division of the National Institute for Occupational Safety and Health Technical Information Centre. The database includes all publications by NIOSH and all records contain abstracts. Information is obtained from more than 400 core journals, monographs and technical reports. These are supplemented by references to articles from other periodicals related to the Occupational Health and Safety sector. The database is a retrospective one, indexing materials dating back into the 1800s.

160 core English-language journals.

All records are indexed with the NIOSH controlled vocabulary.

20:389 Online   ARAMIS

File name	NIOSHTIC
Start year	
Number of records	
Update period	

20:390 Online   CCINFOline

File name	NIOSHTIC
Start year	
Number of records	
Update period	

20:391 Online   CompuServe Information Service

File name	IQUEST File 1035
Start year	1973
Number of records	169,107
Update period	Quarterly
Price/Charges	Subscription: US$8.95 per month
	Database entry fee: US$9/search; some databases carry a surcharge ($2–75)
	Online print: US$10 references free; then $9 per ten; abstracts $3 each

Downloading is allowed

Notes

Accessed via IQUEST or IQMEDICAL, this database is offered by a DIALOG gateway. IQUEST can either search across all databases, a database of the user's choice or selected multiple databases.

20:392 Online   DIALOG

File name	File 161
Start year	1973
Number of records	169,107
Update period	Quarterly
Price/Charges	Connect time: US$72.00
	Online print: US$0.55
	Offline print: US$0.55

Notes

DIALINDEX Categories: POLLUT, REGS, RNMED, SAFETY, TOXICOL.

20:393 Online   ESA-IRS

File name	File 236
Start year	1973
Number of records	162,000
Update period	
Database aids	ESA-QUEST User Manual, ESA-QUEST Mini Manual, ESA-QUEST Pocket Guide, Output Formats on ESA-IRS Infosheet and ESA-QUEST Technical Notes
Price/Charges	Subscription: UK£70.29
	Database entry fee: UK£3.49
	Online print: UK£0.59 – 0.56
	Offline print: UK£0.59
	SDI charge: UK£2.10

Downloading is allowed
Thesaurus is online

Notes

Online ordering of original documents is available through QUESTORDER. The basic index includes the data fields Abstract, Controlled Terms, Single Controlled Terms and Title. The LIMIT command can be used to limit all subsequent sets. This limitation can be cancelled by entering a new LALL or a BEGIN command.

From 1993 ESA-IRS are charging an annual fee of 100 Accounting Units (c.UK£ 70.29) to all users. This is equivalent to the fee for full documentation and will not be charged to customers already paying for documentation.

Record composition

Abstract /AB; Author(s) AU; CAS Registry Number RN; CODEN CO; Controlled Terms /CT; Journal Name JN; Language LA; Native Number NN; Number of Report NR; Publication Date PD; Publication Year PY; Single Controlled Terms /ST; Title /TI and Update UP

20:394 Online   MIC/Karolinska Institute Library and Information Center (MIC KIBIC)

File name	NIOSHTIC
Start year	1974
Number of records	154,000
Update period	Quarterly

20:395 Online   ORBIT

File name	NIOS
Start year	1900
Number of records	170,000
Update period	Quarterly
Database aids	Quick Reference Guide (2/88) Free (single copy)

This database can also be found on:
CCINFOdisc Series C1 – NIOSHTIC
OSH-ROM
Worksafe Disc
TOXLINE

NMD'S Tablettidentifikasjonsdatabase

Arbeids-og administrasjonsdepartementet
Dagens Nöringsliv Norsk Medisinaldepot

20:397 Master record

Alternative name(s)	TABID
Database type	Factual, Textual
Number of journals	
Sources	
Start year	1987
Language	Norwegian and English
Coverage	
Number of records	1,200
Update size	—
Update period	

Keywords

Pharmaceutical Products

Description

Database for identification of unknown tablets and capsules. Description of known products.

Listings on demand.

20:398 Online   AET

File name	Tabid Eregin
Start year	1987
Number of records	1,200
Update period	

20:399 Online   LOVDATA

File name   LOVDATA
Start year   1987
Number of records   1,200
Update period

20:400 Online   Norsk Medisinaldepot (NMD)

File name   Tabid
Start year   1987
Number of records   1,200
Update period
Price/Charges   Subscription: Norwegian krone500.00 (connection fee)
Connect time: Free

Notes

Open to pharmacies and hospitals. Other users may be admitted. Application to the Norwegian Medicinal Depot.

Nuclear Science Abstracts

US Department of Energy, Office of Scientific and Technical Information (OSTI), Integrated Technical Information System (ITIS)

20:401 Master record

Alternative name(s)   NSA
Database type   Bibliographic
Number of journals
Sources   Technical reports, Books, Conference proceedings, Journals, Patents, Dissertations, Technical drawings, Research reports and Government departments
Start year   1948–1976
Language   English
Coverage   International
Number of records   947,000
Update size   —
Update period   Not updated

Keywords

Nuclear Medicine; Physics

Description

Nuclear Science Abstracts is a comprehensive abstract and index collection of international nuclear science and technology literature. Included in the file are scientific and technical reports of the US Atomic Energy Commission, US Energy Research and Development Administrators and associated contractors, and other agencies, universities, and industrial and research organizations. All aspects of nuclear science and technology are covered.

For material from 1977 to date, see Energy Science and Technology database. Corresponds to *Nuclear Science Abstracts*, 1947–1966 and *Nuclear Science Abstracts-II*, 1967–1976. NSA is accessible only in countries which have bilateral exchange agreements with the US Department of Energy, that is, UK and Northern Ireland, Italy, Japan, Spain, France, the Netherlands, Norway, Finland, Denmark, Sweden, Canada and Switzerland.

20:402 Online   DIALOG

File name   File 109
Alternative name(s)   NSA
Start year   1948–1976
Number of records   944,236
Update period   Closed File

Price/Charges   Connect time: US$84.00
Online print: US$0.40
Offline print: US$0.40

Notes

The file is a companion to the DOE Energy Science and Technology File 103 which contains nuclear information processed by the Department of Energy Office of Scientific and Technical Information (OSTI) since 1976.

20:403 Online   US Department of Energy, Office of Scientific and Technical Information (OSTI)

File name
Alternative name(s)   NSA
Start year   1948–1976
Number of records   944,236
Update period   Closed File

Notes

The file is a companion to the DOE Energy Science and Technology File which contains nuclear information processed by the Department of Energy Office of Scientific and Technical Information (OSTI) since 1976.

Occupational Health & Safety: Seven Critical Issues

Bureau of National Affairs Inc

20:404 Master record

Alternative name(s)   BNA Occupational Health & Safety: Seven Critical Issues
Database type   Textual
Number of journals
Sources   Report
Start year   1989 only
Language   English
Coverage   USA
Number of records
Update size   —
Update period   Not updated

Keywords

Criminal Prosecution; Haematology; Hazardous Substances; Legislation; Occupational Health and Safety; Recordkeeping

Description

A special report covering past activities and future concerns of the Occupational Safety and Health Administration. Topics include criminal prosecution, high-risk notification, chemical exposure, recordkeeping, blood-borne diseases and right-to-act legislation. Also includes case studies, court decisions and pending legislation.

Corresponds to *Occupational Health & Safety: Seven Critical Issues*, a special report of the Occupational Safety and Health Administration.

20:405 Online   Executive Telecom System International, Human Resource Information Network (ETSI/HRIN)

File name
Alternative name(s)   BNA Occupational Health & Safety: Seven Critical Issues
Start year   1989 only

Number of records
Update period   Not updated

Notes
Annual subscription to ETSI/HRIN required.

OKU CD-ROM
Accu-MemSystems

20:406 Master record
Database type	Factual, Textual
Number of journals	1
Sources	Books and Journal
Start year	
Language	
Coverage	
Number of records	
Update size	–
Update period	

Keywords
Orthopaedics

Description
Contains three volumes of *Orthopedic Knowledge Update* (published 1984, 1987, and 1990). Also contains the *Journal of Bone and Joint Surgery*.

20:407 CD-ROM   Accu-MemSystems
File name	
Format notes	Mac, IBM
Software	Personal Librarian
Start year	
Number of records	
Update period	

OLIO+
American Osteopathic Association

20:408 Master record
Database type	Bibliographic
Number of journals	
Sources	Monographs, Books, Journals, Associations, Colleges and Clinicians
Start year	1933
Language	English
Coverage	International
Number of records	12,000
Update size	3,600
Update period	Monthly

Keywords
Osteopathy

Description
Citations, with abstracts, to the international literature on osteopathy.

20:409 Online   American Osteopathic Association (AOA)
File name	
Start year	1933

Number of records   12,000
Update period   Monthly

Notes
Annual subscription of $75 required.

Oncodisc
National Cancer Institute, US National Institutes of Health

20:410 Master record
CD-ROM	JB Lippincott Company
Database type	Bibliographic, Directory, Textual
Number of journals	
Sources	Clinicians, directories, conference proceedings, government publications, journals, monographs, research reports, theses and textbooks
Start year	
Language	English
Coverage	International
Number of records	
Update size	–
Update period	Six times per year

Keywords
Cancer

Description
Oncodisc is divided into two databases, Cancerlit and Physicians Data Query (PDQ) both of which are produced by the US National Cancer Institute (NCI).

Cancerlit includes citations from the last three years of the National Cancer Institute's Cancerlit database of over 650,000 citations with abstracts of published cancer literature.

Physicians Data Query is comprised of three files: a protocol file of more than 1,000 active clinical trials; a cancer file containing prognostic and treatment information on all major forms of cancer, including up-to-date information on prognosis, relevant staging and cellular classification systems, and listings of appropriate treatment options by type and stage of cancer; a directory file of 12,000 physicians and 1,400 health care organisations related to cancer care.

The disc also includes the full text of three Lippincott textbooks and reference works: *Cancer: Principles and Practice of Oncology*, 3rd edition; *Important Advances in Oncology* 1985, 1986, 1987, 1988 (four volumes); and *Manual for Staging of Cancer*, 3rd edition.

For more details of constituent databases, see:
Cancerlit
Physician's Data Query – PDQ

Orphan Drug Database
National Organization for Rare Disorders (NORD)

20:412 Master record
Database type	Directory, Textual
Number of journals	
Sources	Government departments and Pharmacopoeias
Start year	1983
Language	English
Coverage	USA

Number of records   400
Update size   –
Update period   Monthly

Keywords

Rare Diseases; Drugs; Therapeutic Agents

Description

Information on over 400 orphan drugs (that is, thera-peutic agents providing treatment for less than 200,000 US residents). Includes US FDA-approved and experimental drugs, giving brand and generic names, indicated diseases and manufacturer data.

20:413 Online   CompuServe Information Service

File name
Start year   1983
Number of records   400
Update period   Monthly
Price/Charges   Subscription: US$8.95 per month
Downloading is allowed

OrthoLine Biomedical Literature Reference Volume 1
Aries Systems Corporation

20:414 Master record

Database type   Bibliographic
Number of journals   70
Sources   Journals
Start year   Most recent ten years
Language   English
Coverage   International
Number of records
Update size   –
Update period   Annually/Quarterly/Monthly
Index unit   Articles

Keywords

Orthopaedics

Description

An archive of references from approximately seventy orthopaedics-related journals which includes material indexed by the National Library of Medicine during the last ten years. Part of a two-volume set: Volume 2 contains a subset of MEDLINE containing ten years of orthopaedics literature.

20:415 CD-ROM   Aries Systems Corporation

File name   OrthoLine Biomedical Literature Reference Volume 1
Format notes   IBM, Mac
Software   Knowledge Finder
Start year   Most recent ten years
Number of records
Update period   Annually/Quarterly/Monthly
Price/Charges   Subscription: US$595 – 2,595

Notes

One of a two-volume/disc set.

Price varies depending on frequency of updates: Monthly, Quarterly, or Annually.

OTC Market Report: Update USA
Nicholas Hall & Company

20:416 Master record

Database type   Textual
Number of journals   1
Sources   Newsletter

Start year   1990
Language   English
Coverage   USA and Canada
Number of records   –
Update size   –
Update period   Monthly

Keywords

Company Profiles; Health Care Products; Hygiene Products; Marketing; Market Reports

Description

Containing the full text of *OTC Market Report*, a news-letter covering the over-the-counter health and hy-giene products market in the USA and Canada. Includes company profiles, product and market re-ports, new product announcements and 'hard data' dealing with the market size and market share in OTC markets.

Corresponds to *OTC Market Report: Update USA* monthly newsletter. On DIALOG and Data-Star this database is available as part of the PTS Newsletter Database.

This database can be found on:
PTS Newsletter Database

OTC News & Market Report
Nicholas Hall & Company

20:418 Master record

Database type   Textual
Number of journals   1
Sources
Start year   1989
Language   English
Coverage   Europe
Number of records
Update size   –
Update period   Monthly

Keywords

Advertising; Company Profiles; Health Care Products; Hygiene Products

Description

Contains the full text of the monthly newsletter cover-ing the over-the-counter health and hygiene products trade in the European market. Includes product re-ports at a country level, company profiles of industry leaders, new products, company mergers and acqui-sitions, expansions, financial performance, advertis-ing and strategic direction.

Corresponds to *OTC News & Market Report* monthly newsletter.On DIALOG and Data-Star this newsletter is made available as part of the PTS Newsletter Database.

This database can be found on:
PTS Newsletter Database

Oxford Textbook of Medicine (OTM)
Oxford Electronic Publishing

20:420 Master record

Database type   Textual
Number of journals
Sources   Monograph

Start year	1987
Language	English
Coverage	International
Number of records	
Update size	–
Update period	Not updated

Keywords

Internal Medicine

Description

The text of the *Oxford Textbook of Medicine*, 2nd edition, acclaimed as the most comprehensive and up-to-date textbook to cover the entire range of internal medicine, on a single compact disc along with 5 electronic indexes. Consists of articles by 396 contributors who are specialists in the many aspects of medicine, contained in 28 sections, concentrating on British practice but with contributions from many international experts. Covers epidemiology, diagnosis, clinical details, treatments and side effects.

20:421 CD-ROM   Oxford Electronic Publishing

File name	Oxford Textbook of Medicine – Electronic edition
Format notes	IBM, Mac
Start year	1987
Number of records	
Update period	Not updated
Price/Charges	Subscription: UK£305 – 395

Notes

Only the text of the printed version is reproduced; figures and tables have not been included. As the database is equivalent to the 2nd edition, the information dates back to 1987 and is not updated, so that with this reasonably dynamic subject, the text may only be useful for background information and other current literature would need to be consulted in addition.

Offers rapid access to text – any word, phrase or combination of words which appear anywhere within the text can be located quickly.

Purchase price for the CD: UK and EEC £305; Rest of the world £395.

PAROL
NIVC AN SSSR

20:422 Master record

Database type	Bibliographic
Number of journals	
Sources	
Start year	1982
Language	English
Coverage	
Number of records	660,000
Update size	–
Update period	

Keywords

Biology; Patents

Description

Patent information to world advances in biology.

20:423 Diskette   NIVC AN SSSR

File name	PAROL
Start year	1982

Number of records	660,000
Update period	

Patient Health Education
Veteran's Administration

20:424 Master record

Database type	Bibliographic
Number of journals	
Sources	Journals, Monographs, Pamphlets and A-V material
Start year	1986
Language	English
Coverage	USA (primarily) and International (some)
Number of records	
Update size	–
Update period	Quarterly

Description

Contains references to health education programmes, designed for Veteran's Administration (VA) patients, on a variety of topics (for example, schizophrenia, weight control). Covers programme goals, methods and strategies, and available print and nonprint materials.

Language is primarily English, with some coverage of materials in other languages.

This database can be found on:
Combined Health Information Database

Pestline
Occupational Health Services Inc (OHS)

20:426 Master record

Database type	Textual, Factual
Number of journals	
Sources	Government departments, Associations and Monograph
Start year	Current information
Language	English
Coverage	International
Number of records	1,100
Update size	–
Update period	Daily

Keywords

Occupational Health and Safety; Hazardous Chemicals; Fire; First Aid; Explosion; Pollution

Description

Material Safety Data Sheets for chemicals used in the manufacture of agricultural chemicals. Each entry gives names (chemical, product, synonyms), chemical family, physical data, components, contaminants, US and international exposure limits, National Fire Protection Association ratings, fire and explosion hazards, transportation, storage and disposal, spill and leak procedures, protective equipment, health effects and first aid procedures.

20:427 Online   Executive Telecom System International, Human Resource Information Network (ETSI/HRIN)

File name	
Start year	Current information

Number of records | 1,100
Update period | Daily

Notes

Annual subscription to ETSI/HRIN required.

20:428 Online — Occupational Health Services Inc (OHS)

File name |
Start year | Current information
Number of records | 1,100
Update period | Daily

Notes

Monthly subscription to OHS required.

Pharma-Digest

Société Suisse de Pharmacie

20:429 Master record

Database type |
Number of journals |
Sources |
Start year |
Language | English
Coverage | Switzerland
Number of records |
Update size | –
Update period |

Keywords

Drugs; Pharmaceuticals; Surgery

Description

This database in the medical and pharmaceutical field forms part of the MediROM and PharmaROM CD-ROMs, originally intended for Swiss pharmacists.

This database can be found on:
PharmaROM

PharmaBiomed Business Journals

Predicasts International Inc

20:431 Master record

Alternative name(s) | PTPB; Predicasts PharmaBiomed Business Journals
Database type | Factual, Textual
Number of journals | 30
Sources | Journals
Start year | 1990
Language | English
Coverage | International
Number of records |
Update size | –
Update period | Weekly
Thesaurus | PTS Company Thesaurus
Database aids | PTS User's Manual, 1989 ed.

Keywords

Biotechnology; Health Care; Marketing; Ophthalmology; Pharmaceuticals

Description

PTPB contains the full text of over thirty journals from international trade publications in pharmaceuticals, biotechnology and healthcare, including *Health Business; Pharmaceutical Manufacturing Review;*

Japan Report: Medical Technology; In Vivo: The Business and Medicine Report; Antiviral Agents Bulletin; and *Ophthalmology Times.* Of use to information professionals, researchers and consultants for information on methods and techniques, business practices, new products, companies, markets, market share, research and development, regulations and applied technology in this field. All documents in the database are full text.

Information is selected from a growing list (currently 30) of trade journals from the pharmaceutical, biotechnology and healthcare industries.

The database is indexed with Predicasts' Product, Event and Country codes.

20:432 Online — Data-Star

File name | PTPB
Alternative name(s) | PTPB; Predicasts PharmaBiomed Business Journals
Start year | 1990
Number of records |
Update period | Weekly
Price/Charges | Subscription: UK£32.00
 | Connect time: UK£80.40
 | Online print: UK£0.00 – 0.49
 | Offline print: UK£0.10 – 0.73
 | SDI charge: UK£4.00

Notes

From June 1993 Data-Star have introduced an annual fee/subscription per contract (that is, not per password) of SFr 80.00 (c.UK£ 32.00) payable every June. For North American customers billed in dollars who also use DIALOG, the DIALOG fee also covers access to Data-Star. Academic customers, 'commitment' customers and customers currently billed in dollars are exempt.

20:433 Database subset
Online — Data-Star

File name | TRPT – PharmaBiomed Business Journals Training database
Alternative name(s) | PTPB; Predicasts PharmaBiomed Business Journals.
Start year | 1990
Number of records |
Update period | Weekly
Price/Charges | Connect time: UK£Free

Notes

Free training database from Data-Star for Pharma-Biomed Business Journals.

PharmaROM

OFAC
Bureau van Dijk
Galenica
Médecine et Hygiéne
OVP – Editions du Vidal
Société Suisse de Pharmacie
Telmed
Georg Thieme Verlag

20:434 Master record

Database type | Factual
Number of journals |
Sources |

Start year
Language — French, English and German
Coverage — Switzerland
Number of records
Update size
Update period — Twice a year

Keywords

Drugs; Drug Therapy; Pharmaceuticals; Surgery; Travel

Description

Primarily destined for the Swiss pharmacists.

Notes

Twelve databases in the pharmaceutical and health care fields, including: Dictionnaire Vidal; Index Nominum; Interactions of the Medical Letter; Interactions de la Société Suisse de Pharmacie; Pharma-Digest; Phytotherapie; Teledoc Galenica; Thermalisme; Vergiftungen; Voyages et Santé. Logical links are possible within the data of some databases.

For more details of constituent databases, see:
Dictionnaire Vidal
Index Nominum
Interactions of the Medical Letter
Interactions de la Société Suisse de Pharmacie
Pharma-Digest
Phytotherapie
Teledoc Galenica
Thermalisme
Vergiftungen
Voyages et Santé

Physician Library
Ellis Enterprises

20:436 Master record

Database type — Factual, Bibliographic
Number of journals
Sources
Start year
Language — English
Coverage
Number of records
Update size — —
Update period

Description

Collected full texts of medical manuals and textbooks in specialty and subspecialty domains.

20:437 CD-ROM — Ellis Enterprises

File name — Physician Library
Format notes — IBM
Start year
Number of records
Update period
Price/Charges — Subscription: US$1,000

This database can also be found on:
Home Reference Library

Physician's Desk Reference
Medical Economics Company Inc

20:439 Master record

Alternative name(s) — PDR
Database type — Factual
Number of journals
Sources — Pharmacopoeias and Monographs

Start year — Current information
Language — English
Coverage — USA
Number of records — 2,750
Update size — —
Update period — Monthly

Keywords

Drugs; Ophthalmology; Pharmaceutical Products

Description

Contains the complete text of the current year's edition of three important reference works: *Physician's Desk Reference, Physician's Desk Reference for Non-Prescribed Drugs* and *Physicians Desk Reference for Ophthalmology*, together with the entire contents of PDR's Drug Interactions and Side Effects Index. Also includes all official FDA- approved labelling in the PDR and companion volumes. Contains full, official prescribing information on prescription and over-the-counter pharmaceuticals plus drug interactions and side effects, as found in the *Drug Interactions and Side Effects Index* and the *Indications Index*. Features include interactions checks, split-screen comparisons and free-text searching. Prescribing information for trade name pharmaceutical products, over-the-counter products and ophthalmological preparations, including manufacturer, generic description, indications, precautions, interactions, adverse reactions, dosage and administration, overdose management, contraindications and patient instructions.

Corresponds to all five volumes: *Physicians' Desk Reference, Physicians' Desk Reference for Nonprescription Drugs, Physicians' Desk Reference for Ophthalmology, Physicians' Desk Reference Drug Information and Side Effects Index,* and *Physicians' Desk Reference Indications Index.*

20:440 Online — Chemical Information Systems Inc (CIS)

File name — Physician's Desk Reference
Alternative name(s) — PDR
Start year — Current information
Number of records — 2,750
Update period — Monthly

Notes

Annual subscription of $300 to CIS required.

20:441 CD-ROM — Medical Economics Company Inc

File name — Physician's Desk Reference
Alternative name(s) — PDR
Format notes — IBM
Start year — Current information
Number of records — 2,750
Update period — Annually
Price/Charges — Subscription: UK£330 – 595

Notes

Contains the full text of PDR, plus all the prescribing information in PDR for Nonprescription Drugs and PDR for Ophthalmology, and the entire contents of PDR's Drug Interactions and Side Effects Index on a single disc, without illustrations. While the print volumes serve as a handy reference work for the health consumer, the CD-ROM is aimed at the health professional. The user is offered a product look-up blank which is the easiest and quickest means of retrieving information on a specific drug. The beginning of each monograph states 'Information based on official labeling in effect date'.

Also features a facility for creating patient files containing treatment regimens, allowing automatic screening for drug interactions.

A version additionally containing the *Merck Manual* of diagnosis and therapy is also available, cost is: for annual subscription £595, subscription renewal £530. Searching possible by brand name, generic ingredient, therapeutic category, interaction potential, side effect or manufacturer.

In an overview of general health CD-ROMs, Nicholas Tomaiuolo noted that the major difference between Physicians' Desk Reference and USP DI is that 'the latter is the only published reference work that uses a structured review system contributed to by experts. The PDR contains basically recapitulated drug package inserts provided by pharmaceutical manufacturers' (*CD-ROM World* 8(1) January 1993 p 38–49).

20:442 CD-ROM   Medical Economics Company Inc

File name	Physician's Desk Reference with Merck Manual
Alternative name(s)	PDR
Format notes	IBM
Start year	Current information
Number of records	2,750
Update period	Monthly
Price/Charges	Subscription: US$895

Notes
Contains the full text without illustrations. While the print volumes serve as a handy reference work for the health consumer, the CD-ROM is aimed at the health professional. The user is offered with a product look-up blank which is the easiest and quickest means of retrieving information on a specific drug. The beginning of each monograph states 'Information based on official labeling in effect date'. Enhanced with the *Merck Manual* on the same disc, this version allows users to locate a disorder in Merck and zoom directly to the proper medication entry in PDR.

Also features a facility for creating patient files containing treatment regimens, allowing automatic screening for drug interactions.

Phytotherapie
Telmed

20:443 Master record

Database type	
Number of journals	
Sources	
Start year	
Language	French
Coverage	Switzerland
Number of records	
Update size	—
Update period	

Keywords
Drugs; Pharmaceuticals; Surgery

Description
This database in the medical and pharmaceutical field forms part of the MediROM and PharmaROM CD-ROMs, originally intended for Swiss pharmacists.

This database can be found on:
MediROM
PharmaROM

Plantas Medicinales
Ministerio de Sanidad y Consumo de España, Dirección General de Farmacia y Productos Sanitarios, Servicio de Gestión del Banco de Datos de Medicamentos

20:445 Master record

Alternative name(s)	Herbal Remedies
Database type	Textual
Number of journals	
Sources	Pharmacopoeias and Government departments
Start year	1988
Language	Spanish
Coverage	Spain
Number of records	3,100
Update size	—
Update period	Daily, as new data become available

Keywords
Alternative Medicine; Medicinal Plants; Herbal Remedies

Description
Descriptions of medicinal plants registered or awaiting registration for use in Spain, giving name, therapeutic group, active and excipient ingredients, dosage and administration, producing laboartory, price and administrative information.

20:446 Online   Ministerio de Sanidad y Consumo de España, Dirección General de Farmacia y Productos Sanitarios, Servicio de Gestión del Banco de Datos de Medicamentos

File name	
Alternative name(s)	Herbal Remedies
Start year	1988
Number of records	3,100
Update period	Daily, as new data become available

PLASTBASE
Arbejdsmiljoinstituttet

20:447 Master record

Database type	Bibliographic
Number of journals	
Sources	

Start year   1987
Language   Danish
Coverage   Denmark
Number of records   1,000
Update size   —
Update period

Keywords

Chemical Substances; Occupational Health and Safety; Air Pollution; Ophthalmology; Plastics; Respiration; Rhinology

Description

Information on the chemical and toxicological aspects of air pollution in the plastics industry, with emphasis on the eye, the nose, and respiration. 64 types of plastic with 465 product names are registered on the database.

Available only in diskette format.

Plastics products in Denmark.

20:448 Diskette   Arbejdsmiljofonden, Denmark

File name   PLASTBASE
Start year   1987
Number of records   1,000
Update period

Population Bibliography
Carolina Population Center, University of North Carolina

20:449 Master record

Database type   Bibliographic
Number of journals
Sources   Monographs, Journals, Technical reports, Government documents, Conference proceedings, Dissertations and Grey literature
Start year   1966 to 1984
Language   English
Coverage
Number of records   67,827
Update size   —
Update period   Not Applicable

Keywords

Demography; Population

Description

Population Bibliography is one of the world's major databases covering monographs, journals, technical reports, government documents, conference proceedings, dissertations, and many unpublished reports on population. Population Bibliography is a principal source for information on abortion, demography, migration, family planning, fertility studies, and all general areas of population research, such as population policy and law, population education, and population research methodology. More comprehensive coverage is given to materials dealing with the socioeconomic aspects than the biomedical aspects of population, and emphasis is on developing countries and the United States. This is a closed file.

20:450 Online   DIALOG

File name   File 91
Start year   1966 to 1984

Number of records   67,827
Update period   Closed File

PRIS
Agriculture Canada

20:451 Master record

Alternative name(s)   Pest Management Research Information System; SILD; Systeme d'Information sur la Lutte Dirigée .
Database type   Textual, Factual, Computer software, Numeric
Number of journals
Sources   Thesaurus, Government departments, Monograph, Research reports and Laws/regulations
Start year   Current information
Language   English
Coverage   Canada
Number of records
Update size   —
Update period   Periodically, as new data become available

Keywords

Biological Control; First Aid; Herbicides; Occupational Health and Safety; Pest Control; Pesticide Residues; Pesticides; Weed Control

Description

Contains five databases and a registration system on pest management products, pesticide research, and biological control methods in use or registered in Canada.

Thesaurus contains cross-references to synonyms used in specific research on agricultural pest control products, covering formulated mixtures and residues, agricultural commodities, pests, biological control agents and other organisms.

Experimental Pest Control Products contains data on current research into new experimental pest control products, giving details on the formulation, biological activity, toxicology, first aid, suggested areas of research and supplier.

Pest Management Research Data contains annual reports from Canadian scientists on the results of efficacy testing of pest control products, covering testing of new and registered products on insect and plant disease pests of agricultural commodities.

Maximum Residue Limits in Foods gives residue limits in agricultural commodities as set by Health and Welfare Canada in the Regulations of the Food and Drugs Act.

Parasitic and Predatory Insect Releases gives records of biological control agent releases in Canada, providing data on the target pest and biological control agent species and the locality of the release, from 1959 to date.

Minor Use Program allows Canadian agricultural users to register for necessary additional use of pest control products, a process not normally addressed in the standard registration procedure.

French-language equivalent database is Systeme d'Information sur la Lutte Dirigée (SILD).

20:452 Online CCINFOline

File name	
Alternative name(s)	Pest Management Research Information System; SILD; Systeme d'Information sur la Lutte Dirigée .
Start year	Current information
Number of records	
Update period	Periodically, as new data become available

Notes

Annual subscription of $C400 in Canada or $US400 elsewhere required.

This database can also be found on:
CCINFOdisc Series A2 – CHEM Data

PROJEKT
Sweden Statens Naturvårdsverk (SNV)

20:454 Master record

Database type	Bibliographic, Textual
Number of journals	
Sources	Research reports
Start year	1970
Language	Original language (titles), Swedish and English (keywords/abstracts)
Coverage	Sweden
Number of records	
Update size	–
Update period	Daily

Keywords

Air Pollution; Civil Engineering; Conservation; Environmental Hygiene; Epidemiology; Ergonomics; Hazardous Waste; Environmental Hygiene; Natural Resources; Noise Pollution; Occupational Health and Safety; Soil Pollution; Toxic Waste; Water Pollution; Wildlife

Description

PROJEKT gives descriptions of environmental research projects Topics covered include: air, noise, water and soil pollution; toxic wastes; natural resources and wildlife; environmental monitoring and technology; environmental hygiene, epidemiology, ergonomics, occupational health and safety and hygiene. This is part of the NATUR database.

This database can be found on:
NATUR

PTS Newsletter Database
Predicasts International Inc

20:456 Master record

Alternative name(s)	Predicasts Newsletter Database
Database type	Textual
Number of journals	
Sources	
Start year	1988
Language	German and English
Coverage	International
Number of records	722,656
Update size	63,000
Update period	Daily
Database aids	PTS Users Manual, Cleveland, Ohio, Predicasts
Hosts have included	CORIS (Thomson Financial Network) (Until 1/92)

Keywords

Acid Rain; Advertising; Air Pollution; Alcohol Abuse; Antiviral Drugs; Asbestos; Asbestosis; Automation and Control; Beauty Care; Beauty Care; Beverages; Biotechnology; Biotechnology Industries; Brewing; Cancer; Ceramics; Chemical Industry; Chromatography; Composites; Computer Data Security; Computer Ergonomics; Company Profiles; Consumer Products; Cosmetics; Data Security; Defence Waste Disposal; Diagnosis; Diagnostic Equipment; Diagnostic Products; Drug Abuse; Drug Treatment; Drugs; Education – Cancer; Electrodialysis; Employee Benefits; Environmental Policy; Ergonomics; Explosion; Filtration; Fire; Food and Drink; Food Additives; Food Processing; Food Technology; Genetic Engineering; Greenhouse Effect; Hazardous Chemicals; Hazardous Substances; Hazardous Substances Transport; Hazardous Waste; Health and Safety; Health Care; Health Care Management; Health Care Products; Health Insurance; Health Services; HIV; Household Products; Hygiene Products; Information Services; Information Systems; Legal Liability; Legislation; Liability Insurance; Manufacturing; Marketing; Market Reports; Materials Industry; Medicare; Medical Equipment; Medical Textiles; Medical Waste Management; Membrane Technology; Metals; Nuclear Waste; Occupational Health and Safety; Packaging; Patents; Personal Hygiene; Pesticides; Pets; Pharmaceutical Industry; Pharmaceutical Products; Pharmaceuticals; Pollution; Polymers; Product Catalogues; Product Liability; Prosthetics; Public Health; Radiation; Research and Development; Separation Technology; Smoking; Standards; Textiles; Waste Management; Water Pollution; Water Purification

Description

Produced by Predicasts, PTS Newsletter is a multi-industry database providing concise information on company activities, new technologies, emerging industry trends, government regulations and international trade opportunities. It consists of the full text of over 500 business and industry newsletters covering almost fifty different industries and subject areas. It is international in scope, covering all major economic and political regions of the world, including Eastern and Western Europe, the USA, the Pacific Rim, Latin America, Asia and the Middle East. Facts, figures and analyses are provided on the following industrial and geographical areas: advanced materials, biotechnology, broadcasting and publishing, computers and electronics, chemicals, defense and aerospace, energy, environment, financial services and markets, instrumentation, international trade, general technology, Japan, Middle East, manufacturing, medical and health, materials packaging, research and development, telecommunications and transportation.

Newsletters include *Multinational Service* which covers decisions and policies affecting corporations operating worldwide; and *Europe Report* which offers broad coverage of EC activities relating to economic and monetary affairs, the internal market and legislation and regulations relating to business. Both Newsletters are published by the Europe Information Service of Cooper's & Lybrand Europe. Middle East coverage includes the *Israel High-Tech Report; The Middle East News Network*; and *The Middle East Consultants' Newsletter*.

20:457 Online Data-Star

File name	PTBN
Alternative name(s)	Predicasts Newsletter Database

Start year	January 1988
Number of records	533,000
Update period	Weekly
Database aids	Data-Star Business Manual, Berne and Online manual (search for NEWS-PTBN in NEWS)
Price/Charges	Subscription: UK£32.00
	Connect time: UK£80.40
	Online print: UK£0.28 – 0.55
	Offline print: UK£0.26 – 1.00
	SDI charge: UK£4.00

Also available on FIZ Technik via a gateway from Data-Star

Notes

From June 1993 Data-Star have introduced an annual fee/subscription per contract (that is, not per password) of SFr 80.00 (c.UK£ 32.00) payable every June. For North American customers billed in dollars who also use DIALOG, the DIALOG fee also covers access to Data-Star. Academic customers, 'commitment' customers and customers currently billed in dollars are exempt.

20:458 Online   DIALOG

File name	File 636
Alternative name(s)	Predicasts Newsletter Database
Start year	1989
Number of records	722,656
Update period	Daily
Price/Charges	Connect time: US$126.00
	Online print: US$0.90
	Offline print: US$0.90
	SDI charge: US$1.00 (daily) – 3.00 (weekly)

Notes

This is the main file of PTS on DIALOG. There is also a menu access version – PTSNL, which enables the user to retrieve the latest issue of a newsletter, print the full text of newspaper articles, etc. It does not have the full range of DIALOG search commands.

20:459 Online   DIALOG

File name	PTSNL
Alternative name(s)	Predicasts Newsletter Database
Start year	1989
Number of records	722,656
Update period	Daily
Price/Charges	Connect time: US$126.00
	Online print: US$0.90

Notes

PTSNL is a menu-access version of the PTS Newsletter Database. PTSNL provides users with the unique capability to easily retrieve the latest issue (or any available issue) of a newsletter, display a Table of Contents listing articles contained in a selected issue, and print the full text of newsletter articles selected by title. To search newsletters for information on specific subjects, use File 636 (the main PTS file), which utilises the full range of DIALOG search commands.

20:460 Online   Dow Jones News/Retrieval

File name	
Alternative name(s)	Predicasts Newsletter Database
Start year	
Number of records	
Update period	Weekly

20:461 Online   FIZ Technik (gateway)

File name	PTBN
Alternative name(s)	Predicasts Newsletter Database
Start year	1988 (January)

Number of records	Volume 1: 159,000
Update period	Weekly
Price/Charges	Connect time: SFr201.00
	Online print: SFr0.61 – 1.22
	Offline print: SFr0.24 – 1.83
	SDI charge: SFr10.00

Available via a gateway to Data-Star

For more details of constituent databases, see:
AIDS Weekly
Air/Water Pollution Report
Alliance Alert – Medical Health
Antiviral Agents Bulletin
Applied Genetics News
Asbestos Control Report
BBI Newsletter
Biomedical Materials
Biomedical Polymers
Cancer Weekly
Cosmetic Insiders' Report
Diagnostics Business-Matters
Environment Week
European Cosmetic Markets
FDA Medical Bulletin
Food Chemical News
Genetic Technology News
Hazmat Transport News
Health Business
Health Daily
Industrial Health and Hazards Update
International Product Alert
Japan Report: Medical Technology
Japan Science Scan
Managed Care Law Outlook
Managed Care Outlook
Managed Care Report
Medical Bulletin
Medical Scan
Medical Waste News
Medical Textiles
Membrane and Separation Technology News
National Report on Computers and Health
Nuclear Waste News
Occupational Health and Safety Letter
OTC Market Report: Update USA
OTC News and Market Report
Pesticide and Toxic Chemical News
Pharmaceutical Business News
Product Alert
PRODUCTSCAN
Report on Defense Plant Wastes
Soviet Bio/Medical Report
Toxic Materials News
Worldwide Biotech

Radiology, Journal of
CMC ReSearch

20:462 Master record

Database type	Textual
Number of journals	1
Sources	Journal
Start year	
Language	
Coverage	
Number of records	
Update size	–
Update period	

Keywords
Radiology

Description
Full text of newsletter.

20:463 CD-ROM   **CMC ReSearch**

File name
Format notes   IBM
Start year
Number of records
Update period

Rare Disease Database
National Organization for Rare
   Disorders (NORD)

20:464 Master record

Database type	Textual, Bibliographic, Directory
Number of journals	
Sources	
Start year	1985
Language	English
Coverage	USA (primarily) and International
Number of records	900 diseases
Update size	—
Update period	Weekly
Thesaurus	Current Medical Information and Terminology (CMIT)

Keywords

Rare Diseases; Support Groups

Description

Gives information on about 900 rare diseases, including description, nomenclature, symptoms, etiology, related disorders, standard and experimental therapies, and for some diseases, bibliographical references. Also provides information on research in progress (including contact information) and lists of organisations offering support to victims and their families or serving as information clearinghouses. Data are accessible by a 15,000-word thesaurus including 1,500 disease names and CMIT numbers.

20:465 Online   CompuServe Information Service

File name	
Start year	1985
Number of records	900 diseases
Update period	Weekly
Price/Charges	Subscription: US$8.95 per month
Downloading is allowed	

Red Sage
University of California, Los Angeles
Springer-Verlag

20:466 Master record

Database type	Image, Textual, Factual
Number of journals	29
Sources	Journals
Start year	1993
Language	English
Coverage	USA, Germany and International
Number of records	
Update size	—
Update period	
Index unit	Articles, Letters and Editorials

Keywords

Radiology; Microbiology

Description

Red Sage places text, graphics and photographs of nine radiology journals, and by the end of 1993, twenty microbiology journals online.

The project is functioning for students at the University of California initially; if the Californian installation is successful, the service will be introduced to other US colleges and universities. Export to Europe is ultimately possible.

Centres on journals published by Springer-Verlag.

20:467 Online   University of California, Los Angeles

File name	
Software	RightPages
Start year	1993
Number of records	
Update period	

Notes

The Red Sage project with AT&T Laboratories' RightPages software aims to pass on the look and feel of a library at the terminal; thus users are first offered an array of journal covers on their screen from which they select an issue. This then shows the Table of Contents page from which an article may be selected. Issues may also be browsed page by page and individuals may create personal interest profiles so that they are e-mailed every time a matching article enters the database. The software also supports 'hyper-paper' features which allow users to point to a certain reference in the text, for example to a figure on another page, and view the image.

Reisemedizin

20:468 Master record

Database type	Textual, Factual
Number of journals	
Sources	
Start year	
Language	German
Coverage	Switzerland
Number of records	
Update size	—
Update period	
Hosts have included	AEK (AerzteKasse)

Keywords

Drugs; Pharmaceuticals; Surgery

Description

This is one of ten databases in the medical and pharmaceutical fields on the MediROM database. It is possible to establish logical links between the data of some of the databases.

This database can be found on:
MediROM

SARATEXT
Micromedex Inc

20:470 Master record

Database type	Factual, Bibliographic
Number of journals	
Sources	Standards and Laws/regulations

Start year
Language   English
Coverage   USA
Number of records   366 chemicals
Update size   —
Update period

Keywords

Chemical Substances; Clinical Medicine; Dangerous Chemicals; Hazardous Substances; Occupational Health and Safety

Description

The SARATEXT chemical database module offers a complete source of information on the acute and chronic health effects and recommendations for medical treatment for individuals exposed to any of the chemicals listed on the SARA Title III Extremely Hazardous Substances (EHS) list. The possibility of such accidents makes it necessary for organisations that handle chemicals to comply with specific reporting requirements for such substances. This is the complete source for SARA TITLE III Mandated Health Effects and Medical treatment Information Reporting. Sara Title III (the Superfund Amendments and Reauthorization Act) specifies reporting of medical evaluation and treatmnt information when the amount of chemical accidentally released exceeds a predetermined Reportable Quantity (RQ). For many of these chemicals, a statutory RQ of only 1 pound is established. In addition to the identity and amount of material released, information regarding the acute and chronic health effects of exposure to the substance, as well as recommended medical treatment information, must be reported to the National Respone Center (NRC), the appropriate State Emergency Response Commission (SERC) and the Local Emergency Planning Committee (LEPC). Notification may also be made to local emergency response organizations such as Fire and Police departments, HAZMAT teams, Emergency Medical Services responders and hospital emergency departments. SARATEXT was specifically designed to be a rapidly accesible reference in emergency accidental chemical release situations. It contains a chemical-specific detailed monograph for each of the 366 chemicals currently on the SARA Title III (EHS) list. Monographs for all chemicals on the CERCLA Hazardous Substances (HS) list will be added in the future. Acute and chronic health effects are summarised, as well as listed by organ system. Relevant laboratory tests on clinical and environmental samples are described. Thorough detailed recommended medical treatment information is provided for all routes of exposure: inhalation, dermal, eye, ingestion and range of toxicity is discussed, allowing assessment of the actual human health impact of a release. Relevant occupational and environmental standards and regulations are also included. There is also a user-defined Notifications file, where users can enter the organisation, telephone number, address, contact person(s) and comments for each organization that must be notified should a reportable release occur. It may be revised by the user at any time.

Substance identification and data retrieval are done through chemical name, synonyms and identifying numbers (for example, CAS, NIOSH/RTECS, UN/NA, EPA Hazardous Waste numbers, etc.)

This database can be found on:
TOMES Plus

Scottish Poisons Information Bureau
Royal Infirmary, The Scottish Poisons Information Bureau

20:472 Master record

Database type   Bibliographic, Textual, Factual
Number of journals
Sources
Start year
Language   English
Coverage
Number of records   10,000
Update size   —
Update period   Irregular

Keywords

Biochemistry

Description

The database contains information on ingredients, toxicity, features and treatment of poisonings for about 10,000 products – drugs, household products, plants, pesticides, chemicals and toiletries. It also contains recent references to clinical toxicology literature.

20:473 Online   Royal Infirmary

File name   SPIB
Start year
Number of records   10,000
Update period   Irregular

Search Master Personal Injury Library CD-ROM
Matthew Bender

20:474 Master record

Database type   Factual, Textual
Number of journals
Sources   Books
Start year
Language   English
Coverage   USA
Number of records
Update size   —
Update period   Quarterly

Keywords

Medical Diagnosis

Description

Consists of five publications which cover over 71 volumes of essential legal information. Access to *Attorney's Textbook of Medicine; Personal Injury – Actions, Defenses, Damages; Damages in Tort Actions; Attorney's Dictionary of Medicine;* and *Proving Medical Diagnosis and Prognosis.*

20:475 CD-ROM   Matthew Bender

File name   Search Master Personal Injury
                   Library CD-ROM
Format notes   IBM
Software   Search Master
Start year

Number of records
Update period · · · · Quarterly

SERIX
Sweden National Environmental Protection Board

20:476 Master record
Alternative name(s) · · Swedish Environmental Research Index
Database type · · Bibliographic
Number of journals
Sources · · Grey literature and Research reports
Start year · · 1975
Language · · Swedish and English (titles/abstracts) (about 30%)
Coverage · · Sweden
Number of records · · 17,500
Update size · · SERIX 2,000; PROJOLD 500
Update period · · Daily

Keywords
Air Pollution; Civil Engineering; Conservation; Environmental Hygiene; Epidemiology; Ergonomics; Hazardous Waste; Natural Resources; Noise Pollution; Occupational Medicine; Occupational Hygiene; Soil Pollution; Toxic Waste; Water Pollution; Wildlife

Description
SERIX contains references to environmental research reports, most of which are so called 'grey literature' that is, it is not formally published and therefore hard to retrieve. Contains citations, most with abstracts, to research reports, including descriptions of research projects on environmental issues in Sweden.

Topics covered include: air, noise, water and soil pollution; toxic wastes; natural resources and wildlife; environmental monitoring and technology; environmental hygiene, epidemiology, ergonomics, occupational medicine and hygiene. Each record includes project or report title, project leader or report author, sponsoring organization, research organisation, abstract (when available), and subject and codes for geographic region.

Corresponds to *Swedish Environmental Research*. A backfile, covering 1975 to four years before the present, is available under the name PROJOLD.

20:477 Online · · ARAMIS
File name · · SERIX
Alternative name(s) · · Swedish Environmental Research Index
Start year · · 1975
Number of records · · 17,500
Update period · · Daily

This database can also be found on:
NATUR

Shepard's Catalogue of Teratogen Agents
Micromedex Inc

20:479 Master record
Database type · · Bibliographic, Textual
Number of journals
Sources

Start year · · 1990
Language · · English
Coverage · · International
Number of records · · —
Update size · · —
Update period · · Quarterly

Description
Part of the Reprorisk database, a supplementary product of the Computerized Clinical Information System (CCIS) from Micromedex, which contains several modules addressing the reproductive risk of drugs, chemicals, and physical and environmental agents for females and males.

This database can also be found on:
Reprorisk

Siemens Gefahrstoffdatenbank
Siemens AG

20:480 Master record
Alternative name(s) · · Siemens Database of Dangerous Goods; SIGEDA
Database type · · Factual, Textual
Number of journals
Sources · · Standards, regulations, Research reports and Data sheets
Start year · · 1992 (June)
Language · · German
Coverage · · Germany
Number of records · · 2,828
Update size · · —
Update period · · Quarterly
Index unit · · Chemicals

Keywords
Dangerous Chemicals; Hazardous Substances; Industrial Health and Safety; Occupational Medicine; Toxic Substances

Description
This is a non-bibliographical toxicological database containing information on dangerous substances and mixtures in the industrial area. Covers toxicology, occupational medicine, standards and regulations (mainly German), environmental protection, chemical-physical properties and monitoring methods. Data is derived mainly from security data sheets of chemical companies, research results and listing of substances in mainly German standards and regulations (Gefahrstoffverotdnung, MAK list, etc.). Records include CAS Registry Number, EINECS Number, synonyms, molecular formula, toxicological and occupational health information, standards and regulations, disposal methods, preventive measures, countermeasures in accidents, first medical aid measures and transport regulations.

20:481 Online · · DIMDI
File name · · SG00
Alternative name(s) · · Siemens Database of Dangerous Goods; SIGEDA
Start year · · 1992 (June)
Number of records · · 2,828
Update period · · Quarterly

Price/Charges	Connect time: UK£08.65 – 14.58
	Online print: UK£01.15 – 01.33
	Offline print: UK£01.07 – 01.13
Downloading is allowed	

Notes

Menu driven user guidance is available in both German and English.

SILD
Agriculture Canada

20:482 Master record

Alternative name(s)	Systeme d'Information sur la Lutte Dirigée; PRIS
Database type	Textual, Factual, Computer software, Numeric
Number of journals	
Sources	Thesaurus, Government departments, Monograph and Research reports
Start year	Current information
Language	French
Coverage	Canada
Number of records	
Update size	–
Update period	Periodically, as new data become available

Keywords

Biological Control; First Aid; Herbicides; Occupational Health and Safety; Pest Control; Pesticide Residues; Pesticides; Weed Control

Description

Contains five databases and a registration system on pest management products and biological control methods in use or registered in Canada.

Thesaurus contains cross-references to synonyms used in specific research on agricultural pest control products, covering formulated mixtures and residues, agricultural commodities, pests, biological control agents and other organisms.

Experimental Pest Control Products contains data on current research into new experimental pest control products, giving details on the formulation, biological activity, toxicology, first aid, suggested areas of research and supplier.

Pest Management Research Data contains annual reports from Canadian scientists on the results of efficacy testing of pest control products, covering testing of new and registered products on insect and plant disease pests of agricultural commodities.

Maximum Residue Limits in Foods gives residue limits in agricultural commodities as set by Health and Welfare Canada in the Regulations of the Food and Drugs Act.

Parasitic and Predatory Insect Releases gives records of biological control agent releases in Canada, providing data on the target pest and biological control agent species and the locality of the release, from 1959 to date.

Minor Use Program allows Canadian agricultural users to register for necessary additional use of pest control products, a process not normally addressed in the standard registration procedure.

English-language equivalent database is Pest Management Research Information System.

20:483 Online   CCINFOline

File name	
Alternative name(s)	SILD; PRIS
Start year	Current information
Number of records	
Update period	Periodically, as new data become available

Notes

Annual subscription of $C400 in Canada or $US400 elsewhere required.

This database can also be found on:
CCINFOdisc Series A2 – CHEM Data

Soviet Bio/Medical Report
Newmedia International Japan

20:485 Master record

Database type	Textual
Number of journals	1
Sources	Newsletter
Start year	1991
Language	English
Coverage	Soviet Union
Number of records	
Update size	–
Update period	Monthly

Keywords

Diagnosis; Drug Treatment

Description

Contains the full text of the newsletter *Soviet Bio/Medical Report*. Reviews developments, advances and application of medical treatment, diagnosis, drug treatment and practice in a range of medical specialties in the Soviet Union.

Corresponds to the monthly publication *Soviet Bio/Medical Report* newsletter. Data-Star and DIALOG are supplied with PTS Newsletter Database by Predicast.

This database can be found on:
PTS Newsletter Database

Sports Medicine
Information USA

20:487 Master record

Database type	Factual, Textual
Number of journals	
Sources	
Start year	
Language	English
Coverage	International
Number of records	
Update size	–
Update period	

Keywords

Sport; Sports Medicine

Description

Information is available for all sports people on basic exercise physiology, exercise testing, training, nutrition and general risks versus benefits of exercise. Articles discuss specific sports and give information on each sport's benefits, advantages and disadvantages, and how to get started. Users can keep track of their fitness efforts by using a chart of energy costs for carious activities.

20:488 Online — CompuServe Information Service

File name	INFOUSA
Start year	
Number of records	
Update period	
Price/Charges	Subscription: US$8.95 per month
Downloading is allowed	

STAT!-Ref

Teton Data Systems
Aries Systems Corporation

20:489 Master record
CD-ROM — **Teton Data Systems**

Database type	Textual, Dictionary, Directory, Factual
Number of journals	
Sources	Journals and Books
Start year	
Language	English
Coverage	USA, Europe, Australasia and Asia
Number of records	
Update size	—
Update period	Quarterly
Index unit	Articles

Keywords
Drugs

Description

A library of twenty full-text (plus tables) medical reference textbooks developed by a physician for physicians. Offers instant access to current medical information from a comprehensive range of textbooks, drug references and ten years of selected Clinical MEDLINE abstracts from the National Library of Medicine for either primary care or cardiology.

Contains the full text of twenty leading reference sources for primary care medicine. These include: *Scientific American Medicine* (from Scientific American); *Drug Information* (USP DI Volumes 1 and 2 from US Pharmacopeial Convention Formulary Service); *Current Diagnosis and Treatment – Emergency, Medical, Obstetrics and Gynecology and Surgery* (from Appleton-Lange) *AMA Drug Evaluation*; Honsten's *Drug Interactions; The Medical Letter; Medical Toxicology*; Stedman's *Dictionary; New England Journal of Medicine;* and *Journal of the American Medical Association*. Contains the equivalent of 10,000 to 20,000 printed pages.

One disc contains the user's choice of MEDLINE subset and all the books. The subscription starts at US$ 295 for just the Clinical MEDLINE subset and the books range in price from $40 to $350. A subscription to the entire library is $2,500.

For more details of constituent databases, see:
MEDLINE
USP DI Volume 1: Drug Information for the Health Care Professional
AfterCare Instructions: USP DI Drug Information Leaflets

Summary Files in Ergonomics
Universite de Paris V

20:491 Master record

Database type	Bibliographic, Factual
Number of journals	
Sources	Standards, Monographs, Government documents, Patents and Journals
Start year	Last 30 years
Language	French
Coverage	International
Number of records	
Update size	—
Update period	

Keywords
Anthropology; Ergonomics; Physiology

Description

Contains about 500 citations, with abstracts, to summaries of current or recommended ergonomic standards for environments where humans and machines work together. Documents can be ordered online. Updated as new data become available.

Annual subscription fee of 1200 French francs required.

This database can be found on:
Ergodata

SV
Minitel Publications Ltd

20:493 Master record

Database type	Textual, Factual
Number of journals	
Sources	
Start year	
Language	French
Coverage	International
Number of records	
Update size	—
Update period	
Index unit	Countries

Keywords
Travel; Vaccination

Description

Country by country guide to obligatory and recommended vaccinations. Also contains practical health advice for travelers.

20:494 Videotex — **Minitel**

File name	SV 3615
Start year	

Number of records
Update period

Teledoc Galenica
Galenica

20:495 Master record
Database type
Number of journals
Sources
Start year
Language French
Coverage Switzerland
Number of records
Update size —
Update period

Keywords
Drugs; Pharmaceuticals; Surgery

Description
This database in the medical and pharmaceutical field forms part of the PharmaROM CD-ROM, originally intended for Swiss pharmacists.

This database can be found on:
PharmaROM

Tell Me Why – Volume I and Volume II
Philips Interactive Media of America

20:497 Master record
Database type Multimedia
Number of journals
Sources
Start year
Language English
Coverage International
Number of records
Update size —
Update period

Description
Contains the answers to children's most usual questions, divided into five broad topic areas: Our World; How Things Began; The Human Body; How Things Work; The Zoo. Includes images and sound.

20:498 CD-I   Philips Interactive Media of America
File name Tell Me Why – Volume I and Volume II
Format notes CD-I
Start year
Number of records
Update period

TERIS
Micromedex Inc

20:499 Master record
Alternative name(s) Teratogen Information System
Database type Bibliographic, Textual
Number of journals
Sources

Start year
Language English
Coverage USA and International
Number of records
Update size —
Update period Quarterly

Keywords
Drugs

Description
Teratogen Information System (TERIS) developed by the University of Washington which addresses the teratogenicity of over seven hundred drugs and environmental agents that affect the unborn child.

Part of the Reprorisk database from Micromedex, which contains several modules addressing the reproductive risk of drugs, chemicals, and physical and environmental agents for females and males. Also part of TOMES Plus.

This database can be found on:
Reprorisk

Textbook of Dermatology
Blackwell Scientific Publishing

20:501 Master record
Alternative name(s) Rook's Textbook of Dermatology
Database type Textual, Factual
Number of journals
Sources Monograph
Start year
Language English
Coverage
Number of records
Update size —
Update period

Keywords
Dermatology

Description
The full 3,570 pages and 1,700 illustrations of the fifth edition of the four-volume, world-renowned Rook's *Textbook of Dermatology* are all easily accessible on this single disc. Software allows users to skip from text to reference to illustration at the click of a mouse and to adjust the size of the illustrations.

20:502 CD-ROM   Blackwell Scientific Publishing
File name Textbook of Dermatology on CD-ROM
Alternative name(s) Rook's Textbook of Dermatology
Format notes IBM
Start year
Number of records
Update period
Price UK£275

Notes
Runs under Windows 3.0 or 3.1.

Thermalisme
Telmed

20:503 Master record
Database type
Number of journals
Sources

Start year
Language   French
Coverage   Switzerland
Number of records
Update size   –
Update period

Keywords

Drugs; Pharmaceuticals; Surgery

Description

This database in the medical and pharmaceutical field forms part of the MediROM and PharmaROM CD-ROMs, originally intended for Swiss pharmacists.

This database can be found on:
MediROM
PharmaROM

TOMES
Micromedex Inc

20:505 Master record

Alternative name(s)   Toxicology, Occupational Medicine, Environmental Series; CCIS: TOMES; Computerized Clinical Information System: TOMES
Database type   Factual, Textual, Directory
Number of journals
Sources
Start year   1987
Language   English
Coverage   International
Number of records
Update size   –
Update period   Quarterly

Keywords

Clinical Medicine; Dangerous Chemicals; Occupational Health and Safety; Occupational Medicine

Description

The Toxicology, Occupational Medicine, Environmental Series, a database on over 12,000 chemicals for occupational health and safety is an industrial chemical database with in-depth coverage of clinical effects, range of toxicity, workplace standards, kinetics, and physiochemical parameters. Detailed, comprehensive and referenced protocols for the medical evaluation and treatment of individuals exposed to chemical agents are provided.

Agents are indexed by chemical names, synonyms and commonly associated numbers.

This database can be found on:
CCIS

Toxichem
Info-One International Pty Ltd

20:507 Master record

Database type   Textual, Factual, Directory
Number of journals
Sources
Start year
Language   English
Coverage   Australia

Number of records   50,000
Update size   –
Update period   Quarterly
Index unit   Chemicals

Keywords

Dangerous Chemicals; First Aid

Description

Chemical spillage information for 50,000 chemicals in Australia provided by the West Australian Fire Brigade – details on clean-up, transport, first-aid and emergency action, after-hours details and contacts of 1,000 Australian manufacturers or distributors. Includes 2,000 Material Safety Data Sheets.

Used primarily by fire services throughout Australia.

20:508 CD-ROM   Info-One International Pty Ltd

File name   Toxichem
Format notes   IBM
Software   Fulcrum
Start year
Number of records   50,000
Update period   Quarterly
Price/Charges   Subscription: Australian $6,000

Toxicological Histopathology
Telecity CD-I NV
Open Universiteit Nederland

20:509 Master record

Database type   Multimedia
Number of journals
Sources
Start year
Language   Dutch and English
Coverage
Number of records
Update size   –
Update period   Varies

Keywords

Histopathology.

Description

Multimedia training course for medical students and toxicology specialists.

20:510 CD-I   Telecity CD-I NV

File name   Toxicological Histopathology
Format notes   IBM
Start year
Number of records
Update period   Varies

Travelset
Travelset OY, Finland

20:511 Master record

Database type   Factual
Number of journals
Sources
Start year
Language   Finnish
Coverage   International

1425

Number of records 240,000
Update size –
Update period Daily

Keywords
Immunology; Travel

Description
Travelset contains information about business and holiday trips organised according to subject field and travel destination, including also information about vaccinations and visas.

20:512 Online — Travelset OY, Finland

File name Travelset
Start year
Number of records 240,000
Update period Daily

Notes
Charges according to connect time, no entrance fees or special user agreements needed.

USP DI Volume 1: Drug Information for the Health Care Professional

Micromedex Inc
US Pharmacopeial Convention

20:513 Master record

Alternative name(s)	USP DI Drug Information for the Health Care Professional; Drug Information for the Health Care Professional: USP DI Volume 1; CCIS: USP DI Volume 1
Database type	Factual, Textual
Number of journals	
Sources	Monographs
Start year	1988
Language	English and Spanish
Coverage	USA
Number of records	5,000
Update size	–
Update period	Quarterly

Keywords
Drugs

Description
Published by the US Pharmacopeial Convention, this database provides access to clinically relevant, consensus based, dispensing, prescribing and drug use information, including all medically accepted uses, both labelled and unlabelled, for virtually all US and Canadian medicines. Covers indications, precautions, pharmacology, dosing information and V.A. classifications. It is recognized as a compendium for unlabelled uses, patient counselling, and drug utilisation review in the Medicaid provisions of the Omnibus budget Reconciliation Act of 1990 (OBRA '90). Information is available in Spanish, English and Easy-to-Read (low literacy) versions.

20:514 CD-ROM — Micromedex Inc

File name	CCIS: USP DI Volume 1
Alternative name(s)	USP DI Drug Information for the Health Care Professional; Drug Information for the Health Care Professional: USP DI Volume 1; CCIS: USP DI Volume 1
Start year	1988

Number of records 5,000
Update period Quarterly
Price/Charges Subscription: UK£360

Notes
As part of the CCIS system, this database complements the Drugdex system. The database can be purchased as a standalone product, cost is £360, with a £65 licence fee.

20:515 CD-ROM — SilverPlatter

File name	USP DI Volume 1: Drug Information for the Health Care Professional
Alternative name(s)	USP DI Drug Information for the Health Care Professional; Drug Information for the Health Care Professional: USP DI Volume 1; CCIS: USP DI Volume 1
Start year	1988
Number of records	5,000
Update period	Quarterly

Notes
From 1993, this database is automatically accompanied by USP DI Volume 2, Advice for the Patient.

This database can also be found on:
STAT!-Ref
CCIS
MAXX

Vergiftungen

Georg Thieme Verlag

20:517 Master record

Database type	
Number of journals	
Sources	
Start year	
Language	German
Coverage	
Number of records	
Update size	–
Update period	

Keywords
Drugs; Pharmaceuticals; Surgery

Description
Forms part of the DIAGNOSIS database from Medisoft and the MediROM database from AEK.

This database can also be found on:
DIAGNOSIS, Vergiftungen, Radiolab
MediROM
PharmaROM

Worksafe Disc

Worksafe Australia

20:519 Master record

CD-ROM — Info-One International

Database type	Textual, Directory, Bibliographic
Number of journals	
Sources	
Start year	
Language	English
Coverage	Australia
Number of records	
Update size	–
Update period	Quarterly

Keywords

Accident Prevention; Biological Hazards; Dangerous Chemicals; Epidemiology; Ergonomics; Hazardous Waste; Health Physics; Industrial Materials; Industrial Processes; Metabolism; Occupational Health and Safety; Pathology; Safety Education; Vocational Training; Waste Management

Description

Worksafe contains occupational health and safety data in five databases: Australian Occupational Health and Safety; Australian Exposure Standards; US RTECS and US NIOSHTIC databases; Australia MSDS Repository.

For more details of constituent databases, see:
Australian Occupational Health and Safety
Australian Exposure Standards
RTECS
NIOSHTIC
Australia MSDS Repository

World Atlas v2.01
Software Toolworks
Electromap

20:521 Master record

Alternative name(s)	Software Toolworks World Atlas
Database type	Mapped statistical, Cartographic
Number of journals	
Sources	
Start year	
Language	English
Coverage	International
Number of records	
Update size	—
Update period	

Keywords

Business Travel; Vaccination

Description

Display maps and information that can be displayed as text, maps or graphs. Includes 250 detailed EGA or VGA full colour reference and relief maps; more than 200 world and country reference maps showing major cities, bodies of water and surrounding countries; thirteen world and regional index maps showing the countries within their regions of the world; fifteen world and regional relief maps showing elevations, mountain ranges, deserts, plains, rivers, lakes, etc; three ocean floor relief maps and four ocean surface maps. A software gazeteer allows places to be found on maps. Over 3,300 different statistical maps can be created from the database which includes information from the United Nations, World Health Organisation, CIA, Interpol, World Bank, Population Reference Bureau, US Department of State, World Meteorological Organisation and others. Graphing facilities are limited to a histogram which allows comparisons of statistical data. James Alloway (*CD-ROM World* 8(1) January 1993 p. 73–76) noted that while full-screen bar charts were adequate, the facility allowing the statistical maps to show rectangles of varying sizes to represent the statistic for each country was very limited as frequently there were so many rectangles that they covered the map completely and it was impossible to tell to which country each belonged!

The latest version (early 1993) includes changes in Eastern Europe.

20:522 CD-ROM   Software Toolworks

File name	World Atlas v2.01
Alternative name(s)	Software Toolworks World Atlas
Format notes	IBM, Mac
Start year	
Number of records	
Update period	
Price	UK£85

X-Ray Demonstration
National Library of Medicine

20:523 Master record

Database type	Various data formats included
Number of journals	
Sources	
Start year	
Language	
Coverage	
Number of records	
Update size	—
Update period	

20:524 CD-ROM   National Library of Medicine

File name	X-Ray Demonstration
Format notes	IBM
Start year	
Number of records	
Update period	

ADDRESSES

ADDRESSES

1. 3M Optical Recording Department
Mark Arps (Marketing Manager
   CD-ROM)
Building 223
3M Center
St Paul
MN 55144–1000
USA
Telephone: (612) 736–3274;
         (612) 733–2141
Fax: (612) 733–0158

2. 3T Productions Ltd
Keith Downes (Marketing Director)
Chapel Studio
47/49 Waterloo Road
Stockport
SK1 3BJ
UK
Telephone: 061 476–5553
Fax: 061 476–2988

**3. 3V Multimedia Computersysteme
   GmbH**
Wolfgang Petersen (Managing Director)
Carl-Zeiss-Ring 9
8045 Ismaning
Germany
Telephone: 89 961 3030
Fax: 89 961 3043

4. 3W International
USA
Telephone: (415) 969 0606
Fax: (415) 964 2027

**5. 21st Century Media
   Communications Inc**
548 Cardero Street
Vancouver
BC V6G 2W6
Canada
Telephone: (604) 688–7103

6. 21st Century Media
Seattle
USA

7. 24 New Media
Dr Gnoni
Via Baradiago 19
20152 Milan
Italy
Telephone: 2 38 0000 83
Fax: 2 33 4024 65

8. 24 Ore New Media Spa
Via Lomazzo 52
Milano 20154
Italy
Telephone: 2–294–04810
Fax: 2–276–040

9. A Giuffre Editore SpA
Via Busto Arsizio 40
20151 Milan
Italy
Telephone: 2 38000975

10. A S Forlaget Kompass Danmark
Ina Soerensen; Ole Lilholt
Lyngby Hovedgade
DK-2800 Lyngby
Denmark
Telephone: 45 42 886000
NUA: 2402001487

11. A/N Group Inc
PO Box 895
Melville
NY 11747
USA
Telephone: (516) 549–4090
Fax: (516) 385–9828

12. A/S Forlaget Kompass Denmark
Ina Sörensen
Lyngby Hovedgade 4
2800 Lyngby
Denmark
Telephone: 02 886–000
Fax: 02 931–805

13. A/S/M Communications Inc
49 E 21 Street
New York
NY 10010
USA
Telephone: (212) 995–7323

14. Aalborg Universitetbibliotek
L. Riget; J. Collins
Langagervej 4
Postboks 8200
DK-9220 Aalborg Oest
Denmark
Telephone: 45 98 159111
NUA: 238302121216

**15. Aarhus School of Business
   Library**
CD-ROM Enquiries
4 Fuglesangs Alle
8210 Aarhus V
Denmark
Telephone: 86 15 55 88
Fax: 86 15 01 88

16. Aaron Smith Associates
Electronic Publishing Division
50 Hurt Plaza
Suite 410
Atlanta
GA 30303
USA
Telephone: (404) 330–2100

17. AB Pressurklipp
112 85 Stockholm
Sweden
Telephone: 46 (8) 54 14 20
Telex/E-mail: 8105030 PRESSUR S

18. ABACIS Inc
135 Village Green Drive
Owings Mills
MD 21117
USA
Telephone: (301) 581–0394

**19. ABC der Deutschen Wirtschaft
   Verlagsgesellschaft mbH**
Margit C. Selka (Publisher); G. Kolb
(EDP Manager)
Berliner Allee 8
6100 Darmstadt 1
Germany
Telephone: (6151) 33411/13
Fax: (6151) 33164
Telex/E-mail: 419257 ABC D

20. ABC International
131 Clarendon Street
6th Floor
Boston
MA 02116
USA
Telephone: (617) 262–5000
Telex/E-mail: 4951813

21. ABC News
Moving Image Collection
47 West 66th Street
6th Floor
New York
NY 10023
USA
Telephone: (800) 221–7386 x 2985;
         (212) 887–2985

22. ABC Online
Mr. Labreke
Centre International Rogier
Passage International 6
Bte 10
B-1210 Bruxelles
Belgium
Telephone: 32 (2) 2184414
NUA: 2062243271

23. ABC Verlag
Berliner Allee 8
Darmstadt 6706
Germany
Telephone: 0675 33477 73

24. ABC voor Handel en Industrie CV
Konigin Wilhelminalaan 16
NL-2012 JK Haarlem
Netherlands
Telephone: 023 31 90 31;
         023 32 00 74
Fax: 023 32 70 33
Telex/E-mail: 41393 ABC NL
NUA: 2041250050

25. ABC-CLIO Inc
Euzetta E Williams (Library Director)
130 Cremona
PO Box 1911
Santa Barbara
CA 93116–1911
USA
Telephone: (805) 968–1911;
         (800) 422–2546
Fax: (805) 685–9685
Telex/E-mail: 21984 (DIALMAIL)

26. Abel Electronics
Max Tifi
Sede Sociale
Viale C Casella 48
00122 Rome
Italy
Telephone: 6 844–2338
Fax: 6 844–2338

27. ABI Books Pvt Ltd
Vipen Parwanda (Director)
Vaikunth
82–83 Nehru Place
New Delhi 110019
India
Telephone: 11 643 2653;
         11 646 1682
Fax: 11 644 8917;
         11 644 7347

28. ABK Consultancies BV
Paul Borm
Beeldsnijdersdreef 85
Maastricht
Netherlands
Telephone: 43 475–515
Fax: 43 436–080

29. Abt Books Inc
Dr Clark C Abt (President and
Publisher)
146 Mount Auburn Street
Cambridge
MA 02138
USA
Telephone: (617) 661–1300
Fax: (617) 661–0511

30. AC Croft, Inc
245 Fischer Avenue, B-2
Costa Mesa
CA 92626
USA
Telephone: (714) 751–1883
Fax: (714) 751–4106

32. AC Nielsen
Arlyce Lillegard (Vice President)
Nielsen Plaza
Northbrook
IL 60062
USA
Telephone: (312) 498–6300
Telex/E-mail: 206466

**33. Academic Bookstore (see
Akateeminen Kirjakauppa)**

**34. Academie Suisse des Sciences
Medicales**
c/o Redation RPM
Bibliotheque de la Faculte de Medicine,
CMU
CH-1221 Geneva 4
Switzerland
Telephone: 022 229–268
Telex/E-mail: 24014 LAUC CH

35. Academy of Model Aeronautics
810 Samuel Morse Drive
Reston
VA 22090
USA
Telephone: (703) 435–0750
Fax: (703) 435–0798

36. Acal Auriema Nederland BV
Ing H J Weernink (Divisional Manager);
H Zwartens (Optical Dealer
Manager)
Doornakkersweg 26
5642 MP Eindhoven
Netherlands
Telephone: 40 816–565
Fax: 40 811–815

37. Acal plc
Acal House
Guildford Road
Lightwater
Surrey
GU18 5SA
UK
Telephone: 0276 74406
Fax: 0276 74835

38. Access Dynamics inc
73 Junction Square Drive
Concord
MA 01742
USA
Telephone: (508) 369–1007

39. Access Innovations Inc
Patrick Sauer (Editor); Ed Greenrich
(Technical Marketing Representative)
P.O. Box 40130
Alberquerque
NM 87196
USA
Telephone: (505) 265–3591;
(800) 468–3453
Fax: (505) 256–1080

40. Accolade Inc
Melinda Mongelluzzo (Associate
Publicity Manager)
550 S Winchester Boulevard
Suite 200
San José
CA 95128
USA
Telephone: (408) 985–1700
Fax: (408) 246–0885

41. Accountable List Brokers P/L
Laird Marshall
Level 7
301 Coronation Drive
Milton
Queensland 4064
Australia
Telephone: 7 369–8511
Fax: 7 368–2647

42. Accu-Mem Systems Inc
Theresa Sandell (President)
3125 N Wilke Road
Suite H
Arlington Heights
IL 60004
USA
Telephone: (708) 670–7030
Fax: (708) 670–0866

43. Accu-Weather Inc
619 W College Avenue
State College
PA 16801
USA
Telephone: (814) 237–0309
Fax: (814) 238–1339

44. ACE Paris
M Gaspard
6 rue Rochambeau
F-75009 Paris
France
Telephone: 01 42 85 46 40
Fax: 01 42 81 44 32
Telex/E-mail: 290437 F

45. ACEL Information Pty Ltd
Marketing Department
666 Chapel Street
South Yarra
VIC 3141
Australia
Telephone: 03 826 6099
Fax: 03 826 6886

46. ACI Computer Services
310 Ferntree Gully Road
Clayton
Melbourne
VIC 3168
Australia

**47. Acid Rain Information Clearing
House**
33 South Washington Street
Rochester
NY 14608
USA
Telephone: (716) 546–3796

48. Ackerman Group, The
1666 Kennedy Causeway
Suite 700
Miami Beach
FL 33141
USA
Telephone: (305) 865–0073;
(305) 865–0072
Fax: (305) 865–0218
Telex/E-mail: SprintMail: ADMIN.
RISKNET

49. ACM Press
Margaret Tuttle; Bernard Rous
(Associate Director of Publications)
11 W 42nd Street
New York
NY 10036
USA
Telephone: (212) 869–7440
Fax: (212) 869–0481

50. Acquisitions Monthly
Lonsdale House
7–9 Lonsdale Gardens
Tunbridge Wells
Kent
TN1 1NU
UK
Telephone: 44 (892) 515454

51. ACS Computer Pte Ltd
Philip Teo (Executive Manager)
Block 211
Henderson Road
10–02/03/04 Henderson Ind. Park
Singapore 0315
Singapore
Telephone: 479 3888
Fax: 475 5666

52. ACT Computer Services Limited
11735 170th Street
Edmonton
Alberta
T5M 3W7
Canada
Telephone: (403) 451–5555
Fax: (403) 452–0756

53. ACT Informatique
83–85 bd Vincent Auriol
75013 Paris
France
Telephone: +33 1 44 23 64 88
Fax: +33 1 44 23 68 69

54. ACT Multimedia
Gerard Dahan (Marketing and
Development Manager)
83–85 bd Vincent Auriol
75013 Paris
France
Telephone: +33 1 44 23 64 88
Fax: +33 1 44 23 68 69

55. ACT Systemes
Denis Oudard
2516 River Bend Drive
Louisville
KY 40206
USA
Telephone: (502) 895–0565
Fax: (502) 893–9589

56. Actdivision
Kelly Zmat
4600 Bohannon Drive
Suite 210
Menlo Park
CA 94025–1001
USA
Telephone: (415) 329–0800
Fax: (415) 322–0260

57. Active English Information Systems Inc
Gary Magee (Director of Marketing)
PO Box 459
44 White Court
Canton
IL 61520
USA
Telephone: (309) 647–7668
Fax: (309) 647–5832

58. Activision, Inc
PO Box 3048
Menlo Park
CA 94025–3048
USA
Telephone: (415) 329–0800

59. Ad-Lib Publications
51 North 5th Street
PO Box 1102
Fairfield
IA 52556–1102
USA
Telephone: (515) 472–6617;
(800) 624–5893

60. Adams Engineering Inc
8484 Breen Road
Houston
TX 77064
USA
Telephone: (713) 937–8320
Fax: (713) 937–6503
Telex/E-mail: 701106

61. Addison-Wesley Publishing Company
Advance Book Program
Laura Likely (Marketing Manager)
350 Bridge Parkway
Suite 209
Redwood City
CA 94065
USA
Telephone: (415) 594–4467
Fax: (415) 594–4440

62. addit Datensysteme GmbH
Thomas Lander (General Manager)
Am Stadtrand 35
2000 Hamburg 70
Germany
Telephone: 40 693–70–86
Fax: 40 693–92–53

63. Adis International Inc.
Suite B-30
582 Middletown Blvd.
Langhorne
PA 19047
USA
Telephone: (215) 752–4500
Fax: (215) 752–4541

64. ADIS International Limited
Private Bag
Mairangi Bay
Auckland 10
New Zealand
Telephone: (09) 403–8100
Fax: (09) 479–1418
Telex/E-mail: 21334 NZ

66. ADIS International Ltd
The Old Palace
Little St. John Street
Chester
CH1 1RE
UK
Telephone: 0244 328–328
Fax: 0244 320–787

67. Admedia
Postbus 2216
NL-1180 EE Amstelveen
Netherlands
Telephone: 020 545–5555

68. Administrative Bibliotek, Det
Peter V. Christensen
Slotsholmen 12
1216 Copenhagen K
Denmark
Telephone: 45 33 924696

69. Adobe Systems Europe BV
Alex Steinberger
Office Center
Jozefisraelskarde 48c
1072 SB Amsterdam
Netherlands
Telephone: +31 20 767661
Fax: +31 20 793181

70. Adobe Systems Inc
1585 Charleston
PO Box 7900
Mountain View
CA 94039–7900
USA
Telephone: (415) 961–4400
Fax: (415) 961–3769

71. Adobe Systems UK Ltd
Fiona Coughlan (Marketing Assistant)
10 Princeton Mews
167–169 London Road
Kingston-Upon-Thames
London
KT2 6PT
UK
Telephone: 081 547–1900;
081 944–1298
Fax: 081 547–3515

72. Adone Systeme
19 rue Michael Faraday
78180 Montigny
France
Telephone: 33 (1) 34 60 34 04

73. ADONIS BV
Barrie Stern (Managing Director, Marketing Services); Henk Compier (Manager)
Molenwerf 1
1014 AG Amsterdam
Netherlands
Telephone: 20 684 2206
Fax: 20 688 0241

74. ADP Automotive Claims Services
2010 Crow Canyon Place
San Ramón
CA 94583
USA
Telephone: (415) 866–1100;
(800) 227–2074

75. ADP Brokerage Information Services Group
2 Journal Square Plaza
Jersey City
NJ 07306
USA
Telephone: (201) 714–3000

76. ADP Collision Estimating Service
2380 West Winston Avenue
Hayward
CA 94545
USA
Telephone: (415) 783–4344;
(800) 227–2074

77. ADP Data Services
42 Broadway
17th Floor, Suite 1730
New York
NY 10004
USA
Telephone: (212) 908–5400

78. ADP Network Services
179–193 Great Portland Street
London
W1N 5FD
UK
Telephone: 071 637–1355

79. ADP Network Services
175 Jackson Plaza
Ann Arbor
MI 48106–2190
USA
Telephone: (313) 769–6800;
(800) 521–3166
Fax: (313) 995–6458

80. ADP
1950 Hassell Rd.
Hoffmann Estates
IL 60195–2308
USA
Telephone: (312) 397–1700

81. ADSET
Association for Database Services in Education and Training
Chancery House
Dalkeith Place
Kettering
Northamptonshire
NN16 0BS
UK
Telephone: 0536 410500
Fax: 0536 414274

82. Advance Publishing
1320 SW Broadway
Portland
OR 97201
USA
Telephone: (503) 221–8327

83. Advanced Media Development
Ideon Research Park
S-223 70 Lund
Sweden
Telephone: 46 18 26 60
Fax: 46 12 98 79

84. Advanced Personnel Systems
PO Box 1438
Roseville
CA 95661
USA
Telephone: (916) 781–2900
Fax: (916) 786–7830; (916) 781–2901
Telex/E-mail: 2644455 (MCI Mail)

85. Advanced Strategies Corporation Japan KK
Ira Hata (President)
Sumitomo Minami Aoyama Big, 5F
5–11–5 Minami-Aoyama
Minato-ku
Tokyo
Japan
Telephone: 3 3486–9009
Fax: 3 4386–9017

86. Advanced Strategies Corporation
Harry Fox (President)
60 Cutter Mill Road
Suite 502
Great Neck
NY 11021
USA
Telephone: (516) 482–0088
Fax: (516) 773–0990

Addresses

87. Advanced Television Publishing
PO Box 5247
Portland
OR 97208–5247
USA
Telephone: (503) 222–3343
Fax: (503) 222–2341

88. Advantage Plus Dist. Inc
7113 Halifax Court
Tampa
FL 33615
USA
Telephone: (919) 362–8212
Fax: (919) 362–7273

89. Adventist World Purchasing Service (see Ellen G White Estate)

90. Adviseur Informatisering en Organisatie
Crailoseweg 26
1272 EV Huizen
Netherlands
Telephone: 02152–68973
Fax: 02152–40999

91. AEIDL asbl
34 rue Breydel
B-1040 Brussels
Belgium
Telephone: 02 230 52 34
Fax: 02 230 34 82

92. AEK Ärztekasse
RE Hagenbuch
Jakob Füglistraße 18
8048 Zurich
Switzerland
Telephone: 1 432–6900
Fax: 1 432–1007

93. Aerospatiale
Oleg Lavroff
12 rue Pasteur
BP 76
Suresnes
Cedex 92152
France
Telephone: (1) 40 99 30 00
Fax: (1) 40 00 35 18

94. Ärzte Zeitung Verlagsgesellschaft mbH
Am Forsthaus Gravenbruch 5
D-6078 Neu-Isenburg 2
Germany
Telephone: (06102) 50 61 75
Fax: (06102) 50 61 23
Telex/E-mail: 414944 D

95. Affärsdata AB
Bengt Wall (Managing Director)
PO Box 3188
103 63 Stockholm
Sweden
Telephone: 8 736 5919
Fax: 8 200 212

96. Affaersvaerlden Forlag AB
PO Box 70497
107 26 Stockholm
Sweden

97. AFRC Institute of Food Research
Norwich Laboratory
Colney Lane
Norwich
Norfolk
NR4 7UA
UK
Telephone: 0603 65122
Fax: 0603 507–723
Telex/E-mail: 975453 G 10075:
DB10013 (Dialcom);
JACKMAN UK.AC.AFRC.FRIN (JANET)

98. Africa News Service Inc
PO Box 3851
Durham
NC 27702
USA
Telephone: (919) 286–0747
Fax: (919) 286–0747

99. Africa Telecommunications Report
1000 Connecticut Avenue NW
Suite 9
Washington
DC 20036
USA
Telephone: (202) 667–2111

100. Aftenposten/AET
PO Box 1178 Sentrum
N-0107 Oslo 1
Norway
Telephone: 02 863–000
Fax: 02 863–832
Telex/E-mail: 71230 N

101. Aftonbladets textarkiv
S-105 18 Stockholm
Sweden
Telephone: 08 725–2000
Fax: 08 600–0180
Telex/E-mail: 10065 AFTBLAD S

102. AG Publications Ltd
PO Box 7422
31070 Haifa
Israel
Telephone: 04 25 51 04
Fax: 04 24 75 32

103. Agence de Cooperation Regionale pour la Documentation (ACORD)
971 avenue Victor Hugo
F-26000 Valence
France
Telephone: 75 90 17 77

104. Agence Europe SA
10–13 boulevard St Lazare
B-1210 Brussels
Belgium
Telephone: 02 219–0256

105. Agence France-Presse (AFP)
13 Place de la Bourse
BP 20
F-75061 Paris Cedex 2
France
Telephone: 01 40 41 48 67
Telex/E-mail: 210064 AFP A F

106. Agence Nationale du Logiciel
Campus Scientifique
PO Box 239
F-54500 Vandoeuvre-les-Nancy
France
Telephone: 083 91 21 58
Fax: 083 27 76 43

107. Agence Nationale pour la Recuperation et l'Elimination des Dechets
Centre National de Documentation sur les Dechets
2 Square Lafayette
BP 406
F-49004 Angers Cedex 01
France
Telephone: 41 20 41 20
Fax: 41 87 23 50
Telex/E-mail: 721325 F

108. Agence Telegraphique Suisse AG
Langgaßtrasse 7
Case Postale
CH-3001 Berne
Switzerland
Telephone: 031 243–333
Fax: 031 244–453
Telex/E-mail: 911–500 SDA CH Marc Luethi (DATAMAIL)

109. Agencia Española del ISBN
Carmen Lacambra Moreno (Directora del Centro del Libro y la Lectura)
Santiago Rusiñol 8
28040 Madrid
Spain
Telephone: 1 534–03–61;
1 533–08–02
Fax: 1 553–99–90

110. Agencia General del Marcado de Valores SA
Calle Alfonso XI 6
28014 Madrid
Spain
Telephone: 01 589–1408
Fax: 01 231–290
Telex/E-mail: 49184 E

111. Agenzia ANSA
94 via della Dataria
I-00187 Rome
Italy
Telephone: 06 677 4298
Fax: 06 677 4655
Telex/E-mail: 612220

112. Agfa Corporation
Agfa Compugraphic Division
Peter Miller
90 Industrial Way
Wilmington
USA
Telephone: (508) 658–5600 x5370

113. Agfa-Gevaert (UK) Ltd
Ralph Hilsdon (Marketing Manager)
Sandbeck Way
Wetherby
West Yorkshire
LS22 4DN
UK
Telephone: 0937 61944
Fax: 0937 61174

114. Agora snc
Bruno Boveri
Via Duchessa Jolanda 13/A
10138 Turin
Italy
Telephone: 11 769–857

115. Agra Europe (London) Limited
25 Frant Road
Tunbridge Wells
Kent
TN2 5JT
UK
Telephone: 0892 33813
Fax: 0892 24593
Telex/E-mail: 95114 AGRATW G
AEL001 (Dialcom)

116. Agriculture Canada
Pesticides Directorate
SBI Building, 2nd Floor
2323 Riverside Drive
Ottawa
Ontario
K1A 0C6
Canada
Telephone: (613) 993–4544

117. Agriculture Canada
Research Branch
George Morris
7th Floor
Sir John Carling Building
930 Carling Avenue
Ottawa
Ontario
K1A 0C5
Canada
Telephone: (613) 995–7084
Fax: (613) 943–0440

118. Agriculture Canada
Research Program Service
Central Experimental Farm
KW Neatby Building
Room 1135
Ottawa
Ontario
K1A 0C6
Canada
Telephone: (613) 995–7084
Fax: (613) 992–7909
Telex/E-mail: 053 3283

119. Agridata Limited
1–2 Berners Street
London
W1P 3AG
UK
Telephone: 071 637–1444

120. AgriData Resources Inc
330 East Kilbourn Avenue
Milwaukee
WI 53202
USA
Telephone: (414) 278–7676;
(800) 558–9044
Fax: (414) 273–5580
Telex/E-mail: AT83IL (StarGram)

121. AGRIS Coordinating Center
A Lebowitz (Head Agris Coordinating
Center)
Food and Agriculture Organization of
the United Nations
Via delle Terme di Caracalla
00100 Rome
Italy
Telephone: 6 579 74993
Fax: 6 514 6172

122. AGRONIITEIP
c/o International Centre for Scientific
and Technical Information
Ulitsa Kuusinena 21b
125252 Moscow
Russia
Telephone: 095 198–7460
Fax: 095 943–0089
Telex/E-mail: 411–925 MCNTI SU

123. AIDSQUEST Online
PO Box 5528
Atlanta
GA 30307–0528
USA
Telephone: (404) 377–8895

**124. Aircraft Technical Publishers
(ATP)**
101 South Hill DRive
Brisbane
CA 94005–1203
USA
Telephone: (415) 468–1705;
(800) 227–4610
Fax: (415) 468–1596
Telex/E-mail: 171048 AIRTECH SFO

**125. Airline Tariff Publishing
Company (ATPCO)**
Dulles International Airport
PO Box 17415
Washington
DC 20041
USA
Telephone: (703) 471–7510

126. AIR
J H Rufer
Gevers Deynootweghome
1130 F Scheveningen
Netherlands
Telephone: +31 70 354 8043
Fax: +31 70 354 9003

**127. Airport Operators Council
International (AOCI)**
1220 19th Street NW
Suite 200
Washington
DC 20036
USA
Telephone: (202) 293–8500

128. AIRS Inc
335 Paint Branch Drive
College Park
MD 20742
USA
Telephone: (301) 454–2022

129. Aiseru
Natalie Yoko
2–9–13 Ikebukuro
Toshima-ku
Tokyo 171
Japan
Telephone: 3 3988 6973
Fax: 3 3988 8450

130. Akateeminen Kirjakauppa
Markus Anaja (Buying Manager)
PO Box 220
SF-00100 Helsinki
Finland
Telephone: 0 12141
Fax: 0 121 4441

131. Aktivbanken
Ladegaardsvej 3
DK-7100 Vejle
Denmark
Telephone: 45 75 857100

132. AKZO Coatings BV
S Chiere
PO Box 237
2130 AE Hoofdorp
Netherlands
Telephone: 250 368 122
Fax: 250 339 146

**133. Al Bayan Press – The Arab
Information Bank**
PO Box 2710
Dubai
United Arab Emirates
Telephone: 04 444 400
Fax: 04 441 854
Telex/E-mail: 48734 MERC EM

134. Albert Bonniers Forlag AB
PO Box 3159
S-10363 Stockholm
Sweden
Telephone: 08 22 91 20
Fax: 08 20 21 48
Telex/E-mail: 14546 BONBOOK S

135. Alberta Agriculture
Market Analysis Branch
7000 113th Street
3rd Floor
Edmonton
AB T6H 5T6
Canada
Telephone: (403) 427–8239
Telex/E-mail: 0372666

**136. Alberta Department of the
Attorney General**
Legislative Counsel Office
9833 109 Street
Edmonton
AB T5K 2E8
Canada
Telephone: 403 427–2217

**137. Alberta Oil Sands Technology
and Research Authority**
Library and Information Services
10010 106 Street
6th Floor
Edmonton
AB T5J 3L8
Canada
Telephone: 403 427–8382
Fax: 403 422–9112
Telex/E-mail: 0372147

138. Alberta Treasury
Bureau of Statistics
Sir Frederick W Haultain Building
AB T5K 0C8
Canada
Telephone: 403 427–3058
Fax: 403 427–0409
Telex/E-mail: 037 43237

139. Alberto Peruzzo Editore
Fabio Mantovani (Product Manager)
Viale E Marelli 165
20099 Sesto S Giovanni
Milan
Italy
Telephone: 2 24 20 21
Fax: 2 24 02 723

140. ALBSU
Steve Brain (Field Officer)
Kingsbourne House
229–231 High Holborn
London
WC1 7DA
UK
Telephone: 071 405–4017
Fax: 071 404–5038

141. Alcom Marine Electronics
Tom Rosnaly
Berth D
101 Shipyard Way
Newport Beach
CA 92663
USA
Telephone: (714) 673–1727
Fax: (714) 673–2057

142. ALDE Publishing Inc
Debbie Hagele; Paula Alleven
6520 Edenvale Boulevard
Suite 118
Eden Prarie
MN 55346
USA
Telephone: (612) 934–4239
Fax: (612) 934–2824

Addresses

143. ALDIS Pty Ltd
Robyne Lovelock (Manager); Julie
  Stevens (Library Consultant)
275 Normanby Road
Port Melbourne
VIC 3207
Australia
Telephone: 03 647 9724
Fax: 03 647 9799

144. Aldrich Chemical Company Inc
Steve Schultz (Manager Data Products)
PO Box 355
1001 W St Paul Avenue
Milwaukee
WI 53201–0664
USA
Telephone: (414) 273–3850
Fax: (414) 273–4979

145. Aldrich Chemical Company Ltd
Nigel Mobbs
The Old Brickyard
New Road
Gillingham
Dorset
SP8 4JL
UK
Telephone: 0747 822–211
Fax: 0747 823–779

146. Alea Sistemi
Umberto Cettomai (President)
Lungotevere Flaminio 66
00196 Rome
Italy
Telephone: 6 323–4926
Fax: 6 323–4924

147. Alert International Inc
1460 Brickwell Avenue
Suite 304
Miami
FL 33131
USA
Telephone: (305) 530–1652

148. Alert Publishing Inc
3706 30th Avenue
Long Island City
NY 11103
USA
Telephone: (718) 626–3356

149. ALERT
c/o San José Police Officers Association
1151 N. 4th Street
San José
CA 95110
USA
Telephone: (408) 292–1014

150. Alexander Krislov
3694 Strandhill Road
Shaker Heights
OH 44122
USA
Telephone: (216) 751–1246

151. All My Features Inc
4853 N Ravenswood
Chicago
IL 60640
USA
Telephone: (312) 935–8779

152. All-Quotes Inc
40 Exchange Place
Suite 1500
New York
NY 10005
USA
Telephone: (212) 425–5030
Fax: (212) 425–6895

153. Alldata Corporation
Marketing Department
Arnold Gold (Director of Marketing)
9412 Big Horn Boulevard
Elk Grove
CA 95758
USA
Telephone: (916) 684 5200
Fax: (916) 684 5225

154. Allegro New Media
387 Passaic Avenue
Fairfield
NJ 07004
USA
Telephone: (201) 808–1992
Fax: (201) 808–2645

**155. Allgemeiner Deutscher
  Nachrichtendienst**
Mollstraße 1
D-1026 Berlin
Germany
Telephone: 0037 235–4076
Fax: 0037 235–4474

**156. Allmaenna
  Reklamationsnaemnden**
Box 523
162 15 Vaellingby
Sweden
Telephone: 46 (8) 759 85 50

157. Alpha Communications Ltd
Philip Cassar (Director)
13/18 Vincenti Buildings
Strait Street
Valletta
Malta
Telephone: 230–805; 246–501
Fax: 223–854

**158. Alzheimer's Disease Education
  and Referral Center**
National Institutes of Health
Federal Building, Room 6C12
7550 Wisconsin Avenue
Bethesda
MD 20892
USA
Telephone: (301) 496–1752

159. AM Best Company
Best DataBase Services
Deb Walyga (Marketing Manager)
Ambest Road
Oldwick
NJ 08858
USA
Telephone: (908) 439–2200
Fax: (908) 439–3363;
  (908) 439–3296
Telex/E-mail: AMBSLS (AT&T Mail);
  SLS04DW (AT&T Mail)

160. AMA Advisers Inc
535 North Dearborn Street
Chicago
IL 60610
USA
Telephone: (312) 645–4455

161. AMA/NET
535 North Dearborn Street
Chicago
IL 60610
USA
Telephone: (312) 645–5085

**162. Amateur Radio Research and
  Development Corporation**
11523 Charlton Drive
Silver Spring
MD 20902
USA
Telephone: (301) 681–7372
Telex/E-mail: 650 248 8912
RBARTRH (MCI Mail)

**163. American Academy of
  Pediatrics**
141 N Westpoint Boulevard
Elk Grove
IL 60009
USA
Telephone: (708) 228–5005
Fax: (708) 228–5094

**164. American Agricultural
  Communications Systems Inc**
225 Touhy Avenue
Park Ridge
IL 60068
USA
Telephone: (312) 399–5870

165. American Airlines
SABRE Travel Information Network
MD 1319
PO Box 619616
Dallas-Fort Worth Airport
TX 75261–9616
USA
Telephone: (817) 963–4790;
  (800) 433–7556
Fax: (817) 963–4658

**166. American Appraisal Associates
  Inc**
525 E Michigan Street
PO Box 664
Milwaukee
WI 53201–0664
USA
Telephone: (414) 271–5544

**167. American Association for
  Medical Systems and
  Informatics**
4405 East-West Highway, Suite 402
Bethesda
MD 20814
USA
Telephone: (301) 657–4142

**168. American Association for the
  Advancement of Science**
1330 H Street NW
Washington
DC 20005
USA
Telephone: (202) 326–6500

**169. American Association of Retired
  Persons**
National Gerontology Resource Center
601 E Street NW
Washington
DC 20049
USA
Telephone: (202) 434–6231

170. American Banker-Bond Buyer
Database Services
1 State Street Plaza
30th Floor
New York
NY 10004
USA
Telephone: (212) 943–6303;
  (212) 943–6166;
  (800) 356–4763
Fax: (212) 943–2222
Telex/E-mail: 129233 AMBANK
SVBJAA (DATAMAIL);
14015 (DAILMAIL);
15493 (DIALMAIL)

171. American Bar Association
750 North Lake Shore Drive
Chicago
IL 60611
USA
Telephone: (312) 988–5958;
(312) 988–5154;
(312) 988–5000;
(800) 322–4638;
(800) 435–7342
Fax: (312) 988–4664;
(312) 988–6281;
(703) 631–4565
Telex/E-mail: ABANET.SOS (SprintMail)

172. American Business Information Inc
Optical Products Division
Bill Kerrey (Vice President, OPD)
5711 S 86th Circle
PO Box 27347
Omaha
NE 68127–0347
USA
Telephone: (402) 593–4593;
(402) 593–4565
Fax: (402) 331–5481;
(402) 331–1505

173. American Ceramic Society Inc
Reference Services
Christine Schnitzer (Product Manager Reference Services)
757 Brooksedge Plaza Drive
Westerville
OH 43081–6136
USA
Telephone: (614) 890–4700
Fax: (614) 899–6109

174. American Chemical Society
1155 16th Street NW
Washington
DC 20036
USA
Telephone: (202) 872–4381;
(800) 424–6747
Fax: (202) 872–4615
Telex/E-mail: 440159 ACSPUI

175. American City Business Journals
3527 Broadway
Suite 500
Kansas City
MO 64111
USA
Telephone: (816) 561–5900

176. American College of Obstetricians and Gynecologists
Michael Dodd (Marketing Manager)
409 12th Street SW
Washington
DC 20024–2188
USA
Telephone: (202) 638–5577

177. American Correctional Association
Division of Training & Contracts
8025 Laurel Lakes Court
Laurel
MD 20707
USA
Telephone: (301) 206–5045;
(800) 825–2665
Fax: (301) 206–5061
Telex/E-mail: NETSTAFF (DELPHI)

178. American Databankers Corporation
1820 South Main Street
Broken Arrow
OK 74012–6542
USA
Telephone: (918) 251–7330
Fax: (918) 251–7419

179. American Economic Association
Drucilla Ekwurzel
PO Box 7320
Oakland Station
Pittsburgh
PA 15213
USA
Telephone: (412) 268–3869

180. American Educational Research Association
1230 17th Street NW
Washington
DC 20036
USA
Telephone: (202) 223–9485

181. American Express Information Services Company
Integrated Marketing Services
John Larson (Manager Marketing Services)
2121 N 117th Avenue
Omaha
NE 68164–3600
USA
Telephone: (402) 498–2185;
(800) 338–6073
Fax: (402) 498–2155

182. American Farm Bureau Federation
225 Touhy Avenue
Park Ridge
IL 60068
USA
Telephone: (312) 399–5770

183. American Financial Network Inc
12001 North Central Expressway
Suite 1000
Dallas
TX 75243
USA
Telephone: (214) 233–6800)

184. American Gas Association
Industry Information Services
1515 Wilson Boulevard
Arlington
VA 22209
USA
Telephone: (703) 841–8400
Fax: (703) 841–8406
Telex/E-mail: 710 955 9848 II2002 (KSI)

185. American Gem Market System
1001 Country Club Drive
Moraga
CA 94556
USA
Telephone: (415) 376–8450

186. American Geological Institute
GeoRef Information System
Kay Yost (Assistant to the Director)
4220 King Street
Alexandria
VA 22302–1507
USA
Telephone: (703) 379–2480;
(800) 336–4764
Fax: (703) 379–7563

187. American Helix Technology Corp.
1857 Colonial Village Lane
Lancaster
PA 17601
USA
Telephone: (717) 392–7840;
(800) 525–6576

188. American Hospital Association
Office of Legal Communications
840 North Lake Shore Drive, 8 East
Chicago
IL 60611
USA
Telephone: (312) 280–6594;
(800) 621–6712

189. American Institute of Aeronautics and Astronautics
370 L'Enfant Promenade SW
Washington
DC 20024
USA
Telephone: (202) 646–7400

190. American Institute of Certified Public Accountants
1211 Avenue of the Americas
New York
NY 10036–8775
USA
Telephone: (212) 575–6326;
(212) 575–6393;
(800) 223–4155

191. American Institute of Chemical Engineers
345 E 47th Street
New York
NY 10017
USA
Telephone: (212) 705–7338

192. American Institute of Physics
335 E 45th Street
New York
NY 10017
USA
Telephone: (212) 661–9260
Fax: (212) 661–2036
Telex/E-mail: 960983 AMINSTPHYS NY
ELLEN AIP.BITNET (BITNET);
ELLEN
PINET.AIP.ORG (Internet);
ELLEN (PINET)

193. American Interactive Media (AIM)
Dave McElhatten (Vice President Production)
11111 Santa Monica Boulevard
Suite 700
Los Angeles
CA 90025
USA
Telephone: (213) 473–4136
Fax: (213) 479–5937

194. American Judicature Society
25 E Washington
Suite 1600
Chicago
IL 60602
USA
Telephone: (312) 558–6900

195. American Lawyer, The
600 Third Avenue
New York
NY 10016
USA
Telephone: (212) 973–2800
Fax: (212) 972–6258

196. American Library Association
Rob Carlson (ALANET)
50 E Huron Street
Chicago
IL 60611
USA
Telephone: (312) 944–6780;
(800) 545–2433
Fax: (312) 440–0901
Telex/E-mail: 41:ALA0006 (Dialcom)

197. American Mathematical Society
Database Services Department
Taissa Kusma (Manager, Database
Services)
201 Charles Street
PO Box 6248
Providence
RI 02940
USA
Telephone: (401) 455–4000;
      (401) 272–9500 x328;
      (800) 321–4267
Fax: (401) 331–3842;
      (401) 455–4004
Telex/E-mail: 797192 TTK
MATH.AMS.COM (Internet)

198. American Medical Association
Caty Bidese
515 North State Street
Chicago
IL 60610
USA
Telephone: (312) 464–5000;
      (312) 464–5129;
      (800) 621–8335
Fax: (312) 464–4184

**199. American Medical Informatics
Association**
4915 St Elmo Avenue
Suite 302
Bethesda
MD 20814
USA
Telephone: (301) 657–1291

**200. American Meteorological
Society**
45 Beacon Street
Boston
MA 02108
USA
Telephone: (617) 227–2425
Fax: (617) 742–8718

201. American Nuclear Society
Information Center on Nuclear
Standards
555 N Kensington Avenue
LaGrange Park
IL 60525
USA
Telephone: (312) 352–6611;
      (800) 323–3044
Fax: (312) 352–0499
Telex/E-mail: 4972673

**202. American Osteopathic
Association**
142 E Ontario Street
Chicago
IL 60611–2864
USA
Telephone: (312) 280–5800;
      (800) 621–1773

203. American Petroleum Institute
Finance, Accounting and Statistics
Department
1220 L Street NW
Washington
DC 20005
USA
Telephone: (202) 682–8525

204. American Petroleum Institute
Central Abstracting and Indexing
Services
275 Seventh Avenue
9th Floor
New York
NY 10001
USA
Telephone: (212) 366–4040
Fax: (212) 366–4298
Telex/E-mail: 4938591

205. American Political Network Inc
282 N Washington Street
Falls Church
VA 22046
USA
Telephone: (703) 237–5130

**206. American Psychological
Association**
Division 14
The Society for Industrial and
Oranizational Psychology
1200 17th Street, NW
Washington
DC 20036
USA
Telephone: (202) 833–7600;
      (703) 247–7705
Fax: (703) 525–5081

**207. American Psychological
Association**
Carolyn Gosling
750 First Street NE
Washington
DC 20002–4242
USA
Telephone: (202) 336–5650;
      (800) 336–4980
Fax: (202) 336–5633

**208. American Society for Testing
and Materials**
1916 Race Street
Philadelphia
PA 19103
USA
Telephone: (215) 299–5410
Fax: (215) 977–9679

**209. American Society of Civil
Engineers**
Information Products
345 E 47th Street
New York
NY 10017–2398
USA
Telephone: (212) 705–7520;
      (800) 548–2723
Fax: (212) 705–7712
Telex/E-mail: 422847 ASCEUI

**210. American Society of
Contemporary Ophthalmology**
233 E Erie Street
Suite 710
Chicago
IL 60611
USA
Telephone: (312) 951–1400

**211. American Society of Hospital
Pharmacists**
Dwight Tousignant (Vice President Drug
Information)
4630 Montgomery Avenue
Bethesda
MD 20814
USA
Telephone: (301) 657–3000
Fax: (301) 657–1641
Telex/E-mail: 13997 (DIALMAIL)

**212. American Society of Mechanical
Engineers**
Michael Merker (Director)
United Engineering Center
345 E 47th Street
New York
NY 10017
USA
Telephone: (212) 705–7789;
      (212) 705 7047
Fax: (212) 705–7674;
      (212) 705–7533

213. American TeleWeb Inc
1332 Hermosa Avenue
Suite 7
Hermosa Beach
CA 90254
USA
Telephone: (213) 372–9364
Fax: (213) 374–6588

**214. American Theological Library
Association**
Matthew E Moore (Manager
Database/Technical Services)
820 Church Street
Suite 300
Evanston
IL 60201–3707
USA
Telephone: (708) 869–7788

**215. American Type Culture
Collection**
Bioinformatics Department
Harold D Hatt (Head of Publishing
Department)
12301 Park Lawn Drive
Rockville
MD 20852–1776
USA
Telephone: (301) 881 2600
Fax: (301) 770 2587

**216. American Water Works
Association**
Technical Library
6666 W Quincy Avenue
Denver
CO 80235
USA
Telephone: (303) 794–7711
Fax: (303) 794–7310
Telex/E-mail: 450895 AWWA DVR
11349 (DIALMAIL)

**217. AMIGOS Bibliographic Council
Inc**
Barbara A Radke (Marketing
Representative)
12200 Park Central Drive
Suite 500
Dallas
TX 75215
USA
Telephone: (214) 851–8000;
      (800) 843–8482
Fax: (214) 991–6061

218. Amnesty International
322 8th Avenue
New York
NY 10001
USA
Telephone: (212) 807–8400

219. Amplifor GmbH
Klaus Gritschneider (Geschäftsführer)
Kronwinklerstraße 24
8000 Munich 60
Germany
Telephone: 89 863–2036
Fax: 89 863–2611

220. AMS Corporation
2–6–2 Marunouchi
Chiyoda-ku
Tokyo 100
Japan
Telephone: 03 210–7300
Fax: 03 3210–7385
Telex/E-mail: 2222063 MSKTOK J

221. Amward Publications Inc
2000 National Press Building
Washington
DC 20045
USA
Telephone: (202) 488–7227

222. Analysis Corporation
3rd Floor
Ibex House
42–47 Minories
London
EC3N 1EU
UK
Telephone: 071 702–0284
Fax: 071 702–2067

**223. Analyste-Conseil Systeme
Informatique Ltd**
969 Route de l'Eglise
Sainte-Foy
Québec G1V 3V4
Canada
Telephone: (418) 653–1456

224. Anaya Systems
Carlos Suavos-Rodriques
Telemaco 43
28027 Madrid
Spain
Telephone: 1 320 01 19
Fax: 1 742 66 31

225. Anchorage Daily News
1001 Northway Drive
Anchorage
AK 99514–9001
USA
Telephone: (907) 257–4200

226. AND Technology Ltd
Peter Boult (Director)
4 Yukon Road
London
SW12 9PU
UK
Telephone: 081 673–5330
Fax: 081 673–4983

**227. Andelsbanken
Erhvervsafdelingen**
Mr. Henrik Aunsborg
Staunings Plads 1–3
DK-1643 Koebenhavn V
Denmark
Telephone: 45 33 145114

**228. Animated Pixels (Publishing)
Ltd**
David Wainwright (Software Producer)
Albemarle House
Osborne Road
Southsea
Hampshire
PO5 3LB
UK
Telephone: 0705 291–866
Fax: 0705 821–677

229. Antic Publishing Inc
544 2nd Street
San Francisco
CA 94107
USA
Telephone: (415) 957–0886
Fax: (415) 882–9502
Telex/E-mail: 76703,1052
(CompuServe);
ANTIC (GEnie)

230. AP-Dow Jones/Telerate
12 Norwich Street
London
EC4A 1BP
UK
Telephone: 071 353–6723

231. Apak Systems Ltd
Paul Nixon (President)
Suite 215
Eglinton Cw
Etobeicoke
ON M9C 5K6
Canada
Telephone: (416) 620–5841
Fax: (416) 620–1819

232. Apak Systems Ltd
Bob Bailey
Apak House
Badminton Court
Station Road
Yate
Bristol
BS17 5HZ
UK
Telephone: 0454 316–086

233. Apex Technology Group Inc
Charlene Cook
4384 Lottsford Vista Road
Lanham
MD 20706–9911
USA
Telephone: (301) 459–1930
Fax: (301) 459–1950

234. Apple Computer Australia
Leon Guss
16 Rodborough Road
Frenchs Forest
NSW 2086
Australia
Telephone: 3 686 1252
Fax: 3 686 1232

235. Apple Computer BV
Mr Appel
Postbus 7
3712 ZG Huis ter Heide
Netherlands
Telephone: 3404 86911
Fax: 3404 24406;
3404 17727

236. Apple Computer Europe
Bénédicte Charrue (Multimedia Project
Manager)
10 cours Michelet Cedex 51
92065 Paris La Défense
France
Telephone: 49 01 49 04
Fax: 49 01 90 51

237. Apple Computer Inc
Chandran Cheriyan (Product Marketing
Manager, Optical Storage
Products)
20525 Mariani Avenue
Cupertino
CA 95014
USA
Telephone: (408) 996–1010;
(408) 974–8605;
(408) 862–7188
Fax: (408) 974–5713
Telex/E-mail: 171 576

238. Apple Computer UK Ltd
Pamela Schure (Product Marketing);
Alex Moore (PR)
6 Roundwood Avenue
Stockley Park
Uxbridge
Middlesex
UB11 1BB
UK
Telephone: 081 569–1199
Fax: 081 569–2957

239. Applidata
RM Groot (Managing Director)
De Pinckart 54
5674 CC Nuenen
Netherlands
Telephone: 40 631–218
Fax: 40 839–270

**240. Applied Information Services
Inc**
100 2nd Street East
Riverside Plaza
Whitefish
MT 59937–9983
USA
Telephone: (406) 862–4484;
(800) 826–2135
Fax: (406) 862–6954

**241. Applied Optical Media
Corporation**
Paul Dellevigne (Director Market
Development)
1450 Boot Road
Building 400
West Chester
PA 19380
USA
Telephone: (215) 429–3701
Fax: (215) 429–3810

242. Applied Videotex Systems
Boston CitiNet
World Trade Center, Suite 717
Boston
MA 02210
USA
Telephone: (617) 439–5678
Fax: (617) 439–5678

243. APS Multiedia
Ted Toms
Station House
Manningtree
Essex
CO11 2LH
UK
Telephone: 0206 391–800
Fax: 0206 391–467

244. APT Data Services Ltd
12 Sutton Row
London
W1V 5FH
UK
Telephone: 081 528–7083

245. Aquarium Optical (Pty) Ltd
Anthony Goldstein (Managing Director)
Nedbank Centre
13th Floor
63 Strand Street
Cape Town 8001
South Africa
Telephone: 21 22 28743
Fax: 21 23 8566

**246. Arab Information Bank (See Al
Bayan Press)**

**247. Arab Press Service
Organisation**
PO Box 3896
Nicosia
Cyprus
Telephone: 2 351–778
Fax: 2 350–265
Telex/E-mail: 3712 APS CY

**248. Arbeitsgemeinschaft
Media-Analyse e.V.**
Wolfsgangstrasse 92
6000 Franfurt am Main 1
Germany
Telephone: 49 (69) 55 03 91

Addresses

249. Arbeitsgemeinschaft Sozialwissenschaftlicher Institut
InformationsZentrum
  Sozialwissenschaften
Lennestraße 30
D-5300 Bonn 1
Germany
Telephone: 0228 228–10
Fax: 0228 228–1120

250. Arbetsmiljoinstitutet
Library
S-171 84 Solna
Sweden
Telephone: 08 730–1900
Fax: 08 273–872
Telex/E-mail: 15816 ARBSKY S

251. Arbitron / The SAMI Company
41 E 42nd Street
New York
NY 10017
USA
Telephone: (212) 297–1162

252. Arbitron Ratings Company
142 W 57th Street
New York
NY 10019
USA
Telephone: (212) 887–1300

253. ARC Professional Services Group
Ted Brandhorst (Director)
2440 Research Boulevard
Suite 400
Rockville
MD 20850
USA
Telephone: (301) 258–5500
Fax: (301) 948–3695

254. Archetype Systems Ltd
Keith Taylor (Director)
7 The Courtyards
The Croxley Centre
Hatters Lane
Watford
WD1 8YH
UK
Telephone: 0923 210–280
Fax: 0923 373–90

255. Architech Publishing Limited
Jill McMahon (Office Manager)
57/59 Gloucester Place
London
W1H 3PE
UK
Telephone: 081 992–5800
Fax: 071 935–7979

256. Archivo General de la Nación
Lic Jorge Cabrera Bohorquez (Director
  of Information)
Avenida Eduardo Molina Esq Con
Albanies
Col Pentenciaria Aplicatión CP 15350
Mexico
Telephone: 702 2209
Fax: 789 5296

257. Arctic Institute of North America
University of Calgary
2500 University Drive NW
Calgary
AB T2N 1N4
Canada
Telephone: (403) 220–4036
Fax: (403) 282–4609
Telex/E-mail: 03821545 RGOODWIN
UCDASVM1 (BITNET); astis
(Envoy 100)

258. ARGO Infographie SA
Barnard Jullien (PDG)
181 rue du Général Gouraud
BP 16
67210 Obernai
France
Telephone: 88 95 40 73
Fax: 88 95 02 28

259. Argonne National Laboratory
National Energy Software Center
9700 S Cass Avenue
Argonne
IL 60439
USA
Telephone: (708) 972–7250
Fax: (708) 972–2206
Telex/E-mail: NESCINFO ANLNESC
(BITNET)

260. Argus Research Corporation
17 Battery Place
18th Floor
New York
NY 10004
USA
Telephone: (212) 425–7500
Fax: (212) 943–4635

261. Ariel Research Corporation
7910 Woodmont
Suite 902
Bethesda
MD 20814
USA
Telephone: (301) 907–7771
Fax: (301) 907–7773

262. Aries Systems Corporation
Lyndon Holmes (President)
One Dundee Park
Andover
MA 01810
USA
Telephone: (508) 475–7200
Fax: (508) 474–8860

263. ARIST Rhône-Alpes
Quai Achille Lignon
69459 Lyon Cedex 06
France
Telephone: 078 89 29 29

264. Aristarchus Knowledge Industries Inc
PO Box 12625
Tucson
AZ 85732
USA
Telephone: (602) 620–1240
Telex/E-mail: APAC (DIALMAIL)

265. Aristotle Industries
John Phillips (President)
205 Pennsylvania Avenue SE
Washington
DC 20003
USA
Telephone: (202) 543–8345
Fax: (202) 543–6407

267. Arkansas Gazette
112 W 3rd Avenue
Little Rock
AR 72203
USA
Telephone: (501) 371–3700

268. Arkansas University Press
Elizabeth Hudgens
University of Arkansas
Fayetteville
AR 72701
USA
Telephone: (501) 575–3246
Fax: (501) 575–6044

269. Arlen Communications Inc
7315 Wisconsin Avenue, Suite 600E
Bethesda
MD 20814
USA
Telephone: (301) 656–7940

270. Art Sales Index Ltd
1 Thames Street
Weybridge
Surrey
KT13 8JG
UK
Telephone: 0932 856–426
Fax: 0932 842–482
Telex/E-mail: 94017217 ASIL G

271. ARTA
Leo Osheroff
83 Nachalat Binyamin Street
PO Box 606
Tel Aviv
Israel
Telephone: 3 611–921
Fax: 3 624–722

272. ArtBeats
Phil Bates (President)
PO Box 20083
San Bernardino
CA 92406
USA
Telephone: (714) 881 1200
Fax: (714) 881 4833

273. ARTFL Project
Mark Olsen (Assistant Director)
University of Chicago
Department of Romance Languages
1010 E 59th Street
Chicago
IL 60637
USA
Telephone: (312) 702–8488
Fax: (312) 702–0775

274. Arthur Andersen & Company
Hilary Dalton
33 West Monroe Street
Chicago
IL 60603
USA
Telephone: (312) 507–2866;
         (312) 507–4801 (Hilary Dalton)
Fax: (312) 507–6748

275. Artificial Intelligence Publishing (See Alberto Peruzzo Editore)

276. Asahi-Shimbun, The
New Electronic Media Division
5–3–2 Tsukiji
Chuo-ku
Tokyo 104–11
Japan
Telephone: 03 3545–0131

277. Asia Pacific Foundation of Canada
999 Canada Place
Room 666
Vancouver
BC V6V 3E1
Canada
Telephone: (604) 684–5986
Fax: (604) 681–1370
Telex/E-mail: 0453332 DM.BROOME
(Envoy 100)

278. Asian Classics Input Project
Washington Area Office
Robert J Taylor (Assistant Director)
11911 Marmary Road
Gaithersburg
MD 20878–1839
USA
Telephone: (301) 948–5569

279. Asian Institute of Technology
Library and Regional Documentation
   Center
PO Box 2754
Bangkok 10501
Thailand
Telephone: 02 516–0110
Fax: 02 529–0374
Telex/E-mail: 84276 AIT TH

280. Asian Institute of Technology
Asian Geotechnical Engineering
   Information Center
PO Box2 2754
Bangkok 10501
Thailand
Telephone: 66 (2) 5290100–13 x2869
Fax: 66 (2) 5290374
Telex/E-mail: 84276 AIT TH

281. Asian Institute of Technology
Environmental Sanitation Information
   Center
PO Box 2754
Bangkok 10501
Thailand
Telephone: 66 (2) 5290100–13 x2870
Fax: 66 (2) 5290374
Telex/E-mail: 84276 AIT TH

282. Asian Institute of Technology
International Ferrocement Information
   Center
PO Box 2754
Bangkok 10501
Thailand
Telephone: 02 516–0110
Fax: 02 529–0374
Telex/E-mail: 84276 AIT BANGKOK TH

283. Asian Institute of Technology
Renewable Energy Resources
   Information Center
PO Box 2754
Bangkok 10501
Thailand
Telephone: 02 516–0110
Fax: 02 516–2126
Telex/E-mail: 84276 AIT TH

284. Asian Wall Street Journal, The
AIA Building
2nd Floor
GPO Box 9825
Hong Kong
Telephone: 05 737–121

285. ASK Kodansha Company Ltd
Harvo Ogawa (Production Manager)
2–1 Shimomiyabi
Shinjuku
Tokyo 162–01
Japan
Telephone: 3 3267–6864
Fax: 3 3267–4471

286. Aslib
Roger Bowes (Chief Executive); Sherry
   Jespersen (Deputy Chief
   Executive)
20–24 Old Street
London
EC1V 9AP
UK
Telephone: 071 253–4488
Fax: 071 430–0814

287. ASM Group Coporation
345 Park Avenue
New York
NY 10154
USA
Telephone: (212) 888–3157

**288. ASM International (See Materials
   Information)**

289. Assemblée Nationale
126 rue de l'Université
F-75355 Paris Cedex 6
France
Telephone: 01 40 63 83 93

**290. Associated Banks of Europe
   Corporation**
Barclay's Bank International Ltd
75 Wall Street
New York
NY 10265
USA
Telephone: (212) 412–4000

291. Associated Press
50 Rockefeller Plaza
New York
NY 10020
USA
Telephone: (212) 621–1500

292. Association Dentaire Française
92 avenue de Wagram
F-75017 Paris
France
Telephone: 01 42 27 89 00

**293. Association for Computing
   Machinery**
Margaret Tuttle (Publishing Manager);
   Bernice Holtzman (Sales
   Associate)
11 W 42nd Street
3rd Floor
New York
NY 10036
USA
Telephone: (212) 869–7440
Fax: (212) 869–0481

**294. Association for Unmanned
   Vehicle Systems**
1101 14th Street NW
Room 1100
Washington
DC 20005
USA
Telephone: (202) 371–1170

**295. Association Française de
   Normalisation**
Nicole West (Head of Information
   Department)
Tour Europe
F-92049 Paris la Défense Cedex 7
France
Telephone: 01 42 91 55 55
Fax: 01 42 91 56 56
Telex/E-mail: 61 19 74 AFNOR F

**296. Association Française pour
   l'Étude des Eaux**
Centre Nationale de Documentation et
   d'Information sur l'Eau
21 rue Madrid
Sophia Antipolis
F-75010 Paris
France
Telephone: 01 45 22 14 67

297. Association IBISCUS
1 bis, avenue de Villars
F-75007 Paris
France
Telephone: 01 45 51 93 12
Telex/E-mail: 214235 ATTNMIX IBISC

**298. Association Nationale de la
   Recherche Technique**
101 avenue Raymond Poincare
F-75116 Paris
France
Telephone: 01 45 01 72 27
Telex/E-mail: 642632 F

**299. Association of European
   Airlines**
B.P. 4
350 Avenue Louise
1050 Brussels
Belgium
Telephone: 32 (2) 640 31 75
Fax: 32 (2) 648 40 17
Telex/E-mail: 22918 BRURBSN B

**300. Association of Home Appliance
   Manufacturers**
20 North Wacker Drive
Chicago
IL 60606
USA
Telephone: (312) 984–5800

**301. Association of International
   Bond Dealers**
Rigistraße 60
CH-8033 Zurich
Switzerland
Telephone: 01 363–4222

**302. Association of Official
   Analytical Chemists**
2200 Wilson Boulevard
Suite 400
Arlington
VA 22201–3301
USA
Telephone: (703) 522–3032

**303. Association of Proprietors of
   Gas Companies in Netherlands
   (VEGIN)**
L J van den Brink (Advertising Manager)
Wilmersdorf 50
Postbox 137
7300 AC Apeldoorn
Netherlands
Telephone: 55 49 49 49
Fax: 55 41 89 63

**304. Association pour la Diffusion de
   l'Information Juridique**
Rue de la Victoire 26
B-1060 Brussels
Belgium
Telephone: 02 539–0253
Fax: 02 539–0068

**305. Association pour la Recherche
   et le Developement en
   Informatique Chimique**
Mrs Panaye
25 rue Jussieu
F-75005 Paris
France
Telephone: +33 143362525 ex 4412

Addresses

306. Association pour le Developpement de l'Information Sociale
37 rue de Moulin
F-94210 St Maur
France
Telephone: 01 48 85 20 00

307. Association pour le Developpement de la Documentation Medicale dans les Hopitaux de Paris
17 Rue du Fer a Moulin
F-75005 Paris
France
Telephone: 01 43 37 93 23
01 43 31 30 08

308. Association RAMIS
Centre Hospitalier Universitaire St Antoine
27 rue de Chaligny
F-75571 Paris Cedex 12
France
Telephone: 01 43 45 10 49

309. Association Technique de l'Industrie des Liants Hydrauliques
Centre de Documentation
8 rue Villiot
F-75012 Paris
France
Telephone: 01 43 46 00 70
Fax: 01 43 44 78 11
Telex/E-mail: 240020 ATILH F

310. Association Télexport
Philippe Do (Product Manager)
92 Bis Rue Cardinet
75017 Paris
France
Telephone: 1 47 63 14 15
Fax: 1 42 67 99 69

311. Assolombarda
Via Pantano 9
I-20122 Milan
Italy
Telephone: 02 882 31
Telex/E-mail: 315648 I

312. Astro Mailing Limited
9 Elmdon Road
Marston Green
Birmingham
B37 7BS
UK
Telephone: 44 (21) 779 3336

313. Astronomical Data Center
Lee E Brotzman
NASA Goddard Space Flight Center
Code 630
Greenbelt
MD 20771
USA
Telephone: (301) 286–6953

314. Astronomical Society of the Pacific
HST Orders Department
CD-ROM Enquiries
390 Ashton Avenue
San Francisco
CA 94112
USA
Telephone: (415) 337–1100
Fax: (415) 337–5205

315. Atari Computer Corporation
Don Mandell (Vice President of Sales & Marketing)
1196 Borregas Avenue
Sunnyvale
CA 94089
USA
Telephone: (408) 745–2000
Fax: (408) 745–2088

316. Atari Computer GmbH
Dr Hens Reidel (Director of Software Support)
Frankfurter Strasse 89–91
6096 Raunheim
Germany
Telephone: 61 42–2090
Fax: 61 42–209–180

317. ATEC GmbH
Herr Gröne (President); Herr Menssen (Chief Software Division)
Niedstraße 22
1000 Berlin 41
Germany
Telephone: 30 859 2958
Fax: 30 851 4615

318. Athlete's Outfitter
M. Handelsman Company
1325 South Michigan Avenue
Chicago
IL 60605
USA
Telephone: (312) 427–0787

319. Atlanta Journal-Constitution
72 Marietta Street
PO Box 4689
Atlanta
GA 30303
USA
Telephone: (404) 526–5193

320. Atlantic City Press
1000 West Washington Avenue
Pleasantville
NJ 08232–3816
USA
Telephone: (609) 645–1234

321. Atlantic Information Services Inc
1050 17th Street NW
Suite 480
Washington
DC 20036
USA
Telephone: (202) 775–9008; (800) 521–4323
Fax: (202) 331–9542

322. Atlis
6011 Executive Blvd
Rockville
MD 20852
USA
Telephone: (301) 770–3000; (800) 638–6595

323. Atoll
42 bis, rue de l'Est
F-92100 Boulogne
France
Telephone: 01 46 03 00 99

324. ATPAC
41 E 42nd Street
Suite 1715
New York
NY 10017
USA
Telephone: (212) 697–6560
Fax: (212) 697–6693

325. Attard & Company
Edward Martin (Technical Sales Executive)
67 South Street
Valletta
Malta
Telephone: 228–857
Fax: 220–186

326. ATTICA Cybernetics Ltd
Caroline Hewson (Marketing Assistant)
Unit 2
King's Meadow
Ferry Hinksey Road
Oxford
OX2 0PD
UK
Telephone: 0865 791 346
Fax: 0865 794 561

327. Attorney General's Department
Robert Garran Offices
National Circuit
Barton
ACT 2600
Australia
Telephone: 062 719–064
Fax: 062 719–053

328. Auckland, Wellington and Canterbury District Law Society Libraries
PO Box 58
Auckland
New Zealand
Telephone: 09 303–1040

329. Audit Bureau of Circulations (ABC)
900 North Meachham Road
Schaumburg
IL 60173–4968
USA
Telephone: (708) 605–0909

330. Aus Corp Serve Inc
155 King George Street
Annapolis
MD 21401
USA
Telephone: (301) 268–4991
Telex/E-mail: 62765939

331. AUSINET (See Ferntree Computer Corporation Ltd)

332. Austin American-Statesman
166 E Riverside Drive
PO Box 670
Austin
TX 78767
USA
Telephone: (512) 445–3745

333. Australasian Digital Video Interactive Technology
Vince Blackburn (Managing Director)
PO Box 653
North Adelaide
SA 5006
Australia
Telephone: 8 269–4811
Fax: 8 269–5435; 8 224–0464

334. Australia Bureau of Transport and Communications Economics
BTCE Information Systems
GPO Box 501
Canberra
ACT 2601
Australia
Telephone: 062 746–846
Fax: 062 746–814
Telex/E-mail: 61733 AA

335. Australia Council Library
PO Box 302
168 Walker Street
North Sydney
NSW 2060
Australia
Telephone: 61 (2) 923–3333;
(008) 22–6912
Fax: 61 (2) 922–7560
Telex/E-mail: 26023 AA

336. Australian Associated Press
364 Sussex Street
PO Box 3888
Sydney
NSW 2001
Australia
Telephone: 02 236–8865

337. Australian Associated Stock Exchanges
Plaza Building
Australia Square
Sydney
NSW 2000
Australia
Telephone: 61 (2) 233–5266

338. Australian Bibliographic Network
National Library of Australia
Parkes Place
Canberra
ACT 2600
Australia
Telephone: 61 62–1484
Telex/E-mail: 62100 LIBAUST AA

339. Australian Bureau of Agricultural and Resource Economics
Economics Statistics System
McArthur House
6th Floor
North Bourne Avenue
Lyneham
ACT 2602
Australia

340. Australian Bureau of Statistics
Information Services
Cameron Offices
PO Box 10
Belconnen
ACT 2616
Australia
Telephone: 062 527–911;
062 526–017;
062 526–627;
062 526–295
Fax: 062 516–009;
062 531–404
Telex/E-mail: 62020 ABOST AA
AUSSTATS (CSIRONET);
ABS880 (Keylink)

341. Australian Business Index
421 Riverside Road
East Hawthorn
VIC 3123
Australia
Telephone: 03 882–7344
Fax: 03 882–6837

342. Australian Business Information Pty Ltd
Neville Bullard (National Sales Director)
128 Little Lonsdale Street
Melbourne
VIC 3000
Australia
Telephone: 3 663 7533
Fax: 3 663 4590

343. Australian Commonwealth Scientific and Industrial Research Organisation
Energy Information Service
314 Albert Street
PO Box 89
East Melbourne
VIC 3002
Australia
Telephone: 03 418–7333
Fax: 03 419–0459
Telex/E-mail: 30236 AA ENERGY
(CSIROMAIL)

344. Australian Commonwealth Scientific and Industrial Research Organisation
Information Services Branch
314 Albert Street
PO Box 89
East Melbourne
VIC 3002
Australia
Telephone: 03 418–7333
Fax: 03 419–0459
Telex/E-mail: 30236 AA

345. Australian Commonwealth Scientific and Industrial Research Organisation
AUSTRALIS
Mary Turner; Lea Giles-Peters
(Manager CSIRO Australis)
314 Albert Street
PO Box 89
East Melbourne
VIC 3002
Australia
Telephone: 03 418–7333;
03 418–7307
Fax: 03 419–0459
Telex/E-mail: 30236 AA

346. Australian Consolidated Press Ltd
54–58 Park Street
Sydney
NSW 2000
Australia
Telephone: 02 267–2150

347. Australian Council for Educational Research
Library and Information Services Unit
9 Frederick Street
PO Box 210
Hawthorn
VIC 3122
Australia
Telephone: 03 819–1400
Fax: 03 819–5502
Telex/E-mail: MLN301450 (ILANET)

348. Australian Database Development Association
PO Box 53
Hawthorn
VIC 3122
Australia
Telephone: 03 867–7426

349. Australian Heritage Commission
GPO Box 1567
Canberra
ACT 2601
Australia
Telephone: 062 271–2119
Fax: 062 732–395

350. Australian Institute of Criminology
JV Barry Library
John Myrtle (Librarian)
PO Box 2944
Canberra
ACT 2601
Australia
Telephone: 062 740–264;
062 274–0200
Fax: 062 740–201
Telex/E-mail: 61340 AUCRIM AA
MLN600350 (ILANET);
TCN4014 (TNC)

351. Australian Institute of Family Studies
Family Information Centre
Deborah A Whithear (Editor, Australian Family and Society Abstracts)
300 Queen Street
Melbourne
VIC 3000
Australia
Telephone: 3 608–6888
Fax: 3 600–0886

352. Australian Leisure Index
FIT Library
PO Box 64
Footscray
VIC 3011
Australia
Telephone: 61 (3) 688–4544
Telex/E-mail: 36596 FITLEX AA

353. Australian MEDLINE Network
National Library of Australia
Parkes Place
Canberra
ACT 2600
Australia
Telephone: 06 262–1523
Fax: 06 257–1703
Telex/E-mail: 62100 LIBAUST AA

354. Australian Mineral Foundation
63 Conyngham Street
Glenside
SA 5065
Australia
Telephone: 08 379–0444
Fax: 08 379–4634
Telex/E-mail: 87437 AMFINC AA

355. Australian Nuclear Science & Technology Oranization
Lucas Heights Research Laboratories
Private Mail Bag 1
Menai
NSW 2234
Australia
Telephone: 61 (2) 543–3111
Fax: 61 (2) 543–5097

356. Australian Road Research Board
500 Burwood Highway
Vermont South
VIC 3131
Australia
Telephone: 03 881–1560
Fax: 03 803–8878
Telex/E-mail: 33113 CUSTUL AA

357. Australian Schools Cataloguing Information Service
CD-ROM Enquiries
325 Camberwell Road
Camberwell
VIC 3124
Australia
Telephone: 3 882–8108
Fax: 3 882–8101

358. Australian Sports Commission
PO Box 176
Belconnen
ACT 2616
Australia

359. Australian Stock Exchange Ltd
Exchange Center
20 Bond Street
POB H224
Australia Square
Sydney
NSW 2000
Australia
Telephone: 02 227–0000
Telex/E-mail: 20630 AA

**360. Australian Trade Practices
    Commission**
PO Box 19
Belconnen
ACT 2616
Australia
Telephone: 062 641–166
Telex/E-mail: 62626 AA

**361. Australian Wine Research
    Institute**
John Fornachon Memorial Library
Waite Road
Urrbrae
SA 5064
Australia
Telephone: 08 799–681
Fax: 08 795–200
Telex/E-mail: 88657 WINRES AA

**362. Australis (See Australian
    Commonwelath Scientific and
    Industrial Research
    Organisation)**

363. Authorware Europe Ltd
Nick Corston (Marketing Consultant)
4 Wellington Business Park
Dukes Ride
Crowthorne
Berkshire
RG11 6LS
UK
Telephone: 0344 761–111
Fax: 0344 761–149

364. Authorware Inc
Roger Llewellyn (Vice President Europe);
    Joe Fantuzzi (Vice President
    Worldwide Marketing)
275 Shoreline Boulevard
Suite 535
Redwood City
CA 94065
USA
Telephone: (415) 595–3107
Fax: (415) 595–3077

365. Auto-Grafica Export Company
Steve Dritschel (Purchasing)
58A Hobart Street
Hackensack
NJ 07601
USA
Telephone: (201) 343–8585
Fax: (201) 343–0711

366. Auto-Graphics Inc
Joel M Lee (Marketing Manager)
3201 Temple Avenue
Pomona
CA 91768–3200
USA
Telephone: (714) 595–7204;
          (800) 325–7961;
          (800) 776–6939
Fax: (714) 595–3506

367. AutoComp
PO Box 32
Fond du Lac
WI 54935
USA

368. Autofacts Inc
63 Chestnut Road
Paoli
PA 19301
USA
Telephone: (215) 644–4747
Fax: (215) 644–4853

369. Automated Archives Inc
Lyman Platt (President); John Whitaker
    (Marketing/Sales)
University Plaza
1160 S State Street
Suite 250
Orem
UT 84058
USA
Telephone: (801) 226–6066
Fax: (801) 224–4510

**370. Automated Marketing Systems
    Inc (see National Research
    Bureau)**

371. Automated Sciences Group
700 Roeder Rd.
Silver Springs
MD 20910–4405
USA

372. Avantext Inc
Includes: Flighline Electronic Publishing
PO Box 366
Honey Brook
PA 19344
USA
Telephone: (215) 273–7410

373. Aviation Data Service Inc
312 E Murdock
Wichita
KS 67214
USA
Telephone: (316) 262–1491
Fax: (316) 262–5333

374. Aviation Safety Institute
PO Box 304
Worthington
OH 43085
USA
Telephone: (614) 885–4242
Fax: (614) 885–5891
Telex/E-mail: 76703,402 (CompuServe
Information Service)

375. Aviation/Aerospace Online
Washington
DC 20005
USA
Telephone: (202) 822–4625
Fax: (202) 293–2682
Telex/E-mail: 892447

376. Axirom
Groupement Canope-Sédinov-UNSFA
Bernard Longhi (CEO)
9 rue Dupré
92600 Asnières
France
Telephone: 1 47 93 29 75
Fax: 1 40 86 18 84

377. Axon Group
LRP Publications
PO Box 980
747 Dresher Road, Horsham
PA 19044–0980
USA
Telephone: (215) 784–0860
Fax: (215) 784–0870

378. Axses Inc
Ian Clayton (President)
Boutiliers Point
Halifax
NS B0J 1G0
Canada
Telephone: (902) 826–2440
Fax: (902) 826–7274

**379. AZ Bertelsmann (See also
    Bertelsmann; eps Bertelsmann)**

380. AZ Bertelsmann GmbH
Carl-Bertelsmann-Straße 161
D-4830 Gütersloh 1
Germany
Telephone: 05241 80 54 73
Fax: 05241 769 84
Telex/E-mail: 933752 D

381. AZtec Hotel Information Service
444 Madison Avenue
New York
NY 10022
USA
Telephone: (212) 980–8320

382. AZtec Inc
220 5th Avenue
7th Floor
New York
NY 10001
USA
Telephone: (212) 557–0055

383. B Breidenstein GmbH
B team
Untermainkai 83
D-6000 Frankfurt am Main 1
Germany
Telephone: 069 23 09 05
Fax: 069 23 52 79

384. B Ticino
Viale Borri
21100 Varese
Italy
Telephone: +39 332 279111
Fax: +39 332 265661

385. Bacchus Data Services
6085 Venice Boulevard, No 16
Los Angeles
CA 90034
USA
Telephone: (213) 558–3281

386. Baker & Taylor Books
Christian K. Larew (Director Customer
Electronic Services)
652 E Main Street
PO Box 6920
Bridgewater
NJ 08807–0920
USA
Telephone: (908) 218–0400
Fax: (908) 722–7420

387. Balslev Publikationer
Jette Balslev
Fosgaarden 14
DK-2620 Albertslund
Denmark
Telephone: 45 04 224020

388. Baltimore County Public Library
Charles Robinson
320 York Road
Towson
MD 21204–5179
USA
Telephone: (301) 296–8500;
          (301) 296–3139

389. Baltimore Sun, The
501 N Calvert Street
Baltimore
MD 21278
USA
Telephone: (301) 332–6300

390. Banca Popolare di Sondrio
Piergiorgio Picceni (Direttore Centrale)
Piazza Garibaldi 16
23100 Sondrio SO
Italy
Telephone: 0342 528–323
Fax: 0342 528–365

391. Bancroft-Parkman Inc
Bookline
PO Box 1236
Washington
CT 06793
USA
Telephone: (212) 737–2715
Fax: (203) 868–0080

392. Bancroft-Whitney Company
301 Brannan Street
San Francisco
CA 94107
USA
Telephone: (415) 986–4410

393. Bank Administration Institute
60 Gould Center
Rolling Meadows
IL 60008
USA
Telephone: (312) 228–6200

394. Bank Marketing Association
309 W Washington Street
Chicago
IL 60606
USA
Telephone: (312) 782–1442;
(800) 433–9013
Fax: (312) 782–0321
Telex/E-mail: 910–221–2897

**395. Bank of America's World
Information Services**
Ellen Bates
BA Plaza Library
335 Madison Avenue
New York
NY 10017
USA
Telephone: (212) 503–8007

396. Bank of America
Emanuel Frenkel
555 California Street
San Francisco
CA 94104
USA
Telephone: (800) 645–6667

397. Bank of England
Financial Statistics Division
Princess Street
Bank Buildings
London
EC2R 8AH
UK
Telephone: 071 601–4311

399. Bank Valuation
2130 Jackson Street
San Francisco
CA 94115
USA
Telephone: (415) 922–0441

400. Banker & Tradesman
Ray Parenteau
210 South Street
5th Floor
Boston
MA 02111
USA
Telephone: (617) 426–4495
Fax: (617) 423–1335

**401. Banker, a Financial Times
Business Publication**
102–108 Ackerwell Road
London
EC1M 5SA
UK
Telephone: 071 251–9321
Fax: 071 251–4686
Telex/E-mail: 23700 FINBI G

**402. Bankers Trust Global Operating
& Information Services**
1 Bankers Trust Plaza
130 Liberty Street
9th Floor
New York
NY 10015
USA
Telephone: (212) 250–3832

**403. Banque d'Information
Automatisee sur les
Medicaments**
Secretariat Technique
15 rue Rieux
F-92100 Boulogne
France
Telephone: 1 48 25 39 52

404. Banque de Donnée Médicale
B Kempf
46 rue des Martyrs
75009 Paris
France
Telephone: 1 48 78 78 88

405. Banque de France
BP 140–01
F-75049 Paris Cedex 01
France
Telephone: 1 42 61 56 72
Telex/E-mail: 220932 F

**406. Banque Internationale
d'Information sur les Etats
Francophones**
Secretary of State of Canada
Room 7E8
Ottawa
ON K1A 0M5
Canada
Telephone: (819) 953–6902
Fax: (819) 997–7836
Telex/E-mail: 0533384

407. Banque Nationale de Belgique
Mr Rubens
Boulevard de Berlaimont 5
B-1000 Brussels
Belgium
Telephone: 02 221 21 11
Fax: 02 221 31 17;
02 221 31 00

408. Barclays Law Publishers
400 Oyster Point Boulevard
Suite 500
PO Box 3066
South San Francisco
CA 94083
USA
Telephone: (415) 244–6611

409. Barnes and Thornburg
11 S Meriadian Street
Indianapolis
IN 46204
USA
Telephone: (317) 638–1313

410. Barter Worldwide Inc
14221 Petaluma Court
Victorville
CA 92392
USA
Telephone: (619) 951–2444
Fax: (619) 951–2442
Telex/E-mail: 466807 BARTER WW/IBC

411. BASELINE II Inc
838 Broadway
4th Floor
New York
NY 10003
USA
Telephone: (212) 254–8235;
(800) 242–7546;
(800) 254–8235
Fax: (212) 529–3330
Telex/E-mail: BASELINE (MCI Mail)

412. BASF AG
Carl-Bosch-Straße 38
D-6700 Ludwigshafen T
Germany
Telephone: 0621 60 28 401
Telex/E-mail: 464990 BAS D

413. BatiDoc SA
JP Matz (Technical Director)
11 bis Place de la Nation
75011 Paris
France
Telephone: 1 43 56 72 72
Fax: 1 43 56 22 31

**414. Baton Rouge State-Times and
Morning Advocate**
525 Lafayette Street
Baton Rouge
LA 70821
USA
Telephone: (504) 383–1111

415. Battelle Memorial Institute
505 King Avenue
Columbus
OH 43201–2693
USA
Telephone: (614) 424–6424
Fax: (614) 424–5263
Telex/E-mail: 245454

416. Battelle, Centre de Recherches
7 route de Drize
12277 Carouge/Geneva
Switzerland
Telephone: 41 (22) 27 02 70
Telex/E-mail: 423472 BATEL CH

417. Bayer AG
Ingenieur-wissenschaftliche Abteilung
Bayerwerk
D-5090 Leverkusen
Germany
Telephone: 0214 30 71 763
Fax: 0214 30 71 367
Telex/E-mail: 85103 285 BY D

**418. Bayerische Staatsbibliothek
Muenchen**
PO Box 340150
8000 Munich 34
Germany
Telephone: 49 (89) 21 98 – 3 96
Telex/E-mail: 897248 BSB D

419. BBC Enterprises Limited
Woodlands
80 Wood Lane
London
W12 0TT
UK
Telephone: 081 743–5588

420. BBC Interactive Television Unit
Elstree Court
Clarendon Road
Boreham Wood
WD6 1JF
UK
Telephone: 081–953 6100

421. BBC
BBC Monitoring
Caversham Park
Reading
Berkshire
RG4 8TZ
UK
Telephone: 0734 472–742
Fax: 0734 461–105

422. BBM Bureau of Measurement
1500 Don Mills Road, Suite 305
Don Mills
ON M3B 3L7
Canada
Telephone: (416) 445–9800
Fax: (416) 445–8644
Telex/E-mail: 06986198

423. BCB – Bertelsmann Computer Beratundienst GmbH
Marketing Department
Heidenkampsweg 44
2000 Hamburg 1
Germany
Telephone: 49 (40) 237001–0

424. BDC Technical Services Ltd
Felicity Coxon (Marketing Manager)
Slack Lane
Derby
DE3 3FL
UK
Telephone: 0332 471–23
Fax: 0332 290–820
Telex/E-mail: 377017

425. Beacham Publishing
2100 South Street N.W.
Washington
DC 20008–4011
USA
Telephone: (202) 234–0877

426. Beacon Journal Publishing Company
44 E Exchange Street
Akron
OH 44328
USA
Telephone: (216) 375–8111

427. Beacon Technology
3550 Stevens Creek Boulevard
San Jose
CA 95117
USA
Telephone: (408) 296–4884

428. Bechelli, Harris & Asociados
Tte. Gral. J.D. Peron 729 piso 9
1038 Buenos Aires
Argentina
Telephone: 54 (1) 46–8976
Telex/E-mail: 823340 SGM UF

429. Bechtel Information Services Inc
9430 Key West Avenue, Suite 200
Rockville
MD 20850
USA
Telephone: (301) 258–4300;
(301) 738–1400
Fax: (301) 279–0511

430. Beeldwerke BV
Ferenc Nemeth
Ringlaan 4
3743 DA Baarn
Netherlands
Telephone: 2154 114–98
Fax: 2154 240–22

431. Begotel
PO Box 2188
4800 CB Breda
Netherlands
Telephone: 76 480890

432. Behavioral Measurement Database Services
PO Box 110287
Pittsburgh
PA 15232–0787
USA
Telephone: (412) 687–6850

433. Beilstein-Institute für Literatur der Organischen Chemie
Clemens Jochum
Varrentrappstraße 40–42
D-6000 Frankfurt am Main 90
Germany
Telephone: 069 791–7251;
069 791–70
Fax: 069 791–7321
Telex/E-mail: 416969 BLSTN D

434. Belgian National Bank
Boulevard de Berlaimont 5
1000 Brussels
Belgium
Telephone: 32 02 219 46 00

435. BELINDIS
Jacques Lauwerys (French); De Waele (Dutch)
Belgian Ministry of Economic Affairs
Centre de Traitement de l'Information
30 rue JA de Mot
B-1040 Brussels
Belgium
Telephone: 02 233–6111;
02–233–6737;
02–233–6696
Fax: 02 230–4619
Telex/E-mail: 23509 ENERGI B
NUA: 2062221012

436. Bell & Howell Publications Systems Company
David Webb (General Manager)
Telford Road
Bicester
Oxfordshire OX6 0UP
UK
Telephone: 0869 245–711
Fax: 0869 240–982

437. Bell & Howell Publications Systems Company
Linda Baron (Marketing Services Specialist)
5700 Lombardo Center
Suite 220
Seven Hills
OH 44131–2531
USA
Telephone: (216) 642–9060
Fax: (216) 642–4308

438. Belser Knowledge Services
New York
NY
USA
Telephone: 212–727–3888

439. Bergen Bank
Bedriftsservice
PO Box 1170
N-0107 Oslo 1
Norway
Telephone: 02 40 06 86
Fax: 02 41 08 32

440. Berkeley Mac User's Group
CD-ROM Enquiries
Suite 62
1442A Walnut Street
Berkeley
CA 94709
USA
Telephone: (510) 549–2684
Fax: (510) 849–9026

441. Bertelsmann (See also AZ Bertelsmann; eps Bertelsmann)

442. Bertelsmann Informations Service GmbH
Renate Mayerhof (Kendenbetreuung)
Landsberger Straße 191a
D-8000 Munich 21
Germany
Telephone: 089 57 95 220;
089 57 95 221
Fax: 089 57 06 693
Telex/E-mail: 521 2943 WILA D
NUA: Available on application

443. Bertrand Narvesens vei 2 (SilverPlatter Agent)
PO Box 6125 Etterstad
N-0602 Oslo 6
Norway
Telephone: 472–678310

444. BetaCorp Technologies Inc
John J Bekto (Director of Sales)
5716–11 Coopers Avenue
Mississauga
ON L4Z 2B9
Canada
Telephone: (416) 890–5441
Fax: (416) 890–5458

445. Beth Israel Hospital
Center for Clinical Computing (PaperChase)
350 Longwood Avenue
Boston
MA 02115
USA
Telephone: (617) 278–3900;
(800) 722–2075
Fax: (617) 277–9792
Telex/E-mail: 76703,2003
(CompuServe)

446. Betriebswirtschaftlicher Verlag Dr Th Gabler
Peter Eichhorn (Marketing)
Taunusstraße 54
6200 Wiesbaden 1
Germany
Telephone: 611 534 69
Fax: 611 534 89

447. Bezugsquellennachweis für den Einkauf GmbH
Rainer Schulte
Normannenweg 18–20
Postfach 100549
D-2000 Hamburg 1
Germany
Telephone: 040 2515–080
Fax: 040 2515–0838
Telex/E-mail: 2173886 WLW D

448. BHRA
The Fluid Engineering Centre
Cranfield
Bedfordshire
MK43 0AJ
UK
Telephone: 44 (234) 750422
Fax: 44 (234) 750074
Telex/E-mail: 825059 G

449. Bibliographic Information on Southeast Asia
University of Sydney Library
Sydney
NSW 2006
Australia
Telephone: 02 692–2222
Fax: 02 692–4203
Telex/E-mail: 20056 AA

450. Biblioteca Nacional de España
Paseo de Recoletos 20
28001 Madrid
Spain
Telephone: 01 275–6800
Fax: 01 564–1550

451. Biblioteca Nacional de Portugal
Campo Grande 83
1751 Lisbon Codex
Portugal
Telephone: 1 76 77 86
Fax: 7393607
Telex/E-mail: 62803 P

452. Biblioteca Nacional
Juan Alvarez (Manager of Computer Department)
c/ Paris Con Caroni
Las Mercedes
EDF Macanao
Venezuela
Telephone: 572–7923 572–0301
Fax: 574–8824

453. Biblioteca Nazionale Centrale
Carla Guiducci Bonanni (Director);
Giovanni Bergamin (Head of Automation Department)
Piazza Cavallegerri 1B
I-50122 Florence
Italy
Telephone: 055 241–187;
055 244–441
Fax: 055 232–2482

454. Bibliotekscentralen
Anders Ravn; Suzanne Christoffersen; Poul Jensen
Tempovej 7–11
DK-2750 Ballerup
Denmark
Telephone: 45 42 974000
Fax: 45 44 681355
NUA: 23830106234600

455. Bibliotekscentrum Sverige AB (See BiC)

456. Biblioteksentralen A/L
PO Box 6142
Etterstad
N-0602 Oslo 6
Norway
Telephone: 02 673–480
Fax: 02 196–443
Telex/E-mail: 19233 BSN N

457. Bibliotekstjanst AB
Svante Hallgren
PO Box 200
S-221 00 Lund
Sweden
Telephone: 046 180–000
Fax: 046 180–125
Telex/E-mail: 32200 BTJLUND S

458. Bibliotheksrechenzentrum Niedersachsen
Prinzenstrasse 1
3400 Goettingen
Germany
Telephone: 49 (551) 39 – 52 64

459. Bibliotheksstelle der Düsseldorfer Kulturinstitute
Stadverwaltung Amt 41/217
PO Box 11 20
4000 Duuesseldorf 1
Germany
Telephone: 49 (211) 899–5573;
49 (211) 899–5589

460. Bibliothèque Cantonale et Universitaire
Secretariat RPM/VMZ
1015 Lausanne-Dorigny
Switzerland
Telephone: 41 (21) 692 32 29
Telex/E-mail: 24014 LAUC CH

461. Bibliothèque de la Sorbonne
Martine Lussier (Chef du Département)
47 rue des Ecoloes
75230 Paris Cedex 5
France
Telephone: 1 40 46 22 11
Fax: 1 40 46 30 44

462. Bibliothèque de Sainte-Geneviève
Isabelle Nectoux (Conservateur Chargé des Nouvelles Technologies)
10 place du Panthéon
75005 Paris
France
Telephone: 1 43 29 61 00
Fax: 1 40 51 73 58

463. Bibliothèque Interuniversitaire Cujas
Dominique Marcillaud (Conservateur)
2 rue Cujas
75005 Paris
France
Telephone: 1 46 34 99 71;
1 43 54 74 44
Fax: 1 46 33 82 61

464. Bibliothèque Nationale du Québec
125 Sherbrook West
Montreal
PQ H2X 1X4
Canada
Telephone: (514) 873–5695
Fax: (514) 873–4310
Telex/E-mail: 05561294

465. Bibliothèque Nationale Universitaire de Strasbourg
Section des Alsatiques
3a Rue de Marechal Joffre
BP 1029 F
F-67070 Strasbourg Cedex
France
Telephone: 88 25 28 46

466. Bibliothèque Nationale
Département de la Phonothèque Nationale
2 rue Louvois
F-75084 Paris Cedex 02
France
Telephone: 1 47 03 88 17

467. Bibliothèque Nationale
2 rue Vivienne
Paris
F-75084 Paris Cedex 02
France
Telephone: 1 47 03 81 26
Fax: 1 42 97 84 47

468. BIBSYS
Library Automation System
7055 Dragvoll
Norway
Telephone: 47 (7) 9 70 67
Fax: 47 (7) 59 68 48
Telex/E-mail: 55620 SINTF N

469. BiC – Bibliotekscentrum Svierge AB
P/O/ Box 113
Norrgatan 17
S-251 04 Växjö
Sweden
Telephone: 470 450 78
Fax: 470 400 45

470. Bielefeld Universitätsbibliothek
Herr Binder (Commissioner for Information)
Postfach 8620
Universitätsstraße 25
4800 Bielefeld 1
Germany
Telephone: 521 106–4051
Fax: 521 106–4052

471. BIIC Technology
Gerald Mulder (General Manager)
14E St Paul's Terrace
London
SE17 3QH
UK
Telephone: 071 582–0488
Fax: 071 582–0488

472. Billboard Publications Inc
1515 Broadway
New York
NY 10036
USA
Telephone: (212) 764–7300
Fax: (212) 536–5310
Telex/E-mail: 710–581–6279

473. BioCommerce Data Ltd
Prudential Buildings
95 High Street
Slough
Berkshire
SL1 1DH
UK
Telephone: 0753 511–777
Fax: 0753 512–239

474. Biologische Bundesanstalt für Land- und Forstwirtschaft
Dokumentationsstelle für Phytomedizin
Königin-Luise-Straße 19
D-1000 Berlin 33
Germany
Telephone: 030 830–4215
Fax: 030 830–4284

475. Biomedical Business International
1524 Brookhollow Drive
Santa Ana
CA 92705
USA
Telephone: (714) 755–5757
Fax: (714) 755–5704

476. BIOSIS UK
Garforth House
54 Mickelgate
York
North Yorkshire
YO1 1LF
UK

477. BIOSIS
Arthus Elias (Director Marketing and Distribution)
2100 Arch Street
Philadelphia
PA 19103–1399
USA
Telephone: (215) 587–4800;
(212) 318–2200;
(800) 523–4806
Fax: (215) 587–2016
Telex/E-mail: 831739 G 2889584 (EasyLink)

478. BioWorld
217 South B Street
San Mateo
CA 94401–9806
USA
Telephone: (415) 696–6590;
(800) 879–8790

479. BIREME (See also Pan American Health Organization)

480. BIREME
Abel Laerte Packer (Systems & Data Processing)
Rua Botucato 862
SP 04023 Sao Paulo
Brazil
Telephone: 011 549 26 11
Fax: 011 571 19 19

481. Bistel
Rue de la Loi 18
1000 Brussels
Belgium
Telephone: (2) 513 80 20

482. Bitstream Inc
Stefan Wennik (Graphic Arts Marketing & PR)
Athenaeum House
215 First Street
Cambridge
MA 02142
USA
Telephone: (617) 497–6222
Fax: (617) 868–4732

483. Black Box Corporation
Mayview Road at Park Drive
Pittsburgh
PA 15241
USA
Telephone: (412) 746–6368
Fax: (412) 746–0746

484. Blackwell Scientific Publications
Osney Mead
Oxford
OX 2 0EL
UK
Telephone: 0865 240–201
Fax: 0865 721–205

485. Blaupunkt-Werke GmbH
Bosch Telecom
Werner Wilmes (Product Manager Navigation Systems)
Robert-Bosch Straße 200
W-3200 Hildesheim
Germany
Telephone: 51 21 49 4779
Fax: 51 21 49 4154

486. Blendon Information Services
126 Willowdale Avenue
Suite 1
Willowdale
ON M2N 4Y2
Canada
Telephone: (416) 223–5397

487. Bloodstock Research Information Services Inc
801 Corporate Drive
Third floor
PO Box 4097
Lexington
KY 40544
USA
Telephone: (606) 223–4444

488. Bloomberg Financial Markets
499 Park Avenue
15th Floor
New York
NY 10022
USA
Telephone: (212) 318–2000

489. Blue Sail Software
Jim Wallace
451 Moody Street, Suite 206
Waltham
MA 02154
USA
Telephone: (617) 899–8474

490. BMT Cortec Ltd
Library
Wallsend
Tyne and Wear
NE28 6UY
UK
Telephone: 091 262–5242
Telex/E-mail: 53476 G

491. BNF Metals Technology Centre
Denchworth Road
Wantage
Oxfordshire
OX12 9BJ
UK
Telephone: 0235 772–992
Telex/E-mail: 837166 G

492. Boersinformation Telecom
Frederiksberggade 2
PO Box 1156
DK-1010 Copenhagen K
Denmark
Telephone: 033 12332
Fax: 033 324–232
Telex/E-mail: 19732 DK

493. Bokfoeringsnaemnden
PO Box 2134
103 14 Stockholm
Sweden
Telephone: 46 (8) 791 06 71

494. Boletín Oficial del Estado
Calle Trafalgar 29
28010 Madrid
Spain
Telephone: 01 446–6000;
01 538–2100
Fax: 01 593–3760

495. Bolsa Oficial de Commercio de Madrid
Plaza de la Lealtad 1
E-28014 Madrid
Spain
Telephone: 01 589–1405
Fax: 01 589–1755
Telex/E-mail: 49184
NUA: Available on application

496. Bonnier Business Publishing Group (See Affärsdata AB)

497. Book Data
Vesna Nall (Customer Services)
Northumberland House
2 King Street
Twickenham
TW1 3RZ
UK
Telephone: 081 892–2272
Fax: 081 892–9109

498. Book Promotion & Service Ltd
Lee Itia (Production Manager)
2220/31 Soi
Ramkhamhanegn 36/1
Huamark
Bangkok 10240
Thailand
Telephone: 2 375–2685
Fax: 2 375–2669

499. Booklink
A division of Sydney Kramer Books Inc
Library Wholesale Services
1722 H Street, NW
Washington
DC 20006
USA
Telephone: (202) 298–8015;
(800) 423–2665

500. Booth Newspapers Inc
155 Michigan Street NW
Grand Rapids
MI 49503
USA
Telephone: (616) 459–1567

501. Bord Cadre
7 rue Sainte Croix de Bretonnerie
Paris 75004
France
Telephone: 33–1–4029–0018

502. Boreal Institute for Northern Studies
CW401 Bio. Sci. Building
The University of Alberta
Edmonton
AB T6G 2E9
Canada
Telephone: (403) 432–4409
Fax: (403) 492–1153

503. Boris Kidric Institute
Hajdrihova 19
61000 Ljubljana
Yugoslavia
Telephone: 38 (61) 263–061
Telex/E-mail: 32121 KIBKLJ YU

504. Borsu International BV
Jacob Rassers (Vice President
    Research and Development)
Bloemendalerweg 43–45
1382 KB Weesp
Netherlands
Telephone: 02940 61111
Fax: 02940 14253

505. Boston Computer Society
Macintosh User Group
Stefan Pagacik (Project Director) Ward
    Poor Rob Graham (Marketing
Management)
48 Grove Street
Somerville
MA 02144
USA
Telephone: (617) 625–7080

506. Boston Spa Training Ltd
CR Fussey (Business Manager)
Clifford Moor Road
Boston Spa
Wetherby
West Yorkshire
LS23 6RW
UK
Telephone: 0937 541–440
Fax: 0937 541–296

507. Boston University
School of Education
605 Commonwealth Avenue
Boston
MA 02215
USA
Telephone: (617) 353–3295

508. Bottin SA
28 rue du Docteur-Finlay
F-75738 Paris Cedex 15
France
Telephone: 1 45 78 61 66
Telex/E-mail: 204286 F

509. Bowker A & I Publishing
121 Chanlon Road
New Providence
NJ 07974
USA
Telephone: (908) 665–6688;
    (800) 322–5006

510. Bowker Business Research
121 Chanlon Road
New Providence
NJ 07974
USA
Telephone: (908) 464–6800;
    (800) 323–3288

511. Bowker Electronic Publishing
Donna Payerle (Sales Coordinator)
121 Chanlon Road
New Providence
New Jersey
NJ 07974
USA
Telephone: (908) 665–2866;
    (800) 323–3288
Fax: (212) 645–0475;
    (908) 665–6688
Telex/E-mail: 127703

512. Bowker-Saur Ltd
Special Sales Department
59/60 Grosvenor Street
London
W1X 9DA
UK
Telephone: 071 493–5841
Fax: 071 580–4089

513. Bowling Green State University
Philosophy Documentation Center
Bowling Green
OH 43403–0189
USA
Telephone: (419) 372–2419;
    (800) 444–2419
Fax: (419) 372–6987

514. BPS Inc
Henk B Rolters (President)
5F Union Building
3–1–3 Kamoi
Midori-ku 226
Yokohama
Japan
Telephone: 45 931–5815
Fax: 45 931–5767

**515. Bradshaw Financial Network,
    The**
253 Channing Way
Suite 13
PO Box 3517
San Rafael
CA 94912–3517
USA
Telephone: (415) 479–3815
Fax: (415) 479–2730

516. Brewing Research Foundation
Lyttel Hall
Nutfield
Redhill
Surrey
RH1 4HY
UK
Telephone: 0737 822–272
Fax: 0737 822–747

517. Bridge Information Systems Inc
717 Office Parkway
St Louis
MO 63141
USA
Telephone: (314) 567–8100;
    (800) 325–3282
Fax: (314) 432–5391

518. Bright Star Technology Inc
Tina Thomsen
1450 114th Ave SE
Suite 200
Bellevue
WA 98004
USA
Telephone: (206) 451–3697
Fax: (206) 454–1062

**519. Brisbane College of Advanced
    Education**
Resource Centre
PO Box 117
Kedron
QLD 4031
Australia
Telephone: 61 (7) 357–7077 x225
Fax: 61 (7) 357–7067

520. Bristol University
Health Care Evaluation Unit
Alex Faulkner
Canynge Hall
Whiteladies Road
Bristol
BS8 2PR
UK
Telephone: 0272 738223
Fax: 0272 238568

521. Britannica Software Inc
Lynn P Batts (Public Relations
    Administrator)
345 Fourth Street
San Francisco
CA 94107
USA
Telephone: (415) 597–5555
Fax: (415) 546–1887

522. British Airways
John Skipsey (Business Analyst)
PO Box 10
Heathrow Airport
Hounslow
Middlesex
TW6 2JA
UK
Telephone: 081 562–1588
Fax: 081 562–1581

523. British Ceramic Research Ltd
Queen's Road
Penkhull
Stoke-on-Trent
ST4 7LQ
UK
Telephone: 0782 45431
Fax: 0782 412–331
Telex/E-mail: 36228 G

**524. British Columbia Ministry of
    Attorney General**
Parliament Buildings
Victoria
BC V8V 1X4
Canada
Telephone: (604) 356–8464;
    (604) 356–8461
Fax: (604) 387–1010

525. British Institute of Management
Cottingham Road
Corby
Northamptonshire
NN14 2AT
UK
Telephone: 0536 204–222
Fax: 0536 201–651

**526. British Library Bibliographic
    Services**
BLAISE-LINE
P Dale
2 Sheraton Street
London
W1V 4BH
UK
Telephone: 071 636–1544 ex 242
NUA: 234227900102

527. British Library
Humanities and Social Sciences
M J Crump (Managing Editor, ESTC);
    L J Carr (Head of Marketing and
Publications)
Great Russell Street
London
WC1B 3DG
UK
Telephone: 071 323–7608
Fax: 071 323–7782

528. British Library
National Bibliographic Service
James Elliot (Manager Record Supply)
Boston Spa
Wetherby
West Yorkshire
LS23 7BQ
UK
Telephone: 0937 546–585;
    0937 843–434
Fax: 0937 546–586

Addresses

529. British Library
Document Supply Centre
Mike Curston (CD-ROM Development)
Boston Spa
Weatherby
West Yorkshire
LS23 7BQ
UK
Telephone: 0937 546–061;
           0937 843–434
Fax: 0937 546–333
Telex/E-mail: 557381 G

530. British Library
National Preservation Office
Great Russell Street
London
WC1B 3DG
UK

531. British Library
National Serials Data Centre
2 Sherman Street
London
W1VB 3DG
UK

532. British Library
Science Reference and Information
  Service
25 Southampton Buildings
Chancery Lane
London
WC2A 1AW
UK
Telephone: 071 323–7494
Fax: 071 323–7930
Telex/E-mail: 266959 SCIREF G; 81:
BLI404 (Telecom Gold)

533. British Market Research Bureau
  Ltd
John Rousay (Choices Manager)
Saunders House
53 The Mall
Ealing
London
W5 3TE
UK
Telephone: 081 567–3060
Fax: 081 579–9809
Telex/E-mail: 935526 G

534. British Medical Association
Tavistock Square
London
WC1H 9JP
UK
Telephone: 071 387–4499
Fax: 071 388–2544
Telex/E-mail: 10074: BMX030 (Dialcom)

535. British Non-Ferrous Metals
  Technology Centre
Grove Laboratories
Denchworth Road
Wantage
Oxfordshire OX12 9BJ
UK
Telephone: 44 (2357) 2992
Telex/E-mail: 837166 G

536. British Olivetti
17–29 Sun Street
London
EC2M 2PU
UK
Telephone: 071 377–8644

537. British Overseas Trade Board
Department of Trade
1 Victoria Street
London
SW1H DET
UK

538. British Standards Institution
Information Department
Joe McLelland
Linford Wood
Milton Keynes
Buckinghamshire
MK14 6LE
UK
Telephone: 0908 220–022
Fax: 0908 320–856
Telex/E-mail: 825777 BSI MK G

539. British Telecom Business
  Direction
Telephone House
Temple Avenue
London
EC4Y 0HL
UK
Telephone: 071 822–1322
Fax: 071 583–6262
Telex/E-mail: 261040 PRSTL G

540. British Telecom Directory
  Products Unit
W Leslie McAllister (Project Manager,
  Phone Disc)
Columbia Centre
Market Street
Bracknell
Berkshire
RG12 1JG
UK
Telephone: 0344 861–961
Fax: 0344 860–872

541. British Universities Film & Video
  Council
55 Greek Street
London
W1V 5LR
UK
Telephone: 071 734–3687
Fax: 071 287–3914

542. Broadcast Advertiser Reports
  Inc
800 2nd Avenue, Room 803
New York
NY 10017
USA
Telephone: (212) 682–8500

543. Broadcast Data Systems
1515 Broadway
37th Floor
New York
NY 10036
USA
Telephone: (212) 536–5341
Fax: (212) 536–5310

544. Broadcast Interview Source
2233 Wisconsin Avenue, NW, #406
Washington
DC 20007–4104
USA
Telephone: (202) 333–4904
Fax: (202) 342–5411

545. Broadcasters Audience
  Research Board
Glenthorne House
Hammersmith Grove
London
W6 0ND
UK
Telephone: 081 741–9110

546. Brocacef B.V.
Dr. H. Gryseels
PO Box 75
3600 Maarssen AA
Netherlands
Telephone: 31 (030) 452654

547. Brock University Library
Sid Fosdick
St Catherines
ON L2S 3A1
Canada
Telephone: (416) 688–5550

548. Brodart Automation
10983 via Frontera
San Diego
CA 92127
USA
Telephone: (619) 451–0250

549. Brodart Company
109 Roy Boulevard
Brantford
Ontario
N3T 5N3
Canada

550. Brodart Company
500 Arch Street
Williamsport
PA 17705–9977
USA
Telephone: (717) 326–2461;
           (800) 233–8467;
           (800) 666–9162 (in Canada)
Fax: (717) 326–6769
Telex/E-mail: 510–655–5523

551. Broderbund Software
81 Rue de la Procession
92500 Rueil Malmaison
France
Telephone: 1 4777 0952

552. Broderbund Software
Softline
London
UK
Telephone: 081 642–2255

553. Broderbund Software
Feyna de Clerq (Export Manager)
17 Paul Drive
San Rafael
CA 94904–2101
USA
Telephone: (415) 492–3200
Fax: (415) 499–8661

554. Broker Services Inc
5950 South Willow Drive, #206
Englewood
CO 80111
USA
Telephone: (303) 779–8930

555. Brookdale Foundation, The
126 E 56th Street
New York
NY 10022
USA
Telephone: (212) 308–7355

556. Brookhaven National Laboratory
Chemistry Department
Upton
NY 11973
USA
Telephone: (516) 282–4382
Fax: (516) 282–5815
Telex/E-mail: 6852516 BNL DOE PDB
NLCHM (BITNET)

557. Brookhaven National Laboratory
National Nuclear Data Center
Building 1970
Upton
NY 11973
USA
Telephone: (516) 282–2901
Fax: (516) 282–2806
Telex/E-mail: 6852516 BNL DOE NNDC
BNL (BITNET);
BNL:NNDC (ESNET)

558. BRS Europe
EPI-Centre
Irwin House
118 Southwark Street
London
SE1 0SW
UK
Telephone: 071 928–1404
Fax: 071 583–3887

559. BRS Information Technologies
Julian Taylor, Marketing Executive
Achilles House
Western Avenue
London
W3 0UA
UK
Telephone: 081 992–3456
Fax: 081 993–7335
Telex/E-mail: 8814614

560. BRS Information Technologies
8000 Westpark Drive
McLean
VA 22102
USA
Telephone: (703) 442–0900;
　　　　　 (800) 289–4277;
　　　　　 (800) 955–0906
Fax: (703) 893–4632
Telex/E-mail: (710) 444–4965

561. BRS Information Technologies
1200 Route 7
Latham
New York
NY 12110
USA
Telephone: (215) 254–0233;
　　　　　 (800) 468–0908

562. Brumberg Publications Inc
124 Harvard Street
Brookline
MA 02146
USA
Telephone: (617) 734–1979
Fax: (617) 734–1989

563. Brylar Pty Ltd
Peter Scarfo (Managing Director); Lynn
　May (Sales Marketing Manager)
Unit 5A
186–188 Canterbury Road
Canterbury
NSW 2193
Australia
Telephone: 2 787–4255
Fax: 2 787–3539

564. BT Distance Learning
BT Training
Stephen Brown
Derby House
219 Queensway
Bletchley
MK2 2DQ
UK
Telephone: +44 (0)908 366166 x378
Fax: +44 (0)908 271557

565. BT North America Inc
2560 N First Street
PO Box 49019
San José
CA 95161–9019
USA
Telephone: (408) 922–0250 (CGS,
　　　　　 Dialcom);
　　　　　 (800) 872–7654 (CGS) ;
　　　　　 (800) 435–7342 (Dialcom)
Fax: (301) 881–9016 (CGS)
Telex/E-mail: 710–825–9601 (Dialcom)

566. Bticino SpA
Ing Brianza
Corso Porta Vittoria 9
20125 Milan
Italy
Telephone: 2 57901

567. BTJ System AB
Anita Daun
PO Box 200
Traktorvägen 11
221 00 Lund
Sweden
Telephone: 46 180 000
Fax: 46 180 125;
　　　 46 180 333

568. BTShare
1 Bankers Trust Plaza
39th Floor
130 Liberty Street
New York
NY 10006
USA
Telephone: (212) 250–3833

569. BUC International Corporation
BUC Information Services
1314 NE 17th Court
Fort Lauderdale
FL 33305
USA
Telephone: (305) 565–6715;
　　　　　 (800) 327–6929
Fax: (305) 561–3095

570. Buchhändler-Vereinigung GmbH
Wilfried H Schinzel (Director
　Documentation & EDP Services)
Grosser Hirschgraben 17–21
Postfach 10 04 42
D-6000 Frankfurt am Main 1
Germany
Telephone: 69 13060
Fax: 69 1306–201

571. Buckmaster Publishing
Jack Speer (President)
PO Box 56
Route 3
Mineral
VA 23117
USA
Telephone: (703) 894–5777
Fax: (703) 894–9141

572. Budget Byte
1647 South West 41st Street
Topeka
KA 66609
USA
Telephone: (913) 266–0444

573. Buffalo News, The
Box 100
1 News Plaza
Buffalo
NY 14240
USA
Telephone: (716) 849–3434

**574. Building Cost Information
　　 Service**
Royal Institution of Chartered Surveyors
85/87 Clarence Street
Kingston upon Thames
Surrey
KT1 1RB
UK
Telephone: 44 (1) 546–7554

**575. Building Services Research and
　　 Information Association**
Old Bracknell Lane West
Bracknell
Berkshire
RG12 4AH
UK
Telephone: 0344 426–511
Fax: 0344 487–575
Telex/E-mail: 848288 BSRIAC G

576. Bull SA
Jeanne El Andaloussi (Documentation
　Groupe)
94 Avenue Gambetta
75020 Paris
France
Telephone: 1 43 56 44 78
Fax: 1 43 56 44 92

577. Bundesanstalt für Arbeitsschutz
Informations- und Dokumentations-
　zentrum für Arbeitsschutz
PO Box 17 02 02
Vogelpothsweg 50–52
D-4600 Dortmund 1
Germany
Telephone: 0231 176–3341
Telex/E-mail: 822153 D

**578. Bundesanstalt für
　　 Geowissenschaften und
　　 Rohstoffe**
Informationszentrum
　Rohstoffgewinnung,
　Geowissenschaften,
Wasserwirtschaft
Stilleweg 2
Postfach 510 153
D-3000 Hannover 51
Germany
Telephone: 0511 643–2819
Telex/E-mail: 923730 BGR HA D

**579. Bundesanstalt für
　　 Materialforschung und -prüfung**
Unter den Eichen 87
D-1000 Berlin 45
Germany
Telephone: 030 8104–6101
Fax: 030 811–2029
Telex/E-mail: 183261 BAMB D

**580. Bundesforschunganstalt für
　　 Rebenzueschung**
Geilweilerhof
6741 Siebeldingen (Pfalz)
Germany
Telephone: 49 (6345) 410
Fax: 49 (6345) 41177

**581. Bundesforschungsanstalt für
　　 Fischerei**
Informations- und Dokumentationsstelle
Dr WP Kirchner (Scientist); Dr U Brüll
　(Scientist)
Palmaille 9
2000 Hamburg 50
Germany
Telephone: 20 389 05 113
Fax: 38 905 129

582. Bundesinstitut für Sportwissenschaft
Fachbereich Dokumentation und Information
Carl-Diem-Weg 4
5000 Cologne 41
Germany
Telephone: 0221 49790
Telex/E-mail: 8881178 BISP D

583. Bundesministerium für das Post und Fernmeldewesen
Dienststelle 701–3
Postfach 8001
5300 Bonn 1
Germany
Telephone: 49 (228) 147013

584. Bundesministerium für Forschung und Technologie
Referat Hausinterne Datenverarbeitung und Dokumentation
PO Box 200240
5300 Bonn 40
Germany

585. Bundesministerium für Gesundheit
Kennedyallee 105–107
D-5300 Bonn 2
Germany
Telephone: 0228 9300

586. Bundesstelle für Außenhandelsinformation
Agrippastraße 87–93
Postfach 108007
D-5000 Cologne 1
Germany
Telephone: 0221 20570

587. Bundesvereinigung Deutscher Apothekerverbände
Postfach 970108
D-6000 Frankfurt am Main 97
Germany
Telephone: 069 75441
Fax: 069 74 92 68
Telex/E-mail: 414804 D

588. Buraff Publications
A division of the Bureau of National Affairs Inc
1350 Connecticut Avenue, NW
Washington
DC 20036
USA
Telephone: (202) 862–0990

589. Burda GmbH
Abteilung Marketing-Service
Postfach 12 30
7600 Offenburg
Germany
Telephone: 49 (781) 84 28 83

590. Bureau de Recherches Geologiques et Minieres
B.P. 6009
45060 Orleans Cedex
France
Telephone: 33 (38) 64 30 98;
33 (38) 64 38 09
Telex/E-mail: 780258 BRGMA F

591. Bureau Development Inc
Barry Cinnamon
141 New Road
Parsippany
NJ 07054
USA
Telephone: (201) 808–2700;
(800) 828–4766
Fax: (201) 808–2676

592. Bureau of Electronic Publishing (See Bureau Development Inc)

593. Bureau of Hygiene and Tropical Diseases
E.W. Fitzsimmons
Keppel Street
London
WC1E 7HT
UK
Telephone: 071 636–8636
Fax: 071 580–6756
Telex/E-mail: 8953474 LSHTML G

594. Bureau of Land Management
Dave Traudt
Eastern States Office, MS 972
350 South Pickett Street
Alexandria
VA 22304
USA
Telephone: (703) 461–1347

595. Bureau of National Affairs Inc
1231 25th Street NW
Washington
DC 20037
USA
Telephone: (202) 452–4132;
(800) 452–7773
Fax: (202) 822–8092
Telex/E-mail: 892692

596. Bureau of Transport and Communications Economics
PO Box 501
Canberra
ACT 2601
Australia
Telephone: 61 (62) 67–9725
Fax: 61 (62) 67–9816
Telex/E-mail: 61773 AA

597. Bureau van Dijk SA
Bernard Van Ommeslaghe (Managing Director); Pierre Gatz (Manager CD-ROM Projects)
Avenue Louise 250
1050 Brussels
Belgium
Telephone: 02 648 66 97
Fax: 02 648 82 30
Telex/E-mail: 20605 MVDBRU

598. Burrelle's Information Services
75 E Northfield Road
Livingston
NJ 07039–9873
USA
Telephone: (201) 992–6600;
(800) 631–1160
Fax: (201) 992–5122

599. Business and Legal Reports Inc
39 Academy Street
Madison
CT 06443–9988
USA
Telephone: (203) 245–7448;
(800) 553–4569
Fax: (203) 245–2559

600. Business and Trade Statistics Ltd
Ian Maclean (Managing Director); H Mirza (Technical Director)
Lancaster House
More Lane
Esher
Surrey
KT10 8AP
UK
Telephone: 0372 63121
Fax: 0372 469847

601. Business Communications Centre
Tallinn
Estonia
Telephone: +7 0142 423420

602. Business Communications Company Inc
25 Van Zant Street
Suite 13
Norwalk
CT 06855
USA
Telephone: (203) 853–4266

603. Business Datenbanken GmbH
Poststraße 42
D-6900 Heidelberg 1
Germany
Telephone: 6221 16 60 61
Fax: 6221 21 53 6
Telex/E-mail: 461 782 D GEO1
ONLINE-GMBH (GEONET)

604. Business Information & Solutions Ltd
Japan Report Division
Kirkman House
12–14 Whitfield Street
London
W1P 4RD
UK
Telephone: 071 435–4050
Fax: 071 436–8451

605. Business Information Publsihers BV
Gustaaf van Ditzhuyzen (General Manager)
Slochterenlaan 7
1405 AL Bussum
Netherlands
Telephone: 02159 51014
Fax: 02159 51568

606. Business International Corporation
215 Park Avenue S
New York
NY 10003
USA
Telephone: (212) 460–0600
Telex/E-mail: 234767

607. Business International S/A
12–14 chemin Reiu
CH-1211 Geneva 17
Switzerland
Telephone: 022 47 53 55
Fax: 022 47 81 18
Telex/E-mail: 422669 CH

608. Business People Publications Ltd
234 Kings Rd
London
SW3 5UA
UK
Telephone: 071 351–7351
Fax: 071 351–2794

609. Business Publishers Inc
951 Pershing Drive
Silver Spring
MD 20910–4464
USA
Telephone: (301) 587–6300
Fax: (301) 587–1081

610. Business Research Publications Inc
1036 National Press Building
Washington
DC 20045
USA

611. Business Surveys Limited
PO Box 21
Dorking
Surrey
RH4 2YU
UK
Telephone: 44 (306) 712867

612. Business Wire
44 Montgomery Street
Suite 2185
San Francisco
CA 94104
USA
Telephone: (415) 986–4422
Telex/E-mail: 34728

613. Business
An associate company of the Financial
   Times Ltd. and Conde Nast
   Publications
London
UK
Telephone: 071 351–7351
Fax: 071 351–2794

**614. Butterworth (Telepublishing)
   Limited**
4–5 Bell Yard
London
WC2A 2JR
UK
Telephone: 071 404–4097;
             071–405–9691 (LEXIS)
Fax: 071 831–1463
Telex/E-mail: 95678 G

615. Butterworth Canada
Salvy Trojman
75 Clegg Road
ON L6G 1A1
Canada
Telephone: (416) 479–2665
Fax: (416) 479–2826

616. Butterworths Pty Ltd
PO Box 345
North Ryde
New South Wales 2113
Australia
Telephone: (612) 887–3444

617. BUY-PHONE Inc
PO Box 29307
Los Angeles
CA 90029
USA
Telephone: (213) 279–1074

**618. BYGGDOK (See Institutet for
   Byggdokumentation)**

619. Byggecentrum
Mrs. Susane; Stig Merrild Hansen
Vester Voldgade 94
DK-1552 Koebenhavn V
Denmark
Telephone: 45 33 127373

**620. Byggeriets
   Realkreditfondkonsulentafd**
Klampenborgvej 205
DK-2800 Lyngby
Denmark
Telephone: 45 45 939393

621. BYTE Information Exchange
One Phoenix Mill Lane
Peterborough
NH 03458
USA
Telephone: (603) 924–7681;
             (800) 227–2983

622. C-CORE
Ocean Engineeering Information Centre
Judy Whittick (Senior Manager
   Business/Information Systems)
Memorial University of Newfoundland
Bartlett Building
St Johns
Newfoundland A1B 3X5
Canada
Telephone: (709) 737–8377
Fax: (709) 737–4706

623. C.BIC
Miguel Jimenez (Manager)
Jorge Manrique 27
28006 Madrid
Spain
Telephone: 1 585 44 43
Fax: 1 564 42 02

624. C.D.ROM & Associates
Caroline Beatty (Product Manager)
648 Whitehorse Road
Mitcham
VIC 3132
Australia
Telephone: 3 872 3211
Fax: 3 872 4814

**625. C.T.DEC (See Centre Technique
   de l'Industrie du Decolletage)**

626. C2H Telematique
64 rue du Creuzat
Parc d'Affaires Saint-Hubert
F-38080 L'Isle d'Abeau
France
Telephone: 974 27 19 89

627. CAB International (CABI)
Sue Hill (Marketing Executive CD-ROM)
Wallingford
Oxfordshire
OX10 8DE
UK
Telephone: 0491 32111
Fax: 0491 33508
Telex/E-mail: 847964 COMAGG G 84:
CAU001 (Dialcom)

628. CAB International
Carla Casler (North American
   Representative)
845 North Park Avenue
Tucson
AZ 85719
USA
Telephone: (800) 528–4841;
             (602) 621–7897
Fax: (602) 621–3816

629. Cabinet Beugnette
Christian Beugnette (Director)
rue Poincaré 19
88210 Senones
France
Telephone: 29 57 64 97
Fax: 29 57 81 19

630. Cable Publishing Group
600 S Cherry Street
Suite 400
Denver
CO 80222
USA
Telephone: (303) 393–7449

631. CACI Inc. – Federal
CACI Marketing Systems
9302 Lee Highway
Fairfax
VA 22031
USA
Telephone: (703) 218–4400;
             (800) 292–2224
Fax: (703) 273–8169

632. CACI Ltd
59/62 High Holborn
London
WC1V 6DX
UK
Telephone: 071 404–0834

633. CAD Information Systems Inc
Ed Green (Executive Vice President)
6551 South Revere Parkway
Suite 220
Englewood
CO 80111
USA
Telephone: (303) 799–1311
Fax: (303) 799–1356

**634. Cahners Technical Information
   Service**
David H Miller (President)
275 Washington Street
Newton
MA 02158–1630
USA
Telephone: (617) 558 4960
Fax: (617) 630 2168

**635. Caisse Nationale de Credit
   Agricole**
91–93 boulevard Pasteur
75710 Paris Brune
France

636. Caja de Ahorros de Valencia
c/o Universidad de Valencia, Facultad
   de Medicina
Centro de Documentación e Informatica
   Biomedica
Avenida Blasco Ibanez 17
46010 Valencia
Spain
Telephone: 34 (6) 369 24 66

637. California Data Solutions
Mike Keyes
2226 Vista Rodeo Drive
El Cajon
CA 92019
USA
Telephone: (619) 447–5959

**638. California Institute of
   International Studies**
766 Santa Ynez
Stanford
CA 94305–8441
USA
Telephone: (415) 322–2026

**639. California Planning and
   Development Report**
1275 Sunnycrest Avenue
Ventura
CA 93003
USA
Telephone: (805) 642–7838

640. CALI
526 East Quail Road
Orem
UT 84057
USA
Telephone: (801) 226–6886

Addresses

641. Call-Chronicle Newspapers Inc
Sixth and Linden Streets
PO Box 1260
Allentown
PA 18105
USA
Telephone: (215) 820–6646

642. Cambridge Information Group
7200 Wisconsin Avenue
Bethesda
MD 20814
USA
Telephone: (301) 961–6750

643. Cambridge Multimedia Systems
Robin Sewell
St. Andrews
North Street
Burwell
Cambridge
CB5 0BB
UK
Telephone: 0638 743 121
Fax: 0638 743 572

**644. Cambridge Planning and
    Analytics Inc**
55 Wheeler Street
PO Box 276
Cambridge
MA 02138
USA
Telephone: (617) 576–6465

645. Cambridge Reports Inc
955 Massachusetts Avenue
Cambridge
MA 02139–9990
USA
Telephone: (617) 661–0110

646. Cambridge Scientific Abstracts
7200 Wisconsin Avenue
Bethesda
MD 20814
USA
Telephone: (301) 961–6750;
            (800) 843–7751
Fax: (301) 961–6720
Telex/E-mail: 910 250 7547 CAMBMD

**647. Cambridge Training and
    Development Ltd**
Lesley Crichton (Project Manager)
43 Clifton Road
Cambridge
CB1 4FB
UK
Telephone: 0223 411–464
Fax: 0223 412–275

648. Cameo Interactive Ltd
Seiji Murai (Director of Marketing)
2–3–21 Nishiwasepa
Shinjuku
Tokyo
Japan
Telephone: 3 5273–1871
Fax: 3 5273–1879

649. Camera dei Deputati d'Italia
Servizio per la Documentazione
    Automatica
Piazza Montecitorio
I-00186 Rome
Italy
Telephone: 06 6760

650. Camerdata SA
Calle Alfonso XI 3
28014 Madrid
Spain
Telephone: 01 521 29 84
Fax: 01 522 88 73
Telex/E-mail: 47140 E

651. CAMIF
Mr Martinez
Trevins de Chauray
79000 Niort
France
Telephone: 49 34 50 72
Fax: 49 34 57 77

652. Campus Informatico SA, El
Juan Manuel Abad
Luis Vives
8 Bajos
50006 Zaragoza
Spain
Telephone: 76 56 72 27
Fax: 76 56 31 85

653. CAN Publishing
Boston Online
29 Wareham Street
Boston
MA 02118
USA
Telephone: (617) 423–9501

**654. Canada Institute for Scientific
    and Technical Information
    (CISTI)**
CAN/OLE
Montréal Road
Ottawa
ON K1A 0S2
Canada
Telephone: (613) 993–1210;
            (613) 993–9225
Fax: (613) 952–8244
Telex/E-mail: 0533115 CA
CISTI.CLIENT.SERV (ENVOY 100);
B.Bullock (iNet 2000)

**655. Canada Institute for Scientific
    and Technical Information
    (CISTI)**
Metals Crystallographic Data Centre
Montréal Road
Ottawa
ON K1A 0S2
Canada
Telephone: (613) 993–3294
Fax: (613) 952–8246
Telex/E-mail: 0533115 CA CANSND
NRCVM01 (BITNET);
CISTI.SND (Envoy 100)
CANSND VM.NRC.CA (Internet)

**656. Canada Institute for Scientific
    and Technical Information
    (CISTI)**
Montréal Road
Ottawa
ON K1A 0S2
Canada
Telephone: (613) 993–1600
Fax: (613) 952–9112
Telex/E-mail: 053 3115 CISTI.INFO
(ENVOY 100)

658. Canada Law Book Inc
240 Edward Street
Aurora
ON L4G 3S9
Canada
Telephone: (416) 841–6472
Fax: (416) 773–2103

659. Canada News-Wire Ltd
10 Bay Street
Suite 914
Toronto
ON M5J 2R8
Canada
Telephone: (416) 863–9350

660. Canada Online Limited
38 Fulton Avenue
Toronto
Ontario
M4K 1X5
Canada
Telephone: (416) 467–0388

661. Canada Patent Office
Department of Consumer and Corporate
    Affairs
Ed Remick
Place du Portage
Tower One
Ottawa
ON K1A 0C9
Canada
Telephone: (819) 997–1936
Fax: (819) 953–7620

662. Canada Remote Systems Ltd
1331 Crestlawn Drive
Mississauga
ON L4W 2P9
Canada
Telephone: (416) 620–1439;
            (800) 465–7562;
            (800) 465 6443 (in
                Canada)
Fax: (416) 624–8064

**663. Canadian Centre for
    Occupational Health and Safety**
250 Main Street E
Hamilton
ON L8N 1H6
Canada
Telephone: (416) 572–2981;
            (800) 263–8276
Fax: (416) 572–2206
Telex/E-mail: 0618532

**664. Canadian Centre for
    Occupational Health and Safety**
CCINFOline
250 Main Street E
Hamilton
ON L8N 1H6
Canada
Telephone: (416) 572–2981;
            (800) 263–8340 (in Canada)
Fax: (416) 572–2206

**665. Canadian Circumpolar Institute
    Library**
Elaine Simpson (Head Librarian)
Cameron Library B-03
Ground Floor
University of Alberta
Edmonton
AB T6G 2J8
Canada
Telephone: (403) 492–4515;
            (403) 492–4409;
            (403) 492–7324
Fax: (403) 492–4327;
     (403) 492–1153
Telex/E-mail: BINS UALTAMTS
(BITNET);
ILL.Boreal (Envoy 100)

666. Canadian Conservation institute
1030 Innes Road
Ottawa
ON K1A 0C8
Canada
Telephone: (613) 998–3721

667. Canadian Institute of Chartered Accountants
150 Bloor Street W
Toronto
ON M5S 2Y2
Canada
Telephone: (416) 962–1242
Fax: (416) 962–3375
Telex/E-mail: 2023: ACA002 (Dialcom)

668. Canadian Museum of Civilization
100 Laurier Street
PO Box 3100
Station B
Hull
PQ J8X 4H2
Canada
Telephone: (819) 776–8365
Fax: (819) 776–8300

669. Canadian Petroleum Association
150 6th Avenue SW
Suite 3800
Calgary
AB T2P 3Y7
Canada
Telephone: (403) 269–6721
Fax: (403) 261–4622

670. Canadian Press, The
36 King Street E
Toronto
ON M5C 2L9
Canada
Telephone: (416) 364–0321

671. Canadian Standards Association
178 Rexdale Boulevard
Rexdale
ON M9W 1R3
Canada
Telephone: (416) 747–4058
Fax: (416) 747–2475

672. Canadian Telebook Agency
Theresa Forrest (Eastern Representative)
301 Donlands Avenue
Toronto
ON M4J 3R8
Canada
Telephone: (416) 467–7887
Fax: (416) 467–7886

673. CANCERNET/Centre National de la Recherche Scientifique
15 quai Anatole France
F-75700 Paris
France
Telephone: 01 46 77 16 16
Telex/E-mail: 220880 CNRS DOC F

674. CANCERQUEST Online
PO Box 5528
Atlanta
GA 30307–0528
USA
Telephone: (404) 377–8895

675. CANNEX Financial Exchanges Ltd
102 Bloor Street W
14th Floor
Toronto
ON M5S 1M8
Canada
Telephone: (416) 926–0882;
              (800) 387–1269 (in Canada)
Fax: (416) 926–0706

676. Cannon & Eger
Bill Eger (Partner)
HCR 5146
Keaau
HI 96749
USA
Telephone: (808) 966–8565

677. CAP. Electronic Sweet's
Pat McGraw (Marketing)
169 Monroe NW
Grand Rapids
MI 49503
USA
Telephone: (616) 454–0000;
              (800) 227–0038
Fax: (616) 454–4140

678. Capital City Press
525 Lafayette Street
Baton Rouge
LA 70802
USA
Telephone: (504) 383–1111

679. Capital Gazette Communications Inc
PO Box 911
2000 Capital Drive
Annapolis
MD 21404
USA
Telephone: (301) 268–5000

680. Capitol Disc Interactive
John Gray; Don Godwin; John Hight (Technical)
2121 Wisconsin Avenue NW
Washington
DC 20007
USA
Telephone: (202) 965–7800
Fax: (202) 625–0210;
      (202) 965–7815

681. Capitol Information Management
11060 White Rock Road
Rancho Cordova
CA 95670
USA
Telephone: (916) 636–4400

682. Capitol Publications Inc
Capitol Publishing Group
PO Box 1453
Alexandria
VA 22313–4100
USA
Telephone: (703) 683–4100
Fax: (703) 739–6490

683. Capitol Reports
921 11th Street
Suite 701
Sacramento
CA 95814–2814
USA
Telephone: (916) 441–4427
Fax: (916) 441–4560

684. Capstone Entertainment Software
Linda Zack (Sales)
14202 SW 136th Court
Miami
FL 33189
USA
Telephone: (305) 252–9040
Fax: (305) 255–1205

685. Cardiff Publishing Company
1170 East Meadow Drive
Palo Alto
CA 94303
USA
Telephone: (415) 494–2800

686. Care Connectors Inc
PO Box 14452
Research Triangle Park
NC 27709
USA
Telephone: (919) 544–7300;
              (800) 635–7986

687. Career Information System
1787 Agate Street
Eugene
OR 97403
USA
Telephone: (503) 686–3872

688. Career Placement Registry Inc
302 Swann Avenue
Alexandria
VA 22301
USA
Telephone: (703) 683–1085;
              (800) 368–3093
Telex/E-mail: 901834

689. CARINET Inc
50 F Street NW
Suite 900
Washington
DC 20001
USA
Telephone: (202) 626–8720
Telex/E-mail: 160923

690. Carl Heymanns Verlag KG
Marketing Department
Frau Kruppa (Product Manager); Frau Raesch (Marketing Department)
Luxemburgerstraße 449
5000 Cologne 41
Germany
Telephone: 221 460 1067
Fax: 221 460 1069

691. CARL Systems Inc
777 Grant
Suite 304
Denver
CO 80203
USA
Telephone: (303) 861–5319
Fax: (303) 830–0103

692. Carswell Company Ltd
2330 Midland Avenue
Agincourt
ON M1S 1P7
Canada
Telephone: (416) 291–8421;
              (800) 387–5143;
              (800) 387–5164
              (in Canada)
Fax: (416) 291–4326
Telex/E-mail: 06525289

693. Caseys' Page Mill
6528 Oneida Court
Englewood
CO 80111
USA
Telephone: (303) 220–1463
Fax: (303) 220–1477

694. CAT Benelux bv
Ton Zellstra
PO Box 557
1620 AH Hoorn
Netherlands
Telephone: 2293 1682
Fax: 2293 1572

695. Cat-Cia Ltd
Stephen Jordan (Managing Director)
Enkolon Industrial Estate
25 Randalstown Road
Antrim BT41 4LJ
Northern Ireland
Telephone: 084 946–0550
Fax: 084 946–5733

696. Cátalogue Collectif National
 (See Centre National du CCN)

697. Catholic News Service
3211 4th Street NE
Washington
DC 20017–1100
USA
Telephone: (202) 541–3266

698. CB Society: Cupcake's Column
53 Brook Road
Valley Stream
NY 11581
USA
Telephone: (516) 791–6174

699. CBANET
Canadian Bar Association
50 O'Connor, Suite 902
Ottawa
ON K1P 6L2
Canada
Telephone: (613) 237–2925

700. CCH Australia Ltd
Cnr Talavera & Khartoum Roads
PO Box 230
North Ryde
NSW 2113
Australia
Telephone: 02 888–2555

701. CCH Canadian Ltd
6 Garamond Court
Don Mills
ON M3C 1Z5
Canada
Telephone: (416) 441–2992
Fax: (416) 441–3418

702. CCMI/McGraw-Hill
500 North Franklin Turnpike
Ramsey
NJ 07446
USA
Telephone: (201) 825–3311;
 (800) 526–5307
Fax: (201) 825–8731

703. CCN Systems Ltd
Richard Webber
Talbot House
Talbot Street
Nottingham
NG1 5HF
UK
Telephone: 44 (602) 410888
Telex/E-mail: 377355 CCNSYS G

704. CD Base Ltd
Michelle Green (Product Development
 Manager)
Tranley House
Tranley Mews
Fleet Road
London
NW3 2QW
UK
Telephone: 071 267–7055
Fax: 071 267–2745
Telex/E-mail: 76: WJJ198 (Dialcom)
NUA: Available on application

705. CD Base
Laboratory II
95164 Lulea
Sweden
Telephone: 46–920–97–302

706. CD Book Publishers
767 Arbolado Drive
Fullerton
CA 92635
USA
Telephone: (714) 526–6434

707. CD Enterprises
Uddbyvagen 14B
S-135 55 Tyreso
Sweden
Telephone: +46 8 712 3620

708. CD Eureka Inc
4643 Nagle Avenue
Sherman Oaks
CA 91423
USA
Telephone: (818) 789–0269
Fax: (818) 789–2647

709. CD Folios
6754 Eton Avenue
Canoga Park
CA 91303
USA
Telephone: (800) 688–FOTO;
 (818) 887–2003

710. CD Forlags AB
Gustavslundsv 137
S-161 36 Bromma
Sweden
Telephone: 8 80 8758

711. CD Guide
Forest Road
Hancock
NH 03449
USA
Telephone: (603) 525–4201

712. CD Plus Inc
Erin Sullivan
333 7th Avenue
6th floor
New York
NY 10001
USA
Telephone: (212) 563–3006;
 (800) 950–2030
Fax: (212) 563–3784

713. CD Plus Ltd
Andrew Cunngingham
16 Connaught Street
London
W2 2AG
UK
Telephone: 071 433–3834
Fax: 071 433–3984

714. CD Productions
CD-ROM Enquiries
1101 Amador Avenue
Berkeley
CA 94707
USA
Telephone: (415) 524–8450

715. CD Products
223 East 85th Street
New York
NY 10028
USA
Telephone: (212) 737–8400

716. CD PubCo Inc
Joseph O Breslawski (President)
777 8 Avenue SW
Suite 2050
Calgary
AB T2P 3R5
Canada
Telephone: (403) 294–0080
Fax: (403) 294–0082

717. CD Resources Inc
Bettina Corke (President/Editor)
1123 Broadway
Suite 902
New York
NY 10010
USA
Telephone: (212) 929–8044
Fax: (212) 877–1276
Telex/E-mail: 238198

718. CD Resources
87 Borge Vittorio
Rome 00193
Italy

719. CD ROM Inc
Dr Roger Hutchison (President)
1667 Cole Boulevard
Suite 400
Golden
CO 80401
USA
Telephone: (303) 231–9373
Fax: (303) 231–9581

720. CD Romics
Dr D Dean Davisson (President)
PO Box 221085
San Diego
CA 92122
USA
Telephone: (619) 546–8278

721. CD Solutions
Dawn Russell (Sales)
Gouring House
Market Street
Bracknell
Berkshire
RG12 1JG
UK
Telephone: 0344 867–706
Fax: 0344 867–714

722. CD Technology Inc
William Liu (President)
766 San Aleso Avenue
Sunnyvale
CA 94086
USA
Telephone: (408) 752–8500
Fax: (408) 752–8501

723. CD-Fiche (Distributors) Ltd
James Phillips (Managing Director);
 Robin Fitton (Product Manager)
Unit 4
Lloyds Court
Manor Royal
Crawley
West Sussex
RH10 2XT
UK
Telephone: 0293 525–271
Fax: 0293 562–066

724. CD-I Training Ltd
Spin UK Ltd
Lombard House
2 Purley Way
Croydon
CR0 3JP
UK
Telephone: +44 81 665 5990
Fax: +44 81 665 6105

725. CD-Information Systems
Staffan Hillberg (President/Owner)
Luntantugatan 2, II
411 20 Göteborg
Sweden
Telephone: 31 11 76 07
Fax: 31 11 26 17

726. CD-ROM de México SA de CV
Leonardo Pasquel # 22
Col. Modelo
Xalapa
Veracruz
CP 91040
Mexico
Telephone: (281) 804–29
Fax: (281) 861–95

727. CD-ROM Edition et Diffusion SA
Vincent Leray (Sales & Marketing
    Manager); Julien Roux
57 boulevard Montmorency
75016 Paris
France
Telephone: 1 45 24 37 95
Fax: 1 45 25 08 04

**728. CD-ROM Publishing Company
    Ltd**
Graham Randles (Sales & Marketing
    Manager); Pauls Goodale
Premier House
10 Greycoat Place
London
SW1P 1SB
UK
Telephone: 071 222–8866;
        071 222–1765
Fax: 071 222–8612; 071 222–5358

729. CD-ROM Resource Group Inc
Marc Rose (President)
1310 Wadsworth Road
Suite 200
Lakewood
CO 80215
USA
Telephone: (303) 232–0210
Fax: (303) 233–2874

730. CD-ROM Resource Group
1045 Lincoln Street
Suite 300
Denver
CO 80203
USA
Telephone: (303) 894–8140

731. CD-ROM Users Club (UK)
Anne Collins
University of Leeds
Medical and Dental Library
Leeds LS2 9JT
UK
Telephone: 44 (532) 335549
Fax: 44 (532) 334381

732. CD-ROM Users Group (US)
Fred Bellomy
PO Box 2400
Santa Barbara
CA 93120
USA
Telephone: (805) 965–0265
Fax: (805) 965–5415

**733. CD-ROM Verlag & Vertrieb
    GmbH**
Business Centre
Claus Schneider (Sales Executive);
    Erik-Jan van Kleef (Sales
Executive)
Merkurhaus
Am Hauptbahnhof 12
6000 Frankfurt 1
Germany
Telephone: 069 27 10 02 58
Fax: 069 27 10 02 10

**734. CD-ROM Verlag GmbH & Co
    KG**
Werner Schäl (Manager)
Im Grund 11
5210 Troisdorf
Germany
Telephone: 2241 7 50 61
Fax: 2241 7 21 28

735. CD/Law Reports
CD-ROM Enquiries
305 S Hale
Suite 1
Wheaton
IL 60187
USA
Telephone: (408) 668–8895

**736. CDA Investment Technologies
    Inc**
1355 Piccard Drive
Rockville
MD 20850
USA
Telephone: (301) 975–9600
Fax: (301) 590–1350

**737. CDC AIDS WEEKLY/NCI
    CANCER WEEKLY**
206 Rogers Street NE
Suite 104
PO Box 5528
Atlanta
GA 30317
USA
Telephone: (404) 377–8895

**738. CDI – Compact Disc
    International Ltd**
Moshe Chasid (Development and
    Marketing Consultant)
Gan Galram Industrial Zone
PO Box 6
Karmiel 20101
Israel
Telephone: 4 983 121
Fax: 4 983 124

739. CDR-Informatique
Sylvain Dietrich (Manager)
BP 32
91470 Limours
France
Telephone: 1 64 91 26 76
Fax: 1 64 91 47 69

740. CDTV Publishing
Curtiz Gangi (Director Sales/Marketing)
1200 Wilson Drive
West Chester
PA 19380
USA
Telephone: (215) 431–9163
Fax: (215) 429–0643

741. CDWord Library Inc
Bill Grubbs
Two Lincoln Centre
5420 LBJ Freeway LB7
Dallas
TX 75240–6215
USA
Telephone: (214) 770–2414
Fax: (214) 770–2345

742. CDX GmbH
Stenzelring 33
D-2102 Hamburg 93
Germany

**743. CEDIB (See Universidad de
    Valencia)**

744. CEDIS Srl
Rolando Dubini (Chief Editor)
Palazzo E/2 Milanofiori
20090 Assago
Milan
Italy
Telephone: 2 824 14 51
Fax: 2 825 41 33

**745. CEDOCAR (See Ministere de
    Defense)**

746. CEDROM Technologies Inc
Philippe Gelinas (President)
1290 Van Horne Avenue
Suite 209
Outremont
PQ H2V 4S2
Canada
Telephone: (514) 278–3373;
        (514) 270–8675
Fax: (514) 270–4162

747. CEDROM Technologies
Bernard C Prost (President)
30 avenue de l'Observatoire
750195 Paris
France
Telephone: 1 43 35 13 84
Fax: 1 43 22 03 41

**748. CEGET (See Centre d'Études de
    Géographie Tropicale)**

749. CEIT Systems Inc
John Nicoletti (President)
4800 Great America Parkway, 200
Santa Clara
CA 95054
USA
Telephone: (408) 986–1101
Fax: (408) 986–1107

**750. CELADE (See Centro
    Latinoamericano de
    Demografía)**

**751. Center for Birth Defects
    Information Services Inc**
Dover Medical Building
Box 1776
Dover
MA 02030
USA
Telephone: (617) 785–2525

**752. Center for Central American
    Studies**
PO Box 11095
Takoma Park
MD 20913
USA
Telephone: (301) 270–9577
Fax: (301) 270–2748

**753. Center for Chronic Disease
    Prevention and Health
    Promotion**
Building 1 South
Room SSB-249
1699 Clifton Rd. NE
Atlanta
GA 30333
USA
Telephone: (404) 639–3492
Fax: (404) 639–1552

**754. Center for Continuing Study of
    California Economy**
610 University Avenue
Palo Alto
CA 94301
USA
Telephone: (415) 321–8550

755. Center for International Financial Analysis and Research (CIFAR)
Sanjiv Vyas (Senior Manager, Information Services)
211 College Road E
Princeton
NJ 08540
USA
Telephone: (609) 520–9333
Fax: (609) 520–0905

756. Center on Education and Training for Employment
The Ohio State University
1900 Kenny Road
Columbus
OH 43210–1090
USA
Telephone: (614) 292–4353;
    (800) 848–4815
Fax: (614) 292–1260

757. Central Institute for Scientific and Technical Information
52–A G.A. Nasser Str.
Sofia 1040
Bulgaria
Telephone: (359) 71 89 46
Telex/E-mail: 22404 ZINTI BG

758. Central Medical Library
Haartmaninkatu
SF-00290 Helsinki
Finland
Telephone: 358 (90) 43461
Fax: 358 (90) 410385
Telex/E-mail: 121498 LKK SF

759. Central News Agency
Daily News Building
Room 1400
220 E 42nd Street
New York
NY 10017
USA
Telephone: (212) 227–7555

760. Central Scientific Medical Library
Automization Technology of Information Services
NPO SOYUZMEDINFORM
Ulitsa Krasikova 30
117418 Moscow
Russia
Telephone: 095 128–3346
Telex/E-mail: 412128 MEDIN SU

761. Central Statistical Office of Finland
PO Box 504
SF-00101 Helsinki 10
Finland
Telephone: 90 173–41

762. Centrale dei Bilanci srl
Corso Vittorio Emanuele II, 93
10128 Turin
Italy
Telephone: 39 (11) 51 73 66
Telex/E-mail: 224210 I

763. Centralforbundet for Alkohol-och Narkotikaupplysning
PO Box 27302
S-102 54 Stockholm
Sweden
Telephone: 08 667–9720
Fax: 08 661–6484

764. Centre Audiovisuel de Royan pour l'Étude des Langues
Patrick Amigouet; Yannick Pellot; Sigrid Ohland; Jacky Karp
48 boulevard Frank Lamy
17200 Royan Cedex
France
Telephone: 46 39 50 00
Fax: 46 05 27 68

765. Centre d'Étude des Supports de Publicité
32 avenue Georges-Mandel
F-75116 Paris
France
Telephone: 1 45 53 22 10

767. Centre d'Études de Géographie Tropicale (CEGET)
Centre de Documentation
Domaine Universitaire de Bordeaux
F-33405 Talence
France
Telephone: 56 80 60 00

769. Centre d'Etudes Prospectives et d'Informations Internationales
M Branur
9 rue Georges Pitard
75015 Paris
France
Telephone: 1 48 42 64 64
Fax: 1 48 42 59 12

770. Centre d'Information Textile Habillement
24 rue Montoyer
B-1040 Brussels
Belgium
Telephone: 02 230–7629

771. Centre d'Informatique Generale Liege
Avenue de l'Informatique 9
B-4430 Alleur
Belgium
Telephone: 41 633–990
NUA: 2062220003

772. Centre de Coopération Internationale en Recherce
Agronomique pour le Développement
Jean François Giovannetti (Head of Information)
Avenue du Val Montferrand
BP 5035
34032 Montpellier Cedex 1
France
Telephone: 67 61 58 00
Fax: 67 61 58 20

773. Centre de Documentation Internationales des Industries
Utilisatrices des Produits Agricoles
1 avenue des Olympiades
F-91300 Massy Cedex
France
Telephone: 6 20 97 38
Fax: 6 01 17 585

774. Centre de Donnees Astronomiques de Strasbourg
Observatoire Astronomique
11 rue de l'Université
F-67000 Strasbourg
France
Telephone: 88 35 82 00

775. Centre de l'Industrie Française des Travaux Publics
3 rue de Berri
F-75008 Paris
France
Telephone: 1 45 63 11 44
Fax: 1 45 61 04 47
Telex/E-mail: 640675 F

776. Centre de Recherches de Pont-a-Mousson
Service de Documentation Industrielle
BP 109
F-54704 Pont-a-Mousson
France
Telephone: 83 80 73 00
Fax: 83 81 74 00
Telex/E-mail: 961330 F

777. Centre de Recherches Documentaire (CREDOC)
PO Box 11
Rue de la Montagne 34
B-1000 Brussels
Belgium
Telephone: 02 511–6941
Fax: 02 513–3195

778. Centre des Utilisateurs de Progiciels
5 rue de Monceau
F-75008 Paris
France
Telephone: 1 42 25 19 60
Fax: 1 45 61 46 76
Telex/E-mail: 642617 F

779. Centre Europeén de Recherches Documentaires sur les Immunoclones
2eme CAI
avenue des Maurettes
F-06270 Villeneuve-Loubet
France
Telephone: 93 20 01 80
Fax: 93 94 22 94

780. Centre for Cold Ocean Resources Engineering (See C-CORE)

781. Centre for the Study of Public Policy
EUROLOC
University of Strathclyde
Livingstone Tower
26 Richmond Street
Glasgow
G1 1XH
Scotland, UK
Telephone: 44 (41) 552–4400

782. Centre Française du Commerce Exterieur
Direction des Produits Agro-alimentaires
10 avenue d'Iena
F-75783 Paris Cedex 16
France
Telephone: 1 40 73 30 00
Fax: 1 40 73 39 79
Telex/E-mail: 611934 CFCEA F

783. Centre Inter-regional d'Informatique de Lorraine
Rue du Doten Roubault
54500 Vandoeuvre
France
Telephone: 33 (83) 55 15 45

784. Centre Inter-Regional de Calcul Electronique
Mr Salzedo
BP 63
F-92406 Orsay Cedex
France
Telephone: 1 69 82 41 41
Telex/E-mail: 692166 F SACORS
NUA: 2080910006931

785. Centre International de l'Enfance
Anne Parrical (Head of Documentation Services)
Château de Longchamp
Bois de Boulogne
75016 Paris
France
Telephone: 1 45 20 79 92
Fax: 1 45 25 73 67

786. Centre Interuniversitaire de Calcul de Nice et Toulon
28 avenue Valrose
F-06034 Nice Cedex
France
Telephone: 93 52 99 52
Fax: 93 52 99 19

787. Centre Medical Universitaire
Department de Biochemie Medicale
CH-1211 Geneva 4
Switzerland
Telephone: 022 468–758

788. Centre National d'Enseignement à Distance
Mme le Delais
7 rue du Clos Courte
35050 Rennes
France
Telephone: 99 63 11 88

789. Centre National d'Études des Telecommunications (CNET)
Service de Documentation Interministerielle (SDI)
38–40 rue du General Leclerc
F-92131 Issy-les-Moulineaux
France
Telephone: 1 45 29 44 44
Telex/E-mail: 250317 CNETLEC F

790. Centre National d'Information Juridique
R Zanatta; Stanislas Zalinski (Deputy Director)
26 rue Desaix
75727 Paris Cedex 15
France
Telephone: 1 40 58 78 50
Fax: 1 40 58 77 80

791. Centre National de la Recherche Scientifique (CNRS)
Centre de Recherche sur les Traitements Automatises en Archeologie Classique
Université de Paris X
200 avenue de la Republique
F-92001 Nanterre Cedex
France
Telephone: 1 40 97 76 84

792. Centre National de la Recherche Scientifique (CNRS)
Greco Programmation
351 Cours de la Liberation
F-33405 Talence Cedex
France
Telephone: 1 56 84 60 89

793. Centre National de la Recherche Scientifique (CNRS)
Groupement Scientifique Isard
Université Toulouse-le-Mirail
5 alleés Antonio-Machado
F-31058 Toulouse Cedex
France
Telephone: 61 40 70 34

794. Centre National de la Recherche Scientifique (CNRS)
Institut de l'Information Scientifique et Technique (INIST)
Anne Lhermitte (Responsable Communication Externe); François Ramon
2 allée du Parc de Brabois
F-54514 Vandoeuvre-les-Nancy Cedex
France
Telephone: 83 50 46 00; 83 50 46 64
Fax: 83 50 46 50
Telex/E-mail: 220880 CNRSDOC F

795. Centre National de la Recherche Scientifique (CNRS)
Institut National de la Langue Français (INaLF)
Bernard Quemada (Directeur de l'InaLF)
52 boulevard Magenta
75010 Paris
France
Telephone: 1 42 45 00 77
Fax: 1 42 45 92 30

796. Centre National de la Recherche Scientifique (CNRS)
Reseau d'Information sur les Migrations Internationales – IRESCO
59–61 rue Pouchet
F-75849 Paris Cedex 17
France
Telephone: 1 40 25 11 18

797. Centre National de la Recherche Scientifique (CNRS)
INTERGEO – Laboratoire de Communication et de Documentation en Geographie
191 rue Saint-Jacques
75005 Paris
France
Telephone: 1 46 33 74 31

798. Centre National du CCN
Mmn Chazal (Promotion)
5 rue Auguste Vacquerie
F-75116 Paris
France
Telephone: 1 47 20 82 33

799. Centre pour le Developpement de l'Information sur la Formation Professionnelle
Tour Europe
F-92080 Paris La Defense Cedex 07
France
Telephone: 1 47 78 13 50
Fax: 1 47 73 74 20
Telex/E-mail: 615383 INFFO F

800. Centre Scientifique et Technique de la Construction-Bruxelles
41 rue du Lombard
1000 Brussels
Belgium
Telephone: 32 (2) 511 06 83

801. Centre Scientifique et Technique du Bâtiment
M André
4 avenue du Recteur-Poincaré
75782 Paris Cedex 16
France
Telephone: 1 40 50 28 28
Fax: 1 45 25 61 51
Telex/E-mail: 610710 PAR F

802. Centre Serveur Duplex/BOTTIN TELEMATIQUE
28 rue du Docteur Finlay
F-75738 Paris Cedex 15
France
Telephone: 1 45 78 61 66
Fax: 1 45 79 39 38
Telex/E-mail: 204286 F

803. Centre Technique de l'Industrie du Decolletage (C.T.DEC)
BP 65
F-74301 Cluses Cedex
France
Telephone: 50 98 20 44
Fax: 50 98 38 98
Telex/E-mail: 385213 F

804. Centre Technique des Industries de la Fonderie
Service Documentation
44 avenue de la Division Leclerc
B.P. 78
92312 Sevres Cedex
France
Telephone: 33 (1) 45 34 27 54
Fax: 33 (1) 45 34 14 34
Telex/E-mail: 270953 CTIF SE F

805. Centre Technique des Industries Mecaniques
Centre d'Information Technologique
52 avenue Felix Loust
PO Box 67
60304 Senlis
France
Telephone: 33 (4) 458 31 31
Fax: 33 (4) 458 34 00
Telex/E-mail: 140006 CETIM SENLI F

806. Centre Textile de Conjoncture et d'Observation Economique
37/39 rue de Neuilly
PO Box 249
F-92113 Clichy Cedex
France
Telephone: 1 47 56 30 30
Telex/E-mail: 613738 F

807. Centro de Estudios em Economia da Energia dos Transportes e
Ambiente
Rua Tiguel Lupi 20
1200 Lisbon
Portugal
Telephone: 1 601–043

808. Centro Internacional de Méjoramiento de Maíz y Trigo
Dr Edith Hesse de Polanco (Head Scientific Information Unit)
Lisboa 27
06600 Mexico City DF
Mexico
Telephone: 595 761 33 11
Fax: 595 41069

809. Centro Latinoamericano de Demografía
Betty Johnson de Vodanovic (Head DOCPAL)
Avenida Dag Hammarskjold s/n
Casilla 91
Santiago
Chile
Telephone: 2 208–5051
Fax: 2 208–0252

810. Century Hutchinson
Brookmount House
62–65 Chandos Place
London
WC2N 4NW
UK
Telephone: 071 240–3411

811. Century Research Center Corporation
Micky Ikeda (General Manager)
4677 Old Ironsides Drive
Suite 200
Santa Clara
CA 95054
USA
Telephone: (408) 727–0766
Fax: (408) 727–7314

812. CeQuadrat
Gesellschaft für Computer und
  Communication mbH
Metzgerstrasse 1–3
5100 Aachen
Germany
Telephone: 0241 1822260
Fax: 0241 162501

813. Ceram Research
Queens Road, Penkhull
Stoke-on-Trent
Staffordshire
ST4 7LQ
UK
Telephone: 44 (782) 45431
Fax: 44 (782) 412331
Telex/E-mail: 36228 G

814. CERCI Communications
19 Store Street
London
WC1E 7BT
UK

815. Cercle de la Librairie
Michele Aderhold (Sales Manager)
35 rue Grégoire de Tours
75006 Paris
France
Telephone: 1 43 29 10 00
Fax: 1 43 29 68 95

816. CERIS/NPIRS
Virginia Walters (User Services
  Specialist)
Purdue University
1231 Cumberland Avenue
West Lafayette
IN 47906–1317
USA
Telephone: (317) 494–6614
Fax: (317) 494–9727

**817. CERVED (Società Nazionale di
  Informatica delle Camere di
  Commercio Italiane)**
Ormelle Speggiorim
Via Staderini 93
I-00155 Rome
Italy
Telephone: 6 225 911
Fax: 6 22 59 12 55
Telex/E-mail: 620061 CERVED I
NUA: Available on application

818. CETIM
Pierre Devalan
52 avenue Felix Louat
BP 67
60304 Senlis Cedex
France
Telephone: 44 58 31 76
Fax: 44 58 31 80

819. CGNET Services International
Georg Lindsey (Managing Director);
  Julie Duffield (CD-ROM Project
  Manager)
1024 Hamilton Court
Menlo Park
CA 94025
USA
Telephone: (415) 325–3061
Fax: (415) 325–2313

**820. CH Beck'sche
  Verlagsbuchhandlung**
Dr Rainer Dechsling
Wilhelmstraße 9
8000 Munich 40
Germany
Telephone: 089 381 89 423
Fax: 089 381 89 398

821. Chadwyck-Healey Inc
Eric Calaluca (Vice President Sales &
  Marketing)
1101 King Street
Alexandria
VA 22314
USA
Telephone: (703) 683–4890;
           (800) 752–0515;
           (800) 535–0228
           (from Canada)
Fax: (703) 683–7589

822. Chadwyck-Healey Ltd
Duncan Christelow (Sales Executive);
  John Russell
Cambridge Place
Cambridge
Cambridgeshire
CB2 1NR
UK
Telephone: 0223 311–479
Fax: 0223 664–40
Telex/E-mail: 9312102281 CH G

**823. Chambre de Commerce et
  d'Industrie de Colmar**
1 place de la Gare
PO Box 7
F-68001 Colmar Cedex
France
Telephone: 89 23 99 40
Fax: 89 41 27 43
Telex/E-mail: 880979 F

**824. Chambre de Commerce et
  d'Industrie de Paris (See Paris
  Chamber of Commerce and
  Industry)**

**825. Chambre Regionale de
  Commerce et d'Industrie de
  Bourgogne**
68 rue Chevreul
PO Box 209
F-21006 Dijon Cedex
France
Telephone: 80 63 52 52
Fax: 80 63 52 53
Telex/E-mail: 350795 CRCIBOU F

**826. Chambre Regionale de
  Commerce et d'Industrie
  Languedoc-Roussillon**
Immeuble du Mas d'Alco
1467 avenue Louis Ravas
BP 6076
F-34030 Montpellier Cedex 1
France
Telephone: 67 61 10 00
Telex/E-mail: 480116 CHAMRECI F

827. Chambre Regionale de l'Energie
55 avenue d'Alsace
F-68000 Colmar Cedex
France
Telephone: 89 24 25 45

**828. Changchun Optical and
  Mechanical Institute**
Chinese Academy of Sciences
Li Shifan
PO Box 1024
Changchun
Jilin 130022
China
Telephone: 0431–684692 x2228
Fax: 0431–682346

829. Chapman and Hall Ltd
Scientific Data Division
Jack Lee (Senior Marketing Manager)
2–6 Boundary Row
London
SE1 8HN
UK
Telephone: 071 865–0066;
           071 410–6916
Fax: 071 522–9623; 071 522–9621
Telex/E-mail: 12070 (DIALMAIL)

830. Charles E. Simon and Company
A company of Prentice-Hall Legal and
  Financial Services
1300 New York Avenue, NW, Suite
  205E
Washington
DC 20005
USA
Telephone: (202) 289–5300;
           (800) 543–4502
Fax: (202) 289–3551

831. Charles Schwab & Company Inc
101 Montgomery Street
San Francisco
CA 94104
USA
Telephone: (415) 398–1000;
           (800) 334–4455

832. Charlotte Observer, The
600 S Tyron Street
PO Box 32188
Charlotte
NC 28202
USA
Telephone: (704) 379–6300

833. CHEM-INTELL
39A Bowling Green Lane
London
EC1R 0BJ
UK
Telephone: 071 833–3812
Fax: 071 833–1563
Telex/E-mail: 28339 CPLCDP G

**834. Chemical Abstracts Service
  (CAS)**
2540 Olentangy River Road
PO Box 3012
Columbus
OH 43210–0012
USA
Telephone: (614) 447–3600;
           (800) 848–6533
Fax: (614) 447–3709
Telex/E-mail: 6842086 CHMAB

**835. Chemical Exchange Directory
  SA (CED)**
Marianne Mowat
9 rue de la Gabelle
CH-1227 Geneva
Switzerland
Telephone: 22 42 20 70
Fax: 22 42 20 79
Telex/E-mail: 428066 CED CH

**836. Chemical Information Systems
  Inc**
7215 York Road
Baltimore
MD 21212
USA
Telephone: (301) 321–8440;
           (800) 247–8737
Fax: (301) 296–0712
Telex/E-mail: 910–380–1738

837. Chemical Intelligence Services
Kevin Cunningham
39A Bowling Green Lane
London EC1R 0BJ
UK
Telephone: 44 (71) 833–3812
Fax: 44 (71) 833–1563
Telex/E-mail: 28339 CPLCDP G

838. Chemical Market Associates Inc
11757 Katy Freeway
Suite 750
Houston
TX 77079
USA
Telephone: (713) 531–4660
Telex/E-mail: 792318

839. Chemical Monitor, The
PO Box 314
Lindenhurst
NY 11757
USA
Telephone: (516) 669–8147

840. Chemical Sources International Inc
PO Box 1824
Clemson
SC 29633
USA
Telephone: (803) 646–7840
Fax: (803) 646–9938

841. Chemical Technologies Corporation
380 Madison Avenue, 12th Floor
New York
NY 10017
USA
Telephone: (212) 309–5000

842. Chemical Week Associates
810 7th Avenue
New York
NY 10018
USA
Telephone: (212) 586–3430
Fax: (212) 586–3147

843. Chemron Inc
Ronald G Oldham (President)
431 Isom Road
Suite 135
San Antonio
TX 78216–5141
USA
Telephone: (512) 340–8121
Fax: (512) 340–8123; (512) 691–2076

844. ChemShare Corporation
PO Box 1885
Houston
TX 77251–1885
USA
Telephone: (713) 627–8945
Fax: (713) 965–0968

845. CHERMETINFORMACIA
c/o International Centre for Scientific
and Technical Information
Ulitsa Kuusinena 21b
125252 Moscow
Russia
Telephone: 095 198–7460
Fax: 095 943–0089
Telex/E-mail: 411925 MCNTI SU

846. CHEST
Computing Services
University of Bath
Claverton Down
Bath
BA2 7AY
UK
Telephone: 0225 826282
Fax: 0225 826176
Telex/E-mail: CHEST SWURCC
(JANET E-mail)

847. Chibret International Documentation Centre
Huguette Legrand
Laboratories MSD-Chibret
200 boulevard E Clementel
63018 Clermont-Ferrand
France
Telephone: 73 23 42 84
Fax: 73 25 62 39

848. Chicago Board of Trade
Information Systems &
Telecommunications Group
141 W Jackson Boulevard
Chicago
IL 60604
USA
Telephone: (312) 435–3732

849. Chicago Sun-Times
401 N Wabash Avenue
Chicago
IL 60604
USA
Telephone: (312) 321–2593

850. Chicago Tribune Company
435 N Michigan Avenue
Chicago
IL 60611
USA
Telephone: (312) 222–3232

851. Chicano Studies Library
Carolyn Soto (Publications Coordinator);
Lillian Castillo Speed
(Database Manager)
University of Berkeley
Dwinelle Hall 3404
Berkeley
CA 94720
USA
Telephone: (510) 642–3859
Fax: (510) 642–6456

852. Children's Hospital, The
Scott Rattray
1056 E 19th Avenue & Downing
Denver
CO 80218
USA
Telephone: (303) 861–8888
Fax: (303) 837–2577

853. China Educational Publications Import & Export Corporation
15 Xueyuan Lu
Beijing 100083
China
Telephone: 1 202 3014

854. Christian Science Publishing Society
1 Norway Street
Boston
MA 02115
USA
Telephone: (617) 450–2000

855. Chronicle Publishing Company, The
20 Franklin Street
PO Box 15012
Worcester
MA 01615–0012
USA
Telephone: (508) 793–9100
Fax: (508) 753–3142

856. Chronometrics Inc
1901 Raymond Drive, [hash]7
Northbrook
IL 60062–6714
USA
Telephone: (708) 272–0949

857. Chuck Lynd
2840 Medary Avenue
Columbus
OH 43202
USA
Telephone: (614) 262–2730

858. Chunichi Shimbun
1 Chome
Sannomaru
Naka-ku
Nagoya 460–11
Japan
Telephone: 52 201–8811

859. CIGL (See Centre d'Information General Liege)

860. CINAHL Information Systems (See Cumulative Index to Nursing & Allied Health Literature)

861. Cincinnati Enquirer, The
617 Vine Street
Cincinnati
OH 45292
USA
Telephone: (513) 721–2700

862. Cineman Syndicate
7 Charles Court
Middletown
NY 10940
USA
Telephone: (914) 692–4572
Telex/E-mail: EasyLink: 62186280 MCI
Mail: 213–9111

863. Cinemaware Corporation
Sam Poole
4165 Thousand Oaks Blvd
Westlake Village
CA 91362
USA
Telephone: (805) 495–6515

864. CIRAD (See Centre de Coopération Internationale en Recherche Agronomique pour le Développement)

865. Circle for Information Company Ltd, The
Woody Puray; Said Hassan Ghaled
(CD-ROM Information Department)
Al-Arbaein Street
The Circle for Information Building
Malaz
Riyadh 11545
Saudi Arabia
Telephone: 1 479 0060
Fax: 1 476 4624

866. CISCO
327 S LaSalle
Suite 800
Chicago
IL 60604
USA
Telephone: (312) 922–3661;
        (800) 666–1223

**867. CISI-Wharton Econometric
    Forecasting Associates**
Ebury Gate
23 Lower Belgrave Street
London
SW1W 0NW
UK
Telephone: 071 730–8171

868. CISI
35 boulevard Brune
75680 Paris Cedex 14
France
Telephone: 33 (1) 45 45 80 00

869. CITI2 Université
Christian Fondrat (Engineer)
45 rue des Saintes Pères
75276 Paris Cedex
France
Telephone: 1 42 96 24 89
Fax: 1 42 96 34 97

870. Citibank N.A.
Richard Cobb
111 Wall Street
17th Floor
New York
NY 10043
USA
Telephone: (212) 657–0885

871. Citibase Database Services
77 Water Street
7th Floor
New York
NY 10043
USA
Telephone: (212) 898–7200
Fax: (212) 688–6689

873. Citicorp
77 Water Street
2nd Floor
New York
NY 10043
USA
Telephone: (212) 898–7425;
        (800) 842–8405
Fax: (212) 742–8769

874. CITIS Inc
Zoë Redmond (Marketing Manager)
80 8th Avenue
Suite 303
New York
NY 10010
USA
Telephone: (212) 683–9221

875. CITIS Ltd
D Murphy
2 Rosemount Terrace
Blackrock
Dublin
Ireland
Telephone: 1 2886–227
Fax: 1 2885–971

876. City University of New York
International RILM Center
33 West 42nd Street
New York
NY 10036
USA
Telephone: (212) 642–2709

877. City-Informations System
Warzburg
Germany
Telephone: +49 31 287099

878. Cityscope Publications Pty Ltd
7/98 Alfred Street
Milsons Point
NSW 2061
Australia
Telephone: 2 957–4811

879. Clarinet Systems Ltd
Stephen Scholefield (Director)
White Hart House
London Road
Blackwater
Camberley
Surrey
GU17 9AD
UK
Telephone: 0276 600–398
Fax: 0276 600–596

880. Claritas Corporation
520 Broadway, Suite 520
Santa Monica
CA 90401
USA
Telephone: (213) 394–6897
Fax: (213) 393–6230

881. Clark Boardman Callaghan
375 Hudson Street
New York
NY 10014
USA
Telephone: (212) 929–7500

882. Clarke School for the Deaf
The Mainstream Center
46 Round Hill Road
Northampton
MA 01060–2199
USA
Telephone: (413) 584–3450
Fax: (413) 586–6654

883. Clarkson, Tetrault
275 Sparks Street
Ottawa
ON K1R 7X9
Canada
Telephone: (613) 238–2000

884. Clinical Communications Inc
132 Hutchin Hill
Shady
NY 12409
USA
Telephone: (914) 679–2217

885. Clinical Informatics, Inc
William M Bates, Jr
11 Newbury Street
Providence
RI
USA
Telephone: (401) 421–3399
Fax: (401) 831–5464
Telex/E-mail: 76456,2012
(CompuServe Information Service)

886. Clinical Reference Systems Ltd
Marketing Department
c/o Information Access Company
362 Lakeside Drive
Foster City
CA 94404–9888
USA
Telephone: (415) 378–5000;
        (800) 227–8431
Fax: (415) 378–5369

887. CLSI
Axis Centre
3 Burlington Lane
London
W4 2TH
UK
Telephone: 081 742–2024

888. CLSI
320 Nevada Street
Newtonville
MA 02160
USA
Telephone: (617) 965–6310;
        (800) 365–0085
Fax: (617) 969–1928

889. CMC ReSearch Inc
Chris Kitze (Publisher); Judith Grillo
    (Marketing Manager)
7150 SW Hampton
Suite C-120
Portland
OR 97223
USA
Telephone: (503) 639–3395
Fax: (503) 639–1796

890. CML Data
Greg Spafford; James Duffy
40 Mill Green Road
Mitcham
Surrey
CR4 4HY
UK
Telephone: +44 (0)81 640 6722

891. CMP Publications Inc
600 Community Drive
Manhasset
NY 11030
USA
Telephone: (516) 562–5000
Fax: (516) 562–5718
Telex/E-mail: 450–4685 (MCI MAIL)

892. CNDP
Direction Documentaire
15 rue des Irlandais
F-75005 Paris
France
Telephone: 1 43 34 94 18

893. CNDST
4 Bd de L'Empereur
B-1000 Bruxelles
Belgium

**894. CNEL – Consiglio Nazionale
    dell'Economia e del Lavoro**
Maurizio Potente
Viale David Lubin 2
Rome 00196
Italy
Telephone: 6 36921

**895. CNERTA – Centre National
    d'Études et de Ressource en
    Technologie**
Avancée
Odile Hologne (Ingénieur, Chef de
    Project)
26 boulevard du Docteur Petitjean
21000 Dijon
France
Telephone: 80 65 41 20
Fax: 80 67 42 05

896. CNUCE Institute
Via Santa Maria 36
I-56100 Pisa
Italy
Telephone: 50 59 32 30
Telex/E-mail: 500371 CNUCE I

897. COBIDOC BV
PO Box 16601
Amsterdam
NL-1001 RC Amsterdam
Netherlands

898. Codehigh Ltd.
Michael Harper
Harrow Way
Whitchurch
Hampshire
RG28 7QT
UK
Telephone: 0256–893539

899. Codus Ltd
196–198 West Street
Sheffield
S1 4ET
UK
Telephone: 0742 761–252
Fax: 0742 750–318
Telex/E-mail: 547216 UGSHEF G

900. Coffee Anyone ???
5673 W Las Positas Boulevard
Suite 215
Pleasanton
CA 94588
USA
Telephone: (415) 734–8355
Fax: (415) 734–8359
Telex/E-mail: COFFEEANYONE
(Delphi)

901. Cogespe srl
Via Taranto 44
I-00182 Rome
Italy
Telephone: 6 77 40 70

902. Cognitive Applications Ltd
4 Sillwood Terrace
Brighton
BN1 2LR
UK
Telephone: 0273 821600
Fax: 0273 728866

903. Coin Base Locator
PO Box 76476
Atlanta
GA 30358
USA
Telephone: (404) 979–6501

904. Colex Data SA (Mapfre Lex)
Antonio Adam
c/ Echegaray 25
28014 Madrid
Spain
Telephone: 1 429–0468
Fax: 1 369–3927

905. Colleague Gateway Service
BT-Tymnet Inc
6120 Executive Blvd, Suite 500
Rockville
MD 20852
USA
Telephone: (301) 881–9020
Fax: (301) 881–9016

906. College Press Service
2505 W 2nd Avenue
Suite 7
Denver
CO 80219
USA
Telephone: (303) 936–9930;
          (800) 521–7525

907. Collets Holdings Ltd
Denington Estate
Wellingborough
Northamptonshire
NN8 2QT
UK
Telephone: 0933 224–351
Fax: 0933 76–402

**908. Colorado Alliance of Research
    Libraries**
777 Grant
Suite 304
Denver
CO 80203
USA
Telephone: (303) 861–5319
Fax: (303) 830–0103

**909. Colorado Springs Gazette
    Telegraph**
30 South Prospect Street
Colorado Springs
CO 80901
USA
Telephone: (719) 632–5511

910. Columbia University Press
Beverley Hauser (Customer Service
    Manager)
136 S Broadway
Irvington
NY 10533
USA
Telephone: (914) 591–9111
Fax: (914) 591–9201

911. Columbia University
Avery Architectural and Fine Arts
    Library
116th and Broadway
New York
NY 10027
USA
Telephone: (212) 280–8404
Telex/E-mail: GIRAL
CUNIXF.CC.COLUMBIA.EDU (Internet)

912. Columbia University
Center for Population and Family Health
Library/Information Program
60 Haven Avenue
New York
NY 10032
USA
Telephone: (212) 305–6960
Fax: (212) 305–7024
Telex/E-mail: 971913

913. Columbia University
Graduate School of Business
Center for International Business Cycle
    Research
Uris Hall
New York
NY 10027
USA
Telephone: (212) 280–2916
Fax: (212) 280–8706

914. Columbus Information
Tim Smith (Technical Manager); P
    Barklem (Sales Manager)
5–7 Luke Street
London
EC2A 4PX
UK
Telephone: 071 729–4535
Fax: 071 729–1156

**915. Comargus Information Service
    GmbH**
Hindenburgdamm 85
D-1000 Berlin 45
Germany
Telephone: 030 834–9057
Fax: 03– 834–1831
Telex/E-mail: 186566 COMBO D

**916. Combined Health Information
    Database**
National Institutes of Health
PO Box NDIC (CHID)
Bethesda
MD 20892
USA
Telephone: (301) 468–2162
Fax: (301) 770–5164

**917. ComCenter Disc & Database
    GmbH**
Fr Bühl
Holzofallee 38
Postfach 11 04 52
6100 Darmstadt
Germany
Telephone: 61 513–910
Fax: 61 513–91200

**918. COMLINE International
    Corporation**
H Morimoto (General Manager)
Shugetsu Building 2F
3–12–7 Kita-Aoyama
Minato-ku
Tokyo 107
Japan
Telephone: 03 3486–0696
Fax: 03 3400–7704
Telex/E-mail: 2428134 COMLIN J

**919. COMLINE International
    Corporation**
T Silveria (US Sales Manager); Michael
McCoy (Account Executive)
10601 S DeAnza Boulevard 216
Cupertino
CA 95014
USA
Telephone: (408) 257–9956
Fax: (408) 257–0695

920. COMMARS International AB
Box 27112
Gyllenstiernsgatan 4
105 52 Stockholm
Sweden
Telephone: 08 67 94 80
Telex/E-mail: 8106099 EXPOCOM S

**921. CommCenter Disc & Database
    GmbH**
Holzhofallee 38
Box 1105452
D-6100 Darmstadt
Germany
Telephone: 06151 3910
Fax: 06151 391–200
Telex/E-mail: 419548 DAV D

922. Commerce Clearing House Inc
Marketing Department
4025 W Peterson Avenue
Chicago
IL 60646
USA
Telephone: (312) 583–8500;
          (800) 835–0105

**923. Commerce Management
Services**
PO Box E162
Queen Victoria Terrace
ACT 2600
Australia
Telephone: 61 (62) 95–1961
Fax: 61 (62) 95–0170

924. Commerzbank AG
Economic Research and Corporate
    Communication Department
Postfach 100505
D-6000 Frankfurt am Main 1
Germany
Telephone: 069 13620
Fax: 069 1362–3422

**925. Commissariat a l'Energie
Atomique**
Centre d'Etudes de Ripault
29–33 rue de la Federation
F-75752 Paris Cedex 15
France
Telephone: 1 40 56 10 00

**926. Commissariat a l'Energie
Atomique**
Centre d'Études Nucleaires de Saclay
F-91191 Gif-sur-Yvette Cedex
France
Telephone: 1 69 08 88 98
Fax: 1 69 08 71 73
Telex/E-mail: 604641 ENERG X F

**927. Commissariat a l'Energie
Atomique**
31–33 rue de la Federation
BP 510
F-75752 Paris Cedex 15
France
Telephone: 1 40 56 17 42
Fax: 1 40 56 18 73

**928. Commissie van het Nationaal
Fonds voor Wetenschappelijk
Onderzoek (See Conference des
Bibliothecaires en Chef)**

**929. Commission de la Santé et de la
Securité du Travail**
1199 rue de Bleury
4th Floor
CP 6067, Succurasale A
Montréal
Québec H3C 4E1
Canada
Telephone: (514) 873–3160
Fax: (514) 873–6593

**930. Commission of the European
Communities**
EUROBASES
Christian de Bruyne
200 rue de la Loi
B-1049 Brussels
Belgium
Telephone: 02 235 00 01;
        02 235 00 03
Fax: 02 236 06 24
Telex/E-mail: 21877 COMEU B
NUA: 270429200

**932. Commission of the European
Communities**
Central Library
200 rue de la Loi
B-1049 Brussels
Belgium
Telephone: 02 235–0001
Fax: 02 236–0624
Telex/E-mail: 21877 COMEU B

**933. Commission of the European
Communities**
Directorate General for Agriculture
    Division VI/FII.3
200 rue de la Loi
B-1049 Brussels
Belgium
Telephone: 02 235–8612

**934. Commission of the European
Communities**
Directorate General for Energy
200 rue de la Loi
B-1049 Bressels
Belgium
Telephone: 02 235–9105

**935. Commission of the European
Communities**
Directorate General for Personnel and
    Administration
200 rue de la Loi
B-1049 Brussels
Belgium
Telephone: 02 235–0001

**936. Commission of the European
Communities**
Joint Research Centre Environmental
    Institute
Dr M Boni (ECDIN Team Leader)
21020 Comunità Ispra
Italy
Telephone: 0332 78 97 20;
        0332 78 91 11
Fax: 0332 789 963
Telex/E-mail: 380042 EURI I
NUA: 2222220051

**937. Commission of the European
Communities**
Statistical Office of the European
    Communities (Eurostat)
Bâtiment Jean Monnet
BP 1907
Rue Alcide de Gaspari
L-2920 Luxembourg
Luxembourg
Telephone: 4301–14567
Fax: 4301–3015
Telex/E-mail: 3423 COMEUR LU

**938. Commission of the European
Communities**
Directorate General for Information
University Information Division
Bâtiment Jean Lonnet
BP 1907
Rue Alcide de Gasperi
L-2920 Luxembourg
Luxembourg

**939. Commission of the European
Communities**
Specialized Department for Terminology
    and Computer Applications
Bâtiment Jean Monnet A2/101
L-2920 Luxembourg
Luxembourg
Telephone: 4301–2389

**940. Commission of the European
Communities**
ECHO
Mr R Haber
BP 2373
L-1023 Luxembourg
Luxembourg
Telephone: 488–041
Fax: 488–040
Telex/E-mail: 2181 EUROL LU
NUA: 270448112;
Dial up connection (300 baud):
    +352 436428;
Dial up connection (1200 baud):
    +352 420347

**941. Commodity Information
Services Company (See CISCO)**

942. Commodity Systems Inc
200 W Palmetto Park Road
Boca Ratón
FL 33432–3788
USA
Telephone: (407) 392–8663;
        (800) 327–0175
Fax: (407) 392–1379
Telex/E-mail: 522107

**943. Commodore Business Machines
Inc**
Computer Systems Division
1200 Wilson Drive
West Chester
PA 19380
USA
Telephone: (215) 431–9100
Telex/E-mail: 6105530008

944. Commodore
Peter Talbot (Educational Sales
    Manager)
Commodore House
The Switchback
Gardener Road
Maidenhead
Berkshire
SL6 7XA
UK
Telephone: 0628 770–088
Fax: 0628 71456

945. Common Knowledge
Jefferson
MD 21755
USA
Telephone: (301) 695–3100

**946. Commonwealth Agricultural
Bureau (See CAB International)**

**947. Commonwealth Bank of
Australia**
GPO Box 2719
Sydney
NSW 2001
Australia
Telephone: 02 227–7111
Telex/E-mail: 20345 COMBANK AA

**948. Commonwealth Department of
Education**
PO Box 826
Woden
ACT 2606
Australia
Telephone: 61 (62) 89–1333

949. Communications Canada
Canadian Heritage Information Network
Journal Tower South
12th Floor
365 Laurier Avenue W
Ottawa
ON K1A 0C8
Canada
Telephone: (613) 952–2318

**950. Community Development
Foundation**
60 Highbury Grove
London
N5 2AG
UK
Telephone: 071 226–5375
Fax: 071 704–0313

951. Comp-U-Card Ltd
1 Eton Court
Eton
Windsor
Berkshire
SL4 6BY
UK
Telephone: +44 753–853553

952. Compact Cambridge
Ted Caris (Publisher); Jenny McGee
    (Director of Electronic Publishing)
7200 Wisconsin Avenue
Suite 601
Bethesda
MD 20814
USA
Telephone: (301) 961–6750
Fax: (301) 961–6720

953. Compact Data (SilverPlatter Agent)
Forchhammersvej 19
DK-1920 Frederiksberg C
Denmark
Telephone: 45–31210005
Fax: 45–31214605

954. Compact Disc Inc
Bob Rager (President)
1908 Rainbow Drive
Silver Spring
MD 20905
USA
Telephone: (301) 384–0012
Fax: (301) 384–0012

955. Compact Disc Technologies Corp
Manuel G Diaz Ruiz
421 Muñoz Rivera Avenue
Midtown Plaza
Suite 06–07
Hato Rey
PR 00918
USA
Telephone: 767–8418
Fax: 767–8421

956. Compact Discoveries
1050 South Federal Highway
Delray Beach
FL 33483
USA
Telephone: (305) 243–1453

957. Compact Disk Products
223 E. 85 St.
New York
NY 10028
USA
Telephone: (212) 737–8400;
    (800) 634–2298
Fax: (212) 737–8289

958. Compact Publications Inc
8 Doaks Lane
Little Harbor
Marblehead
MA 01945–3533
USA
Telephone: (617) 630–1100
Fax: (617) 639–2980

959. Compact Publishing Inc
Robert Ellis (Publisher)
4958 Ashby Street NW
Washington
DC 20007
USA
Telephone: (202) 965–2718;
    (202) 244–4770
Fax: (202) 298–8487

960. Compagnie Europeenne d'Edition et de Publications Periodiques
120 avenue des Champs Elysees
75008 Paris
France
Telephone: 33 (1) 45 62 62 95

961. Company of Science and Art (See CoSA)

962. Compaq Computer Corporation
Catherine Macora
20555 State Highway 249
Houston
TX 77070
USA
Telephone: (713) 370–0670
Fax: (713) 374–1462

963. Compaq Computer Ltd
Lee Johns (Software Marketing); Nick
    Fright (Technical Planning Manager)
Hotham House
1 Heron Square
Richmond
Surrey
TW9 1EJ
UK
Telephone: 081 332–3000
Fax: 081 332–1952

964. Compton New Media
c/o Brittanica Software
345 Fourth Street
San Francisco
CA 94107
USA
Telephone: (800) 533–0130;
    (415) 597–5555
Fax: (415) 546–0153

965. Compu-Mark (UK) Limited
New Premier House
Suite 3
150 Southampton Row
London
WC1B 5AL
UK
Telephone: 071 278–4646
Fax: 071 278–5934
Telex/E-mail: 25105 COMPUK G

966. Compu-Mark US
500 Victory Drive
North Quincy
MA 02171–1545
USA
Telephone: (800) 421–7881
Fax: (301) 907–9414
Telex/E-mail: 440388 COMUS

967. Compu-Mark
St Pietersvliet 7
B-2000 Antwerp
Belgium
Telephone: 3 220 7211
Fax: 3 220 7390
Telex/E-mail: 32741 COMPU B

968. CompuCraft
UK
Telephone: 0908 342154

969. Compuflight Operations Service Inc
48 Harbor Park Drive
Port Washington
NY 11050
USA
Telephone: (516) 625–0202

970. CompuKennel Information Service Inc
599 Boggs Run
Benwood
WV 26031
USA
Telephone: (304) 232–5773

971. Compunication GmbH
Gerhard Klaes
Datenbankdienste
PO Box 100708
4300 Essen 1
Germany
Telephone: 201 267 282;
    201 8127 233
Fax: 201 251 506

972. Compusearch Corporation
Michele Darnell (Sales)
7926 Jones Branch Drive
Suite 260
McLean
VA 22102
USA
Telephone: (703) 893–7200
Fax: (703) 893–7499

973. CompuServe Inc
1 Redcliffe Street
Bristol
BS1 6NP
UK
Telephone: 0800 289458;
    0272 255111

974. CompuServe Inc
5000 Arlington Centre Blvd
PO Box 20212
Columbus
OH 43220
USA
Telephone: (614) 457–8600;
    (800) 848–8990
Telex/E-mail: 810 482 1709 CPS A C

975. Computaprint
39A Bowling Green Lane
London
EC1R 0BJ
UK
Telephone: 071 278–8981
Fax: 071 833–1563

976. Computer Access Corporation
26 Brighton St.
Suite 324
Belmont
MA 02178
USA
Telephone: (617) 484–2412

977. Computer Aided Marketing Programs Inc
4131 NW 13th Street
Gainesville
FL 32609
USA
Telephone: (904) 376–5769

978. Computer Aided Planning Inc (See CAP Electronic Sweet's)

979. Computer Brokers Exchange BV
PO Box 3124
NL-2001 DC Haarlem
Netherlands
Telephone: 23 31 91 75
Fax: 23 31 12 47
Telex/E-mail: 41749 CBE NL

980. Computer Company, The
PO Box 6987
Richmond
VA 23230
USA
Telephone: (804) 965–7400;
(800) 446–2612

**981. Computer Equipment
Information Bureau**
50 Fairhaven Road
Concord
MA 01742
USA
Telephone: (508) 493–9550
Telex/E-mail: 949329 CEIB

982. Computer Express
31D Union Avenue
Sudbury
MA 01776
USA
Telephone: (508) 443–6125
Fax: (508) 443–5645
Telex/E-mail: 70007,1534 (Compuserve
Information Service)

983. Computer Intelligence
3344 N Torrey Pines Court
La Jolla
CA 92037
USA
Telephone: (619) 450–1667
Fax: (619) 452–7491

984. Computer Microfilm Corporation
3900 Wheeler Avenue
Alexandria
VA 22304
USA
Telephone: (800) 227–3742

985. Computer Music Consortium Inc
David Barnett (President)
145 W 28 Street
6th Floor
New York
NY 10001
USA
Telephone: (212) 629–4365
Fax: (212) 564–5433

**986. Computer Petroleum
Corporation**
6949 Valley Creek Road
St Paul
MN 55125
USA
Telephone: (612) 738–1088;
(800) 328–7353

987. Computer Products Directory
520 Puscy Avenue
PO Box 439
Collingdale
PA 19073–0539
USA
Telephone: (215) 522–1400;
(800) 873–2731
Fax: (215) 353–0402

988. Computer Research Group Inc
2112 Broadway
Suite 305
New York
NY 10023
USA
Telephone: (212) 496–7774

989. Computer Review
594 Marrett Rd.
Lexington
MA 02173
USA
Telephone: (617) 861–0515

990. Computer Sciences of Australia
André Michau
460 Pacific Highway
Saint Leonards
NSW 2065
Australia
Telephone: 2901 1111
Fax: 2901 1122
Telex/E-mail: 22453 CSASYD AA

**991. Computer Search International
Corporation**
7926 Jones Branch Drive
Suite 305
McLean
VA 22102
USA
Telephone: (302) 749–1735

992. Computer Sports World
1005 Elm Street
Boulder City
NV 89005
USA
Telephone: (702) 294–0191;
(800) 321–5562
Fax: (702) 294–1322

**993. Computer Users Survival
Electronic Magazine**
J Walman (Director)
400 E 59th Street
Suite 9F
New York
NY 10022
USA
Telephone: (212) 755–4363
Fax: (212) 755–4365
Telex/E-mail: PUNCHIN (DELPHI)

994. Computerized Bizmart Systems
451 Moody Street
Suite 206
Waltham
MA 02154
USA
Telephone: (615) 894–4452

995. Computers Unlimited
2 The Business Centre
Colindeep Lane
London
NW9 6DV
UK
Telephone: 081 200–8282

996. Comshare Inc
3001 S State Street
Ann Arbor
MI 48108
USA
Telephone: (313) 994–4800

997. Comstock
Kathy Mullins (Director of Marketing)
30 Irving Place
New York
NY 10003
USA
Telephone: (212) 353–8686
Fax: (212) 353–3383
Telex/E-mail: 6503209859

998. Comtex Scientific Corporation
911 Hope Street
PO Box 4838
Stamford
CT 06907
USA
Telephone: (203) 358–0007;
(800) 624–5089
Fax: (203) 358–0236
Telex/E-mail: 5101011152

999. Comunicación y Calculo SA
Paseo de Gracia 49 1.1
08007 Barcelona
Spain
Telephone: +34 3 215 7641

1000. Conceptual Arts
Gainesville
Florida
USA

1001. Conference Board Inc, The
845 3rd Avenue
New York
NY 10022
USA
Telephone: (212) 759–0900
Telex/E-mail: 234465 CONF UR

**1002. Conference Board of Canada,
The**
Applied Economic Research and
Information Centre
225 Smyth Road
Ottawa
ON K1H 8M7
Canada
Telephone: (613) 526–3280
Fax: (613) 526–4857
Telex/E-mail: 0533043

**1003. Conference des Bibliothecaires
en Chef**
c/o Reseau Libis
Mgr. Ladeuzeplein 21
B-3000 Louvain
Belgium
Telephone: 16 28 46 01
Fax: 18 20 22 48
Telex/E-mail: 33646 B

**1004. Conference des Grandes
Ecoles**
60 Boulevard Saint Michel
75272 Paris Cedex 06
France
Telephone: 33 (1) 43 26 25 57

**1005. Conferentie van Universitaire
Hoofdbibliothecarissen (See
Conference des Bibliothecaires
en Chef)**

1006. Confindustria
Viale dell'Astronomia 30
I-00100 Rome
Italy
Telephone: 06 590 31
Telex/E-mail: 611393 CONFIN I

**1007. Congressional Information
Service**
Jack Carey (Marketing Manager)
4520 East-West Highway
Suite 800
Bethesda
MD 20814–3389
USA
Telephone: (301) 654–1550;
(800) 638–8380
Fax: (301) 657–3203
Telex/E-mail: 292386 DIALMAIL: 12425

1008. Congressional Quarterly Inc
Washington Alert Service
1414 22nd Street NW
Washington
DC 20037
USA
Telephone: (202) 887–6253

1009. Connect Inc
10101 Bubb Road
Cupertino
CA 95014
USA
Telephone: (408) 973–0110;
      (800) 262–2638
Fax: (408) 973–0497
Telex/E-mail: Connect: CONNECT INC

1010. Connecticut State Department of Environmental Protection
Michael Prisloe
National Resource Center
165 Capitol Avenue
Hartford
CT 06106
USA
Telephone: (203) 566–3450

1011. Conseil des Ministres de l'Education du Canada
252 Bloor Street W
Toronto
ON M5S 1V5
Canada
Telephone: (416) 964–2551
Fax: (416) 964–2296

1012. Conseil International de la Langue Française
103 rue de Lille
F-75007 Paris
France
Telephone: 1 47 05 07 93

1013. Consejo General de Colegios Oficiales de Farmaceuticos de España
Calle Villanueva 11
28001 Madrid
Spain
Telephone: 1 431 25 60

1014. Consejo Superior de Investigaciones Científicas
Instituto de Información y
   Documentación en Ciencias Sociales
   y Humanidades
Concha Alvaro Bermejo
Calle Pinar 25, 3o
6 Madrid
Spain
Telephone: 1 262 77 55
Fax: 5645069
Telex/E-mail: 42182 CSIC E
NUA: 2145215063232

1015. Consejo Superior de Investigaciones Científicas
Servicio de Distribución e Información
Consuelo Ruiz
Calle Pinar 19
28006 Madrid
Spain
Fax: 1 261 61 93

1016. Conservation Information Network
Getty Conservation Institute
4503 Glencoe Avenue
Marina del Rey
CA 90292–6537
USA
Telephone: (213) 822–2299
Fax: (213) 301–4931
Telex/E-mail: GCI.KM (Envoy 100)

1017. Consiglio Nazionale dell'Economia e del Lavoro (See CNEL)

1018. Consiglio Nazionale delle Ricerche d'Italia
Center for Stratigraphy and Petrology of
   the Central Alps
Via Botticelli 23
20133 Milano
Italy
Telephone: 39 (2) 29 39 94

1019. Consiglio Nazionale delle Ricerche d'Italia
Istituto per la Documentazione Giuridica
Via Panciatichi 56/16
I-50127 Florence
Italy
Telephone: 055 431 722
Telex/E-mail: 574593 IDGFI I

1020. Consiglio Nazionale delle Ricerche d'Italia
Istituto per la Documentazione Giuridica
Servizio Elaborazione Dati
Via Vasco de Gama 223
50127 Florence
Italy
Telephone: 055 41 09 77
Telex/E-mail: 574593 IDGFI I

1021. Consorcio de Informacion y Documentacion de Cataluna
Calabria 168
E-08015 Barcelona
Spain
Telephone: 3 321 8000
Telex/E-mail: 54310 CIDC E
NUA: Available on application

1022. Consortium of University Research Libraries (CURL)
John Rylands University Library of
   Manchester
Shirley Perry (Project Officer)
Oxford Road
Manchester
M13 9PP
UK
Telephone: 061 275 3786
Fax: 061 273 7488
Telex/E-mail: Janet email: CURLSYS
UK.AC.MCC.CMS

1023. Consorzio Interuniversitario Lombardo per l'Elaborazione Automatica
Via R Sanzio 4
I-20090 Segrate/Milan
Italy
Telephone: 2 223 2541
Telex/E-mail: 310330 CILEAM I
NUA: 2222260139

1024. Consorzio S.I.NO.DO.
Via Pomba 23
I-10123 Turin
Italy
Telephone: 011 561 20 79
Fax: 011 561 56 91

1025. Construction Industries Technical Information Service (See CITIS)

1026. Construction Industry Press
PO Box 9838
San Rafael
CA 94912
USA
Telephone: (415) 731–1913

1027. Construction Information Center Company Ltd
Data-base System Division
Tachibana Building
2–26 Nishi-shinjuku
3–Chome
Shinjuku-ku
Tokyo 160
Japan
Telephone: 03 3342–2811

1028. Construction Information Services Group, Sweet's Group
McGraw-Hill Inc
1221 Avenue of the Americas
New York
NY 10020
USA
Telephone: (212) 512–2000;
      (800) 848–9002
Fax: (212) 512–4302
Telex/E-mail: 12 7960 MCGRAWH NYK

1029. Consulplano SA
Joao Luis de Ayala Boaventura
(Technical Director)
Av Frei Miguel Contreiras 54–3
1700 Lisbon
Portugal
Telephone: 351 189 1187
Fax: 351 189–6738

1030. Consult Srl
Umberto Jovine
Via Mauro Macchi 63
20124 Milan
Italy
Telephone: 39 (2) 67 00 791
Fax: 39 (2) 66 93 742

1031. Consultative Group on International Agricultural Research
Pauline Zoellick (Consultant)
924 Kelly Road W
Boulder
CO 80302
USA
Telephone: (303) 449–3134
Fax: (303) 440–6766

1032. Consumer Industries Press
Quadrant House
The Quadrant
Sutton
Surrey
SM2 5AS
UK

1033. Consumer Network Inc, The
3624 Science Centere
Philadelphia
PA 19104
USA
Telephone: (215) 386–5890
Fax: (215) 557–7692

1034. Consumers Union of the US Inc
Wendy Goldman (Assistant Editor)
101 Truman Avenue
Yonkers
NY 10703
USA
Telephone: (914) 378–2562
Fax: (914) 378–2907
Telex/E-mail: 710 562 0102 CONSUME

1035. Contactgroep Audiovisuele Centra Wetenschappelijk Onderwijs
c/o Pica Centrum voor
  Bibliotheekautomatisering
PO Box 876
NL-2300 AW Leiden
Netherlands
Telephone: 071 257–257
Fax: 071 223–119
Telex/E-mail: 34402 NL

1036. Context Systems Inc
Paul J Kelly (Vice President)
The Technology Center
333 Byberry Road
Hatboro
PA 19040
USA
Telephone: (215) 675–5000
Fax: (215) 957–1218

1037. Control Data Corporation/Business Information Services
500 W Putnam Avenue
PO Box 7100
Greenwich
CT 06836
USA
Telephone: (203) 622–2000

1038. Control Data Ltd
Abraham Fullard
3 Roundwood Avenue
Stockley Park
Uxbridge
UB1 1AG
UK
Telephone: 081 848–1919
Fax: 081 848–3133

1039. Control Data
130 Albert Street
Suite 1105
Ottawa
ON K1P 5G4
Canada
Telephone: (613) 598–0212;
              (613) 598–0200
Fax: (613) 563–1716

1040. Control Risks Information Services
83 Victoria Street
London
SW1H 0HW
UK
Telephone: 071 222–1552

1041. Control Risks Limited
4350 East-West Highway, Suite 900
Bethesda
MD 20814
USA
Telephone: (301) 654–2075
Fax: (301) 654–4645
Telex/E-mail: 256502 CRW UR

1042. Conway Data Inc
40 Technology Park/Atlanta
Norcross
GA 30092
USA
Telephone: (404) 446–6996;
              (800) 554–5686
Fax: (404) 263–8825
Telex/E-mail: 804468 ATL

1043. Coopers and Lybrand Europe
European Community Office
Av. de Tervuren 2
1040 Brussels
Belgium
Telephone: 02 735 9065

1044. Copenhagen School of Economics and Business Administration
Hans Engstrom
Rosenoerns Alle 31
1970 Copenhagen V
Denmark
Telephone: 33 144–414
Fax: 23 141–128

1045. Copper Development Association Inc
PO Box 1840
Greenwich
CT 06836
USA
Telephone: (203) 625–8210
Fax: (203) 625–0174
Telex/E-mail: 643784

1046. COREF
Tour Vendome
204 Rond-point du Pont-de-Sevres
F-92516 Boulogne-Billancourt Cedex
France
Telephone: 91 46 08 90 82

1047. Corel Systems Corporation
1600 Carling Ave
Ottawa
Ontario
K1Z 8R7
Canada
Telephone: +1 613 728 8200
Fax: +1 613 728 2891

1048. Cornell Laboratory of Ornithology
Library of Natural Sounds
Greg Budney
159 Sapsucker Woods Road
Ithaca
NY 14850
USA
Telephone: (607) 254–2404
Fax: (607) 254–2415

1049. Cornell University
Chemistry Department
FW McLafferty
Baker Laboratory
Ithaca
NY 14853–1301
USA
Telephone: (607) 255–4699
Fax: (607) 255–7880

1050. Corporate Agents Inc
PO Box 1281
Wilmington
DE 19899
USA
Telephone: (302) 998–0598;
              (800) 441–9975

1051. Corporate Jobs Outlook Inc
PO Drawer 100
Boerne
TX 78006
USA
Telephone: (512) 755–8810;
              (800) 325–8808
Fax: (512) 755–2410

1052. Corporate Technology Information Services Inc
12 Alfred Street
Suite 200
Woburn
MA 01801–9998
USA
Telephone: (617) 932–3939
Fax: (617) 932–6335
Telex/E-mail: 4972961 CRPTECH

1053. CorpTech (See Corporate Technology Information Services Inc)

1054. Corte Suprema di Cassazione d'Italia
Centro Elettronico di Documentazione
E Giannantonio
Via Damiano Chiesa 24
I-00136 Rome
Italy
Telephone: 6 330 81
Fax: 6 330 83 38
Telex/E-mail: 620461
NUA: available on application

1055. CoSA (Company of Science and Art)
Gregory Deocampo (CEO)
14 Imperial Place
Suite 203
Providence
RI 02903
USA
Telephone: (401) 831–2672
Fax: (401) 274–7517

1056. Cosmos
19530 Pacific Highway South
Seattle
WA 98188
USA
Telephone: (206) 842–9942

1057. Council for Exceptional Children
Department of Information Services
1920 Association Drive
Reston
VA 22091
USA
Telephone: (703) 620–3660
Fax: (703) 264–9494
Telex/E-mail: Specialnet: CEC.RESTON

1058. Council of Europe
Directorate of Education, Culture and
  Sport
B.P. 431 R6
67006 Strasbourg Cedex
France
Telephone: 33 (88) 61 49 61
Fax: 33 (88) 36 70 57
Telex/E-mail: 870943 EUR F

1059. Council of Europe
European Documentation and
  Information System for Education
BP 431 R6
F-67006 Strasbourg Cedex
France
Telephone: 88 41 20 00
Fax: 88 41 27 81
Telex/E-mail: 870943 EUR F

1060. Council of Ministers of Education of Canada (See Conseil des Ministres de l'Education du Canada)

1061. Council of Scientific Research
Scientific Documentation Center
Jadiriyah
P.O.B. 2241
Baghdad
Iraq
Telephone: 964 (1) 776–0023
Telex/E-mail: 2187

1062. Council on Foreign Relations Inc
58 E 68th Street
New York
NY 10021
USA
Telephone: (212) 734–0400
Fax: (212) 861–1789

1063. Counterpoint Publishing
Sanford Friedman
20 William Street
Suite G-70
PO Box 9135
Wellesley
MA 02181–9135
USA
Telephone: (617) 235–4667
Fax: (617) 235–5467

1064. Countryside Information Systems
East Close
Ditcheat
Shepton Mallet
Somerset BA4 6PS
UK
Telephone: 44 (74) 986358

1065. Courier-Journal Company
525 W Broadway
Louisville
KY 40202
USA
Telephone: (502) 582–4011

1066. COURTHOUSE Records Inc
James W Burneson (President)
12375 E Cornell Avenue
Unit 7
Aurora
CO 80014
USA
Telephone: (303) 695–1111 x27;
(800) 950–3232
Fax: (203) 695–0182

1067. Cowles Publishing Company
PO Box 2160
Spokane
WA 99210
USA
Telephone: (509) 459–5060
Fax: (509) 459–5234

1068. Cox Texas Publications Inc
166 E. Riverside
Austin
TX 78704
USA
Telephone: (512) 445–3500

1069. Cox, Matthews & Associates Inc
10520 Warwick Avenue Suite B-8
Fairfax
VA 22030
USA
Telephone: (703) 385–2981

1070. CPS Online
2505 West 2nd Avenue, Suite 7
Denver
CO 80219
USA
Telephone: (303) 936–9930;
(800) 521–7525

1071. CPU Peripherals Ltd
Copse Road
St Johns
Woking
Surrey
GU21 1SX
UK
Telephone: 0483 723–411

1072. Crain Communications Inc
740 N Rush Street
Chicago
IL 60611
USA
Telephone: (312) 649–5411

1073. Crain Communications Inc
1400 Woodbridge
Detroit
MI 48207
USA
Telephone: (313) 446–6000

1074. CRC Press Inc
CD-ROM Enquiries
2000 Corporate Boulevard NW
Boca Ratón
FL 33431
USA
Telephone: (407) 994–0555
Fax: (407) 997–0949
Telex/E-mail: 568689 CRC PRESS

1075. CRC Research Institute
Jimmy Nakamura (Department Officer)
3–6–2 Nihombashi Honcho
Chuo-ku
Tokyo 103
Japan
Telephone: 3 3665 9817
Fax: 3 3664 4044

1076. CRC Systems Inc
4020 Williamsburg Court
Fairfax
VA 22032
USA
Telephone: (703) 385–0440

1077. Creative Communications Inc
PO Box 1519–GRI
Herndon
VA 22070
USA
Telephone: (703) 787–4647
Fax: (703) 742–9696

1078. Creative Information Systems Inc
PO Box 30567
Portland
OR 97230
USA
Telephone: (503) 253–6812

1079. Creditel of Canada Ltd
PO Box 532
Station F
Toronto
ON M4Y 2N1
Canada
Telephone: (416) 922–4660
Fax: (416) 922–9734

1080. Creditreform
Werner Strahler (Controller)
Hellersbergstraße 12
4040 Neuss
Germany
Telephone: 2101 109–100
Fax: 2101 109–140
NUA: Available on application

1081. CREDOC (See also Centre de Recherche Documentaire)

1082. CREDOC a.s.b.l.
Rue de la Montagne 34
Box 11
1000 Brussels
Belgium
Telephone: 33 (2) 511 69 41
Fax: 33 (2) 513 31 95

1083. CRESM/IREMAM
3 et 5, Avenue Pasteur
13100 Aix-en-Provence
France
Telephone: 33 (42) 21 59 88

1084. CrimeBooks Inc
Bill Young
1213 Wilmette Avenue
Suite 203
Wilmette
IL 60091–2557
USA
Telephone: (708) 256–9813
Fax: (708) 251–5289

1085. CSA
Mike Niswonger
2–H David Street
Fort Walton Beach
FL 32548
USA
Telephone: (904) 862–7127

1086. CSIRO (See Australian Commonwealth Scientific and Industrial Research Organisation)

1087. CSK Research Institute Corporation
Koji Yada (President)
2–5–1, Suwa
Tama-Shi
Tokyo 206
Japan
Telephone: 3 4237–51271
Fax: 3 4237–50095

1088. CSPP – Centre for the Study of Public Policy
Prof. Kevin Allen
Livingstone Tower
Richmond Street
Glasgow
G1 1XH
UK
Telephone: +44 041–5524400 ex 3908/3910
NUA: 23424126010604

1089. CSR Inc
1400 I Street, NW, Suite 600
Washington
DC 20005
USA
Telephone: (202) 842–7600

1090. CT Whipple Company USA
PO Box 6713
Mesa
AZ 85216
USA
Telephone: (602) 641–9789
Fax: (602) 641–0747

1091. CTL
16 rue de la Michaudiere
75002 Paris
France
Telephone: 33 (1) 47 42 86 59

1092. CTU, University of Milan
Dr Patrizia Ghislandi
Via Celoria 20
Settore Didattico
20133 Milan
Italy
Telephone: 2 2364–504
Fax: 2 2668–1051

1469

1093. Cuadra/Elsevier
11835 West Olympic Blvd, Suite 855
Los Angeles
CA 90064
USA
Telephone: (213) 478–0066
Fax: (213) 477–1078
Telex/E-mail: 755814 CUADRA SNM

1094. CUC International Inc
707 Summer Street
PO Box 10049
Stamford
CT 06904–2094
USA
Telephone: (203) 324–9261;
(800) 843–7777
Fax: (203) 348–4528
Telex/E-mail: 643100

1095. Cultural Resources Inc
7 Little Falls Way
Scotch Plains
NJ 07076
USA
Telephone: (201) 232–4333
Fax: (201) 232–3683

**1096. Cumulative Index to Nursing &
Allied Health Literature**
Caroline Fischel (Electronic Information
Specialist)
1509 Wilson Terrace
PO Box 871
Glendale
CA 91209–0871
USA
Telephone: (818) 409–8005
Fax: (818) 546–5679
Telex/E-mail: GAMCL (DOCLINE)

1097. Cumulus Systems Limited
1 High Street
Rickmansworth
Hertfordshire
WD3 1ET
UK
Telephone: 44 (923) 720477

**1098. Current Awareness in
Biological Sciences**
132 New Walk
Leicester
LE1 7QQ
UK
Telephone: 44 (533) 548707
Fax: 44 (533) 471001

**1099. Current Digest of the Soviet
Press**
3857 N High Street
Columbus
OH 43214
USA
Telephone: (614) 292–4234
Fax: (614) 267–6310

1100. Current Drugs Ltd
Middlesex House
34–42 Cleveland Street
London
W1P 5FB
UK
Telephone: 071 631–0341;
071 580–8393
Fax: 071 580–1938;
071 580–5646

1101. Curtis Development Company
1000 Waterway Boulevard
Indianapolis
IN 46202
USA
Telephone: (317) 633–2045

1102. Cutter Information Corporation
37 Broadway
Arlington
MA 02174–5539
USA
Telephone: (617) 648–8700

1103. CVC Online Inc
801 2nd Avenue
New York
NY 10017
USA
Telephone: (212) 986–5100

1104. CW Credit Abstract Company
c/o Trans Union Credit Information
Company
Litigations Division
8th Floor
95–25 Queens Boulevard
Rego Park
NY 11374
USA
Telephone: (718) 459–3614
Fax: (718) 830–5329

**1105. Cynetics Data Modelling
Technologies BV**
JJ van Vliet R van Leeuwen
Gebouw Blue Wings
Paasheuvelweg 39
1105 BJ Amsterdam Zuid-Oost
Netherlands
Telephone: 20 696–5436
Fax: 20 691–9921

1106. D A T A Group
St. James Court
PO Box 34
King's Lynn
Norfolk
UK
Telephone: 44 (553) 691459
Fax: 44 (553) 691457
Telex/E-mail: 818461 G

1107. D-S Marketing GmbH
Ostbahnhofstrasse 13
D-6000 Frankfurt/Main
Germany

1108. D-S Marketing Inc.
Suite 110
485 Devon Park Drive
Wayne
PA 19087
USA

1109. DAFA Data AB
Box 34101
S-100 26 Stockholm
Sweden
Telephone: 08 738–5000
Fax: 08 509–772

1110. DAFSA Division Entreprises
7 rue Bergere
F-75009 Paris
France
Telephone: 1 45 23 19 19

1111. DAFSA News
10 Cite Paradis
75010 Paris
France

1112. DAFSA
125 rue Montmartre
F-75081 Paris Cedex 02
France
Telephone: 1 42 33 21 23
Telex/E-mail: 640472 DAF DOC F

1113. Dagens Naeringsliv
PO Box 1182 Sentrum
0107 Oslo 1
Norway
Telephone: 47 (2) 41 36 90

**1114. Dai Nippon Printing Company
Ltd**
Yasutaka Yoshida (General Manager)
1–1 Ichigaya-Kagacho 1–chome
Shinjuku-ku
Tokyo 162–01
Japan
Telephone: 3266–2910
Fax: 3266–4599

**1115. Daikei Data Processing
Company**
Kawaguchi 339
Nishi-Ku
Osaka
Japan
Telephone: 6584 0444

1116. Daily News
PO Box 4200
21221 Oxnard Street
Woodland Hills
CA 91365
USA
Telephone: (818) 713–3000

1117. Daily Oklahoman
PO Box 25125
Oklahoma City
OK 73125
USA
Telephone: (405) 457–3311

1118. Daily Press and Times-Herald
7505 Warwick Blvd
Newport News
VA 23607
USA
Telephone: (804) 247–4600

1119. Daily Reporter, The
PO Box 33999
Milwaukee
WI 53233–0999
USA
Telephone: (414) 276–0273

1120. Daily Telegraph plc
Petersborough Court
South Quay
181 Marsh Wall
London
E14 9SR
UK
Telephone: 071 353–4242

1121. Daily Texan
26th and White
Austin
TX 73713–7209
USA
Telephone: (512) 471–6221

1122. Dainippon Ink & Chemicals Inc
Takamu Yao (Manager Business
Development Department)
3–7–20 Nihonbashi
Chuo-ku
Tokyo 103
Japan
Telephone: 3 3272–4511
Fax: 3 3273–5680

1123. DAIS Group Inc, The
60 Broad Street
New York
NY 10004
USA
Telephone: (212) 422–4200
Fax: (212) 422–7036

1124. Daiwa Securities Research Institute
1–2–1 Kyobashi
Chuo-ku
Tokyo
Japan
Telephone: 03 3553–6014

1125. DAK Industries
8200 Remmet Avenue
Canogo Park
CA 91304
USA
Telephone: (800) 325–0800

1126. DALCTRAF Inc
Box 5815
10248 Stockholm
Sweden
Telephone: 46 (8) 663 67 95
Fax: 46 (8) 661 64 84

1127. Dallas Morning News
508 Young Street
PO Box 655237
Dallas
TX 75265
USA
Telephone: (214) 977–8222

1128. Dallas Theological Seminary
3909 Swiss Avenue
Dallas
TX 75204
USA
Telephone: 214–824–3094

1129. DAMAR Real Estate Information Service
3550 W Temple Street
Los Angeles
CA 90004
USA
Telephone: (213) 380–7105;
        (800) 873–2627
Fax: (213) 386–8476

1130. Danish National Institute of Occupational Health
Produktregistret
Lerso Parkalle 105
DK-2100 Copenhagen 0
Denmark
Telephone: 031 299–711

1131. Danish Standards Association
Strandvejen 203
DK-2900 Hellerup
Denmark
Telephone: 01 62 32 00
Fax: 01 62 36 44
Telex/E-mail: 119203 DSSTAND DK

1132. Danmarks Patentdirektoratet
Helheshoj Alle 81
DK-2630 Taastrup
Denmark
Telephone: 43 71 71 71
Fax: 43 71 71 70
Telex/E-mail: 16046 DPO DK

1133. Danmarks Radio
Bent Sorensen (Chief Int Departments)
TV-Byen
DK-2860 Soborg
Denmark
Telephone: 31 671–233
Fax: 31 672–997

1134. Danmarks Statistik
Sejrogade 11
Bostboks 2550
DK-2100 Copenhagen 0
Denmark
Telephone: 31 298–222
Fax: 31 184–801
Telex/E-mail: 16236 DASTAT DK

1135. Danmarks Tekniske Bibliotek
Dokumentationsafdelingen
Durga S. Nag; Niels Berg Olsen; Mrs. Betty Vedel
Anker Engelunds Vej 1
DK-2800 Lyngby
Denmark
Telephone: 42 883–088
Fax: 42 883–040
Telex/E-mail: 37148 DTBC DK
NUA: 238242126400

1136. Danmarks Tekniske Hoejskole
Kurt Kielsgaard Hansen
Laboratoriet for Bygningsmaterialer; Bygn. 118
DK-2800 Lyngby
Denmark
Telephone: 45 42 883511

1137. Danmarks Turistraad
Poul Michael Linnebelle; Finn Larsen; Dorte Skjoldager
Vesterbrogade 6D
DK-1620 Koebenhavn V
Denmark
Telephone: 45 33 111415
NUA: 23824119420000

1138. Dansk Byplanlaboratorium Biblioteket
Lisa La Cour
Peder Skramsgade 2B
DK-1054 Koebenhavn V
Denmark
Telephone: 45 33 137281

1139. Dansk Data Arkiv
Karsten Boye Rasmussen; Per Nielsen
Odense Universitet
Munkebjerguaenget 48
DK-5230 Odense M
Denmark
Telephone: 66 157–920
Fax: 66 158–320
Telex/E-mail: DDA VM1 (EARN)

1140. Dansk Diane Center
Sigurdsgade 41
DK-2200 Koebenhavn N
Denmark
Telephone: 45 31 181711

1141. Dansk Teknisk Oplysningstjenste
Mogens Bertung
Rygaards Allee 131A
DK-2900 Hallerup
Denmark
Telephone: 45 31 181711

1142. Danske Bank, Den
Dick Meng; Gunnar Wedan; Pia Johansen; Ole Larsen
Holmens Kanal 12
1092 Koebenhavn K
Denmark
Telephone: 45 33 156500

1143. Dartmouth College
Social Science Computing
Hinman Box 6121
Hanover
NH 03755
USA
Telephone: (603) 646–3114

1144. Dartmouth Medical School
Project CORK Institute
Department of Pharmacology and Toxicology
Hanover
NH 03756
USA
Telephone: (603) 646–7540
Fax: (603) 646–2810

1145. Data Base Products Inc
Earl Doolin (President)
12770 Coit Road
Suite 1218
Dallas
TX 75251
USA
Telephone: (214) 233–0595;
        (800) 345–2876
Fax: (214) 233–0594

1146. DATA Business Publishing
15 Inverness Way E
PO Box 6510
Englewood
CO 80155–6510
Telephone: (303) 799–0381;
        (800) 447–4666;
        (800) 241–7824

1147. Data Communications Corporation of Korea
DACOM
Sales and Marketing Division
10th Floor
Insong Building
194–45 Hoehyundong 1 GA
Choong-Ku
Seoul
Korea

1148. Data Development Inc
Steve Swan (Vice President)
3595 SW Corporate Parkway
Palm City
FL 34990
USA
Telephone: (407) 288–7226
Fax: (407) 288–2775

1149. Data Disc System Inc
Takashi Nishi (Managing Director)
2–16–2 Sotokanda
Chiyoda-ku
Tokyo 101
Japan
Telephone: 03 3257–9334
Fax: 03 3257–9338

1150. Data Program Gruppen
Ulf Vasstrom
Nordiska Minister Rådet
Vester Brogade 72
1629 Copenhagen
Denmark
Telephone: 3123–7111
Fax: 3123–7153

1151. Data Services Ltd
PO Box 33–1125
Takapuna
Auckland 9
New Zealand
Telephone: 09 460–703
Fax: 09 949–6349

1152. Data West Inc
Naokazu Akita (Manager)
3–8–28 Hanatenhigashi
Turumi-ku
Osaka 538
Japan
Telephone: 6 968–1236
Fax: 6 968–2792

Addresses

1153. Data-Star
Karen Pierce; Jane Westwater
Plaza Suite
114 Jermyn Street
London
SW1Y 6HJ
UK
Telephone: 071 930–5503
Fax: 071 930–2581
Telex/E-mail: 94012671 STAR G
NUA: 22846431007014

1154. DataArkiv AB
Soina Torg 19
PO Box 1502
S-171 29 Solna
Sweden
Telephone: 08 705 1300
Fax: 08 82 82 96
Telex/E-mail: 8828296 S

1155. DATABANK SpA
Via Dei Piatti 11
I-20123 Milan
Italy
Telephone: 02 80 95 56
Fax: 02 86 55 79
Telex/E-mail: 324217 DTBK I

1156. Database International Limited
Box 62
Maidstone
Kent
UK
Telephone: 44 (622) 65743

1157. Database Publishing Company
PO Box 7440
Newport Beach
CA 92658–7440
USA
Telephone: (714) 646–1623;
　　　　　　(800) 824–9896

1158. DATABASE SC
BP 111
B-1410 Waterloo
Belgium
Telephone: 02 354 82 49
Fax: 02 354 69 83

1159. Database Software Ltd
Europa House
Adlington Park
Macclesfield
SK10 4NP
UK

1160. Datacentralen
Retorvej 6–8
25000 Valby
Copenhagen
Denmark
Telephone: 45 (31) 46 81 22
Fax: 45 (31) 16 88 05
Telex/E-mail: 27122 DC DK

1161. Datalex SA
Paseo de la Castellana 83–85
28046 Madrid
Spain
Telephone: 01 455 69 65

1162. Dataline Inc
67 Richmond Street, West, Suite 700
Toronto
ON M5H 1Z5
Canada
Telephone: (416) 365–1515
Telex/E-mail: 06219661

1163. Datalink Computer Sales Ltd
88 Jane Street
Leith
Edinburgh
EH6 5HG
UK
Telephone: 031 555–0400

1164. Datamonitor
106 Baker Street
London
W1M 1LA
UK
Telephone: 071 625–8548
Fax: 071 625–5080

1165. DATANETWORK
A division of Applied Business Systems
　Inc
400 Embassy Square
Louisville
KY 40299
USA
Telephone: (502) 491–1050;
　　　　　　(800) 626–2358

**1166. DataPro Information Services
　　　Group**
Rebecca Shepherd (Product Manager)
600 Delran Parkway
Delran
NJ 08075
USA
Telephone: (609) 764–0100
Fax: (609) 764–2811

1167. Dataquest Inc
Robert R Gaskin (Staff Analyst)
1290 Ridder Park Drive
San José
CA 95131
USA
Telephone: (408) 437–8000
Fax: (408) 437–0292

**1168. DataQuick Information
　　　Systems Inc**
13160 Mindanao Way
Suite 240
Marina Del Rey
CA 90292
USA
Telephone: (213) 306–4295

1169. Datastream International Ltd
Monmouth House
58–64 City Road
London
EC1Y 2AL
UK
Telephone: 071 250–3000
Fax: 071 253–0171
Telex/E-mail: 916001 G

1170. Datatek Corporation
14000 Quail Springs Parkway
Suite 450
Oklahoma City
OK 73134
USA
Telephone: (405) 751–6400

1171. DataTimes Corporation
Parkway Plaza
Suite 450
1400 Quail Springs Parkway
Oklahoma City
OK 73134
USA
Telephone: (405) 751–6400;
　　　　　　(800) 642–2525

1172. DataTrends Publications Inc
8130 Boone Boulevard
Suite 210
Vienna
VA 22182–2608
USA
Telephone: (703) 760–0660;
　　　　　　(800) 766–8130
Fax: (703) 760–9365
Telex/E-mail: 7401009 DATA UC
RIBM/DATA.TRENDS (Sprintmail)

1174. Dataware Technologies GmbH
(includes Dataware 2000 GmbH)
Barthstrasse 24
D-8000 Munchen 22
Germany
Telephone: 49 89 540924–0
Fax: 49 89 540924–10

1175. Dataware Technologies Inc
David Wilcox (Vice President Sales &
　Marketing)
Suite 3300
222 Third Street
Cambridge
MA 02142–1188
USA
Telephone: (617) 621–0820
Fax: (617) 621–0307

1176. Datex Services Ltd
PO Box 30–988
Lower Hutt
New Zealand
Telephone: 04 693–293
Fax: 04 697–997

**1177. DAV Publishing House (See
　　　ComCenter Disc & Database
　　　GmbH)**

1178. David Aldstadt
PO Box 16080
Columbus
OH 43216
USA
Telephone: (614) 228–1488;
　　　　　　(614) 878–2075

1179. Davidson & Associates Inc
Julie Gibbs (Educational Sales
　Manager)
3135 Kashiwa Street
Torrance
CA 90505
USA
Telephone: (800) 556–6141;
　　　　　　(213) 534–4070
Fax: (213) 534–3169

1180. DBMIST
Ministere de l'Education Nationale, de la
　Jeunesse et des Sports
Direction des Bibliotheques, des
　Musees et de l'Info. Sci. Tech.
3–5 boulevard Pasteur
75015 Paris
France
Telephone: 33 (1) 45 39 25 75

**1181. DC Host Centre, I/S
　　　Datacentralen af 1959**
Mr Torben Friis
Retortvej 6–8
DK-2500 Valby
Denmark
Telephone: +45 31–468122
Fax: +45 31–168805
NUA: 238241592400 (1200 baud);
　　　238241594500 (300 baud)

1183. DCA Publications
217 E 86th Street
Suite 322
New York
NY 10028
USA
Telephone: (212) 535–3336

1184. DDRI – Diversified Data Resources
6609 Rosecroft Place
Falls Church
VA 22043–1828
USA
Telephone: (703) 237–0682
Fax: (703) 532–5447

1185. De Agostini
Guido Bucciotti (Electronic Publishing Manager)
Via Giovanni da Verrazano 15
28100 Novara
Italy
Telephone: 0321 422–477
Fax: 0321 422–451

1186. Dea Librerie Internazionali
Via Lima 28
00198 Rome
Italy
Telephone: +39 6 8551441
Fax: +39 6 8543228

1187. DECHEMA
Theodor-Heuss-Allee 25
Postfach 97 01 46
D-6000 Frankfurt am Main 97
Germany
Telephone: 069 756–4244
Fax: 069 756–4201
Telex/E-mail: 412490 DCHA D

1188. Decision Resources
17 New England Executive Park
Burlington
MA 01803
USA
Telephone: (617) 270–1207
Fax: (617) 273–3048
Telex/E-mail: 921436 14237
(DIALMAIL)

1189. Deemar Company Limited
6th Floor, Anglo-Thai Building
64 Silom Road, P.O. 2732
Bangkok
Thailand
Telephone: 66 (2) 2344521;
66 (2) 2344520
Telex/E-mail: 87258 DEEMAR TH

1190. Defense Systems Management College
Paulette Langlas (Commandant Secretary)
Fort Belvoir
VA 22060–5426
USA
Telephone: (703) 664–6323
Fax: (703) 780–1785

1191. Del Mar Group
722 Genviere Street
Suite M
Solana Beach
CA 92014
USA
Telephone: (619) 259–0444

1192. Delcas (Pty) Ltd
301 Research House
178 Fox Street
Johannesburg 2001
Republic of South Africa
Telephone: 011 3376–7067
Telex/E-mail: 83598 SA

1193. Deloitte & Touche
10 Westport Road
Wilton
CT 06897–0820
USA
Telephone: (203) 761–3212
Fax: (203) 834–2200

1194. Deloitte Haskins & Sells
Kortenberglaan 79
Brussels
Belgium
Telephone: 32 (2) 736 20 58

1195. DeLorme Mapping Systems
Charles Hinds
PO Box 298
Freeport
ME 04032
USA
Telephone: (207) 865–4171
Fax: (207) 865–9628

1196. Delwel Uitgeverij
Mr Wit
Alexanderstraat 26
Postbus 19110
2500 CC's-Gravenhagen
Netherlands
Telephone: 070 362 48 00
Fax: 070 360 56 06

1197. Demand Research Corporation
625 N Michigan Avenue
Chicago
IL 60611
USA
Telephone: (312) 664–6500
Telex/E-mail: 73207,3434 (CompuServe Information Service)

1198. Demografiska Databasen
Carl-Johan Ruisniemi
Box 94
Storgatan 69
953 22 Haparanda
Sweden
Telephone: 922 11450;
922 11480
Fax: 922 13682

1199. Denshi Media Services Company Ltd
Norihiko Kato (General Manager)
Toppan Yaesu Building 3F
2–7 Yaesu 2–chome
Chuo-ku
Tokyo 104
Japan
Telephone: 3 3276–8071
Fax: 3 3276–0951

1200. Denver Children's Hospital
1056 East 19th Avenue & Downing
Denver
CO 80218
USA
Telephone: (303) 861–8888

1201. Denver Post Corporation
PO Box 1709
Denver
CO 80201
USA
Telephone: (303) 820–1010

1202. Department of Agriculture and Rural Affairs, Victoria
PO Box 500
East Melbourne
VIC 3002
Australia
Telephone: 61 (3) 651–7233
Fax: 61 (3) 651–7009
Telex/E-mail: 34261 AGVIC AA

1203. Department of Community Services and Health
Library and Information Service
Woden
ACT 2606
Australia
Telephone: 61 (62) 89–7395
Telex/E-mail: 62149 AA

1204. Department of Consumer and Corporate Affairs
Information Systems Branch
Place du Portage, Phase II, 5th Floor
Hull
PQ K1A 0C9
Canada
Telephone: (819) 997–2938

1205. Department of Defence
Defence Central Library
Campbell Park Offices
Canberra
ACT 2601
Australia
Telephone: 06 266–2346

1206. Department of Employment, Education and Training
64 Northbourne Avenue
Canberra
ACT 2601
Australia
Telephone: 062 768–330

1207. Department of Employment, Training Agency
Room W815
Moorfoot
Sheffield
South Yorkshire
S1 4PQ
UK
Telephone: 44 (742) 594174
Fax: 44 (742) 594713

1208. Department of Energy, Mines and Resources
Canada Centre for Mineral and Energy Technology
Library & Documentation Services Division
555 Booth Street
Ottawa
ON K1A 0G1
Canada
Telephone: (613) 995–4059
Fax: (613) 952–2587
Telex/E-mail: 0533395 TECHINFO OTT

1209. Department of Energy, Mines and Resources
Canada Centre for Remote Sensing
588 Booth Street
3rd Floor
Ottawa
ON K1A 0Y7
Canada
Telephone: (613) 943–8833
Fax: (613) 952–7353;
(613) 996–9843
Telex/E-mail: 0533777

1210. Department of Finance
Barbara Lohitnvy (Toolbox Coordinator)
Newlands Street
Parkes
ACT 2600
Australia
Telephone: 62 632–318
Fax: 62 733–021

1211. Department of Fisheries and Oceans
Scientific Publications
Heather Cameron (Manager Library Services)
200 Kent Street
Ottawa
ON K1A 0E6
Canada
Telephone: (613) 993–2950
Fax: (613) 996–9055

1212. Department of Foreign Affairs
Parkes
ACT 2600
Australia
Telephone: 61 (62) 61–9111

1213. Department of Health and Social Security
Library
Alexander Fleming House
Elephant and Castle
London SE1 6BY
UK
Telephone: 44 (1) 407–5522 x7233;
44 (1) 407–5522 x7680
Telex/E-mail: 883669 G

1214. Department of Insurance
Office of the Superintendent of Financial Institutions
255 Albert Street
13th Floor
Ottawa
ON K1A 0H2
Canada
Telephone: (613) 990–7788

1215. Department of Justice
West Memorial Building
344 Wellington Street
Room 2117
Ottawa
ON K1A 0H8
Canada
Telephone: (613) 952–1618

1216. Department of National Revenue
Taxation
Ottawa
ON K1A 0L8
Canada

1218. Department of Primary Industries and Energy (Australia)
Water Branch
GPO Box 858
Canberra
ACT 2601
Australia
Telephone: 062 724–751
Fax: 062 724–526
Telex/E-mail: 62188 AA

1219. Department of Supply and Services
15 Eddy Street
Hull
Quebec
K1A 0M5
Canada
Telephone: (819) 997–2891

1220. Department of the Environment
Building Research Establishment Library
Bucknall's Lane
Garston
Watford
Hertfordshire
WD2 7JR
UK
Telephone: 0923 894–040
Fax: 0923 664–010
Telex/E-mail: 923220 G

1221. Department of the Prime Minister and Cabinet
Office of Multicultural Affairs
Canberra
ACT 2600
Australia
Telephone: 062 715–658

1222. Department of the Secretary of State of Canada
Promotion and Client Services
John Carey (Project Officer)
Ottawa
ON K1A 0M5
Canada
Telephone: (819) 997–9727
Fax: (819) 994–3670

1223. Department of Trade and Industry
Central Office of Information
Hercules Road
London SE1 7DU
UK
Telephone: 44 (71) 928–2345;
071–215–4720 (Spearhead)

1224. Department of Trade and Industry
Room 392
Ashdown House
123 Victoria Street
London
SW1E 6RB
UK

1225. Department of Trade and Industry
Internal European Policy Division
1–19 Victoria Street
London
SW1H 0ET
UK
Telephone: 071 215–7877

1226. Department of Transport and Communications
Transport Group Library
GPO Box 594
Civic Square
ACT 2608
Australia
Telephone: 062 679–780
Fax: 062 572–505
Telex/E-mail: 62018 AA

1227. Departments of Health and Social Security
Library
Hannibal House
Elephant and Castle
London
SE1 6TE
UK
Telephone: 071 403–2609

1228. Departments of the Environment and Transport Library
Room P3/008E
2 Marsham Street
London
SW1P 3EB
UK
Telephone: 071 276–5673
Fax: 071 276–5713

1229. Derwent Inc
1313 Dolley Madison Boulevard
Suite 303
McLean
VA 22101
USA
Telephone: (703) 790–0400;
(800) 451–3451
Fax: (703) 790–1426
Telex/E-mail: DIALMAIL; 11592

1230. Derwent Publications Ltd
Dr Mike Harvey (Director Product Development); Paul Dixon (Director Product Development)
Rochdale House
128 Theobalds Road
London
WC1X 8RP
UK
Telephone: 071 242–5823
Fax: 071 405–3630
Telex/E-mail: 267487 DERPUB G
LONDON DERWENT (DIALMAIL)

1231. Des Moines Register & Tribune Company
715 Locust Street
Des Moines
IA 50304
Telephone: (515) 284–8000

1232. Desktop Direct Mail
PO Box 12944
Fresno
CA 93779–2944
USA
Telephone: (209) 237–3801

1233. Detroit Free Press
321 W Lafayette Boulevard
Detroit
MI 48231
USA
Telephone: (313) 222–6400

1234. Deutsche Automobil Treuhand GmbH
Mr Jülich (Sales Manager)
Wollgrasweg 43
D-7000 Stuttgart 70
Germany
Telephone: 0711 45030
Fax: 0711 451–340
Telex/E-mail: 723722 D

1235. Deutsche Bank AG
Volkswirtschaftliche Abteilung
Bockenheimer Landstraße 42
D-6000 Frankfurt am Main 1
Germany
Telephone: 069 7150–3144
Fax: 069 7150–422
Telex/E-mail: 417300 FM D

1237. Deutsche Bibelgesellschaft
Roland Kober (Product Manager Software)
Balinger Stra[e1]e 31
D-7000 Stuttgart 80
Germany
Telephone: 711 71810
Fax: 711 7181 126
Telex/E-mail: 7255299 BIBL D

1238. Deutsche Bibliothek
Werner Stephan (Leader Central Bibliographic Services Department)
Zeppelinallee 4–8
D-6000 Frankfurt am Main 1
Germany
Telephone: 069 75661
Fax: 069 7566–476
Telex/E-mail: 416643 DEU BI D

1239. Deutsche Bundesbank
Postfach 100602
D-6000 Frankfurt am Main 1
Germany
Telephone: 069 1581
Telex/E-mail: 41443 BBKF D

1240. Deutsche Bundespost
General Directorate
Hr Michels, 433–2, Executive Officer
PO Box 30001
D-5300 Bonn I
Germany
Telephone: 228 14 70 13
Fax: 228 14 70 16

1241. Deutsche Messe AG
Messegelande
3000 Hannover 82
Germany
Telephone: +49 511 89–0
Fax: +49 511 8932626

1242. Deutsche Postreklame GmbH
Jutta Hegwein (Verkaufsleiterin)
Wiesenhüttenstraße 18
Postfach 16 02 11
6000 Frankfurt am Main 1
Germany
Telephone: 069 26820;
069 2682–464

1243. Deutsche Presse-Agentur GmbH
Mittelweg 38
D-2000 Hamburg 13
Germany
Telephone: 040 411–3327
Telex/E-mail: 212995 DPA D

1244. Deutscher Adressbuch-Verlag für Wirtschaft und Verkehr GmbH
Mr. Rinas
Holzhofallee 38
Postfach 11 04 52
D-6100 Darmstadt 1
Germany
Telephone: 6151 3910
Fax: 6151 391–200
Telex/E-mail: 419548 DAV D

1245. Deutscher Fachverlag
Mainzer Landstraße 251
D-6000 Frankfurt am Main 1
Germany
Telephone: 069 7595–2101
Fax: 069 7595–2100
Telex/E-mail: 411862 D

1246. Deutscher Sparkassenverlag GmbH
Am Wallgraben 115
Postfach 800330
D-7000 Stuttgart 80
Germany
Telephone: 0711 7871–1618
Fax: 0771 7871–1635
Telex/E-mail: 7255530 D

1247. Deutscher Wetterdienst
135 Frankfurterstrasse
6050 Offenbach
Germany
Telephone: 49 (69) 80 62 – 0

1248. Deutsches Bibliotheksinstitut
Frau Traute Braun
Bundesallee 184–185
D-1000 Berlin 31
Germany
Telephone: 030–85050
Telex/E-mail: 2627308512 DBI D
NUA: 26245300040020

1249. Deutsches Institut für Normung eV
Deutsches Informationszentrum für
Technische Regeln
Andrea Hillers
Burggrafenstraße 6
Postfach 1107
D-1000 Berlin 30
Germany
Telephone: 030 260–1260;
030 26011
Fax: 030 260–1231;
030 262–8125
Telex/E-mail: 185269 DITR D

1250. Deutsches Krankenhausinstitut e.V.
Tersteegenstrasse 9
4000 Dusseldorf 30
Germany
Telephone: 49 (211) 45 48 80
Fax: 49 (211) 45 48 850

1251. Deutsches Kunststoff-Institut
Schloßgartenstraße 6
D-6100 Darmstadt
Germany
Telephone: 06151 16 21 06
Fax: 06151 29 28 55

1252. Deutsches Patentamt
Zweibrückenstraße 12
D-8000 Munich 2
Germany
Telephone: 089 21950
Fax: 089 2195–2221
Telex/E-mail: 523534 BPBM D

1253. Dewey Publications Inc
PO Box 3423
Arlington
VA 22203
USA
Telephone: (703) 522–4761

1254. DeWitt & Company Inc
16800 Greenspoint Park
North Atrium
Suite 120
Houston
TX 77060–2386
Telephone: (713) 875–5525
Telex/E-mail: 762854 HOU

1255. DGM Associates
330 Washington Street
Suite 700
PO Box 10639
Marina Del Rey
CA 90292
USA
Telephone: (213) 578–1428

1256. DIAL/DATA
A division of Track Data Corporation
61 Broadway
New York
NY 10006
USA
Telephone: (718) 522–6886

1257. Dialcom Inc
6120 Executive Blvd
Rockville
MD 20852
USA
Telephone: (301) 881–9020;
(800) 435–7342

1258. DIALOG Information Services Europe Ltd
PO Box 188
Oxford
OX1 5AX
UK
Telephone: 0865 730–275
Fax: 0865 736–354

1259. DIALOG Information Services Inc
3460 Hillview Avenue
Palo Alto
CA 94304–1396
USA
Telephone: (415) 858–3785;
(415) 858–4240;
(800) 334–2564;
(800) 387–2689 (in Canada)
Fax: (415) 858–7069
Telex/E-mail: DIALMAIL: MARKETING
334499 DIALOG

1260. Diamond Research Corporation
9850 Old Creek Road
Ventura
CA 93001
USA
Telephone: (805) 649–2209
Fax: (805) 649–1700

1261. Diamond Research Corporation
ATR Division
6256 Pleasant Valley Road
PO Box 80
El Dorado
CA 95623
USA
Telephone: (916) 626–4104
Fax: (916) 626–5560

1262. Diana M. Priestly Law Library
University of Victoria
PO Box 2300
Victoria
British Columbia
V8W 3B1
Canada
Telephone: (604) 721–8566

1263. Dictionnaires Le Robert
Mme Zimmerman
107 avenue Parmentier
75011 Paris
France
Telephone: 1 43 57 73 13
Fax: 1 43 57 36 11

1264. DIDA*El srl
Cristina Chizzoni (Project Manager)
Via Lamarmora 3
20122 Milan
Italy
Telephone: 2 5518–1738;
2 5518–0042
Fax: 2 5518–1751

1265. Diffusione Edizioni Anglo Americane
Bianca Ligi (Manager New Media)
Via Lima 28
00198 Rome
Italy
Telephone: 6 855–1441
Fax: 6 854–3228

1266. Digidesign Inc
Toby Richards (Product Manager)
1360 Willow Road
Suite 101
Menlo Park
CA 94025
USA
Telephone: (415) 688–0600
Fax: (415) 327–0777

1267. Digipress Inc
Denis F Oudard (Director of Marketing
    USA/Canada)
2016 Bainbridge Row Drive
Louisville
KY 40206
USA
Telephone: (502) 895–0565
Fax: (502) 893–9589

1268. Digipress SA
J Mathews (Marketing Director)
18 rue Bailey
14050 Caen Cedex
France
Telephone: 31 47 25 00
Fax: 31 47 25 01

1269. Digita International Ltd
J Rihll (Director)
Black Horse House
Exmouth
Devon
EX8 1JL
UK
Telephone: 0395 270–273
Fax: 0395 268–893

1270. Digital Data Library
Joe Grajewski (Vice President); Craig
    Keilman (Sales Manager); Linda
De Mayo (Director Library Services)
12379 Sunrise Valley Drive
Reston
VA 22091
USA
Telephone: (703) 758–7500
Fax: (703) 648–0882

1271. Digital Diagnostics Inc
601 University Avenue
Suite 255
Sacramento
CA 95825
USA
Telephone: (916) 921–6629;
            (800) 826–5595

**1272. Digital Directory Assistance
    Inc**
Claude Schoch
5161 River Road
Building 6
Bethesda
MD 20816
USA
Telephone: (301) 657–8548
Fax: (301) 652–7810

**1273. Digital Equipment Corporation
    Users' Group**
333 South Street
SHR1–4/D31
Shrewsbury
MA 01545–4195
USA
Telephone: (508) 841–3564
Fax: (508) 841 3357

1274. Digital Equipment Corporation
John Zocchi (Product Manager)
334 South Street
Shrewsbury
MA 01545
USA
Telephone: (508) 841–6625
Fax: (508) 841–6100

1275. Digital Publications Inc
PO Box 1409
Norcross
GA 30091
USA
Telephone: (404) 441–4973

1276. Digital Research Inc
70 Garden Court
Monterey
CA 93940
USA
Telephone: (408) 649–3896

1277. Digital Vision International Ltd
Isobel Pring
Suite 202
Blackfriars Foundry
156 Blackfriars Road
London
SE1 8EN
UK
Telephone: 071 721–7053
Fax: 071 721–7054

1278. Digitized Information
5–26–301 Yoyogi
Shibuya-ku
Tokyo 151
Japan
Telephone: 03 3466–0141
Fax: 03 3468–9229
Telex/E-mail: 28899 SIBINBTH J

1279. DIMDI
(Deutsches Institut für Medizinische
    Dokumentation und Information)
Mr Kurzwelly; Dr Ursula Kueppers
Weißhausstraße 27
Postfach 420580
D-5000 Cologne 41
Germany
Telephone: 0221 47241
Fax: 0221 411–429
Telex/E-mail: 8881364 DIM D
NUA: 26245221040104;
    262452210140901

1280. Dimensions
The WEFA Group
150 Monument Road
Bala Cynwyd
PA 19004
USA
Telephone: (215) 667–6000
Fax: (215) 667–7012
Telex/E-mail: 831609

1281. Diogenes
12315 Wilkins Avenue
Rockville
MD 20852–1877
USA
Telephone: (301) 881–2100
Fax: (301) 881–0415

1282. Dioikema
Palazzo Isolani
Via S. Stefano 16
40125 Bologna
Italy
Telephone: 51 239 728

**1283. Direction Generale des
    Douanes et Droits Indirects**
Bureau C1
8 Rue de la Tour des Dames
75436 Paris Cedex 09
France
Telephone: 33 (1) 42 80 67 22
Telex/E-mail: 660168 DOUAN AA ET B
F

**1284. Direction National des
    Statistiques du Commerce
    Exterieur**
Centre des Pins
161 chemin de Lestang
F-31057 Toulouse Cedex
France
Telephone: 61 41 11 78

**1285. Direction Regionale Jeunesse
    et Sports**
51 rue du Pensionnat
F-69422 Lyon Cedex 03
France
Telephone: 078 60 70 91

**1286. Directories Publishing
    Company Inc**
PO Box 1824
Clemson
SC 29633
USA
Telephone: (803) 646–7840
Fax: (803) 646–9938

1287. DirekTek
London
UK
Telephone: 081 547–0825

**1288. disABILITIES Information
    Services**
PO Box 1086
Arleta
CA 91334
USA
Telephone: (818) 899–1598
Fax: (818) 367–1825
Telex/E-mail: Mari.S (GEnie)

1289. Discimagery
Robert Lehnhardt
18 E 16th Street
4th Floor
New York
NY 10003
USA
Telephone: (212) 675–8500
Fax: (212) 691–7873

**1290. Discis Knowledge Research
    Inc**
Fiona Ferguson (Marketing Coordinator)
45 Sheppard Avenue E
Suite 410
North York
ON M2N 5W9
Canada
Telephone: (800) 567–4321;
            (416) 250–6537
Fax: (416) 250–6540

1291. Disclosure Inc
Doug Schiffman (Vice President
    Marketing and Sales)
5161 River Road
Bethesda
MD 20816
USA
Telephone: (301) 951–1300;
            (800) 843–7747
Fax: (301) 657–1962
Telex/E-mail: 898452

1292. Disclosure Ltd
Guy Maguire (Sales Manager)
London Demand Centre
26–31 Whiskin Street
London
EC1R 0BP
UK
Telephone: 071 278–7848
Fax: 071 278–3898

**1293. Discount Corporation of New
    York**
58 Pine Street
New York
NY 10005
USA
Telephone: (212) 248–8900

1294. Discovery Systems
7001 Discovery Boulevard
Dublin
OH 43017
USA
Telephone: (614) 761–2000
Fax: (614) 761 4258

1295. Disctronics Manufacturing
(UK) Ltd
D Williamson (Plant Manager)
Southwater Business Park
Worthing Road
Southwater
West Sussex
RH1 7YT
UK
Telephone: 0403 732–302
Fax: 0403 732–313

1296. DISKROM Australia
David Eagle (Disc Publishing Manager)
Level 6
2 Bligh Street
Sydney
NSW 2000
Australia
Telephone: 2 223–5911
Fax: 2 223–5174

1297. Dispatch Printing Company,
The
34 S 3rd Street
Columbus
OH 43216
USA
Telephone: (614) 461–5000

1298. Distribuciones de La Ley S.A.
Carlos M. Oliva-Velez Remorino
C.I.F. A08627333
Registro Mercantil de Barcelona
Barcelona
Spain

1299. Distribution Sciences Inc
1700 Higgins Road
Suite 280
Des Plaines
IL 60018
USA
Telephone: (708) 699–6620

1300. Distributor Concepts
PO Box 1508
2460 S Industrial Highway
Ann Arbor
MI 48106
USA
Telephone: (313) 663–4214

1301. Dittler Airline Data Systems
3915 Old Mundy Mill Road
Oakwood
GA 30566
USA
Telephone: (404) 535–2218

1302. Divers & Associates Ltd
1624 Laukahi Street
Honolulu
HI 96821
USA
Telephone: (808) 373–2674
Telex/E-mail: 76703,4377
(CompuServe)

1303. Djanogly City Technology
College
Library and Information Services
Nigel Akers (Director Library and
    Information Services)
Sherwood Rise
Nottingham Road
Nottingham
NG7 7AR
UK
Telephone: 0602 424–422
Fax: 0602 424–034

1304. DNASTAR Inc
Sandra M Maples (Sales Manager)
1228 S Park Street
Madison
WI 53715
USA
Telephone: (608) 258–7420
Fax: (608) 258–7439

1305. DNASTAR Ltd
Dr Patricia Hoyle
St James House
105–113 The Broadway
West Ealing
London
W13 9BL
UK
Telephone: 081 566–1200
Fax: 081 566–3377

1306. Doane Information Services
11701 Borman Drive
Suite 100
St Louis
MO 63146
USA
Telephone: (314) 569–2700

1307. Doane Marketing Research Inc
1807 Park 270 Drive
Suite 300
PO Box 46904
St Louis
MO 63146
USA
Telephone: (314) 878–7707
Telex/E-mail: 447698

1308. Doane-Western Inc
8900 Manchester Road
St Louis
MO 63144
USA
Telephone: (314) 968–1000
Telex/E-mail: 447698

1309. Doc6 SA
Isabel Ramos (Product Manager)
Tuset 21, 6è 3a
08006 Barcelona
Spain
Telephone: 34 3414–0679
Fax: 34 3201–6357

1310. Documentación de Medios SA
Lola Santos (Directora General)
Donoso Cortes 86, 1
28015 Madrid
Spain
Telephone: 1 544 64 94
Fax: 1 544 79 53

1311. Documentation Française, La
CD-ROM Enquiries
29 Quai Voltaire
75007 Paris
France
Telephone: 1 42 96 14 22
Fax: 1 42 61 37 04

1312. Documentation Française, La
Banque d'Information Politique et
    d'Actualite
Lydia Merigot (Sous-Directeur
Documentation)
8 avenue de l'Opéra
F-75001 Paris
France
Telephone: 1 42 96 14 22
Fax: 1 42 61 37 84;
    1 40 15 72 30
Telex/E-mail: 204826 DOC FRAN PARI

1313. Dokumentation Kraftfahrwesen
Ulrichstraße 14
D-7120 Bietigheim-Bissingen
Germany
Telephone: 07142 54011
Fax: 07142 65898

1314. Dokumentations- und
Informationsgesellschaft für
Wirtschaft und Touristik mbH
Langesstraße 94
D-7570 Baden-Baden
Germany
Telephone: 07221 83320

1315. Domark Software Ltd
Russell Ferrier (CD-ROM Product
    Manager)
Ferry House
51–57 Lacy Road
Putney
London
SW15 1PR
UK
Telephone: 081 780–2222
Fax: 081 780–1540

1316. Dominion Software & Design,
Inc
3328 Oakshade Court
Fairfax
VA 22033
USA

1317. Domstolsverket
551 81 Joen Koeping
Sweden
Telephone: 46 (36) 16 94 60

1318. Donaldson, Lufkin & Jenrette
Pershing Division
140 Broadway
New York
NY 10005
USA
Telephone: (212) 504–3000

1319. Donnelley Marketing
Information Services
Chris Cordua (Director of Marketing)
70 Seaview Avenue
PO Box 10250
Stamford
CT 06904
USA
Telephone: (203) 353–7404;
    (203) 353–7595
Fax: (203) 353–7380;
    (203) 353–7291

1320. Donoghue Organization
360 Woodland Street
Holliston
MA 01746
USA
Telephone: (508) 429–5930;
    (800) 343–5413

1321. Donovan Data Systems
Berger House
7 Farm Street
London
W1X 7RB
UK
Telephone: 071 629–7654
Fax: 071 493–0239

1322. Donovan Publishing
2808 Lafayette Avenue
Newport Beach
CA 92663
USA
Telephone: (714) 723–5031
Fax: (714) 723–4011

1323. Dorlig Kindersley Multimedia
Ltd
Alan Buckingham (Managing Director)
36–38 West Street
London
WC2H 9NA
UK
Telephone: 071 836–5411
Fax: 071 379–0057

1324. Douglas R Pratt
10903 Harpers Square Court
Reston
VA 22091
USA
Telephone: (703) 620–2249
Fax: (703) 860–8638
Telex/E-mail: 76703,3041
(CompuServe)

1325. Dover Publications Inc
Clarence Stroubridge
31 E 2nd Street
Mineola
NY 11501
USA
Telephone: (516) 294–4000
Fax: (516) 742–5049

1326. Dow Jones & Company Inc
PO Box 300
Princeton
NJ 08543–0300
USA
Telephone: (609) 520–4000

1327. DR Bolagen
PO Box 1522
S-171 29 Solna
Sweden
Telephone: 08 735–5320
Telex/E-mail: 13704 ADRESS S

1328. Dr Dean Linscott
40 Glen Drive
Mill Valley
CA 94941
USA
Telephone: (415) 383–2666

1329. Dr Dvorkovitz & Associates
PO Box 1748
Ormond Beach
FL 32074
USA
Telephone: (904) 677–7033
Fax: (904) 677–7113

1330. Dr Richard J Roberts
Cold Spring Harbor Laboratory
Box 100
Cold Spring Harbor
NY 11724
USA
Telephone: (516) 367–8461
Telex/E-mail: ROBERTS CSHL.ORG
(Internet)

1331. Dr T's Music Software Inc
Steve Thomas (Marketing Coordinator);
   Jeff Pucci (Director Marketing)
100 Crescent Road
Needham
MA 02194
USA
Telephone: (617) 455–1454
Fax: (617) 455–1460

1332. Dr Wolfram Westmeier
Gesellschaft für Kernspektrometrie mbH
Moeliner Weg 32
3557 Ebsdorfergrund-Moelln
Germany

1333. Drennan Econometric
Forecasting Service
20 Polhemus Place
Brooklyn
NY 11215
USA
Telephone: (718) 783–4049

1334. Dresdner Bank AG
Economic Research Department
Postfach 110661
D-6000 Frankfurt am Main 1
Germany

1335. Drexel, Burnham, Lambert Inc
60 Broad Street
New York
NY 10004
USA
Telephone: (212) 480–6281

1336. DRI Europe Ltd
30 Old Queen Street
St James's Park
London
SW1H 9HP
UK
Telephone: 071 222–9571

1337. DRI/McGraw-Hill
Data Products Division
24 Hartwell Avenue
Lexington
MA 02173
USA
Telephone: (617) 863–5100
Telex/E-mail: 440480 DRI WASHDC

1338. DS Production Limited
St. George's Work
Silver Street
Trowbridge
Wiltshire
BA14 8AA
UK
Telephone: 44 (1) 950–5503

1339. DSI Data Service & Information
Konrad Wilms (General Manager);
   Dr Wilhelm Hennerkes (General
   Manager)
Orsoyerstra[e1]e 4
PO Box 1127
4134 Rheinberg 1
Germany
Telephone: 2843–3220
Fax: 2843–3230

1340. DTB Library
Anker Engelunds Vej 1
DK-2800 Lyngby
Denmark

1341. Duff & Phelps Inc
55 E Monroe Street
Suite 4000
Chicago
IL 60603
USA
Telephone: (312) 263–2610

1342. Dun & Bradstreet (Australia)
Pty Ltd
Chris Pellegrinetti (General Manager)
479 St Kilda Road
Melbourne
VIC 3004
Australia
Telephone: 3 828–3401
Fax: 3 828–3271

1343. Dun & Bradstreet AG
Schoeneggstraße 5
8026 Zurich
Switzerland
Telephone: 01 241 02 30
Fax: 01 242 53 07
Telex/E-mail: 812193 CH

1344. Dun & Bradstreet Canada Ltd
David LaMarche (National Marketing
   Manager)
9th Floor
5770 Hurontario Street
Mississauga
ON L5R 3G5
Canada
Telephone: (416) 568–6151
Fax: (416) 568–6197

1345. Dun & Bradstreet Corporation
1 Diamond Hill Road
Murray Hill
NJ 07974–0027
USA
Telephone: (201) 665–5000;
          (201) 665–5036;
          (800) 362–3425

1346. Dun & Bradstreet Europe Ltd
Nigel Dickinson (Marketing Manager)
Holmers Farm Way
High Wycombe
Buckinghamshire
HP12 4UL
UK
Telephone: 0494 422–000
Fax: 0494 422–260
Telex/E-mail: 83128

1347. Dun & Bradstreet France SA
17 avenue de Choisy
Le Palatino
F-75643 Paris Cedex 13
France
Telephone: 1 45 84 12 83
Fax: 1 45 83 92 34
Telex/E-mail: 270086 F

1348. Dun & Bradstreet International
International Marketing Services
1 World Trade Center
Suite 9069
New York
Telephone: (212) 524–8240;
          (800) 223–1026

1349. Dun & Bradstreet Publications
Corporation
711 3rd Avenue
New York
NY 10022
USA
Telephone: (212) 867–4361

1350. Dun & Bradstreet/Hyidahl
EDP Department
Egegardsvej 32–34
DK-2610 Rodovre
Denmark
Telephone: 031 709–000
Fax: 031 709–129

1351. Dun's Marketing Services
Dawn Adams (Marketing Coordinator)
3 Sylvan Way
Parsippany
NJ 07054–3896
USA
Telephone: (201) 605–6000;
       (800) 223–1026
Fax: (201) 605–6921;
    (201) 605–6911;
    (201) 605–6930

1352. Dunod
Claude H Bardot (Marketing Manager
   New Products)
15 rue Gossin
Montrouge 72543 Cedex
France
Telephone: 1 40 92 65 00
Fax: 1 40 92 65 97

1353. DuPont de Nemours & Co. Inc
E352/129
Wilmington
DE 19898
USA

1354. Dutch Broadcasting Company
Mr van den Born
Postbus 10
1200 JB Hilversum
Netherlands
Telephone: 35 773–636
Fax: 35 773–307

**1355. Dutch Centre for Public
     Libraries and Literature**
Taco Scheltemastraat 5
PO Box 93054
NL-2509 CP The Hague
Netherlands
Telephone: 070 314–1500
Fax: 070 314–1600
Telex/E-mail: 32102 NBLC NL

1356. DW Thorpe
18 Salmon Street
Port Melbourne
VIC 3207
Australia
Telephone: 03 645–1511
Fax: 03 645–3981

1357. Dwight's Energydata Inc
1633 Firman Drive
Suite 100
Richardson
TX 75081
USA
Telephone: (214) 783–8002;
      (800) 468–3381
Fax: (214) 783–0058

1358. Dynamic Graphics Inc
C J Craig (Manager Computer
   Graphics Division); Peter Force
   (Vice President Marketing)
6000 N Forest Park Drive
Peoria
IL 61614
USA
Telephone: (309) 688–8800
Fax: (309) 688–3075

1359. DynEd International
Nicholas Randall (Chief Operating
   Officer)
4370 Alpine Road
Suite 101
Portola Valley
CA 94028
USA
Telephone: (415) 578–8067
Fax: (415) 578–8069

1360. Dynix Library Systems
UK
Telephone: 0895 824091

1361. Eagle Eye Publishers Inc
Timothy D Yeaney (Vice President)
1010 N Glebe Road
Suite 890
Arlington
VA 22201
USA
Telephone: (703) 528–0680
Fax: (703) 528–2991

1362. Earth View Inc
Brian Brewer (President)
6514 18th Avenue NE
Seattle
WA 98115
USA
Telephone: (206) 527–3168
Fax: (206) 524–6803

1363. EarthInfo Inc
June Brennan (Marketing Director);
   John Edwards (President);
   Jill Lerman (Sales Manager)
5541 Central Avenue
Boulder
CO 80301
USA
Telephone: (303) 938–1788
Fax: (303) 938–8183

1364. EasyNet
Telebase Systems Inc
763 West Lancaster Avenue
Bryn Mawr
PA 19010
USA
Telephone: (215) 296–2800;
      (800) 421–7616
Fax: (215) 527–1956

1365. EBook
Jessee Albread
39315 The Zacate Avenue
Fremount
CA 94538
USA
Telephone: (415) 794–4816
Fax: (408) 262–0502

**1366. EBSCO Electronic Information
    (See EBSCO Publishing)**

1367. EBSCO Publishing
Tim Collins (General Manager)
PO Box 325
461 Boston Road
Suite E4
Topsfield
MA 01983
USA
Telephone: (508) 887–6667;
      (800) 221–1826
Fax: (508) 887–3923

1368. EBSCO Subscription Services
Keith Abbott (UK Operations Manager)
3 Tyers Gate
London
SE1 3HX
UK
Telephone: 071 357–7516
Fax: 071 357–7507

1369. EBSCO Subscription Services
3 Waters Park Drive
Suite 211
San Mateo
CA 94403–1149
USA
Telephone: (415) 572–1505;
      (800) 633–4604
Fax: (415) 572–0117

1370. ECCTIS 2000 Ltd
Virginia Isaac (Sales Coordinator); Chris
   West (Chief Executive)
Fulton House
Jessop Avenue
Cheltenham
GL50 3SH
UK
Telephone: 0242 518–724
Fax: 0242 225–914

**1371. ECHO (See Commission of the
    European Communities –
    ECHO)**

1372. Echos, Les
46 rue la Boetie
75381 Paris Cedex 08
France
Telephone: 1 49 53 65 65
Fax: 1 45 62 43 44
Telex/E-mail: 640331 F

1373. Eclat Inc
Bruce Fagin (Vice President Marketing)
7041 Koll Center Parkway
Suite 220
Pleasanton
CA 94566
USA
Telephone: (510) 484–8400
Fax: (510) 484–2210

1374. Eclat Intelligent Systems Inc
14470 Doolittle Avenue
San Leandro
CA 94577
USA
Telephone: (415) 483–2030
Fax: (415) 483–9238

**1375. ECODATA
    Wirtschaftsinformationen
    GmbH**
Oskar-Sommerstraße 15–17
D-6000 Frankfurt am Main 70
Germany
Telephone: 069 630–0050
Fax: 069 6300–0540
NUA: 2284641090814

**1376. Ecole d'Architecture de
    Paris-La Villette**
144 rue de Flandre
75019 Paris
France
Telephone: 33 (1) 42 45 74 91

**1377. Ecole Nationale des Ponts et
    Chaussees**
28 rue des Saints Peres
75007 Paris
France

**1378. Ecole Nationale Superieure des
    Mines**
60 Boulevard St. Michel
75006 Paris
France
Telephone: 33 (1) 43 29 21 05

1379. Econ Verlagsgruppe
D-4000 Dusseldorf
Germany

1380. Economic and Social Research Council
Data Archive
Wivenhoe Park
Colchester
Essex
CO4 3SQ
UK

1381. Economic Documentation and Information Centre Ltd
EDICLINE
Karl H Schumacher
19 Stratford Place
London
W1N 9AF
UK
Telephone: 071 409–8053
Fax: 071 493–8280
Telex/E-mail: EM1:EDICMAIL
026245722193202 (Euromail);
EM1:EDICMAIL 026245722140209
 (EDICMAIL)
NUA: 26245722140209

1382. Economist Intelligence Unit Ltd
40 Duke Street
London
W1A 1DW
UK
Telephone: 071 493–6711
Fax: 071 499–9767
Telex/E-mail: 266353 EIU G

1383. Economist Publications Limited
10 Rockefeller Plaza, 12th Floor
New York
NY 10020
USA
Telephone: (212) 541–5730
Telex/E-mail: 148393

1384. Economist Publications Ltd, The
25 St James Street
London
SW1A 1HG
UK
Telephone: 071 839–7000
Telex/E-mail: 919555 ECOPUB G

1385. ECRI
5200 Butler Pike
Plymouth Meeting
PA 19462
USA
Telephone: (215) 825–6000
Fax: (215) 834–1275
Telex/E-mail: 510 660 8023

1386. Edge Interactive Media
36/38 Southampton Street
Covent Gardens
London
WC2E 7HE
UK

1387. EDGE Publishing Inc
PO Box 471
40 Edinboro Court
Hackettstown
NJ 07840
USA
Telephone: (908) 852–7217
Fax: (908) 850–8304
Telex/E-mail: 150210384 MCI
Mail:EDGE

1388. Edgell Communications Inc
7500 Old Oak Boulevard
Cleveland
OH 44130
USA
Telephone: (216) 826–2839;
 (800) 225–4569
Fax: (212) 891–2726

1389. EDI Data GIE
123 rue d'Alesia
75678 Paris Cedex 14
France
Telephone: 33 (1) 45 39 22 91
Fax: (415) 644–1943
Telex/E-mail: 270737 F

1390. Ediciones Anaya
Ferrer del Rio 35
28028 Madrid
Spain
Telephone: 34 (1) 742 66 31

1391. Edilservice 3B srl
Aldo Besozzi
Via Calzecchi 6
20133 Milan
Italy
Telephone: 02 7010 03 34

1392. Editions de Cercle de la Librairie
35 rue Gregoire de Tours
F-75006 Paris
France
Telephone: 1 43 29 10 00
Fax: 1 43 29 68 95
Telex/E-mail: 270838 LIFRAN F

1393. Editions Francis LeFebvre
Nicole Chebassier
5 rue Jacques Bingen
75854 Paris Cedex 17
France
Telephone: 33 (1) 476–31260
Fax: 33 (1) 462–27264

1394. Editions Sagret
5 rue Plumet
F-75015 Paris
France
Telephone: 1 45 67 46 74
Telex/E-mail: 699559 F

1395. Editions Techniques
JP Esclavard M Griveau
123 rue d'Alésia
F-75014 Paris Cedex 14
France
Telephone: 1 45 39 22 91
Telex/E-mail: 270737 F

1396. Editoria Elettrica Editel srl
E Pentinaro (Managing Director)
Via Argelati 28
20143 Milan
Italy
Telephone: 02 5810–1951
Fax: 02 8940–5630

1397. Editorial Aranzadi SA
Pedra Martin de Hijas (EDP Manager)
Ctra Aoiz, KM10
31486 Elcano (Navarra)
Spain
Telephone: 048 33 14 11
Fax: 048 33 18 60

1398. Editorial Marin
Manuel Marin
Paseo de Gracia 49.1.1
08007 Barcelona
Spain
Telephone: 34 (3) 215 7641
Fax: 34 (3) 215 7148

1399. Editors Only
PO Box 175
Litchfield
CT 06759
USA
Telephone: (203) 283–0769
Telex/E-mail: 208–8305 (MCI Mail)

1400. Editrice Bibliografica srl
Viale Vittorio Veneto 24
I-20124 Milan
Italy
Telephone: 02 659 79 50;
 02 659 72 46
Fax: 02 65 46 24

1401. Editrice Euroitalia srl
Grassi Paolo (Secretary) Albo Rosy
 (Secretary)
Via XX Settembre 37/12
16121 Genoa
Italy
Telephone: 010 593–519;
 010 581–245
Fax: 010 542–320

1402. Edmonton Journal, The
10006 101st Street
Edmonton
AB T5J 2S6
Canada
Telephone: (403) 429–5100

1403. Edmonton Public Library
AJ Davis (Head of Technical Services)
7 Sir Winston Churchill Square
Edmonton
AB T5J 2V4
Canada
Telephone: (403) 423–2331
Fax: (403) 429–9825

1404. Education Group Inc
One Hinde Street
London
W1M 5RH
UK
Telephone: 071 495–8033
Fax: 071 495–5678

1405. Education Systems Corporation
6170 Cornerstone Court East
Suite 300
San Diego
CA 92121–3710
USA
Telephone: (619) 587–0087

1406. Educational Software for Microcomputers
Ysanna Heald (Divisional Director)
Abbeygate House
East Road
Cambridge
CB1 1DB
UK
Telephone: 0223 65445
Fax: 0223 460557

1407. Educational Testing Service
Carter Road
Princeton
NJ 08541
USA
Telephone: (609) 734–5737
Fax: (609) 734–5410

1408. Educators Forum
2840 Medary Avenue
Columbus
OH 43202
USA
Telephone: (614) 262–2730

1409. EduCorp USA
Vache Guzel
531 Stevens Avenue
Suite B
Solana Beach
CA 92075
USA
Telephone: (619) 259–0255;
      (800) 843–9497
Fax: (619) 259–0367

1410. Educorp
Scott Papathakis (Technical Support
   Department)
7434 Trade Street
San Diego
CA 92121
USA
Telephone: (619) 536–9999;
      (800) 843–9497
Fax: (619) 536–2345

1411. Eduvision
Sebastian Levy (President Directory
   General)
31 cours des Juilliottes
94702 Maisons Alfort Cedex
France
Telephone: 1 43 96 75 00
Fax: 1 43 96 75 03

1412. EDV-Fachredaktion Kellerbach
Germany
Telephone: +49 2204 60284

1413. EG&G Idaho
Idaho National Engineering Laboratory
PO Box 1625
Idaho Falls
ID 83415
USA
Telephone: (208) 526–0757

1414. EIC Intelligence Inc
48 West 38th Street
New York
NY 10018
USA
Telephone: (212) 944–8500

1415. Eidetic Knowledge Systems
Elsevier Publishing Group
PO Box 211
1000 AE Amsterdam
Netherlands
Telephone: 20580 3911

1416. Eidetic Knowledge Systems
Alexander M. Grimwade
50 Valley Stream Parkway
Malvern
PA 19355
USA
Telephone: (215) 889–9780
Fax: (215) 889–9788

1417. Eikon S p a
9 Lungotevere Raffaello Sanzio
Rome 00153
Italy
Telephone: 16 5809920

1418. Einstein
Learning Link National Consortium
356 West 58th Street
New York
NY 10019
USA
Telephone: (212) 560–6868

1419. ELC International
Sinclair House
The Avenue
West Ealing
London
W13 8NT
UK
Telephone: 081 998–8812
Fax: 081 998–8318
Telex/E-mail: 938283 G

**1420. Electric Power Research
    Institute**
Technical Information Division
PO Box 10412
3412 Hillview Avenue
Palo Alto
CA 94303
USA
Telephone: (415) 855–2411;
      (415) 855–2343
Fax: (415) 855–2954;
      (415) 856–6621
Telex/E-mail: 910 373 1163 12301
(DIALMAIL)

1421. Electricite de France
Service Informatique et Mathematiques
   Appliquees
Departement Systems d'Information et
   de Documentation
1 avenue du General de Gaulle
F-92141 Clamart Cedex
France
Telephone: 1 47 65 43 21
Fax: 1 47 65 31 24
Telex/E-mail: 204347 EDFNORM F

1422. Electromap Inc
Richard Smith; Joan Smith; Greg
   Mitchell
700 W 20th Street
Fayetteville
AR 72701
USA
Telephone: (501) 442–2309
Fax: (501) 575–7446

**1423. Electronet Information
    Systems Inc**
Electronet Advanced Publishing
   Services
1605 King Street
Suite 200
Alexandria
VA 22314
USA
Telephone: (703) 739–5510
Telex/E-mail: L.Freedman (Electronet)

1424. Electronic Data Expertise
Ouwehand Consultancy
Crailoseweg 26
1272 EV Huizen
Netherlands
Telephone: +31 2152–68973
Fax: +31 2152 40999

1425. Electronic Data Systems (EDS)
3700 Industry Ave.
Lakewood
CA 90714–6050
USA
Telephone: (213) 595–4756

1426. Electronic Data Systems (EDS)
13600 EDS Drive
Herndon
VA 22071
USA
Telephone: 703–742–2000
Fax: 703–742–1239

1427. Electronic Editions
999 West Riverside
Spokane
WA 99210
USA
Telephone: (509) 459–5060;
      (509) 459–5065

**1428. Electronic Information
    Exchange System**
Computerized Conferencing and
   Communications Center
New Jersey Institute of Technology
Newark
NJ 07102
USA
Telephone: (201) 596–3437
Fax: (201) 596–0137

**1429. Electronic Information
    Services Company**
Tom Hamilton
Premier House
10 Greycoat Place
London
SW1P 1SB
UK
Telephone: 071 222–8866

**1430. Electronic Networking
    Association**
Executive Technology Associates Inc
2744 Washington Street
Allentown
PA 18104–4225
USA
Telephone: (215) 821–7777

1431. Electronic Publications Service
Organisation for Economic Cooperation
   and Development (OECD)
2 rue Andre Pascal
F-75775 Paris Cedex 16
France
Telephone: 1 52 48 712

1432. Electronic Text Corporation
778 South 400 East
Orem
UT 84058
USA
Telephone: (801) 226–0616;
      (800) 234–0546
Fax: (801) 226–4278

1433. Elektroson bv
Myrna Sommer (Marketing & Sales)
Huis Groot Velder
Velderseweg 25
5298 LE Liempde
Netherlands
Telephone: 04113 3021
Fax: 04113 2763

1434. Elimia Marc
DP Mgez
TEI of Kozani
50100 Kozani
Greece
Telephone: 30 (461) 39682

1435. Eliot Stein
PO Box 1945
Burbank
CA 91507
USA
Telephone: (818) 843–2837

1436. Elk Horn Publishing
PO Box 126
Aromas
CA 95004
USA
Telephone: (408) 726–3148

1437. Ellen G White Estate
CD-ROM Enquiries
12501 Old Columbia Pike
Silver Spring
MD 20904
USA
Telephone: (301) 680–6552

1438. Ellis Enterprises Inc
Bob Hall (Vice President, CD-ROM
  Technology)
4205 McAuley Boulevard
Suite 385
Oklahoma City
OK 73120
USA
Telephone: (405) 729–0273;
             (800) 729–9500
Fax: (405) 751–5168

**1439. Elsevier Advanced Technology
  Publications**
Mayfield House
256 Banbury Road
Oxford
OX2 7DH
UK
Telephone: 0865 512–242
Fax: 0865 516–120

1440. Elsevier Publishing Group
Postbus 5521
NL-1000 AN Amsterdam
Netherlands
Telephone: 020 586–2751
Fax: 020 586–2850
Telex/E-mail: 10704 ESPOM NL

1441. Elsevier Science Publishers bv
Hans Hoogeweegen (Product Manager)
Molenwerf 1
1014 AG Amsterdam
Netherlands
Telephone: 20 580–3911
Fax: 20 580–3222
Telex/E-mail: 18582 ESPA NL

**1442. Elsevier Science Publishers
  Inc**
North American Database Office
Linda Sacks (Sales Manager)
655 Avenue of the Americas
New York
NY 10010
USA
Telephone: (212) 633–3971;
             (212) 989–5800
Fax: (212) 633–3913

1443. Elsevier/Geo Abstracts
Regency House
34 Duke Street
Norwich
Norfolk
NR3 3AP
UK
Telephone: 0603 626327
Fax: 0603 667934
Telex/E-mail: 975247 CHACOM G
  10079: IRC013 (Dialcom); 14281
  (DIALMAIL)

**1444. Emerging Technology
  Applications**
Colleen Hurley
111 Speen Street
Framingham
Massachusetts 01701–9107
USA
Telephone: (508) 879–0006
Fax: (508) 820–4396

1445. EMI AEROCORP Inc
7 N Brentwood Boulevard
St Louis
MO 63105
USA
Telephone: (314) 727–9600
Telex/E-mail: 70007,345 (CompuServe
Information Service)

**1446. Employee Benefit Research
  Institute**
2121 K Street NW
Suite 600
Washington
DC 20037
USA
Telephone: (202) 775–6349
Fax: (202) 775–6312
Telex/E-mail: EBR075 (EBRI.NET)
IP064A (HRIN)

**1447. Employment Management
  Association**
4101 Lake Boone Trail
Suite 201
Raleigh
NC 27607
USA
Telephone: (919) 828–6614
Fax: (919) 787–4916

**1448. Employment Transition
  Services/ETS Inc**
1255 Drummers Lane, Suite 306
Wayne
PA 19087
USA
Telephone: (215) 687–3900;
             (800) 341–9850
Fax: (215) 687–6814

**1449. Empresa Provincial de
  Informatica de Madrid**
Avenida de los Madronos 29
28043 Madrid
Spain
Telephone: 01 200 81 40

1450. EMS Professional Software
4505 Buckhurst Court
Olney
MD 20832
USA
Telephone: (301) 924–3594
Fax: (301) 963–2708

**1451. Encyclopaedia Britannica
  Educational Corporation**
310 South Michigan Avenue
Chicago
Illinois 60604
USA
Telephone: (312) 347–7128;
             (800) 554–9862

**1452. Energy, Mines and Resources
  Canada**
Peter Turner (Databases and
Information Services)
615 Booth Street
Room 408
Ottawa
ON K1A 0E4
Canada
Telephone: (613) 995–0314
Fax: (613) 991–6001

**1453. Engineering Bulletin Board
  System**
14825 Begonias Lane
Canyon Country
CA 91351
USA
Telephone: (805) 252–2177

1454. Engineering Information Inc
Michael Gannon (Sales Director)
345 E 47th Street
New York
NY 10017–2330
USA
Telephone: (212) 705–7600;
             (800) 221–1044
Fax: (212) 832–1857
Telex/E-mail: 4990438

1455. Engineering Information Inc
(Main office)
Stevens Institute of Technology campus
Castle Point
Hoboken
New Jersey
USA

1456. ENIDATA SpA
Documentazione
Via Medici del Vascello 26
I-20138 Milan
Italy
Telephone: 02 52 02 94 53
Fax: 02 52 02 92 57
Telex/E-mail: 310246 ENI I

**1457. Ente Nazionale per l'Energia
  Elettrica**
Direzione Studi e Ricerche
Via Dalmazia 15
I-00198 Rome
Italy
Telephone: (06) 85 09 27 35
Fax: 06 85 09 25 60
Telex/E-mail: 610518 I

1458. ENTEL SA
Paseo de la Castellana 141
28046 Madrid
Spain
Telephone: 01 450 90 96
Fax: 01 279 10 74
Telex/E-mail: 22019 E

**1459. Entertainment Systems
  International**
183 N Martel Avenue
Suite 205
Los Angeles
CA 90036
USA
Telephone: (213) 937–0347

1460. Environment Canada
Departmental Library
Ottawa
ON K1A 0H3
Canada
Telephone: (819) 997–1767
Fax: (819) 997–1929
Telex/E-mail: 0533799 ILL.OOFF
(Envoy 100)

1461. Environment Canada
National Environmental Emergency
  Centre
Ottawa
ON K1A 0H3
Canada
Telephone: (819) 997–3742

1462. Environment Canada
New Substances Division, Commercial
  Chemicals Branch
Ottawa
ON K1A 0H3
Canada
Telephone: (819) 953–7155
Fax: (819) 953–7155

1463. Environment Canada
Inland Waters Directorate, WATDOC
Ottawa
ON K1A 0H3
Canada
Telephone: (819) 997–3742

**1464. Environment Compliance
Reporter Inc**
3154B College Drive
Suite 522
Baton Rouge
LA 70808
USA
Telephone: (800) 729–1964

1465. Environmental Law Institute
1616 P Street NW
Suite 200
Washington
DC 20036
USA
Telephone: (202) 328–5150
Fax: (202) 328–5002

**1466. Environmental Resources
Management Inc (ERM)**
Computer Services
George T. Esey
855 Springdale Drive
Exton
PA 19341
USA
Telephone: (800) 544–3118;
(215) 524–3600

**1467. Environmental Systems
Research Institute Inc**
Duane Niemeyer (DCW Project
Manager)
380 New York Street
Redlands
CA 92373
USA
Telephone: (714) 793–2853
Fax: (714) 793–5953

1468. Environnement Quebec
Quebec-New York State Clearing
House on Acid Rain
Centre de Documentation
3900 Rue Marly, 6E-57
Sainte-Foy
PQ 61X 4E4
Canada
Telephone: (418) 643–5363
Telex/E-mail: 05131629

1469. EOLAS
Glasnevin
Dublin 9
Eire
Telephone: 01 370–101
Fax: 01 379–620
Telex/E-mail: 32501 OLAS EI

1470. EP DIT
Direction de l'Informatique: Infocentre
European Parliament
2929 Luxembourg
Luxembourg
Telephone: (352) 43004300;
(352) 43001
Fax: (352) 437009
NUA: 2704428901001

**1471. EPIC Interactive Media
Company, The**
Jim Braithwaite (Managing Director)
VPS House
22 Brighton Square
Brighton
East Sussex
BN3 1RF
UK
Telephone: 0273 728–686
Fax: 0273 821–567

1472. EPMS bv
Ellis Publications
Richard Hainebach (Managing Director)
Terhorst 19
6262 NA Banholt
Netherlands
Telephone: 04457–2275
Fax: 04457–2148

1473. EPRC Ltd
141 St James Road
Glasgow
G4 DLT
UK
Telephone: 041 552–4400
Fax: 041 552–0775
Telex/E-mail: 77472 UNSLIB G
NUA: 23424126010604

**1474. eps Bertelsmann (See also
Bertelsmann; AZ Bertelsmann)**

**1475. eps Bertelsmann Electronic
Printing Service GmbH**
Antonius Huerkamp (Manager Sales
Marketing); Dr Anette Kahre
(European Sales Manager)
Dieselstraße 66
4830 Gütersloh 108
Germany
Telephone: 5241 6010
Fax: 5241 68285

1476. EPWING Consortium
(A consortium of Fujitsu, Dai Nippon,
Iwanami Shoten, Sony, Toppan)
Japan

**1477. Equal Employment
Oppurtunity Commission**
2401 E Street, NW
Washington
DC 20507
USA
Telephone: (202) 634–6922;
(800) 872–3362

1478. Equatorial
Patrice Boursier (Scientific Manager)
Les Algoritmes-Université
Bât Aristote Parc Technologie
91194 Saint-Aubin
France
Telephone: 1 45 35 56 71
Fax: 1 45 35 64 02

**1479. Equifax National Decision
Systems**
Tom Holland (Vice President)
539 Encinitas Boulevard
Encinitas
CA 92024–9007
USA
Telephone: (619) 942–7000
Fax: (619) 944–9543

1480. ERGODATA
Prof. A. Coblentz
Universite Paris V Rene Descartes
Rue des Saints-Peres
75270 Paris Cedex 06
France
Telephone: 33 (1) 42862233
NUA: 208091000192

**1481. Erhverve- og
Selskabsstyrelsen**
Kampmannsgade 1
DK-1604 Copenhagen V
Denmark
Telephone: 033 124–280

1482. ERICA Data Center
Chuck Browne (Data Manager)
Department of Physics and Atmospheric
Science
Drexel University
Philadelphia
PA 19104
USA
Telephone: (215) 895–2786
Fax: (215) 895–4989

**1483. Erico Petroleum Information
Ltd**
Erico House
93–99 Upper Richmond Road
London
SW15 2TG
UK
Telephone: 081 789–1812

1484. ERM Computer Services
855 Springdale Drive
Exton
PA 19341
USA
Telephone: (215) 524–3600
Fax: (215) 524–4801

1485. Ernst & Young
1225 Connecticut Avenue NW
Washington
DC 20036
USA
Telephone: (202) 862–6042

**1524. ESA-IRS (see European Space
Agency Information Retrieval
Service)**

1525. ESCAPE
S Cartigny (Director); W Spapens
(Sales Manager)
Apennijnenweg 11
5022 DT Tilburg
Netherlands
Telephone: 013 371–311
Fax: 013 355–595

1526. ESMERK OY
PL 37
Ratapihantie 11
SF-00521 Helsinki
Finland
Telephone: 90 143–311
Fax: 90 147–619

1527. Espial Productions
PO Box 624
Station K
Toronto
ON M4P 2H1
Canada
Telephone: (416) 485–8063

1528. ESRC Data Archive
Economic & Social Research Council
Wivenhoe Park
Colchester
Essex
CO4 3SQ
UK

1529. Esselte Focus
Esselte Ordbok
Tomas Bjoerdorff
PO Box 30125
Nordenflychtsvagen 55
10425 Stockholm
Sweden
Telephone: 46 (8) 789 3400;
46 (8) 789 3357
Fax: 46 (8) 618 7962

1530. Esselte Online
Box 1391
S-171 27 Solna
Sweden

1531. Esselte Studium
Stefan Tiderman
Sunbybergsvagen 1
17176 Solna
Sweden
Telephone: 46 (8) 734 3000
Fax: 46 (8) 838 207

1532. ETAK Inc
Andrew Pitcair (Marketing Manager)
1430 O'Brien Drive
Menlo Park
CA 94025
USA
Telephone: (415) 328–3825
Fax: (415) 328–3148

1533. ETI SpA
Mrs Gollimo
Viale Mazzini 25
00195 Rome
Italy
Telephone: 06 321–7578
Fax: 06 321–7808

1534. EureCom Datenbank GmbH
Pia Dudenhöffer
Hochallee 40
2000 Hamburg 13
Germany
Telephone: 040 44 70 39
Fax: 040 44 70 30

1535. EUREKA Secretariat
c/o ECHO Service
BP 2373
L-1023 Luxembourg
Luxembourg
Telephone: 0352 48 80 41
Fax: 0352 48 80 40
Telex/E-mail: 2181 EUROL LU

1536. EURO DB
18 Place de l'Université
B-1348 Louvain-la-Neuve
Belgium
Telephone: 010 47 67 11

1537. Euro-CD Diffusion
2516 River Bend Drive
Louisville
KY 40206
USA
Telephone: (502) 895–0565

1538. Euro-CD Management
Christian Delacourt (Managing Director);
　Vincent Prevost (Macintosh Area)
13 Cité Voltaire
75011 Paris
France
Telephone: 1 40 09 80 30
Fax: 1 43 67 00 38

1539. Euro-Tender
Wibautstraat 135–139
1097 DN Amsterdam
Netherlands
Telephone: 31 (20) 663 09 41

1540. Eurobases (See Commission of the European Communities)

1541. Eurobrokers SARL
BP 2761
L-1027 Luxembourg
Luxembourg
Telephone: 0352 43 90 97
Fax: 0352 43 32 59

1542. Eurocentre Alexandria
Mike Carrier
101 N Union Street
Alexandria
VA 22314
USA
Telephone: (703) 684–1494
Fax: (703) 684–1495

1543. Eurocentres Learning Service
John Arnold (Head of Learning Service)
Seestraße 247
8038 Zurich
Switzerland
Telephone: 1 482 10 65
Fax: 1 482 50 54

1544. Eurocentres
Glyn Jones
56 Eccleston Square
London
SW1V 1PQ
UK
Telephone: 071 834–4155
Fax: 071 834–1866

1545. Eurokom
Computing Centre
Belfield
Dublin 4
Eire
Telephone: (1) 83 05 55
Fax: (1) 83 86 05

1546. Eurolink
Alain Ottenwaelter (Managing Director)
4 rue Ferou
75006 Paris
France
Telephone: 1 43 26 19 00
Fax: 1 46 34 71 42

1547. Euromoney Publications plc
Whitefriars House
6 Carmelite Street
London
EC4Y 0BN
UK
Telephone: 071 353–6033
Telex/E-mail: 8814985/6 EUROMON G

1548. Euromonitor Online
87–88 Turnmill Street
London
EC1M 5QU
UK
Telephone: 071 251–8024
Fax: 071 608–3149
Telex/E-mail: 21120 MONREF G

1549. Europ Export Edition GmbH
Margit C Selka (Publisher); G Kolb
　(EDP Manager)
Berliner Allee 8
PO Box 4034
D-6100 Darmstadt 1
Germany
Telephone: 06151 33411 3892 0
Fax: 06151 33164
Telex/E-mail: 419257 ABC D

1550. Europa Fachpresse Verlag
Werner Kreitz
Thomas-Dehler-Strasse 27
8000 Munchen 83
Germany
Telephone: 49 (89) 67804–255
Fax: 49 (89) 67804–108

1551. European Association for Grey Literature Exploitation
Bureau Jupiter
Postbus 90407
NL-2509 LK The Hague
Netherlands
Telephone: 070 314–0281

1552. European Association for Health Information and Libraries
Rue de la Concorde, 60
Brussels
1050 Brussels
Belgium
Telephone: +32 2 511 80 63

1553. European Brewery Convention
PO Box 510
NL-2280 BB Zoeterwoude
Netherlands
Telephone: 071 81 40 47

1554. European Business School Librarians Group
London Business School Library
Sussex Place
Regent's Park
London
NW1 4SA
UK
Telephone: 071 262–5050
Telex/E-mail: 27461 LBSKOX G

1555. European Center for Work and Society
PO Box 3073
NL-6202 Maastricht
Netherlands
Telephone: 043 216–724
Fax: 043 255–712
Telex/E-mail: 56164 EUR CW

1556. European Centre for the Development of Vocational Training
Bundesallee 22
D-1000 Berlin 15
Germany
Telephone: 030 884–120
Fax: 030 8841–2222
Telex/E-mail: 184 163

1557. European Chemical News
Quadrant House
The Quadrant
Sutton
Surrey
SM2 5AS
UK
Telephone: 44 (1) 661–8145

1558. European Commission Host Organization (See Commission of the European Communities – ECHO)

1559. European Conference of Ministers of Transport
Documentation Centre
19 Rue de Franqueville
75016 Paris Cedex 16
France
Telephone: 33 (1) 45 (313) 222–68 98

1560. European Molecular Biology Laboratory
Data Library
Peter J Stoehr Graham Cameron
Postfach 10.2209
Meyerhofstra[e1]e 1
D-6900 Heidelberg
Germany
Telephone: 06221 38 72 58
Fax: 06221 38 55 19
Telex/E-mail: DATALIB
EMBL-HEIDELBERG.DE (Internet)

1561. European Multimedia Centre
Paul Fletcher
24 Stephenson Way
London
NW1 2HD
UK
Telephone: 071 387–2233
Fax: 071 387–5373

1562. European Organization of Textile and Clothing Manufacturers
c/o SIRIO
Via Orazio, 2
Milan
Italy
Telephone: 39 (2) 882 31

1563. European Patent Office
Principal Directorate for Patent Information
F Rudolf D Dickinson (Principal Directorate Patent Information)
Erhardtstraße 27
D-8000 Munich 2
Germany
Telephone: 089 2399–2550
Fax: 089 2399–4465 089 2399–5143
Telex/E-mail: 523656 EPMU D

1564. European Space Agency-Information Retrieval Service (ESA-IRS)
George Proca; Marino Saksida (Head of Service)
ESRIN
Via Galileo Galilei
Frascati
00044 Rome
Italy
Telephone: 06 94 18 01
Fax: 06 94 18 03 61
Telex/E-mail: 610637 ESRIN I
NUA: 22226500143

1565. European Space Agency
Commercialisation Office and Contracts Department
8–10 rue Mario Nikis
F-75738 Paris Cedex 15
France
Telephone: 1 42 73 76 54 (Contracts Department);
1 42 73 71 68
(Commercialisation Office)
Telex/E-mail: 202746 ESA F

1566. European Space Agency
Earthnet Programme Office
ESRIN
Via Galileo Galilei
Frascati
I-00044 Rome
Italy
Telephone: 06 94 18 01
Fax: 06 94 18 03 61
Telex/E-mail: 610637 ESRIN I

1567. European Space Agency
IRS-Dialtech
Roy Kitley; Lesley Haji-Gholam
British Library Science Reference and Information Service
25 Southampton Buildings
Chancery Lane
London
WC2A 1AW
UK
Telephone: 071 323–7951
Fax: 071 323–7930
Telex/E-mail: 266959

1568. Européenne de Données, L'
Ms Liliane Grabinski; Mr Denis Berthault
164 ter, rue d'Aguesseau
F-92100 Boulogne-Billancourt
France
Telephone: 1 46 05 29 89;
1 46 05 29 29
Fax: 1 46 05 42 55
NUA: 208077000841; 208077040153

1569. Européenne de Données, L'
1 rue du Boccador
Paris 75008
France
Telephone: 1–47–20–88–34
Fax: 1–47–20–11–43

1570. Europress Software Ltd
Anna Donaldson
Europa House
Adlington Park
Macclesfield
SL10 4NP
UK
Telephone: 0625 859–333
Fax: 0625 879–962

1571. Eurostat (See Commission of the European Communities)

1572. Eurostudy/Stonehart Publications Ltd
Ludgate House
107 Fleet Street
London
EC4A 2AB
UK

1573. Eurosyntheses SC
128 Boulevard Lambermont
B-1030 Brussels
Belgium
Telephone: 02 242 30 07
Fax: 02 245 76 69
Telex/E-mail: 4627035 B

1574. Eurotalk Ltd
315/317 New Kings Rd
London
SW6 4RF
UK
Telephone: 071 371–7711

1575. Eutelsat
Online European Satellite Information System
Paris
France
Telephone: +33 1 4321 2338

1576. Evangelical Lutheran Church in America
8765 W Higgins Road
Chicago
IL 60631–4178
USA
Telephone: (312) 380–2700

1577. Evans Economics Inc
1660 L Street
Suite 207
Washington
DC 20036
USA
Telephone: (202) 467–4900

1578. Evans Research Corporation
2005 Sheppard Avenue East, 4th Floor
Willowdale
ON M2J 5B1
Canada
Telephone: (416) 498–6664
Fax: (416) 498–7275

1579. EventLine
PO Box 521
1000 AN Amsterdam
Netherlands
Telephone: 31 (20) 58 62 751
Fax: 31 (20) 58 62 850
Telex/E-mail: 10704 EPSOM NL

1580. Evergreen Communications Inc
301 W. Washington
Bloomington
IL 61701
USA
Telephone: (309) 829–9411

1581. EVR & Wahlings
Box 1
Danderyd 18211
18211
Sweden
Telephone: 46–8–755–2740
Fax: 46–8–753–4883

1582. EW Scripps Company
125 E Court Street
Cincinnati
OH 45202
USA
Telephone: (513) 352–2000

1583. Excerpta Informatica
Jola G.B. Prinsen
Tilburg University
Postbus 90153
5000 Le Tilburg
Netherlands
Telephone: 31 (13) 662637
Fax: 31 (13) 662996
Telex/E-mail: 52426 KUB
NUA: 14200610200

1584. Excerpta Medica Publishing Group
Hans Hoogeweegen (Product Manager)
Molenwerf 1
PO Box 1527
NL-1014 AG Amsterdam
Netherlands
Telephone: 020 580–3911
Fax: 020 580–3439;
020 580–3222
Telex/E-mail: 18582 ESPA NL 11395
(DIALMAIL)

1585. Exchange Telegraph Company Limited
Financial Services Division
10 Throgmorten Avenue
London
EC2N 2DL
UK
Telephone: 071 628–9361
Telex/E-mail: 886880 G

1586. Executive Speaker
PO Box 292437
Dayton
OH 45429
USA
Telephone: (513) 294–8493

1587. Executive Telecom System International
The Human Resource Information Network
9585 Valparaiso Court
Indianapolis
IN 46268
USA
Telephone: (317) 872–2045;
(317) 421–8884;
(800) 421–8884
Fax: (317) 872–2059

Addresses

1588. EXIS
Pauline Eldred
71–77 Leadenhall Street
London
EC3A 2PQ
UK
Telephone: 071 623–3456
Fax: 071 929–4282
Telex/E-mail: 884380 SRUK G
NUA: 23423500124

1589. ExperNet Ltd
225 W Ohio Street
Suite 325
Chicago
IL 60610
USA
Telephone: (312) 527–0470
Telex/E-mail: 44: ABA375 (Dialcom)

1590. Expert Financial Systems
Connie Brown
Ferry House
48–53 Lower Mount Street
Dublin 2
Eire
Telephone: 212 (9) 385200

1591. Expert Information Ltd
Woodside
Hinksey Hill
Oxford
OX1 5AU
UK
Telephone: 0865 730275

1592. Export Intelligence Service
Department of Trade and Industry
Lime Grove
Eastcote
Ruislip
Middlesex
HA4 8SG
UK
Telephone: 44 (1) 866–8771
Telex/E-mail: 888013 DOTEIS G

1593. Export Network Ltd
Regency House
1–4 Warwick Street
London
W1R 5WA
UK
Telephone: 071 494–4030
Fax: 071 494–1245

1594. Extel Computing Ltd
Lowndes House
1–9 City Road
London
EC1Y 1AA
UK
Telephone: 071 638–5544
Telex/E-mail: 884319 G

1595. Extel Financial Ltd
MR Levy (Business Development
    Manager Company Information)
Fitzroy House
13–17 Epworth Street
London
EC2A 4DL
UK
Telephone: 071 251–3333
Fax: 071 251–1439
Telex/E-mail: 884319 EXTELX G

**1596. Extel Statistical Services
    Limited**
37/45 Paul Street
London
EC2A 4PB
UK
Telephone: 071 253–3400
Telex/E-mail: 262687 STATS G

1597. External Affairs Canada
International Trade Commissions Group
125 Sussex Drive
Ottawa
ONC K1A 062
Canada
Telephone: (613) 996–9134

1598. Fabritius AS
Infobase Department, Fabritius Online
    Service
PO Box 1156 Sentrum
N-0107 Oslo 1
Norway
Telephone: 02 636–4000
Fax: 02 650–200
Telex/E-mail: 78137 FABRI N

**1599. FABS International Inc
    (See Foundation for Advanced
    Biblical Studies)**

**1600. Fachinformationszentrum
    (See FIZ)**

1601. FACT FINDERS
Private Bag
Manukau City
New Zealand
Telephone: 09 525–2181
Fax: 09 525–2372

1602. Facts on File Inc
Michael Goldman
460 Park Avenue S
New York
NY 10016
USA
Telephone: (212) 683–2244;
            (800) 322–8755;
            (800) 443–8323
Fax: (212) 213–4578
Telex/E-mail: 238552

1603. Facts on File Ltd
Alan Goodworth
Collins Street
Oxford
OX4 1XJ
UK
Telephone: 0865 728–399
Fax: 0865 244–839

1604. FactSet Data Systems Inc
1 Greenwich Plaza
Greenwich
CT 06830
USA
Telephone: (203) 863–1500

**1605. Faellesbankens
    Informationsservice**
Knud Larsen
Borgergade 24
1347 Koebenhavn K
Denmark
Telephone: 45 (33) 112733

**1606. Faellesudvalget for Gartneriets
    Informationstjeneste**
Grethe Bjerregaard
Lottenborgvej 21
2800 Lyngby
Denmark
Telephone: 45 (42) 886366

1607. Fairbase Database Ltd
Ihmepassage 4
Postfach 91 04 46
D-3000 Hannover 91
Germany
Telephone: 0511 44 33 30
Fax: 0511 44 27 70

1608. Fairchild Publications Inc
7 E 12th Street
New York
NY 10003
USA
Telephone: (212) 741–4000

**1609. Fairplay Information Systems
    Ltd**
PO Box 96
Coulsdon
Surrey
CR3 2TE
UK
Telephone: 081 660–2811
Fax: 081 660–2824
Telex/E-mail: 884595 G

1610. Falcon Scan Ltd
Oussama Mohtar
263 Laurier Avenue W
Ottawa
ON K1P 5J9
Canada
Telephone: (613) 236–6655
Fax: (613) 236–3348

1611. FAR/SRS INFO HB
Karlavagen 50
S-114 69 Stockholm
Sweden
Telephone: 08 667–5030
Fax: 08 665–3942

1612. Farallon Computing Inc
2000 Powell Street
Emeryville
CA 94608
USA
Telephone: (415) 597–9000;
            (415) 596–9100
Fax: (415) 596–9025

1613. Farallon Computing
Bob McNich
79 Knightsbridge
London
SW1X 7RB
UK
Telephone: 071 245–6919
Fax: 071 245–9248

1614. Faulkner Information Services
William Gaul (National Sales Manager)
114 Cooper Center
7905 Browning Road
Pennsauken
NJ 08109–4319
USA
Telephone: (609) 662–2070;
            (800) 843–0460
Fax: (609) 662–0905

1615. Faxon Company, The
Maureen Maher (Manager); Michael
    Ault (Editor)
15 Southwest Park
Westwood
MA 02090
USA
Telephone: (617) 329–3350;
            (800) 766–0039
Fax: (617) 326–5484;
    (617) 461–1862
Telex/E-mail: 6817238

1616. Faxon UK Ltd
Andrejs Alferovs (Manager)
Dormer House
15 Dormer Place
Leamington Spa
CV32 5AA
UK
Telephone: 0926 450–424
Fax: 0926 450–616

1617. Faxtel Information Systems Ltd
133 Richmond Street W
Suite 405
Toronto
ON M5H 2L3
Canada
Telephone: (416) 365–1899
Fax: (416) 364–6599

1618. Faxtex
Searchcraft Inc
Wayne
PA
USA

1619. FBR Data Base Inc
PO Box 11530
Taipei
Taiwan
Telephone: 03 326–2911
Fax: 03 326–2900
Telex/E-mail: 21496 FBR TAI

1620. FD Inc
Acquired by Information Handling
  Services
Frank Duckworth (President)
600 New Hampshire Avenue NW
Suite 355
Washington
DC 20037
USA
Telephone: (202) 337–0432
Fax: (202) 337–0457

1621. FDC Reports Inc
5550 Friendship Boulevard
Suite 1
Chevy Chase
MD 20815
USA
Telephone: (301) 657–9830
Fax: (301) 656–3094

1622. Federal Bureau of Investigation
FBI Headquarters
10th & Pennsylvania NW
Washington
DC 20535
USA
Telephone: (202) 324–5348

1623. Federal Communications Commission
Office of Congressional and Public
  Affairs
1919 M Street NW
Washington
DC 20554
USA
Telephone: (202) 254–7674

1624. Federal Election Commission
1325 K Street NW
Washington
DC 20463
USA
Telephone: (202) 523–4065

1625. Federal Employee/Retiree News Service
53 Rollingwood Court
Gulfport
MS 39503
USA

1626. Federal Filings Inc
450 5th Street NW
Suite 850 N
Washington
DC 20001
USA
Telephone: (202) 393–2098
Fax: (202) 393–5439

1627. Federal Home Loan Bank Board
320 1st Street
Washington
DC 20552
USA
Telephone: (202) 377–6000

1628. Federal Ministry for Youth, Family Affairs, Women and Health
Postfach 20 04 90
5300 Bonn 2
Germany
Telephone: 49 (228) 33 83 39

1629. Federal News Service
620 National Press Building
Washington
DC 20045
USA
Telephone: (202) 347–1400
Fax: (202) 393–4733

1630. Federation Nationale du Batiment Direction de la Recherche
Domaine de Saint-Paul
BP 1
78470 Saint-Remy-les-Chevreuse
France
Telephone: 33 (1) 30 52 92 00
Fax: 33 (1) 30 52 75 75

1631. Ferguson & Company
Simon G Davidson (Director of
  Marketing)
1667 K Street NW
Suite 640
Washington
DC 20006
USA
Telephone: (202) 659–8300
Fax: (202) 659–4192

1632. Ferntree Computer Corporation Ltd
AUSINET
Dibbie Jotkowitz
310 Ferntree Gully Road
North Clayton
VIC 3168
Australia
Telephone: 03 541–5600
Fax: 03 542–2671;
03 544–6295
Telex/E-mail: 33852 ACICS AA

1633. Fidelity Brokerage Services Inc
161 Devonshire Street
Boston
MA 02110
USA
Telephone: (617) 570–2162;
         (800) 225–5531

1634. Fidelity Investment Southwest
Canal Plaza Buildings
400 E Las Colinas Boulevard
Irving
TX 75039
USA
Telephone: (214) 830–7000;
         (800) 225–5531

1635. Fidelity Investors EXPRESS
161 Devonshire Street
Boston
MA 02110
USA
Telephone: (617) 570–2612;
         (800) 225–5531

1636. Financial Courseware Limited
Leah Kinsella (Client Liason); Padraig
  Cummins (Marketing)
48–53 Lower Mount Street
Dublin 2
Eire
Telephone: 01 602–811
Fax: 01 614–665

1637. Financial Courseware UK Ltd
Simon Bank Robert Lanigan
Hamilton House
1 Temple Avenue
London
EC4Y 0HA
UK
Telephone: 071 353–4212
Fax: 071 353–3325

1638. Financial Interstate Service Corporation
617 West Main Street
Knoxville
TN 37902
USA
Telephone: (615) 637–2035

1639. Financial Post Datagroup, The
333 King Street E
Toronto
ON M5A 4N2
Canada
Telephone: (416) 350–6440
Fax: (416) 596–6075

1640. Financial Times Business Information Ltd
102–108 Clerkenwell Road
London
EC1M 5SA
UK
Telephone: 071 251–9321
Fax: 071 251–4686
Telex/E-mail: 23700 FINBI G

1641. Financial Times Business Information
Financial Times Electronic Publishing
1 Southwark Bridge
London
SE1 9LS
UK
Telephone: 071 873–3000
Fax: 071 925–2125
Telex/E-mail: 8811506 FINFO G

1642. Financial Times of Canada
1231 Yonge Street, Suite 300
Toronto
ON M4T 2Z1
Canada
Telephone: (416) 922–1133

1643. Financial Times
25 St James's Street
London
SW1A 1HG
UK
Telephone: 071 839–7000

1644. Financial World Magazine
1450 Broadway
New York
NY 10018
USA
Telephone: (212) 869–1616

1645. Financieel-Ekonomische Tijd
Christine Copers (Information Manager)
Brouwersvliet 5/3
2000 Antwerp
Belgium
Telephone: 03 231 57 56
Fax: 03 232 88 57

1646. Financieele Dagblad BV, Het
Mr Leeuwen
Weesperstraat 85–87
PO Box 216
NL-1000 AE Amsterdam
Netherlands
Telephone: 020 55 74 300 31;
020 55 74 511
Fax: 020 55 74 200
Telex/E-mail: 14576 NL
NUA: Available on application

1647. FIND/SVP Inc
625 Avenue of the Americas
New York
NY 10011
USA
Telephone: (212) 645–4500

1648. Finland Central Medical Library
Haartmaninkatu 4
SF-00290 Helsinki
Finland
Telephone: 90 43461
Fax: 90 410–385
Telex/E-mail: 121498 LKK SF

1649. Finnish Library Bureau
Kirjastopalvely Oy
PO Box 84
SF-00211 Helsinki
Finland
Fax: 358 0 692 4797

1650. Finnish State Computer Centre
PO Box 40
SF-02101 Espoo
Finland
Telephone: 358 (0) 4571
Fax: 358 (0) 457 3620

1651. Finsbury Data Services Limited
Nicholas Paget-Brown; J. Sanders
68–74 Carter Lane
London
EC4V 5EA
UK
Telephone: 071 248–9828
Telex/E-mail: 892520
NUA: 234219200101

1652. Fire Research Station
Building Research Establishment
Borehamwood
Hertfordshire
WD6 2BL
UK
Telephone: 44 (1) 953–6177

1653. First Boston Corporation, The
55 E 52nd Street
7th Floor
New York
NY 10055
USA
Telephone: (212) 909–2000

1654. First Data Resources
Government Services Division
John Larson
10825 Old Mill Road
Omaha
NE 68154–2606
USA
Telephone: (402) 399–7317;
(800) 338–6073

1655. FIZ Chemie GmbH
Postfach 12 60 50
Steinplatz 2
D-1000 Berlin 12
Germany
Telephone: 030 31 90 030
Fax: 30 31 32 037
Telex/E-mail: 181255 FIZC D

1656. FIZ Karlsruhe
Dr B Jenschke
PO Box 2465
7500 Karlsruhe
Germany
Telephone: 07247 808–555;
07247 8080
Fax: 07247 808–666;
07247 2968
Telex/E-mail: 17724710 D

1657. FIZ Technik
Mr Reiner Pernsteiner
Ostbahnhofstraße 13
Postfach 60 05 47
D-6000 Frankfurt am Main 60
Germany
Telephone: 069 4308–0225
Fax: 069 4308–0200
Telex/E-mail: 4189459 FIZT D
NUA: 26245690010552;
22846431122014

1658. FIZ Werkstoffe
Unter den Eichen 87
D-1000 Berlin 45
Germany
Telephone: 030 83 00 01

1659. FLA Consultants
27 rue de la Vistule
F-75013 Paris
France
Telephone: 1 45 82 75 75
Fax: 1 45 82 46 04
Telex/E-mail: 205231 FLA F

1660. Flightline Electronic Publishing Inc
Now owned by Avantext
Tom Harnish (President)
274 Lancaster Avenue
Suite 204
Malvern
PA 19355
USA
Telephone: (215) 296–9205
Fax: (215) 993–8117

1661. Florida Fruit Shippers
5006 Gulfport Boulevard
Gulfport
FL 33707
USA
Telephone: (813) 323–5412
Telex/E-mail: 70007,1624
(CompuServe)

1662. Florist's Transworld Delivery
William Golden
USA
Telephone: (313) 355–9300

1663. Flysheet Information Services Inc
Peggy Shu-Te Liu (Marketing Manager)
12F-6
171 Ming-Sheng E Road, SEC 5
Taipei 105
Taiwan
Telephone: 02 766–7282;
02 767–3034
Fax: 02 766–7668

1664. FM Waves
Karen Weiss (Marketing Director)
70 Derby Alley
San Francisco
CA 94102
USA
Telephone: (415) 474–7464
Fax: (415) 474–2820

1665. Focus Research Systems
A company of the Dun & Bradstreet
Corporation
342 North Main Street
West Hartford
CT 06117
USA
Telephone: (203) 561–1047
Fax: (203) 561–1713

1666. Focus Research
10 Executive Drive
Farmington
CT 06032
USA
Telephone: (203) 676–2200;
(800) 622–3774
Fax: (203) 676–1656

1667. Focus Uppslagböker / Liber AB
Lars Axelsson
PO Box 30125
104 25 Stockholm
Sweden
Telephone: 08 789–3400
Fax: 08 618–3780

1668. FOI Services Inc
12315 Wilkins Avenue
Rockville
MD 20852–1877
USA
Telephone: (301) 881–0410
Fax: (301) 881–0415

1669. Folkstone Design Inc
Luinda Bleackley (Partner)
Box 44
552 Reed Road
Grantham's Landing
BC V0N 1X0
Canada
Telephone: (604) 886–4502
Fax: (604) 886–9060

1670. Follett Software Company
Kojo Darkwa (Market Research)
809 N Front Street
McHenry
IL 60050–5589
USA
Telephone: (815) 344–8700
Fax: (815) 344–8774

1671. Fondo de Cultura Economica
Mrs Canor
Avenida Universidad 975
Mexico DF
Mexico
Telephone: 05 524–6664
Fax: 05 534–4319

1672. FontWorks
UK
Telephone: 071 490 5390

1673. Food Chemical News Inc
1101 Pennsylvania Avenue SE
Washington
DC 20003
USA
Telephone: (202) 544–1980
Fax: (202) 546–3890

1674. Foodline
Sarah Lambie
Randalls Road
Leatherhead
Surrey
KT2Z 7RY
UK
Telephone: 44 (372) 376761
Telex/E-mail: 929846

1675. FOODS ADLIBRA Publications
9000 Plymouth Avenue N
Minneapolis
MN 55427
USA
Telephone: (612) 540–4759
Fax: (612) 540–3166

**1676. Footscray Institute of
Technology**
Library
PO Box 64
Footscray
VIC 3011
Australia
Telephone: 03 688–4413
Fax: 03 688–4801
Telex/E-mail: 36596 FITLEX AA

1677. Forbes Inc
60 5th Avenue
New York
NY 10011
USA
Telephone: (212) 620–2368

1678. Ford Investor Services Inc
Nancy Furlong
11722 Sorrento Valley Road
Suite I
San Diego
CA 92121
USA
Telephone: (619) 755–1327
Fax: (619) 455–6316

1679. Ford New Holland
500 Diller Ave.
PO Box 1895
New Holland
PA 17557
USA
Telephone: (717) 355–1965

1680. Forecast International Inc/DMS
22 Commerce Road
Newtown
CT 06470
USA
Telephone: (203) 426–0800
Fax: (203) 426–1964
Telex/E-mail: 467615

1681. Forecast Plus
DRI/McGraw-Hill
1750 K Street, NW, Suite 1060
Washington
DC 20006
USA
Telephone: (202) 862–3720
Telex/E-mail: 440480 DRI WASHDC

**1682. Foreningen Afdanske
Eksportvognmaend**
Jo Madsen
Omfartsvejen 1
6330 Padborg
Denmark
Telephone: 45 (74) 571233

**1683. Forest Products Research
Society**
2801 Marshall Court
Madison
WI 53705
USA
Telephone: (608) 231–1361

1684. Forlaget Borsone A/S
Green's Redaktionen
Montergade 19
DK-1116 Copenhagen K
Denmark
Telephone: 033 157–250

1685. Forlaget Impetus
Helge Clausen
Randersvej 15
8544 Moerke
Denmark
Telephone: 45 (86) 377656 (x15)

1686. Forlagsentralen I/S (FS)
PO Box 1 Furuset
N-1001 Oslo 10
Norway
Telephone: 02 326–050
Fax: 02 305–383

**1687. Forschungsinstitut und
Naturmuseum Senckenberg**
Informationszentrum fuer Biologie
Senckenberganlage 25
6000 Frankfurt am Main 1
Germany
Telephone: 49 (69) 75 42 350
Fax: 49 (69) 74 62 38
Telex/E-mail: 413129 D

**1688. Forskningsbibliotekernes
Edb-kontor**
Nyhaven 31E
DK-1051 Copenhagen K
Denmark
Telephone: 033 934–633
NUA: 238242127000; 238242155000

1689. Fort Worth Star-Telegram
StarText
400 W 7th Street
PO Box 1870
Fort Worth
TX 76102
USA
Telephone: (817) 390–7400;
          (817) 390–7463

**1690. Fortia Marketing Consultants
Ltd**
Magpies House
Bottrells Lane
Chalfont St Giles
Buckinghamshire
HP8 4EH
UK
Telephone: 02407 5905
Fax: 02407 3118

1691. Foster Associates Inc
1015 15th Street NW
Suite 1100
Washington
DC 20005
USA
Telephone: (202) 408–7710
Fax: (202) 408–7723

1692. Foster Travel Publishing
PO Box 5715
Berkeley
CA 94705–0715
USA
Telephone: (415) 549–2202

1693. Fototeca Storica Nazionale Snc
Patrizia Piccini (Vice Director Digital
    Archives)
Via Degli Imbriani 31
20158 Milan
Italy
Telephone: 02 3932–0380;
          02 3931–2652
Fax: 02 373–380

1694. Foundation Center, The
79 5th Avenue
New York
NY 10003
USA
Telephone: (212) 620–4230

**1695. Foundation for Advanced
Biblical Studies**
Leyda Lewis (President)
PO Box 427
146 Country Manor Drive
DeFuniak Springs
FL 32433
USA
Telephone: (904) 892–6257

1696. FP ONLINE
A division of the Financial Post
    Information Service
777 Bay Street
Toronto
ON M5G 2E4
Canada
Telephone: (416) 593–3118
Fax: (416) 596–6075
Telex/E-mail: 06219547

**1697. France Bureau de Recherches
Geologiques et Minieres**
Service Geologique National,
    Departement Sevice Public
BP 6009
F-45060 Orleans Cedex 2
France
Telephone: 38 64 38 09
Telex/E-mail: 780258 BRGMA F

**1698. France Direction Generale des
Douanes et Droits Indirects**
Bureau C1
8 rue de la Tour des Dames
F-75436 Paris Cedex 09
France
Telephone: 1 42 80 67 22
Fax: 1 48 74 31 58
Telex/E-mail: 660168

**1699. France Documentation
Organique**
11 rue de Teheran
F-75008 Paris
France
Telephone: 1 45 62 54 35
Fax: 1 45 63 95 51

1700. Frankfurter Allgemeine
Information Services division
Frank Wenz
Germany
Telephone: +49 61 96 96 06 373

1701. Franklin Electronic Publishers
122 Burrs Road
Mt. Holly
NJ 08060
USA
Telephone: (609) 261–4800

1702. Fraunhofer-Gesellschaft
Informationszentrum RAUM und BAU
J Acevedo-Alvarez
Nobelstraße 12
D-7000 Stuttgart 80
Germany
Telephone: 0711 970–2500
Fax: 0711 970–2507
Telex/E-mail: 7255167 IRB D

**1703. Fraunhofer-Institut für
Lebensmitteltechnologie und
Verpackung**
Scragenhofstrasse 35
D-8000 Munich 50
Germany
Telephone: 49 (89) 1 41 10 91

1704. Free Spirit Software
Jim Gracely (Director of Marketing)
58 Noble Street
Kutztown
PA 19530
USA
Telephone: (215) 683–5609
Fax: (215) 683–8567

1705. Freedom Newspapers Inc
30 S Prospect
PO Box 1779
Colorado Springs
CO 80901
USA
Telephone: (719) 632–5511

1706. Freie Universität Berlin
Leitstelle Politischer Dokumentation
Paulinenstraße 22
D-1000 Berlin 45
Germany
Telephone: 030 83 37 027

1707. Frequent Publications
4715–C Town Center Drive
Colorado Springs
CO 80916
USA
Telephone: (719) 597–8889
Fax: (719) 597–6855

1708. FRI Information Services Ltd
1801 McGill College Avenue
Suite 600
Montreal
PQ H3A 2N4
Canada
Telephone: (514) 842–5091

1709. Frick Company, The
Technical Services Department
1260 Andes Boulevard
PO Box 283
St Louis
MO 63166
USA
Telephone: (314) 997–2100;
　　　　　　(314) 878–4121

1710. Friedrich Rauch
Friedrich Rauch (Proprietor)
Stollbergstraße 1
8000 Munich 22
Germany
Telephone: 089 224–484
Fax: 089 291–3258

1711. Fritzes Fackboksföretaget
Mikael Johanson (Product Manager
　　CD-ROM)
Box 16356
S-103 26 Stockholm
Sweden
Telephone: 08 238–900
Fax: 08 205–021

1712. Frost & Sullivan Inc
106 Fulton Street
New York
NY 10038
USA
Telephone: (212) 233–1080
Fax: (212) 619–0831
Telex/E-mail: 235986 FSNY UR

1713. FT Analysis
Ibex House
42/47 Minories
London
EC3 1DY
UK
Telephone: 071 702–0991
Fax: 071 702–2067

1714. FT Profile
Chris Palmer (Business Development
　　Manager); David Lennon
PO Box 12
Sunbury-on-Thames
Middlesex
TW16 7UD
UK
Telephone: 0932 761–444
Fax: 0932 781–425
Telex/E-mail: 8811720; 79:QWE-013
(Dialcom); 79:QWE-014 (Dialcom)
NUA: 234213300124

1715. Fujitsu Ltd
Michael Beirne (Public Relations
　　Division); Tadashi Sekizawa
　　(President)
6–1 Maranouchi 1–chome
Chiyoda-ku
Tokyo 100
Japan
Telephone: 03 3215–5236;
　　　　　　03 3216–3211
Fax: 03 3216–9365

1716. Fujitsu
281 Winter Street
Suite 320
Waltham
MA 02154
USA
Telephone: (617) 890–4833

1717. Fulcrum Technologies Inc
Larry Trenwith (Director, Canadian
　　Operations)
785 Carling Avenue
Ottawa
ON K1S 5H4
Canada
Telephone: (613) 238–1761
Fax: (613) 238–7695

**1718. Fundación para el Desarrollo
　　de la Función Social de
　　las**
Comunicaciones (FUNDESCO)
Calle Alcalá 61
28014 Madrid
Spain
Telephone: 01 431 12 14
Fax: 01 522 74 89
Telex/E-mail: 42608 USEF E

**1719. FUNDESCO (See Fundación
　　para el Desarrollo de la
　　Función Social de las
　　Comunicaciones)**

1720. Futur Vision
Alain Dupuy (President)
186 rue du Faubourg Saint-Martin
Paris
F-75010 Paris
France
Telephone: 1 46 07 00 43
Fax: 1 46 07 09 50

1721. Future Office Systems Ltd
Nicholas Broome (Sales Director)
Firs House
High Street
Whitchurch
Aylesbury
Buckinghamshire
HP22 4JL
UK
Telephone: 0296 641–110
Fax: 0296 641–869

1722. Future Systems Inc
PO Box 26
Falls Church
VA 22046
USA
Telephone: (703) 241–1799
Fax: (703) 532–0529
Telex/E-mail: 75236,1717
(CompuServe Information Service);
　　204–7849 (MCI Mail)

**1723. Futureline Communications /
　　Linedrive Baseball
　　Communications**
Ernie McCullough
120 Eglington Avenue E
Suite 1000
Toronto
ON M4P 1E2
Canada
Telephone: (416) 481–6346
Fax: (416) 481–6246

1724. FutureMedia Ltd
Dr Derek Moore (Managing Director); Dr
　　Peter Copeland
Media House
Arundel Road
Walberton
Arundel
West Sussex
BN18 0QP
UK
Telephone: 0243 555–000
Fax: 0243 555–020

**1725. FW Dodge Group (See
　　McGraw-Hill Inc, Construction
　　Information Services Group,
　　FW Dodge Division)**

1726. G&G Designs/Communications
Rod Swanson (Vice President Graphics
　　Division)
6359 Paseo del Lago
Carlsbad
CA 92009
UK
Telephone: (619) 431–7400;
　　　　　　(800) 828–7707
Fax: (619) 431–7495

1727. G. & C. Merriam Company
47 Federal Street
Springfield
MA 01101
USA
Telephone: (413) 734–3134

1728. G.CAM Serveur
Européenne de Données
1 rue du Boccador
F-75008 Paris
France
Telephone: 1 47 02 88 34
Fax: 1 47 20 11 43

1729. G.CAM Serveur
25–29 High Street
Kingston-upon-Thames
Surrey
KT1 1LN
UK
Telephone: 081 546–1077

1730. Gakken Company
Hideaki Tanaka
4–28–5 Nishi-Gotanda
Shinagawa-Ku
Tokyo 141
Japan
Telephone: 81 (3) 493 3280
Fax: 81 (3) 493 3290

1731. Gale Data Center
Drexel University
Philadelphia
PA
USA
Telephone: (215) 895–2000

1732. Gale Research Inc
Richard McElroy (Electronic Services
    Manager)
835 Penobscot Building
Detroit
MI 48226–4094
USA
Telephone: (313) 961–2242;
        (800) 3474–4253
Fax: (313) 961–6083;
    (313) 961–6815
Telex/E-mail: 810 221 7087

**1733. Gale Research International
    Ltd**
Ian Savage (Marketing Director)
PO Box 699
Cheriton House
North Way
Andover
Hampshire
SP10 5YE
UK
Telephone: 0264 334–446
Fax: 0264 334–158

1734. Galenica AG
Ulrich Schäfer
Untermattweg 8
3001 Berne
Switzerland
Telephone: 031 55 22 22
Fax: 031 56 16 69

1735. Gallup Markedsanalyse AS
Finn W. Kaysfeld Klaus Nielsen
G1. Vartorvvej 6
2900 Hallerup
Denmark
Telephone: 45 (31) 298800

1736. GAMA
Groupe d'Analyse Macroeconomic
    Appliquee
Universite de Paris X
200 Av. de la Republique
92001 Nanterre Cedex
France
Telephone: 33–1–40 97 77 88

1737. Gannett New Media Services
1000 Wilson Boulevard
Arlington
VA 22229
USA
Telephone: (703) 276–5940;
        (800) 222–0990

**1738. Gary Post-Tribune Publishing
    Inc**
1065 Broadway
Gary
IN 46402
USA
Telephone: (219) 881–3000

1739. Gat GbmH
Herr Gotthardt
Carl-Zeiss-Straße 25
3008 Garbsen 4
Germany
Telephone: 05131 700000
Fax: 05131 700–015

1740. Gaylord Information Systems
Connie Sirois (Product Specialist)
PO Box 4901
Syracuse
NY 13221–4901
USA
Telephone: (315) 457–5070;
        (800) 962–9580
Fax: (315) 457–8387;
    (800) 272–3412

1741. Gaz de France
Direction des Etudes et Techniques
    Nouvelles
361 avenue de President Wilson
F-93210 La Plaine Saint-Denis
France
Telephone: 1 49 22 58 00
Fax: 1 49 22 57 60
Telex/E-mail: 236735 GAZDETN F

1742. Gazelle Technologies
7434 Trade Street
San Diego
CA 92121
USA
Telephone: (619) 536–9999;
        (800) 843–9497
Fax: (619) 536–2345

1743. GBM FontCentre
Manchester
UK
Telephone: 061 273 5562

1744. GE Information Services (GEIS)
GEnie
401 N Washington Boulevard
Rockville
MD 20850
Telephone: (301) 340–4000;
        (301) 340–4572;
        (800) 638–9636
Fax: (301) 294–5501
Telex/E-mail: 898431

1745. Geisco Limited
25–29 High Street
Kingston-upon-Thames
Surrey
KT1 1LN
UK
Telephone: 44 (81) 546 1077

**1746. GEM Gesellschaft für
    elektronische Medien**
Online Service
Postfach 710363
6000 Frankfurt am Main 71
Germany
Telephone: 49 (69) 66 87 01
Fax: 49 (69) 66 87 290
Telex/E-mail: 414351 GEMFM D

1747. GenBank On-Line Service
Intelligenetics Inc
700 East El Camino Real
Mountain View
CA 94040
USA
Telephone: (415) 962–7300
Fax: (415) 962–7302
Telex/E-mail: 4937543

1748. General Cellular International
50 California Stree
Suite 470
San Francisco
CA 94111
USA
Telephone: (415) 391–2121

1749. General Drafting Company Inc
PO Box 10117
Houston
TX 77206–0119

1750. General Dynamics
PO Box 85808
San Diego
CA 92186
USA
Telephone: (619) 573–8000

1751. General Electric Canada
1420 Dupont Street
Toronto
ON M6H 2B2
Canada
Telephone: (416) 858–1073

1752. General Information Inc
Steve Miles (Editor)
11715 N Greek Parkway South
Suite 106
Bothell
WA 98011
USA
Telephone: (206) 483–4555
Fax: (206) 485–0666

1753. General Motors Corporation
Information Systems
Detroit
Michigan
USA

1754. General Research Corporation
Library Systems
Darcy Cook (Marketing Director)
5383 Hollister Avenue
PO Box 6770
Santa Barbara
CA 93111
USA
Telephone: (805) 964–7724;
        (800) 933–5383
Fax: (805) 967–7094

1755. General Videotex Corporation
Delphi
3 Blackstone Street
Cambridge
MA 02139–9998
USA
Telephone: (617) 491–3393;
        (800) 544–4005
Telex/E-mail: MAIL (DELPHI)

1756. Generale Bank
Business Information Services
Montagne du Parc 3
B-1000 Brussels
Belgium
Telephone: 02 5164–837
Fax: 02 5162–164
Telex/E-mail: 21283

1757. Generaltullstyrelsen
Box 2267
103 17 Stockholm
Sweden
Telephone: 46 (8) 789 73 00

**1758. GENIOS
    Wirtschaftsdatenbanken**
Mr. Gokl Frau Breunger
PO Box 1102
Kasernenstrasse 67
4000 Dusseldorf 1
Germany
Telephone: 49 (211) 8 38 81 84;
        49 (211) 8 38 81 85
Fax: 49 (211) 37 23 30
Telex/E-mail: 17211308 HBL VERL D
NUA: 26245400030296;
    26245400030566

1759. Genome
Peter Small
3 Lime Walk
Pinkneys Green
Maidenhead
Berkshire
SL6 6QB
UK
Telephone: 44 (628) 23090

1760. Geographic Data Technology Inc
Christopher Sachs (Vice President)
13 Dartmouth College Highway
Lyme
NH 03768–9713
USA
Telephone: (603) 795–2183
Fax: (603) 795–2115

1761. Geographical Software
London
UK
Telephone: 071 638–0287

1762. Georg Olms Verlag AG, Olms New Media
Dr Eberhard Mertens (Director); Uwe Freund (Section Manager)
Hagentorwall 7
3200 Hildesheim
Germany
Telephone: 05121 37007
Fax: 05121 32007

1763. Georg Thieme Verlag
Rüdigerstraße 14
D-7000 Stuttgart 30
Germany
Telephone: 069 77 43 21

1764. George Mason University
Public Choice Center
George's Hall
4400 University Drive
Fairfax
VA 22030
USA
Telephone: (703) 323–3877

1765. George Wells & Associates Inc
1120 Connecticut Avenue NW
Suite 270
Washington
DC 20036
USA
Telephone: (202) 659–1700

1766. Georgetown University
Kennedy Institute of Ethics, Center for Bioethics
Washington
DC 20057
USA
Telephone: (202) 687–3885;
(800) 633–3849

1767. Georgia Griffith
4 Furry Court, Rear
Lancaster
OH 43130
USA
Telex/E-mail: 76703,266
(CompuServe Information Service)

1768. Georgia Technology Research Institute
RAIL/TDD/ITB/CCRF
Atlanta
GA 30332
USA
Telephone: (404) 528–7568
Fax: (404) 528–7728

1769. Geosystems
PO Box 40
Didcot
Oxfordshire
OX11 9BX
UK
Telephone: 0235 813–913

1770. GEOVISION Inc
Kenneth S Shain (President)
Suite B
5680 Peachtree Parkway
Norcross
GA 30092
USA
Telephone: (404) 448–8224
Fax: (404) 447–4525

1771. German American Chamber of Commerce
666 5th Avenue
New York
NY 10103
USA
Telephone: (212) 974–8830
Fax: (212) 974–8867
Telex/E-mail: 234209

1772. German Business Information (See Gesellschaft für Betriebswirtschaftliche Information)

1773. German Information Center
950 3rd Avenue
New York
NY 10022
USA
Telephone: (212) 888–9840
Fax: (212) 752–6691

1774. German Patent Office
Zweibrückenstraße 12
D-8000 München 2
Germany
Telephone: 089/2195–1
Fax: 089/2195–2221
Telex/E-mail: 523534 BPBM D

1775. German Technology Exchange Inc
1 Farragut Square S
Suite 600
Washington
DC 20006
USA
Telephone: (202) 347–0247
Fax: (202) 628–3685
Telex/E-mail: 248652 RCA

1776. Gert Richter
Postfach 4249
D-2900 Oldenburg
Germany
Telephone: 0441 506–499

1777. Gesellschaft für Betriebswirtschaftliche Information
Agnese Marcia
Freischützstraße 96
Postfach 81 03 60
D-8000 Munich 81
Germany
Telephone: 089 957–0064
Fax: 089 954–229

1778. Gesellschaft für Biotechnologische Forschung mbH
Mascheroder Weg 1
D-3300 Braunschweig-Stöckheim
Germany
Telephone: 0531 618–1539
Fax: 0531 618–1515

1779. Gesellschaft für Mathematik und Datenverarbeitung
Informationszentrum für Informationswissenschaft und -Praxis
Dolivostraße 15
PO Box 104326
D-6100 Darmstadt
Germany
Telephone: 06151 875–880
Fax: 06151 875–740
Telex/E-mail: 61513899 GMD DO D

1780. Gesellschaft für Wissenschaftlich-Technische Information (See FIZ Karlsruhe)

1781. Getty Conservation Institute
4503 Glencoe Avenue
Marina del Rey
CA 90292–6537
USA
Telephone: (213) 822–2299

1782. GFFIL (French Association of Online Information Providers)
24 rue de l'Arcade
Paris
75008 Paris
France
Telephone: +33 1 42 65 78 99

1783. GIANO (See Confindustria)

1784. GIANO
Sistema Informatico della Confindustria
Viale dell'Astronomia 30
Rome
Italy
Telephone: 39 (6) 590 31
Telex/E-mail: 611393 CONFIN I

1785. GIDEP
Government-Industry Data Exchange Program
GIDEP Operations Center
Corona
CA 91720
USA
Telephone: (714) 736–4677

1786. Gilbert W Speed and Associates Inc
1801 Avenue of the Stars
Suite 217
Los Angeles
CA 90067
USA
Telephone: (213) 203–9603
Fax: (213) 203–9352
Telex/E-mail: 71292674 SPNWS UR

1787. Giuffrè Editore SpA
Ruggero Carraro
Via Busto Arsizio 40
20151 Milan
Italy
Telephone: 2 38000975;
2 3800 0905;
2 3800 0975
Fax: 2 3800 9582

1788. GK Hall and Company
Patrick Roll (Sales Manager)
70 Lincoln Street
Boston
MA 02111–9985
USA
Telephone: (617) 423–3990;
(800) 343–2806
Fax: (617) 423–3999

1789. GKTC
11 rue Plelo
F-75015 Paris
France
Telephone: 1 62 51 25 84

1790. Glass's Guide Service Ltd
Sales and Marketing
Michael Poole
One Trinity Place
Thames Street
Weybridge
Surrey
KT13 8JQ
UK
Telephone: 0932 853211
Fax: 0932 846564

1791. Glimpse Corporation, The
1101 King Street
Suite 601
Alexandria
VA 22314
USA
Telephone: (703) 838–5529

1792. Global Communications
Albermarle House
Osborne Road
Southsea
PO5 3LB
UK
Telephone: 0705 291866

1793. Global Finance Information Inc
270 Lafayette Street
Suite 1305
New York
NY 10012
USA
Telephone: (212) 925–2300
Fax: (212) 925–3892

1794. Global Information Network Ltd
777 United Nations Plaza
Concourse Level
New York
NY 10017
USA
Telephone: (212) 286–0123
Fax: (212) 818–9249
Telex/E-mail: TCN4100 (Dialcom)

1795. Global Learning Systems
Lonsdale House
Lodge Lane
Derby
DE1 3HB
UK
Telephone: 0332 31132

1796. Global Meeting Line Inc
1345 Oak Ridge Turnpike
Suite 357
Oak Ridge
TN 37830
USA
Telephone: (615) 482–6451

1797. Global Scan
28 Scrutton Street
London
EC2A 4RQ
UK
Telephone: 071 377–8872
Fax: 071 247–4194
Telex/E-mail: 893530 INFO

1798. Global Villages Inc
1 Kendall Square
Building 200
4th Floor
Cambridge
MA 02139
USA
Telephone: (617) 494–5226;
(800) 225–0750

1799. Globe and Mail, The
444 Front Street W
Toronto
ON M5V 2S9
Canada
Telephone: (416) 585–5250
Fax: (416) 585–5249
Telex/E-mail: 06219629

1800. Globe Information Services
Toronto
Canada
Telephone: +1 416 585 5250
Fax: +1 416 585 5249

1801. Globe Newspaper Company
135 Morrissey Boulevard
Boston
MA 02107
USA
Telephone: (617) 929–2000

**1802. Gmelin Institut für
Anorganische Chemie und
Grenzgebiete**
Dr Deplauque; Dr Kirchhof
Varrentrappstraße 40–42
Carl-Bosch-Haus
D-6000 Frankfurt am Main 90
Germany
Telephone: 069 79171;
069 791–7577
Fax: 069 791–7338
Telex/E-mail: 412526 D

**1803. GML Corporation (Computer
Review)**
George Luhowy (President)
594 Marrett Road
Lexington
MA 02173
USA
Telephone: (617) 861–0515

1804. Godiva Chocolatier Inc
260 Madison Avenue
New York
NY 10016
USA
Telephone: (212) 951–2882

1805. Gold Disk
5155 Spectrum Way
Unit 5
Mississaugga
Ontario
L4W 5A1
Canada

1806. GoldMind Publishing
297 Grulla Court
Norco
CA 91760
USA
Telephone: (714) 371–6298

1807. Gorman Publishing Company
8750 W Bryn Mawr Avenue
Chicago
IL 60631
USA
Telephone: (312) 693–3200

**1808. Government Counselling
Limited**
Lynn Bateman; Ed Gauthier; Susan
Baker-Low
6281 B Old Franconia Road
Alexandria
VA 22310
USA
Telephone: (703) 719–7602
Fax: (703) 719–9359

1809. Government Information Office
2 Tientain Street
Taipei
Taiwan
Telephone: 886 (2) 371–8201

**1810. Government National Mortgage
Association**
U.S. Department of Housing and Urban
Development
451 7th Street, SW
Washington
DC 20410
USA
Telephone: (202) 755–5926

**1811. Government-Industry Data
Exchange Program**
GIDEP Operations Center
Corona
CA 91720
USA
Telephone: (714) 736–4677
Fax: (714) 736–5200

1812. Graphitec inc
9101 West 123rd Street
Palos Park
IL 60464
USA
Telephone: (708) 448–6660
Fax: (708) 448–6492

1813. Grasso Giuseppe Informatica
Giuseppe Grasso
Vicolo Parrini 10
90145 Palermo
Italy
Telephone: 091 676–0563
Fax: 091 676–0563;
091 343–499

**1814. Great Barrier Reef Marine Park
Authority**
PO Box 1379
Townsville
QLD 4810
Australia
Telephone: 077 818–811

**1815. Great Britain Central Statistical
Office**
CSO Branch E1
Great George Street
London
SW1P 4AQ
UK
Telephone: 071 270–6387

**1816. Greater Detroit Society for the
Blind**
16625 Grand River Avenue
Detroit
MI 48227
USA
Telephone: (313) 272–3900
Fax: (313) 272–6893

**1817. Greater Orlando Chamber of
Commerce**
Tourism Development Department
75 E Ivanhoe Boulevard
PO Box 1234
Orlando
FL 32802
USA
Telephone: (305) 425–1234

1818. Greensboro News & Record
200 E Market Street
PO Box 20848
Greensboro
NC 27420-5667
USA
Telephone: (919) 373-7111

1819. Greenwood Press Inc
88 Post Road West
PO Box 5007
Westport
CT 06881
USA
Telephone: (203) 226–3571

1820. Grolier Electronic Publishing Inc
Maryanne Piazza (Director of Marketing)
Sherman Turnpike
Danbury
CT 06816
USA
Telephone: (203) 797–3365;
(203) 797–3500;
(800) 356–5590
Fax: (203) 797–3365

1821. Grolier Electronic Publishing
c/o New Media Productions
12 Oval Road
London
NW1 7DH
UK
Telephone: 071 482–5258

1822. Groliers Ltd
20 Torbay Road
Markham
Ontario
L3R 1G6
Canada
Telephone: (416) 474–0333

1823. Group 1 Software
Dick Kirsch (Manager Dealer Sales)
6404 Ivy Lane
Suite 500
Greenbelt
MD 20770–1400
USA
Telephone: (301) 982–2000;
(800) 368–5806
Fax: (301) 982–4069

1824. Groupe d'Analyse Macroeconomique Appliquee
Universite de Paris X
200 avenue de la Republique
92001 Nanterre Cedex
France
Telephone: 33 (1) 40 97 77 88;
33 (1) 47 21 46 89
Telex/E-mail: 638898 UPX NANT F

1825. Groupe DPV
24 rue Morere
F-75014 Paris
France
Telephone: 1 45 41 52 02

1826. Groupe Galande
Chateau de Sens
Rochecorbon
37210 Vouvray
France
Telephone: 33 (47) 52 51 84
Telex/E-mail: 750034 F

1827. Groupe TESTS
5 place du Colonel Fabien
75491 Paris Cedex 10
France
Telephone: 33 (1) 42 40 22 01

1828. Gruner & Jahr AG & Co.
2 Hamburg 36
Postfach 30 20 40
Hamburg 3021
Germany

1829. Gruppo Editoriale Fabbri Bompiani Sonzogno Etas SpA
Jan Miguel Battistoni
Via Mecenate 91
20132 Milan
Italy
Telephone: 02 509–5824
Fax: 02 506–5361

1830. GSI Marketing Economie (GSI-ECO)
Smaïl Metadjer (Consultant)
45 rue de la Procession
F-75015 Paris
France
Telephone: 1 45 66 78 89
Fax: 1 47 34 46 92
Telex/E-mail: 613163 GSIEMS F
250682 F
NUA: 20803802086610

1831. GTE Education Services Inc
SpecialNet
8505 Freeport Parkway
Irving
TX 75063
USA
Telephone: (214) 929–3000
Fax: (214) 929–3020

1832. Guardian Business Information
CCN Systems Ltd
PO Box 39
Bridgewater Place
Manchester
M60 4AA
UK

1833. Guardian Newspapers Ltd
Gerald Knight
119 Farringdon Road
London
EC1R 3ER
UK
Telephone: 071 278–2332
Fax: 071 837–2114;
071 833–8342
Telex/E-mail: 881174178 GUARON G

1834. Guido Monaci SpA
Giancarlo Zapponini
Via Vitorchiano 107–109
I-00189 Rome
Italy
Telephone: 06 333–1333
Fax: 06 333–5555

1835. Guildford Educational Services Ltd
Robin Twining (Director)
32 Castle Street
Guildford
Surrey
GU1 3UW
UK
Telephone: 0483 579–472;
0483 579–454
Fax: 0483 574–277

1836. GuildSoft
Mike Holman
UK
Telephone: 0752 606200

1837. Guinness Publishing Ltd
Sarah Duncan (Marketing Manager)
33 London Road
Enfield
Middlesex
EN2 6DJ
UK
Telephone: 081 367–4567
Fax: 081 367–5912

1838. GWP-Gesellschaft fuer Wirtschaftspublizistik GmbB
Kasernenstrasse 67
4000 Dusseldorf 1
Germany
Telephone: 29 (211) 8 38 81 83
Telex/E-mail: 17211308 HBL VERL D

1839. Gyldendal Publishing
Mogens Wennicke
3 Klareboderne
1001 Copenhagen K
Denmark
Telephone: 33 110–775
Fax: 33 110–323

1840. H & J Price Company
35 Ridgewood Terrace
Maplewood
NJ 07040
USA
Telephone: (201) 762–7516

1841. Hachette SA
24 Boulevard Saint Michel
75006 Paris
France
Telephone: 1 46 34 86 65

1842. Hachette-Filipacchi Telematique
6 rue Ancelle
F-92200 Neuilly-sur-Seine
France
Telephone: 1 42 56 72 72

1843. Hachette
A Pierrot (Director of Educational Engineering)
79 boulevard Saint Germain
75288 Paris
France
Telephone: 1 46 34 87 18;
1 46 34 86 34
Fax: 1 46 34 88 38

1844. Haelso- och sjukvaardens ansvarsnaemnd
PO Box 3539
S-103 69 Stockholm
Sweden
Telephone: 08 786 92 00

1845. Hake Brainware GmbH
Turmstrasse 10
D-6500 Mainz
Germany
Telephone: 49–6131–683 071–4

1846. Hamburg Educational Partnership
Professor MS Wall (Director)
Berliner Tor 21
D-2000 Hamburg
Germany
Telephone: 040 24 88 3014
Fax: 040 24 88 2847;
040 24 88 2599

1847. Hammerhead Publishing
220 South Military Trail
Deerfield Beach
FL 33442
USA
Telephone: (305) 426–8114
Fax: (305) 426–9801

1848. HamNet Online
16440 Rustling Oak Court
Morgan Hill
CA 95037
USA
Telephone: (408) 570–3670

1849. Handelsbanken
Afd. for Teknisk Salg
Holmens Kanal 2
1091 Koebenhavn K
Denmark
Telephone: 45 (33) 128600

1850. Handelsblatt GmbH
Kasernenstraße 67
Postfach 11 02
D-4000 Dusseldorf 1
Germany
Telephone: 0211 887–1524;
0211 83880;
0211 838–8500
Fax: 0211 326–759
Telex/E-mail: 17211308 HBLD;
17211308 HBL VERL D

1851. Handelsblatt GmbH
Redaktion Chemische Industrie
Karlstraße 21
D-6000 Frankfurt am Main 1
Germany
Telephone: 069 255–6454

1852. Handelshoejskolens Regnskabsdatabase Fond
Bodil Pederson
Howitzvej 60, 6.sal
6000 Frederiksberg
Denmark
Telephone: 45 (31) 861149

1853. HandsNet Inc
20195 Stevens Creek Boulevard
Suite 120
Cupertino
CA 95014
USA
Telephone: (408) 427–4500
Fax: (408) 427–4560
Telex/E-mail: HNOOXO (HandsNet)

1854. Hark and Gjellerups Boghandel
Joergen Lauridsen
Fiolstraede 31–33
1171 Koebenhavn K
Denmark
Telephone: 45 (33) 129148

1855. Harper & Row
East Washington Square
Philadelphia
PA 19105
USA
Telephone: (215) 238–4408

1856. Harrap France S.A.
177 rue St. Honore
75001 Paris
France

1857. Harrap Ltd
19–23 Ludgate Hill
London
EC4M 7PD
UK
Telephone: 071 248–6444
Fax: 071 248–3357

1858. Harrap Publishing Group
David Skinner (Editorial Director, Reference)
Chelsea House
26 Market Square
Bromley
Kent
BR1 1NA
UK
Telephone: 081 313–3484
Fax: 081 313–0702

1859. Harris Media Systems Ltd
1835 Yonge Street
5th Floor
Toronto
ON M4S 1X8
Telephone: (416) 487–2119

1860. Harrisburg Patriot and Evening News
812 Market Street
Harrisburg
PA 17105
USA
Telephone: (717) 255–8100

1861. Harrison Scott Publications
1 Riverfront Plaza
Suite 1480
Newark
NJ 07102
USA
Telephone: (201) 596–1300

1862. Hart MacFarlane & Associates Pty Ltd
Dr Charles Hart (Director)
56 Snows Road
Stirling
SA 5152
Australia
Telephone: 08 370–9328
Fax: 08 370–9969

1863. Harvard University Library
Harvard University
Cambridge
MA 02138
USA
Telephone: (617) 495–9025

1864. Harvard University
Department of the Classics
Gregory Crane
319 Boylston Hall
Cambridge
MA 02138
USA
Telephone: (617) 495–9025
Fax: (617) 496–8886

1865. Harvest Information Services Ltd
18–19 Long Lane
London
EC1A 9HE
UK
Telephone: 071 606–4533
Fax: 071 226–6083
Telex/E-mail: 23123 G

1866. Hary & Company
Noburu Toyoshima (Director of International Marketing)
5–4–8 Shimotakaido
Suginami-ku
Tokyo 168
Japan
Telephone: 3 5687–3657;
3 290–6104
Fax: 3 290–6107

1867. Hassan Division
Materials & Design Services (Pvt) Ltd
1 Canal Road
Abdullah Plaza
Abdullah Pur
Faisalabad
Pakistan
Telephone: 0411 713–302;
0411 713–349
Fax: 0411 41599

1868. Hatier Logiciels
T Gibrat
'Nomadic'
Port Debilly
75116 Paris
France
Telephone: 1 47 23 43 43;
1 47 23 40 92

1869. Haver Analytics
60 E 42nd Street
Suite 620
New York
NY 10165
USA
Telephone: (212) 986–9300
Fax: (212) 986–5857

1870. Haymarket Medical Publications Ltd
30 Lancaster Gate
London
W2 3LP
UK
Telephone: 071 402–4200

1871. Haymarket Publications
22 Lancaster Gate
London W2 3LY
UK
Telephone: 44 (71) 434–2233

1872. HBJ Miller Accounting Publications Inc
1250 6th Ave.
San Diego
CA 92101
USA
Telephone: (619) 699–6716

1873. HCI Publications
410 Archibald
Suite 100
Kansas City
MO 64111
USA
Telephone: (816) 931–1311
Fax: (816) 931–2062

1874. HCI Service
P.O. Box 31
Loughborough
Leicestershire
LE11 1QU
UK

1875. HE Corporation
Dennis Steer
Grimsby
UK
Telephone: +44 (0)472 355504
Fax: +44 (0)891 408840

1876. Head Software International
Sue Hyman (Director)
Oxted Mill
Spring Lane
Oxted
Surrey
RH8 9PB
UK
Telephone: 0883 717–057
Fax: 0883 712–327
Telex/E-mail: 957525 (OXMILL G)

1877. Health & Welfare Canada
Room 1C
LCDC Building
Ottawa
ON K1A 0L2
Canada
Telephone: (613) 957–0329
Fax: (613) 941–2057;
(613) 952–7009

1878. Health and Safety Executive
Library and Information Services
Sheila Pantry (Head of Library and
   Information Services)
Broad Lane
Sheffield
South Yorkshire
S3 7HQ
UK
Telephone: 0742 768–141
Fax: 0742 720–006;
   0742 755–792
Telex/E-mail: 54556 HSE RLSD G

**1879. Health Care Literature
   Information Network**
Institu für Krankenhausbau
Straße des 17. Juni 135
D-1000 Berlin 12
Germany
Telephone: 030 3142–3905
Fax: 030 3142–1112
Telex/E-mail: 184262 TUBLN D

1880. Health Promotion Wales
Health Link Wales
Fiona Stobie; Ann Davies
Health Link Wales
Health Promotion Wales
Ffynnon-Lis
Ty Glas Avenue
Llanishen
Cardiff
CF4 5DZ
Wales, UK
Telephone: 0222 752222
Fax: 0222 756000

**1881. Healthcare Information
   Services Inc**
Richard Wertz (President)
2335 American River Drive
Suite 307
Sacramento
CA 95825
USA
Telephone: (916) 648–8075;
   (800) 468–1128
Fax: (916) 648–8078

1882. HealthNet Ltd
716 East Carlisle
Milwaukee
WI 53217
USA
Telephone: (414) 963–8829

**1883. Hearst Business
   Communications Inc**
Armand Villiger (Publisher); Marie Botta
645 Stewart Avenue
Garden City
NY 11530–9854
USA
Telephone: (516) 227–1300
Fax: (516) 227–1901

1884. Hearst Publishing Group
Capital Newspapers Division
News Plaza
Box 1500
Albany
NY 12212
USA
Telephone: (518) 454–5694

1885. HeartBeat Software Solutions
Craig Oka (Partner)
PO Box 4497
Cerritos
CA 90703
USA
Telephone: (213) 404–7083
Fax: (213) 802–1435

**1886. Heat Transfer & Fluid Flow
   Service**
Building 392.7
Harwell Laboratory
Harwell
Oxfordshire
OX11 0RA
UK
Telephone: 44 (235) 24141
Fax: 44 (235) 831981
Telex/E-mail: 83135 ATOMHA G

1887. HEC Software Inc
Leonard Eversole (President)
3471 South 550 West
Bountiful
UT 84010
USA
Telephone: (801) 295–7054;
   (800) 333–0054
Fax: (801) 298–1008

**1888. HECLINET (See Health Care
   Literature Information Network)**

**1889. Hedeselskabet Hydrometriske
   Undersoegelser**
Joergen Erup
Anholtsvej 5
Postboks 4
4200 Slagelse
Denmark
Telephone: 45 (53) 521701

1890. Heery International Inc
Susan McClerndon
999 Peachtree Street NE
Atlanta
GA 30367–5401
USA
Telephone: (404) 881–9880
Fax: (404) 875–1283

1891. Hein, William S. & Co. Inc.
Daniel P. Rosati
1285 Main Street
Buffalo
NY 14209–1987
USA
Telephone: (716) 882–2600
Fax: (716) 883–8100

**1892. Heiwa Information Center
   Company Ltd**
Shinjuku Green Tower Building
19th Floor
6–14–1 Nishi-Shinjuku Shinjuku-ku
Tokyo 160
Japan
Telephone: 03 3349–7771
Fax: 03 3343–4080

1893. Helen Adam & Associates Inc
Benjamin Fox Pavillion
Suite 824
Jenkintown
PA 19046
USA
Telephone: (215) 572–6410
Telex/E-mail: Site 123 (RSA)

1894. Helgerson Associates Inc
Betsy Perrin
6609 Rosecroft Place
Falls Church
VA 22043–1828
USA
Telephone: (703) 237–0682
Fax: (703) 532–5447

1895. Helicon Publishing Ltd
(previously Random Century's
   Reference Division)
Michael Upsall (Reference Editor)
20 Vauxhall Bridge Road
London
SW1V 2SA
UK
Telephone: 07) 973–9700
Fax: 071 931–7672

1896. Hellas PTT
Hellenic Telecom Administration
99 Kifisias Av.
Athinai 15124
Greece
Telephone: +30 1 6118562
Fax: +30 1 6826499
Telex/E-mail: 219797 ote

**1897. Hellenic Organisation for
   Standardisation**
E Melagrakis (Managere)
313 Acharnon Street
11145 Athens
Greece
Telephone: 01 201 5025
Fax: 01 202 5917

1898. Help for Health Trust
Information Services
Maria Cook; Robert Gann
The Help for Health Trust
Highcroft Cottage
Romsey Road
Winchester
SO22 5DH
UK
Telephone: 0962 844825;
   0962 949100
Fax: 0962 849079

1899. Helsinki Commission
Baltic Sea Environment Protection
   Commission
Mannerheimintie 12 A
SF-00100 Helsinki
Finland
Telephone: 0 602366

**1900. Helsinki School of Economics
   Library**
Information Services
Kyllikki Ruokonen (Director of
   Information Services)
Runeberginkatu 22–24
SF-00100 Helsinki 10
Finland
Telephone: 0 431–3413;
   0 431–3418
Fax: 0 431–3539
Telex/E-mail: 122220 ECON SF
NUA: 224202006

1901. Helsinki University Library
Science Library
Teollisuukatu 23
SF-00510 Helsinki
Finland
Telephone: 0 43131
Fax: 0 43135
Telex/E-mail: 122220 ECON SF

1902. Helsinki University Library
National Bibliography Office
Eeva Murtomaa (Librarian)
Teollisuusk 23
SF-00510 Helsinki
Finland
Telephone: 0 7084335;
0 70851
Fax: 0 1912719;
0 7084441

1903. Hemmington Scott
City Innovation Centre
26–31 Whiskin Street
London
EC1R 0BP
UK
Telephone: 071 278–7769
Fax: 071 278–9808

**1904. Henley Centre for Forecasting
Ltd**
2 Tudor Street
Blackfriars
London
EC4Y 0AA
UK
Telephone: 071 353–9961
Telex/E-mail: 298817 G

1905. Heritage Foundation, The
214 Massachusetts Avenue NE
Washington
DC 20002
USA
Telephone: (202) 546–4400

1906. Hermeneutika
Mark Rice (Marketing)
PO Box 98563
Seattle
WA 98198
USA
Telephone: (206) 824–9673
Fax: (206) 824–7160

1907. Herner and Company
1700 North Moore Street
Arlington
VA 22209
USA
Telephone: (703) 558–8200

**1908. HEROLD – Fachverlag für
Wirtschaftsinformation**
Christian Wagner
Wipplingerstraße 14
A-1013 Vienna
Austria
Telephone: 0222 533 262 630
Fax: 0222 533 262 68

1909. Hewitt Associates
100 Half Day Road
Lincolnshire
IL 60015
USA
Telephone: (708) 295–5000

1910. Hewlett-Packard Company
Cindy Kennaugh (Product Managere)
100 Mayfield Avenue
Mountain View
CA 94043
USA
Telephone: (415) 968–5600;
(415) 691–5688
Fax: (415) 691–5484

1911. High Society Magazine
801 2nd Avenue
New York
NY 10017
USA
Telephone: (212) 986–5100

**1912. High Tech Publishing
Company**
PO Box 1923
Brattleboro
VT 05301
USA
Telephone: (802) 254–3539

1913. High Tech Verlag GmbH
Leopoldstraße 70
D-8000 Munich 40
Germany
Telephone: 089 39 10 11

1914. High Technology Magazine
214 Lewis Wharf
Boston
MA 02110
USA
Telephone: (617) 723–6611

1915. Highlighted Data Inc
Jim Tracy (Office Manager)
4350 N Fairfax Drive
Suite 450
Arlington
VA 22203
USA
Telephone: (703) 516–9211
Fax: (703) 516–9216

1916. HighTech Lab Japan Inc
Takeshi Yoshizaki (President)
1–4–1 Higashiyama
Meguro-ku
Tokyo 153
Japan
Telephone: 03 3711–5111
Fax: 03 3711–5110

1917. Hilfe Ltd
Nick Hill
84 Long Lane
London
SE1 4QE
UK
Telephone: 071 407–6414

1918. Hitachi New Media
James Dunkason (Customer Liaison
Engineer)
Hitachi House
Station Road
Hayes
Middlesex
UB3 4DR
UK
Telephone: 081 848–8787;
081 561–4565
Fax: 081 569–2763

1919. Hitachi Pharmacia
800 Centennial Avenue
PO Box 1327
Piscataway
NJ 08855–1327
USA

**1920. Hitachi Software Engineering
America Ltd**
Kathy Padgett (Product Manager)
2000 Sierra Point Parkway
MS 580
Brisbane
CA 94005–1819
USA
Telephone: (415) 244–7551;
(415) 244–7593

**1921. Hitachi Software Engineering
Company Ltd**
Yoshiya Fukuma (Representative
International Sales & Marketing)
6–81 Onoe-cho Naka-ku
Yokohama 231
Japan
Telephone: 045 681–2111
Fax: 045 681–4914

1922. HMSO Books
Peter Raggett (Bibliographics Manager)
Publications Centre
51 Nine Elms Lane
London
SW8 5DR
UK
Telephone: 071 873–8401;
071 873–0011
Fax: 071 873–8463
Telex/E-mail: 297138 G

1923. HMSO New Media Publishing
David Martin (Publishing Manager);
Marion Maxwell; Ann Brock (New
Media Project Officer)
St Crispins
Duke Street
Norwich
NR3 1PD
UK
Telephone: 0603 695–550;
0603 695–726;
0603 695–498
Fax: 0603 695–317

1924. Hodos Ltd
Stefan Nowak (Technical Director)
New Caledonian Wharf
Odessa Street
London
SE16 1LU
UK
Telephone: 071 252–3122
Fax: 071 231–3114

**1925. Holger Mayer
Unternehmensberatung für
Informationsverarbeitung**
Elisabethenstraße 18
D-6368 Bad Vilbel 1
Germany
Telephone: 06161 8331

1926. Hollywood Hotline
PO Box 2510
Sparks
NV 89432
USA
Telephone: (702) 331–0991

1927. Home Management Systems
485 Maddison
Winnepeg
MB R3J 1J2
Canada
Telephone: (204) 885–2558

**1928. Home Office Forensic Science
Service**
Central Research Establishment and
Support, Information Services
Aldermaston
Reading
Berkshire
RG7 4PN
UK
Telephone: 0734 814–100
Fax: 0734 815–490
Telex/E-mail: 847082 G

1929. Honeywell Inc
Honeywell Plaza
PO Box 524
Minneapolis
MN 55408–5440
USA
Telephone: (612) 870–5200
Fax: (612) 870–6231

1930. Hong Kong Government
Census and Statistics Department
Donna Shum (Senior Statistician)
21/F Wanchai Tower I
12 Harbour Road
Wanchai
Hong Kong
Telephone: 823–4701
Fax: 865–2900

1931. Hooksett Publishing Inc
PO Box 895
Melville
NY 11747
USA
Telephone: (516) 549–4090
Fax: (516) 385–9828

1932. Hopewell Agency
154 2nd Street
Trenton
NJ 08611–2204
USA
Telephone: (609) 394–0370

1933. Hopital Charles-Lemoyne
25 Taschereau Boulevard
Suite 100
Greenfield Park
PQ J4V 2G8
Canada
Telephone: (514) 466–5696
Fax: (514) 465–0816

1934. Hopkins Technology
Carol Dun (Marketing)
421 Hazel Lane
Suite 240
Hopkins
MN 55343–7117
USA
Telephone: (612) 931–9376;
          (800) 397–9211
Fax: (612) 931–9377

**1935. Hoppenstedt
    Wirtschaftsdatenbank GmbH**
Wolfgang Benscheck (Managing
Director)
Havelstraße 9
Postfach 4006
D-6100 Darmstadt 1
Germany
Telephone: 6151 3800;
          6151 380–357
Fax: 6151 380–360
Telex/E-mail: 4 19 258 HOPP D 13652
(DIALMAIL)

1936. Horler Information Inc
Emerald Plaza
1547 Merivale Road, 4th Floor
Ottawa
ON K1A 0Y7
Canada
Telephone: (613) 952–2706
Fax: (613) 952–7353
Telex/E-mail: 0533777

1937. Houghton Mifflin Company
Educational Software Division
Steven Vana-Paxhia (Vice President);
   Win Carus (Editorial Department)
1 Memorial Drive
Cambridge
MA 02142–1301
USA
Telephone: (617) 252–3000
Fax: (617) 252–3145
Telex/E-mail: 4430255HMHQUI

1938. House of Commons
Room A-001
Wellington Building
Ottawa
ON K1A 0A6

1939. House of Commons Library
Palace of Westminster
London
SW1A 0AA
UK
Telephone: 071 219–5714
Fax: 071 219–5910
Telex/E-mail: 76: LRF001 (Dialcom)

1940. Houston Chronicle
801 Texas Avenue
Houston
TX 77002
USA
Telephone: (713) 220–7171

1941. HTE Research Inc
400 Oyster Point Boulevard
Suite 220
South San Francisco
CA 94080
USA
Telephone: (415) 871–4377
Telex/E-mail: 296667 HTEM

1942. HUD User
Sue Ellen Hersh (Referencee
   Supervisor)
PO Box 6091
Rockville
MD 20850
USA
Telephone: (301) 251–5183;
          (301) 251–5154;
          (800) 245–2691
Fax: (301) 251–5747

1943. Huddinge University Hospital
Drug Information Center
S-141 86 Huddinge
Sweden
Telephone: 08 746 10 60
Fax: 08 746 88 21

1944. Hughes Tool Company
PO Box 2539
Houston
TX 77252–2539
USA
Telephone: (713) 924–2222
Fax: (713) 924–2009
Telex/E-mail: 3730688 HUGHES

1945. Human Relations Area Files
David Levenson (Vice President)
PO Box 2054
Yale Station
755 Prospect Street
New Haven
CT 06520–2054
USA
Telephone: (203) 777–2334
Fax: (203) 777–2337

**1946. Human Resource Selection
    Network Inc**
3 Cabot Place
Stoughton
MA 02072
USA
Telephone: (617) 341–1968

**1947. Hungarian Central Statistical
    Office**
Keleti Karoly u 5–7
1525 Budapest 11
Hungary
Telephone: 01 358–530;
          01 115–9640
Fax: 01 115–9640

1948. HW Wilson Company
Betty Clarke
950 University Avenue
Bronx
NY 10452
USA
Telephone: (212) 588–8400;
          (800) 367–6770;
          (800) 462–6060
Fax: (212) 538–2716;
     (212) 538–7507;
     (212) 590–1617

**1949. HWWA Institut für
    Wirtschaftsforschung,
    Hamburg**
Informationszentrum
Neuer Jungfernsteig 21
D-2000 Hamburg 36
Germany
Telephone: 040 35620

**1950. HY-System Datenservice
    GmbH**
Essen
Germany
Telephone: +49 211 310010

1951. Hydrocomp Inc
201 San Antonio Circle
Mountain View
CA 94040
USA
Telephone: (415) 948–3919
Telex/E-mail: 348357

1952. Hyperdoc plc
Alrich Kaun (Sales Director)
Kingsgate Business Centre
Kingsgate Road
Kingston-upon-Thames
Surrey
KT2 5AA
UK
Telephone: 081 541–1877
Fax: 081 541–4697

1953. HyperGlot – Validata Australia
Bob Cann (Managing Director)
43 Beaufort Road
Terrigal
NSW 2260
Australia
Telephone: 043 852–091
Fax: 043 842–323

**1954. HyperGlot Software Company
    Inc**
Leigh Wood (Customer Service
   Manager)
PO Box 10746
5108D Kingston Pike
Knoxville
TN 37939–0746
USA
Telephone: (800) 726–5087;
          (617) 558–8270
Fax: (617) 588–6569

1955. HyperMedia Group, The
Tim Boyle (Director of Business
   Development)
5900 Hollis Street
Suite O
Emeryville
CA 94608
USA
Telephone: (415) 601–0900
Fax: (415) 601–0933

1956. i P Sharp Associates Limited
Heron House
10 Dean Farrar Street
London
SW1H 0DX
UK
Telephone: 071 222–7033

1958. I see!
L.D.C., Ministerie van Sociale
Zaken en Werkgelegenheid
Muzenstraat 30
2511 VW Den Haag
Netherlands
Telephone: 70 624 611

1959. I.E. Informazioni Editoriali
Mavro Zerbini; Simonetta Pillon
Via Filippino Lippi 19
20131 Milan
Italy
Telephone: 02 70 60 19 28
Fax: 02 70 60 19 32

**1960. I.P. Sharp Associates, Hong
Kong Limited**
1801 Bank of America Tower
12 Harcourt Road
Hong Kong
Telephone: 852 (5) 266 341

1961. I.P. Sharp Associates
A Reuter Company
Suite 1900, Exchange Tower
2 First Canadian Place
Toronto
ON M5X 1E3
Canada
Telephone: (416) 364–5361;
(800) 387–1588
Fax: (416) 364–0646
Telex/E-mail: 0622259

1962. I.S. Grupe Inc
Peter B. Schipma (President)
948 Springer Drive
Lombard
IL 60148
USA
Telephone: (312) 627–0550
Fax: (312) 627–4086

1963. I/S Datacentralenn
Retortvej 6–8
DK-2500 Valby Copenhagen
Denmark
Telephone: 031 468–122
Fax: 031 168–805
Telex/E-mail: 27122 DC DK

**1964. IBC/Donoghue Organization
Inc**
360 Woodland Street
PO Box 540
Holliston
MA 01746
USA
Telephone: (508) 429–5930;
(800) 343–5413
Fax: (508) 429–2452

1965. Ibericom SA
E Suja (Director Tecnico)
Manuel Gonzalez Longoria 7
28010 Madrid
Spain
Telephone: 01 447–9056
Fax: 01 447–8225

1966. Ibis Enterprises
4866 NW 95th Avenue
Sunrise
FL 33351
USA
Telephone: (305) 749–1213

1967. IBIS Service AG
Peter Kubli (President of Board of
Directors)
Muehlegasse 11
8001 Zurich
Switzerland
Telephone: 01 252 17 71
Fax: 01 252 18 30

1968. IBM Deutschland
Informations- und Netzwerkservice
DEP. 3670
7000–75 Schlossstrasse 70
7000 Stuttgart 1
Germany
Telephone: 49 (7) 117 85 – 0
Telex/E-mail: 413245 IBMG D

**1969. IBM Information Network
Services-Europe**
Avenue Louise 523
B-1050 Brussels
Belgium
Telephone: 02 214–2111
Telex/E-mail: 62465580 UITHONE B

1970. IBM Information Network
PO Box 30104
Tampa
FL 33630–3104
USA
Telephone: (813) 872–2111;
(800) 426–3333

1971. IBM PCS
Eurocoordination
Tour Pascal, Cedex 40
92075 Paris la Defense
France
Telephone: 33 (1) 47 67 60 00

1972. IBM United Kingdom Limited
Information Network Services
389 Chiswick High Road
London W4 4AL
UK
Telephone: 44 (71) 995–1441
Telex/E-mail: 23295 IBM CHI G

1973. IBM
Old Orchard Road
Armonk
NY 10504
USA
Telephone: (914) 765–1900

1974. iBS Systemvertrieb
Rolf Cotthardt (Product Manager)
Carl-Zeiss-Straße 25
3008 Garbsen 4
Germany
Telephone: 05131 7000–17
Fax: 05131 7000–15

1975. ICC Business Publications
Duncan Mackinnon
Field House
72 Oldfield Road
Hampton
Middlesex
TW12 2HQ
UK
Telephone: 081 783–0922
Fax: 081 783–1940
Telex/E-mail: 296090 ICC G

1976. ICC Information Group Ltd
Karen Chandler
Field House
72 Oldfield Road
Hampton
Middlesex
TW12 2HQ
UK
Telephone: 081 783–1122
Fax: 081 783–0049
Telex/E-mail: 296090 ICC G 11627
(Dialmail)

1977. ICC Online Ltd
Sandra Whiteman
Field House
72 Oldfield Road
Hampton
Middlesex
TW12 2HQ
UK
Telephone: 081 783–1122
Fax: 081 783–0049

**1978. ICD Mutual Fund Information
Services**
406 Merle Hay Tower
Des Moines
IA 50310
USA
Telephone: (515) 270–8600;
(800) 255–2255 x 5222
Fax: (515) 270–9022

**1979. ICEX (See Instituto Español de
Comercio Exterior)**

1980. ICIS-LOR Group Ltd
18 Upper Grosvenor Street
London
W1X 9PD
UK
Telephone: 071 493–3040
Fax: 071 499–8200
Telex/E-mail: 296557 LOR G

1981. ICL
Office Systems Division
Product Marketing Manager
Lovelace Rd.
Bracknell
Berks.
RG12 4SN
UK
Telephone: 0344 424842

1982. ICOM Simulations Inc
Michele Boeding (Marketing Director)
648 S Wheeling Road
Wheeling
IL 60090
USA
Telephone: (708) 520–4440
Fax: (708) 459–3418

**1983. ICP (Institut de la
Communication Parlée)**
Jean-François Serignat
INPG
46 avenue Félic Viallet
38031 Grenoble Cedex
France
Telephone: 76 57 45 00
Fax: 76 57 47 10

**1984. ICP (International Computer
Programs)**
Stephen F Bowers (Director, Software
Information Database)
8900 Keystone Crossing
Suite 1100
Indianapolis
IN 46240
USA
Telephone: (317) 844–7461;
(800) 428–6179
Fax: (317) 574–0571

**1985. ICSTI International Centre for
Scientific and Technical
Information**
A W Butrimenko
ul. Kuusinenena 21 b
125252 Moscow
Russia
Telex/E-mail: 064 41 1925

1986. ID/Farma BV
Dr H Gryseels
Molenweg 34
3981 CC Bunnik
Netherlands
Telephone: 03405 71068
Fax: 03405 71068

**1987. Idaps Information Services Pty
Ltd**
30 Bowden Street
Postal Bag 30
Alexandria 2015
Australia
Telephone: 02 699–9955
Fax: 02 699–7495
Telex/E-mail: 72394 CIDSCB AA

1988. IDC-KTHB
Valhallavaegen 81
S-10044 Stockholm
Sweden

**1989. IDD Information Services
(Waltham)**
100 5th Avenue
Waltham
MA 02154
USA
Telephone: (617) 890–7227
Telex/E-mail: 6987392

1990. IDD Information Services
c/o Extel Financial Ltd
Fitzroy House
13–17 Epworth Street
London
EC2A 4DL
UK
Telephone: 071 251–3333

1991. IDD Information Services
Thomas E Ferb (Vice President)
Two World Trade Center
18th Floor
New York
NY 10048
USA
Telephone: (212) 432–0045
Fax: (212) 321–9617
Telex/E-mail: 261251

**1992. IDD Verlag für Internationale
Dokumentation**
Werner Flach KG
Heddernheimer Landstra[e1]e 78a
D-6000 Frankfurt am Main 50
Germany
Telephone: 069 57 77 77

1993. IDG Communications
PO Box 9171
375 Cochituate Road
Framingham
MA 01701–9171
USA
Telephone: (508) 875–9831
Telex/E-mail: COMPUTERWORLD
(MCI Mail)

1994. IEA Coal Research
Robert Davidson (Head of Information
Services)
Gemini House
10–18 Putney Hill
London
SW15 6AA
UK
Telephone: 081 780–2111
Fax: 081 780–1746;
081 828–9508
Telex/E-mail: 917624 NICEBA G

1995. IFI/Plenum Data Company
H Alcock
302 Swann Avenue
Alexandria
VA 22301
USA
Telephone: (703) 683–1085;
(800) 368–3093
Fax: (703) 683–0246
Telex/E-mail: 901834

1996. IFIS Publishing
SH Hill
Lane End House
Shinfield
Reading
RG2 9BB
UK
Telephone: 0734 883–895
Fax: 0734 885–065

**1997. IFO-Institut für
Wortschaftsforschung**
Abteilung Ökonometric und
Datenverarbeitung
Poschingerstraße 5
D-8000 Munich
Germany
Telephone: 089 922–420

**1998. IFREMER (See Institut Français
de Recherche pour
l'Exploitation
de la Mer)**

1999. IFS Publications
35–39 High Street
Kempston
Bedfordshire
MK42 7BT
UK
Telephone: 0234 953–605
Fax: 0234 854–499
Telex/E-mail: 825489 G

2000. Igaku Chuo Zasshi Kanko-kai
2–5–18 Takaido Higashi
Suginami-ku
Tokyo 168
Japan
Telephone: 03 3334–7625

2001. IGTnet
3424 S State Street
Room 244 N
Chicago
IL 60616–3896
USA
Telephone: (312) 567–3663
Fax: (312) 567–5209
Telex/E-mail: 256189 INSTGASCO
JJ.KRUSE (iNet)

2002. IHS Regulatory Products Inc
Sherry Koch (Sales Representative)
4909 Pearl East Circle
Suite 104
Boulder
CO 80301
USA
Telephone: (303) 444–8535
Fax: (303) 444–8954

**2003. IInstituto de Información y
Documentación en Ciencia y
Tecnología**
Rose de la Viesca
Joaquin Costa 22
28002 Madrid
Spain
Telephone: 01 563 54 82;
01 563 54 87
Fax: 01 564 26 44

2004. IKONA Srl
Mario Taccini (Manager)
Via Montebello 37
00185 Rome
Italy
Telephone: 06 529–1742
Fax: 06 529–0932

**2005. IKS (See Institut für
Angewandte Kommunikations-
und Sprachforschung)**

2006. Il Sole 24 Ore
Mr Migli
Via Paolo Lomazzo 52
20129 Milan
Italy
Telephone: 02 31031
Fax: 02 310–3436

**2007. ILI (Informe London
Information)**
Richard Boden (Publishing Manager)
Index House
Ascot
Berkshire
SL5 7EU
UK
Telephone: 0344 874–343;
0344 233–77
Fax: 0344 291–194

**2008. Illinois Institute of
Technology**
National Institute for Petroleum and
Energy Research
PO Box 2128
Bartlesville
OK 74005
USA
Telephone: (918) 336–2400

**2009. Illinois State Legislative
Information System**
705 Stratton Office Building
Springfield
IL 62706
USA
Telephone: (217) 782–3944

2010. Image Club Graphics Inc
Danielle Dawson (Marketing Assistant)
Suite 5
1902 11th Street SE
Calgary
AB T2G 3G2
Canada
Telephone: (403) 262–8008
Fax: (403) 261–7014;
(403) 261–4013
Telex/E-mail: APPLE-LINK CDA0573

2011. Images + Data
Peter Martin (CD-ROM Sales)
Berkeley Farm House
Swindon Road
Wroughton
Swindon
SN4 9AQ
UK
Telephone: 0793 815–022
Fax: 0793 815–075

2012. Imagetects
Alan Reed (Principal)
7200 Bollinger Road
802 San José
CA 95129
USA
Telephone: (408) 252–5487
Fax: (408) 252–7409

2013. IMP Interactive Media Publishers
C Mastenbroek (Director); J G L Janssen (Director/General Manager)
Oostmaaslaan 71
3063 AN Rotterdam
Netherlands
Telephone: 010 424–4330
Fax: 010 424–4353

2014. Impact Partnership Services
16040 NE 103rd
Redmond
WA 98052
USA
Telephone: (206) 882–4506

2015. Imperial College of Science and Technology (See University of London)

2016. IMS AG
International Services Division
364 Euston Road
London
NW1 3BL
UK
Telephone: 071 387–8434
Telex/E-mail: 868953 CH

2017. IMS America Ltd
PO Box 905
Plymouth Meeting
PA 19462–0905
USA
Telephone: (215) 834–5000; (800) 523–5333
Telex/E-mail: 685–1007

2018. Imsmarq AG
Industriestraße 9
CH-6301 Zug
Switzerland
Telephone: 042 21 16 66
Fax: 042 21 07 55
Telex/E-mail: 865356

2019. IMSworld Publications Ltd
Helena Westcott-Weaver
11–13 Melton Street
London
NW1 2EH
UK
Telephone: 071 387–9880
Fax: 071 388–0036
Telex/E-mail: 295526 G

2020. In-Cat System Srl
Fabrizio Caffarelli (President)
Via Carnevali 109
20158 Milan
Italy
Telephone: 02 393–1134; 02 393–11335
Fax: 02 393–11374

2021. INaLF (Institut National de la Langue Française)
Bernard Quemada (Directeur de l'INaLF)
52 boulevard de Magenta
75010 Paris
France
Telephone: 1 42 45 00 77
Fax: 1 42 45 92 30

2022. Inc. Publishing Corporation
38 Commercial Wharf
Boston
MA 02110
USA
Telephone: (617) 227–4700

2023. INCITE
Daniel Re'em (Director)
Suite 202
Blackfriars Foundry
156 Blackfriars Road
London
SE1 8EN
UK
Telephone: 071 721–7121
Fax: 071 721–7122

2024. INCOM Information und Computer GmbH
G Frackenpohl (President)
Poppelsdorfer Allee 114
5300 Bonn 1
Germany
Telephone: 0228 63 03 16
Fax: 0228 65 63 64

2025. Incorporated News Inc
1000 E William Street
Suite 100
Carson City
NV 89701
USA
Telephone: (702) 885–9748

2026. Independant Computer Consultants Association
933 Gardenview Office Parkway
St Louis
MO 63141–5917
USA
Telephone: (314) 997–4633; (800) 438–4222

2027. Independent Insurance Agents of America
127 Peyton
Alexandria
VA 22314
USA
Telephone: (703) 683–4422

2028. Industrial Bank of Japan Limited
5–1–1 Yaesu
Chuo-ku
Tokyo 104
Japan
Telephone: 81 (3) 216–0251

2029. Industrialization Fund of Finland
Fabianinkatu 34
SF-00100 Helsinki
Finland

2030. Industriedatenbank Sachon Verlag GmbH & Co
Herr Düda (Advertising Manager)
Postfach 1213
Schlo[e1] Mindelburg
D-8948 Mindelheim
Germany
Telephone: 08261 99971; 08261 9990
Fax: 08261 999–132
Telex/E-mail: 539624 SACH D

2031. Industrielle-Services Techniques Inc
1611 Cremazie E
Montreal
PQ H2M 2P2
Canada
Telephone: (514) 383–1611

2032. Industry, Science and Technology Canada
235 Queen Street
Ottawa
ON K1A 0H5
Canada
Telephone: (613) 954–5031
Fax: (613) 954–1894
Telex/E-mail: 053 5123

2033. iNet 2000
160 Elgin Street, Room 2535
Ottawa
ON K1G 3J4
Canada
Telephone: (613) 781–5128; (800) 267–8480

2034. iNet Company of America
Westfields
4795 Meadow Wood Lane
Suite 300
Chantilly
VA 22021
USA
Telephone: (703) 631–6500; (800) 366–4638
Fax: (703) 631–4565

2035. Info Access & Distribution Pte Ltd
Lee Pit Teong (Director)
113 Eunos Avenue
3 Industrial Building 07–03
Singapore 1440
Telephone: 226–0865; 741–8422
Fax: 741–8821

2036. Info Globe
The Globe and Mail
444 Front Street West
Toronto
ON M5V 2S9
Canada
Telephone: (416) 585–5250
Fax: (416) 585–5249
Telex/E-mail: 06219629

2037. Info-Marketing Verlagsgesellschaft für Bürosysteme mbH
Grafenberger Allee 368
D-4000 Dusseldorf 1
Germany
Telephone: 0211 669–070

2038. INFO-ONE International Pty Ltd
Eddie Tracey
Level 7
77 Pacific Highway
North Sydney
NSW 2060
Australia
Telephone: 02 959–5075; 02 959–6075
Fax: 02 929–5127
Telex/E-mail: 21885 FHP AA

2039. Infobases International Inc
1875 South State Street
Orem
UT 85058
USA
Telephone: (800) 274–1048; (801) 224–2223
Fax: (801) 224–3888

2040. Infocheck Group Limited
Global Scan
Martin Bromboszcz
Godmersham Park
Godmersham
Nr Canterbury
Kent
UK
Telephone: 0227 813000
Fax: 0227 813100

2041. Infocheck Limited
D Clark (Managing Director)
28 Scrutton Street
London
EC2A 4RQ
UK
Telephone: 071 377–8872
Fax: 071 247–4194
Telex/E-mail: 892530 INFOCR G

2042. INFOCUE
N.I.F. Corporation
Kojimachi Koyo Building
1–10 Kojimachi
Chiyoda-Ku
Tokyo 102
Japan
Telephone: 81 (3) 221–0219
Fax: 81 (3) 238–9819

2043. Infodidact
Jean-Luc Arfi
5 bis rue du Louvre
75001 Paris
France
Telephone: 1 42 60 01 70
Fax: 1 42 61 72 97

2044. Infogrames Ltd
Henri Coron
18a Old Town
Clapham
London
SW4 0LB
UK
Telephone: 071 738–8199
Fax: 071 498–7593

2045. Infogrames SA
Veronique Genot (Product Manager)
84 rue du 1er Mars 1943
69628 Villeurbanne cedex
France
Telephone: 78 03 18 46
Fax: 78 03 18 40

2046. Infolink Ltd
Coombe Cross
2–4 South End
Croyden
Surrey
CR0 1DL
UK
Telephone: 081 686–7777;
081 686–5644
Fax: 081 680–8295
Telex/E-mail: 928088 UAPT G

2047. Infomart Online
1450 Don Mills Road
Don Mills
ON M3B 2X7
Canada
Telephone: (416) 445–6641;
(800) 668–9215
Fax: (416) 445–3508

2048. Infomat Ltd
VoTec Centre
Hambridge Lane
Newbury
Berkshire RG14 5HA
UK
Telephone: 0635 34867
Telex/E-mail: 265871 WQQ:363
MONREF G

2049. Infonet Inc
112 W 9th Street
Suite 102
Kansas City
MO 64105
USA
Telephone: (816) 842–8227

2050. InfoPro
8000 Westpark Drive, Suite 400
McLean
VA 22102
USA
Telephone: (703) 442–0900;
(800) 456–7248
Fax: (703) 893–4632
Telex/E-mail: 901811

2051. Infordata International Inc
4927 N Barnard
Chicago
IL 60625
USA
Telephone: (312) 583–2610

2052. Inform II Microfor
Marc André Ledoux (President)
801 Sherbrooke Street E
Suite 615
Montreal
PQ H2L 1K7
Canada
Telephone: (514) 524–7722
Fax: (514) 524 5441;
(514) 484–4223

2053. Informaat BV
GCJ Bourgonje (Commercial Manager)
Larixlaan 1
PO Box 5
1200 AA Hilversum
Netherlands
Telephone: 035 238–201
Fax: 035 239–663

2054. Informacijski Center
Kardeljava Ploscad 17
Y-61000 Ljubljana
Yugoslavia

2055. Informatics (India) Private Ltd
NV Sathyanarayana (Managing Director)
PB No 360
No 87, 2nd Floor, 11th Cross
Malleswaram
Bangalore 560003
India
Telephone: 0812 344–598
Fax: 0812 320–840

2056. Information Access Company
Peter Reardon
13 Baywell
Leybourne
West Malling
Kent
ME19 5QQ
UK
Telephone: 0732 871587
Fax: 0732 871589

2057. Information Access Company
Sandy Thorpe (Manager, Basic Products)
362 Lakeside Drive
Foster City
CA 94404–9888
USA
Telephone: (415) 591–2333;
(415) 378–5000;
(415) 378–5200;
(800) 227–8431
Fax: (415) 358–4609;
(415) 378–5420
Telex/E-mail: 12603 (DIALMAIL)

2058. Information Access Group
(a subsidiary of Ziff – includes IAC, Predicasts and Infomat)

2059. Information America
1 Georgia Center
600 W Peachtree Street NW
Atlanta
GA 30308
USA
Telephone: (404) 892–1800
Fax: (404) 881–0278

2060. Information Analytics
Moorestown
New Jersey
USA
Telephone: (215) 443 9824

2061. Information Centre for European Culture Collections
Mascheroder Weg 1b
D-3300 Braunschweig
Germany
Telephone: 0531 618–715

2062. Information Design Inc
PO Box 7130
1300 Charleston Road
Mountain View
CA 94039–7130
USA
Telephone: (415) 969–7990

2063. Information Dimensions
15 Hanover Square
London
W1R 9AJ
UK
Telephone: 071 409–1443

2064. Information Dimensions
655 Metro Place South
Dublin
OH 43017–1396
USA
Telephone: (614) 761–7303

2065. Information Express
1155 Malvern Road
Malvern
VIC 3144
Australia
Telephone: 03 823–2222
Fax: 03 823–2227
Telex/E-mail: 151224 AA 1E999C
(STARGRAM/INFOGRAM)

2066. Information for Public Affairs Inc
State Net
1900 14th Street
Sacramento
CA 95814
USA
Telephone: (916) 444–0840

2067. Information Handling Services
Department 438
Liz Maynard Prigge (Senior Manager Corporate Relations)
15 Inverness Way E
PO Box 1154
Englewood
CO 80150
USA
Telephone: (303) 790–0600;
(800) 241–7824;
(800) 525–7052
Fax: (303) 799–4085;
(303) 790–0686
Telex/E-mail: 4322083 IHSUI

2068. Information Handling Services
HAYSTACK Operations
Patricia Wimberly
80 Blanchard Road
Burlington
MA 01803
USA
Telephone: (617) 272–5560

2069. Information Inc
1725 K Street NW
Suite 1414
Washington
DC 20006
USA
Telephone: (202) 833–1174

2070. Information Indexing Inc
Chris E Nuñez (Publisher)
12872 Valley View Street
Suite 10
Garden Grove
CA 92645
USA
Telephone: (714) 893–2471
Fax: (714) 893–4856

2071. Information Industry Association
Liz Dechert (Database & Publishing Division Liaison)
555 New Jersey Avenue NW
Suite 800
Washington
DC 20001
USA
Telephone: (202) 639–8262
Fax: (202) 638–4403

2072. Information Institute of Medical Science and Technology
State Medicine and Drug Administration Bureau
38A North Lishi Road
Xicheng District
Beijing 100810
China
Telephone: (83) 13344–1804

2073. Information Intelligence Inc
Richard S Huleatt (President/Publisher)
PO Box 31098
Phoenix
AZ 85046
USA
Telephone: (602) 996–2283;
          (800) 228–9982

2074. Information North
Michael Long (Manager)
Quaker Meeting House
1 Archibold Terrace
Newcastle-Upon-Tyne
NE2 1DB
UK
Telephone: 091 281–8887
Fax: 091 212–0922

2075. Information Plus
DRI/McGraw Hill
1750 K Street NW, Suite 1060
Washington
DC 20006
USA
Telephone: (202) 862–3720
Telex/E-mail: 440480 DRI WASHDC

2076. Information Products Europe
Mergenthaler Allec 31–33
W-6236 Eschborn/TS
Germany
Telephone: +49 6196 496175

2077. Information Resources Inc
150 N Clinton Street
Chicago
IL 60606
USA
Telephone: (312) 726–1221

2078. Information Resources Inc
499 South Capitol Street SW
Suite 406
Washington
DC 20003
USA
Telephone: (202) 554–0614
Fax: (202) 554–0613

2079. Information Services Corporation
Sofia
Bulgaria
Telephone: +3592 442249
Fax: +3592 463247

2080. Information Services Inc
2852 Bluebill Drive
Virginia Beach
VA 23456
USA
Telephone: (804) 427–3659;
          (804) 427–3665

2081. Information Services Limited
Windsor Court
East Grinstead House
East Grinstead
West Sussex
RH19 1XE
UK
Telephone: 44 (342) 26972

2082. Information Sources Inc
Ruth Koolish (President)
1173 Colusa Avenue
PO Box 7848
Berkeley
CA 94707
USA
Telephone: (415) 525–6220;
          (800) 433–6107
Fax: (415) 525–1568

2083. Information Update Inc
Dennis Beaumont (Executive Vice President)
101 First Street
Suite 432
Los Altos
CA 94022–2792
USA
Telephone: (408) 720–0804
Fax: (415) 941–5208

2084. Information USA Inc
10335 Kensington Parkway
PO Box E
Kensington
MD 20895
USA
Telephone: (301) 369–1519;
          (800) 545–3758
Fax: (301) 929–8970

2085. Information Ventures Inc
Dr Robert Goldberg (Project Director)
1500 Locust Street
Suite 3213
Philadelphia
PA 19102
USA
Telephone: (215) 732–9083
Fax: (215) 732–3754

2086. Informationszentrum für Biologie
Forschungsinstitut Senckenberg
Senckenberganlage 25
D-6000 Frankfurt am Main 1
Germany
Telephone: 069 754–2350
Fax: 069 746–238
Telex/E-mail: 413129 D

2087. Informationszentrum RAUM und BAU
Nobelstrasse 12
D-7000 Stuttgart 80
Germany
Telephone: 0711/970–2555
Fax: 0711/970–2700
Telex/E-mail: 7255167 IRB D

2088. Informationszentrum Sozialwissenschaften
Lennestrasse 30
5000 Bonn 1
Germany
Telephone: 49 (228) 22 81 – 0
Fax: 49 (228) 22 81 – 120

2089. Informcenter VNIRO
Dr Ivan Bukhanevich (Director); Vera Ulanova (Assistant)
V Krasnoselskaya 17
107140 Moscow
Russia
Telephone: 264–9367
          264–6533
Fax: 264–9187

2090. Informed Communications Inc
510 E 23rd Street
New York
NY 10010
USA
Telephone: (212) 979–7881

2091. INFORMENERGO
c/o International Centre for Scientific and Technical Information
Ulitsa Kuusinena 21b
125252 Moscow
Russia
Telephone: 095 198–7460
Fax: 095 943–0089
Telex/E-mail: 411925 MCNTI SU

2092. INFORMIT
Jan Swinburne
GPO Box 2476V
Melbourne
VIC 3001
Australia
Telephone: 03 660–2062
Fax: 03 663–3047

2093. Inforonics Inc
550 Newtown Road
PO Box 458
Littleton
MA 01460
USA
Telephone: (617) 486–8976

2094. Infoscan – M. Nissen LIE A/S
Morten Groseth
PO Box 35 BYGDOY
Dronningen
0211 Oslo 2
Norway
Telephone: 47 (2) 556–220
Fax: 47 (2) 434–702

2095. Infosearch
Istel Limited
PO Box 5
Grosvenor House
Prospect Hill
Redditch
Worcestershire
B97 4DQ
UK
Telephone: 44 (527) 64274 x4632
Fax: 44 (527) 63360
Telex/E-mail: 339954 ISTEL G

2096. Infotap
Infopartners
2, rue A. Borschette
BP 262
2012 Luxembourg
Luxembourg
Telephone: (352) 43 61 65

2097. InfoTeam Inc, The
PO Box 15640
Plantation
FL 33318–5640
USA
Telephone: (305) 473–9560
Fax: (305) 473–0544

2098. Infotech Research
Trumanstede 9320
Amsterdam
4463 WE GOES
Netherlands

**2099. Infotechnology Publishing
     Corporation**
9990 Lee Highway
Room 301
Fairfax
VA 22030–1720
USA

2100. Infotouch
Hib Broekman
PO Box 81
8200 AB Lelystad
Netherlands
Telephone: 03200 33225
Fax: 03200 33880

2101. INFOTRADE NV
Jos Schepens
A Gossetlaan 32a
B-1720 Groot-Bijgaarden
Belgium
Telephone: 02 466 64 80
Fax: 02 466 69 70
Telex/E-mail: 62862 DGROUP B
NUA: Available on application

2102. InfoWorld Magazine
1060 Marsh Road
Suite C-200
Menlo Park
CA 94025
USA

2103. Ingram Customer Systems Inc
Art Carson (Vice President Field Sales)
1125 Heil Quaker Boulevard
La Vergne
TN 37086
USA
Telephone: (615) 793–5000;
            (800) 937–7978
Fax: (615) 793–3825

2104. Ingram Distribution Group Inc
347 Reedwood Drive
Nashville
TN 37217
USA
Telephone: (800) 251–5902

2105. Ingram Micro D
Softeurop
Avenue des Eglantiers 14
B-1180 Brussels
Belgium
Telephone: 2 722 9511

2106. Ingram Micro
Barry Evleth (Product Manager)
2801 S Yale Street
Santa Ana
CA 92704
USA
Telephone: (714) 540–4781 x2713
Fax: (714) 540–0932

2107. INION RAN
Online Service Group
Lada Gromova
Ul. Krasikova 28/21
117418 Moscow
Russia

**2108. INIST (See Centre National de
     la Recherche Scientifique,
     Institut de l'Information
     Scientifique et Technique)**

2109. INKADAT
Dr B Jenschke
c/o KIZ Karslruhe
D-7514 Eggenstein-Leopoldshafen 2
Germany
Telephone: 07247 808–555
Fax: 07247 808–666
Telex/E-mail: 17724710 D
NUA: 26245724740141;
     26245724740001

2110. Innotech Inc
Simon Arnison (Director, CD-ROM
     Services)
110 Silver Star Boulevard
Unit 107
Scarborough
Toronto
ON M1V 5A2
Canada
Telephone: (416) 321–3838
Fax: (416) 321–0095

**2111. Innovationstechnik GmbH &
     Company**
Subvent Datenbank Systeme
Heinrich-Hertz-Straße 15
D-2000 Hamburg 76
Germany
Telephone: 040 229–0008

**2112. Innovative Technologies
     Inc**
7927 Jones Branch Drive
Suite 500
McLean
VA 22102
USA
Telephone: (703) 734–3000;
            (800) 327–6514
Fax: (703) 734–3210

2113. Innovest Systems Inc
111 Broadway
Suite 1400
New York
NY 10006
USA
Telephone: (212) 608–4650

**2114. INSERM – Institut National de
     la Santé et de la Recherche**
Médicale
IMA
Hôpital de Bicêtre
80 Rue du Général Leclerc
94276 Le Kremlin Bicêtre
France
Telephone: (33) 1–49 59 19 21
Fax: (33) 1–46 58 40 57
NUA: 36 29 00 36; 36 13 INSERM

2115. INSERM-IMA
Anne Sarjeant (CD-MED Service);
Jacques Halpern
Hôpital de Bicêtre
94270 Le Kremlin Bicêtre
France
Telephone: 1 45 21 10 44
Fax: 1 46 58 40 57

2116. INSPEC
Diane Richards (New Products
     Manager)
Michael Faraday House
Six Hills Way
Stevenage
Hertfordshire
SG1 2AY
UK
Telephone: 0438 313–311
Fax: 0438 742–840
Telex/E-mail: 825578 IEESTV G;
11472 INSPEC UK (DIALMAIL);
     INSPEC (DATAMAIL)

2117. INSPEC
IEEE Service Center
Jim Ashling
445 Hoes Lane
PO Box 1331
Piscataway
NJ 08855–1331
USA
Telephone: (908) 562–5549
Fax: (908) 981–0027
Telex/E-mail: 833233 IEEE PWAY

2118. Instant Software Generation
98 Battery St.
Fourth Floor
San Francisco
CA 94111
USA
Telephone: (415) 434–2122

2119. Institut Belge de Normalisation
29 Avenue de la Brabanconne
B-1040 Brussels
Belgium
Telephone: 02 734 92 05
Fax: 02 733 42 64
Telex/E-mail: 23877 BENOR B

2120. Institut Boiron
20 rue de le Liberation
F-69110 Sainte Foy-les-Lyon
France
Telephone: 72 32 41 31

**2121. Institut d'Amenagement et
     d'Urbanisme de la Region
     d'Ile-de-France**
Micette Hercelin
Secretariat Permanent 1990
251 rue de Vaugirard
75740 Paris Cedex 15
France
Telephone: 40 43 79 66
Fax: 40 43 76 02

**2122. Institut d'Estadistica de
     Catalunya**
Xavier Lopez
Calabria 168
08015 Barcelona
Spain
Telephone: 093 425 21 11
Fax: 093 425 04 06
Telex/E-mail: 54310 E

2123. Institut d'Etudes Politiques
Centre Regional d'Informations
     Politiques, Economiques et Sociales
1 rue Raulin
F-69007 Lyon
France
Telephone: 78 72 85 63

2124. Institut de l'Audiovisuel et des Telecommunications en Europe
Bureaux de Polygone
34000 Montpelier
France
Telephone: 33 (67) 65 48 48
Fax: 33 (67) 65 57 19
Telex/E-mail: 490290 IDATE F

2125. Institut de l'Information Scientifique et Technique (See Centre National de la Recherche Scientifique, Institute de l'Information Scientifique et Technique)

2126. Institut de Recherches et d'Études sur le Monde Arabe et Musulman
Maison de la Mediterranée
3–7 avenue Pasteur
F-13100 Aix-en-Provence
France
Telephone: 042 245–988

2127. Institut de Recherches Mediterraniennes
Reseau d'Information en Sciences Humaines de la Santé
3–5 avenue Pasteur
13100 Aix en Provence
France
Telephone: 33 (42) 21 59 88

2128. Institut de Recherches sur les Fruits et Agrumes
6 rue du Clergerie
75116 Paris
France
Telephone: 33 (1) 45 53 16 92
Telex/E-mail: 610992 F

2129. Institut der Deutschen Wirtschaft
PO Box 51 06 69
Gustav-Heinemann-Ufer 84–88
D-5000 Cologne 51
Germany
Telephone: 0221 375–550
Fax: 0221 376–5555
Telex/E-mail: 8882768 IWK D GEO3 1WDAT (GEONET)

2130. Institut Français de Recherche pour l'Exploitation de la Mer
Mme Proehonne
SDP
Centre de Brest
BP 70
29263 Plouzane
France
Telephone: 98 22 40 40
Fax: 98 22 45 45

2131. Institut Français du Petrole
Direction de l'Economie et de la Documentation
1–4 avenue de Bois-Preau
BP 311
F-92506 Rueil-Malmaison
France
Telephone: 1 47 49 02 14
Fax: 1 47 52 64 29
Telex/E-mail: 203050 IFP A F

2132. Institut für Angewandte Kommunikations- und Sprachforschung eV
J Brustkern (Executive Director)
Poppelsdorfer Allee 47
5300 Bonn 1
Germany
Telephone: 0228 735–645
Fax: 0228 735–639

2133. Institut für Dokumentation und Information, Sozialmedizin und Öffentliches Gesundheitswesen
Postfach 20 10 12
Westerfeldstraße 35–37
D-4800 Bielefeld 1
Germany
Telephone: 0521 86033

2134. Institut für Wirtschaftsforschung
HWWA
Jungfernstieg 21
2000 Hamburg 36
Germany
Telephone: 49 40 3562–0
Fax: 49 40 351900

2135. Institut International du Froid
Documentary Service
177 boulevard Malesherbes
F-75017 Paris
France
Telephone: 1 42 27 32 35
Fax: 1 47 63 17 98
Telex/E-mail: 643269 ININFRI F

2136. Institut National de la Langue Française (See INaLF)

2137. Institut National de la Propriété Industrielle
Catherine Pagis (Marketing Manager)
26 bis rue de Léningrad
F-75800 Paris Cedex 08
France
Telephone: 1 42 94 52 60;
  1 42 94 52 61;
  1 42 93 21 20
Fax: 1 42 93 59 30
Telex/E-mail: 290368 F

2138. Institut National de la Recherche Agronomique
147 rue de l'Université
75328 Paris
France
Telephone: 1 42 97 90 00
Fax: 1 47 05 99 66
Telex/E-mail: 695269 INFRAVER F

2139. Institut National de la Statistique et des Etudes Economiques
18 boulevard Adolphe Pinard
F-75675 Paris Cedex 14
France
Telephone: 1 45 40 06 14
Telex/E-mail: 204924 INSEE F

2140. Institut National de Recherche en Informatique et Automatique
Domaine de Voluceau-Rocquencourt
PO Box 105
78153 Le Chesnay Cedex
France
Telephone: 33 (1) 39 63 55 11
Telex/E-mail: 697033 F

2141. Institut National de Recherche et de Sécurité
Service de Documentation
M Le Ruz
30 rue Oliver Noyer
F-75680 Paris Cedex 14
France
Telephone: 1 40 44 30 26;
  1 40 44 30 00
Fax: 1 40 44 30 99

2142. Institut Quebeçois de Recherche sur la Culture
14 rue Haldimand
Quebec City
PQ G1R 4N4
Canada
Telephone: (418) 643–4695

2143. Institut Technique du Batiment
Centre d'Assistance Technique et de Documentation
Domaine de St Paul
F-78470 Saint Remy-les-Chevreuse
France
Telephone: 1 30 85 24 72
Fax: 1 30 85 24 66
Telex/E-mail: 611975 FEDEBAT F
NUA: 208075000155DAT

2144. Institut Textile de France
PO Box 141
F-92223 Bagneux Cedex
France
Telephone: 1 46 64 15 40
Telex/E-mail: 250940 ITEXFRA F

2145. Institut za Nuklearne Nauke Boris Kidric
PO Box 522
YU-11000 Belgrade
Yugoslavia
Telephone: 011 440–871
Telex/E-mail: 32121 KIBKLJ YU

2146. Institute for Fermentation
Hakko Kenkyujo
17–85 Juso-honmachi 2–chome
Yodogawa-ku
Osaka 532
Japan
Telephone: 06 302–7281
Fax: 06 300–6814

2147. Institute for Industrial Research & Standards
Balymun Rd.
Dublin 9
Eire

2148. Institute for Research in Constuction
National Research Council Canada
Building M-20
Ottawa
ON K1A 0R6
Canada
Telephone: (613) 993–3773
Fax: (613) 954–5984
Telex/E-mail: 0533145 CA

2149. Institute for Scientific Information
European Branch
Robert Kimberly (Managing Director)
Brunel Science Park
Brunel University
Uxbridge
Middlesex
UB8 3PQ
UK
Telephone: 0895 270–016
Fax: 0895 256–710
Telex/E-mail: 933693 UKISI

2150. Institute for Scientific Information
Barabara Negy-Teti (CD-ROM Index Products)
3501 Market Street
Philadelphia
PA 19104
USA
Telephone: (215) 386–0100;
  (800) 336–4474;
  (800) 523–1857
Fax: (215) 386–6362
Telex/E-mail: 845305 15010 (DIALMAIL)

2151. Institute of Chartered Accountants in Australia
Level 11
37 York Street
PO Box 3921
Sydney
NSW 2000
Australia
Telephone: 02 290–1344
Fax: 02 299–1689
Telex/E-mail: 26534 AA

2152. Institute of Cultural Affairs International
8 rue Amadee Lynen
B-1050 Brussels
Belgium
Telephone: 02 219–0087
Telex/E-mail: 62035 ICABRU B

2153. Institute of Electrical and Electronics Engineers Inc
Jim Ashling
445 Hoess Lane
PO Box 1331
Piscataway
NJ 08855–1331
USA
Telephone: (908) 562–5550
Fax: (908) 981–0027

2154. Institute of Energy Economics
Energy Data and Modeling Center
No 10 Mori Building
1–18–1 Toranomon
Minato-ku
Tokyo 105
Japan
Telephone: 03 3501–7864
         03 3501–2901
Telex/E-mail: 2225427 IEETKY J

2155. Institute of Freight Forwarders Limited
Redfern House
Browells LAne
Saltham
Middlesex
TW13 7EP
UK
Telephone: 44 (1) 844–2266

2156. Institute of Gas Technology
Technical Information Services
3424 S State Street
Room 244 N
Chicago
IL 60616–3896
USA
Telephone: (312) 567–3650
Fax: (312) 567–5209
Telex/E-mail: 256189 INSTGASCO

2157. Institute of Inorganic Chemistry
University of Bonn
Gerhard-Domagk-Strasse 1
5300 Bonn 1
Germany
Telephone: 49 (228) 73 26 57

2158. Institute of International Finance
2000 Pennsylvania Avenue NW
Suite 8500
Washington
DC 20006
USA
Telephone: (202) 857–3600

2159. Institute of Journal Industrial Titles, The
Library Department
1–9–4 Otemachi
Chiyoda-ku
Tokyo 100
Japan

2160. Institute of Metals, The
Materials Information
1 Carlton House Terrace
London
SW1Y 5DB
UK
Telephone: 071 839–4071
Fax: 071 839–2289
Telex/E-mail: 8814813 METSOC G

2161. Institute of Microbiology
Chinese Academy of Sciences
Song Da Kang (Director)
Zhongguancun
Haidlan District
Beijing 100080
China
Telephone: 282057

2162. Institute of Paper Science and Technology Inc
575 14th Street NW
Atlanta
GA 30318
USA
Telephone: (404) 853–9500
Fax: (404) 853–9510
Telex/E-mail: 25526 (DIALMAIL)

2163. Institute of Petroleum
61 New Cavendish Street
London
W1M 8AR
UK
Telephone: 071 636–1004

2164. Institute of Scientific and Technical Information of China
Chongging Branch
Huo Lipu; Wang Shide
PO Box 2104
Chongging
Sichuan 630013
China
Telephone: (86) 811–357022 x4085
Fax: (86) 811–352473
Telex/E-mail: 62128 CBIST CN

2165. Institute of Textile Technology
Textile Information Center
PO Box 391
Charlottesville
VA 22902
USA
Telephone: (804) 296–5511
Fax: (804) 977–5400

2166. Institutet for Byggdokumentation
Halsingegatan 47
S-113 31 Stockholm
Sweden
Telephone: 08 340–170
Fax: 08 324–859
Telex/E-mail: 12563 BYGGDOK S

2167. Institutet for Lärarutbildning (See Interactive Media Group)

2168. Institution of Chemical Engineers
George E Davies Building
165–171 Railway Terrace
Rugby
Warwickshire
CV21 3HQ
UK
Telephone: 0788 78214
Fax: 0788 60833
Telex/E-mail: 311780 ICHEME G

2169. Institution of Electrical Engineers (See also INSPEC)

2170. Institution of Electrical Engineers (IEE)
Technical Information Unit
Savoy Place
London
WC2R 0BL
UK
Telephone: 071 240–1871
Fax: 071 240–7735
Telex/E-mail: 261176 IEELDN G

2171. Institution of Engineers, Australia
11 National Circuit
Barton
ACT 2600
Australia
Telephone: 6 270–6555
Fax: 6 273–1488
Telex/E-mail: 62758 AA

2172. Institution of Mining and Metallurgy
Library and Information Services
44 Portland Place
London
W1N 4BR
UK
Telephone: 071 580–3802
Fax: 071 436–5388
Telex/E-mail: 261410 IMM G

2173. Institutional Investor
488 Madison Avenue
New York
NY 10022
USA
Telephone: (212) 303–3300;
         (212) 303–3368
Fax: (212) 303–3592

2174. Institutionen for Lararutbildning
Box 2136
75002 Uppsala
Sweden
Telephone: 18 18 24 65

2175. Instituto de Centro Nazionale ricerche
CNUCE
Mr G Argentieri
Via Santa Maria 36
I-56100 Pisa
Italy
Telephone: +39 5–0593111
NUA: Available on application

2176. Instituto de la Mujer
Almagro 36
28071 Madrid
Spain
Telephone: 01 410 39 74

2177. Instituto de la Pequena y Mediana Empresa Industrial
Fermin Montero
Paseo de la Castellana 141
E-28046 Madrid
Spain
Telephone: 01 582 93 00;
01 582 93 38;
01 582 93 36
Fax: 01 571 28 31
NUA: 213022023; 213022024;
212020429; 212024415

2178. Instituto Español de Comercio Exterior
Antonio Rodriques (Jefe de Departemento de Encuestas y Bases de Datos)
Paseo de la Castellana 14
28046 Madrid
Spain
Telephone: 01 431–1240
Fax: 01 431–6128
Telex/E-mail: 44838 IECE E

2179. Instituto Geográfico Nacional
Calle General Ibanez de Ibero 3
28003 Madrid
Spain
Telephone: 01 233 38 00
Telex/E-mail: 23465 ICG E

2180. Instituto Nacional de Estadistica
Paseo de la Castellana 183
28046 Madrid
Spain
Telephone: 01 270 06 37

2181. Instituto Nacional de Fomento de la Exportación
Amporo Vera
Paeso de la Castellana 14
E-28046 Madrid
Spain
Telephone: +34 1–4311240
Fax: +34 1–4316128
NUA: Available on application

2182. Instituto Nacional de la Administracion Publica
Centro de Estudios y Documentacion
Calle Zurbano 42
28003 Madrid
Spain
Telephone: 34 (1) 410 60 41

2183. Instituto Nacional de Seguridad e Higiene en el Trabajo
Centro Nacional de Condiciones de Trabajo
Calle Dulcet s/n
08034 Barcelona
Spain
Telephone: 34 (3) 204 45 00
Fax: 34 (3) 204 46 55

2184. Instituto National de Investigacao Cientifica
Centro de Documentacao Cientifica e Tecnica
Av Prof Gama Pinto 2
1699 Lisbon Codex
Portugal
Telephone: 01 793–1300
Fax: 01 765–622
Telex/E-mail: 63593 TIFM P G. Lopez
DASILVA (DataMail)

2185. Instituto para la Diversificación y Ahorro de la Energia
Paseo de la Castellana 95
Edificio Torre Europa
28046 Madrid
Spain
Telephone: 01 442 90 22
Fax: 01 455 13 89
Telex/E-mail: 42885 SEID E

2186. Instituto Tecnologico GeoMinero de España
Calle Rios Rosas 23
28003 Madrid
Spain
Telephone: 01 441–6500
Fax: 01 442–6216

2187. Insurance Information Institute
110 William Street
New York
NY 10038
USA
Telephone: (212) 669–9200
Fax: (212) 732–1916

2188. Insurance Marketing Services
525 Broadway
Suite 300
PO Box 2440
Santa Monica
CA 90407–2440
Telephone: (213) 458–3222;
(800) 753–4467
Fax: (213) 395–9018

2189. INTA
Torrejon de Ardoz
Madrid
Spain

2190. Intechnica International Inc
Stan Bolin (President)
PO Box 30877
Midwest City
OK 73140
USA
Telephone: (405) 732–0138;
(800) 788–8730
Fax: (405) 732–4574

2191. Integrated Digital Services Ltd
93–99 Upper Richmond Road
London
SW15 2TG
UK
Telephone: 081 789–1200

2192. Integrated Information Private Ltd.
456 Alexandra Road
18 NOL Building
0511
Singapore

2193. Integrated Marketing Services (see American Express Information Services Company)

2194. Integrierte Business Systems
Carl-Zeiss-Strasse 25
3008 Garbsen 4
Germany
Telephone: +49 5131 7000 17
Fax: +49 5131 7000 15

2195. Intel Corporation
Microcomputer Components Group
3065 Bowers Ave.
NW1–17
Santa Clara
CA 95052
USA
Telephone: (408) 765–4758

2196. Intellibanc Corporation
8220 Delmar Boulevard
Suite 260
St Louis
MO 63214
USA
Telephone: (314) 567–6009

2197. Intelligate
Bell Atlantic
181 North Lane
Conshohocken
PA 19428
USA
Telephone: (800) 543–8843

2198. IntelliGenetics Inc
A Akhtari
Amocolaan 2
B-2440 Geel
Belgium
Telephone: 014 57 83 35
Fax: 014 58 50 78

2199. IntelliGenetics Inc
Yuki Abe (GenBank Administrator)
700 East El Camino Real
Mountain View
CA 94040
USA
Telephone: (415) 962–7300;
(415) 962–7364
Fax: (415) 962–7302
Telex/E-mail: 4937543

2200. Intelligent Information (ii)
INFOTAP SA
B.P. 262
2012 Luxembourg
Luxembourg
Telephone: (352) 436165
Fax: (352) 433159
Telex/E-mail: 60468 ILUX LU

2201. Inter-University Consortium for Political and Social Research
Consortium Data Network
University of Michigan
Institute for Social Research
PO Box 1248
Ann Arbor
MI 48106
USA
Telephone: (313) 763–5010;
(313) 764–2570

2202. Interactive Biological Information System Group
University of Nottingham, Department of Life Science
Dr Peter Davies; Dr Susan Scarborough
IBIS Development Group
Nottingham
NG7 2RD
UK
Telephone: 0602 484–848 x 2056
Fax: 0602 790–782

2203. Interactive Data Corporation
12–15 Fetter Lane
6th Floor
London
EC4A 1BR
UK
Telephone: 071 583–0765

2204. Interactive Data Corporation
95 Hayden Avenue
Lexington
MA 02173–9144
USA
Telephone: (617) 863–8100

2205. Interactive Data GmbH
Taunusanlage 11
D-6000 Frankfurt am Main 1
Germany
Telephone: 069 253–077

2206. Interactive Data Services Inc
Larry Jacobsen (Director of Marketing)
14 Wall Street
12th Floor
New York
NY 10005
USA
Telephone: (212) 285–0700
Fax: (212) 306–6962

**2207. Interactive Design and
Development Inc**
Teresa M Hypes (Assistant Director);
Mary G Miller (Director)
105 Colony Park
2001 S Main Street
Blacksburg
VA 24060
USA
Telephone: (703) 951–9836
Fax: (703) 951–9839

**2208. Interactive Market Systems
(UK) Limited**
Grosvenor Gardens House
Grosvenor Gardens
London
SW1W 0BS
UK
Telephone: 071 630–5033

2209. Interactive Market Systems Inc
Kelly Smith (Publications)
11 W 42nd Street
11th Floor
New York
NY 10036–8088
USA
Telephone: (212) 789–3600;
(800) 223–7942
Fax: (212) 789–3636

2210. Interactive Media Group
Arne Lindquist (Project Coordinator)
Institutet for Lärarutbildning
PO Box 2136
750 02 Uppsala
Sweden
Telephone: 01818 2465
Fax: 01818 2400

**2211. Interactive Media Publications
Ltd**
IM Publications Ltd
104a St. John Street
London
EC1M 4EH
UK
Telephone: 071 490–1185
Fax: 071 490–4706

2212. Interactive Office Services
3 Blackstone Street
Cambridge
MA 02139
USA
Telephone: (617) 876–5551
Fax: (617) 661–3354
Telex/E-mail: TRAVEL (DELPHI)

2213. Interavia Publishing
A part of Jane's Information Group
4201 Wilshire Blvd, Suite 406
Los Angeles
CA 90010
USA
Telephone: (213) 933–4600

**2214. Intercom Information
Resources**
PO Box 180231
Austin
TX 78718–0231
USA
Telephone: (512) 339–6383
Telex/E-mail: 6502506618 Via WUI

**2215. Intercontinental Marketing
Corp.**
Warren Ball, President
Japan
Telephone: +81 3 6618373
Fax: +81 3 6679646

**2216. Intercontinental Medical
Statistics Limited**
364 Euston Road
London
NW1 3BL
UK
Telephone: 071 387–8434

2217. Intercorp
86 Viaduct Road
PO Box 4430
Stamford
CT 06907
USA
Telephone: (203) 278–3800

2218. Interests Ltd
8512 Cedar Sireet
Silver Spring
MD 20910
USA
Telephone: (301) 588–7916
Fax: (301) 588–2085
Telex/E-mail: 6501701421; 71067,1407
(CompuServe Information Service);
170–1412 (MCI Mail)

2219. Interfoto-Pressebild-Agentur
Mr Rauch
Stollbergstrasse 1
D-8000 Munchen 22
Germany
Telephone: 089 224484

**2220. Intergovernmental
Oceanographic Commission**
Trevor Sankey (Assistant Secretary)
Unesco
7 place de Fontenoy
75700 Paris
France
Telephone: 1 45 68 40 08
Fax: 1 45 67 16 90
Telex/E-mail: 204461 F

2221. Interlink
Telephone: +7 (95) 192 8834
Fax: +7 (95) 943 0087

**2222. International Academy at Santa
Barbara**
Peggy Cordero
800 Garden Street
Suite D
Santa Barbara
CA 93101–1552
USA
Telephone: (805) 965–5010
Fax: (805) 965–6071
Telex/E-mail: JSTJOHN (Sprintmail and
NOTICE)

2223. International Advancement Inc
14825 Begonias Lane
Canyon Country
CA 91351
USA
Telephone: (805) 252–2177

**2224. International Air Transport
Association**
1730 K Street, NW
Washington
DC 20006
USA
Telephone: (202) 822–3929

**2225. International Archives Institute
Inc**
William W Buchanan (President)
105 B Douglas Court
Sterling
VA 22170
USA
Telephone: (703) 318–7768;
(800) 833–3627
Fax: (703) 318–7319

**2226. International Association of
Corporate Real Estate
Executives Inc**
471 Spencer Drive South, Suite 8
West Palm Beach
FL 33409–6685
USA
Telephone: (305) 683–8111

**2227. International Atomic Energy
Agency**
Wagramerstraße 5
PO Box 100
A-1400 Vienna
Austria
Telephone: 01 2360–2883
Fax: 01 234–564
Telex/E-mail: 112645 A NIU IAEA1
(EARN/BITNET)

**2228. International Blind Users
Group**
PO Box 1352
Roseville
CA 95661–1352
USA
Telephone: (916) 783–0364

2229. International Brainware
Dr Eric Melse
PO Box 423
NL-2270 CK Voorburg
Netherlands
Telephone: 70 475 993
Fax: 70 459 290

2230. International Brainware
Jim Rosenvall
Electronic Text Corporation
778 South 400 East
Orem
UT 84058
USA
Telephone: (801) 226–0616
Fax: (801) 226–4278

**2231. International Bureau of Fiscal
Documentation**
Alexander T Dek (Sales Manager)
PO Box 20237
NL-1000 HE Amsterdam
Netherlands
Telephone: 020 626–7726;
020 626–7728
Fax: 020 622–8658;
020 208–626
Telex/E-mail: 13217 INTAX NL

**2232. International BusinessMan
News Bureau**
485 5th Avenue
Suite 1042
New York
NY 10017
USA
Telephone: (212) 503–0802

2233. International Center for Scientific and Technical Information
Ulitsa Kuusinena 21b
125252 Moscow
Russia
Telephone: 095 198–7460
Fax: 095 943–0089
Telex/E-mail: 411925 MCNTI SU

2234. International Centre for Diffraction Data
Mark Holomany (Systems Manager)
1601 Park Lane
Swarthmore
PA 19081–2389
USA
Telephone: (215) 328–9400
Fax: (215) 328–2503

2235. International Civil Aviation Organization
1000 Sherbrooke Street W
Suite 400
Montreal
PQ H3A 2R2
Canada
Telephone: (514) 286–4816;
(514) 285–6716;
(514) 286–6292
Fax: (514) 288–4772
Telex/E-mail: 0524513 CA

2236. International Coffee Organization
22 Berners Street
London
W1P 4DD
UK
Telephone: 071 580–8591
Fax: 071 580–6129
Telex/E-mail: 267659 INTCAF G 18759
(DIALMAIL)

2237. International Commission on Glass
Pool d'Abstracts
Stazione Sperimentale del Vetro
Via Briati 10
I-30141 Murano-Venezia
Italy
Telephone: 041 739–422
Fax: 041 739–420
Telex/E-mail: 420698 SPEVET I

2238. International Committee for Social Science Information and Documentation
27 rue Saint-Guillaume
F-75341 Paris Cedex 7
France
Telex/E-mail: 201002 SCIPOL F

2239. International Commodities Clearing House
10 Spring Street
Sydney
NSW 2000
Australia
Fax: 02 251–5152
Telex/E-mail: 122142 AA

2240. International Computaprint Corporation
Jim Krull (Marketing)
475 Virginia Drive
Fort Washington
PA 19034
USA
Telephone: (215) 641–6000
Fax: (215) 641–6067;
(215) 641–6227

2241. International Conference of Building Officials
5360 South Workman Mill Road
Whittier
CA 90601
USA
Telephone: (213) 699–0541
Fax: (213) 692–3853

2242. International Data Corporation
5 Speen Street
PO Box 9015
Framingham
MA 01701–9908
USA
Telephone: (508) 872–8200
Fax: (508) 935–4015
Telex/E-mail: 951168

2243. International Data Group
Germany
Telephone: +49 89 224676
Fax: +49 89 295249

2244. International Data Media (UK) Limited
Dunster House
Mincing Lane
London
EC3R 7BQ
UK
Telephone: 071 283–4445

2245. International Data Pty Ltd
Greg Bullard
258 Little Bourke Street
4th Floor
Melbourne
Victoria 3000
Australia
Telephone: +61 03 663 7533
Fax: +61 3 663 4590

2246. International Energy Agency
Organization for Economic Cooperation
and Development (OECD)
2 rue Andre-Pascal
75775 Paris Cedex 16
France
Telephone: 33 (1) 45 24 82 00
Telex/E-mail: 630190 ENERG A F

2247. International Executive Reports Ltd
717 D Street NW
Suite 300
Washington
DC 20004–2807
USA
Telephone: (202) 628–6900
Fax: (202) 628–6618
Telex/E-mail: 440462

2248. International Federation of Multiple Sclerosis Societies
309 Heddon Street
London
W1R 7LE
UK
Telephone: 071 734–9120

2249. International Federation of the Societies of Cosmetic Chemists
Delaport House
57 Guilford Street
Luton
Bedfordshire
LU1 2NL
UK
Telephone: 0582 26661
Fax: 0582 405–217
Telex/E-mail: 826314 G

2250. International Food Information Service GmbH
IFIS
Günther Kalbskopf (Managing Director)
Melibocusstraße 52
D-6000 Frankfurt am Main 71
Germany
Telephone: 069 669–0070
Fax: 069 669–00710
Telex/E-mail: 14423 (DIALMAIL)
DIFISFRG (DATAMAIL)

2251. International Food Information Service
IFIS
c/o National Food Lab Inc.
6363 Clark Avenue
Dublin
CA 94568
USA
Telephone: (800) 336 3782
Fax: (415) 833 8795

2252. International Foundation of Employee Benefit Plans
PO Box 69
18700 W Bluemound Road
Brookfield
WI 53008–0069
USA
Telephone: (414) 786–6700
Fax: (414) 786–2990

2253. International Freedom Foundation
200 G Street
Suite 300
Washington
DC 20002
USA
Telephone: (202) 546–5788

2254. International Halley Watch
Jet Propulsion Laboratories
4800 Oak Grove Drive
Mail Stop 169–237
Pasadena
CA 91109
USA
Telephone: (818) 354–8751

2255. International Industrial Information Ltd
PO Box 12
Monmouth
Gwent
NP5 3YL
UK
Telephone: 0600 890–274
Telex/E-mail: 497104 LINDLY G

2256. International Institute of Refrigeration
177 Boulevard Malesherbes
75017 Paris
France
Telephone: 33 (1) 42 27 32 35
Fax: 33 (1) 47 63 17 98
Telex/E-mail: 643269 ININFRI F

2257. International Labour Organisation (See CIS)

2258. International Labour Organisation (See UN International Labour Organisation)

2259. International Marine Banking Company Limited
401 North Washington Street
Rockville
MD 20850
USA
Telephone: (301) 340–4000
Telex/E-mail: 898360

**2260. International Media
    Corporation**
110 N Royal Street
Suite 307
Alexandria
VA 22314
USA
Telephone: (703) 684–8455

**2261. International Medical Tribune
    Syndicate**
257 Park Avenue S
19th Floor
New York
NY 10010
USA
Telephone: (212) 674–8500

2262. International Monetary Fund
Bureau of Statistics
James McKee (Statistics Department)
700 19th Street NW
Washington
DC 20431
USA
Telephone: (202) 473–7904;
        (202) 623–7900;
        (202) 623–7988
Fax: (202) 623–6460;
    (202) 623–4661
Telex/E-mail: 248 331 IMF UR

**2263. International Museum of
    Photography**
George Eastman House
900 East Avenue
Rochester
NY 14607
USA
Telephone: (716) 271–3361
Telex/E-mail: ANDY UORMVS
(BITNET)

**2264. International Occupational
    Safety and Health Information
    Centre (See CIS)**

**2265. International Patent
    Documentation Center**
Dipl-KFM Norbert Fux
Möllwaldplatz 4
Postfach 163
A-1040 Vienna
Austria
Telephone: 0222 50155
        0222 658–784
Fax: 01 505–3386
Telex/E-mail: 136337 A
NUA: 232911602323

2266. International Reports Inc
14 E 60th Street
Suite 1206
New York
NY 10022
USA
Telephone: (212) 888–1505
Fax: (212) 888–3566
Telex/E-mail: 233139 RPTUR

**2267. International Research and
    Evaluation**
21098 IRE Control Center
Eagan
MN 55121
USA
Telephone: (612) 888–9635
Fax: (612) 854–8180
Telex/E-mail: 291008 131425 (ITTD)

2268. International RILM Center
33 W 42nd Street
Room 1009
New York
NY 10036
USA
Telephone: (212) 642–2709
Fax: (212) 642–2642
Telex/E-mail: ETF2 CUNYVMS1
(BITNET)

**2269. International Society of
    Appraisers**
PO Box 726
Hoffman Estates
IL 60195
USA
Telephone: (312) 882–0706

2270. International Software Ltd
John Gray
7 Ryan Drive (off Shield Drive)
Great West Road
Brentford
Middlesex
TW8 9ER
UK
Telephone: 081 847–3761;
        081 479–0049
Fax: 081 847 5232;
    081 479–0076

**2271. International Stock Exchange
    (London) Inc, The**
Quoted Companies Data Service
Publications Unit
London
EC2N 1HP
UK
Telephone: 071 588–2355
Fax: 071 796–3319

**2272. International
    Telecommunications Union**
Laszlo I Mercz; Klaus Ohms
Place des Nations
CH-1211 Geneva 20
Switzerland
Telephone: 022 730 51 11;
        022 730 55 01;
        022 730 53 18
Fax: 022 730 53 37;
    022 730 57 85;
    022 730 72 56

**2273. International Translations
    Centre**
Schuttersveld 2
NL-2611 WE Delft
Netherlands
Telephone: 015 14 22 42
Fax: 015 15 85 35
Telex/E-mail: 38104 NL

2274. InterNetwork Inc
Payson R Stevens (President)
411 7th Street
Del Mar
CA 92014
USA
Telephone: (619) 755–0439
Fax: (619) 481–8181

2275. InterOptica Publishing Ltd
Catherine Winchester (Managing
Director)
1213 Shui On Centre
6 Harbour Rd
Hong Kong
Telephone: 824–2868
Fax: 824–2508

2276. InterOptica Publishing Ltd
300 Montgomery Street
San Francisco
CA 94104
USA
Telephone: (415) 788–8788
Fax: (415) 788–8886

2277. Interplay Productions
Anita Lauer (PR Coordinator)
3710 S Susan
Suite 100
Santa Ana
CA 92704
USA
Telephone: (714) 545–9001
Fax: (714) 549–5075

2278. Interpol Ottawa
National Central Bureau
1200 Vanier Parkway
Ottawa
ON K1A 0R2
Canada
Telephone: (613) 993–8305
Fax: (613) 993–8309

2279. Intersearch Systems Ltd
Tony Blake (Director); Roger Kendrick
    (Director)
Combs Tannery
Stowmarket
Suffolk
IP14 2EN
UK
Telephone: 0449 770–662
Fax: 0449 677–600

2280. Inventory Locator Service Inc
3965 Mendenhall Road
Memphis
TN 38115
USA
Telephone: (901) 794–4784;
        (800) 233–3414
Fax: (901) 794–1760
Telex/E-mail: 882179 WU

2281. Invest/Net Inc
3265 Meridian Parkway
Suite 130
Fort Lauderdale
FL 33331
USA
Telephone: (305) 384–1500
Fax: (305) 384–1540

**2282. Investext (Thomson Financial
    Networks)**
Andrea Hirschfeld (Marketing Manager)
11 Farnsworth Street
Boston
MA 02210
USA
Telephone: (617) 330–7878;
        (800) 662–7878;
        (617) 345–2000
Fax: (617) 330–1986;
    (617) 350–5011;
    (617) 426–3957
Telex/E-mail: 466199

2283. Investment Company Data Inc
2600 72nd Street
Suite A
Des Moines
IA 50322
USA
Telephone: (515) 270–8600;
        (800) 735–4234
Fax: (515) 270–9022

2284. Investment Technologies Inc
510 Thornall Street
Edison
NJ 08837
USA
Telephone: (908) 494–1200;
        (800) 524–0831

2285. Investor's Daily Inc
1941 Armacost Avenue
Los Angeles
CA 90025
USA
Telephone: (213) 207–1832

2286. InVision Interactive
Denny Mayer (Vice President Sales)
269 Mt Hermon Road
Suite 105
Scotts Valley
CA 95066–4029
USA
Telephone: (408) 438–5530;
(800) 468–5530
Fax: (408) 438–6784

2287. Invittox
Dr Krys Ungar
Eastgate House
34 Stoney Street
Nottingham
NG1 1NB
UK

2288. Iopis Corporation
Jock Johnson
590 E Rich Street
Columbus
OH 43215
USA
Telephone: (614) 461–6565
Fax: (614) 461–8060

2289. Iowa Drug Information Service
Westlawn
PO Box 330
Iowa City
IA 52242
USA
Telephone: (319) 335–8913
Telex/E-mail: 62008097

2290. Iowa State Library
East 12th Street and Grand
Des Moines
IA 50319
USA
Telephone: (515) 281–4499;
(515) 281–4118

2291. Ipacri Spa
Instituto per l'Automazione delle Casse
di Risparmio Italiane
Dott. Claudio Mazi
Via Adolfo Rava 124
00142 Rome
Italy
Telephone: 6 548–11;
6 547–901
Fax: 6 548–12225

2292. IPMC
Cite de la Musique
Etablissement Public du Parc de la
Villette
211 avenue J Jaures
F-75019 Paris
France

2293. IPSOA Editore SpA
Giulia Fasciolo (Product Manager);
Bruno Ortolani (Software
Development)
Strada 3 – Palazzo F6 Assago
20090 Milan
Italy
Telephone: 02 824–76962;
02 824–761;
02 824–76992
Fax: 02 824–76968

**2294. IPU – Instituttet for
Produktudvikling**
Niels Frees
DTH, Bygn. 423
2800 Lyngby
Denmark
Telephone: 45 (42) 882522

2295. IQuest
CompuServe Inc
5000 Arlington Center Blvd
Columbus
OH 43220
USA
Telephone: (614) 457–8600;
(800) 848–8990

**2296. IRB (See
Fraunhofer-Gesellschaft)**

2297. IRI/ABA Inc.
USA
Telephone: (213) 376–8081

2298. Iris Technology Ltd
Steve Horne (Director)
The Old Forge
Chapel Lane
Charwelton
Daventry
NN11 6YU
UK
Telephone: 0327 60594
Fax: 0327 60049

2299. Isabelle Seguy
20 avenue du Chateau
F-33400 Talence
France
Telephone: 56 48 09 66

2300. ISA
Ted Sluymer
PO Box 47
1740 AA Schagen
Netherlands
Telephone: 02240 14842
Fax: 02240 96303

2301. Ise Cegos
C Marquèze (Product Manager)
Tour Amboise
204 Rond Point du Pont de Sèvres
92516 Boulogne Cedex
France
Telephone: 46 09 28 28
Fax: 46 09 28 00

2302. Ishiyaku Shuppan
1–7–10 Moto-Komagome
Bunkyo-ku
Tokyo 130
Japan
Telephone: 03 3944–3143
Fax: 03 3827–2585

2303. ISP Ltd
1st Floor
Fountain House
Great Cornbow
Halesowen
West Midlands
UK
Telephone: 021 550 8887
Fax: 021 501 3917

2304. Israel Government Press Office
Beit Agron
37 Hillel Street
94581 Jerusalem
Israel
Telephone: 02 244–684
Fax: 02 244–448

**2305. Israel National Center of
Scientific and Technological**
Information
Ministry of Energy and Infrastructure
Atidim Industrial Park
PO Box 43074
61430 Tel-Aviv
Israel
Telephone: 03 492–037;
03 492–038
Fax: 03 492033
Telex/E-mail: 32332 IL

2306. Istituto Centrale di Statistica
Via Cesare Balbo 16
I-00100 Rome
Italy
Telephone: 06 46731
Fax: 06 464–797
Telex/E-mail: 610338 I

2307. Istituto Geografico De Agostini
v. Giovanni da Verrazano 15
28100 Novara
Italy
Telephone: +39 321 422477
Fax: +39 321 422451

**2308. Istituto Nazionale per il
Commercio Estero**
Via Liszt 21
Rome
Italy
Telephone: 06 59921
Telex/E-mail: 610178 I

2309. Isvor – Fiat spa
Marco Vergeat
Corso Dante 103
10126 Turin
Italy
Telephone: 011 65 221
Fax: 011 652–2461

2310. Italeco
Lucio Cavazza
Via Carlo Pesenti 109–111
00156 Rome
Italy
Telephone: 06 439–971
Fax: 06 451–2948

**2311. ITBTP-CATED – Institut
Technique de Batiment et des
Travaux Publics**
Centre d'Assistance Technique et de
Documentation
Mr Clavel
9 Rue Laperouse
F-75784 Paris Cedex 16
France
Telephone: +33 1–4720 8800
NUA: 208075000155DAT

2312. Itelis Limited
9 D'Olier Street
Dublin 2
Eire
Telephone: 353 (1) 717035

**2313. ITG Innovationstechnik GmbH
& Co HG**
SDS Subvent Datenbank Systeme
Heinrich-Hertz Strasse 15
2000 Hamburg 76
Germany
Telephone: 49 (40) 2 29 00 08

2314. Iwanami Shoten Publishers
Atsushi Aiba (Deputy General Manager,
New Media Department)
2–5–5 Hitotsubashi
Chiyoda-Ku
Tokyo
Japan
Telephone: 03 265–4111
Fax: 03 221–8998

2315. J Paul Getty Trust
Clark Art Institute
Williamstown
MA 01267
USA
Telephone: (413) 458–8260
Fax: (413) 458–8503

2316. J Whitaker & Sons Ltd
12 Dyott Street
London
WC1A 1DF
UK
Telephone: 071 836–8911
Fax: 071 836–2909

2317. J.W. Cappelens Forlag AS
Pal Steigen
Postboxs 350
Sentrum 0101 Oslo 1
Norway
Telephone: 47 242 9440

2318. JA Micropublishing Inc
Rita DeSimone
271 Main Street
PO Box 218
Eastchester
NY 10707
USA
Telephone: (914) 793–2130;
          (800) 227–2477

2319. Ja Ne't Global
931 Austin Avenue
Salt Lake City
UT 84106
USA
Telephone: (801) 485–9585

2320. Jaeger + Waldmann (See Telex-Verlag Jaeger + Waldmann)

2321. Jaguar
Reed Travel Group
Sally Little
Francis House
11 Francis Street
Victoria
London
SW1P 1BB
UK
Telephone: 071 798–9766
Fax: 071 798–9720
Telex/E-mail: 4951813

2322. James R. LymBurner & Sons Ltd
PO Box 289
Station A
Toronto
ON M5W 1B2
Canada
Telephone: (416) 964–0789
Fax: (416) 323–1961

2323. James S. Teicher
7000 Blvd East, Suite 35E
Guttenberg
NJ 07093
USA
Telephone: (201) 854–0920

2324. Jane's Information Group (USA)
Rahul Belani (Applications Programmer Analyst)
1340 Braddock Place
Suite 300 PO Box 1436
Alexandria
VA 22313–2036
USA
Telephone: (703) 683–3700;
          (800) 544–3678
Fax: (703) 836–0029

2325. Jane's Information Group
Aine Molloy (CD-ROM Product Manager); Lynne Samuel (Marketing Assistant)
Sentinel House
163 Brighton Road
Couldson
Surrey
CR5 2NX
UK
Telephone: 081 763–1030
Fax: 081 763–1005

2326. Janet Greco
Luxembourg
Telephone: +352 34981 370
Fax: +352 34981 389

2327. Janet Matthews Information Services
David Thew
19 Hatherley Road
Sidcup
Kent
DA14 4BH
UK
Telephone: 081 300–3661
Fax: 081 300–7367

2328. Janssen Chimica
Turnhoutsebaan 30
B-2340 Beerse
Belgium
Telephone: 014 60 21 11
Telex/E-mail: 32540 B

2329. Japan Computer Technology Company Ltd
4–3 Kanda Surugadai
Chiyoda-ku
Tokyo 101
Japan
Telephone: 03 3233–1111

2330. Japan External Trade Organization
Information Coordination Division
2–5 Toranomon
2–Chrome
Minato-ku
Tokyo 105
Japan
Telephone: 03 3582–5549
Fax: 03 3589–4179

2331. Japan Fisheries Resource Conservation Association
Ms Masako Ikenouye
Tokyo Suisan Building 6F
4–18 Toyomi
Chuo-ku
Tokyo 104
Japan

2332. Japan Food Industry Center
3–22 Toranomon
2–Chome
Minato-ku
Tokyo 105
Japan
Telephone: 03 3591–7451
Fax: 03 3592–2869

2333. Japan Information Center of Science and Technology
2–5 Nagatacho
2–Chome
Chiyado-ku
CPO Box 1478
Tokyo 100
Japan
Telephone: 03 3581–6411
Fax: 03 3593–3375
Telex/E-mail: 02223604 JOCST J;
  JICSTECH TOKYO J

2334. Japan Library Association
Katsuaki Tohya
1–10 Taishido 1–Chome
Setagaya-ku
Tokyo 154
Japan
Telephone: 03 410–6411
Fax: 03 421–7588

2335. Japan National Diet Library
Library Automation Systems
1–10, 1–Chome
Nagato-cho
Chiyoda-ku
Tokyo 100
Japan
Telephone: 03 3581–2331

2336. Japan Patent Information Organization
5–16–1 Toranomon
Minato-ku
Tokyo 105
Japan
Telephone: 03 3503–6181
Fax: 03 3580–7164
Telex/E-mail: 2224152 JAPATI J

2337. Japan Travel Bureau Inc
Publishing Division
R Nakashima (Manager)
1–10–8 Dogenzaka
Shibuyaku
Tokyo 150
Japan
Telephone: 03 3477–9546
Fax: 03 3477–9587

2338. Japanese Database Industry Association (DINA)
2–7 Kagurazaka
Shinjuku-ku
Tokyo 162
Japan
Telephone: (81) 3 3235–5966
Fax: (81) 3 3235–5976

2339. Jaques Cattel Press
A division of R.R. Bowker Company
245 West 17th Street
New York
NY 10011
USA
Telephone: (212) 916–1727;
          (800) 323–3288 (in NY)
Telex/E-mail: 127703

2340. Jay C White
PO Box 1148
Redwood City
CA 94064
USA
Telephone: (415) 594–9300

2341. JB Business Information
Nyhavn 20
PO Box 1507
1020 Copenhagen K
Denmark
Telephone: 45 (33) 32 10 03

2342. JB Lippincott Company
Maria Zacierka (Manager Media & Information Services)
227 E Washington Square
Philadelphia
PA 19106–3780
USA
Telephone: (215) 238–4221;
          (800) 523–2945
Fax: (215) 238–4227;
     (215) 238–4216

2343. JD Power and Associates
30401 Agoura Road
Suite 200
Agoura Hills
CA 91301
USA
Telephone: (818) 889–6330

2344. Jeppesen Sanderson, Inc
H Bergmann
55 Inverness Drive
Englewood
CO 80112
USA
Telephone: (303) 799–9090

2345. Jeriko
5 Boulevard Poissoniere
75002 Paris
France

2346. Jerusalem Post Publications Ltd
PO Box 81
Romema
Jerusalem 91000
Israel
Telephone: 02 551–616
Fax: 02 537–527
Telex/E-mail: 26121 IL

2347. Jet Propulsion Laboratory (See NASA)

2348. Jiji Press Ltd
1–3 Hibiya Koen
Chiyoda-ku
Tokyo 100
Japan
Telephone
Telex/E-mail: 22270 J

2349. JK Publishing Company
4008 N Morris Boulevard
Suite 2
Shorewood
WI 53211
USA
Telephone: (414) 332–1625

2350. JM Dent & Sons Ltd
91 Clapham High Street
London
SW4A 7TA
UK
Telephone: 071 622–9933
Fax: 071 627–3361
Telex/E-mail: 8954130 ALDINE G

2351. JMA Research Institute Inc
4–3–13 Toranomon
Minato-ku
Tokyo 105
Japan
Telephone: 03 3434–1721
Fax: 03 3434–1721

2352. John Fairfax and Sons Ltd
235 Jones Street
GPO Box 506
Sydney
NSW 2001
Australia
Telephone: 02 282–2833
Fax: 02 212–2424

2353. John Wiley & Sons Inc
Wiley Electronic Publishing
Karen Kroboth
605 3rd Avenue
5th Floor
New York
NY 10158–0012
USA
Telephone: (212) 850–6000;
(212) 850–6194;
(212) 850–6360;
(212) 850–6487
Fax: (212) 850–6362
Telex/E-mail: 127063

2354. John Wiley & Sons Limited
Helen Ramsey (Software & Mathematics Editor)
Baffins Lane
Chichester
West Sussex
PO19 1UD
UK
Telephone: 0243 770–215;
0243 779–777
Fax: 0243 775–878
Telex/E-mail: 86290 WIBOOK G
83:JWP001 (Dialcom)

2355. Johns Hopkins University
Population Information Program
Anne W Compton (Associate Director)
527 St Pauls Place
Baltimore
MD 21202
USA
Telephone: (301) 659–6300;
(301) 659–6341
Fax: (301) 659–6266
Telex/E-mail: 240430 JHUPCS UR

2356. Johnston & Company
Catherine Johnston (President); James W Johnston (Director)
PO Box 446
American Fork
UT 84003
USA
Telephone: (801) 756–1111
Fax: (801) 756–0242

2357. Joint Industry Committee for National Readership Surveys
44 Belgrave Square
London
SW1X 8QS
UK
Telephone: 071 235–7020
Fax: 071 245–9904
Telex/E-mail: 918352 G

2358. Jordan & Sons Ltd
Sally Harlow (Customer Support Manager)
Jordan House
47 Brunswick Place
London
N1 6EE
UK
Telephone: 071 253–3030
Fax: 071 251–0825
Telex/E-mail: 261010 G 74:JOR001 (Dialcom)

2359. Jostens Learning Corporation
6150 North 16th Street
Phoenix
AZ 85016
USA
Telephone: (602) 230–7030

2360. Jostens Learning Corporation
John Kernan (CEO)
6170 Cornerstone Court E
Suite 300
San Diego
CA 92121–3170
USA
Telephone: (619) 587–0087;
(800) 548–8372
Fax: (619) 587–1629

2361. Journal Graphics Inc
267 Broadway
New York
NY 10007–2361
USA
Telephone: (212) 732–8552

2362. Journal of Commerce Inc
2 World Trade Center
27th Floor
New York
NY 10048–0662
USA
Telephone: (212) 837–7000
Fax: (212) 208–0393

2363. Journal of Economic Literature
American Economic Association
PO Box 7320
Oakland Station
Pittsburgh
PA 15213–0320
USA
Telephone: (412) 621–2291;
(412) 268–3869

2364. Journal Record
621 N Robinson
Oklahoma City
OK 73102
USA
Telephone: (405) 235–3100

2365. Journal/Sentinel Inc
333 W State Street
PO Box 661
Milwaukee
WI 53201–0661
USA
Telephone: (414) 224–2472

2366. Jouve Systemes d'Information
Nathalie Rabin (Promotion Communication)
18 rue Saint-Denis
75025 Paris Cedex 01
France
Telephone: 1 42 33 17 99
Fax: 1 40 28 04 55

2367. JR O'Dwyer Company
271 Madison Avenue
New York
NY 10016
USA
Telephone: (212) 679–2471

2368. JR Publishing Inc
PO Box 6654
McLean
VA 22106
USA
Telephone: (703) 532–2235

2369. JT Baker Inc
222 Red School Lane
Phillipsburg
NJ 08865
USA
Telephone: (908) 859–2151
Fax: (908) 859–9318

2370. JTB
Mr Nakajima
3–3 Kanda-Kajimachi
Chiyoda-ku
Tokyo 101
Japan
Telephone: 03 3257–8303

2371. Jupiter Communications
594 Broadway
Suite 1003
New York
NY 10012
USA
Telephone: (212) 941–9252

2372. Juridial
1 rue du Boccador
75008 Paris
France
Telephone: 33 (1) 47 20 88 34

Addresses

2373. Juris Data GiE
123 rue d'Alesia
75014 Paris Cedex 14
France
Telephone: 33 (1) 45 39 22 91
Fax: 33 (1) 45 42 81 55
Telex/E-mail: 270737 F

2374. Juris GmbH
Mr Walker Mr Kuhlmann
Gutenbergstraße 23
PO Box 552
D-6600 Saarbrücken
Germany
Telephone: 0681 5866–180;
　　　　　　0681 5866–234
Fax: 0681 5866–239
Telex/E-mail: 8869679
NUA: Available on application

2375. Justitiedepartementet
103 33 Stockholm
Sweden
Telephone: 46 (8) 763 47 80

2376. Jutastat (Pty) Ltd
SP Sephton (Manager)
PO Box 14373
Kenwyn 7790
Howard Place 7450
Cape Town
Republic of South Africa
Telephone: 021 531–8004;
　　　　　　021 797–5101
Fax: 021 761–5010

2377. Jydsk Telefon
K. Allerman S. Villumsen
Sletvej 30
8310 Tranbjerg
Denmark
Telephone: 45 (86) 293366

2378. Jyske Bank
Peter Helle
Vestergade 8–10
8600 Silkeborg
Denmark
Telephone: 45 (86) 821122

**2379. Jyukokumin-Sha Publishing
　　　Company Ltd**
Hideki Hasegawa
2–4–12 Kyobashi
Chuo-Ku
Tokyo 104
Japan
Telephone: 03 3281–1271
Fax: 03 3281–9815

**2380. Kadokawa Shoten Publishing
　　　Inc**
Kadokawa Hongo Building
5–24–5 Hongo
Bunkyo-Ku
Tokyo 113
Japan
Telephone: 03 817–8521

2381. Kahn Enterprises
1538 Markan Drive
Atlanta
GA 30306
USA
Telephone: (404) 876–6027

2382. Kaihatsu Computing Center
1–8–2 Marunouchi
Chiyoda-ku
Tokyo 100
Japan
Telephone: 03 3213–0921

2383. Kalo Communications Inc
10 Valley Drive
Greenwich
CT 06831
USA
Telephone: (203) 869–8200
Fax: (203) 869–9235

2384. Kansas City Star
1729 Grand Avenue
Kansas City
MO 64108
USA
Telephone: (816) 234–4141

2385. Kansas State Library
Capitol Building
3rd Floor
Topeka
KS 66612–1593
USA
Telephone: (913) 296–3296

2386. Kapital
Slemdalsveien 72
N-0373 Oslo 3
Norway
Telephone: 02 14 84 50

**2387. Karolinska Institutets Bibliotek
　　　och Informationscentral**
Medical Information Center (MIC-KIBIC)
Mrs Christine Wickman
Box 60201
Doktorsringen 21 C
S-104 01 Stockholm
Sweden
Telephone: 08 23 22 70;
　　　　　　08 34 05 60
Fax: 08 34 87 93 KAROLINST
Telex/E-mail: 17179 KIBIC S
NUA: 240200100130; 240200101904

2388. Kauppakaari Yhtymae Oy
Uudenmaankatu 4–6 A
SF-00120 Helsinki
Finland
Telephone: 358 (0) 64 71 01

2389. Kauppalehti
PO Box 189
SF-00101 Helsinki
Finland
Telephone: 09 50781
Fax: 09 563–0001
Telex/E-mail: 125827 KAUP SF

2390. Keep In Touch
Mr Burette (Directeur Commercial –
　　Lyon); Mr Soty (Directeur
　　Commercial – Paris)
Tour Credit Lyonnais
129 rue Servient
69431 Lyon Cedex 03
France
Telephone: 78 63 61 00
Fax: 78 62 07 61

**2391. Keller International Publishing
　　　Corporation**
150 Great Neck Road
Great Neck
NY 11021
USA
Telephone: (516) 829–9210

2392. Kemikalieinspektionen
Library
PO Box 1384
S-171 27 Solna
Sweden
Telephone: 08 730–5700

2393. Kenney Communications Inc
4303 Vineland Road
Suite F-15
Orlando
FL 32811
USA
Telephone: (407) 422–8333

**2394. Kenny S & P Information
　　　Services**
Patricia Wyle (Director of Sales)
65 Broadway
New York
NY 10006
USA
Telephone: (212) 208–8339;
　　　　　　(212) 208–8021
Fax: (212) 344–4185;
　　　　　　(212) 412–0498

**2395. Kernforschungszentrum
　　　Karlsruhe GmbH**
Abteiung fuer Angewandte
　　Systemanalyse
Postfach 3640
7500 Karlsruhe 1
Germany
Telephone: 49 (7247) 8 21
Telex/E-mail: 7826484 D

2396. Keskuslaboratorio Oy
Teknisk Information
PO Box 136
SF-00101 Helsinki
Finland
Telephone: 0 43711
Fax: 0 464–305
Telex/E-mail: 1001522 KCL SF

2397. Keystroke Knowledge
TACIN Ltd.
Orcop
Hereford
HR2 8SF
UK
Telephone: 0981 540263;
　　　　　　0981 540127

2398. Keystroke Knowledge
Queens Chambers
Queen Street
Penzance
Cornwall
TR18 4BH
UK
Telephone: 0736 51631
Fax: 0736 64278

2399. KH Services BV
Jan Kloos (Director)
Utrechtsweg 8
1213 TS Hilversum
Netherlands
Telephone: 035 238–835
Fax: 035 239–307

2400. KIDSNET
6856 Eastern Avenue NW
Room 208
Washington
DC 20012
USA
Telephone: (202) 291–1400
Telex/E-mail: 41:KDS001 (Dialcom)

2401. KimTec UK
Fairways House
8 Highland Road
Wimborne
Dorset
BH21 2QN
UK
Telephone: 0202 888–873
Fax: 0202 888–863

2402. King Communications Group Inc
627 National Press Building
Washington
DC 20045
USA
Telephone: (202) 638–4260
Fax: (202) 662–9744

2403. Kingswood Ltd
Mary Short
London
UK
Telephone: 081 994–5404

2404. Kinki University
Industrial and Law Information Institute
Kowakae 3–4–1
Higashiosaka-shi
Osaka 577
Japan
Telephone: 06 721–2332

2405. Kinokuniya Company Ltd (UK)
Mr Toliyama
Radnor House
93–97 Regent Street
London
W1R 7TG
UK
Telephone: 071 734–3074
Fax: 071 734–1804

2406. Kinokuniya Company Ltd.
ASK Information Retrieval Services
P.O. Box 55
Chitose
Tokyo 56
Japan

2407. Kinokuniya Company Ltd
T Totsuka
38–1 Sakuragaoka
5–chome
Setagaya-ku
Tokyo 156
Japan
Telephone: 03 3439–0123
Fax: 03 3439–1093

2408. Kirjastopalvelu Oy Biblioteksservice
Riitta Valtonen
Särkiniementie 5
PO Box 84
SF-00211 Helsinki
Finland
Telephone: 0 692–6266
Fax: 0 692–4797

2409. Kiwinet
PO Box 696
Wellington
New Zealand
Telephone: 64 (4) 743–000
Fax: 64 (4) 743–042
Telex/E-mail: 30076 NATLIB NZ

2410. Kluwer Bedrijfswetenschappen
Hubert Krekels
Postbus 23
7400 GA Deventer
Netherlands
Telephone: 05700 48999
Fax: 05700 11504

2411. Kluwer Datalex
Peter van Wegen (Manager)
Postbus 23
NL-7400 GA Deventer
Netherlands
Telephone: 05700 91243 05700 47141
Fax: 05700 34740
Telex/E-mail: 49295 KLUD NL
NUA: 2041570020

2412. Kluwer Rechtswetenschappen
Guy Van Peel (Publisher); Dirk Smets
(Product Manager)
Santvoortbeeklaan 21–25
2100 Deurne (Antwerp)
Belgium
Telephone: 033 600–354
Fax: 033 600–467

2413. Kluwer Technische Boeken BV
NHL van Herk (Managing Director)
Postbus 23
7400 GA Deventer
Netherlands
Telephone: 05700 48321
Fax: 05700 10918

2414. Knight Publishing Company
600 Tyron Street
PO Box 32188
Charlotte
NC 28232
USA
Telephone: (704) 379–3600

2415. Knight-Ridder Commodity Information
100 Church Street
Suite 1850
New York
NY 10007
USA
Telephone: (212) 233–9420;
(800) 762–3243
Fax: (212) 227–4835

2416. Knight-Ridder Financial
75 Wall Street
22nd Floor
New York
NY 10005
USA
Telephone: (212) 269–1110;
(800) 433–8930

2417. Knight-Ridder Financial
2100 W 89th Street
PO Box 6053
Leawood
KS 66206
USA
Telephone: (913) 642–7373;
(800) 255–6490
Fax: (913) 967–5966

2418. Knight-Ridder MoneyCenter
75 Wall Street
23rd Floor
New York
NY 10005
USA
Telephone: (800) 433–8930

2419. Knight-Ridder Tribune News
790 National Press Building
Washington
DC 20045
USA
Telephone: (202) 383–6080

2420. Knowledge Access International
Julian Olson (Sales); William Paisley
(Business Development)
2685 Marine Way
Suite 1305
Mountain View
CA 94043
USA
Telephone: (415) 969–0606
Fax: (415) 964–2027

2421. Knowledge Index
DIALOG Information Services Inc
3460 Hillview Avenue
Palo Alto
CA 94304
USA
Telephone: (415) 858–3785;
(800) 334–2564
Fax: (415) 858–4069
Telex/E-mail: 334499DIALOG

2422. Knowledge Industry Publications Inc
701 Westchester Avenue
White Plains
NY 10604
USA
Telephone: (914) 328–9157;
(800) 248–5474
Fax: (914) 328–9093

2423. Knowledge Research Ltd
2 All Saints Street
London
N1 9RL
UK
Telephone: 071 833–1162

2424. KnowledgeSet Corporation
Martin Miller (Product Marketing
Manager)
888 Villa Street
Suite 410
Mountain View
CA 94041
USA
Telephone: (415) 968–9888;
(800) 456–0469
Fax: (415) 968–9962

2425. Knoxville News-Sentinel Company
208 W Church Avenue
PO Box 59038
Knoxville
TN 37950–9038
USA
Telephone: (615) 523–3131

2426. Kobmandstanden A/S
Michael Goth (Divisional Manager)
Gammel Mont 4
DK-1117 Copenhagen K
Denmark
Telephone: 33 11 12 00
Fax: 33 11 16 29
Telex/E-mail: 27571 SOLID DK

2427. Koch Digitaldisc GmbH & Company KG
Abteilung Datentechnik
Dr Georg Hittmair (Marketing)
Langer Weg 28
6020 Innsbruck
Austria
Telephone: 0512 47950
Fax: 0512 47975

2428. Koch International
Langer Weg 28
A-6020 Innsbruck
Austria
Telephone: +43 512 47950
Fax: +43 512 47975

2429. Koda Online
P Cangley
Windsor Court
East Grinstead House
East Grinstead
West Sussex
RH19 1XA
UK
Telephone: +44 342–26972
NUA: 228468114080

Addresses

2430. Kodex Inc
139 Chestnut Street
PO Box 626
Nutley
NJ 07110
USA
Telephone: (201) 235–0041
Fax: (201) 235–0132
Telex/E-mail: 133551 DEFENSE

2431. Kokusai Information Service Company Limited
9th Floor, Shibuya Sumitomo Shintaku Building
22–3 Jinnan 1–chome
Shubuya-ku
Tokyo 150
Japan
Telephone: 81 (3) 463–7181
Fax: 03-3770–1865
Telex/E-mail: 2423526 KOKIMF J

2432. Kommunedata
Brigitte Hansen
Hadsundsvej 184
9100 Aalborg
Denmark
Telephone: 45 (08) 135511

2433. Kompass Belgium SA-NV
Guy Verneirsch (Product Manager)
Avenue Molière 256
1060 Brussels
Belgium
Telephone: 02 345 19 83
Fax: 02 347 33 40

2434. Kompass Deutschland Verlags- und Vertriebsgesellschaft mbH
Norbert Schütze
Postfach 964
Wilhelmstraße 1
7800 Freiburg im Breisgau
Germany
Telephone: 0761 31331
Fax: 0761 24492

2435. Kompass France SA
Josiane Belkechout (Product Manager)
22 avenue Franklin Roosevelt
75008 Paris
France
Telephone: 1 43 59 37 59
Fax: 1 45 63 83 49

2436. Kompass Israel Ltd
118 Ahad Haam Street
64253 Tel-Aviv
Israel
Telephone: 03 561–9374

2437. Kompass Italia SpA
Ezio Pennisi (Manager Electronic Media)
Via G Servals 125
10146 Turin
Italy
Telephone: 011 779–2337
Fax: 011 794–919

2438. Kompass Luxembourg SARL
Giovanni Carola (Director)
Rue Ste Zithe 12
2763 Luxembourg
Luxembourg
Telephone: 496–051
Fax: 496–056

2439. Kompass Nederland BV
Dion Brocken (EDP Department)
Hogehilweg 15
Gebouw "California"
1101 CB Amsterdam ZO
Netherlands
Telephone: 020 974–041
Fax: 020 965–603

2440. Kompass Norge A/S
H Tangen
Postboks 40
Linderud
0517 Oslo 5
Norway
Telephone: 02 640–575
Fax: 02 647–712

2441. Kompass Sverige
Tore Thallaug (Director)
Saltmätargaten 8
Box 3223
103 64 Stockholm
Sweden
Telephone: 08 736–3000
Fax: 08 31–1898

2442. Kompass UK (Reed Information Services)
Patrick Cangley (General Manager, Electronic Publishing)
East Grinstead House
East Grinstead
West Sussex
RH19 1XA
UK
Telephone: 0342 326–972
Fax: 0342 315–130
Telex/E-mail: 95127 INFSER G
NUA: 228468114080

2443. Kompass
Centre d'Information et de Demonstrations
World Trade Center #
2 place de la Defense
PO Box 421
F-92090 Paris le Defense
France
Telephone: 1 46 92 25 20

2444. Kongelige Bibliotek, Det
Susane Sugar Barbara Melchior
Chr. Brygge 8
1219 Copenhagen K
Denmark
Telephone: 45 01 930111
NUA: 24824125080000

2445. Koninkijke Bibliotheek
Trudi Noordermeer (Library Research & Development)
Prins Willem Alexanderhof 5
PO Box 90407
NL-2509 LK The Hague
Netherlands
Telephone: 070 314–0911;
070 314–0597
Fax: 070 314–0450;
070 314–0440

2446. Koninklijke Nederlandse Akademie van Wetenschappen
Bureau voor de Bibliographie van de Neerlandistiek
PO Box 90407
NL-2509 LK The Hague
Netherlands
Telephone: 070 14 02 84;
070 14 04 13

2447. Koninklijke Nederlandse Maatschappij ter Bevordering der
Pharmacie
Alexanderstraat 11
Postbus 30460
2500 GL Den Haag
Netherlands
Telephone: 070 362–4111
Fax: 070 310–6530

2448. Koninklijke Vermande BV
Platinastraat 33
PO Box 20
NL-8200 AA Lelystad
Netherlands
Telephone: 032 22944
Fax: 032 226–334

2449. Korda and Company Ltd
Charterhouse Walk
78 St John Street
London
EC1 4HR
UK
Telephone: 071 253–0089

2450. Korea Economic Daily, The
441 Chungnim-dong
Chung-gu
CPO Box 960
Seoul
Republic of Korea
Telephone: 02 313–5511
Fax: 02 312–6610

2451. Kreditforeningen Danmark
Mrs. Mary Louise Tonning
Jarmers Plads 2
1590 Koebenhavn V
Denmark
Telephone: 45 (33) 125300

2452. Kreditschutzverband von 1870
Zelinkgasse 10
A-1010 Vienna
Austria
Telephone: 01 5348–46
Fax: 01 5348–4380

2453. Kriminalvaardsstyrelsen
601 80 Norrkoeping
Sweden
Telephone: 46 (11) 19 30 00

2454. Krishnamurti Foundation Trust Ltd.
Brockwood Park
Bramdean
Alresford
Hants.
SO24 0LQ
UK

2455. Krist & Ketel
Fokko Ketel
Pres. Rooseveltlaan 4B
5707 GD Helmond
Netherlands
Telephone: 04920 38444
Fax: 04920 38444

2456. Kronos Europea
Paolo Cellini
Via Castello Della Magliana 75B
I-00148 Rome
Italy
Telephone: 6 6855551

2457. KTAS
Inger Antonsen
Rentemestervej 8
2400 Koebenhavn NV
Denmark
Telephone: 45 (38) 993010

2458. Kubli & Partners
IBIS Service
Peter Kubli
Airgate
Thurgauerstrasse 40
CH-8050 Zurich
Switzerland
Telephone: 41 (1) 302 11 17
Fax: 41 (1) 302 32 91

2459. Kunnskapsforlaget
Sehesteds Gate 1
Postboks 6736
St Olavs plass 0130
N-0130 Oslo 1
Norway
Telephone: 02 20 52 15
Fax: 02 33 34 43;
02 11 21 22

2460. Kuraray Co Ltd
Newbury Park
CA
USA
Telephone: (805) 499–6789

2461. Kuraray Company Ltd
Katsuhiko Hayashi
Shin-Nihonbashi Building 8–2
3–chome Nihonbashi
Chuo-ku
Tokyo 103
Japan
Telephone: 03 3277–3100
Fax: 03 3277–3363

2462. Kvinnohistoriska Samlingarna
Goteborgs Universitetsbibliotek
PO Box 5096
S-402 22 Gothenburg
Sweden
Telephone: 031 631–000

2463. Kwang Hwa Publishing Company
3 Chung Hsiao East Road
Section 1
Taipei
Taiwan
Telephone: 02 331–6753
Fax: 02 356–8233

2464. Kyodo Keikaku Company Ltd
Publishing Department
Minoru Nakamura (Editor in Chief)
Futaba Building, 3–4–18–901
Mita
Minato-ku
Tokyo 108
Japan
Telephone: 03 3452–8080
Fax: 03 3452–5728

2465. Kyodo News International Inc
50 Rockefeller Plaza
Room 803
New York
NY 10020
USA
Telephone: (212) 397–3726;
(212) 586–0152
Fax: (212) 307–1532;
(212) 397–3721
Telex/E-mail: PSTEIN (MCI Mail)

2466. L & B Ltd
19 Rock Creek Church Road NW
Washington
DC 20011–6005
USA
Telephone: (202) 723–1600;
(202) 723–5031
Fax: (202) 723–5031

2467. L'Industrielle-Services Techniques Inc
1611 boulevard Cremazie East
Montreal
PQ H2M 2P2
Canada
Telephone: (514) 383–1611

2468. L'ISOC / CSIC
Adelaida Roman (Manager)
Pinar 25
28006 Madrid
Spain
Telephone: 01 411 22 20
Fax: 01 564 50 69

2469. L'Usine Nouvelle
23 rue Laugier
75017 Paris
France
Telephone: 33 (1) 47 66 01 57 x402
Telex/E-mail: 650485 F

2470. La Ley
División Informatica
Monterrey, 1
Madrid
28230 Las Rozas
Spain
Telephone: 34 1 634 53 62;
34 1 634 22 00
Fax: 34 1 634 41 61

2471. Laboratoire Central des Ponts et Chaussees
58 boulevard Lefebvre
75015 Paris
France
Telephone: 33 (1) 48 56 50 00
Telex/E-mail: 200361 LCPARI F

2472. Laboratoire d'Anthropologie Appliquée
45 rue des Saints-Peres
F-75270 Paris Cedex 6
France
Telephone: 1 42 86 20 38
Fax: 1 42 61 53 80

2473. Laboratoire National d'Essais
1 rue Gaston Boissier
F-75015 Paris
France
Telephone: 1 40 43 37 54
Telex/E-mail: 202319 LNE F

2474. Laboratory of the Government Chemist
Biotechnology Group
Cornwall House
Waterloo Road
London
SE1 8XY
UK
Telephone: 071 211–8834

2475. Labour Canada
Federal-Provincial Relations Branch
Ottawa
ON K1A 0J2
Canada

2476. LaFountain Research Corporation
1 Palmer Square
Suite 300
Princeton
NJ 08542
USA
Telephone: (609) 683–9191

2477. Lakewood Publications Inc
50 S 9th Street
Minneapolis
MN 55402
USA
Telephone: (612) 333–0471;
(800) 324–4329
Fax: (612) 333–6526

2478. Landbrugets Edb Center
Karin Kuehl
Bytofen
8240 Risskov
Denmark
Telephone: 45 (86) 214000

2479. Landesamt für Datenverarbeitung und Statistik Nordrhein-Westfalen
Mr Plewa; Mr Pricking
Mauerstraße 51
4000 Dusseldorf 1
Germany
Telephone: 0211 9449 01
Fax: 0211 4420 06

2480. Landmark Communications Inc
150 W Brambleton Avenue
Norfolk
VA 23510
USA
Telephone: (804) 446–2000

2481. Landscentralen for Undervisninger
Jutta Eskildsen
Oernevej 30
2400 Koebenhavn NV
Denmark
Telephone: 45 (31) 107733

2482. Lang Learning Systems
Minervastraat 2
1930 Zaventem
Brussels
Belgium
Telephone: 32–2–720 50 06/07

2483. Lange & Springer (Italy)
Eva Lindenmayer
Libreria Scientifica
Via San Vitale 13
I-40125 Bologna
Italy
Telephone: 051 238–069;
051 262–696
Fax: 051 262–982

2484. Lange & Springer
Claudia Ittner (Sales Manager);
Annette Naprahi (Sales Manager)
Otto-Suhr-Allee 26–28
1000 Berlin 10
Germany
Telephone: 030 34005–0;
030 34005–211
Fax: 030–34206–11

2485. Langley Publications
1350 Beverly Road
PO Box 115–354
McLean
VA 22101
USA
Telephone: (703) 241–2131

2486. Larkspur Digital Inc
Cathy Pawelczyk (President)
70 Walnut Street
Arlington
MA 02174
USA
Telephone: (617) 643–6264
Fax: (617) 641–1125

2487. Las Vegas Hotline
3426 Biela Avenue
Las Vegas
NV 89120
USA
Telephone: (702) 456–0621

2488. Lasec Datenbank Technologien GmbH & Company
Gabriele Häuser-Allgaier
Fasanenstraße 47
D-1000 Berlin 15
Germany
Telephone: 030 882–7718;
030 882–7719
Fax: 030 881–5394

2489. Laser Magnetic Storage
Robert Brandt Henry Magielse
PO Box 218
Building HWA-1
5600 MD Eindhoven
Netherlands
Telephone: 040 758–753;
040 758–742
Fax: 040 758–817

2490. Laser Media
Norbert Paquel (Director)
38 rue de l'Ouest
75014 Paris
France
Telephone: 1 43 20 53 45
Fax: 1 43 20 52 90

2491. Laser Optical Technology
1803 Mission Street
Suite 403
Santa Cruz
CA 95060
USA
Telephone: (408) 426–7294;
(408) 426–7171

2492. Laser Plot Inc
Hobie Zeller (Director of Marketing);
Holly Winchester
48 Sword Street
Auburn
MA 01501
USA
Telephone: (508) 757–2831;
(800) 888–0888
Fax: (508) 757–1424

2493. Laserbook
4925 University Drive N.W.
Suite 176–336
Huntsville
AL 35816
USA

2494. LaserData SpA
Gtaetani Savasta (Marketing Manager)
Via S Salvador 3
00040 Pomezia
Italy
Telephone: 06 912–5589;
06 910–8224
Fax: 06 910–6826;
06 910–5260

2495. LaserMedia UK Ltd
Kaye Miller
Media House
Arundel Road
Walberton
Arundel
West Sussex
BN18 0QP
UK
Telephone: 0243 555–005
Fax: 0243 555–025

2496. LaserScan Systems
Leonard Fox (President)
5310 NW 33rd Avenue
Suite 115
Fort Lauderdale
FL 33309
USA
Telephone: (305) 739–7715
Fax: (305) 739–7845

2497. LaserTrak
6235–B Lookout Road
Boulder
CO 80301
USA
Telephone: (303) 530–2711

2498. Lasion Europe NV
Christian Souvereyns (Application
Marketing Manager)
Prins Albertlei 7
2600 Antwerp
Belgium
Telephone: 03 230 16 78
Fax: 03 230 55 36

2499. Latin American & Caribbean Center on Health Sciences Information (See BIREME)

2500. Latin American Newsletters
61 Old Street
London
EC1V 9HX
UK
Telephone: 071 251–0012
Fax: 071 253–8193

2501. Lavis Marketing
PDR International
73 Lime Walk
Headington
Oxford
OX3 7AD
UK
Telephone: 0865 67575

2502. Law & Business Inc
855 Valley Road
Clifton
NJ 07013
USA
Telephone: (201) 472–7400

2503. Law Book Company
44–50 Waterloo Road
North Ryde
NSW 2113
Australia
Telephone: 02 887–0177

2504. Law Library Management Ltd
Wellesley Street
PO Box 5694
Auckland
New Zealand
Telephone: 09 370–928

2505. Law MUG Inc
PO Box 11191
Chicago
IL 60611–0191
USA
Telephone: (312) 951–8451
Telex/E-mail: 44:ESQ007 (Dialcom);
107–5685 (MCI Mail)

2506. Law Office Information Systems
822 Broadway
Van Buren
AK 72956
USA
Telephone: (501) 471–5581
Fax: (501) 471–5635

2507. Lawtel Ltd.
Clarendon House
125 Shenley Road
Borehamwood
Hertfordshire
WD6 1AG
UK
Telephone: 081–905 1315
Fax: 081–905 1274
Telex/E-mail: 94070251 LTEL Telecom
Gold 76: CJJ093
NUA: Prestel *251 #

2508. Lawtomation Inc
PO Box 11191
Chicago
IL 60611–0191

2509. Lawyer's PC Review
2640 W 183rd Street
PO Box 2577
Homewood
IL 60430
USA
Telephone: (708) 957–3322
Fax: (708) 957–3337

2510. Lawyers Co-operative Publishing Company
50 Broad Street E
Rochester
NY 14694
USA
Telephone: (716) 546–5530

2511. Lawyers Weekly Publications
30 Court Square
PO Box 2577
Homewood
IL 60430
USA
Telephone: (708) 957–3322
Fax: (708) 957–3337

2512. LBI International (SilverPlatter Agent)
No 2 Torri Katur
Lourdes Lane
St Georges
St Julians
Malta
Telephone: 356–340761

2513. LD-Lovdata
Niels Juels Gate 16
0272 Oslo 2
Norway
Telephone: 47 (2) 244 97 78

2514. Le Ley SA
Martin Arribalzaga (Head of Law
Information)
Tucuman 1471
1050 Buenos Aires
Argentina
Telephone: 01 495–481;
01 495–489
Fax: 01 322–9231

2515. Learned Information (Europe) Limited
Lee Duddell (CD-ROM Sales)
Woodside
Hinksey Hill
Oxford
OX1 5AU
UK
Telephone: 0865 730–275
Fax: 0865 736–354
Telex/E-mail: 837704 INFORM G

2516. Learned Information Inc
Thomas Hogan (President); Lisa Jasper
(Technical Support
Representative)
143 Old Marlton Pike
Medford
NJ 08055–8707
USA
Telephone: (609) 654–6266
Fax: (609) 654–4309

**2517. Learning Link Educators'
Information Network**
356 W 58th Street
New York
NY 10091
USA
Telephone: (212) 560–6613

**2518. Leatherhead Food Research
Association**
Information Group
Dr Dee Marrable
Randalls Road
Leatherhead
Surrey
KT22 7RY
UK
Telephone: 0372 376–761
Fax: 0372 386228
Telex/E-mail: 929846 FOODRA G
NUA: Available on application

2519. Lee Foster
PO Box 5715
Berkeley
CA 94705
USA
Telephone: (415) 549–2202
Fax: (415) 549–2202
Telex/E-mail: 76703,364 (CompuServe
Information Service)

2520. Legi-Slate Inc
777 N Capital Street
9th Floor
Washington
DC 20002
USA
Telephone: (202) 898–2300;
(800) 366–6363
Fax: (202) 842–4748

2521. Legi-Tech Corporation
1029 J Street
Suite 450
Sacramento
CA 95814
USA
Telephone: (916) 447–1886
Fax: (916) 447–1109

2522. Legislative Retrieval System
State Capitol Building
Room 308
Albany
NY 12224
USA
Telephone: (518) 455–7672;
(800) 356–6566 (in NY)

2523. Lehigh University
Mountaintop Campus
111 Research Drive
Bethlehem
PA 18015
USA
Telephone: (215) 758–3230

2524. Les Tracy
8376 Lichen Drive
Citrus Heights
CA 95621
USA
Telephone: (916) 728–5200
Telex/E-mail: 76703,1061 (CompuServe
Information Service)

2525. Letraset USA
40 Eisenhower Dr.
Paramus
NJ 07653
USA
Telephone: (201) 845–6100
Fax: (201) 845–5351

2526. Level-7 Ltd
Centennial Court
Easthampstead Road
Bracknell
Berkshire
RG12 1YQ
UK
Telephone: 0334 868436
Telex/E-mail: concise
concise.level-7.co.uk
NUA: 23423440019315 (PSS);
20433450399915 (IXI);
000046560015 (JANET)

2527. Lex-C-Rom
451 Moody Street
Suite 266
Waltham
MA 02154
USA
Telephone: (617) 894–4452

**2528. Lexington Herald-Leader
Company**
100 Midland Avenue
Lexington
KY 40508
USA
Telephone: (606) 231–3100

2529. Leybold AG
Wilhelm-Rohn-Straße 25
D-6450 Hanau 1
Germany
Telephone: 06181 340
Fax: 06181 341–690
Telex/E-mail: 4152060 IH D

**2530. Library Association Publishing
Limited**
7 Ridgemount Street
London
WC1E 7AE
UK
Telephone: 071 636–7543
Telex/E-mail: 21897 LALDN G

2531. Library Corporation, The
Doug Storer
Research Park
Inwood
WV 25428–9733
USA
Telephone: (304) 229–0100;
(800) 624–0559
Fax: (304) 229–0295

2532. Library of America, The
Max Rudin (Director of Marketing)
14 E 60th Street
New York
NY 10022
USA
Telephone: (212) 308–3360
Fax: (212) 750–8352

2533. Library of Congress
Cataloging Distribution Service
Deborah Ramsey (Marketing
Supervisor)
Washington
DC 20541–5017
USA
Telephone: (202) 707–6100;
(202) 707–1308
Fax: (202) 707–1334

2534. Library of Congress
Cold Regions Bibliography Project
Science and Technology Division
10 First Street SE
Washington
DC 20540
USA
Telephone: (202) 707–1181;
(202) 287–6171;
(202) 707–5668

2535. Library of Congress
Information System7
101 Independence Avenue SE
Washington
DC 20540
USA
Telephone: (202) 287–6560;
(202) 707–5114

2536. Library Systems & Services Inc
Robert E Windrow (Vice-President)
200 Orchard Ridge Drive
Gaithersburg
MD 20878
USA
Telephone: (301) 975–9800
Fax: (301) 975–9844

2537. Library Wholesale Services
1722 H Street NW
Washington
DC 20006
USA
Telephone: (202) 298–8015;
(800) 423–2665

2538. Light Years Ahead Pty Ltd
Ian Eastman (Managing Director)
PO Box 561
14 Salisbury Road
Hornsby
NSW 2077
Australia
Telephone: 02 477–6666
Fax: 02 477–6655

2539. Lightbinders
Janice Rozier (Admin)
2325 Third Street
Suite 320
San Francisco
CA 94107
USA
Telephone: (415) 621–5746
Fax: (415) 621–5898

2540. LINC Resources Inc
4820 Indianola Avenue
Columbus
OH 43214
USA
Telephone: (614) 885–5599

**2541. Linedrive Baseball
Communications (See
Futureline Communications)**

2542. LINK Resources Corporation
79 5th Avenue
12th Floor
New York
NY 10003
USA
Telephone: (212) 627–1500
Fax: (212) 620–3099

2543. Linotype-Hell
UK
Telephone: 0242 222333

2544. LIST Foundation
800 Smithe Street
Vancouver
BC V6Z 2E1
Canada
Telephone: (604) 660–3296

2545. Little, Brown and Company
Electronic Library of Medicine
Janet Carlson
34 Beacon Street
Boston
MA 02108
USA
Telephone: (617) 227–0730;
          (617) 859–5643;
          (800) 289–MAXX
Fax: (617) 859–1269;
     (617) 859–0629

2546. Livingstone Hire
Teddington
Middlesex
UK

**2547. Lloyd's Maritime Information
      Services Inc**
1200 Summer Street
Stamford
CT 06905
USA
Telephone: (203) 359–8383;
          (800) 423–8672
Fax: (203) 358–0437
Telex/E-mail: 509788

**2548. Lloyd's Maritime Information
      Services Ltd**
1 Singer Street
London
EC2A 4LQ
UK
Telephone: 071 490–1720
Fax: 071 250–3142
Telex/E-mail: 987321 LLOYDS G

2549. Lloyd's Transpotel
Lloyd's of London Press Limited
Collwyn House
Sheepen Place
Colchester
Essex
CO3 3LP
UK
Telephone: 44 (206) 772277

2550. Log Corporation
Masayuki Sugiura (Chief of
  Development Section)
Matumoto Building 4F
2–4–3 Taito
Taito-ku
Tokyo 110
Japan
Telephone: 03 3837–2595
Fax: 03 3833–3991

2551. Logic Associates
Chicago
IL
USA
Telephone: (312) 274–0531

2552. Login Services Corporation
245 E 6th Street
Suite 809
St Paul
MN 55101–9006
USA
Telephone: (612) 297–9006;
          (800) 328–1921
Fax: (612) 225–1484

2553. Logistics Systems
95 Wells Avenue
Newton Centre
MA 02159–3321
USA
Telephone: (617) 965–1111

2554. Logitec Informatica SL
Pilar de Brugada (Director)
c/o Emilio Vargas, 17 4o, D0
28043 Madrid
Spain
Telephone: 01 416–4481
Fax: 01 519–6505

2555. Logo-A
Dr. Ph. B Frank
Mercator plein 2
Apeldoorn 7316 HL
Netherlands

2556. Logos Progetti
Str. 4 Palazzo Q8
Milano-Fiori
20089 Rozzano
Italy
Telephone: +39 2 8244177

2557. London Partnership Limited
Giltspur House
6 Giltspur Street
London
EC1A 9DE
UK
Telephone: 071 975–9977
Fax: 071 975–9982
Telex/E-mail: 28509 TLP G

2558. London Property Database Ltd
Glen House
200–208 Tottenham Court Road
London
W1P 9LA
UK
Telephone: 071 323–4770
Fax: 071 627–9606

2559. London Research Centre
Research Library
Annabel Davies (Deputy Director
  Research Library); Richard Golland
  (Director Research Library)
Parliament House
81 Black Prince Road
London
SE1 7SZ
UK
Telephone: 071 735–4250;
          071 627–9660;
          071 627–9661
Fax: 071 627–9674

2560. Long Distance Roses
804 E Nichols Boulevard
Colorado Springs
CO 80907
USA
Telephone: (800) 537–6737

2561. Longman Cartermill Ltd
Hugh Look (Commercial Director);
Gill Joy (Business Development
  Manager)
Technology Centre
St Andrews
Fife
KY16 9EA
UK
Telephone: 0334 77660
Fax: 0334 77180
NUA: 234233400101

2562. Longman Group UK Ltd
J Banfield (Senior Editor);
  K Larkin (Editor)
Westgate House
6th Floor
Burnt Mill
The High
Harlow
Essex
CM20 1YR
UK
Telephone: 0279 442–601
Fax: 0279 444–501
Telex/E-mail: 817484 G

2563. Lonrho Group
Chelsea Bridge House
Queenstown Road
Battersea
London
SW8 4NN
UK
Telephone: 071 627–0700
Telex/E-mail: 888963

**2564. Loren D Jones & Associates
      Ltd**
Loren D Jones (President)
PO Box 127
LaGrange
IL 60525
USA
Telephone: (708) 352–1005

**2565. Los Angeles Gay and Lesbian
      Community Services Center**
1213 N Highland Avenue
Los Angeles
CA 90038
USA
Telephone: (213) 464–7400
Fax: (213) 469–2689
Telex/E-mail: LACAIN (Delphi)

2566. Los Angeles Times, The
Times Mirror Square
Los Angeles
CA 90038
USA
Telephone: (213) 237–3000

**2567. Lotus Development
      Corporation**
Bryan Simmons (Manager Public
  Resources)
55 Cambridge Parkway
Cambridge
MA 02142
USA
Telephone: (617) 577–8500;
          (800) 554–5501
Fax: (617) 225–1293;
     (617) 693–1197

**2568. Lotus Information Services
      Group**
Philip Garlick (Marketing
  Communications Executive)
Lotus Park
The Causeway
Staines
Middlesex
TW18 3AG
UK
Telephone: 0784 455–445
Fax: 0784 469–342;
     0784 469–344

2569. Louisiana State Library
Michael McCann (Deputy State
  Librarian)
760 Riverside N
Baton Rouge
LA 70802
USA
Telephone: (504) 342–3389;
          (504) 342–4923
Fax: (504) 342–3547

2570. Lovdata / Lawdata
VE Henning (System Manager)
Rådhusgaten 7b
0151 Oslo
Norway
Telephone: 02 41 82 00
Fax: 02 41 81 80

2571. Loyola College
Department of Computer Science
Dr Dwayne Shelton
Baltimore
MD 21210
USA
Telephone: (301) 323–1010

2572. LRP Publications
PO Box 579
Fort Washington
PA 19034
USA
Telephone: (215) 628–3113
Fax: (215) 784–0870

2573. LSI Systems Lin
11A Village Green
Crofton
MD 21114
USA
Telephone: (301) 721–3838

2574. Luciano Bosio
33 rue des Jeuneurs
75002 Paris
France
Telephone: 33 (1) 42 36 12 13

2575. Lundberg Survey Inc
PO Box 3996
North Hollywood
CA 91609–0996
USA
Telephone: (818) 768–5111
Telex/E-mail: 910 498 2739

2576. Lynch, Jones & Ryan
Laura Alpent (Marketing)
345 Hudson Street
New York
NY 10014
USA
Telephone: (212) 243–3137
Fax: (212) 645–0698
Telex/E-mail: 420150

2577. M TEK
Majdalen 9
8210 Aarhus
Denmark
Telephone: 45 (86) 105572;
45 (06) 107098

2578. ma Verlag für Messen, Ausstellungen und Kongresse GmbH
Mainzer Landstrasse 251
Postfach 101 528
D-6000 Frankfurt am Main 1
Germany
Telephone: 069 75 95 02
Fax: 069 75 95 1280
Telex/E-mail: 411699 MUA D

2579. Maatschappy voor Informatica Diensten (MID)
Utrechtseweg 15–17
3704 4A Zeist
Netherlands
Telephone: +31 3404 41411

2580. MABB Sistemas Interactivos SA
Josep Monguet (Projects Director)
Tarradellas 123–127 3 C
08029 Barcelona
Spain
Telephone: 03 410 61 15
Fax: 03 419 20 01

2581. MacGuide Advanced Technology
550 South Wadsworth Boulevard
Suite 411
Lakewood
CO 80226
USA
Telephone: (303) 936–0076;
(800) 777–5382
Fax: (303) 936–8232

2582. MacGuide Magazine Inc
Brian Hayashi (Chief Information Officer)
444 17th Street
Suite 200
Denver
CO 80202
USA
Telephone: (303) 893–1454;
(800) 873–1454
Fax: (303) 893–9340

2583. Machon Otzar HaTorah HaMemuchshav – ATM
59 Rabbi Akiva Street
B'nei B'raq
Israel
Telephone: (972) 3–783–262

2584. Mack Trucks Inc
Dave Covey (Specifications Department)
2100 Mac Boulevard
Allentown
PA 18103
USA
Telephone: (215) 439–3011
Fax: (215) 439–2676

2585. MacLean Hunter Limited
MacLean Hunter Building
777 Bay Street
Toronto
ON M5W 1A7
Canada
Telephone: (416) 596–2696
Fax: (416) 596–7730

2586. MacLean Hunter Publishing Company
29 N Wacker Drive
Chicago
IL 60606
USA
Telephone: (312) 726–2802
Fax: (312) 726–2574

2587. Macmillan Inc
Macmillan Directory Division
3002 Glenview Road
Wilmette
IL 60091
USA
Telephone: (312) 441–2387;
(800) 621–9669
Telex/E-mail: 181162 52:MWWOO1 (Dialcom)

2588. Macmillan New Media
(represented in the UK by Microinfo's CD-ROM department – see Microinfo)

2589. Macmillan New Media
Frederick Bowes
124 Mount Auburn Street
Cambridge
MA 02138
USA
Telephone: (800) 342–1388;
(617) 661–2955
Fax: (617) 868–7738

2590. MacMillan Publishing Company
Phil Friedman; Thomas M Wright (The College Blue Book)
866 3rd Avenue
New York
NY 10022
USA
Telephone: (800) 257–5755;
(212) 702–4296
Fax: (202) 6055–9368

2591. MacNeil-Lehrer-Gannett Productions
356 W 58th Street
New York
NY 10019
USA
Telephone: (212) 560–2000

2592. Macromedia Europe
4 Wellington Business Park
Dukes Ride
Crowthorne
Berks
RG11 6LS
UK
Telephone: 0344 761111
Fax: 0344 761149

2593. Macromind Europe
David Jones
19 Manor Place
Edinburgh
EH3 7DX
UK
Telephone: 031 226–5143
Fax: 031 220–4385

2594. MacroMind Inc
Lori Sutherland (Vice President of International Sales); Dave Kleinberg (Director of International Sales)
600 Townsend
San Francisco
CA 94103
USA
Telephone: (415) 442–0200
Fax: (415) 442–0190

2595. MacTutor
Laura Schenk (Owner); Kirk Chase (Editor)
1250 N Lakeview
Suite O
Anaheim
CA 92807
USA
Telephone: (714) 777–1255
Fax: (714) 777–6972

2596. MacWarehouse
Teledirect House
Queens Road
Barnet
Hertforshire
EN5 4DL
UK
Telephone: 0800 181332

2597. MacWeek Inc
301 Howard Street
15th Floor
San Francisco
CA 94105
USA
Telephone: (415) 882–7370

2598. Madison Newspapers Inc
1901 Fish Hatchery Road
PO Box 8058
Madison
WI 53708
USA
Telephone: (608) 252–6200;
         (608) 252–6238

2599. Maersk Data Incom
Sten Bertelsen; Peter Stougaard;
   Behrndt Andersen
Titangade 11
2200 Koebenhavn N
Denmark
Telephone: 45 (31) 838211

2600. Maeventec
735 Ekekela Place
Honolulu
HI 96817
USA
Telephone: (808) 595–7089

2601. Magazine Article Summaries
   (See EBSCO Publishing)

2602. Maggie Mae's Gourmet Pet
   Products Inc
PO Box 4245
Mountain View
CA 94040
USA
Telephone: (415) 967–9492
Fax: (415) 941–2704
Telex/E-mail: MAGGIEMAE (GEnie)

2603. Magnum Software
Moorend House
Sampford Peverell
Tiverton
EX16 7EQ
UK
Telephone: 0884 820240
Fax: 0884 821497

2604. MAID Systems Ltd
MAID House
26 Baker Street
London
W1M 1DF
UK
Telephone: 071 935–6460

2605. Maine State Library
Karl Beifer
Statheouse Section 64
Augusta
ME 04333
USA
Telephone: (207) 289–5600;
         (207) 581–1656

2606. Mainichi Newspapers, The
1–1–1 Hitotsubashi
Chiyoda-ku
Tokyo 100
Japan
Telephone: 03 3212–3358
Fax: 03 3284–1601
Telex/E-mail: 22324 J

2607. Makrolog GmbH
A Herberger
von-Leyden-Stra[e1]e 46
6200 Wiesbaden
Germany
Telephone: 0611 5620–45
Fax: 0611 5620–49

2608. Mallinckrodt Inc
Science Products Division
PO Box 800
Paris
KY 40361
USA
Telephone: (606) 987–7000

2609. Mallory International
Norman J Guthrie (Partner)
Potters Market
West Hill
Ottery St Mary
Devon
EX11 1TY
UK
Telephone: 0404 815–310
Fax: 0404 812–245

2610. Mammoth Micro Productions
Thomas Lopez (Chairman); Barbara
   Witt (Corporate Communications)
1700 Westlake Avenue N
Seattle
WA 98109
USA
Telephone: (206) 281–7500
Fax: (206) 281–7734

2611. Management Association of
   Illinois, The
2400 S Downing
Westchester
IL 60154–5194
USA
Telephone: (708) 562–9063
Fax: (708) 562–8436

2612. Management Directions
PO Box 26987
Austin
TX 78755
USA
Telephone: (512) 331–0224

2613. Management Science
   Associates Inc
6565 Penn Avenue at Fifth
Pittsburgh
PA 15206–4490
USA
Telephone: (412) 362–2000
Fax: (412) 363–8878

2614. Mandarin Communications Ltd
Greenaway
London Road
Balcombe
Haywards Heath
RH17 6HS
UK
Telephone: 0444 811 519

2615. Manitoba Legislative Counsel
   Office
444 St Mary Avenue
Room 350
Winnipeg
MB R3C 3T1
Canada
Telephone: (204) 945–3758

2616. ManLabs Inc
21 Erie Street
Cambridge
MA 02139
USA
Telephone: (617) 491–2900

2617. MARCIVE Inc
Janifer Meldrum (Director of Marketing)
PO Box 47508
San Antonio
TX 78265–7508
USA
Telephone: (800) 531–7678;
         (512) 646–6161
Fax: (512) 646–0167

2618. Maridean Mansfield Shepard
9840 Stanwin Avenue
Arleta
CA 91331–5303
USA
Telephone: (818) 899–1598

2619. MARIS ON-LINE Ltd
D Draper (Managing Director)
Bank House
1 St Mary's Street
Ely
Cambridgeshire
CB7 4ER
UK
Telephone: 0353 661–284
Fax: 0353 663–279

2620. Maritime Law Book Company
   Ltd
PO Box 302
Fredericton
NB E3B 4Y9
Canada
Telephone: (506) 453–9921

2621. Maritime Technical Information
   Facility
National Maritime Research Center
Kings Point
NY 11024–1699
USA
Telephone: (516) 773–5577

2622. Market Buy Market
Division of Golden West Broadcasters
5858 Sunset Blvd
Los Abgeles
CA 90028
USA
Telephone: (213) 469–5341

2623. Market Data Retrieval
16 Progress Drive
Shelton
CT 06484–2117
USA
Telephone: (203) 926–4800;
         (800) 243–5538
Fax: (203) 926–0721

2624. Market Guide Inc
John D Case (President)
49 Glen Head Road
Glen Head
NY 11545
USA
Telephone: (516) 759–1253;
         (800) 642–3840
Fax: (516) 676–9240

2625. Market Intelligence Research
   Company
Michael Galvin (Account Executive)
2525 Charleston Road
Mountain View
CA 94043
USA
Telephone: (415) 961–9000
Fax: (415) 961–5042
Telex/E-mail: 804294 62776943
(EasyLink)

2626. Market Location Ltd
1 Warwick Street
Leamington Spa
Warwickshire
CV32 5LW
UK
Telephone: 0926 450–388
Fax: 0926 450–592

2627. Market Research Africa (Pty) Ltd
178 Fox Street
Johannesburg 2001
Republic of South Africa
Telephone: 011 292–544
Telex/E-mail: 483598 SA

2628. Market Science Associates Inc
1560 Broadway
3rd Floor
New York
NY 10036
USA
Telephone: (212) 398–9100

2629. Market Statistics
Bob Katz
633 Third Avenue
New York
NY 10017
USA
Telephone: (212) 986–4800
Fax: (212) 983–6930

2630. Marketing Data
W.F. Verweel
Koninginneweg 20a
Postbus 1188
1000 BD Amsterdam
Netherlands
Telephone: 31 (20) 626081
Telex/E-mail: 18424
NUA: 2041290340

2631. Marketing Intelligence Corporation
14–11, 2–Chome Yatomachi
Tanashi-shi
Tokyo 188
Japan
Telephone: 0424 3231–111
Fax: 03 3981–9109
Telex/E-mail: 2822545 MIC J

2632. Marketing Intelligence Service Ltd
33 Academy Street
Naples
NY 14512
USA
Telephone: (716) 374–6326;
              (800) 836–5710
Fax: (716) 374–5217

2633. Marketing Publications Ltd
22 Lancaster Gate
London
W2 3LY
UK
Telephone: 071 402–4200

2634. Marketing Strategies for Industry (UK) Ltd
Heathmans House
19 Heathmans Road
Parsons Green
London
SW6 4TJ
UK
Telephone: 071 371–0955
Fax: 071 371–5284
Telex/E-mail: 27950 G

2635. MarketPlace Information Corporation
Douglas C Burchard (President);
    Catherine J Engelke (Marketing
    Communications Manager)
1 Canal Park
Cambridge
MA 02141–2228
USA
Telephone: (617) 225–7853;
              (617) 225–7850
Fax: (617) 225–7860

2636. Markets Advisory
601 Lake Avenue
Racine
WI 53403
USA
Telephone: (414) 634–3373

2637. Marknadsdomstolen
Box 2217
S-103 15 Stockholm
Sweden
Telephone: 08 24 41 55
Fax: 08 21 23 35

2638. Marmen Computing Inc
123 6th Street
Menominee
MI 49858
USA
Telephone: (906) 863–2611

2639. Marshall & Swift
1617 Beverly Boulevard
PO Box 26307
Los Angeles
CA 90026–0307
USA
Telephone: (213) 250–2222;
              (800) 526–2756

2640. Martin Marietta Data Systems
6303 Ivy Lane
Greenbelt
MD 20770
USA
Telephone: (301) 982–6877

2641. Martin Marietta Information Systems Group
4795 Meadow Wood Lane
Chantilly
VA 22021
UK
Telephone: (703) 802–5000

2642. Martindale-Hubbell Electronic Publishing
Lenora Luciano (Sales Coordinator)
121 Chanlon Road
New Providence
NJ 07974
USA
Telephone: (908) 665–6717;
              (800) 526–4902
Fax: (908) 665–6688

2643. Martindale-Hubbell Inc
PO Box 1001
Summit
NJ 07901
USA
Telephone: (908) 464–6800;
              (800) 526–4902
Telex/E-mail: 138755

2644. Maruzen Company Ltd
Maruzen Scientific Information Service
    Center
Masahiro Nishi (Deputy General
    Manager, New Media Department)
PO Box 5335
Tokyo International 100–31
Japan
Telephone: 03 3271–6068;
              03 3272–7211
Fax: 03 3271–6082; 03 3274–3072
Telex/E-mail: 26630 MARUZEN J
11511 (DIALMAIL)

2645. Maryland Center for Public Broadcasting
11767 Bonita Avenue
Baltimore
MD 21117
USA
Telephone: (301) 356–5600

2646. Maryland Public Television
11767 Bonita Avenue
Baltimore
MD 21117
USA
Telephone: (301) 337–4190

2647. Maryland University Advanced Development Laboratory
Virgil Davis (Director of Electronic
    Programs)
6411 Ivy Lane
Suite 110
Greenbelt
MD 20770
USA
Telephone: (301) 345–8664
Fax: (301) 345–7305

2648. Marymac Industries
22511 Katy Freeway
Katy
TX 77450
USA
Telephone: (713) 392–0747;
              (800) 231–3680

2649. Massachusetts General Hospital
Laboratory of Computer Science
55 Fruit Street
Boston
MA 02114
USA
Telephone: (617) 726–3950

2650. Massachusetts Institute of Technology
Information Services
Room 11–315
Cambridge
MA 02139
USA
Telephone: (617) 253–8421

2651. Massachusetts Medical Society
Publishing Division
1440 Main Street
Waltham
MA 02254
USA
Telephone: (617) 890–0385;
              (617) 893–3800;
              (617) 893–4610;
              (800) 342–1338
Fax: (617) 893–8103;
              (617) 647–5785

2652. Masterclips Inc
5201 Ravenswood Road
Suite 111
Fort Lauderdale
FL 33312
USA
Telephone: (800) 292–2547
Fax: (305) 967–9452

2653. Materials Information
Barbara Sanduleak (Manager
    Information Services)
ASM International
Materials Park
OH 44073
Telephone: (216) 338–5151
Fax: (216) 338–4634
Telex/E-mail: 980619 ASMINT 13073
    (DIALMAIL); MSDASM01
    (ORBIT)

2654. Materials Information
Mark Furneaux (Marketing Manager);
    Jill Feldt (Info Retrieval Specialist)
The Institute of Metals
1 Carlton House Terrace
London
SW1Y 5DB
UK
Telephone: 071 839–4071
Fax: 071 839–2289

2655. Materials Properties Council
345 E 47th Street
New York
NY 10017
USA
Telephone: (212) 705–7693

2656. MathSoft
c/o Adept Scientific Micro Systems
    Ltd
Letchworth
Hertfordshire
UK
Telephone: +44 (0)462 480055

2657. Matrikeldirektoratet
Ole Anderson
Titangade 13
2200 Koebenhavn N
Denmark
Telephone: 45 (31) 837733

**2658. Matthew Bender & Company
    Inc**
Don Eddy (Manager of Marketing
    Projects)
11 Penn Plaza
New York
NY 10001
USA
Telephone: (212) 216–8025;
          (212) 216–8094;
          (212) 216–8058;
          (800) 223–1940
Fax: (212) 239–2082

2659. Matthew Bender & Company
Promotions
Melissa Lande; David Ouellette
134 West 29th Street
New York
NY 10001
USA
Telephone: (212) 344–0930;
          (800) 424–4200

2660. Max Ule & Company Inc
26 Broadway
Suite 200
New York
NY 10004
USA
Telephone: (212) 766–2610

2661. Maxis
1042 Country Club Drive
Suite C
Moraga
CA 94556
USA

2662. Maxwell Data Management Inc
Don Bissell (Director Product
    Development); C Richard Gray
    (Senior Vice President)
275 E Baker
Suite A
Costa Mesa
CA 92626
USA
Telephone: (714) 435–7700
Fax: (714) 751–1442

2663. Maxwell Data Management
Slack Lane
Derby
DE3 3FL
UK
Telephone: 0332 47123

**2664. Maxwell Electronic
    Publishing**
Frederick Bowes III (President); Randi
    Straus (Director of Marketing)
124 Mount Auburn Street
Cambridge
MA 02138
USA
Telephone: (617) 576–5737;
          (800) 342–1338
Fax: (617) 868–7738

2665. Maxwell Macmillan
Professional and Business Division
920 Sylvan Avenue
Englewood Cliffs
NJ 07632
USA
Telephone: (201) 569–4000

2666. Maxwell Multi Media Inc
Pat Call
4820 Riverbend Road
Suite 200
Boulder
CO 80301
USA
Telephone: (303) 440–0669
Fax: (303) 443–8247

2667. Maxwell Multi Media Ltd
Marketing Department
Marc Deschamps (Director Marketing &
    Sales); Alison Turner (Marketing
    Communications)
Knowsley House
176 Sloane Street
London
SW1X 9QJ
UK
Telephone: 071 235–5992
Fax: 071 235–6191

2668. MBC Information Services Ltd
Paulton House
8 Shepherdess Walk
London
N1 7LB
UK
Telephone: 071 490–0049
Fax: 071 490–2979

2669. McCarthy Information Ltd
Manor House
Ash Walk
Warminster
Wiltshire
BA12 8PY
UK
Telephone: 0985 215–151
Fax: 0985 217–479

2670. McCarthy, Crisanti & Maffei Inc
Electronic Information Services
71 Broadway
New York
NY 10006
USA
Telephone: (212) 509–5800
Fax: (212) 509–7389
Telex/E-mail: 423720 MCMUI

2671. McCarthy, Tetrault
275 Sparks Street
Suite 1000
Ottawa
ON K1R 7X9
USA
Telephone: (613) 238–2000
Fax: (613) 563–7813

2672. McClatchy Newspapers
1626 E Street
Fresno
CA 93786
USA
Telephone: (209) 441–6111

2673. McClelland & Stewart Inc
380 Esna Park Drive
Markham
L3R 1H5
Canada
Telephone: (416) 940–8855
Fax: (416) 940–3642

**2674. McClure Lundberg Associates
    Inc**
1515 U Street NW
Washington
DC 20009
USA
Telephone: (202) 483–4107

**2675. McDonnel Douglas
    Cegi-Tymshare**
106 Bureau de la Colline
92213 Saint-Cloud
Paris
France
Telephone: 33 (1) 46 02 70 12
Telex/E-mail: 270315 F

2676. McGill University
Computing Center
805 Sherbrooke Street W
Montreal
PQ H3A 2K6
Canada
Telephone: (514) 398–3702

**2677. McGraw-Hill Book Company
    Europe**
Stephen Rickard (Multimedia Contact);
    Juliette Ward (Product Manager
    Marketing)
Shoppenhangers Road
Maidenhead
Berkshire
SL6 2QL
UK
Telephone: 0628 23432
Fax: 0628 770–224

2678. McGraw-Hill Book Company
Rachel Handler (Senior Marketing
    Manager)
11 W 19th Street
4th Floor
New York
NY 10011
USA
Telephone: (212) 337–5904;
          (212) 337–5916;
          (212) 337–6010;
          (800) 722–ISBN;
          (800) 262–4729
Fax: (212) 337–4092

2679. McGraw-Hill Financial Services Company
25 Broadway
New York
NY 10004
USA
Telephone: (212) 208–8880
Fax: (212) 208–1718

2680. McGraw-Hill Inc
Construction Information Services Group, FW Dodge Division
1221 Avenue of the Americas
New York
NY 10020
USA
Telephone: (212) 512–2000;
(800) 426–7766
Fax: (212) 512–6204

2681. McGraw-Hill Inc
Princeton-Hightstown Road
North-1
Hightstown
NJ 08520
USA
Telephone: (609) 426–5523;
(609) 426–5000
Fax: (609) 426–7352
Telex/E-mail: 13957
(DIALMAIL)

2682. McGraw-Hill Inc
1 Phoenix Mill Lane
Peterborough
NH 03458
USA
Telephone: (603) 924–7681;
(800) 227–2983
Fax: (603) 924–2530
Telex/E-mail: Liberty (BIX)

2683. McGraw-Hill Inc
Electronic Markets and Information Systems
1221 Avenue of the Americas
42nd Floor
New York
NY 10020–1095
USA
Telephone: (212) 512–4091;
(212) 512–2000
Fax: (212) 208–1718

2684. McGraw-Hill Publications Company
Aviation Week Group
1156 15th Street NW
Suite 600
Washington
DC 20005
USA
Telephone: (202) 822–4675;
(800) 877–6236
Fax: (202) 293–2682
Telex/E-mail: 892447

2685. MCI International
MCI IInsight
2 International Drive
Rye Brook
NY 10573–1098
USA
Telephone: (914) 934–6166;
(914) 937–3444;
(800) 444–6245;
(800) 876–4030
Telex/E-mail: 6712472

2686. McMillan UK
2 Lindsay Street
Arbroath
Tayside
DD11 1RP
UK
Telephone: 0241 78411
Fax: 0241 70560

2687. MCN (Muziek Catalogus Nederland)
Muziekdokumentatie
Postbus 119
1200 AC Hilversum
Netherlands
Telephone: 035 772–450
Fax: 035 775–228

2688. McNaught Syndicate
537 Steamboat Road
Greenwich
CT 06830
USA
Telephone: (203) 661–4990

2689. MDX (See Medical Data Exchange)

2690. Mead Data Central International
International House
1 St. Katharine's Way
London
E1 9UN
UK
Telephone: 071 488–9187
Fax: 071 480–7228

2691. Mead Data Central
Park Avenue 17
New York
NY 10166
USA
Telephone: (212) 309–8169;
(212) 309–8187

2692. Mead Data Central
9443 Springboro Pike
PO Box 933
Dayton
OH 45401–9964
USA
Telephone: (513) 865–6800;
(513) 865–6889;
(800) 227–4908
Fax: (513) 865–6909

2693. Mead Ventures Inc
3800 North Central Avenue
Suite 1601
PO Box 44952
Phoenix
AZ 85064
USA
Telephone: (602) 234–0044;
(800) 669–6323
Fax: (602) 234–0076

2694. Meckler Corporation
11 Ferry Lane W
Westport
CT 06880–5808
USA
Telephone: (203) 226–6967
Fax: (203) 454–5840
Telex/E-mail: ALA 0961 (ALANET);
CLASS MECKLER/JPE (OnTyme)

2695. Meckler
247–249 Vauxhall Bridge Road
London
SW1V 1HQ
UK
Telephone: 071 931–8908

2696. Media Access Inc
150 E 58th Street
35th Floor
New York
NY 10155
USA
Telephone: (212) 826–2800;
(800) 242–2463
Fax: (212) 826–0069

2697. Media Clip Art Inc
Scott Gross (Sales); Hugh Maguire (Sales); Susan Gross (Sales)
411 Narragansett Drive
Cherry Hill
NJ 08002
USA
Telephone: (609) 795–5993;
(609) 667–5044
Fax: (609) 667–5690

2698. Media Design Interactive Ltd
Philip Nash (Publisher); Philip Devin (Director)
Alexandra House
Station Road
Aldershot
Hampshire
GU11 1BQ
UK
Telephone: 0252 344–454;
0252 851–405
Fax: 0252 318–775

2699. Media Expenditure Analysis Ltd
110 St Martin's Lane
London
WC2N 4BH
UK
Telephone: 071 240–1903

2700. Media General Financial Services Inc
Horace Dowdy (Director of Project Development)
PO Box C-32333
301 E Grace Street
Richmond
VA 23219
USA
Telephone: (804) 649–6736
Fax: (804) 649–6097

2701. Media Group Srl
Annalisa Borgia (General Manager); Glauco Ferrari
Via Bessarione 29
20139 Milan
Italy
Telephone: 02 539–7575
Fax: 02 539–7575;
02 574–03680

2702. Media Technology (Pvt) Ltd
200 Herbert Chitepo Avenue
PO Box HG 328
Highlands
Harare
Zimbabwe
Telephone: 04 702–009
Fax: 04 702–006

2703. Media Week Ltd
20–27 Wellington Street
London
WC2E 7DD
UK
Telephone: 071 240–9851

2704. Media-Service GmbH (MS)
Bahnhofstraße 1
D-6084 Gernsheim
Germany
Telephone: 06258 3073
Fax: 06258 51536

2705. Mediagenic
3885 Bohannon Drive
Menlo Park
CA 94025
USA
Telephone: (415) 329–0800

2706. Medialink International Corporation
200 East Del Mar Blvd, Suite 100
Pasadena
CA 91105–2544
USA
Telephone: (818) 304–1122;
  (800) 451–0360
Fax: (818) 577–7970

2707. Mediamark Research Inc
David C Arpin (Vice President Product Development)
708 3rd Avenue
New York
NY 10017
USA
Telephone: (212) 599–0444
Fax: (212) 682–6284

2708. MediaNews Group Inc
1560 Broadway
Denver
CO 80202
USA
Telephone: (303) 820–1010

2709. Médias Communication Production
Bernard Dudoignon (Responsable Produits)
13 rue Etienne Marcel
75001 Paris
France
Telephone: 1 40 26 90 37
Fax: 1 40 26 90 43

2710. MediaTel Limited
52 Poland Street
London
W1V 3DF
UK
Telephone: 071 439–7575

2711. Mediavision
Bert Harenberg (Managing Director)
PO Box 441
1250 AK Laren
Netherlands
Telephone: 02153 12637

2712. Medical Data Exchange (MDX)
445 S San Antonio Road
Los Altos
CA 94022
USA
Telephone: (415) 941–3600
Fax: (415) 941–3683
Telex/E-mail: 62910349 (EasyLink)

2713. Medical Economics Data Inc
(Part of Thomson Corporation)
5 Targon Drive
Oradell
Montvale
NJ 07645
USA
Telephone: (201) 358–7200;
  (201) 262–3030;
  (800) 526–4870
Fax: (201) 664–1902; (201) 573–4956

2714. Medical Information Systems
Reference and Index Services Inc
3845 North Meridian Street
Indianapolis
IN 46208
USA
Telephone: (317) 923–1575

2715. Medical Malpractice Verdicts, Settlements & Experts
901 Church Street
Nashville
TN 37203
USA
Telephone: (615) 255–6288

2716. Medical Publishing Group
Saxon Way
Melbourn
Royston
Hertfordshire
SG8 6NJ
UK
Telephone: 07636 2401

2717. Medical Publishing Group
1440 Main Street
Waltham
MA 02154
USA
Telephone: (617) 893–3800

2718. Medicindata
Box 33031
400 33 Goeteborg
Sweden
Telephone: 46 (31) 41 11 10

2719. Médicine et Hygiène
P-Y Balavoine
78 rue de la Roseraie
Case Postale 456
1211 Geneva 4
Switzerland
Telephone: 022 46 93 55
Fax: 022 47 56 10

2720. Mediconsult GmbH
Andreas M Herberger
von-Leyden-Straße 46
6200 Wiesbaden
Germany
Telephone: 0611 5620 45;
  0611 5620 46
Fax: 0611 5260 49

2721. Mediothek der Medizinischen Fakultät der Universität Basel Foundation Neocortex
Prof Dr Med Hanspeter Rohr (Medical Director)
Kantonsspital Basel
Holsteinerhof
Hebelstraße 32
4031 Basel
Switzerland
Telephone: 061 265–2450
Fax: 061 261–4868

2722. Medisoft Gesellschaft für Medizinische Datenbanken mbH
Herman Schultze
Georg-Speyr-Straße 42
D-6000 Frankfurt 90
Germany
Telephone: 069 77 43 21;
  069 77 43 74
Fax: 069 77 23 41

2723. MedMedia bv
Delistraat 41
2585 Den Haag
Netherlands
Telephone: 0865 200972
Fax: 0865 200747

2724. Megalith Technologies Inc
Sandra Hovey (Sales Manager)
1 Antares Drive
Suite 510
Nepean
ON K2E 8C4
Canada
Telephone: (613) 225–2300
Fax: (613) 225–2304

2725. Melissa Data Company
Nicole Luck (Marketing Manager)
32122 Paseo Adelanto 2B
San Juan Capistrano
CA 92675
USA
Telephone: (714) 661–5885
Fax: (714) 661–5002

2726. Mellon InvestData Corporation (See Muller Data Corporation)

2727. Memphis Publishing Company
495 Union Avenue
Memphis
TN 38103
USA
Telephone: (901) 529–2211

2728. Mendelsohn Media Research Inc
352 Park Avenue S
New York
NY 10010
USA
Telephone: (212) 684–6350

2729. Mentor Graphics Corporation
8005 SW Boeckman Road
Wilsonville
OR 97070–7777
USA
Telephone: (503) 685–7000
Fax: (503) 685–1202

2730. Menu International
Françoise Quenon (Manager)
14 rue des Pavilions
92800 Puteaux
France
Telephone: 1 47 75 30 72
Fax: 1 49 06 05 71

2731. Menu Publishing
PO Box MENU
Mayview Road at Park Drive
Pittsburg
PA 15241
USA
Telephone: (412) 746–6368;
  (800) THE-MENU

2732. Mercersburg Academy
Science Department
Rick Needham
Mercersburg
PA 17236
USA
Telephone: (717) 328–2151

2733. Merck Sharp & Dohme Research Laboratories
Dr Asa Mays (Associate Editor)
PO Box 2000
Building 86–215
Rahway
NJ 07065–0900
USA
Telephone: (908) 750–7512;
  (908) 594–4890
Fax: (908) 594–3868;
  (908) 750–7513
Telex/E-mail: 16530 (DIALMAIL)

2734. Mercury Electronic Publishing Corporation (See METCO)

2735. Mercury Link 7500
1 Brentside Executive Centre
Great West Road
Brentford
Middlesex
TW8 9DS
UK
Telephone: 44 (1) 528–2500
Fax: 44 (1) 528–2366

2736. Meridian Data Europe BV
Aad Proeme (General Manager)
Mierloseweg 53
5667 JB Geldrop
Netherlands
Telephone: 040 863–082
Fax: 040 859–455

2737. Meridian Data Inc
5615 Scotts Valley Drive
Scotts Valley
CA 95066
USA
Telephone: (408) 438–3100;
            (800) 755–8324
Fax: (408) 438–6816

2738. Meridian Systems Management Limited
Bromley Data Centre
18 Elmfield Road
Bromley
Kent
BR1 1LR
UK
Telephone: 44 (1) 313–0178
Fax: 44 (1) 313–0813

2739. Merit Software
J Roddy McGinnis (Director Product Development)
13635 Gamma Road
Dallas
TX 75244
USA
Telephone: (214) 385–2353
Fax: (214) 385–8205

2740. Merit Systems Protection Board
Marcus Wood
1120 Vermont Avenue NW
Washington
DC 20419
USA
Telephone: (202) 653–7124
Fax: (202) 65333–7130

2741. Merkur Direktwerbegesellschaft mbH
Mr Rehborn
Kapellenstraße 44
3352 Einbeck
Germany
Telephone: 05561 314–0
Fax: 05561 314–33

2742. Merlin Gerin
Documentation
38050 Grenoble Cedex
France
Telephone: 33 (76) 57 94 60
Telex/E-mail: 320842 F

2743. Merton Allen Associates
PO Box 15640
Plantation
FL 33318–5640
USA
Telephone: (305) 473–9560
Fax: (305) 473–0544

2744. Messaggerie Libri SpA
Alberto Ottieri (Product Manager)
Via G Carcano 32
20141 Milan
Italy
Telephone: 02 84 38 141
Fax: 02 64 63 169; 02 89 50 0298

2745. Metals Economics Group Ltd
Cogswell Tower
Suite 804
2000 Barrington Street
PO Box 2206
Halifax
NS B3J 3C4
Canada
Telephone: (902) 429–2880
Fax: (902) 429–6593
Telex/E-mail: 0636700485 MBX CA

2746. Metatec / Discovery Systems
Mary Vaughn (Director of Marketing)
7001 Discovery Boulevard
Dublin
OH 43017
USA
Telephone: (614) 761–2000
Fax: (614) 761–4258
Telex/E-mail: 70673,20 (CompuServe Information Service); 71216,1271 (CompuServe Information Service)

2747. METCO
Warren T Stone
PO Box 447
Elizabethtown
PA 17022
USA
Telephone: (800) 669–2441;
            (717) 367–4200
Fax: (717) 367–9120

2748. Metracom Inc
PO Box 23498
Oklahoma City
OK 73132
USA
Telephone: (405) 721–0207

2749. Metromail Corporation
360 E 22nd Street
Lombard
IL 60148–4989
USA
Telephone: (708) 620–3012

2750. Metromail Inc
901 West Bond
Lincoln
NE 68521
USA
Telephone: (402) 475–4591

2751. Meyer & Siegers
Wim Siegers
Pietersbergseweg 14
6862 BV Oosterbeek
Netherlands
Telephone: 085 341–045
Fax: 085 337–514

2752. MI-Iran
Nader Naghshineh (Manager)
PO Box 3993
Tehran 14155
Iran
Telephone: 021 623–728
Fax: 021 890–178

2753. Miami Herald Publishing Company, The
1 Herald Plaza
Miami
FL 33132–1693
USA
Telephone: (305) 350–2111

2754. Miami News
PO Box 6175
Miami
FL 33152
USA
Telephone: (305) 376–3100

2755. Michael Linden Agency
PO Box 1319
Ashland
OR 97520
USA
Telephone: (503) 488–2326
Telex/E-mail: 62804934

2756. Michael Naver
PO Box 11966
Baltimore
MD 21207
USA
Telephone: (301) 747–8241

2757. Michie Company, The
Andrew Wyszkowski (Vice President Information Resources Management)
PO Box 7587
Charlottesville
VA 22906–7587
USA
Telephone: (804) 295–6171;
            (804) 972–7600;
            (804) 972–7614;
            (800) 446–3410
Fax: (804) 972–7656

2758. Michigan Department of Natural Resources Surface Water Quality Division
Great Lakes and Environmental Assessment Section
Robert Sills (Senior Toxicologist); Gary Hurlburt (Unit Supervisor)
Knapp's Office Center
PO Box 30028
Lansing
MI 48909
USA
Telephone: (517) 373–2190
Fax: (517) 373–9958

2759. Micro Haus Ltd
Derek Davidson (Managing Director); Andrew McBride (General Manager)
PO Box 149
Gloucester
GL3 4EG
UK
Telephone: 0452 371–707;
            0452 864–298
Fax: 0452 864–293

2760. Micro Map & CAD
PO Box 621135
Littleton
CO 80162
USA

2761. Micro Progettazione Avanzata SRL
Nicola Sgarra
Via del Boschetto 40c
00184 Rome
Italy
Telephone: 06 474–6683
Fax: 06 487–1459

2762. Microbial Culture Information Service
Laboratory of the Government Chemist
Room C004
Queens Road
Teddington
Middlesex
TW11 0LY
UK
Telephone: 44 (81) 943–7612;
            44 (81) 943–7384
Fax: 44 (81) 943–2767

2763. Microbial Strain Data Network
Cambridge University
MSDN Secretariat, Institute of
  Biotechnology
307 Huntingdon Road
Girton
Cambridge
CB3 0JX
UK
Telephone: 44 (223) 276622
Fax: 44 (223) 277605
Telex/E-mail: 81240 CAMSPL G

2764. Microcell Communications
170 Broadway
Suite 1515
New York
NY 10038
USA
Telephone: (212) 385–0280

2765. Microcomputers in Education
Custom Publishing Service
85 Beach Street
Westerly
RI -2891
USA
Telephone: (401) 596–6080

2766. Microinfo Ltd
Roy Selwyn (Director)
PO Box 3
Omega Park
Alton
Hampshire
GU34 2PG
UK
Telephone: 0420 86848
Fax: 0420 89889
Telex/E-mail: 858431 MINFO G

2767. Micromedex Inc
Phillip Bird (International Sales
  Manager)
600 Grant Street
Denver
CO 80203–3527
USA
Telephone: (303) 831–1400;
        (800) 525–9083
Fax: (303) 837–1717
Telex/E-mail: 703618 MEDEX UD

2768. Micromedia Ltd
June Ann Cole (Customer Service
  Representative)
20 Victoria Street
Toronto
ON M5C 2N8
Canada
Telephone: (416) 362–5211;
        (800) 387–2689 (in Canada)
Fax: (416) 362–6161
Telex/E-mail: 06524668; DIALOG
CANADA (DIALMAIL);
ADMIN/MICROMEDIA
  (Envoy 100)

2769. Micronet SA
José Antonio Cerezo
Maria Tubau no 7
Edifico Auge III
6th Floor
28049 Madrid
Spain
Telephone: 01 372–0517;
        01 358–9625
Fax: 01 372–0562;
        01 308–0975;
        01 358–9544

2770. MicroPatent
Elizabeth Hearle
Cambridge Place
Cambridge
CB2 1NR
UK
Telephone: 0223 311–479
Fax: 0223 66440

2771. MicroPatent
Judy Hickey (Marketing Director)
25 Science Park
New Haven
CT 06511
USA
Telephone: (203) 786–5500;
        (800) 648–6787
Fax: (203) 786–5499

2772. Microsoft Corporation
Customer Services
1 Microsoft Way
PO Box 97017
Redmond
WA 98052–6394
USA
Telephone: (206) 882–8080;
        (800) 426–9400
Fax: (206) 883–8101
Telex/E-mail: 160520

2773. Microsoft Ltd
David Svendsen (Managing Director)
Excel House
84 Caversham Road
Reading
Berkshire
RG1 8LP
UK
Telephone: 0734 391–123
Fax: 0734 507–624

2774. MicroTrends
650 Woodfield Drive
Suite 730
Schaumburg
IL 60173
USA
Telephone: (312) 310–8928

**2775. Middle East Executive Reports
Limited**
717 D Street, NW, Suite 300
Washington
DC 20004–2807
USA
Telephone: (202) 628–6900
Telex/E-mail: 440462

2776. Military Data Corporation
1745 Jefferson Davis Highway
Crystal Square 4, Suite 501
Arlington
VA 22202
USA
Telephone: (703) 553–0208;
        (800) 443–7216
Fax: (703) 521–7447

2777. Military Forum
1041 Carnation Drive
Rockville
MD 20850
USA
Telephone: (301) 340–9617
Telex/E-mail: 76703,603 (Compuserve
Information Service)

2778. MILITRAN Inc
1255 Drummers Lane
Suite 306
Wayne
PA 19087
USA
Telephone: (215) 687–3900;
        (800) 426–9954
Fax: (215) 687–6814

2779. Mill Hollow Corporation
19 W 21st Street
8th Floor
New York
NY 10010
USA
Telephone: (212) 741–2095

2780. Mindscape
Software Toolworks
Debbie King (Press Relations)
The Coach House
Hooklands Estate
Scaynes Hill
West Sussex
RH17 7NG
UK
Telephone: 0444 831–761
Fax: 0444 831–688

2781. Mining Journal Ltd, The
60 Worship Street
London
EC2A 2HD
UK
Telephone: 071 377–2020
Fax: 071 247–4100

2782. Ministere de Defense
Delegation Generale pour l'Armement
Centre de Documentation de
  l'Armement (CEDOCAR)
26 boulevard Victor
F-00460 Paris-Armeés
France
Telephone: 1 45 52 45 04
Fax: 1 45 52 60 47
Telex/E-mail: 202778 CEDOCAR F
NUA: 208075060238

**2783. Ministere de l'Agriculture et de
la Foret**
RESAGRI
78 rue de Varenne
F-75700 Paris
France
Telephone: 1 45 44 95 50

2784. Ministere de l'Agriculture
Sous-direction de l'Informatique
33 rue de Picpus
75012 Paris
France
Telephone: 1 43 44 53 00

2785. Ministere de l'Agriculture
Service Central des Enquetes et Etudes
  Statistiques
4 avenue de Saint-Mande
75570 Paris Cedex 12
France
Telephone: 1 43 44 53 00

**2786. Ministere de l'Education
Nationale, de la Jeunesse et
des Sports**
DBMIST
3–5 boulevard Pasteur
F-75015 Paris
France
Telephone: 1 45 39 25 75
Fax: 1 47 34 21 98

2787. Ministere de l'Education Nationale
Comite des Travaux Historiques et
  Scientifiques
3–5 boulevard Pasteur
F-75015 Paris
France
Telephone: 1 45 39 25 75

2788. Ministere de la Recherche et de la Technologie
Martine Comberousse (Chargée de
  Mission)
1 rue Descartes
F-75231 Paris Cedex 5
France
Telephone: 1 46 34 35 77;
           1 46 43 30 28
Fax: 1 46 34 34 02

2789. Ministere des Communications
Bibliotheque administrative
Building DIFICE G
1056 Conroy Street, Quebec
PQ G1R 5E6
Canada
Telephone: (418) 643–9927
Telex/E-mail: 0513542

2790. Ministere du Developpement Industriel Scientifique
110 rue de Grenelle
F-75700 Paris
France
Telephone: 1 45 56 36 36

2791. Ministerie van Economische Zaken
Bezuidenhoutseweg 30
Postbus 20 101
2500 's-Gravenhage
Netherlands
Telephone: 31 (70) 79 89 11;
          31 (70) 47 40 81

2792. Ministerie van Verkeer en Waterstaat
Afdeling Documentie en Bibliotheek
PO Box 20901
NL-2500 EX The Hague
Netherlands
Telephone: 070 351 70 89
Fax: 070 351 78 95
Telex/E-mail: 32562 MINVW NL

2793. Ministerio da Industria e Energia de Portugal
Laboratorio Nacional de Engenharia e
  Tecnologia Industrial
Azinghaga dos Lameiros a Estrada do
  Paco do Lumiar
Centro de Informacao Tecnica para a
  Industria
Building A
First Floor
1699 Lisbon Codex
Portugal
Telephone: 1 75 82 712
Fax: 1 75 96 732
Telex/E-mail: 42486 LNETI P

2794. Ministerio de Cultura de España
Centro del Libro y de la Lectura,
  Agencia Española del ISBN
Santiago Rusinol 8
28040 Madrid
Spain
Telephone: 01 253 93 29;
         01 233 08 02

2795. Ministerio de Cultura de España
Biblioteca Nacional
Recoletos 20 and 22, 1st Floor
28004 Madrid
Spain
Telephone: 34 (1) 275 68 00
Fax: 34 (1) 564 15 50

2796. Ministerio de Cultura de España
Consejo Superior de Deportes
Martin Fierro s/n
28040 Madrid
Spain
Telephone: 01 449 39 24

2797. Ministerio de Cultura de España
Centro de Información Documental de
  Archivos
Museo Español de Arte Contemporaneo
Avenida Juan de Herrera 2
28040 Madrid
Spain
Telephone: 01 243 70 48
Telex/E-mail: 27286 CULTU E

2798. Ministerio de Cultura de España
Dirección de Museos Estatales
Plaza del Rey s/n
28010 Madrid
Spain
Telephone: 01 521 56 28

2799. Ministerio de Cultura de España
Dirección General de Bellas Artes y
  Archivos
Avenida Juan de Herrera s/n
28040 Madrid
Spain
Telephone: 01 449 71 50

2800. Ministerio de Cultura de España
Instituto de la Cinematografía y de las
  Artes Audiovisuales
Ctra. Dehesa de la Villa s/n
28040 Madrid
Spain
Telephone: 01 449 00 11

2801. Ministerio de Cultura de España
Instituto Nacional de las Artes
  Escénicas y de la Musica
Centro de Documentación Musical
Capitán Haya 44
28020 Madrid
Spain
Telephone: 01 279 32 96

2802. Ministerio de Cultura de España
Instituto Nacional de las Artes
  Escénicas y de la Musica
Centro de Documentación Teatral
Capitán Haya 44
28020 Madrid
Spain
Telephone: 01 270 57 49

2803. Ministerio de Cultura de España
Secretaria General Tecnica Puntos de
  Información Cultural
Plaza de Rey 1
28071 Madrid
Spain
Telephone: 01 429 24 44;
        01 429 77 11
Fax: 01 531 92 12
Telex/E-mail: 27286 CULTURA E

2804. Ministerio de Cultura
Hemeroteco Nacional
Magdalena 10
28071 Madrid
Spain
Telephone: 34 (1) 468 54 99

2805. Ministerio de Educación y Ciencia de España
Centro de Proceso de Datos
Calle Vitruvio 6
28006 Madrid
Spain
Telephone: 091 262–6900
Fax: 091 262–3602

2806. Ministerio de Sanidad y Consumo de España
Dirección General de Farmacia y
  Productos Sanitarios
Servicio de Gestión del Banco de Datos
  de Medicamentos
Paseo del Prado 18–20
Planta 9
28014 Madrid
Spain
Telephone: 01 420–0417

2807. Ministerio de Trabajo de España
Instituto Nacional de Seguridad e
  Higiene en el Trabajo
Programa de Información y
  Documentación
Calle Dulcet s/n
08034 Barcelona
Spain
Telephone: 932044500

2808. Ministry of Civil Affairs
Computer Centre
Chen Yi
147
Beiheyan Street
Beijing 100721
China
Telephone: 512–1882;
        513–5644 x1246
Fax: 512–1882

2809. Ministry of Economic Affairs
Department of Metrology
24–26 Rue JA de Mot
B-1040 Brussels
Belgium
Telephone: 02 233–6111

2810. Ministry of Economic Affairs
DIE-OPRI
24–26 Rue JA de Mot
B-1040 Brussels
Belgium
Telephone: 02 233–6426;
        02 233–6111
Fax: 02 231–0256
Telex/E-mail: 20627 COMHAN B

2811. Ministry of Economic Affairs
Fond Quetelet
Guy de Saedleer (Head of the Library)
Rue de l'Industrie 6
1040 Brussels
Belgium
Telephone: 02 506–5111
Fax: 02 513–4657

2812. Ministry of Foreign Affairs
External Trade and Development
  Cooperation
African Library
Place Royale 7
B-1000 Brussels
Belgium
Telephone: 02 511–5870

2813. Ministry of Foreign Affairs
External Trade and Development
    Cooperation Central Library
2 rue Quatre-Bras
B-1000 Brussels
Belgium
Telephone: 02 516–8111

2814. Ministry of Trade and Industry
Library
Rue de l'Industrie 6
B-1040 Brussels
Belgium
Telephone: 02 506–5111; 02 511–1930
Telex/E-mail: 21262 MINECO B

2815. Minnesota Department of
    Education
Dan Bryan (Education Specialist)
Capital Square Building
555 Cedar Street
St Paul
MN 55101
USA
Telephone: (612) 296–2970
Fax: (612) 297–7201

2816. Minnesota Extension Service
University of Minnesota
475 Coffey Hall
1420 Eckles Avenue
St Paul
MN 55108
USA
Telephone: (612) 624–2708
Fax: (612) 625–2207

2817. Minnesota State Revisor of
    Statutes Office
Marcia Valencour (Deputy Revisor)
700 State Office Building
100 Constitution Avenue
St Paul
MN 55155–1297
USA
Telephone: (612) 296–2868
Fax: (612) 296–0569

2818. Mintel International Group
18–19 Long Lane
London
EC1A 9HE
UK
Telephone: 071 606–4533
Fax: 071 836–1682
Telex/E-mail: 21405 KAEMIN G

2819. Mintel Publications Ltd
KAE House
7 Arundel Street
London WC2R 3DR
UK
Telephone: 44 (71) 836–1814
Fax: 44 (71) 836–1682
Telex/E-mail: 21405 KAEMIN G

2820. Mirrorsoft Ltd
Peter Bilotta
Irwin House
118 Southwark Street
London
SE1 0SW
UK
Telephone: 071 928–1404;
071 928–1454
Fax: 071 583–3494

2821. Misawa Homes R&D
Kazuo Ohno
2–5–10 Kichijoji Honcho
Musashino
Tokyo 180
Japan
Telephone: 0422 20 5193
Fax: 0422 20 5199

2822. Missouri State Library
Stan Gardner (Assistant State Librarian)
2002 Missouri Boulevard
PO Box 387
Jefferson City
Missouri 65102
USA
Telephone: (314) 751–3615;
            (314) 751–0331;
            (314) 751–2768
Fax: (314) 751–3612

2823. MIT Press Journals
55 Hayward Street
Cambridge
MA 02142
USA
Telephone: (617) 253–2889
Fax: (617) 258–6779
Telex/E-mail: 921473 MITCAM

2824. Mitchell International
Bob Gradijan (Director of Marketing);
    Amy Kuhn (Marketing Operations
Analyst)
PO Box 26260
9889 Willow Creek Road
San Diego
CA 92131
USA
Telephone: (800) 854–7030;
            (619) 578–6550
Fax: (619) 549–0629;
            (619) 578–4652

2825. MIT
Hannelore Zumbruch
Am Zollstock 1
6382 Friedrichsdorf 1
Germany
Telephone: 06172 7100–0
Fax: 06172 7100–10

2826. Mitsui & Company (USA) Inc
200 Park Avenue, 39th Floor
New York
NY 10166–0130
USA
Telephone: (212) 878–0938;
            (212) 878–0939
Fax: (212) 878–2788
Telex/E-mail: 012056

2827. MJK Associates
Commodities Data Information Service
1885 Lundy Avenue
Suite 207B
San José
CA 95131
USA
Telephone: (408) 456–5000

2828. MK Technology Associates Ltd
1920 N Street
Suite 650
Washington
DC 20036
USA
Telephone: (202) 463–0904

2829. MLR Publishing Company
229 S 18th Street
3rd Floor
Philadelphia
PA 19103
USA
Telephone: (215) 875–2631;
            (215) 790–7000;
            (800) 637–4464
Fax: (215) 875–8873;
            (215) 790–7005

2830. MLS
Mast Learning Systems
26 Warwick Road
London
SW5 9UD
UK
Telephone: 071 373–9489
Fax: 071 835–2163

2831. MMS International
1301 Shoreway Road
Suite 300
Belmont
CA 94002
USA
Telephone: (415) 595–0610

2832. Mnematics Inc
722 Main Street
PO Box 19
Sparkill
NY 10976
USA
Telephone: (914) 365–0184;
            (800) 322–3633;
            (800) 374–3633

2833. Mobil Oil Corporation
3225 Gallows Road
Fairfax
VA 22037
USA
Telephone: (703) 849–3964;
            (703) 849–3979

2834. ModelVision Inc
William Hanson (President)
Miller Plaza
Suite 11B
8006 Madison Pike
Madison
AL 35758–1458
USA
Telephone: (205) 461–0878
Fax: (205) 461–0879

2835. Modern Language Association
    of America
Daniel Uchitelle
10 Astor Place
New York
NY 10003–6981
USA
Telephone: (212) 614–6350;
            (212) 475–9500
Fax: (212) 477–9863
Telex/E-mail: MLAOD CUVMB
(BITNET); 13945 (DIALMAIL); BB.MLA
(RLIN)

2836. Moessbauer Effect Data Center
University of North Carolina
Ashville
NC 28804–3299
USA
Telephone: (704) 258–0200 x273

2837. Molecular Design Ltd
2132 Farallon Road
San Leandro
CA 94577
USA
Telephone: (415) 895–1313;
            (800) 635–0064
Fax: (415) 352–2870

2838. Monash University
National Centre for Research &
    Development in Australian Studies
Clayton
VIC 3168
Australia
Telephone: 03 565–5232
Fax: 03 565–5238

2839. Monde, Le
François Luquit
5 rue des Italiens
75427 Paris
France
Telephone: 1 40 65 25 25
Fax: 1 40 65 25 99

2840. Monotype Typography Inc
Steve Kuhlman (Sales & Marketing
    Manager)
Suite 504
53 W Jackson Boulevard
Chicago
IL 60604
USA
Telephone: (312) 855–1440
Fax: (312) 939–0378

2841. Monotype Typography
Ian Buller (Sales & Marketing Manager);
    Pauline Dubber (Sales &
    Marketing Administrator)
Honeycrock Lane
Salfords
Redhill
Surrey
RH1 5JP
UK
Telephone: 0737 765–959
Fax: 0737 769–243

**2842. Montage Information Systems
    Inc**
Jim McAndrew
1650 Oakbrook Drive
Suite 435
Norcross
GA 30093
USA
Telephone: (404) 840–0183
Fax: (404) 840–9463

**2843. Monterey Bay Area
    Cooperative Library System**
Ellen Pastore (Coordinator)
MPC
Library Building
980 Fremont Boulevard
Monterey
CA 93940
USA
Telephone: (408) 646–4256
Fax: (408) 646–4111

2844. Moody Press
820 North LaSalle Drive
Chicago
IL 60610
USA
Telephone: (800) 621–5111

2845. Moody's Investors Service Inc
Subsidiary of the Dun & Bradstreet
    Corporation
Edmund J Moeller (Assistant Vice
    President International Sales)
99 Church Street
New York
NY 10007
USA
Telephone: (212) 553–0442;
                (212) 553–0857;
                (212) 553–0494;
                (212) 553–0546;
                (800) 342–5647
Fax: (212) 553–4700
Telex/E-mail: 421889 7607447

2846. Mope, Lda
Rua de Santa Marta 43 E/F 4
1100 Lisbon
Portugal
Telephone: 01 522–996
Fax: 01 529–867
Telex/E-mail: 64060 MOPE P

**2847. Morgan Guaranty Trust
    Company of New York**
23 Wall Street
New York
NY 10015
USA
Telephone: (212) 483–2323

2848. Morgan-Rand Publications Inc
2200 Sansom Street
Philadelphia
PA 19103–4350
USA
Telephone: (215) 557–8200
Fax: (215) 259–4810

2849. Morning Call Newspaper
PO Box 1260
Allentown
PA 18105
USA
Telephone: (215) 820–6523

2850. Morningstar
Liz Michaels (Product Manager)
53 W Jackson Boulevard
Chicago
IL 60604
USA
Telephone: (312) 427–1985
Fax: (312) 427–9215

2851. Mosby Year-Book Inc
Marketing Department
11830 Westline Industrial Drive
St Louis
MO 63146
USA
Telephone: (800) 633–6699
Fax: (314) 432–5471

2852. MotherLode Inc
Lea Léon (Sales Manager)
2001 E Lohman
Suite 236
Las Cruces
NM 88001
USA
Telephone: (505) 524–4043
Fax: (505) 523–9509

**2853. Motor Industry Research
    Association**
Watling Street
Nuneaton
Warwickshire
CV10 0TU
UK
Telephone: 0203 348–541
Fax: 0203 343–772
Telex/E-mail: 311277 MIRA G

2854. MPO
Bruno d'Orgeval (Commercial Manager)
195 avenue Charles de Gaulle
92200 Neuilly-sur-Seine
France
Telephone: 1 47 22 20 00
Fax: 1 47 22 60 77

2855. MPT Review
PO Box 5695
Incline Village
NV 89450–5695
USA
Telephone: (702) 831–7800
Fax: (702) 831–1359

2856. MS MEDIA-SERVICE GmbH
Johannishofweg 7
6084 Gernsheim-Allmendfeld
Germany
Telephone: 49 (6258) 5 15 36

2857. Münzinger-Archiv GmbH
Hans-Züricher-Weg 7
D-7980 Ravensburg
Germany
Telephone: 0751 31916
Fax: 0751 17261

2858. Muller Data Corporation
161 William Street
New York
NY 10038–2607
USA
Telephone: (212) 766–2700

2859. Muller Data Corporation
Chris Kennedy
90 5th Avenue
New York
NY 10011
USA
Telephone: (212) 807–3840
Fax: (212) 989–1938

2860. Multi-Ad Services Inc
Perry Rice
1720 W Detweiller Drive
Peoria
IL 61615–1695
USA
Telephone: (309) 692–1530
Fax: (309) 692–5444

2861. Multiconsult SC
Harry Sorum
Insurgentes Sur 949–9
Col Napoles
03810 Mexico DF
Mexico
Telephone: 5543 7706;
                5536 8672
Fax: 5687 7482

2862. MultiMedia Corporation, The
Jan Maulden (Managing Director); Peter
    Armstrong (Production
    Director/Chairman)
109X Regent's Park Road
London
NW5 1BL
UK
Telephone: 071 722–7595
Fax: 071 722–7027

**2863. Multimedia Products
    Corporation**
Lois Whitman
300 Airport Executive Park
Spring Valley
NY 10977
USA
Telephone: (212) 355–5049

**2864. Multinational Computer Models
    Inc**
333 Fairfield Road
Fairfield
NJ 07004
USA
Telephone: (201) 575–8333
Fax: (201) 783–1194

2865. Municipal Market Data Inc
155 Federal Street
4th Floor
Boston
MA 02110
USA
Telephone: (617) 542–2277

2866. Murdoch Magazines
1156 15th Street N.W.
Suite 600
Washington
DC 20005
USA

1531

Addresses

2867. Museo Cerralbo
Venture Rodrigues 17
28008 Madrid
Spain
Telephone: 01 449–7150

2868. Music Bank, The
PO Box 3150
Saratoga
CA 95070
USA
Telephone: (408) 867–4756

2869. Music Information Service
PO Box 14012
Fort Lauderdale
FL 33312
USA
Telephone: (305) 463–7954

2870. Mutual Fund Education Alliance
11 Penn Plaza, Suite 2204
New York
NY 10001
USA
Telephone: (212) 563–4540

2871. NAK
Jean-Marc Quilbé
12 avenue des Près
78180 Montigny le Bretonneux
France
Telephone: +33 1 30 57 17 08
Fax: +33 1 30 57 18 63

2872. Nantucket Corporation
12555 W Jefferson Boulevard
Suite 300
Los Angeles
CA 90066
USA
Telephone: (213) 390–7923

2873. Narvesen Info Center
Bertrand Narvesensvei 2
PO Box 6125
Etterstad
N-0602 Oslo 6
Norway
Telephone: +47 2 573300
Fax: +47 2 681901

2874. NASA Newsroom
Office of Public Affairs
Code LM
NASA Headquarters
Washington
DC 20546
USA
Telephone: (202) 453–8400
Fax: (202) 472–2309

2875. NASA/RECON
Scientific and Technical Information
   Division
Code NTT
NASA Headquarters
Washington
DC 20546
USA
Telephone: (703) 271–5640
Fax: (703) 271–5605

2876. NASA
Jet Propulsion Laboratory
Jason Hyon
4800 Oak Grove Drive
Mail Stop 233–208
Pasadena
CA 91109
USA
Telephone: (818) 354–8751;
          (818) 354–7050
Fax: (818) 393–6962

2877. NASA
Goddard Space Flight Center
Code 743
Greenbelt
MD 20771
USA
Telephone: (301) 344–9156

2878. NASA
Scientific and Technical Information
   Division (NIT-2)
Washington
DC 20546
USA
Telephone: (202) 453–2910
Fax: (202) 453–0134

2879. NASA
Technology Utilization Division
Washington
DC 20546
USA
Telephone: (202) 453–1910

2880. NASA
Ames Research Centre
Steve Hipskind
M/S 245–3
Moffett Field
CA 94035
USA
Telephone: (415) 604–5076
Fax: (415) 605–3625

2881. NASA
Industrial Applications Center
University of Pittsburg
823 William Pitt Union
Pittsburgh
PA 15260
USA
Telephone: (412) 648–7000

2882. NASA
Scientific and Technical Information
   Facility
PO Box 8757
BWI Airport
MD 21240
USA
Telephone: (703) 271–5640

2883. Nathan Logiciels
Christophe Vital Durand
6/10 Boulevard Jourdan
75014 Paris
France
Telephone: 1 45 65 06 06
Fax: 1 45 89 87 89

2884. Nathan Logiciels
Michael Bussac
3–5 Avenue Galliéni
94257 Gentilly Cedex
France
Telephone: 1 47 40 66 66
Fax: 1 47 40 65 77

2885. National Academy of Sciences
Transportation Research Information
   Services
2101 Constitution Avenue NW
Washington
DC 20418
USA
Telephone: (202) 334–3250
Fax: (202) 334–2003
Telex/E-mail: NARECO

2886. National Adoption Center
1218 Chestnut Street
Philadelphia
PA 19107
USA
Telephone: (215) 925–0200
Fax: (215) 925–3445
Telex/E-mail: NAE.ADMIN
(CompuServe Information Service)

2887. National American Sports Communications LP
15 W 52nd Street
New York
NY 10019
USA
Telephone: (212) 730–1374;
          (800) 642–2525

2888. National Arthritis and Musculoskeletal and Skin Disease
Information Clearing House
PO Box AMS
Bethesda
MD 20892
USA
Telephone: (301) 468–3235

2889. National Association for Law Placement
1666 Connecticut Avenue
Suite 450
Washington
DC 20009
USA
Telephone: (202) 667–1666
Fax: (202) 265–6735

2890. National Association of Blind and Visually Impaired Computer
Users
PO Box 1352
Roseville
CA 95661–1352
USA
Telephone: (916) 783–0364

2891. National Association of Credit Management of Kentucky
PO Box 1062
Louisville
KY 40201
USA
Telephone: (502) 583–4471

2892. National Association of Home Builders of the US
15th & M Streets NW
Washington
DC 20005
USA
Telephone: (202) 822–0477;
          (202) 822–0200

2893. National Association of Insurance Commissioners
120 W 12th Street
Suite 1100
Kansas City
MO 64105–1925
USA
Telephone: (816) 842–3600;
          (816) 374–7194

2894. National Association of Manufacturers
Suite 1500N
1331 Pennsylvania Avenue NW
Washington
DC 20004–1703
USA
Telephone: (202) 637–3082

2895. National Association of Realtors
430 N Michigan Avenue
Chicago
IL 60611–4087
USA
Telephone: (312) 329–8200

2896. National Association of Social Workers
Lori B Gardner (Marketing Manager)
7981 Eastern Avenue
Silver Spring
MD 20910
USA
Telephone: (301) 565–0333;
         (800) 638–8799
Fax: (301) 587–1321

2897. National Bank of Belgium
P Van Overwaelle
Boulevard de Berlaimont 5
Brussels 1000
Belgium
Telephone: 02–221 42 63

2898. National Biomedical Research Foundation
Protein Identification Resource
Georgetown University Medical Center
3900 Reservoir Road NW
Washington
DC 20007
USA
Telephone: (202) 687–2121
Fax: (202) 687–1662
Telex/E-mail: PIRMAIL GUNBRF (BITNET)

2899. National Board of Patents and Registration
Albertinkatu 25
SF-00180 Helsinki
Finland
Telephone: 0 69531
Fax: 0 695–3204

2900. National Center for Research in Vocational Education
1995 University Avenue, Suite 375
Berkeley
CA 94704–1058
USA
Telephone: (415) 642–4004
Fax: (415) 642–2124

2901. National Center of Scientific and Technological Information
Ministry of Energy and Infrastructure
Atidim Industrial Park
PO Box 43074
Tel-Aviv 61430
Israel
Telephone: 972 (3) 492037;
         972 (3) 492038
Fax: 972 (3) 492033
Telex/E-mail: 32332 IL

2902. National Centre for Atmospheric Research (NCAR)
Roy Jenne
PO Box 3000
Boulder
CO 80303–3000
USA
Telephone: (303) 497–1000
Fax: (303) 497 1137

2903. National Centre for Australian Studies
Monash University
Clayton
VIC 3168
Australia

2904. National Child Safety Council
Missing Children Division
4065 Page Avenue
PO Box 1368
Jackson
MI 49204
USA
Telephone: (517) 764–6070;
         (800) 222–1464;
         (800) 248–1464 (in Canada)
Fax: (517) 764–3068
Telex/E-mail: 70007,2356 (CompuServe Information Service)

2905. National Clearinghouse for Bilingual Education
1118 22nd Street NW
Washington
DC 20031
USA
Telephone: (202) 467–0867;
(800) 336–4560

2906. National Climatic Data Center
Tom Ross
Federal Building
Asheville
NC 28801
USA
Telephone: (704) 259–0682
Fax: (704) 259–0246

2907. National Collection of Yeast Cultures
Agricultural and Food Research Council
Institute of Food Research
Colney Lane
Norwich
Norfolk
NR4 7UA
UK
Telephone: 44 (603) 56122
Fax: 44 (603) 58939
Telex/E-mail: 975453 G

2908. National Companies and Securities Commission
31 Queen Street
17th Floor
Melbourne
VIC 3000
Australia
Telephone: 03 616–1811

2909. National Computer Network Corporation
1929 N Harlem Avenue
Chicago
IL 60635
USA
Telephone: (312) 622–6666;
         (800) 942–NCNC
Fax: (312) 622–6889

2910. National Computing Centre Ltd
Oxford Road
Manchester
M1 7ED
UK

2911. National Council for Research on Women
Sarah Delano Roosevelt Memorial House
47–49 East 65th Street
New York
NY 10021
USA
Telephone: (212) 570–5001

2912. National Council on Family Relations
Mary-Jo Czaplewski
Family Resources Database
3989 Central Avenue NE
Suite 550
Minneapolis
MN 55421
USA
Telephone: (612) 781–9331
Fax: (612) 781–9348

2913. National Credit Union Administration
1776 G Street NW
Washington
DC 20456
USA
Telephone: (202) 357–1100

2914. National Data Corporation
Corporate Financial Services Division
Corporate Square
Atlanta
GA 30329
USA
Telephone: (404) 329–8500

2915. National Data Corporation
Health Care Data Services Division
National Data Plaza
Corporate Square
Atlanta
GA 30329
USA
Telephone: (404) 728–2430;
         (800) 225–5632
Telex/E-mail: 542785

2916. National Decision Systems
Tom Holland
539 Encinitas Boulevard
Box 9007
Encinitas
CA 92024–9007
USA
Telephone: (619) 942–7000

2917. National Demonstration Laboratory for Interactive Educational Technologies
Jacqueline Hess
Library of Congress
Madison Building
101 Independence Avenue South East
Washington DC 20540
USA
Telephone: (202) 357 4749
Fax: (202) 786 2304

2918. National Diabetes Information Clearinghouse
Box NDIC
Bethesda
MD 20892
USA
Telephone: (301) 468–2162

2919. National Diet Library
Somu-bu Denshi Keisan-ka Division
1–10–1 Nagato-cho
Chiyoda-ku
Tokyo 100
Japan
Telephone: 81 (3) 581–2331 x284

2920. National E-Mail Registry
Two Neshaminy Interplex
Suite 110
Trevose
PA 19147–9905
USA
Telephone: (215) 245–4018;
　　　　　　(800) 843–6088
Fax: (215) 639–4911
Telex/E-mail: 9102501684; 1NEMR
(AT&T Mail); 72147,126 (CompuServe
　Information Service); 62023102
　(EasyLink); 349–6145 (MCI Mail)

**2921. National Electrical
　　　　Manufacturers Association**
2101 L Street NW
Suite 300
Washington
DC 20037
USA
Telephone: (202) 457–8400

2922. National Film Board of Canada
150 Kent Street
Ottawa K1A 0M9
Canada
Telephone: (613) 996–4863

2923. National Film Board of Canada
Audiovisual Information Services
PO Box 6100
Station A
Montreal
PQ H3C CH5
Canada
Telephone: (613) 283–9427

2924. National Forensic Center
17 Temple Terrace
Lawrenceville
NJ 08648
USA
Telephone: (609) 883–0550;
　　　　　　(800) 526–5177

2925. National Gallery of Canada
Library
PO Box 427
Station A
Ottawa
ON K1N 9N4
Canada
Telephone: (613) 990–0588
Fax: (613) 993–4385

2926. National Geographic Society
Educational Media Division
Betty Kotcher Sarah Clark
1145 17th Street, NW
Washington
DC 20036
USA
Telephone: (800) 368–2728;
　　　　　　(202) 775–6583;
　　　　　　(202) 828–5664
Fax: (202) 429–5770

**2927. National Geomagnetic
　　　　Information Center**
Donald C Herzog; Charles W Lupica
USGS
Box 25046, MS 968
Denver Federal Center
Denver
CO 80225–0046
USA
Telephone: (303) 236 1365
Fax: (303) 236 1519

**2928. National Geophysical Data
　　　　Center**
Carla Moore; Dr Peter Sloss; Mai
　Edwards; J Allen
325 Broadway
Boulder
CO 80303–3328
USA
Telephone: (303) 497–6276;
　　　　　　(303) 497–6339;
　　　　　　(303) 497–6119;
　　　　　　(303) 497–6346;
　　　　　　(303) 497–6323
Fax: (303) 497–6958; (303) 497–6513

**2929. National Ground Water
　　　　Information Center**
6375 Riverside Drive
Dublin
OH 43017–3536
USA
Telephone: (614) 761–3222
Fax: (614) 761–3446
Telex/E-mail: 241302

**2930. National Health Information
　　　　Clearinghouse**
PO Box 1133
Washington
DC 20013–1133
USA
Telephone: (301) 496–3583

2931. National Health Service
Regional Drug Information Service
The London Hospital
London
E1 1BB
UK
Telephone: 071 247–5976

**2932. National Heart, Lung and
　　　　Blood Institute**
Information Center
4733 Bethesda Avenue, Suite 530
Bethesda
MD 20814
USA
Telephone: (301) 951–3260

**2933. National Information Centre for
　　　　Educational Media (NICEM)**
Division of Access Innovations, Inc
Stephanie Korney
PO Box 40130
4314 Mesa Grande SE
Albuquerque
NM 87196
USA
Telephone: (505) 265–3591;
　　　　　　(800) 421–8711

**2934. National Information Services
　　　　Corporation – NISC**
Fred Dürr
Suite 6, Wyman Towers
3100 St Paul Street
Baltimore
MD 21218
USA
Telephone: (301) 243–0797
Fax: (301) 243–0982

**2935. National Information Standards
　　　　Organisation (NISO)**
Patricia Harris
PO Box 1056
Bethesda
MD 20827
USA
Telephone: (301) 975 2814

**2936. National Institute for
　　　　Educational Research**
6–5–22 Shimomeguro
Meguro-ku
Tokyo 153
Japan
Telephone: 03 3714–0111

**2937. National Institute of Building
　　　　Sciences**
Attn: CCB
Layne Evans
1201 L Street NW
Suite 400
Washington
DC 20005
USA
Telephone: (202) 289–7800
Fax: (202) 289–1092

2938. National Institute of Health
Earl Henderson
Lister Hill Center
8600 Rockville Pike
Bethesda
MD 20209
USA
Telephone: (301) 496–4441

2939. National Journal
1730 M Street NW
Washington
DC 20036
USA
Telephone: (202) 857–1400;
　　　　　　(800) 424–2921
Fax: (202) 833–8069

**2940. National Kidney and Urologic
　　　　Diseases Information
　　　　Clearinghouse**
National Institutes of Health
Box NKUDIC
Bethesda
MD 20892
USA
Telephone: (301) 468–6345

**2941. National Land Survey of
　　　　Sweden**
Bengt Rystedt; Karin Persson; Erik
　Normann
801 92 Gävle
Sweden
Telephone: 026 100340;
　　　　　　026 153000
Fax: 026 653160
NUA: 026 187594

**2942. National Legal Databases
　　　　Corporation**
Ed Enquist
PO Box 701764
Tulsa
OK 74170–1764
USA
Telephone: (918) 492 5275
Fax: (918) 492 0306

2943. National Library for Education
Bankplassen 3
PO Box 8194 Dep.
0034 Oslo 1
Norway
Telephone: 47 (2) 42 03 39

2944. National Library of Australia
Network Services Branch
Sandra Henderson
Canberra
ACT 2600
Australia
Telephone: 61 (62) 262–1484
Fax: 61 (62) 57–1703
Telex/E-mail: 62100 LIBAUST AA

2945. National Library of Australia
OZLINE: Australian Information Network
Parkes Place
Canberra
ACT 2600
Australia
Telephone: 062 621–484;
          062 621–524
Fax: 062 571–703
Telex/E-mail: 62100 LIBAUST AA

2947. National Library of Australia
Australian Bibliographic Network
Parkes Place
Canberra
ACT 2600
Australia
Telephone: 06 262–1111
Fax: 06 273–3648
Telex/E-mail: 62100 LIBAUST AA

2948. National Library of Canada
Acquisition & Bibliographic Branch
David Balatti
395 Wellington Street
Room 224
Ottawa
Ontario
K1A 0N4
Canada
Telephone: (819) 994 6882
Fax: (819) 952 0291
Telex/E-mail: 0534312

2949. National Library of Canada
395 Wellington Street
Ottawa
Canada
Telephone: (613) 992–0474
Telex/E-mail: 0534312

2950. National Library of Canada
Public Services Breanch, Union
    Catalogue Division
395 Wellington Street
Ottawa
ON K1A 0N4
Canada
Telephone: (613) 996–7507

2951. National Library of Canada
Reference Services
395 Wellington Street
Ottawa
ON K1A 0N4
Canada
Telephone: (613) 992–0474
Telex/E-mail: 0534311

2952. National Library of Canada
Information Technology Services
395 Wellington Street
Ottawa
ON K1A 0N4
Canada
Telephone: (819) 997–7000
Fax: (819) 994–6835
Telex/E-mail: 053 4311;
CANCON.SS (Envoy 100)

2953. National Library of Denmark
Computer Department
Nyhavn 31 E
DK-1051 Copenhagen
Denmark
Telephone: 33 934–633

2954. National Library of Medicine
MEDLARS Management Section
Robert Mehnert
8600 Rockville Pike
Bethesda
MD 20894
USA
Telephone: (301) 496–6308;
          (301) 496–6193;
          (800) 638–8480;
          (301) 496–6531
Fax: (301) 496 4450
Telex/E-mail: JJL NINCU (BITNET);
FERGUSON NLM.NIK.GOVS
(Internet)

2955. National Library of Medicine
Toxicology Information Program
8600 Rockville Pike
Bethesda
MD 20894
USA
Telephone: (301) 496–1131;
          (800) 638–8480

**2956. National Library of New
    Zealand**
Collections Management
Database Development Unit
Private Bag
Wellington
New Zealand
Telephone: 64 (4) 743–098
Fax: 64 (4) 743–035

**2957. National Library of New
    Zealand**
Cnr Molesworth and Aitken Streets
PO Box 1476
Wellington
New Zealand
Telephone: 04 743–098
Fax: 04 743–035
Telex/E-mail: 30076

**2958. National Library of New
    Zealand**
Kiwinet
Cnr Molesworth and Aitken Streets
PO Box 12–264
Wellington
New Zealand
Telephone: 04 743–000
Fax: 04 743042
Telex/E-mail: 30076 NATLIB NZ;
LWN095 (Starnet)

**2959. National Library of the
    Netherlands (See Koninklijke
    Bibliotheek)**

2960. National Meteorological Library
London Road
Bracknell
Berkshire
RG12 2SZ
UK
Telephone: 0344 854–844;
          0344 654–842
Fax: 0344 854–840
Telex/E-mail: 849801 G

**2961. National Oceanographic Data
    Center**
Robert C Lockerman
1825 Connecticut Avenue NW
Washington
DC 20235
USA
Telephone: (202) 673–5600
Fax: (202) 673 5586

**2962. National Online Legislative
    Associates**
c/o Legi-Tech Corporation
1029 J Street
Suite 450
Sacramento
CA 95814
USA
Telephone: (916) 447–1886
Fax: (916) 447–1109

**2963. National Organization for Rare
    Disorders**
PO Box 8923
New Fairfield
CT 06812
USA
Telephone: (203) 746–6518;
          (800) 999–6673
Fax: (203) 746–6481
Telex/E-mail: 76703,3014 (CompuServe
Information Service)

**2964. National Pesticide Information
    Retrieval Service**
Ed Ramsey
Purdue University
Entomology Hall
West Lafayette
IN 47907
USA
Telephone: (317) 494–6614
Fax: (317) 494–0535

**2965. National Planning Data
    Corporation**
John Behler
PO Box 610
20 Terrace Hill
Ithaca
NY 14851–0610
USA
Telephone: (607) 273–8208;
          (800) 876–NPDC
Fax: (607) 273–1266

2966. National Poisons Unit
Guy's Hospital
St Thomas Street
London
SE1 9RT
UK
Telephone: 071 639–9653

2967. National Portrait Gallery
Margo Kabel
Smithsonian Institute
Room 311
8th & F Street NW
Washington
DC 20560
USA
Telephone: (202) 786–2343
Fax: (202) 357–2753

**2968. National Public Employer
    Labor Relations Association**
1620 Eye Street NW
4th Floor
Washington
DC 20006
USA
Telephone: (202) 296–2230

2969. National Quotation Bureau
600 Plaza Three
Harborside Financial Center
Jersey City
NJ 07311–3895
USA
Telephone: (201) 435–9000

2970. National Reference Centre for Environmental Information (CIMI)
Ir P.K. Koster
PO Box 1
3720 BA Bilthoven
Netherlands
Telephone: +31 30 743085
Fax: +31 30 250740

2971. National Register Publishing Company
Reference Marketing
MacMillan Directory Division
3004 Glenview Road
Wilmette
IL 60091
USA
Telephone: (708) 441–2267;
(800) 323–6772;
(708) 256–6067

2972. National Rehabilitation Information Center
Macro Systems Inc
8455 Colesville Road
Suite 935
Silver Springs
MD 20910–3319
USA
Telephone: (301) 588–9284;
(800) 346–2742

2973. National Research Bureau
Renee Milan
225 West Wacker Drive
Suite 2275
Chicago
IL 60606
USA
Telephone: (312) 346 9097
Fax: (312) 246 9097

2974. National Research Corporation
Jon Bournstein
1033 "O" Street
Lincoln
NE 68508
USA
Telephone: (402) 475–2525
Fax: (402) 475–9061

2975. National Research Council of Canada
Institute for Research in Construction
Building M-20
Ottawa
ON K1A 0R6
Canada
Telephone: (613) 993–3773
Fax: (613) 954–5984
Telex/E-mail: 0533145 CA;
Cisti.irc (Envoy 100)

2976. National Safety Data Corporation (NSDC)
Michael Shea
259 West Road
Salem
CT 06415
USA
Telephone: (203) 859–1162

2977. National School Public Relations Association
1501 Lee Highway
Suite 201
Arlington
VA 22209
USA
Telephone: (703) 528–5840

2978. National Science Council
Science and Technology Information Center
PO Box 91–37
Taipei
Taiwan
Telephone: 02 737–7631
Fax: 02 737–7663
Telex/E-mail: 29674 STIC ROC

2979. National Science Foundation
Division of Polar Programs
Guy Guthridge
1800 G Street, NW, Rm 620
Washington
DC 20550
USA
Telephone: (202) 357 7817
Fax: (202) 357 9422

2980. National Snow and Ice Data Center
Claire Hanson
CIRES
Campus Box 449
University of Colorado
Boulder
CO 80309
USA
Telephone: (303) 492–1834;
(303) 492 5171
Fax: (303) 492–1149

2981. National Sport Information Centre
Greg Blood
PO Box 176
Belconnen
ACT 2616
Australia
Telephone: 06 252–1369
Fax: 06 252–1681

2982. National Sports Committee
Jianzhong Zhao
9 Tiyuguan Road
Chongwen Qu
Beijing 100763
China
Telephone: (70) 12233–2497

2983. National Standards Association Inc
Geoffrey Smith
1200 Quince Orchard Boulevard
Gaithersburg
MD 20878
USA
Telephone: (301) 590–2300;
(800) 638–8094
Fax: (301) 990–8378
Telex/E-mail: 446194 NATSTA GAIT

2984. National Systems Management Inc
2021 K Street, NW, Suite 315
Washington
DC 20006
USA
Telephone: (202) 296–1800

2985. National Technical Information Service (NTIS)
Center for the Utilization of Federal Technology
5285 Port Royal Road
Springfield
VA 22161
USA
Telephone: (703) 487–4838;
(703) 487–4929
Fax: (703) 321–8199
Telex/E-mail: 899405

2986. National Technological Library of Denmark
Anker Engelundsvej 1
2800 Lyngby
Denmark
Telephone: 45 (2) 88 30 88
Fax: 45 (2) 88 30 40
Telex/E-mail: 37148 DTBC DK

2987. National Underwriter Company
505 Gest Street
Cincinnati
OH 45203
USA
Telephone: (513) 721–2140

2988. National Weather Service
National Meteorological Center
Climate Analysis Center
Room 808 World Weather Building
Washington
DC 20233
USA
Telephone: (301) 763–4670

2989. National Weather Service
National Meteorological Center
5200 Auth Road
Suite 101
Camp Springs
MD 20233
USA
Telephone: (301) 763–8016

2990. Naval Facilities Engineering Command
Louise McMonegal
Code DSO-1E
200 Stovall Street
Alexandria
VA 22332–2300
USA
Telephone: (703) 325 0450

2991. NBD Product-Informationsystems BV
Gedempte Gracht 4
PO Box 23
7400 GA Deventer
Netherlands
Telephone: +31 5700 48601
Fax: +31 5700 42761

2992. NBLC – Nederlands Bibliothek en Lektuur Centrum
Taco Scheltemastraat 5
PO Box 93054
2597 CP The Hague
Netherlands
Telephone: +31 70 3141500
Fax: +31 70 3141600

2993. NBLC Systemen BV
Randstad 22 01
1316 BN Almere-Stad
Netherlands
Telephone: +31 3240 90611
Fax: +31 3240 90639

2994. NCB (IEA Services) Limited
14/15 Lower Grosvenor Place
London
SW1W 0EX
UK
Telephone: 071 828–4661

2995. NCC Samenwerkingsverband
PO Box 90407
NL-2509 LK The Hague
Netherlands
Telephone: 070 14 04 60

2996. NDL Direct Marketing
Judy Bishop
London
UK
Telephone: 071 738–0522

2997. Nebraska Department of Health
Nebraska HealthNetwork
301 Centennial Mall S
PO Box 95007
Lincoln
NE 68509–5007
USA
Telephone: (402) 471–3495
Telex/E-mail: 177000,649 (CompuServe
    Information Service)

2998. NEC (UK) Ltd
Russell Cole
Computer Peripherals Dept
NEC House
1 Victoria Road
LONDON
W3 6UL
UK
Telephone: 081 993 8111
Fax: 081 992 7161

2999. NEC Canada
6711 Mississauga Road
Suite 200
Mississauga
Ontario
L5N 2W3
Canada
Telephone: (416) 858–3500

3000. NEC Computer Peripherals
NEC House
1 Victoria Road
Acton
London
W3 6BR
UK
Telephone: 081 993–8111

3001. NEC France SA
Tour Gan Cedex 13
92082 Paris La Defense
France
Telephone: 1 49 00 07 07

3002. NEC Technologies (USA)
William Wegmann
1255 Michael Drive
Wooddale 0108
IL 60191
USA
Telephone: (708) 860–9500;
          (800) 826–2255
Fax: (708) 860 7794

**3003. Nedbook International BV
    (SilverPlatter Agent)**
PO Box 3113
Amsterdam 1003 AC
Netherlands
Telephone: 20–340963

**3004. Nedbook Scandinavia BV
    (SilverPlatter Agent)**
Hollandargatan 31
S113 59, Stockholm
Sweden
Telephone: 8–33–2613

**3005. Nederlands Centrum voor
    Bibliotheekautomatisering Pica**
Schipholweg 99
NL-2316 XA Leiden
Netherlands
Telephone: 071 257–257
Fax: 071 223–119
Telex/E-mail: 34402 NL

**3006. Nederlands Organisatie voor
    Toegepast-
    Natuurwetenschappelijk
    Onderzoek**
Centrum voor Informatie en
    Documentatie
PO Box 6063
97 Schoemakerstraat 97
NL-2600 JA Delft
Netherlands
Telephone: 015 696–6800
Fax: 015 560–825
Telex/E-mail: 38071 ZPTNP NL

3007. NEFA NORD NYT
Nordisk Etnologisk Folkloristisk
    Arbejdsgruppe
Joergen Burchardt
Nyborgvej 13 Soedinge
5750 Ringe
Denmark
Telephone: 45 (62) 623617

3008. Neilsen
Sharon Sims
Neilsen House
Headington
Oxford
OX3 9RX
UK
Telephone: 0865 742742
Fax: 0865 742222

**3009. Nelson B Heller and
    Associates**
707 Skokie Boulevard
Suite 600
Northbrook
IL 60062
USA
Telephone: (708) 205–4390

3010. NERAC Inc
1 Technology Drive
Tolland
CT 06084
USA
Telephone: (203) 872–7000

3012. NESTOR
Plein 26
NL-2511 CS The Hague
Netherlands
Telephone: 070 361–7070
Fax: 070 364–6680

**3013. Netherlands Foreign Trade
    Agency Library**
Ministry of Economic Affairs
Bezuidenhoutseweg 151
NL-2594 AG The Hague
Netherlands
Telephone: 070 79 72 09
Fax: 070 79 78 78
Telex/E-mail: 31099 ECZA NL

**3014. Netherlands Information
    Combine**
PO Box 36
2600 AA Delft
Netherlands
Telex/E-mail: 38071 ZPTNO NL

**3015. Netherlands Information
    Service**
Dorine Rijkers
Anna Paulownastraat 76
2518 BJ The Hague
Netherlands
Telephone: 70 564 284;
          +31 70 356 40 00
Fax: 70 463 585;
          +31 70 356 46 81

**3016. Netherlands Maritime
    Information Centre/CMO**
PO Box 21873
NL-3001 AW Rotterdam
Netherlands
Telephone: 010 413 09 60
Fax: 010 411 28 57
Telex/E-mail: 26585 CMO NL

**3017. Netherlands Ministry of
    Housing, Physical
    Planning and Environment**
PO Box 20951
2500 EX The Hague
Netherlands
Telephone: 070 335–3535;
          070 326–4201
Fax: 070 335–3360

**3018. Netherlands Ministry of
    Welfare, Health and Cultural
    Affairs**
Sir Winston Churchillaan 362
PO Box 5406
NL-2280 HK Rijswijk
Netherlands
Telephone: 070 40 56 76
Fax: 070 40 50 44
Telex/E-mail: 32347 WVCRW NL

3019. Netwits
PO Box 6010
Suite 431
Sherman Oaks
CA 91413
USA

**3020. Network Cybernetics
    Corporation**
4201 Wingren Road
Suite 202
Irving
TX 75062–2763
USA
Telephone: (214) 650–2002
Fax: (214) 650–1929

**3021. Network Management Inc/CRC
    Systems Inc**
11242 Waples Mill Road
Fairfax
VA 22030
USA
Telephone: (703) 359–9400

**3022. Network Technology
    Corporation**
Ann Richards
7401–F Fullerton Road
Springfield
VA 22153–3122
USA
Telephone: (703) 866–9000
Fax: (703) 866 9007

**3023. Networking and World
    Information Inc**
333 East River Drive
East Hartford
CT 06108
USA
Telephone: (203) 282–3700

**3024. Neurofibromatosis Institute
    Inc, The**
5415 Briggs Avenue
La Crescenta
CA 91214
USA
Telephone: (818) 957–3508
Fax: (818) 405–9708

Addresses

3025. New Brunswick Department of Justice
Law Reform Division
Centennial Building
Room 416
PO Box 6000
Fredericton
NB E3B 5H1
Canada
Telephone: (506) 453–2668
Fax: (506) 453–3275

3026. New England Law Library Consortium
Martha Berglund Crane
Langdell Hall
Cambridge
MA 02138
USA
Telephone: (617) 495–9918
Fax: (617) 495–4449

3027. New Jersey Institute of Technology
Computerized Conferencing and Communications Center
Electronic Information Exchange System
323 Martin Luther King Boulevard
Newark
NJ 07102
USA
Telephone: (201) 596–3437
Fax: (201) 596–0137

3028. New Laboratory for Teaching & Learning, The
The Dalton School
108 East 89th Street
New York
NY 10128
USA
Telephone: (212) 722 5160
Fax: (212) 348 5885

3029. New Media
12 Oval Road
Camden Town
London
NW1 7DH
UK
Telephone: 071 482–5258
Fax: 071 482–4957

3030. New Scientist
IPC Magazines Ltd
Kings Reach Tower
Stamford Street
London
SE1 9LS
UK
Telephone: 071 261–5568
Fax: 071 261–5041
Telex/E-mail: 915748 MAGDIV G

3031. New South Wales Corporate Affairs Commission
Stockland House
175 Castlereagh Street
Sydney
NSW 2000
Australia
Telephone: 02 266–0635

3032. New South Wales Department of Minerals and Energy
Information Delivery and Service Branch
Minerals & Energy House
50–55 Christie Street
Saint Leonardos
NSW 2065
Australia
Telephone: 02 901–8888

3033. New South Wales Department of Water Resources
David C Malone (Project Manager)
PO Box 3720
Parramatta
NSW 2150
Australia
Telephone: 2 895–7577
Fax: 2 891–5884

3034. New South Wales Land Titles Office
Queens Square
Sydney
NSW 2000
Australia
Telephone: 02 228–6666

3035. New York Amateur Computer Club
Jan Warner
PO Box 3442
Church Street Station
New York
NY 10010
USA
Telephone: (212) 505–6021

3036. New York Law Publishing Company
111 8th Avenue
New York
NY 10011
USA
Telephone: (212) 741–8300

3037. New York On-Line
PO Box 829
Brooklyn
NY 11202–6018
USA
Telephone: (718) 875–8949
Fax: (718) 852–2662
Telex/E-mail: WBOWLES (MCI Mail)

3038. New York Society of Security Analysts
71 Broadway
New York
NY 10006
USA
Telephone: (212) 344–8450

3039. New York Stock Exchange
20 Broad Street, 22nd Floor
New York
NY 10005
USA
Telephone: (212) 656–3800

3040. New York Times Company
New York Times Index Department
229 West 43rd Street
New York
NY 10036
USA
Telephone: (212) 556–1234;
(212) 556–1573;
(800) 543–6862
Fax: (212) 556–4603
Telex/E-mail: 12207

3041. New York Times Company
Times On-Line Services
1719A Route 10
Parsippany
NJ 07054
USA
Telephone: (201) 267–2268

3042. New York Times Syndication Sales Corporation
130 5th Avenue
New York
NY 10011
USA
Telephone: (212) 645–3000

3043. New Zealand Court of Appeal
Cnr Molesworth and Aitken Streets
PO Box 1606
Wellington
New Zealand
Telephone: 04 727–370
Fax: 04 734–147

3044. New Zealand Department of Scientific and Industrial Research
Sandra Young
Head Office
PO Box 2922
Wellington
New Zealand
Telephone: 04 729–919
Fax: 04 729–135
Telex/E-mail: 31313 STATSWN NZ

3045. New Zealand Department of Scientific and Industrial Research
DSIR Library Centre
Private Bag 13
Petone
New Zealand
Telephone: 666–919
Fax: 694–500
Telex/E-mail: 3814 PHYSICS

3046. New Zealand Department of Statistics
Information Network for Official Statistics
PO Box 2922
Wellington
New Zealand
Telephone: 04 729–119
Fax: 04 729–135
Telex/E-mail: 31313 STATSWN NZ

3047. New Zealand Government Printing Office
Greg Comfort
Private Bag
Wellington 1
New Zealand
Telephone: 04 737–320
Fax: 04 734–943;
04 732–900
Telex/E-mail: 31370 GOVPRNT NZ

3048. New Zealand Labour Court
Arbitration Commission
PO Box 596
Wellington
New Zealand
Telephone: 04 739–804
Fax: 04 712–094

3049. Newark Morning Ledger Company
One Star Ledger Plaza
Newark
NJ 07101
USA
Telephone: (201) 877–4141

3050. Newington Children's Hospital
Marian Hall
Adaptive Equipment Center
181 E Cedar Street
Newington
CT 06111
USA
Telephone: (203) 667–5405;
(800) 344–5405

3051. Newmedia International Japan
Avenida Infanta Carlota 74 5.1
08029 Barcelona
Spain
Telephone: 03 410 70 34

3052. Newport Associates Ltd
Kathleen Moynihan
7400 E Orchard Road
Suite 320
Englewood
CO 80111
USA
Telephone: (303) 779–5515;
  (800) 733–5515
Fax: (303) 220–9045;
  (303) 779–0908

3053. News & Observer, The
215 S McDowell Street
PO Box 191
Raleigh
NC 27602
USA
Telephone: (919) 829–4500

3054. News and Sun-Sentinel Company
101 North New River Drive E
Fort Lauderdale
FL 33301–2293
USA
Telephone: (305) 761–4060

3055. News International plc
1 Pennington Street
Wapping
London
E1 9XN
UK
Telephone: 081 782–5000

3056. News$ource
Infomart Online
1450 Don Mills Road
Don Mills
ON M3B 2X7
Canada
Telephone: (416) 445–6641
Fax: (416) 442–2077

3057. News-a-tron Corporation
1 Peabody Street
Salem
MA 01970
USA
Telephone: (617) 744–4744

3058. News-Sentinal, The
600 W Main Street
PO Box 102
Fort Wayne
IN 46801
USA
Telephone: (219) 461–8222

3059. NewsBank Inc
Readex
Jane Kelly
58 Pine Street
New Canaan
CT 06840–5408
USA
Telephone: (203) 966–1100;
  (800) 223–4739;
  (800) 762–8182
Fax: (203) 966–6254

3060. Newsbytes
822 Arkansas Street
San Francisco
CA 94107
USA
Telephone: (415) 550–7334
Fax: (415) 648–2550
Telex/E-mail: NEWSBYTES (GEnie);
WWOODS (MCI Mail)

3061. Newscan Services Limited
PO Box 39363
Auckland West
New Zealand
Telephone: 64 (9) 370–440
Fax: 64 (9) 370–399

3062. Newscan Services Ltd
PO Box 39363
Auckland West
New Zealand
Telephone: 09 370–440
Fax: 09 370–399
Telex/E-mail: N2N1340 (Synet)

3063. Newsday Inc
235 Pinelawn Road
New York
NY 11747
USA
Telephone: (516) 454–2020

3064. NewsNet Inc
945 Haverford Road
Bryn Mawr
PA 19010
USA
Telephone: (215) 527–8030;
  (800) 345–1301
Fax: (215) 527–0338

3065. Newspaper Marketing Bureau Inc
21 King Street E
Suite 2100
Toronto
ON M5C 1A2
Canada
Telephone: (416) 364–3744
Fax: (416) 363–2568

3066. Newspaper Publishing plc
Rose Siggers
40 City Road
London
EC1Y 2DB
UK
Telephone: 071 253–1222
Fax: 071 608–1552

3067. Newsreel Access Systems
150 East 58th Street
53rd Floor
New York
NY 10155
USA
Telephone: (212) 826–2800;
  (800) 242–2463

3068. Newsweek Inc
444 Madison Avenue
New York
NY 10022
USA
Telephone: (212) 350–4000

3069. Nexpri Nederlands Expertisecentrum voor Ruimtelijke Informat.
Boyke Hiralal; Erna van den Doel
Heidelberglaan 2
PO Box 80115
35008 TC Utrecht
Netherlands
Telephone: +31 30 534261
Fax: +31 30 523699

3070. Next Technology Corporation Ltd
Graham Brown-Martin; Nik Baker
St John's Innovation Centre
Cambridge
CB4 4WS
UK
Telephone: 0223 420222;
  0223 341180
Fax: 0223 420015

3071. NGB Corporation
Kasumigaseki Building. 32F
2–5 Kasumigaskei 3–chome
Chiyoda-ku
Tokyo 100
Japan
Telephone: (03) 3581 7711
Fax: (03) 3503 0513

3072. NHK Enterprises Inc
2–1–1 Jinnan
Shibuya-ku
150–01 Tokyo
Japan
Telephone: +3 3481 1658

3073. NHK Joho Network Inc
Kazuo Yoshino
5–5 Kamiyama Cho
Shibuyaku
Tokyo
Japan
Telephone: +81 3 3481 1771
Fax: +81 3 3481 1777

3074. NIAM
Pieter Burghart
Neuhuyskade 94
2596 XM The Hague
Netherlands
Telephone: +31 70 3143500
Fax: +31 70 3143588

3075. Nichigai Associates
1–23–8 Ohmori-kita
Ohta-ku
Tokyo 143
Japan
Telephone: 03–763–7581;
  03–763–5241

3076. Nicholas Hall & Company
35 Alexandra Street
Southend-on-Sea
Essex
SS1 1BW
UK
Telephone: 0702 433–422
Fax: 0702 430–787

3077. Nicola Zanichelli SpA
Lorenzo Enriques
Editore
Via Irnerio 34
40126 Bologna
Italy
Telephone: 051 293111
Fax: 051 249782

3078. Nielsen Media Research
1290 Avenue of the Americas
New York
NY 10104
USA
Telephone: (212) 708–7500
Fax: (212) 708–7724

3079. Nielsen (See also AC Nielsen)

3080. Nielsen
Sharon Sims
Nielsen House
Headington
Oxford
OX3 9RX
UK
Telephone: 0865 742–742
Fax: 0865 742–222

3081. NIFTY Corporation
NIFTY-Serve
26–1 Minami-oi
6–chome
Shinagawa-ku
Tokyo 140
Japan
Telephone: 03 5471–5800

3082. Nihon Keizai Shimbun America Inc
Databank Representative
1221 Avenue of the Americas
Suite 1802
New York
NY 10020
USA
Telephone: (212) 512–3600
Fax: (212) 512–4550

3083. Nihon Keizai Shimbun Europe Ltd
Databank Representative
Bush House
London
WC2B 4PJ
UK
Telephone: 071 379–4994
Fax: 071 379–0378

3084. Nihon Keizai Shimbun Inc
Databank Representative Databank Bureau
1–9–5 Otemachi
Chiyoda-ku
Tokyo 100
Japan
Telephone: 81 (3) 270–0251;
81 (3) 5294–2407
Fax: 81 (3) 270–8555;
81 (3) 5294–2411
Telex/E-mail: 22308 NIKKEI J

3085. Nihon Keizai Shimbun Inc
Databank Bureau
2–11–2 Hishigaoka Building
Nagata-cho
Chiyoda-ku
Tokyo 100
Japan
Telephone: 03 3506–8323
Fax: 03 3270–8555
Telex/E-mail: 22308 NIKKEI J

3086. Nihon Micon Hambai KK
4–8–15 Fukushima
Fukushima-ku
Osaka 553
Japan
Telephone: +81 6 452 0023
Fax: +81 6 452 5351

3087. NIITECHIM
c/o International Center for Scientific and Technical Information
Ulitsa Kuusinena 21b
125252 Moscow
Russia
Telephone: 095 198–7460
Fax: 095 943–0089
Telex/E-mail: 411925 MCNTI SI

3088. Nijgh Periodieken PV
B Th van Ette
PO Box 122
3100 AC Schiedam
Netherlands
Telephone: 0034 10 4732000
Fax: 0034 10 4739911

3089. Nikkan Kogyo Shimbunsha
1–8–10 Kudan-kita
Chiyoda-ku
Tokyo 107
Japan
Telephone: 03 3263–2311;
03 3222–7142

3090. NIKKEI (See Nihon Keizai Shimbun Inc)

3092. Nikko Research Center
1–1–3 Marunouchi
Chiyoda-ku
Tokyo 100
Japan

3093. NILS Publishing Company
PO Box 2507
21625 Prairie Street
Chatsworth
CA 91311
USA
Telephone: (818) 998–8830;
(800) 423–5910
Fax: (818) 718–8482

3094. Nimbus Information Systems
(CD-ROM division of Nimbus Records Ltd.)
Emil J Dudek; John Metcalf; Steve Conolly
Wyastone Leys
Monmouth
Gwent
NP5 3SR
UK
Telephone: 0600 890682
Fax: 0600 890779

3095. Nimbus Records Ltd
200 West 57th Street
New York
NY 10019
USA
Telephone: (212) 262–5400

3096. Nimbus Records
Joe Cannariato
PO Box 7305
Charlottesville
VA 22906
USA
Telephone: (804) 985–1100;
(800) 782–0778

3097. Nims Associates Inc
12200 Ford Road
Suite 200
Dallas
TX 75234–7264
USA
Telephone: (214) 241–0292
Fax: (214) 241–0308

3098. Nippon Columbia Company
International Trade Dept. 1
14–14 Akasaka 4–Chome
Minato-Ku
Tokyo 107
Japan
Telephone: 3 584 8111

3099. Nippon Courseware
c/o Stalk-Kuramae M & K
4–16–6, Kuramae,
Taito-ku
Tokyo 111
Japan
Telephone: +81 3 35687 9800
Fax: +81 3 35687 9822

3100. Nippon Kankoo Kyokai
CD-ROM Enquiries
Kokusai Kankoo Kaikan Building
1–8–2 Marunouchi
Chiyoda-ku
Tokyo 100
Japan
Telephone: +81 3 3287 2745
Fax: +81 3 3287 2747

3101. Nippon Office Systems
c/o Hibaya Park Building, 932
1–8–1 Yuraku-cho
Chiyoda-ku
Tokyo
Tokyo 100
Japan

3102. Nippon Shuppan Hanbai Inc
4–3 Surugadai
Kanda
Chiyoda-ku
Tokyo 101
Japan
Telephone: 03 3233–1111
Fax: 03 3292–8521

3103. Nippon Telegraph and Telephone Corporation
1–6–6 Uchisaiwai-cho
Chiyoda-ku
Tokyo
Japan
Telephone: 81 (3) 509–5111;
81 (3) 509–3051
Telex/E-mail: 2225300 J

3104. Nissan
Parts Information
6–17–1, Ginza
Chuo-ku
Tokyo 104
Japan

3105. Nite-Line
National Computer Network Corporation
1929 North Harlem Avenue
Chicago
IL 60635
USA
Telephone: (312) 622–6666

3106. Nix Pix Windy City
Hot Pix Disk Info
Northbrook
Illinois
IL
USA
Telex/E-mail: (708) 564–1069 (Bulletin Board); 70521,666 (CompuServe Information System)

3107. NOB Nederlands Omroepproduktie Bedrijf NV
Mr van den Born
Postbus 10
1200 JB Hilversum
Netherlands
Telephone: +31 35 773636
Fax: +31 35 773307

3108. Noel D Adler
PO Box 150
East Setauket
NY 11733
USA

3109. Nomina Gesellschaft für Wirtschafts- und Verwaltungsregister mbH
Hansastraße 28
D-8000 Munich 21
Germany
Telephone: 089 578–310
Fax: 089 578–311–11;
089 560–0500
Telex/E-mail: 5212689 INF D

3110. NOMOS Datapool/EDICLINE
Waldseestraße 3–5
D-7570 Baden-Baden
Germany
Telephone: 07221 2104;
EM1:NOMOS (EuroMail)
Fax: 07221 210–427

3111. Nomura Research Institute
Edobashi Building
1–11–1 Nihonbashi
Chuo-ku
Tokyo 103
Japan
Telephone: 81 (3) 276–4762
Telex/E-mail: 27586 NRITKY J

3112. Nomura Research Institute
Systems Research Department, Data
    Bank Section
Dai-Ni Yamaman Building
6–7 Koami-Cho
Nihonbashi Chuo-Ku
Tokyo 103
Japan
Telephone: 03 3297–8234
Telex/E-mail: 27586 NRITKY J

**3113. Nomura Securities Company
    Ltd**
1–9–1 Nihonbashi
Chuo-ku
Tokyo 103
Japan
Telephone: 03 3211–1811;
    03 3211–3811

3114. NONOS Datapool
Nomos Verlagsgesellschaft
Waldsee Strasse 3–5
Postfach 610
7570 Baden-Baden
Germany
Telephone: 49 (7221) 34 41;
    49 (7221) 21 04 – 0
Fax: 49 (7221) 21 04 27

3115. Nordens folkiga akademi
Box 1004
442 25 Kungalv
Sweden
Telephone: 46 (9) 303 114 85
Fax: 46 (9) 303 121 13

**3116. Nordic Atomic Libraries Joint
    Secretariat**
Riso Library
PO Box 49
DK-4000 Roskilde
Denmark
Telephone: 42 371–212
Fax: 42 755–627
Telex/E-mail: 43116 RISOE DK

**3117. NORDICOM (See Nordisk
    Dokumentationscentral for
    Massekommunikations-
    forskning)**

**3119. Nordisk
    Dokumentationscentral for
    Massekommunikations-
    forskning**
State and University Library
Universitetsparken
DK-8000 Aarhus C
Denmark
Telephone: 06 122–022
Fax: 06 132–704

3120. Norelem Informatique
Z.I. de la Vigne aux Loups
Rue Blaise Pascal
PO Box 21
Chilly-Maxarin
CEDEX 91380
France
Telephone: 33 1 64 48 64 70
Fax: 33 1 64 48 10 01

**3121. Norges
    Standardiseringsforbund**
Postboks 7072 Homansbyen
N-0306 Oslo 3
Norway
Telephone: 02 466–094
Fax: 02 464–457
Telex/E-mail: 19050 NSF N

3122. Norman Ross Publishing Inc
Sandra Surrette
330 West 58th Street
New York
NY 10019
USA
Telephone: (212) 765 8200
Fax: (212) 765 2393

3123. Norminfo
Jean-Louis Huot
RN 20
PA du Moulin n 41
91882 Massy Cedex
France
Telephone: +33 1 64 47 11 00
Fax: +33 1 69 30 97 43

3124. Norsk Mediesentral
Ovre Slottsgate 7
0157 Oslo 1
Norway
Telephone: 47 (2) 41 82 75

**3125. Norsk Oseanografisk
    Datasenter,
    Fiskeridirektoratets**
Havforskningsinstitutt
Mr Leinebö
Postboks 1870/72
5024 Bergen
Norway
Telephone: +47 5 23 84 00
Fax: +47 5 23 85 31

**3126. Norsk Samfunnsvitenskapelig
    Datatjeneste**
Hans Homboesgate 22
N-5007 Bergen
Norway
Telephone: 05 212–118
Fax: 05 960–660

**3127. Norsk Senter for Informatikk
    A/S**
Brobekkveien 80
Postboks 1156 Sentrum
0107 Oslo 1
Norway
Telephone: 47 (2) 64 08 88

3128. Norsk Telegrambyra AS
Holbergsgt 1
PO Box 6817
St Olavs Place
N-0130 Oslo 1
Norway
Telephone: 02 20 16 70

**3129. Norsk Voksenpedagogisk
    Institutt**
Jonsvannsvn 82
N-7017 Trondheim
Norway
Telephone: 07 941–100

3130. Norske Creditbank, Den
PO Box 1171 Sentrum
N-0107 Oslo 1
Norway
Telephone: 02 482–790
Fax: 02 481–855
Telex/E-mail: 78175 N

3131. Norske Veritas, Det
Box 300
N-1322 Hovik
Norway
Telephone: 02 47 99 00
Telex/E-mail: 76192 VERIT N

3132. Norstedts Förlag
Eva Rudmann
Box 2052
103 12 Stockholm
Sweden
Telephone: +46 8 789 3000
Fax: +46 8 796 4905

**3133. North American Investment
    Corporation**
800 Connecticut Boulevard
East Hartford
CT 06108
USA
Telephone: (203) 528–9021;
    (800) 243–4322;
    (800) 842–8771 (in CT)
Telex/E-mail: 759522

**3134. North Atlantic Treaty
    Organization**
NATO ASI Series Publication
    Coordination Office
Dr Tilo Kester
Elcerlyclaan 2
B-1900 Overijssel
Belgium
Telephone: 02 687 66 36
Fax: 02 687 98 82
Telex/E-mail: 04026105831 B;
    051 933524 GEONET G

3135. North Carolina State University
School of Humanities and Social
    Sciences
PO Box 8101
Raleigh
NC 27695–8101
USA
Telephone: (919) 737–3791
Telex/E-mail: POLINET (DELPHI)

**3136. North of England Newspapers
    (NEN)**
Peter Chapman
Priestgate
Darlington
DL2 1NF
UK
Telephone: 0325 381–313
Fax: 0325 380–539

**3137. North Sea Information Centre
    AS**
B. Holst Andersen; Agnete Tram
Hvidovre Stationscentre 151
2650 Hvidovre
Denmark
Telephone: 45 (31) 473229

3138. Northamber plc
Lion Park Avenue
Chessington
Surrey
KT9 1SU
UK
Telephone: 081–391 2066

3139. Northeast Industrial Waste Exchange Inc
90 Presidential Plaza
Suite 122
Syracuse
NY 13202
USA
Telephone: (315) 422–6572
Fax: (315) 422–9051

3140. Northern Echo
Catherine Edwards
Library
Darlington
DL1 1NF
UK
Telephone: 0325 381 313 x2468
Fax: 0325 380 539

3141. Northern Ireland News Service
PO Box 11057
Albany
NY 12211–0057
USA
Telephone: (518) 329–3003
Telex/E-mail: 270–1457 (MCI Mail)

3142. Northern Miner
7 Labatt Avenue
Toronto
ON M5A 3P2
Canada
Telephone: (416) 368–3481

3143. Northern Telecom Canada Ltd
Michael Kinrys
8200 Dixie Road
PO Box 3000
Brompton
Ontario
L6V 2M6
Canada
Telephone: (416) 452–5133
Fax: (416) 452–5423

3144. Northern Telecom Europe Ltd
STC Digital Switching Division
Julie Shields
Meridian House
134 Bridge Road
Maidenhead
Berkshire
SL6 8DJ
UK
Telephone: 0628 795000
Fax: 0628 795001

3145. Northern Telecom/DMR Group
Tony van Atta
200 Athens Way
Nashville
TN 37228–1803
USA
Telephone: (615) 734 4000
Fax: (615) 734 4771

3146. Northfield Information Services Inc
PO Box 181164
99 Summer Street
Suite 1620
Boston
MA 02110
USA
Telephone: (617) 737–8360;
         (800) 262–6085
Telex/E-mail: 72620,22 (CompuServe Information Service)

3147. Northumberland Press Corporation
1717 Boulevard of the Allies
Pittsburgh
PA 15219
USA
Telephone: (412) 281–6179

3148. Northwest Regional Educational Laboratory
101 SW Main Street
Suite 500
Portland
OR 97204–3212
USA
Telephone: (503) 275–9628;
         (800) 547–6339
Telex/E-mail: 701716

3149. Norwegian Computing Centre
Maartmann Moe
Postboks 114
Blindern 0314
Oslo 3
Norway
Telephone: 47 246 6930;
         47 245 3500

3150. Norwegian Petroleum Directorate
PO Box 600
4001 Stavanger
Norway
Telephone: 47 (4) 87 60 00
Fax: 47 (4) 55 15 71
Telex/E-mail: 42863 NOPED N

3151. Norwegian School of Economics and Business Administration
Mr Steen
Library
Helleveien 30
5035 Bergen Sandviken
Norway
Telephone: 47 (5) 95 94 11
Fax: 47 (5) 25 83 00

3152. Norwegian Standards Association
PO Box 7020 HO
0306 Oslo 3
Norway
Telephone: 47 (2) 46 60 94
Fax: 47 (2) 46 44 57
Telex/E-mail: 19050 NSF N

3153. Norwich County Council
Library and Information Services
Mr. D Jones
County Hall
Martineau Lane
Norwich
NR1 2DH
UK
Telephone: 0603 222395

3154. Nottingham Polytechnic
Library and Information Services
  Consultancy Unit
Burton Street
Nottingham
NG1 4BU
UK
Telephone: 0602 258–837

3155. Nova Idea
Bergisch Gladbacher Strasse 978
5000 Cologne 80
Germany
Telephone: +49 221 680 4053
Fax: +49 221 680 4013

3156. Nova Scotia Research Foundation Corporation
PO Box 790
101 Research Drive
Woodside Industrial Park
Dartmouth
NS B2Y 3Z7
Canada
Telephone: (902) 424–8670
Fax: (902) 424–4679
Telex/E-mail: 01922719

3157. Novamedias
27 rue Garnier
F-92200 Neuilly
France
Telephone: 1 47 38 10 09
Fax: 1 46 24 08 98

3158. Novell Inc
Cal Call
122 E 1700 South
Provo
UT 84606
USA
Telephone: (801) 429 7000
Fax: (801) 429 5200

3159. Novosti Press Agency
Oleg Polyschuk
4 Zoubovsky Bd
119021 Moscow
Russia
Fax: +7 (095) 2302667

3160. NPA Data Services Inc
1424 16th Street NW
Suite 700
Washington
DC 20036
USA
Telephone: (202) 265–7685
Fax: (202) 797–5516

3161. NPK Technology Services (SilverPlatter Agent)
14 Esser Tachanot Street
Box 10117
Tel Aviv 61100
Israel
Telephone: 972–3 497802/3
Fax: 972–3 497812

3162. NSI – Norsk Senter for Informatikks A/S
Brobekkveien 80
Postboks 1156 Sentrum
N-0107 Oslos 1
Norway
Telephone: +47 2 640888

3163. NTC Publishing Group
Gail Cassel
4255 West Touhy Avenue
Lincolnwood
IL 60646–1975
USA
Telephone: (708) 679–5500;
         (708) 323–4900
Fax: (312) 679–2494

3164. NTT Data Communications Systems Corporation
1–6–6 Uchisaiwai-cho
Chiyoda-ku
Tokyo
Japan
Telephone: 03 3509–5111
Telex/E-mail: 2225300 J

3165. NTT Joho-Kaihatsu
Tokyo
Japan
Telephone: +8 1 3662–0151

3166. NTT Nippon Telegraph and Telephone Corporation
Kuniomi Sakurai
1–6 1 chome Uschisaiwai-cho
Chiyoda-Ku
Tokyo 100
Japan
Telephone: 03 3509–5925
Fax: 03 3508–1080

3167. NTUB
Documentation Department
Hoegskoleringen 1
7034 Trondheim
Norway

3168. Numerax Inc
615 Winters Avenue
Paramus
NJ 07652
USA
Telephone: (201) 967–9318

3169. NYKredit
Systemsektionen
Tiendeladen 7
9000 Aalborg
Denmark
Telephone: 45 (98) 168200

3170. Nymott AG
Switzerland
Telephone: +41 1 29 12040

**3171. Nynex Information
      Technologies Company**
Mark Remmer
100 Church Street
9th Floor
New York
NY 10007–2670
USA
Telephone: (212) 513–9700;
          (800) 338–0646
Fax: (212) 513–9788

3172. Oak Ridge National Laboratory
John S Watson
Environmental Mutagen Information
Building 2001
PO Box 2008
Oak Ridge
TN 37831–6050
USA
Telephone: (615) 574–7871;
          (615) 576–1746

3173. Oak Ridge National Laboratory
Biomedical and Environmental
   Information Analysis Section
Environmental Teratology Information
PO Box 2008
Oak Ridge
TN 37831–6050
USA
Telephone: (615) 574–7871

3174. Oak Ridge National Laboratory
Toxicology Information Response
   Center
PO Box 2008
Building 2001
Oak Ridge
TN 37831–6050
USA
Telephone: (615) 576–1746

3175. Oakland Tribune, The
409 13th Street
PO Box 24304
Oakland
CA 24304
USA
Telephone: (510) 645–2000

**3176. Observatoire det Matieres
      Premieres**
120 rue du Cherche Midi
75006 Paris
France
Telephone: 33 (1) 45 56 47 17

**3177. Occupational Health Services
      Inc**
Richard Cohen
11 W 42nd Street
12th Floor
New York
NY 10036
USA
Telephone: (212) 789 3535
Fax: (212) 789 3646
Telex/E-mail: 4754124

**3178. Occupational Health Services
      Inc**
450 7th Avenue
Suite 2407
New York
NY 10123
USA
Telephone: (212) 967–1100;
          (800) 445–6737

**3179. Ocean Resources Engineering
      Center**
St. Johns
Newfoundland
Canada

3180. Oceandril Inc
777 N Eldridge
Suite 640
Houston
TX 77079
USA
Telephone: (713) 558–9018

3181. OCLC Europe
7th Floor
Tricorn House
51–53 Hagley Road
Birmingham
B16 3TP
UK
Telephone: 021–456 4656

**3182. OCLC Online Computer Library
      Center Inc**
CD-ROM Enquiries
6565 Frantz Road
Dublin
OH 43017–0702
USA
Telephone: (614) 764–6000;
          (800) 848–5878;
          (800) 848–8266 (in OH)
Fax: (614) 764–6096
Telex/E-mail: 810 339 2026

**3183. ODAV Datenverarbeitung
      GmbH**
Josef Bielmeier
Ernst-Heinkel-Straße 11
D-8440 Straubing
Germany
Telephone: 09421 610 52;
          09421 70 50
NUA: Available on application

3184. Odense Universitetsbibliotek
Ingelise Staehr
Campusvej 55
5230 Odense M
Denmark
Telephone: 45 (66) 158600

3185. ODIS BV
Eric van Lubeek
Piazza 403
5611 AG Eindhoven
Netherlands
Telephone: +31 40 433605
Fax: +31 40 434145

3186. OEMF spa
Elene Trezza
Via Edolo 42
Milan 20125
Italy
Telephone: +39 2 675051
Fax: +39 2 67505223

3187. OERI Toll Free Bulletin Board
555 New Jersey Avenue
Washington
DC 20208
USA
Telephone: (202) 357–6524;
          (202) 626–9853

**3188. Österreichische
      Apotheker-Verlagsgesellschaft
      mbH**
Dr Helmut Rücker
Spitolgasse 31
1094 Vienna
Austria
Telephone: +43 222 4023588
Fax: +43 222 4085355

**3189. Österreichische
      Nationalbibliothek**
Austrian National Library
H Ortner
Planungsstelle
Josefsplatz 1
1015 Vienna
Austria
Telephone: 43 1 533 70 49 87;
          43 1 534 10353
Fax: 43 1 53370 4983

**3190. Österreichische
      Normunginstitut**
Austrian Standards Institute
Manfred Görlich
Heinestrasse 38
1021 Vienna
Austria
Telephone: +43 222 26 75 35
Fax: +43 222 26 75 52

**3191. Österreichisches
      Staatdruckerel**
Austrian State Print Office
Dr Andreas Manak
Rennweg 12a
1038 Vienna
Austria
Telephone: 43 (222) 797 89 235
Fax: 43 (222) 797 89 419

**3192. Österreichisches Statistisches
      Zentralamt**
Technisch-Methodische Abteilung
Hintere Zollamtsstraße 2B
Postfach 8000
A-1033 Vienna
Austria
Telephone: 01 71128
Fax: 01 71127

3193. OFAC
Claudine Magnin-Leuthold M Madada
Rue Pedro-Meylan 7
1211 Geneva 17
Switzerland
Telephone: 22 736 46 02
Fax: 22 718 9801

**3194. Office for Official Publications
      of the European Communities**
Database Section
John Mortier
2 rue Mercier
2985 Luxembourg
Luxembourg
Telephone: (352) 499281
Fax: (352) 488573
Telex/E-mail: 1324B PUBOF LU

3195. Office of Multicultural Affairs
Department of the Prime Minister and
    Cabinet
Canberra
ACT 2600
Australia
Telephone: 61 (62) 71–5658

**3196. Office of Personnel
    Management**
1900 East Street NW
Washington
DC 20415
USA
Telephone: (202) 632–5491

**3197. Office of the Attorney General,
    New Brunswick**
Law Reform Branch
Centennial Building, Room 414
PO Box 6000
Fredericton
New Brunswick
E3B 5H1
Canada
Telephone: (506) 453–2854
Fax: (506) 453–3275

**3198. Office of the President of the
    United States**
1600 Pennsylvania Avenue NW
Washington
DC 20500
USA
Telephone: (202) 456–1414

**3199. Office of the Superintendant of
    Financial Institutions**
140 O'Connor Street
Esplanade Laurier, 15th Floor
Ottawa
ON K1A 0H2
Canada
Telephone: (613) 996–8665

3200. Official Airline Guides
2000 Clearwater Drive
Oak Brook
IL 60521
USA
Telephone: (708) 574–6000;
        (800) 323–4000
Fax: (708) 574–6091
Telex/E-mail: QHOAGXD; 210144

3201. Ohio State University
Department of Chemistry
Martin Caffrey
Columbus
OH 43210
USA

3202. Ohmsha Ltd
Mr Takeo
3–1 Kanda Nishiki-cho
Chiyoda-ku
Tokyo 101
Japan
Telephone: +81 3 3233 0641
Fax: +81 3 3293 2824

3203. Oil & Gas Journal
PO Box 1260
Tulsa
OK 74101
USA
Telephone: (918) 832–9346
Fax: (918) 831–9497
Telex/E-mail: 203604

**3204. Oil Pipeline Research Institute
    Inc**
PO Box 1433
Manhatten Beach
CA 90266
USA
Telephone: (310) 372–0722
Fax: (310) 374–0259

**3205. Oliphant Washington News
    Service**
1819 H Street NW
Suite 330
Washington
DC 20006–3677
USA
Telephone: (202) 296–0924

3206. Olivetti Research Ltd
CD-ROM Enquiries
24A Trumpington Street
Cambridge
CB2 1QA
UK
Telephone: 0223 343000
Fax: 0223 313542

3207. Olivetti Systems & Networks
Mr Grauata
Via Jervis 77
10015 Ivrea
Italy
Telephone: 0125 522–130
Fax: 0125 523–390

3208. Oljedirektoratet
PO Box 600
Prof Olav Hanssens vei 10
N-4001 Stavanger
Norway
Telephone: 04 876–000
Fax: 04 551–571
Telex/E-mail: 42863 NOPED N

3209. OLMS Microform System
Georg OLMS Verlag
Hagentorwall 7
Hildesheim
W-3200
Germany
Telephone: 05121–37007

3210. Omaha World-Herald Company
World-Herald Square
Omaha
NE 68102
USA
Telephone: (402) 444–1000

3211. OMEC International Inc
727 15th Street NW
Washington
DC 20005
USA
Telephone: (202) 639–8900
Fax: (202) 639–8993

3213. Omega Corporation
Via Murri 39
40137 Bologna
Italy
Telephone: +39 51 306644
Fax: +39 51 398654

**3214. Omo Middelbaar
        Onderwijs/ESCAPE**
OMO/ESCAPE
Postbus 574
5000 AN Tilburg
Netherlands
Telephone: 013 371311

3215. On-Line Entertainment Ltd
Michael Hodges
642a Lea Bridge Road
Leyton
London
E10 6AP
UK
Telephone: 081 558–6114
Fax: 081 558–3914

3216. On-Line Kredittkontroll
PO Box 5387
Majorstua
N-0303 Oslo 3
Norway
Telephone: 02 468–900
Fax: 02 465–390
Telex/E-mail: 11093 CINFO N

3217. On-Line Research Inc
200 Railroad Avenue
Greenwich
CT 06830
USA
Telephone: (203) 661–1395
Fax: (203) 869–8326

3218. One to One
Scorpio House
102 Sydney Street
Chelsea
London
SW3 6NL
UK
Telephone: 071 351–2468
Fax: 071 351–2075
Telex/E-mail: 8950511 ONEONE G

3219. Online Computer Systems Inc
William Ford; Lisa Huber
20251 Century Boulevard
Germantown
MD 20874
USA
Telephone: (301) 428–3700
Fax: (301) 428–2903
Telex/E-mail: 3746439

3220. Online Inc
11 Tannery Lane
Weston
CT 06883
USA
Telephone: (203) 227–8466
Telex/E-mail: 23337 (DialMail);
    CLASS ONLINE/SV (OnTyme)

3221. Online Information Network
A division of American Business
    Information Inc
5711 South 86th Circle
PO Box 27347
Omaha
NE 68127
USA
Telephone: (402) 593–4593
Fax: (402) 331–1505

3222. Online Research Systems
2901 Broadway
Suite 154
New York
NY 10025
USA
Telephone: (212) 408–3311;
        (212) 932–1486

3223. Online Resource Exchange Inc
1800 Bering Drive
Suite 850
Houston
TX 77057
USA
Telephone: (713) 975–1111

3224. Ons Middlebaar Onderwijs
Apennijnenweg 11
5022 DT Tilburg
Netherlands
Telephone: 013 371–311
Fax: 013 355–595

3225. Ontario Legislative Assmebly
Parliament Building
Room 104
Toronto
ON M7A 1A2
Canada
Telephone: (416) 965–2700

3226. Ontario Ministry of Culture and Communications
77 Bloor Street W
10th Floor
Toronto
ON M7A 1L2
Canada
Telephone: (416) 324–7061

3227. Ontario Ministry of Education
Centre for Curriculum Resources and Technologies
Mowat Block
24th Floor
Queens Park
Toronto
ON M7A 1L2
Canada
Telephone: (416) 965–4110
Fax: (416) 965–0383

3228. Ontario Ministry of Housing
Buildings Branch
Ali Arlani (Manager Code Services);
   Ralph Di Gartano (Code Advisor)
777 Bay Street
2nd Floor
Toronto
ON M5G 2E5
Canada
Telephone: (416) 585–6666
Fax: (416) 585–4029

3229. Ontario Museum Association
George Brown House
50 Baldwin Street at Beverley
Toronto
ON M5T 1L4
Canada
Telephone: (416) 348–8672
Fax: (416) 348–8689
Telex/E-mail: OMA.1 (Envoy 100)

3230. Ontario Securities Commission
20 Queen Street W
Room 1800
PO Box 55
Toronto
ON M5H 3S8
Canada
Telephone: (416) 597–0681

3231. Opdirom Optical Disc Systems GmbH & Co KG
Herbert Ulshöfer
Haupstrasse 49
6308 Butzbach 7
Germany
Telephone: +49 60 33 5297
Fax: +49 60 33 16356

3232. Open University
International Centre for Distance Learning
Dr K Harry
Walton Hall
Milton Keynes
MK7 6AA
UK
Telephone: 0908 653537
Fax: 0908 653744

3233. Opetusministerioe
Tieteellisten Kirjastojen ATK-yksikkoe
PO Box 312
SF-00171 Helsinki
Finland
Telephone: 0 708–4298

3234. OPOCE
Mr. J. Mortimer
Office des Publications
2 Rue Mercier
2985 Luxembourg
Luxembourg
Telephone: (352) 499282563
Telex/E-mail: 1324 PUBOF LU

3235. Opsys
Alain Gagne
3 rue Paul Valerien Perrin
38170 Seyssinet-Pariset
France
Telephone: +33 76 49 04 40
Fax: +33 76 48 35 00

3236. Optech
East Street
Farnham
Surrey
GU9 7XX
UK
Telephone: 0252 714340

3237. Opti-Stora BV
A Proeme; G Vogels
Mierloseweg 53
5667 JB Geldrop
Netherlands
Telephone: +31 40 854411
Fax: +31 40 859455

3238. Optical Media International
Allen Adkins; Susan Wilson
180 Knowles Drive
Los Gatos
CA 95030
USA
Telephone: (408) 376–3511
Fax: (408) 376–3519

3239. Optical Publishing Association
Richard Bowers
PO Box 21268
Columbus
OH 43221
USA
Telephone: (614) 793 9660
Fax: (614) 793 0749

3240. Optical Publishing Inc
Katherine Stubler
155 West Harvard Street
Fort Collins
CO 80525
USA
Telephone: (303) 226–3466;
   (800) 869–7989
Fax: (303) 226–3464

3241. OPTIM Corporation
Barbara Dourma
338 Somerset Street West
Ottawa
Ontario
K2P 0J9
Canada
Telephone: +1 613 232 3766
Fax: +1 613 232 8413

3242. Optimage Interactive Services Company
Dell Wolfensparger; Craig Rispin; Vicki Hictland
1900 NW 114th Street
Des Moines
IA 50325
USA
Telephone: (515) 225 7000;
   (800) CDI 5484
Fax: (515) 225 0252

3243. Optosof
Box 42
S-16493 Kista
Sweden
Telephone: 46 8 750 7950

3244. Opus Species
14 rue de l'Atlas
75019 Paris
France
Telephone: +33 1 42 45 51 23
Fax: +33 1 42 39 60 09

3245. OR Telematique
7 rue de Sens
Rochecorbon
F-37210 Vouvray
France
Telephone: 47 62 62 62
Fax: 43 60 21 57

3246. Oracle Corporation
3 Crestway Road-Knollcrest
New Fairfield
CT 06812
USA
Telephone: (203) 746–7534

3247. Orange County Register, The
PO Box 11626
625 N Grand Avenue
Santa Ana
CA 92711
USA
Telephone: (714) 953–4937;
   (714) 835–1234

3248. ORBIT Search Service
Achilles House
Western Avenue
London
W3 0UA
UK
Telephone: 081 992–3456
Fax: 081 993–7335

3249. ORBIT Search Service
8000 Westpark Drive
Suite 400
McLean
VA 22102
USA
Telephone: (703) 442–0900
Fax: (703) 893–4632
Telex/E-mail: 901811

3250. ORDA-B Nederland
J Gower
Edisonweg 15
3442 AC Woerden
Netherlands
Telephone: +31 3480 11 454
Fax: +31 3480 16 497

3251. ORDA-B NV
Paul Muls
Leuvensesteenweg 384
1932 Zaventum
Belgium
Telephone: 32 2 725 40 20
Fax: 32 2 725 42 62

**3252. Oregon State Legislative
Administration Committee**
S408 State Capitol
Salem
OR 97310
USA
Telephone: (503) 378–8194

**3253. Oregon State Legislative
Administration Committee**
S408 State Capitol
Salem
OR 97310
USA
Telephone: (503) 378–8194

**3254. Oregonian Publishing
Company**
1320 S.W. Broadway
Portland
OR 97201
USA
Telephone: (503) 221–8327

3255. ORFEUS Data Center (ODC)
Instituut voor Aardwetenschappen
Dr B Dost
University of Utrecht
Budapestiaan 4
3584 CD Utrecht
Netherlands
Telephone: +31 30 535143;
030 535115
Fax: +31 30 535030

**3257. Organisation for Economic
Cooperation and Development
(OECD)**
2 rue Andre Pascal
F-75775 Paris Cedex 16
France
Telephone: 1 45 24 98 87

**3258. Organización de Estados
Iberoamericanos para la
Educacion, la**
Ciencia y la Cultura
Cuidad Universitaria s/n
28040 Madrid
Spain
Telephone: 01 449 69 54

3259. ORI Inc
ERIC Processing and Reference Facility
Ted Brandhorst
2440 Research Boulevard
Rockville
MD 20850–3238
USA
Telephone: (301) 590–1420;
(301) 258–5500

**3260. Orlando Sentinel
Communications Company**
633 North Orange Avenue
Orlando
FL 32801
USA
Telephone: (305) 420–5000

3261. ORS Publishing
Dennis Gilbert
1342 Timberlane Road
Suite 201A
Tallahassee
FL 32312
USA
Telephone: (904) 668 9922;
(800) 462 8913

3262. Oryx Press
Customer Service
4041 N Central Avenue
Suite 700
Phoenix
AZ 85012–3399
USA
Telephone: (602) 265–6250;
(602) 265–6251;
(800) 279–6799;
(800) 279–4663
Fax: (602) 265–6250
Telex/E-mail: 910 951 1333

3263. Osaka City Hall
Comprehensive Planning Bureau
Urban Engineering Information Center
1–3–20 Nakoshima
Kita
Osaka
Japan
Telephone: 06 208–7858

**3264. Oscar Brandstetter Verlag
GmbH &Company KG**
Mr Froehlen
Postfach 1708
Stiftsrasse 30
Postfach 1708
D-6200 Wiesbaden
Germany
Telephone: +49 611 580913
Fax: +49 611 580938

3265. OSEC
Stampfenbachstrasse 85
8035 Zürich
Switzerland
Telephone: 41 (1) 365 51 51
Fax: 41 (1) 365 52 21

**3266. OSS Optical Storage Systems
Inc**
7 West 7th Avenue
Suite 300
Vancouver
British Columbia
V54 1C4
Canada
Telephone: 604–876–3838
Fax: 604 876 3255

**3267. Oster Communications
Inc**
219 Parkade
Cedar Falls
IA 50613
USA
Telephone: (319) 277–6341;
(800) 553–1781;
(800) 553–2910
Fax: (319) 277–7892
Telex/E-mail: 439034

3268. OTC IntelNet
OTC Limited
231 Eliabeth Street
Sydney
NSW 2000
Australia
Telephone: 61 (612) 287–5000

3269. OTE/Telephone Directories
A Koutsorodis
24 Sygrou Avenue
11742 Athens
Greece
Telephone: +301 923 9499
Fax: +301 923 6599

3270. Ouwehand Consultancy
Ye Olde Hand Consultancy
H T A Ouwehand
Crailoseweg 26
1272 EV Huizen
Netherlands
Telephone: +31 2152–68973
Fax: +31 2152 40999

3271. OVP – Editions du Vidal
Nadine Pedreau; F DuFour
11 rue Quentin Bauchart
75384 Paris Cedex 08
France
Telephone: 1 47 23 90 91
Fax: 1 47 20 72 89

3272. OWL International Inc
Luann Garwood
2800 156th Avenue SE
Bellvue
WA 98007
USA
Telephone: (206) 747 3203
Fax: (206) 641 9367

3273. OWL International Ltd
Tom McCallum
144 Broughton Road
Edinburgh
E47 4LE
UK
Telephone: 031 557 5720
Fax: 031 557 5721

3274. Oxford University Press
Electronic Publishing Division
Janet Caldwell (Customer Services)
Walton Street
Oxford
OX2 6DP
UK
Telephone: 0865 56767;
0344 369369
Fax: 0865 56646

3275. Oxford University Press
Oxford Electronic Publishing
Royalynn O'Connor
200 Madison Avenue
New York
NY 10016
USA
Telephone: (212) 679–7300;
(800) 872–2828
Fax: (212) 725–2972

3276. Oxko Corporation
Steven W Oxman
175 Admiral Cochrane Drive
North Lobby
Annapolis
MD 21401
USA
Telephone: (301) 266 1671
Fax: (301) 266 6572

3277. P/K Associates Inc
3006 Gregory Street
Madison
WI 53711–1847
USA
Telephone: (608) 231–1003

3278. Pace Publications
443 Park Avenue South
New York
NY 10016
USA
Telephone: (212) 685–5450

3279. Pacific CD Corporation
John M Bond
PO Box 31328
Honolulu
Hawaii
96820
USA
Telephone: (808) 949 4594

3280. Pacific Press Ltd
2250 Granville Street
Vncouver
BC V6H 3G2
Canada
Telephone: (604) 732–2111

**3281. Pacific Rim Specialists
(SilverPlatter Agent)**
PO Box 4992
Irvine
CA 92716
USA
Telephone: (714) 641–6645

3282. Pacific Veterinary Services
1526 Crespi Drive
Pacifica
CA 94044–3608
USA
Telephone: (415) 355–2720
Telex/E-mail: DR.RICH (GEnie)

3283. Packard Humanities Institute
300 Second St.
Suite 201
Los Altos
CA 94022
USA
Telephone: (415) 948–0150

3284. Packard Press
606 South Olive St.
Suite 707
Los Angeles
CA 90014
USA
Telephone: (213) 239–8335

3285. Paint Research Association
Information Department
Waldegrave Road
Teddington
Middlesex
TW11 8LD
UK
Telephone: 081 977–4427
Fax: 081 943–4705
Telex/E-mail: 928720 OPRA G

3286. Palm Beach Newspapers Inc
2751 S Dixie Highway
PO Box 24700
West Palm Beach
FL 33405–4700
USA
Telephone: (407) 837–4100;
(407) 837–4277

**3287. Pan American Health
Organization (PAHO)**
Centro Latino-Americano e do Caribe
de Informacao em Ciencias de Saude
Rua Botucatu 862
CP 20381
04023 Sao Paulo
Brazil
Telephone: 011 549–2611
Fax: 011 571–1919
Telex/E-mail: 22143 OPAS BR

**3288. Pan American Health
Organization (PAHO)**
525 23rd St. NW
Washington
DC 20037
USA
Telephone: (202) 861–3365

3289. Pantagraph, The
301 W Washington Street
Bloomington
IL 61701
USA
Telephone: (309) 829–9411

3290. PaperChase
Beth Israel Hospital
350 Longwood Avenue
Boston
MA 02115
USA
Telephone: (617) 732–4800;
(800) 722–2075

3291. Papiertechnische Stiftung
Heßstraße 130 A
D-8000 Munich 40
Germany
Telephone: 089 1260–0146
Fax: 089 123–6592
Telex/E-mail: 5213088 PTS D

3292. Paracomp Inc
Alane Bowling
1725 Montgomery Street
2nd Floor
San Francisco
CA 94111
USA
Telephone: (415) 956 4091
Fax: (415) 956 9525

3293. Paribas
3 rue d'Antin
75002 Paris
France
Telephone: 33 (1) 42 98 05 75

**3294. Paris Chamber of Commerce
and Industry**
Department of International Trade
2 rue de Viarmes
F-75002 Paris
France
Telephone: 1 45 08 36 00
Fax: 1 45 08 35 80
Telex/E-mail: 230823 DRICCIP F

**3295. Paris Chamber of Commerce
and Industry**
Economic Documentation Center
27 avenue de Friedland
F-75382 Paris Cedex 8
France
Telephone: 1 42 89 70 00
Fax: 1 42 89 78 68
Telex/E-mail: 650 100 CCI PARIS F
230 823 DRICCIP F

**3296. Paris Chamber of Commerce
and Industry**
Office for Information, Orientation and
Improvement
Direction de l'Enseignement
47 rue de Tocqueville
F-75017 Paris
France
Telephone: 1 47 66 72 73

**3297. Paris Chamber of Commerce
and Industry**
PMI Division
2 rue de Viarmes
F-75001 Paris
France
Telephone: 1 45 08 35 96

3299. Paris Gestion Informatique
5 place Salvador Allende
BP 98
F-94011 Creteil Cedex
France
Telephone: 1 48 98 91 02
Fax: 1 47 74 61 56

**3300. PARS Travel Information
Systems**
7310 Tiffany Springs Parkway
Kansas City
MO 64153
USA
Telephone: (816) 891–5300

3301. Particulier, Le
21 boulevard Montmartre
F-75082 Paris
France
Telephone: 1 40 20 70 00
Telex/E-mail: 220700 F

3302. Pasha Publications Inc
1401 Wilson Boulevard
Suite 900
Arlington
VA 22209
USA
Telephone: (703) 528–1244;
(800) 424–2908
Fax: (703) 528–1243
Telex/E-mail: 248852 PASUR

3303. Passport Designs Inc
Anastasia Lanier
625 Miramontes Street
Half Moon Bay
CA 94019
USA
Telephone: (415) 726–0280
Fax: (415) 726–2254

3304. Patent Office
State House
66–71 High Holborn
London
WC1R 4TP
UK
Telephone: 071 829–6474;
071 831–2525

3305. Patent Office
25 Southampton Buildings
London
WC21 1AW
UK
Telephone: 071 438 4700

3306. Patent Search Systems, Inc
R Macdonald
2001 Jefferson Davis Highway
Suite 802
Arlington
VA 22202
USA
Telephone: (703) 521–9030

3307. Patentdirektoratet
J.P. Schougaard Henny Lohse
Helgeshoej Allee 81
2630 Taastrup
Denmark
Telephone: 45 (4) 3717171

3308. Patriot-News, The
812 King Boulevard
PO Box 2265
Harrisburg
PA 17105
USA
Telephone: (717) 255–8100

3309. Patscan Service
Science Division
Ronald V Simmer
University of British Columbia
1956 Main Mall
Vancouver
British Columbia
V6T 1Z1
Canada
Telephone: (604) 228–5404
Fax: (604) 228–6465

3310. Paul Bernstein
333 East Ontario Street 2102B
Chicago
IL 60611
USA
Telephone: (312) 951–8264

3311. Paul de Haen International Inc
2750 S Shoshone Street
Englewood
CO 80110
USA
Telephone: (303) 781–6683;
(800) 438–0296
Fax: (303) 789–2534

3312. PAXUS ComNet
PO Box 1800
Canberra
ACT 2601
Australia
Fax: 062 478–985

3313. PC Connections
Wigan
UK
Telephone: 0706 222–988
Fax: 0706 222–989

3314. PC Resources
180 Wilson Street
Fairfield
CT 06432
USA
Telephone: (203) 371–6062

3315. PC-SIG
Kim Washington
1030 East Duane Avenue
Suite D
Sunnyvale
CA 94086
USA
Telephone: (408) 730–9291;
(800) 245–6117
Fax: (408) 730–2107

3316. PCI
80 Bloor Street West
11th Floor
Toronto
ON M5S 2V1
Canada
Telephone: (416) 928–6733

**3317. PComm Information Systems
Inc**
1411 Fort Street
Suite 2001
Montreal
PQ H3H 2N7
Canada
Telephone: (514) 937–1114
Telex/E-mail: 167/1 (FidoNet)

3318. PDO Company
Robert Fisher
Building EF-5
PO Box 218
5600 MD Eindhoven
Netherlands
Telephone: +31 40 751120
Fax: +31 40 757866

3319. PDO Company
Lawrence Walker
Queen Anne House
11 The Green
Richmond Upon Thames
Surrey
TW9 1PX
UK
Telephone: 081 948–7368
Fax: 081 940–7137

**3320. PDSC – Publishers Data
Service Corporation**
Division of Sony
D Quarnstrom
1 Lower Ragsdale Drive
Suite 160
Monterey
CA 93940
USA
Telephone: (408) 372–2812
Fax: (408) 375 7130

3321. Peat Marwick McLintock
1 Puddle Dock
Blackfriars
London
EC4V 3PD
UK
Telephone: 071 236–8000
Fax: 071 248–6552
Telex/E-mail: 8811541 PMM LON G

3322. Peking Union Medical College
Chinese Academy of Medical Sciences
9 Dongdan 3rd Lane
Beijing 100730
China
Telephone: 512–7733

3323. Peking University
CHINALAW Computer-Assisted Legal
Research Center
Hai Dian
Beijing 100871
China

3324. Pendragon Optical Media Ltd
36 Sciberras Road
Unionville
Ontario
L3R 2J3
Canada
Telephone: (416) 477–9707

3325. Pennsylvania State Library
School Library Media Services Division
Margaret Goodlin
333 Market Street
Harrisburg
PA 17126–0333
USA
Telephone: (717) 783–4414
Fax: (717) 783–5420

3326. PennWell Publishing Company
PO Box 1260
Tulsa
OK 74101
USA
Telephone: (918) 835–3161
Fax: (918) 831–9497
Telex/E-mail: 203604 PPUB UR

3327. PennWell Publishing Company
1421 S Sheridan Road
PO Box 1260
Tulsa
OK 74101
USA
Telephone: (918) 832–9346
Fax: (918) 831–9497
Telex/E-mail: 203604

**3328. Pennyslvania Department of
Education**
State Library
Dr Doris Epler
11th Floor
33 Market Street
Harrisburg
PA 17126–0333
USA
Telephone: (717) 787 6704
Fax: (717) 783 5420

3329. Pentagon Library
Carol J Bursik
Room 1A518
The Pentagon
Washington
DC 20310–6000
USA
Telephone: (703) 697 4658
Fax: (703) 693 3731

3330. Penton Publishing Company
1100 Superior Avenue
Cleveland
OH 44114
USA
Telephone: (216) 696–7000

3331. Penton Publishing Inc
611 Route 46 W
Hasbrouck Heights
NJ 07604
USA
Telephone: (201) 393–6060

3332. Perceptronics Inc
Tom Lubaczewski
21135 Erwin Street
Woodland Hills
CA 91367
USA
Telephone: (818) 884 3485
Fax: (818) 348 0540

3333. PEREMEDIA AG
Elizabeth Pilet
Gfellerstrasse 1
3175 Flamatt
Switzerland
Telephone: 31 744 52 48
Fax: 31 744 52 47

3334. Pergamon Press Inc
Rebecca Rich
Maxwell House
Fairview Park
Emsford
NY 10523
USA
Telephone: (914) 592–7700
Fax: (914) 592–3625

3335. Pergamon Press Ltd
Dinah Bott
Headington Hill Hall
Headington
Oxford
OX3 0BW
UK
Telephone: 0865 64881;
0865 794–141
Fax: 0865 743–951;
0865 60285
Telex/E-mail: 83177 G; 76:GAM002
(Dialcom)

**3336. Personal Employee Profiling
Inc**
601 Lee Street
Des Plaines
IL 60016
USA
Telephone: (708) 803–2890

3337. Personnel Journal
245 Fisher Avenue, B-2
Costa Mesa
CA 92626
USA
Telephone: (714) 751–1883
Fax: (714) 751–4106

3338. Personnel Policy Service Inc
PO Box 7697
Louisville
KY 40257–0697
USA
Telephone: (502) 897–6782

3339. Personnel Research Associates
49 Oakridge Road
Verona
NJ 07044
USA
Telephone: (201) 239–6154
Fax: (201) 239–1013

3340. Peruzzo
Viale E. Marelli 165
Sesto S. Giovanni
20099 Milan
Italy
Telephone: +39 2 24 07 800
Fax: +39 2 24 02 723

3341. Peter J Phethean Ltd
Peter Phethean
1640 East Brookdale Avenue
La Habra
CA 90631
USA
Telephone: (213) 694–2112
Fax: (213) 691 8248

3342. Peterson's Guides Inc
Eric A Suber
PO Box 2123
202 Carnegie Center
Princeton
NJ 08543–2123
USA
Telephone: (609) 243–9111;
        (800) 338–3282
Fax: (609) 243–9150;
        (609) 452–0966

3343. Petroconsultants (CES) Ltd
Helen Newport
Europa House
266 Upper Richmond Road
Putney
London
SW15 6TQ
UK
Telephone: 081 780–2500
Fax: 081 780–9707

3344. Petroflash! Inc
PO Box 798
Lakewood
NJ 08701
USA
Telephone: (201) 367–1600
Telex/E-mail: 132435

3345. Petroleum Abstracts
The University of Tulsa
600 South College/Harwell 101
Tulsa
OK 74104
USA
Telephone: (918) 631–2296;
        (800) 247–8678
Fax: (918) 631–3823
Telex/E-mail: 497543 INFOSVC TU
    TUL

3346. Petroleum Argus Ltd
83–93 Shepperton Road
London
N1 3DF
UK
Telephone: 081 359–8792
Fax: 081 226–0695
Telex/E-mail: 21277 ARGUS G

3347. Petroleum Information Corporation
4100 East Dry Creek Road
Littleton
CO 80122
USA
Telephone: (303) 740–7100;
        (800) 525–5569
Telex/E-mail: 450244

3348. Petroleum Information
PI On-Line Services
PO Box 2612
Denver
CO 80201
USA
Telephone: (303) 740–7100;
        (800) 525–5569
Telex/E-mail: 45044

3349. Petroleum Intelligence Weekly
575 Broadway
4th Floor
New York
NY 10012–3230
USA
Telephone: (212) 941–5500
Telex/E-mail: 62371 PETROIN

3350. Petroleum Registry Inc
6565 West Loop South, Suite 115
Houston
TX 77401
USA
Telephone: (713) 668–5596
Fax: (713) 669–0314

3351. PetroScan
A division of United Communications
    Group
4550 Montgomery Avenue, Suite 700N
Bethesda
MD 20814
USA
Telephone: (301) 961–8700
Fax: (301) 961–8666

3352. PGI/ICT Corporation Harman Cadis
1555 West 10th Place
Suite 106
Tempe
AZ 85281
USA
Telephone: (602) 967 1421
Fax: (602) 968 0177

3353. Pharma Daig & Laur
Herr Herzog; Herr Deppner
Gebhardstraße 41–45
D-8510 Furth/Bayern
Germany
Telephone: 0911 7432–274
Fax: 0911 7432–100

3354. Pharma Marketing Service
A section of Aerzte Zeitun
    Verlagsgesellschaft mbH
Am Forsthaus Gravenbruch 5
6078 Neu-Isenburg 2
Germany
Telephone: 49 (6102) 50 61 45
Fax: 49 (6102) 50 61 23
Telex/E-mail: 414944 D

3385. Pharmaprojects PJB Publications Ltd
18–20 Hill Rise
Richmond
Surrey
TW10 6UA
UK
Telephone: 081 948–0751;
        081 948–3262
Fax: 081 948–6866;
        081 322–1245
Telex/E-mail: 263124 G; 926700 PJB;
    PJB (Data-Mail); 81–MMU124
    (Telecom Gold)

3355. Philadelphia Newspapers Inc
400 N Broad Street
PO Box 8527
Philadelphia
PA 19130
USA
Telephone: (215) 854–5000

3356. Philipps-Universitaet Marbur
Fachbereich Physikalische Chemie
Hans-Meerwein-Strasse
3550 Marburg/Lahn
Germany

3357. Philips Analytical
Dr E Y Fantner
Lelyweg 1
7602 EA Almelo
Netherlands
Telephone: +31 5790 39448
Fax: +31 5490 39599

3358. Philips Electronic Instruments, Inc
Dr James Edmonds
85 McKee Drive
Mahwah
NJ 07430
USA
Telephone: (201) 529–3800

3359. Philips Electronics
Interactive Media Systems Div.
City House
420–430 London Road
Croydon
CR9 3QR
UK
Telephone: 081–689 2166

3360. Philips IMS
Ugo Rietmann
Viale Fulvio Testi 327
20162 Milan
Italy
Telephone: +39 2 6752 3164
Fax: +39 2 6752 3023

3361. Philips Interactive Media of America (see American Interactive Media)

3362. Philips Interactive Media Systems (UK)
K George
Freeland House
Station Road
Dorking
Surrey
RH4 1UL
UK
Telephone: 0306 76777
Fax: 0306 75789

3363. Philips Interactive Media Systems
P Hermans
Building SFH-6
PO Box 80002
5600 JB Eindhoven
Netherlands
Telephone: +31 40 735 961
Fax: +31 40 735 932

3364. Philips International Telecommunications & Data Systems
PO Box 245
7300AE Apeldoorn
Netherlands
Telephone: +31 55 433441

3365. Philips New Media Systems
Mr Levnis
De Brouckére Plein 2 (B8)
1000 Brussels
Belgium
Telephone: +32 2 211 96 03
Fax: +32 2 211 98 11

3366. Philips Telecommunications & Data Systems Ltd
Guy Norman
43 Waterloo Road
North Ryde
NSW 2113
Australia
Telephone: 2 805 4444

3367. Philips-DuPont Optical Company
Greyhound House
23–24 George Street
Richmond
Surrey
TW7 1JY
UK
Telephone: 081 948–7368

3368. Philips-DuPont Optical Company
Pamela Sansbury
19360 Rinaldi Street
Suite 329
Northridge
CA 91326
USA
Telephone: (818) 363–5991

3369. Philips-DuPont Optical Company
1409 Foulk Road
Suite 200
Wilmington
DE 19803
USA
Telephone: (800) 433–DISK

3370. Phillips Publishing Inc
7811 Montrose Road
Potomac
MD 20854–3363
USA
Telephone: (301) 340–2100
Fax: (202) 659–5927
Telex/E-mail: 358149

3371. Phoenix Newspapers Inc
Library
PO Box 1950
Phoenix
AZ 85001
USA
Telephone: (602) 271–8115;
          (602) 271–8000
Fax: (602) 271–8914

3372. PhoneDisc USA Corporation
Digital Directory Assistance
Scott Beatty; Dante Tuccero
70 Atlantic Avenue
Marblehead
MA 01945
USA
Telephone: (617) 639–2900
Fax: (800) 284–8355;
     (617) 639–2980

3373. PhotoDisc Inc
Sally von Bargen
2101 4th Avenue
Suite 200
Seattle
WA 98121
USA
Telephone: (206) 441–9355
Fax: (206) 441–9379

3374. Photonet Computer Corporation
Suite 1714
1001 South Bayshore Drive
Miami
FL 33131
USA
Telephone: (305) 374–0074;
          (800) 368–6638

3375. PhotoSource International
Pine Lake Farm
Osceola
WI 54020
USA
Telephone: (715) 248–3800
Fax: (715) 248–7394
Telex/E-mail: PSI (GEnie); 189–2053
     (MCI Mail)

3376. Pica Centrum voor Bibliotheekautomatisering
PO Box 90412
2509 The Hague
Netherlands
Telephone: 31 (15) 69 72 83
NUA: 204117302400

3377. PICTEL – Picardie Telematique
19 Espace les Oriels
Place de l'Hotel de Ville
F-02100 Saint Quentin
France
Telephone: 23 09 23 09
Telex/E-mail: 140584 F

3378. Pielle Sistemi Spa
Via PGA Filippini 119
Rome 00144
Italy
Telephone: 39–6–5981–742
Fax: 39–6–5980–932

3379. Pinpoint Analysis
Nigel Wilson
London
UK
Telephone: 071 836–1511

3380. Pioneer Hi-Bred International Inc
Business Information Services
Carla Cain
11153 Aurora Avenue
Des Moines
IA 50322
USA
Telephone: (515) 253–5848;
          (800) 826–5944
Fax: (515) 253–5793

3381. PIRA International
Information Services
Randalls Road
Leatherhead
Surrey
KT22 7RU
UK
Telephone: 0372 376–161
Fax: 0372 377–526

3382. Pirelli
H Becker
Grosse Umstadtterstrasse 4
Hochst Odenwald 6128
Germany
Telephone: 06163 712872;
          06163 71280;
          06163 710
Fax: 06163 712539

3383. Pitagora
Mr. N. Mandarino
Pitagora Spa
Contrada Santo Stefano
87030 Rende (Provence Di Cosenza)
Italy
Telephone: 39 (9848) 33320
NUA: Available on application

3384. Pittsburgh Press, The
34 Boulevard of the Allies
PO Box 566
Pittsburgh
PA 15230
USA
Telephone: (412) 263–1100

3386. PJS Enterprises
1240 N Ogden Drive
Suite 9
Los Angeles
CA 90046
USA
Telephone: (213) 650–1195

3387. Plain Dealer Publishing Company
1801 Superior Avenue
Cleveland
OH 44114
USA
Telephone: (216) 344–4500

3388. Planning Exchange
Jacqueline Chalmers
186 Bath Street
Glasgow
G2 4HG
Scotland, UK
Telephone: 44 (41) 332–9317
Fax: 44 (41) 332–8277

3389. Planning Research Corporation
1500 Planning Research Drive
McLean
VA 22102
USA
Telephone: (703) 556–1000

3390. PLATO
11 West 42nd Street
20th Floor
New York
NY 10036
USA
Telephone: (212) 944–4680

3391. Plenum Publishing Co Ltd
J Curtis
88–90 Middlesex Street
London
E1 7EZ
UK
Telephone: 071 377–0686
Fax: 071 247–0555

3392. Plesman Publications Ltd
2005 Sheppard Avenue E
4th Floor
Willowdale
ON M2J 5B1
USA
Telephone: (416) 497–9562
Fax: (416) 497–9427

3393. Plexus Publishing Inc
143 Old Mariton Pike
Medford
NJ 08055
USA
Telephone: (609) 654–6500

3394. Plymouth Marine Laboratory
Library and Information Services
A Varley; D Moulder
Citadel Hill
Plymouth
PL1 2PB
UK
Telephone: 0752 222772
Fax: 0752 226865

3395. PMB Print Measurement Bureau
77 Bloor Street W
Suite 1502
Toronto
ON M5S 1M2
Canada
Telephone: (416) 961–3205

3396. PME Services
2–4 Ville au Hôchard
93380 Beurrfitte
France
Telephone: +33 1 48 29 52 52
Fax: +33 1 48 29 80 95

3397. Point Foundation
27 Gate 5 Road
Sausalito
CA 94965
USA
Telephone: (415) 332–1717

3398. POLINFO
Johs. Chr. Johansen
Raadhuspladsen 37
1585 Koebenhavn V
Denmark
Telephone: 45 (31) 118511

3399. Political Reference Service Pty Ltd
Civic Square
PO Box 607
Canberra
ACT 2608
Australia
Telephone: 062 476–950
Fax: 062 488–169
Telex/E-mail: 62614 AA

3400. Political Risk Services
407 University Avenue
Suite 210
Syracuse
NY 13210
USA
Telephone: (315) 472–1224
Fax: (315) 472–1235
Telex/E-mail: MARYLOU WALSH
    (DATAMAIL); FSI (MCI Mail)

3401. Polycom Systems Ltd
90 Nolan Court
Suite 50
Markham
ON L3R 4L9
Canada
Telephone: (416) 429–0440

3402. Polygram Records Inc
Mark Fine
Worldwide Plaza
825 Eighth Avenue
New York
NY 10019
USA
Telephone: (212) 333 8000

3403. Pomona College Medicinal Chemistry Project
Seaver Chemistry Laboratory
Claremont
CA 91711
USA
Telephone: (714) 621–8000

3404. Popular Computing Inc
1060 Marsh Road, Suite C-200
Menlo Park
CA 94075
USA

3405. Portugal Centro de Estudos em Economia da Energia dos Transportes e Ambiente
Rua Miguel Lupi 20
1200 Lisbon
Portugal
Telephone: 01 601–043

3406. Portugal Departamento Central de Planeamento
Avenida Don Carlos I, 126
1293 Lisbon Codex
Portugal
Telephone: 01 60 30 81
Fax: 01 67 69 88
Telex/E-mail: 16044 P

3407. Post Office
National Postcode Centre
Room 302
8 Surrey Street
Portsmouth
PO1 1AX
UK
Telephone: 0705 835251

3408. Post- und Ortsbuchverlag Postmeister
Friedrich Müller
PO Box 18 01 30
D-5600 Wuppertal 1
Germany

3409. Post-Tribune Publishing Inc
1065 Broadway
Gary
IN 46402
USA
Telephone: (219) 881–3187

3410. Postamt
Mr Schneider
Dienstelle 113–21
PO Box 1100
3550 Marburg
Germany
Telephone: +49 6421 2 04

3411. Poulter Communications Ltd
Graham Poulter; David Evans
Poulter House
2 Burley Road
Leeds
LS3 1NJ
UK
Telephone: 0532 832832
Fax: 0532 343574

3412. Power Computing
2525 Washington Street
Kansas City
MO 64108
USA
Telephone: (816) 221–9700

3413. PR Newswire Inc
National Press Communications Service
150 E 58th Street
31st Floor
New York
NY 10155
USA
Telephone: (212) 832–9400;
    (800) 832–5522
Fax: (212) 832–9406
Telex/E-mail: 12284

3414. Practising Law Institute
810 7th Avenue
New York
NY 10019
USA
Telephone: (212) 765–5700

3415. Predicasts
Sue Rhodes
8–10 Denman Street
London
W1V 7RF
UK
Telephone: 071 494–3817
Fax: 071 734–5935

3416. Predicasts
Emily Melton
11001 Cedar Avenue
Cleveland
OH 44106
USA
Telephone: (216) 795–3000;
    (800) 321–6388
Fax: (216) 229–9944
Telex/E-mail: 985604; 14294
    (DIALMAIL)

3417. Prentice Hall
PHINet
Thomas Speyer
1 Golf and Western Plaza
18th Floor
New York
NY 10023
USA
Telephone: (212) 373–8600

3418. Prentice-Hall Law & Business
270 Sylvan Avenue
Englewood Cliffs
NJ 07632
USA
Telephone: (201) 1894–8833;
    (800) 447–1717

3419. Prentice-Hall Online Services
1900 E 4th Street
Suite 130
Santa Ana
CA 92705
USA
Telephone: (714) 547–0590

3420. Presentation Graphics Group
Rich Cook; Steve Deming
270 North Cannon Street
Suite 103
Beverley Hills
CA 90210
USA
Telephone: (213) 277 3050
Fax: (213) 465 2407

3421. Press Association, The
85 Fleet Street
London
EC4P 4BE
UK
Telephone: 071 353–7440
Fax: 071 353–9838

3422. Presscom Australia
121 King William Street
Adelaide
SA 5000
Australia
Telephone: 08 218–9559
Fax: 08 231–5374

3423. PressText News Service
1200 N Street NW
Suite 216
Washington
DC 20005
USA
Telephone: (202) 223–8444

3424. Prestel
Telephone House
Temple Avenue
London EC4Y 0HL
UK
Telephone: 44 (71) 822 1122

3425. Presto Studios Inc
Eric Hook
PO Box 262535
San Diego
CA 92196–2535
USA
Telephone: (619) 689–4895

3426. Preston Publications
S Tinsley Preston
PO Box 48312
7800 Merrimac Avenue
Niles
IL 60645
USA
Telephone: (708) 965–0566
Fax: (708) 965–7639

3427. Prime Time/Martin Enterprises
PO Box 6997
Burbank
CA 91505
USA
Telephone: (818) 982–4152
Fax: (818) 765–5472

3428. Princeton University
Office of Population Research
Princeton
NJ 08544
USA

3429. Print Measurement Bureau (PMB)
Joanne Vandenburg
77 Bloor Street West
Suite 1502
Toronto
Ontario
M5S 1M2
Canada
Telephone: +1 416 961 3205
Fax: +1 416 961 5052

3430. Printing Bureau
Ministry of Finance
Shigeru Okada
2–2–4 Toranomon
Minato-ku
Tokyo 105
Japan
Telephone: +81 3 3587 4444;
        +81 3 3587 4445
Fax: +81 3 3586 3210

3431. Privatbanken AS
Annett Petersen
Postboks 1000
2400 Koebenhavn NV
Denmark
Telephone: 45 (31) 112344

3432. Probe Economics Inc
Millwood Business Center
Route 100
Postal Drawer M
Millwood
NY 10546–0909
USA
Telephone: (914) 923–4505

3433. Procuradoria-Geral da Republica
Rua da Escola Politecnica 140
1294 Lisbon Codex
Portugal
Telephone: 01 609–319
Fax: 01 675–255
Telex/E-mail: 42701 PROCUR P

3434. Prodigy Services Company
455 Hamilton Avenue
White Plains
NY 10601
USA
Telephone: (914) 993–8000

3435. Profectus
CD-ROMs
Vesa Sihvola
c/o Paritet AB
Företagscentrum
953 33 Haparanda
Sweden
Telephone: +46 922 11480
Fax: +46 922 14790

3436. Professional Farmers of America
219 Parkade
Cedar Falls
IA 50613
USA
Telephone: (319) 277–1278;
        (800) 553–1781;
        (800) 772–2920 (in IA)
Telex/E-mail: 439034

3437. Profit Press
2956 N. Campbell Avenue
Tucson
AZ 85719
USA
Telephone: (800) 843–7990;
        (602) 577–9696
Fax: (602) 577–9624
Telex/E-mail: (602) 299–0693
    (Bulletin Board); (602) 577–6969
    (Bulletin Board – For Adults Only)

3438. Proinfo
1133 13th Street NW
Suite 2A
Washington
DC 20005
USA
Telephone: (202) 289–3893
Fax: (202) 347–1566

3439. Project Associates
USA
Telex/E-mail: (203) 938–8469 (Online)
NUA: PA + PA01

3440. Project Database Ltd.
Weymouth
UK
Telephone: 0305–761102

3441. Projektsamvirket
Johan Jacobsen
Skoleforvaltningen
2750 Ballerup
Denmark
Telephone: 45 (42) 970501

3442. PROMPT
150 N Clinton Street
Chicago
IL 60606
USA
Telephone: (312) 726–1221

3443. ProNet, The Packer Produce Network
7950 College Boulevard
Overland Park
KS 66210
USA
Telephone: (913) 451–2200;
        (800) 255–5113
Telex/E-mail: 4941149

3444. Proscope Inc
Takeshi Itou, CEO
932 Hibiya Park Building
1–8–1 Yurakuchyou
Chiyoda-ku
Tokyo 100
Japan
Telephone: +81 3 214 3423
Fax: +81 3 214 3423

3445. Prous Science Publishers
Electronic Publications
Ann L Wescott
Apartado de Correos 540
08080 Barcelona
Spain
Telephone: +34 3 459 2220
Fax: +34 3 258 1535

3446. Provinciale Bibliotheek Centrale voor Noord-Brabant
Mr Bruurmijn
Statenlaan 4
Postbus 90114
5000 LA Tilburg
Netherlands
Telephone: +31 13 685951
Fax: +31 13 630218

3447. Provinsbanken
Edwin Rahrs Vej 40
8220 Brabrand
Denmark
Telephone: 45 (86) 122522

3448. PRS Corporate Information Services Ltd
100 Hutton Garden
London
EC1N 8NX
UK
Telephone: 071 430–9265

3449. PSSI – Patent Search Systems Inc
Stafford
Virginia
USA
Telephone: (703) 659–7235

3450. PsyComNet
1346 Lexington Avenue
New York
NY 10028
USA
Telephone: (212) 876–7800
Telex/E-mail: 76010,727
    (CompuServe Information Service);
    IGOLDBERG (MCI Mail)

3451. Public Affairs Information Service (PAIS)
Barbara Preschel
512 W 43rd Street
New York
NY 10036–4396
USA
Telephone: (212) 736–6629;
        (800) 288–7247
Fax: (212) 643–2848
Telex/E-mail: ALA 1857 (ALANET)

3452. Public Priority Systems Inc
W L Bainbridge
5027 Pine Creek Drive
Blendonview Office Park
Westerville
OH 43081
USA
Telephone: (614) 890–1573

3453. Public Relations Society of America
33 Irving Place
New York
NY 10022
USA
Telephone: (212) 995–2230

3454. Public Utilities Reports Inc
2111 Wilson Boulevard
Suite 200
Arlington
VA 22201
USA
Telephone: (703) 243–7000;
(800) 368–5001
Fax: (703) 527–5829

3455. Publications du Moniteur
17 rue d'Uzes
PO Box 486
F-75067 Paris Cedex 02
France
Telephone: 1 40 41 05 50

3456. Publications Transcontinental Inc
465 rue St Jean
9e etage
Montreal
PQ H2Y 3S4
Canada
Telephone: (514) 842–6491

3457. Publinet BV
ITT World Directories
Hoekenrode 1
NL-1102 BR Amsterdam
Netherlands
Telephone: 020 567–6665
Fax: 020 911–700

3458. Punch In International
J Walman
400 E 59th Street
Suite 9F
New York
NY 10022
USA
Telephone: (212) 755–4363
Fax: (212) 755–4365
Telex/E-mail: PUNCH IN (DELPHI)

3459. Puntos de Información Cultural (See Ministerio de Cultural de España)

3460. Puntos de Información Cultural
Ricardo Jerez
Ministerio de Cultura
Plaza del Rey 1
E-28071 Madrid
Spain
Telephone: 01 532–5089;
01 429–2944
Telex/E-mail: 27286 CULTURA

3461. Purdue University
National Pesticide Information Retrieval System
Entomology Hall
West Lafayette
IN 47907
USA
Telephone: (317) 494–6616

3462. Pure Data Holdings plc
St James Court
King's Lynn
UK
Telephone: 0553 691–459
Fax: 0553 691–459
Telex/E-mail: 818461 G

3463. QL Systems Ltd
901 St Andrew's Tower
275 Sparks Street
Ottawa
ON K1R 7X9
Canada
Telephone: (613) 238–3499
Fax: (613) 548–4260

3464. Quadrant Communicate NV
Koos Witteveen
PO Box 9549
3506 GM Utrecht
Netherlands
Telephone: +31 30 736565
Fax: +31 30 732166

3465. Quali-Data
Mr Van Hecke
Pater Kenislaan 6
2970 Schilde
Belgium
Telephone: +32 3383 6027

3466. Quanta Press
Dennis E Burke
1313 Fifth Street
Suite 208C
Minneapolis
MN 55414
USA
Telephone: (612) 379 3956
Fax: (612) 623–4570

3467. Quantum Access Inc
1700 West Loop South
Suite 1460
Houston
TX 77027
USA
Telephone: (713) 622–3211
Fax: (713) 622–6454

3468. Quantum Computer Services Inc
8619 Westwood Center Drive
Vienna
VA 22182
USA
Telephone: (703) 448–8700;
(800) 227–6364

3469. Quantum Leap Technologies (QLTech)
Robert A Burr; Robin Vee
1399 SE 9 Avenue
Hialeah
FL 33010–5999
USA
Telephone: (305) 885 9985
Fax: (305) 447–0745

3470. Quantum Research Corporation
Fabrizio R Golino
7300 Pearl Street
Suite 210
Bethesda
MD 20814
USA
Telephone: (301) 657 3070
Fax: (301) 657 3862

3471. Quebec Ministere de l'Education
Department of Education
Research Service Department
1035 de la Chevrotiere Street, 8th Floor
Quebec
PQ G1R 5A5
Canada
Telephone: (418) 643–1723
Telex/E-mail: 0513848

3472. Quebec Ministere de l'Energie et des Ressources
Division des Donnees Geoscientifiques
Centre de Diffusion
5700 4c avenue Ouest
Local A-201
Charlesbourg
PQ G1H 6R1
Canada
Telephone: (418) 643–4601
Fax: (418) 644–3814

3473. Quebec Ministere de l'Environnement
Centre de Documentation
3900 rue Marly
Box 57
Sainte-Foy
PQ G1X 4E4
Canada
Telephone: (418) 643–5363
Telex/E-mail: 05131629

3474. Queensland Newspapers Pty Ltd
GPO Box 130
Brisbane
QLD 4001
Australia
Telephone: 07 252–6011
Fax: 07 252–6697
Telex/E-mail: 40110 AA

3475. Queensland University of Technology
Library
PO Box 117
Kedron
QLD 4031
Australia
Telephone: 07 864–4077
Fax: 07 357–7067

3476. Questel SA
Osman Sultan
Le Capitole
55 avenue des Champs Pierreux
F-92000 Nanterre
France
Telephone: 1 46 14 55 55
Fax: 1 46 14 55 11;
1 83 50 46 50
NUA: 208006040201

3477. Quevillon Editions
Gregory Quevillon
PO Box 306
South Dennis
MA 02660
USA
Telephone: (508) 362–8744

3478. Quick Source, Inc
James O Brown
1010 Wayne Avenue
Suite 510
Silver Spring
MD 20910
USA
Telephone: (301) 650–8865;
(800) 888–0736
Fax: (301) 565–9412

3479. Quotron Systems Inc
12731 W Jefferson Boulevard
PO Box 66914
Los Angeles
CA 90066
USA
Telephone: (213) 827–4600

3480. Radarsoft
De Meeten 10
4706 NG Roosendaal
Netherlands
Telephone: +31 1650 51020
Fax: +31 1650 68074

3481. Radio Advertising Bureau
304 Park Avenue
New York
NY 10010
USA
Telephone: (212) 254–4800;
(800) 232–3131

3482. Radio-Suisse Marketing AB
Mässans gata 18
PO Box 5278
S-402 25 Göteborg
Sweden
Telephone: 031–83–59–75
Fax: 031–83–59–36

3483. Radiotelevisione Italiana
Verifiche Qualitative Prodotto e
    Immagine
Plazza Monte Grappa 4
I-00195 Rome
Italy
Telephone: 06 3686–5324
Fax: 06 322–6070
Telex/E-mail: 614432 RAI RM I

**3484. RAI (See Radiotelevisione
    Italiana)**

3485. Rainbo Electronic Reviews
8 Duran Court
Pacifica
CA 94044
USA
Telephone: (415) 993–6029

3486. Ramware
Rob Neary
PO Box 500
Alderley
Queensland 44051
Australia
Telephone: 61–7–356–1166
Fax: 61–7–856–4702

3487. Rand McNally-TDM Inc
8255 N Central Park Avenue
Skokie
IL 60076–2970
USA
Telephone: (708) 673–9100;
        (708) 673–0470
Fax: (708) 673–9109
Telex/E-mail: 210041 RMCNUR

3488. Random Century
Michael Upshall
20 Vauxhall Bridge Road
London
SW1V 2SA
UK
Telephone: 071 973–9700
Fax: 071 931–7672

**3489. Random Lengths Publications
    Inc**
PO Box 867
Eugene
OR 97440–0867
USA
Telephone: (503) 686–9925

3490. Rapaport Diamond Corporation
15 W 47th Street
Suite 700
New York
NY 10036
USA
Telephone: (212) 354–0575
Fax: (212) 840–0243
Telex/E-mail: 428 349

3491. RAPRA Technology Ltd
Shawbury
Shrewsbury
Shropshire
SY4 4NR
UK
Telephone: 0939 250–383
Fax: 0939 251–118
Telex/E-mail: 35134 RAPRA G

3492. Ratings Bureau Pty Ltd, The
Plante & Associates
140A Cressy Road
North Ryde
NSW 2113
Australia
Telephone: 02 881–340;
        02 452–2898

3493. Raymond Software Inc
James Raymond
347 Massol Avenue
Suite 105
Los Gatos
CA 95030
USA
Telephone: (408) 395 6157
Fax: (408) 395 6157

**3494. RCA Global Communications
    Inc**
201 Centennial Avenue
Piscataway
NJ 08854
USA
Telephone: (201) 885–4310;
        (800) 526–3969
Telex/E-mail: 219901 RCAC UR

3495. RCC
F R Hengeveld
Postbus
7300 HN Apeldoorn
Netherlands
Telephone: +31 (55) 778822
Fax: +31 55 215960
Telex/E-mail: 30435
NUA: Available on application

3496. RDB
Rechtsdatenbank Gesellschaft
Wiedner Haupstrasse 18/14
1040 Vienna
Austria
Telephone: 43 (222) 5873620
NUA: Available on application

3497. Reactor
Mike Saenz
3110 North Sheffield Avenue
Chicago
IL 60657
USA
Telephone: (312) 528 1600
Fax: (312) 528 9562

3498. Read Only Memory Pty Ltd
Con Mitropoulos
127 Lawrence Street
Alexandria
NSW 2015
Australia
Telephone: 61 2 550 3938
Fax: 61 2 550 1195

3499. Readag
Hans Burren
Rue Zaehringen 98
CH-1700 Fribourg
Switzerland
Telephone: 37 23 13 46;
        37 23 13 47
Fax: 37 23 13 18

3500. Reading Eagle/Reading Times
PO Box 582
Reading
PA 19603–0582
USA
Telephone: (215) 371–5000

3501. ReadySoft, Inc
Elizabeth Arnold
30 Wertheim Court
Unit 2
Richmond Hill
Ontario
L4B 1B9
Canada
Telephone: (414) 731 4175
Fax: (416) 764 8867

3502. Real Estate Data
2398 N W 119th Street
Miama
FL 33167
USA
Telephone: (305) 685–5731

3503. Real Property Data, Inc
Dan Levison
1570 Northside Drive
Atlanta
GA 30318
USA
Telephone: (404) 355–2630

3504. Rechtsdocumentatie
Guy Van Peel
Eekhout 2
9000 Ghent
Belgium
Telephone: 32–91–253–112
Fax: 32–91–238–212

3505. Record
150 River Street
Hackensack
NJ 07602
USA
Telephone: (201) 646–4000

3506. Red Box Publishers
Herr Gebert
Abteistrasse 49
2000 Hamburg 13
Germany
Telephone: +49 40 410 8081
Fax: +49 40 440 214

**3507. Redgate Communications
    Corporation**
660 Beachland Boulevard
Vero Beach
FL 32963
USA
Telephone: 407–231–6904

3508. Reed Business Publishing Ltd
Quadrant House
Room 501
The Quadrant
Sutton
Surrey
SM2 5AS
UK
Telephone: 081 661–3500

3509. Reed Information Services Ltd
Jean Cangley; Ken Finch
Windsor Court
East Grinstead House
East Grinstead
West Sussex
RH10 1XA
UK
Telephone: 0342 326–972
Fax: 0342 315–130
Telex/E-mail: 95127 INFSER G

3510. Reed Opti-Ware
Alex Papps
Church Street
Dunstable
LU5 4HB
UK
Telephone: +44 0582 472744
Fax: +44 0582 695123

3511. Reference Technology Inc.
A part of Dataware Technologies
Bill Thornburg
5775 Flatiron Parkway
Suite 220
Boulder
CO 80301
USA
Telephone: (303) 449–4157
Fax: (303) 442–1816

3512. Reflective Arts International
485 Alberto Way
Los Gatos
CA 95032
USA
Telephone: (408) 395–4332

3513. Regie Multi-media Service BO
6 rue Masperan
75116 Paris
France
Telephone: 1 40 13 01 02
Telex/E-mail: 230560 F

3514. Regional Drug Information Service
The London Hospital
Whitechapel Road
London
E1 1BB
UK
Telephone: 071 377–7489

3515. Registro de la Propiedad Industrial de España
Oficina de Difusión
Ana Maria Moreno
Calle Panama 1
28071 Madrid
Spain
Telephone: 01 458 22 00
Fax: 01 259 24 28
Telex/E-mail: 47020 RPI E

3516. Religious and Theological Abstracts, Inc
Janet Dorsey
PO Box 215
Myerstown
PA 17067
USA
Telephone: (717) 866–6734;
           (717) 866–4667

3517. Religious News Service Inc
PO Box 1015
Radio City Station
New York
NY 10101
USA
Telephone: (212) 315–0870
Fax: (212) 315–5850
Telex/E-mail: 290–2861 (MCI Mail);
           4158 (TCN)

3518. Renault
Bernard Pargamin
34 Quai du Point du Jour
92109 Boulogne
France
Telephone: +33 1 46 09 52 97
Fax: +33 1 46 09 64 64

3519. Repair-Tech Publishing, Inc
Ykio Ishino
1–2–13 Kawaramachi Chuoh-ku
Osaka 541
Japan
Telephone: 81–6–227–5661
Fax: 81–6–227–5664

3520. Repertoire International de Litterature Musicale
RILM
Adam O'Connor
City University of New York
33 West 42nd Street
New York
NY 10036
USA
Telephone: (212) 642 2709
Fax: (212) 642 2642

3521. Research Institute of America
90 5th Avenue
New York
NY 10011
USA
Telephone: (212) 645–4800;
           (800) 431–9025

3522. Research Institute of High Temperatures
Thermophysical Centre of the USSR
   Academy of Sciences
c/o International Center for Scientific
   and Technical Information
Ulitsa Kuusinena 21b
125252 Moscow
Russia
Telephone: 095 198–7460
Fax: 095 943–0089
Telex/E-mail: 411925 MCNTI SU

3523. Research Libraries Group Inc
Art and Architecture Program
Jordan Quadrangle
Stanford
CA 94305
USA
Telephone: (415) 328–0920

3525. Research Libraries Group Inc
Research Libraries Information Network
1200 Villa Street
Mountain View
CA 94041–1100
USA
Telephone: (415) 962–9951
Fax: (415) 964–0943
Telex/E-mail: BL.RIC RLG (BITNET)

3526. Research Publications Inc
Frank Faxio
12 Lunar Drive
Drawer AB
Woodbridge
CT 06525
USA
Telephone: (203) 397–2600;
           (800) 444–0799;
           (800) 336–5010
Fax: (203) 397–3893
Telex/E-mail: 892362

3527. Research Publications, Inc
Mark Holland; Nicola Furrie
50 Milford Road
Reading
RG1 8LG
UK
Telephone: 0734 583–247
Fax: 0734 591–325

3528. Research Services Ltd
Research Services House
Elmgrove Road
Harrow
Middlesex
HA1 2QG
UK
Telephone: 081 861–6000

3529. Reseau des Organismes Agricoles pour un Documentation Technique,
Socio-Economique, Juridique, et
   Financiere
78 rue de Varenne
F-75700 Paris
France
Telephone: 1 45 55 95 50

3530. Réseau URBAMET
Miccette Hercelin
STU
64 Rue de la Fédération
75015 Paris
France
Telephone: 33–1–4567–3536
Fax: 33–1–4567–1220

3531. Reserve Bank of Australia
65 Martin Place
GPO Box 3947
Sydney
NSW 2001
Australia
Telephone: 02 551–8111

3532. Resource Consultants Inc.
The Chemtox System
7121 CrossRoads Boulevard
PO Box 1848
Brentwood
TN 37024–1848
USA
Telephone: (615) 373–5040
Fax: (615) 370–4339

3533. Resource Group, The
11 Reynolds Road
Hove
East Sussex
BN3 5RJ
UK
Telephone: 0273 206–121
Fax: 0273 204–447

3534. Resource Information Systems Inc
110 Great Road
Bedford
MA 01730
USA
Telephone: (617) 271–0030
Fax: (617) 271–0037
Telex/E-mail: 265634 RISI U

3535. Resources for Communication
341 Mark West Station Road
Windsor
CA 95492–9620
USA
Telephone: (707) 542–7819

3536. Reteaco Inc
Nathan Leslie
716 Gordon Baker Road
Willowdale
Ontario
M2H 3B4
Canada
Telephone: (416) 497–0579;
           (800) 387–5002

Addresses

3537. Retrieval Technologies
1 Kendall Square
Building 100
Cambridge
MA 02139
USA
Telephone: (616) 577–1574
Fax: (617) 577–9517

3538. Reuter Textline
Reuter:file Ltd
Albert House
1 Singer Street
London
EC2A 4BQ
UK
Telephone: 071 867–1155
Fax: 071 253–6134

3539. Reuters Australia Pty Ltd
National Press Club Building
16 National Circuit
Canberra
ACT 2600
Australia
Telephone: 02 733–700

3540. Reuters Holdings plc
85 Fleet Street
London
EC4P 4AJ
UK
Telephone: 071 250–1122;
            071 324–6892 (Textline)

**3541. Reuters Information Services
(Canada) Ltd**
Data User Services Division
Exchange Tower
Suite 1900
2 First Canadian Place
Toronto
ON M5X 1E3
Canada
Telephone: (416) 364–5361;
            (800) 387–1588
Fax: (416) 364–0646
Telex/E-mail: 0622259

**3542. Reuters Information Services
Inc**
1333 H Street NW
Washington
DC 20005
USA
Telephone: (202) 898–8300

3543. Revenue Canada
Customs & Excise
Connaught Building
2nd Floor
Ottawa
ON K1A 0L5
Canada
Telephone: (613) 957–0275

3544. Revenue Canada
Taxation
875 Heron Road
Ottawa
ON K1A 0L8
Canada
Telephone: (613) 957–3503

3545. Review Journal
1111 W Bonanza
PO Box
Las Vegas
NV 89125
USA
Telephone: (702) 383–0211

3546. Rhône-Poulenc Interservices
Jacques Boudon
25 quai Paul du-Mer
92408 Courbevoie
France
Telephone: 33–1 47 68 12 34
Fax: 33–1 47 68 14 66

**3547. Ricardo Consulting Engineers
Ltd**
Bridge Works
Shoreham-by-Sea
West Sussex
BN43 5FG
UK
Telephone: 0273 455–611
Fax: 0273 464–124
Telex/E-mail: 87383 RICSHM G

3548. Richmond Newspapers Inc
333 E Grace Street
Richmond
VA 23219
USA
Telephone: (804) 649–6000

3549. Riddell Publishing Pty Ltd
100 Alexander Street
Crows Nest
NSW 2065
Australia
Telephone: 02 438–2833
Fax: 02 438–1024

3550. Riga Chamber of Commerce
Mr Gavars
Riga
Latvia
Telephone: +7 0132 332205
Fax: +7 0132 372276

3551. Rijks Computer Centrum
Fauststraat 1
NL-7323 BA Apeldoorn
Netherlands
Telephone: 055 77 88 22
Fax: 055 21 59 60
Telex/E-mail: 30435 NL

**3552. Riksdagens Utredningstjaenst
Registersektionen**
100 12 Stockholm
Sweden
Telephone: 46 (8) 14 20 20

3553. Riksskatteverket
Raettsenheten
171 94 Solna
Sweden
Telephone: 46 (8) 764 80 00

**3554. Risk and Insurance Manaement
Society**
205 E 42nd Street
Suite 1504
New York
NY 10017
USA
Telephone: (212) 286–9292
Fax: (212) 986–9716
Telex/E-mail: 968289

3555. Riso Library
DK-4000 Roskilde
Denmark
Telephone: 42 371–212
Fax: 46 755–627
Telex/E-mail: 43116 RISOE DK

3556. RKI Kredit information A/S
Glarmestervej 2
Postboks 259
DK-8600 Silkeborg
Denmark
Telephone: 086 800–344

**3557. RMIT-INFORMIT: Royal
Melbourne Institute of
Technology**
INFORMIT
Don Schauder
GPO Box 2476V
Melbourne
Victoria 3000
Australia
Telephone: 61–3 663–3440
Fax: 61–3 663–3047

**3558. RNR International Marketing
Group**
Chris Pellegrinetti
140 Arthur Street
6th Floor
North Sydney
NSW 2060
Australia

**3559. Road Transport Research
Program**
Organisation for Economic Cooperation
and Development (OECD)
2 rue Andre Pascal
F-75775 Paris Cedex 16
France
Telephone: 1 45 24 82 00
Fax: 1 45 24 79 60
Telex/E-mail: 620 160 OCDE Paris

3560. Roanoke Times & World-News
201–09 W Campbell Avenue SW
Roanoke
VA 24011
USA
Telephone: (703) 981–3100

3561. Robert Colbert
1958 Poinciana Road
Winterpark
FL 32792
USA
Telephone: (305) 671–3530

3562. Robin Hood Distribusjon A/S
Kongens Gate 16
N-0153 Oslo 1
Norway
Telephone: 2 429911

**3563. Robinson Black-more Printing
and Publishing**
Box 8330
Station A
Halifax
NS B3K 5M1
Canada
Telephone: (902) 465–1222

3564. Robnor Group Ltd
PO Box 112
Coudersport
PA 16915–0112
USA
Telephone: (814) 274–7602
Fax: (814) 274–7159
Telex/E-mail: 910 250 5232 ROBNOR

**3565. Rock Mechanics Information
Service**
Department of Mineral Resources
Engineering
Imperial College of Science, Technology
and Medicine
Royal School of Mines
Prince Consort Road
London
SW7 2BP
UK
Telephone: 071 589–5111 x6436
Telex/E-mail: 071 589–6806

3566. Rocky Mountain Communications Inc
Marc Miller
2023 Montane Drive East
Golden
CO 80401–9123
USA
Telephone: (303) 526 5454
Fax: (303) 526 2662

3567. Rocky Mountain Mineral Law Foundation
Porter Administration Building
7039 E 18th Avenue
Denver
CO 80220
USA
Telephone: (303) 321–8100

3568. Rocky Mountain News
400 W Colfax Avenue
Denver
CO 80204
USA
Telephone: (303) 892–5000

3569. ROM Pty
Railway Square
PO Box 11
Sydney
NSW 2000
Australia
Telephone: 61–2–550–3938
Fax: 61–2–319–0015

3570. ROM Publishers
1033 "O" Street
Suite 300
Lincoln
NE 68508
USA
Telephone: (402) 476–2965

3571. Roper Center for Public Opinion Research, The
PO Box 440
Storrs
CT 06268–0440
USA
Telephone: (203) 486–4440

3572. Roper Organization
205 E 42nd Street
New York
NY 10017
USA
Telephone: (212) 599–0700

3573. Rossipaul Verlagsgesellschaft mbH
Michael Mackel
Menzinger Strasse 37
8000 Munich 19
Munich
Germany
Telephone: +49 89 1791060
Fax: +49 89 17910622

3574. Roth Publishing, Inc.
Kevin Moran
185 Great Neck Road
Great Neck
NY 11021
USA
Telephone: (800) 327–0295
Fax: (516) 829–7746

3575. Roy Morgan Research Centre Pty LLtd
411 Collins Street
GPO Box 2282U
Melbourne
VIC 3001
Australia
Telephone: 03 629–6888
Telex/E-mail: 36720 AA

3576. Royal Bank of Canada
PO Box 6001
Montreal
PQ H3C 3A9
Canada
Telephone: (514) 874–5206
Fax: (514) 874–5993

3577. Royal Institute of British Architects
British Architectural Library
66 Portland Place
London
W1N 4AD
UK
Telephone: 071 580–5533
Fax: 071 255–1541
Telex/E-mail: 24224

3578. Royal Institution of Chartered Surveyors
Building Cost Information Service
85/87 Clarence Street
Kingston upon Thames
Surrey
KT1 1RB
UK
Telephone: 081 546–7554

3579. Royal Library
Box 5039
102 41 Stockholm
Sweden
Telephone: 46 (8) 783 39 00
Fax: 46 (8) 783 39 30
Telex/E-mail: 19640 KBS S

3580. Royal Mail
Post Office Headquarters
Anne Wine
Postal Headquarters
148–166 Old Street
London
EC1V 9HQ
UK
Telephone: 071 245–7951;
071 250–2307
Fax: 071 250–2366

3581. Royal Melbourne Institute of Technology Libraries (See INFORMIT)

3582. Royal Netherlands Academy of Arts and Sciences
Joan Muyskenweg 25
PO Box 41950
NL-1009 DD Amsterdam
Netherlands
Telephone: 020 668–5511

3583. Royal Pharmaceutical Society of Great Britain
J McGlashan
1 Lambeth High Street
London
SE1 7JN
UK
Telephone: 071 735–9141;
071 582–8455
Fax: 071 735–7629

3584. Royal Photographic Society of Great Britain
The Octagon
Milsom Street
Bath
Avon
BA1 1DN
UK
Telephone: 0225 62841

3585. Royal School of Mines (See University of London)

3586. Royal Society of Chemistry Information Services
Mass Spectrometry Data Centre
Frances Powers; Judith Barnsby
(Help Desk)
Thomas Graham House
Science Park
Milton Road
Cambridge
CB4 4WF
UK
Telephone: 0223 423–623;
0223 420–066
Fax: 0223 423–623
Telex/E-mail: 818293 ROYAL G; CBNB
(DATAMAIL); 84:BUR5000 (Dialcom);
13012 (DIALMAIL)

3587. Royal Tropical Institute
Information and Documentation
Marc Keylard
Mauritskade 63
NL-1092 AD Amsterdam
Netherlands
Telephone: 020 568 85 08;
020 568 83 78;
020 568 87 11
Fax: 020 568 84 44
Telex/E-mail: 15080 KIT NL

3588. Roytech Publications Inc
840 Hinckley Road, Suite 147
Burlingame
CA 94010
USA
Telephone: (415) 697–0541
Fax: (415) 697–6255

3589. RPI – Registro de la Propriedad Industrial
Departemento de Informacion
Technologica
Panama 1
E-28036 Madrid
Spain
Telephone: +34 1–4582200
Fax: +34 1–2592428
NUA: Available on application

3590. RR Bowker Comapny
Donna Payerle (Sales Coordinator)
121 Chanlon Road
New Providence
NJ 07974
USA
Telephone: (908) 464–6800;
(908) 665–2866;
(800) 323–3288
Fax: (908) 665–6688
Telex/E-mail: 127703 12804
(DIALMAIL)

3591. RR Donnelley & Sons Company
Richard P Thorn (General Manager)
1815 S Prairie Avenue
Chicago
IL 60616
USA
Telephone: (312) 567–0300
Fax: (312) 567–0337

3592. Ruder, Finn & Rotman
301 East 57th Street
New York
NY 10022
USA
Telephone: (212) 593–6400

3593. RunTime Innovations Ltd
1.02 Kelvin Campus
West of Scotland Science Park
Glasgow
G20 0SP
UK
Telephone: 041 945 2491

3594. Runzheimer International
Publications Division
555 Skokie Blvd, Suite 340
Northbrook
IL 60062
USA
Telephone: (312) 291–9011;
(800) 942–9949
Fax: (312) 291–9581

3595. Rutgers University
Department of History, CN 5059
Medieval and Early Modern Data Bank
NJ 08903
USA
Telephone: (201) 932–8316;
(201) 932–8335

3596. Rutgers University
Department of History
New Brunswick
NJ 08903
USA
Telephone: (908) 932–8316
Fax: (908) 932–6763
Telex/E-mail: BB.MXC RLG.BITNET
(BITNET)

**3597. Ryerson Polytechnical Institute
Library**
Rita Murphy
350 Victoria Street
Toronto
ON M5B 2K3
Canada
Telephone: (416) 979–5000;
(416) 979–5083

3598. S & S Enterprises
Marketing Department
Steven Peskaitis
PO Box 552
Lemont
IL 60439
USA
Telephone: (708) 257 7616;
(800) ROM DISC
Fax: (708) 257 7616

3599. SAAB Automation AB
Klas Melander
Box 1017
551 11 Jönköping
Sweden
Telephone: +46 36 1942 00
Fax: +46 36 1661 57

3600. Saarbrücker Zeitung
Gutenbergstrasse 11–23
6600 Saarbrücken
Germany
Telephone: 49 (681) 50210;
49 (681) 50211
Fax: 49 (681) 502300

3601. Saddleback Graphics
Hal Lafferty
1281 Garden Grove Blvd, Unit P
Garden Grove
CA 92643
USA
Telephone: (714) 741 7093
Fax: (714) 741 7095

3602. SAE-Agenturer AB
Arne Eriksson
Ångskärsgatan 4
115 29 Stockholm
Sweden
Telephone: +46 8 6653250;
+46 8 6653252
Fax: +46 8 6675566

3603. Saen Software Development
Guus Hildesheim
Czaar Peterstraat 19
1506 SL Zaandam
Netherlands
Telephone: +31 75 178257

3604. SAE
Electronic Publishing Division
400 Commonwealth Drive
Warrendale
PA 15096
USA
Telephone: (412) 776–4841
Fax: (412) 776–5760
Telex/E-mail: 866355

3605. Sage Data Inc
104 Carnegie Center
Princeton
NJ 08540
USA
Telephone: (609) 987–0012

**3606. Sagit Publishing International
Limited**
PO Box 30617
61 306 Tel Aviv
Israel
Telephone: 972 (3) 383322
Fax: 972 (3) 384291

3607. Sahovski Informator
Milutin Kostic
Francuska 31
PO Box 739
Beograd
11001 Beograd
Yugoslavia
Telephone: +38 11 186 498
Fax: +38 11 626 583

3608. Salem Press Inc
150 S Los Robles Avenue
Suite 720
Pasadena
CA 91101
USA
Telephone: (818) 584–0106
Fax: (818) 584–1525

**3609. Sales and Marketing
Information Ltd**
1 Warwick Street
Leamington Spa
Warwickshire
CV32 5LW
UK
Telephone: 0926 451–199
Fax: 0926 450–592;
0926 886–967

3610. Salomon Brothers Inc
One New York Plaza
New York
NY 10004
USA
Telephone: (212) 747–7947

3611. SAMI
800 Broadway
Cincinnati
OH 45202
USA
Telephone: (513) 852–3888

**3612. Samsom H.D. Tjeenk Willink
B.V.**
A C H M Henderickx
Prinses Margrietlaan 3
2404 AH Alphen a/d Rijn
Netherlands
Telephone: +31 1720 66619
Fax: +31 1720 93270

3613. Samson-Veldkamp
F van Boetzelaer
Wibautstaat 129
1091 GL Amsterdam
Netherlands
Telephone: 020–6683191
Fax: 020–6651253

**3614. Samsung Advanced Institute of
Technology**
Hye K Kwag
PO Box Suwon 111
San 14 Nong Seo-Ri, Kihung-Eup
Yongin-Gun, Kyung Ki-Do
Korea
Telephone: +82 2 744 0011;
+82 331 281 3721
Fax: +82 2 744 6217

3615. San Antonio Light, The
PO Box 161
420 Broadway
San Antonio
TX 78291
USA
Telephone: (512) 271–2700

3616. San Diego Union and Tribune
350 Camino De La Reina
San Diego
CA 92108
USA
Telephone: (619) 299–3131
Fax: (619) 293–2333

3617. San Francisco Chronicle
901 Mission Street
San Francisco
CA 94103
USA
Telephone: (415) 777–1111

3618. San Francisco Examiner, The
925 Mission Street
San Francisco
CA 94103
USA
Telephone: (415) 777–5700

**3619. San Francisco Newspaper
Agency**
Marketing Research Department
925 Mission Street
San Francisco
CA 94103
USA
Telephone: (415) 777–7291;
(800) 227–4423

3620. San José Mercury News
CD-ROM Enquiries
750 Ridder Park Drive
San José
CA 95190
USA
Telephone: (408) 920–5000;
(408) 920–5444
Fax: (408) 288–8060

3621. Sandpiper Services Limited
Haddon House
2–4 Fitzroy Street
London
W1P 5AD
UK
Telephone: 071 637–7361

3622. Sanseido Co Ltd
2–22–14 Misaki-Cho
Chiyoda 101
Tokyo
Japan
Telephone: 03–3230–9412
Fax: 03 323095969

3623. Sansyusya Publishing Company
K Maeda
1–5–34 Shitaya
Taito-Ku
Tokyo 110
Japan
Telephone: 03 3842 1711;
                03 3842 1631;
                03 3847 2581
Fax: 03 3845 3965;
        03 3841 8125

3624. Sanyo Information System Corp.
Koho Bldg 11–8
1–Chome, Kayabacho
Nihonbashi Chuo-ku
Tokyo 103
Japan
Telephone: 03–661–2290

3625. SARIN SpA
SS 148 Pontina KM 29,100
I-00040 Rome
Italy
Telephone: 06 91 19 71
Telex/E-mail: 616436 SARIN I

3626. SARITEL SpA
Via Aurelio Saffi 18
CP 512
I-10138 Torino
Italy
Telephone: 011 33301

3627. Saskatchewan Legislative Counsel Office
1874 Scarth Street
Regina
SK S4P 3V7
Canada
Telephone: (306) 787–7872

3628. Satori Enterprises Inc
10909 Trotting Ridge Way
Columbia
MD 21044
USA
Telephone: (301) 596–6427

3629. SAZTEC Europe Ltd.
Robert Martin
Tangier Lane
Eton
Windsor
Berkshire
SL4 6BB
UK
Telephone: 071 753 833131
Fax: 071 753 832454

3630. Saztec International Inc
Donald E Mack; Elvin Smith
6700 Corporate Drive
Lakeside Building 11
Kansas City
MO 64120
USA
Telephone: (816) 483 6900
Fax: (816) 241 4966

3631. Scalaire
Jean-Mark Pouyot
41 rue Lafaurie de Monbadon
33000 Bordeaux
France
Telephone: +33 56 52 47 18
Fax: +33 56 51 39 16

3632. Scan C2C Inc
Tina Bosse; Glenn Hoetker
500 E Street SW
Suite 800
Washington
DC 20024
USA
Telephone: (202) 863–3850;
                (800) 525–3965
Fax: (202) 863–3855

3633. Scannet
c/o Helsinki University of Technology
    Library
Otanimentie 9
SF-02150 Espoo
Finland
Telephone: 0 4552633
Fax: 0 4514132
Telex/E-mail: 121591 SF

3634. ScanRom Publications
555 Chestnut Street
Cedarhurst
NY 11516
USA
Telephone: (516) 295–2237

3635. Scarborough Research Corporation
989 6th Avenue
New York
NY 10018
USA
Telephone: (212) 736–1990

3636. Scheltema Holkema Vermeulen BV
Jaap Büchli; Robert Windrich
Koningsplein 20
Postbox 271
1000AB Amsterdam
Netherlands
Telephone: +31 20 5231411
Fax: +31 20 6227684

3637. Schweizerische Depeschenagentur AG
Laenggassstrasse 7
3001 Bern
Switzerland
Telephone: 41 (31) 24 33 33
Fax: 41 (31) 23 85 38
Telex/E-mail: 911500 SDA CH

3638. Schweizerische Volksbank
Departement Documentation
PO Box 5323
CH-3G001 Berne
Switzerland
Telephone: 031 32 75 20;
                031 32 88 86
Fax: 031 32 75 03;
        031 32 89 00
Telex/E-mail: SVBI (DATAMAIL)

3639. Schweizerischer Gesamtkatalog
Landesbibliothek
Hallwylstrasse 15
3003 Bern
Switzerland
Telephone: 41 (31) 61 89 49

3640. Scicon Limited
Brick Close
Kiln Farm
Milton Keynes
MK11 3EJ
UK
Telephone: 44 (908) 565656

3641. Scicon
Mike Bunbury
Sanderson House
49 Berners Street
London
W1P 4AQ
UK
Telephone: 071 580–5599
Fax: SCICON M KEYNES
NUA: 234290840111

3642. Science and Engineering Information Center Company
6F CENT-FOR Building
12–6, 2–Chome
Shinjuku-ku
Tokyo 160
Japan
Telephone: 03 3356–7971

3643. Science Applications International Corporation
800 Oak Ridge Turnpike
PO Box 2501
Oak Ridge
TN 37831
USA
Telephone: (615) 482–9031

3644. Science for Kids
9950 Concord Church Road
Lewisville
NC 27023
USA
Telephone: (919) 945–9000
Fax: (919) 945–2500

3645. Scientific American Inc
Janet Zinn
415 Madison Avenue
New York
NY 10017–1111
USA
Telephone: (212) 754–0805;
                (212) 754–0801;
                (212) 754–0550
Fax: (212) 980–3062

3646. Scientific Consulting
Dr Schulte-Hillen
Mathias-Bruggen-Strasse 87–89
D-5000 Köln 30
Germany
Telephone: 49–221 597000
Fax: 49–221 59700 90

3647. Scientific Consulting
1735 New York Avenue
Washington
DC 20006
USA

3648. Scientific Database System
Computing Centre
Senliang Li; Nianhu Xiao; Shizhen
    Zhang
Chinese Academy of Sciences
Zhongguancun
Beijing 100080
China
Telephone: 285023
Fax: 2562485

3649. SCIX Corporation
PO Box 3244
Williamsport
PA 17701–0244
USA
Telephone: (717) 323–3276

3650. Scott Loftesness
16440 Rustling Oak Court
Morgan Hill
CA 95037
USA

3651. Scottish Council for Educational Technology
SEND
Stuart Beresford; Peter Brannan
Dowanhill
74 Victoria Crescent Road
Glasgow
G12 9JN
Scotland, UK
Telephone: 041 334–9314;
　　　　　041 357–0340
Fax: 041 334–6519

3652. Scottish HCI Centre
George House
36 N Hanover Street
Glasgow
G1 2AD
UK
Telephone: 041 552–1576
Fax: 041 552–1415
Telex/E-mail: ANNE UK.AC.TURING
　　　(JANET); ANNE UK.AC.TURING
　　　(UUCP)

3653. Scottish Poisons Information Bureau
Royal Infirmary
Edinburgh
EH3 9YW
UK
Telephone: 031 228–6907
Fax: 031 228–3332

3654. Screen Digest Ltd
37 Gower Street
London
W1CE 6HH
UK
Telephone: 071 580–2842
Fax: 071 580–0060

3655. Scripps Howard News Service
1090 Vermont Avenue NW
Suite 1000
Washington
DC 20005
USA
Telephone: (202) 408–1484

3656. SCRL (Société Commerciale de Recouvrement Litigieux)
Jean-Michel Joly
5 Quai Jayr
F-69255 Lyon Cedex 9
France
Telephone: 72 20 10 00
Fax: 72 20 10 50;
　　　78 47 14 49
Telex/E-mail: 330903 F

3657. Scuola Normale Superiore
Piazza dei Cavalieri 7
I-56100 Pisa
Italy
Telephone: 050 59 72 68
Telex/E-mail: SNSPI 590 5481

3658. SDC Informatique
Pascale Berthault M Sylvestre
9 rue Jeoffroy de St Hilaire
75005 Paris
France
Telephone: +33 1 40 51 00 11
Fax: +33 1 43 25 34 67

3659. SDT
Sevicios de teledocumentacion S.A.
Rachel Lauziere
Gatztambide 61
3–e 1.a Puerta
E-28015 Madrid
Spain
Telephone: +34 1–4492048
Fax: +34 1–2444650
NUA: 212022032

3660. SDU Uitgeverij Plantijnstraat
SDLI Uitgeverij Plantijnstraat
Christaffel Plantijnstraat 2
Postbus 20014
The Hague
Netherlands
Telephone: +31 70 3709911
Fax: +31 70 3475770

3661. Search Systems Ltd
Christopher Durant
High Holborn House
52–54 High Holborn
London
WC1V 6RL
UK
Telephone: 071 430–1685
Fax: 071 430–1685

3662. SEAT Divisione STET SpA
Dr Giorio Caniglia
Viale del Policlinico 147
I-00161 Rome
Italy
Telephone: 06 84941
Fax: 06 849–4421
Telex/E-mail: 212248 I

3663. Seattle Post-Intelligencer, The
101 Elliot Avenue W
Seattle
WA 98119
USA
Telephone: (206) 448–8173;
　　　　　(206) 448–8000
Fax: (206) 448–8165
Telex/E-mail: 329549 SEATTLE PI

3664. Seattle Times
Fairview Avenue N & John Street
PO Box 70
Seattle
WA 98111
USA
Telephone: (206) 624–8484;
　　　　　(206) 464–2994

3665. SEC Online Inc
Robert Galvin
201 Moreland Road
Suite 2
Hauppauge
NY 11788
USA
Telephone: (516) 864–7200;
　　　　　(800) 832–3282
Fax: (516) 864–7215

3666. SECODIP
Department Pige Publicitaire
2 rue Francis-Pedron
PO Box 3
F-78241 Chambourcy
France
Telephone: 1 30 74 60 11;
　　　　　1 39 65 56 56
Fax: 1 39 65 12 19
Telex/E-mail: 698370 F

3667. Secretaria General del Plan Nacional de Investigacion Cientifica y Desarrollo Tecnologico
Vicesecretaria de Informacion Cientifica
　y Tecnica
Rosario Pino 14–16
28020 Madrid
Spain
Telephone: 34 (1) 450 05 02
Telex/E-mail: 46962 E

3668. Secretariat of the Nordic Energy Information Libraries
Risoe Library
Risoe National Laboratory
4000 Roskilde
Denmark
Telephone: 45 (2) 37 12 12
Fax: 45 (2) 75 56 27
Telex/E-mail: 43116 RISOE DK

3669. Securities Data Company Inc
1180 Raymond Boulevard
5th Floor
Newark
NJ 07102
USA
Telephone: (201) 668–0940

3670. Securities Industry Association
120 Broadway
35th Floor
New York
NY 10271
USA
Telephone: (212) 608–1500

3671. Securities Objective Services
17175 N Lake Drive
Bay Minette
AL 36507
USA
Telephone: (205) 937–6308

3672. Security Pacific/Market Information
127 John Street
20th Floor
New York
NY 10038
USA
Telephone: (212) 809–3000;
　　　　　(800) 824–7755

3673. SEDES
15 rue Bleue
F-75009 Paris
France
Telephone: 1 47 70 61 61
Telex/E-mail: 641 755 SEDESOC F

3674. SEDOC
283 rue de la Miniere
Zone Industrielle Nord BP 6
Buc 78530
France
Telephone: 33–3956–8055
Fax: 33–39–561151

3675. SEFLIN Inc
SouthEast Florida Library Information
　Network
Cindy Ansell
100 South Andrews Avenue
Fort Lauderdale
FL 33301
USA
Telephone: (305) 357 7318
Fax: (305) 357 6998

3676. SEIBT Verlag Gmbh
Leopoldstrasse 208
8000 Munchen 40
Germany
Telephone: +49 89 363067
Fax: +49 89 364317

3677. Seidl Datenbank Service GmbH
Gudrun H Seidl
Tannenweg 5
6052 Muhlheim/Main
Germany
Telephone: +49 6108 753 96
Fax: +49 6108 7 34 32

3678. Sekretariatet for Retsinformation Justitsministeriet
Vaegtergarden
Axeltorv 6
DK-1609 Copenhagen V
Denmark
Telephone: 033 325–222

3679. SelectWare Technologies Inc.
29200 Vassar
Suite 200
Livonia
MI 48152
USA
Telephone: (313) 477–7340;
(800) 342–3366
Fax: (313) 477–6488

3680. Semaphore Corporation
207 Granada Drive
Aptos
CA 95003
USA
Telephone: (408) 688–9200

3681. Semiconductor Industry Association
4300 Stevens Creek Boulevard
Suite 271
San José
CA 95129
USA
Telephone: (408) 246–2711

3682. Seminar Clearinghouse International Inc
350 N Robert Street
Suite 598
St Paul
MN 55101
USA
Telephone: (612) 293–1044
Fax: (612) 293–0492
Telex/E-mail: IP002 (HRIN)

3683. Seminar Information Service Inc
17752 Skypark Circle
Suite 210
Irvine
CA 92714
USA
Telephone: (714) 261–9104
Fax: (714) 261–1963

3684. Senat du France
Service des Impressions de la
Documentation Parlementaire et de
l'Informatique
15 rue de Vaugirard
F-75291 Paris Cedex 6
France
Telephone: 1 42 34 21 38;
1 42 34 20 70;
1 42 34 20 14
Fax: 1 42 34 25 52
Telex/E-mail: 260 430 SENAT PARIS

3685. Sentinel Communications Company
633 N Orange Avenue
PO Box 2833
Orlando
FL 32801
USA
Telephone: (407) 420–5000

3686. Sequoia Data Corporation
875 Mahler Road
Suite 261
Burlingame
CA 94010
USA
Telephone: (415) 697–0955;
(800) 359–8131

3687. Sercresa
50–006 Zaragoza
Supervia 26
Spain
Telephone: 76 439043

3688. Serveur Universitaire National de l'Information Scientifique et Technologique
Mr. Jean Louis Duclos
Chemin Saint-Hubert
L'Isle d'Abeau, B.P. 112
38303 Bourgoin-Jallieu Cedex
France
Telephone: 33 (74) 27 28 10
NUA: 2080138001731

3689. Services Documentaires Multimedia Inc
Marielle Boucher; Reine Guérin
1685 rue Fleury est
Montreal
PQ H2C 1T1
Canada
Telephone: (514) 382–0895
Fax: (514) 384–9139

3690. Services du Premier Ministre
Direction des Journaux Officiels,
Service des Bulletins Annexes
26 rue Desaix
F-75727 Paris Cedex 15
France
Telephone: 1 40 58 75 00
Fax: 1 40 58 77 80
Telex/E-mail: 201176 DIRJO F

3691. Services du Premier Ministre
Centre National de l'Informatique
Juridique
26 rue Desaix
F-75727 Paris Cedex 15
France
Telephone: 1 45 79 80 78

3692. Servicio Publico de Videotex
Avenida Fontes Pereira de Melo 38/9
1000 Lisbon
Portugal
Telephone: 01 540–020
Fax: 01 543–843
Telex/E-mail: 64200 TDATA P

3693. Servicios de Teledocumentación
Rachel Lauziere
Calle Luchana 4, 2 A-B
28010 Madrid
Spain
Telephone: 01 593 96 12
Fax: 01 593 98 21
NUA: 212022032

3694. Servicos de Telematica, SA
Rua Joao Black, 18
Sobreda da Caparica
2825 Monte da Caparica
Portugal
Telephone: 351 (1) 295 17 45
Fax: 351 (1) 168 91 19

3695. SHARE Systems Ltd
Mark Beeley
2a High Street
Yeadon
Leeds
LS19 7PP
UK
Telephone: 0532 500055
Fax: 0532 502153

3696. Shaw Data Services Inc
122 E 42nd Street
New York
NY 10168
USA
Telephone: (212) 682–8877

3697. Shell International Petroleum
Maatschappij
PO Box 650
2501 The Hague CR
Netherlands

3698. Shepard's/McGraw-Hill Inc
420 N Cascade Avenue
PO Box 35300
Colorado Springs
CO 80921
USA
Telephone: (719) 488–3000

3699. Sherburne Knowledge Systems Inc
Frankie Dune; Woody Edstrom
12220 Riverwood Drive
Burnsville
MN 55337
USA
Telephone: (612) 895 6099
Fax: (612) 895 1792

3700. Sheshunoff Information Services Inc
Laurel Toth
One Texas Center
505 Barton Springs Road
Austin
TX 78704
USA
Telephone: (512) 472–2244
Fax: (512) 476 1251

3701. Shin-Nippon Hooki Pub. Co. Ltd.
1–23–20 Sakae
Naka-Ku
Nagoya
Nagoya 460–11
Japan
Telephone: +81 52 211 5781
Fax: +81 52 211 1530

3702. Shinnippon-hoki Publishing Co Ltd
Media Development Department
1–23–20 Sakae
Naka-ku
Nagoya 460
Japan
Telephone: +81 52 211 5781
Fax: +81 52 211 1520

3703. Shirley Institute
Didsbury
Manchester
M20 8RX
UK
Telephone: 44 (61) 445–8141
Fax: 44 (61) 434–9957
Telex/E-mail: 668417 SHIRLY G

3704. Shufunotomo Co Ltd
Book Publishing Department for Health
and Medical
Haruo Nagoaka
2–9 Kanda Surugadai
Chiyoda-ku
Tokyo 101
Japan
Telephone: +81 3 3294 1119
Fax: +81 3 3294 0492

Addresses

3705. SIDAC
Bruno Cerboni; Filippo Fantasia
S S 148 Pontina Km 29100
Rome
00040 Pomezia
Italy
Telephone: +39 6 91198201;
                   +39 6 91198219
Fax: +39 6 91198500

3706. Sierra On-Line Inc.
Rick Cavin Srini Vasan
PO Box 485
Coarsegold
CA 93614
USA
Telephone: (209) 683 4468
Fax: (209) 683 3633

3707. Sigenhogo-Kyokai (See Japan
         Fisheries Resource
         Conservation Association)

3708. Silicon Valley Information
         Center
San José Public Library
180 W San Carlos Street
San José
CA 95113
USA
Telephone: (408) 277-5754

3709. Silory Graph Snc
Mrs. Loredana Apolloni; Mrs. Silvana
    Cecchi; Mrs. Simona Ravano
Via Maurizio Quuadrio 15
00152 Rome
Italy
Telephone: 39 (6) 5898040
NUA: 22226100340

3710. SilverPlatter Information
Jane Niemi
One Newton Executive Park
Newton Lower Falls
MA 02162-1449
USA
Telephone: (617) 969-2332
Fax: (617) 969-5554

3711. SilverPlatter
Susan Day; Ruth Hudson
10 Barley Mow Passage
Chiswick
London
W4 4PH
UK
Telephone: 081 995-8242
Fax: 081 995-5159

3712. SIMBA Information Inc
PO Box 7430
Wilton
CT 06897
USA
Telephone: (203) 834-0033
Fax: (203) 834-1771

3713. Simmons Market Research
         Bureau Inc
380 Madison Avenue
New York
NY 10017
USA
Telephone: (212) 916-8900
Fax: (212) 916-8918

3714. Simmons-Boardman
         Publishing Corporation
345 Hudson Street
New York
NY 10014
USA
Telephone: (212) 620-7200
Fax: (212) 633-1165

3715. Sininen Kirja Oy
Uudenmaankatu 16-20
SF-00120 Helsinki
Finland
Telephone: 358 (0) 1221
Fax: 358 (0) 601875
Telex/E-mail: 125368 SINFO SF

3716. Sintrom Electronics
Arkwright Road
Reading
Berkshire
RG2 0LS
UK
Telephone: 0734 311088

3717. SIRIO
Via Orazio 2
Milan
Italy
Telephone: 02 882 31

3719. SIS Standardiseringskom-
         missionen I Sverige
Swedish Standards Institution
Gunnar Arnoldsson
Box 3295
103 66 Stockholm
Sweden
Telephone: +46 8 613 52 00
Fax: +46 8 11 70 35

3721. SiteSelex On-Line
80024 Benjamin Fox Pavilion, Suite 824
Jenkintown
PA 19046
USA
Telephone: (215) 572-6410

3722. Sittelle
Jean C Roche
Châteaubois
38350 La Mure
France
Telephone: +33 76 81 10 01;
                   +33 76 81 23 95
Fax: +33 76 30 96 95

3723. SJ Rundt & Associates
130 E 63rd Street
New York
NY 10021
USA
Fax: (212) 838-0141

3724. Sjukvardens och
         Socialvardens Planerings- och
Rationaliserings-Institut
SPRI Biblioteket och Utredningsbanken
PO Box 27310
S-102 54 Stockholm
Sweden
Telephone: 08 663-0560
Fax: 08 702-4799

3725. Skillchange Systems Ltd
Alistair Morrison; Derek Hay
Ardent House
Gates Way
Stevenage
Herts
SG1 3NS
UK
Telephone: 0438 741441
Fax: 0438 741339

3726. Slater Hall Information
         Products
George Hall
1522 K Street NW
Suite 522
Washington
DC 20005
USA
Telephone: (202) 682-1350
Fax: (202) 898 0181

3727. Sleigh Corporation
EURASTAR Division
Jan D Slee
PO Box 591
Franklin Lakes
NJ 07417
USA
Telephone: (201) 891-7528
Fax: (201) 891-7528

3728. SLEUTH
TRAC Inc
282 North Washington Street, Suite 100
Falls Church
VA 22046
USA
Telephone: (703) 538-6181

3729. SLIGOS
Mr Estapa
91 rue Jean-Jaures
F-92807 Puteaux Cedex
France
Telephone: 1 47 76 42 42
Telex/E-mail: 610677 SLIGO F
NUA: 208092020028

3730. Smart Communications Inc
885 3rd Avenue
29th Floor
PO Box 963
FDR Station
New York
NY 10022
USA
Telephone: (212) 486-1894
Fax: (212) 752-6441;
        (212) 826-9775
Telex/E-mail: 220883 TAUR

3731. Smithsonian Astrophysical
         Observatory
Einstein Data Products Office
Elizabeth Bohlen
CFA, 60 Garden Street
Cambridge
MA 02138
USA
Telephone: (617) 495 7164
Fax: (617) 495 7356

3732. SNEI sa
Mari Jose Cocquyt; Josiane Belkechout
22 avenue Franklin D Roosevelt
Paris 75008
France
Telephone: 1 43 59 37 59;
                   1 46 92 25 20
Fax: 1 45 63 83 49

3733. Sociaal-Wetenschappelijk
         Informatie- en
         Documentatiecentrum
Herengracht 410
NL-1017 BX Amsterdam
Netherlands
Telephone: 020 225061
Fax: 020 62 38 374
Telex/E-mail: STEINM SARA.NL
    (EARN)

3734. Social Issues Resources Series, Inc (SIRS)
Paula Jackson
PO Box 2348
Boca Raton
FL 33427
USA
Telephone: (407) 994 0079;
　　　　　(800) 232 SIRS
Fax: (407) 994 4704

3735. Sociedade Portuguesa de Computadores em Tempo Divido Sarl
R. Almeida Brandao 24–A
P-1200 Lisbon
Portugal
Telephone: +351 1–603181/2/3/4
NUA: 268006010313

3736. Societe de Diffusion d'Informations Boursieres
17 rue Monsigny
F-75002 Paris
France
Telephone: 1 42 65 47 32
Telex/E-mail: 217630 F

3737. Societe Française de Biologie Clinique
Hopital Necker
149 Rue de Sevres
75743 Paris Cedex 15
France
Telephone: 33 (1) 273 80 00

3738. Societe Generale de Banque
Centre de Documentation
Montagne du Parc 3
1000 Brussels
Belgium
Telephone: 32 (2) 516 33 50

3739. Société MERLIN GERIN
Service de Documentation
F-38050 Grenoble Cedex
France
Telephone: 76 57 94 60
Fax: 76 57 75 32
Telex/E-mail: 320 842 F

3740. Societé Nationale d'Etudes et de Constructia de Moteurs d'Aviation
SNECMA
Jacky Pignoux
2 Bd du Gal Martial Valim
75274 Paris Cedex 15
France
Telephone: 1 60 66 87 40
Fax: 1 60 66 89 02

3741. Societe Nouvelle Cirtel
1 Impasse Clemenceau
76230 Bois Guillaume
France
Telephone: 33 (35) 61 70 70
Fax: 33 (35) 61 52 00

3742. Societe Nouvelle de l'Edition pour l'Industrie SA
91 rue du Faubourg St Hoonore
F-75008 Paris
France
Telephone: 1 43 59 37 59
Fax: 1 42 66 18 97
Telex/E-mail: 660911 SNEI F

3743. Société Suisse de Pharmacie
Stationsstrasse 12
Case Postale 226
3097 Berne-Liebefeld
Switzerland
Telephone: 41 31 53 58 58
Fax: 41 31 59 15 69

3744. Society for Human Resource Management
606 N Washington Street
Alexandria
VA 22314
USA
Telephone: (703) 548–3440
Fax: (703) 836–0367
Telex/E-mail: IP041 (HRIN)

3745. Society for Industrial and Organizational Psychology Inc
617 E Golf Road
Suite 103
Arlington Heights
VA 60005
USA
Telephone: (708) 640–0068

3746. Society of Automotive Engineers
SAE International
Gina Rape
Electronic Publishing Division
400 Commonwealth Drive
Warrendale
PA 15096–0001
USA
Telephone: (412) 772–7144;
　　　　　(412) 776–4970
Fax: (412) 776–5760
Telex/E-mail: 866355

3747. Society of Exploration Geophysicists
PO Box 702740
Tulsa
OK 74170
USA
Telephone: (918) 493–3516

3748. Society of Manufacturing Engineers
One SME Drive
Dearborn
MI 48121
USA
Telephone: (313) 271–1500
Telex/E-mail: 297742 SMEUR

3749. Society of Petroleum Engineers
PO Box 833836
Richardson
TX 75083–3836
USA
Telephone: (214) 669–3377;
　　　　　(800) 527–6863

3750. Sociological Abstracts Inc
Database Services
Miriam Chall
PO Box 22206
San Diego
CA 92192–0206
USA
Telephone: (800) 752–3945;
　　　　　(619) 565–6603;
　　　　　(619) 695–8803
Fax: (619) 565–0132;
　　　　　(619) 695–0416
Telex/E-mail: OWENT SDSC (BITNET);
　　　　　14217 (DIALMAIL)

3751. Sociometrics Corporation
Sachi Mizuno
170 State Street
Suite 260
Los Altos
CA 94022
USA
Telephone: (415) 949–3282
Fax: (415) 949–3299

3752. Softissimo
Laurent Schuhl
129 Boulevard de Sabastopol
Paris 75002
France
Telephone: 1 42 33 77 10
Fax: 1 42 36 62 63

3753. Softline Information Inc.
Ralph Ferragamo
Eastchester
New York
USA

3754. SoftSearch Inc
1 Civic Center Plaza
1560 Broadway
Suite 900
Denver
CO 80202
USA
Telephone: (303) 831–3400;
　　　　　(800) 525–9851;
　　　　　(800) 468–3381;
　　　　　(800) 443–2475 (in Texas)
Fax: (303) 831–3466

3755. Softsel Computer Products Ltd
Softsel House
941 Great West Road
Brentford
Middlesex
TW8 9DD
Telephone: 081–568 8866

3756. Software Club
London
UK
Telephone: 081 205–4548

3757. Software Development Co
CD-ROM Enquiries
8–12 Shibuya 3–chrome
Shibuya-ku 150
Tokyo
Japan
Telephone: +81 3 3406 3711
Fax: +81 3 3406 6850

3758. Software Law Bulletin
7721 Kalohelani
Honolulu
HI 96825
USA

3759. Software Mart Inc
Richard Smith
Suite E-100
3933 Spicewood Springs Road
Austin
TX 78759
USA
Telephone: (512) 346 1393
Fax: (512) 346 1393

3760. Software Toolworks
Janet Shirley Faul
60 Leveroni Court
Novato
CA 94949
USA
Telephone: (415) 883–3000;
　　　　　(800) 231–3088
Fax: (415) 883–3303

3761. SoftWright
791 South Holly Street
Denver
CO 80222
USA
Telephone: (303) 329–6388
Fax: (303) 329–0901

3762. Sola Publishing Group
Fabrizio Caffarelli
Via Carnevali 109
20158 Milan
Italy
Telephone: +39 2 39311341;
　　　　　+39 2 39311325
Fax: +39 2 39311374

3763. Somak Software Inc
535 Encinitas Blvd.
Suite 113
Encinitas
CA 92024
USA
Telephone: 619–942–2556
Fax: 619–632–9087

3764. Sonic Images Productions Inc
John Ramo
4590 MacArthur Boulevard NW
Washington
DC 20007
USA
Telephone: (202) 333 1063
Fax: (202) 338 1386

3765. Sonopress Data-replication
Carl Bertelsmann-Strasse 161
W-4830 Gutersloh
Germany
Telephone: +49 5241 80 3912

**3766. Sony Electronic Publishing
　　　 Company**
Columbia Tri-Star
Paul Ayscough
London
UK
Telephone: 081 748–6000
Fax: 081 748–4546

**3767. Sony Electronic Publishing
　　　 Company**
Multimedia Productions
One Lower Ragsdale Drive
Monterey
CA 93940
USA
Telephone: (408) 372 7141
Fax: (408) 375 7130

**3768. Sony Electronic Publishing
　　　 Company**
Olaf J. Olafsson, President
9 West 57th Street, 43rd Floor
New York
NY 10019
USA
Telephone: (212) 418–9439
Fax: (212) 308–9841

3769. SONY Europa GmbH
Marketing Department
Sony House
South Street
Staines
Middlesex
TW18 4PF
UK
Telephone: 0784 67000;
　　　　　0784 67208

3770. Sony
SB/UK
Janet Whitaker
Jays Close
Viables
Basingstoke
Hants.
RG22 4SB
UK
Telephone: 0256 474011
Fax: 0256 816397

3771. Sorefi Ile de France
Caisses d'Espagne
Mme Donati; Mme Bassez
7 rue Mornay
75004 Paris
France
Telephone: +33 1 48 04 97 97
Fax: +33 1 48 04 98 50

3772. Source, The
1616 Anderson Road
McLean
VA 22102
USA

**3773. South African Consulate
　　　 General**
333 E 38th Street
9th Floor
New York
NY 10016
USA
Telephone: (212) 213–7997
Fax: (212) 371–7577

**3774. South Australian Department
　　　 of Mines and Energy**
191 Greenhill Road
Parkside
SA 5063
Australia
Telephone: 08 274–7500
Fax: 08 272–7597

**3775. South Jersey Publishing
　　　 Company**
1000 W Washington Avenue
Pleasantville
NJ 08232
USA
Telephone: (609) 272–1100

**3776. Southam Business Information
　　　 and Communications Group
　　　 Inc**
1450 Don Mills Road
Don Mills
ON M3B 2X7
Canada
Telephone: (416) 445–6641
Fax: (416) 445–3508

3777. Southam Communications
1231 Yonge Street
Suite 300
Toronto
ON M4TW 2Z1
Canada
Telephone: (416) 922–1133

3778. Southam Electronic Publishing
Dennis Ablett
1450 Don Mills Road
Don Mills
Ontario
M3B 2X7
Canada
Telephone: (416) 445–6641
Fax: (416) 442–2077

3779. Southam Inc
250 St Antoine Street W
Montreal
PQ H2Y 3R7
Canada
Telephone: (514) 282–2750

3781. Southeastern Library Network
Plaza Level
400 Colony Square
1201 Peachtree Street, NE
Atlanta
GA 30361
USA
Telephone: (404) 892–0943

3782. Southscan Ltd
PO Box 724
London
N16 5RZ
UK
Telephone: 081 800–7654

3783. Southwest Newswire Inc
2301 N Akard
Suite 110
Dallas
TX 75201
USA
Telephone: (214) 871–2940

3784. Soutraitel Interregional
10 place Gutenberg
F-67000 Strasbourg
France
Telephone: 88 32 12 55

3785. SovInfoLink
Stuart Merrill
440 S. La Salle
Suite 3300
Chicago
IL 60605
USA
Telephone: (312) 431–3553
Fax: (312) 922–3476

**3786. Space Age Publishing
　　　 Company**
20431 Stevens Creek
Cupertino
CA 95014–2225
USA
Telephone: (408) 996–9210

3787. Space Base Inc
200 Railroad Avenue
Greenwich
CT 06830
USA
Telephone: (203) 661–1877
Fax: (203) 869–8326

**3788. Space Telescope Science
　　　 Institution**
Dr Brian McLean
3700 San Martin Drive
Baltimore
MD 21218
USA
Telephone: (301) 338–4700
Fax: (301) 338–4767

3789. Space-Time Research
Jack Massey
668 Burwood Road
Hawthorn East
Melbourne
Victoria 3123
Australia
Telephone: +61 3 813 3211
Fax: +61 3 883 4029

3790. Spang Robinson Wiley
830 Menlo Avenue
Suite 100
Menlo Park
CA 94025
USA
Telephone: (415) 328–0302

3791. Spear Securities Inc
505 North Brand Blvd, 16th Floor
Glendale
CA 91203
USA
Telephone: (818) 242–1466;
　　　　　(800) 252–9011
Fax: (818) 242–9525

3792. Speednews
1801 Avenue of the Stars
Los Angeles
CA 90067–5904
USA
Telephone: (213) 203–9603
Fax: (213) 203–9352
Telex/E-mail: 71292674 SPNWS UR

3793. Spicers Centre for Europe Ltd
17 Marina Court
Hull
HU1 1TJ
UK
Telephone: 0482 589–022
Fax: 0482 589–008

3794. Spin UK Ltd
Shell Philips Interactive
Stephen Weil
Lombard House
2 Purley Way
Croydon
CR0 3JP
UK
Telephone: +44 81 665 5990
Fax: +44 81 665 6105

3795. Spinnaker Software
1 Kendall Square
Cambridge
MA 02139
USA
Telephone: (617) 494–1200

**3796. Sport Information Resource
Centre**
Linda Wheeler
1600 James Naismith Drive
Gloucester
Ontario
K1B 5N4
Canada
Telephone: (613) 748–5658
Fax: (613) 748–5706;
(613) 748–5701
Telex/E-mail: 0533660

3797. Sportdoc
11 avenue du Tremblay
F-75012 Paris
France
Telephone: 1 43 74 11 21

**3798. Sportel Communications
Network**
PO Box 1182
Las Vegas
NV 89125
USA
Telephone: (702) 871–6529;
(800) 634–3112

**3799. Sporting News Publishing
Company**
Joan Kardasz
PO Box 56
1212 N Lindbergh Boulevard
St Louis
MO 63132
USA
Telephone: (314) 997–7111
Fax: (314) 993–7726

3800. Sports Council
Information Centre
16 Upper Woburn Place
London WC1H 0QP
UK
Telephone: 44 (71) 388–1277

3801. Sports Network, The
701 Mason's Mill Business Park
Huntington Valley
PA 19006
USA
Telephone: (215) 947–2400

3802. SportsTicker Inc
Harborside Financial Center
600 Plaza Two
Jersey City
NJ 07311
USA
Telephone: (201) 309–1200

3803. SPRI SA
Gran Via 35 – 3 Planta
48009 Bilbao
Spain
Telephone: 34 (4) 415 82 88

**3804. Springer-Verlag GmbH &
Company KG**
Gertraud Griepke
PO Box 105280
Tiergartenstrasse 17
6900 Heidelberg 1
Germany
Telephone: 49 (6221) 487 665;
49 (6221) 487 457
Fax: 49 (6221) 413982

3805. Springer-Verlag New York Inc
Dr R Badger
175 Fifth Avenue
New York
NY 10010
USA
Telephone: (212) 460–1683
Fax: (212) 473–6272

3806. SPRITEL
Sociedad Para la Promocion y
Reconversion Industrial Sprit
Sr. Jose Maria Fernandez
Gran Via 2–4a planta
48001 Bilbao
Spain
Telephone: 34 (4) 4236319
Fax: 34 (4) 4243591
Telex/E-mail: 31047 SPRM E

3807. SRI International
Business Intelligence Center
333 Ravenswood Avenue
Menlo Park
CA 94025
USA
Telephone: (415) 859–6300;
(415) 859–3695;
(415) 859–4600
Fax: (415) 859–6028
Telex/E-mail: 334486

3808. SRI International
Chemical Economics Handbook
Program
333 Ravenswood Avenue AE208
Menlo Park
CA 94025–3493
USA
Telephone: (415) 859–5039
Fax: (415) 326–5512;
(415) 415–2182
Telex/E-mail: STEVEN READ
(DIALMAIL); MSDCEH02 (ORBIT)

**3809. St Elizabeth Hospital Medical
Center**
1044 Belmont Avenue
Youngstown
OH 44501
USA
Telephone: (216) 746–7211

3810. St Louis Post-Dispatch
900 N Tucker Boulevard
St Louis
MO 63101–9990
USA
Telephone: (314) 622–7148;
(314) 622–7000

3811. St Paul Pioneer Press Dispatch
345 Cedar Street
St Paul
MN 55101–1057
USA
Telephone: (612) 222–5011

3812. St Petersburg Times
PO Box 1121
St Petersburg
FL 33731
USA
Telephone: (813) 893–8111

**3813. Staatsbibliothek Preussischer
Kulturbesitz**
Postdamer Straß]e 33
1000 Berlin 30
Germany
Telephone: 49 (30) 2 66 – 24 78

**3814. Stadt- und Universitaets-
bibliothek Frankfurt**
Bockenheimer Landstrasse 134–138
6000 Frankfurt am Main 1
Germany
Telephone: 49 (69) 79 07 – 1;
49 (69) 79 07 – 235
Telex/E-mail: 4104 24 STUB D

3815. Staff Directories Ltd
Bruce Brownson
PO Box 62
Mount Vernon
VA 22121–0062
USA
Telephone: (703) 739–0900
Fax: (703) 739–0234

**3816. Staffordshire Open Learning
Centre**
Telephone: 0785 52313

3817. Stamm Publishing Ltd
389–810 W Broadway
Vancouver
BC V5Z 4C9
Canada
Telephone: (604) 873–4247
Fax: (604) 873–4347
Telex/E-mail: 04508338 REGENT VCR;
USSR BUSINESS MINDLINK.UUCP

**3818. Standard and Poor's
Compustat Services Inc**
Frank Hermes
7400 S Alton Court
Englewood
CO 80112
USA
Telephone: (303) 771–6510;
(800) 525–8640
Fax: (303) 740–4652;
(303) 740–4548

**3819. Standard and Poor's
Compustat Services**
John Fildes
Wimbledon Bridge House
1 Hartfield Road
London
SW19 3RU
UK
Telephone: 081 543–2555
Fax: 081 545–6292

**3820. Standard and Poor's
Corporation**
Lucy Llanos
25 Broadway
New York
NY 10004
USA
Telephone: (212) 208–0052;
(212) 208–8300
Fax: (212) 412–0498
Telex/E-mail: 226634

3821. Standard and Poor's/McGraw-Hill
25 Broadway
New York
NY 10004
USA
Telephone: (212) 208–8000;
(800) 233–2310
Telex/E-mail: 235145

3822. Standard International Consulting
12 place Henry Pate
F-75016 Paris
France
Telephone: 1 45 20 85 21
Fax: 1 47 07 20 47

3823. Standards Council of Canada
Standards Information Service
350 Sparks Street
Suite 1200
Ottawa
ON K1P 6N7
Canada
Telephone: (613) 238–3222;
(800) 267–8220 (in Canada)
Fax: (613) 995–4564
Telex/E-mail: 053 4403;
D.c.thompson (iNet)

3824. Stanton Library
Margaret Torrens; Ellen Forsyth
234 Miller Street
North Sydney
NSW 2060
Australia
Telephone: 02 955–5889
Fax: 02 954–5512

3825. Star Data Systems Inc
330 Bay Street
Suite 402
Toronto
ON M5H 2S8
Canada
Telephone: (416) 363–7827
Telex/E-mail: 06219661

3826. Star-Tribune, Newspaper of the Twin Cities
425 Portland Avenue
Minneapolis
MN 55488
USA
Telephone: (612) 372–4141

3827. Starch INRA Hooper Inc
566 E Boston Post Road
Mamaroneck
NY 10543
USA
Telephone: (914) 698–0800
Fax: (914) 698–0485
Telex/E-mail: 996637

3828. Starcom International Inc
One Marquis Plaza
5315 Campbells Run Road
Pittsburgh
PA 15205
USA
Telephone: (412) 788–3100;
(800) 441–9796
Telex/E-mail: 315960

3829. Startel Inc
PO Box 382
SF-00121 Helsinki
Finland
Telephone: 01 22 33 11
Fax: 01 22 48 75;
01 60 18 75
Telex/E-mail: 125368 SINFO SF;
12762: TBX232 (Dialcom)

3830. StarText
A division of the Fort Worth
Star-Telegram
400 W. 7th Street
PO Box 1870
Fort Worth
TX 76101
USA
Telephone: (817) 390–7463

3831. State Net
A service of Information for Public
Affairs
1900 14th Street
Sacramento
CA 95814
USA
Telephone: (916) 444–0840

3832. State-Record Company Inc, The
Stadium Road
PO Box 1333
Columbia
SC 29202
USA
Telephone: (803) 771–6161

3833. Statens arbetsgivarverk (SAV)
PO Box 2243
10 316 Stockholm
Sweden
Telephone: 46 (8) 796 93 16
Fax: 46 (8) 10 15 52

3834. Statens Husdyrbrugsforsoeg Biblioteket
Anne Mette Emdal
Postboks 139
8833 Oerum Soender Lyng
Denmark
Telephone: 45 (86) 652500

3835. Statens Museum for Kunst
Alena Marchwinski
Soelvgade 48–50
1307 Koebenhavn
Denmark
Telephone: 45 (33) 912126

3836. Statens Planteavlforsoegs Afd. for Biometri og Informatik
Ove Hansen; Kim Hansen
Lottenborgvej 24
2800 Lyngby
Denmark
Telephone: 45 (42) 870631

3837. States News Service
1333 F Street NW
4th Floor
Washington
DC 20004
USA
Telephone: (202) 628–3100

3838. Statewide Information Systems
c/o Prentice-Hall Online
1873 Western Avenue
Albany
NY 12203
USA
Telephone: (518) 458–8111
Fax: (714) 543–1879

3839. Statistica
10 boulevard Voltaire
F-75011 Paris
France
Telephone: 1 48 05 10 65
Fax: 1 43 38 34 90

3840. Statistical Bureau of Iceland
Mr Snorrason
Hagstofa Islands
Skuggasundi 3
150 Reykjavik
Iceland
Telephone: +354 (1) 6098 00
Fax: +354 (1) 6288 65

3841. Statistics Canada
Library
RH Coates Building
2nd Floor
Ottawa
ON K1A 0T6
Telephone: (613) 951–8218
Fax: (613) 951–0939
Telex/E-mail: I11:OOS (Envoy 100)

3842. Statistics Canada
Electronic Data Dissemination Division
Marie Parij
RH Coats Building
9th Floor
Tunney's Pasture
Ottawa
ON K1A 0T6
Canada
Telephone: (613) 951–8200
Fax: (613) 951–1134;
(613) 951–8093
Telex/E-mail: 0533585

3843. Statsbiblioteket
Henning Midtgaard
Universitetsparken
8000 Aarhus C
Denmark
Telephone: 45 (86) 122022

3844. Statutes Office of State of Minnesota
700 State Office Building
100 Constitution Ave.
St. Paul
MN 55155–1297
USA
Telephone: (612) 296–2868
Fax: (612) 296–0569

3845. Stazione Sperimentale del Vetro
Pool d'Abstracts
Via Briati 10
30141 Murano (Venezia)
Italy
Telephone: 39 (41) 73 94 22
Fax: 39 (41) 73 94 20
Telex/E-mail: 431447 SPEVET I

3846. Sterling Resources Inc
Robert Klatsky
10 Forest Avenue
Paramus
NJ 07652
USA
Telephone: (201) 368 8725
Fax: (201) 368 9024

3847. Stevens Features
15 Breckinridge Road
Chappaqua
NY 10514
USA
Telephone: (914) 238–3569

3848. Stewart Data Services
11 Broadway
Suite 1768
New York
NY 10004
USA
Telephone: (212) 344–9600

3849. Stichting Nederlandse Informatie Managers Combinatie
PO Box 36
NL-2600 AA Delft
Netherlands
Telephone: 03115 696–800
Fax: 03115 560–825
Telex/E-mail: 38071 ZPTNO NL;
  01520 (ESA/IRS); 737,3 (Chemical
  Information Systems Inc (CIS));
  10141 (DIALMAIL)

3850. STICS Inc
9714 S Rice Avenue
Houston
TX 77096
USA
Telephone: (713) 499–3932;
  (713) 723–3949

3851. Stiftelsen Affärsvarlden
PO Box 1234
S-111 82 Stockholm
Sweden
Telephone: 08 796–6500

3852. Stiftelsen LOVDATA
Niels Juels gate 16
N-0272 Oslo 2
Norway
Telephone: 02 449–773
Fax: 02 558–628

3853. STI
4 Kings Meadow
Ferry Hinksey Road
Oxford
OX2 0DU
UK
Telephone: 0865 798–898
Fax: 0865 798–788
Telex/E-mail: 825059 G

3854. Stjernquist Foretagskonsulter
Magnus Ladulasgatan 53
11627 Stockholm
Sweden
Telephone: 46 (8) 720 03 21
Fax: 46 (8) 20 03 24

3855. STM Systems Corporation
WISDOM Information Services
2300 St Laurent Boulevard
Ottawa
ON K1G 4K1
Canada
Telephone: (613) 737–7373
Fax: (613) 737–9479
Telex/E-mail: (800) 267–7018

3856. STN International
c/o Fachinformationszentrum Energie,
  Physik, Mathematik GmbH
7514 Eggenstein-Leopoldshafen 2
Germany
Telephone: 49 (7247) 82 45 66
Telex/E-mail: 7826487 FIZE D

3857. STN International
Fachinformationszentrum Karlsruhe
PO Box 2465
7500 Karlsruhe 1
Germany
Telephone: 07247 808–555
Fax: 07247 808–666
Telex/E-mail: 17724710+;
  7826487 FIZE D
NUA: 26245724790114

3858. STN International
Japan Association for International
  Chemical Information
Gakkai Center Building
2–4–16 Yayoi
Bunkyo-ku
Tokyo 113
Japan

3859. STN International
c/o Chemical Abstracts Service
2540 Olentangy River Road
PO Box 3012
Columbus
OH 43210
USA
Telephone: (614) 447–3600;
  (800) 848–6533
Fax: (614) 447–3713
Telex/E-mail: 6842086 CHMAB

3860. Stock Exchange (London)
Information Services Division
London
EC2N 1NP
UK
Telephone: 071 588–2355

3861. Stockholm School of Economics
Library
Box 6501
113 83 Stockholm
Sweden
Telephone: 46 (8) 736 01 20

3863. Strategic Mapping
UK
Telephone: 081 994–2780
Fax: 081 994–4467

3864. Strategic Planning Institute
1030 Massachusetts Avenue
Cambridge
MA 02138
USA
Telephone: (617) 491–9200
Fax: (617) 491–1634
Telex/E-mail: 710 320 0893

3865. Stratus
Cherril Smith
Dolina 55
62–081 Przezmierowo
Poznan
Poland
Telephone: +48 61 238998
Fax: +48 61 411760

3866. StreetSense
641 Lexington Avenue
7th Floor
New York
NY 10043
USA
Telephone: (212) 303–0248;
  (800) 241–2476

3867. STSC Inc
2115 E Jefferson Street
Rockville
MD 20852
USA
Telephone: (301) 984–5000;
  (800) 592–0050
Telex/E-mail: 710 828 9790 STSC RO

3868. Studstrup and Oestgaard
Jens Ove Skjaerbaek
Postboks 154
9100 Aalborg
Denmark
Telephone: 45 (98) 188133

3869. Studsvik Biblioteket
S-611 82 Nykoeping
Sweden
Telephone: 0155 21000
Fax: 0155 63044
Telex/E-mail: 64070 STUBIB S

3870. Suicide Information and Education Center
1615 10th Avenue SW
Suite 201
Calary
AB T3C 0J7
Canada
Telephone: (403) 245–3900

3871. Sun Microsystems Ltd
Andrew C MacRae; Dan Gauthier
Watchmoor Park
Riverside Way
Camberley
Surrey
GU15 3YL
UK

3872. Sun Moon Star Group, USA
Michael Wu
1941 Ringwood Avenue
San Jose
CA 95131
USA
Telephone: (408) 452 7811
Fax: (408) 452 1411

3873. SUNIST
Mr Jean Louis Duclos
Parc d'Affaires Saint-Hubert
64 rue du Creuzat
BP 112
F-38081 L'Isle d'Abeau Cedex
France
Telephone: 74 27 28 10
NUA: 2080138001731

3874. SunShine
Steven Schwarzman
PO Box 4351
Austin
TX 78765
USA
Telephone: (512) 453 2334

3875. Suntory Ltd
Distribution Systems Services Section
  Information Division
1–2–3 Motoakasa
Minato-Ku
Tokyo 107
Japan
Telephone: +81 3 3423 1159
Fax: +81 3 3423 9727

3876. Suomen Standardisoimislitto
Information Service
PO Box 205
Bulevardi 5 A 7
SF-00121 Helsinki
Finland
Telephone: 0 645601
Fax: 0 643147
Telex/E-mail: 122303 STAND SF

3877. Surplus Record Information Services
20 N Wacker Drive
Chicago
IL 60606
USA
Telephone: (312) 372–9077

3878. Survey Research Hong Kong Ltd
Paul Hashfield
7th Floor
Warwick House, East Wing
28 Tong Chong Street
Quarry Bay
Hong Kong
Telephone: 5880–3388
Fax: 565–0418
Telex/E-mail: 65122 SRHHX

3879. Survey Research Indonesia
Jalan Nusu Indah 9, Tomang
Tromol POS 3020
Jakarta Barat
Indonesia
Telephone: 62 (21) 591729
Telex/E-mail: 46331 SAHID JKT IA

3880. Survey Research Malaysia Sdn. Bhd.
63c Wisma Kimtoo, 3rd Floor
Jalan Loke Yew
PO Box 12231
50943 Kuala Lumpur
Malaysia
Telephone: 60 (3) 2486122
Telex/E-mail: 30077 ESAREM MA

3881. Survey Research Singapore (Pte) Ltd
51 Newton Road
09–01/12 Goldhill Plaza
Singapore 1130
Singapore
Telephone: 252–8595
Telex/E-mail: 24546 SRS RS

3882. Svensk Byggtjanst
S-171 88 Solna
Sweden
Telephone: 08 734–5000
Fax: 08 734–5099
Telex/E-mail: 8125070 SVEBYGG S

3883. Svensk Konstvetenskaplig Bibliografi
Bastionsplatsen 2
S-411 08 Goeteborg
Sweden
Telephone: 031 634–700
Fax: 031 634–703

3884. Svenska Dagbladet
Ralambsvagen 7
S-105 17 Stockholm
Sweden
Telephone: 08 135–000

3885. Sveriges Tekniska Attacheer
PO Box 5282
S-102 46 Stockholm
Sweden
Telephone: 08 796–7640
Fax: 08 796–7649
Telex/E-mail: 15367 STATT S

3886. Sveriges Verkstadsfoerening
PO Box 5510
S-114 85 Stockholm
Sweden
Telephone: 08 782–0800
Fax: 08 782–0966
Telex/E-mail: 17045 SWEMET S

3887. SVP France
54 rue de Monceau
F-75384 Paris Cedex 8
France
Telephone: 1 47 87 11 11
Fax: 1 45 63 46 95
Telex/E-mail: SVPFR 650 453F;
20128 (DIALMAIL)

3888. Sweden Allmanna Reklamationsnamnden
Box 523
S-162 15 Vaellingby
Sweden
Telephone: 08 759–8550
Fax: 08 759–6211

3889. Sweden Domstolsverket
Kyrkogatan 34
S-551 81 Joenkoeping
Sweden
Telephone: 036 155–300

3890. Sweden Justitiedepartementet
S-103 33 Stockholm
Sweden
Telephone: 08 763–4780

3891. Sweden Kriminalvaardsstyrelsen
S-601 80 Norrkoping
Sweden
Telephone: 011 193–000

3892. Sweden National Board oof Health and Welfare
Department of Drugs
PO Box 607
S-751 25 Uppsala
Sweden
Telephone: 018 174–600

3893. Sweden Riksdagens Upplysningstjanst Registersektionen
S-100 12 Stockholm
Sweden
Telephone: 08 786–4000
Fax: 08 209–573

3894. Sweden Riksskatteverket
S-171 94 Solna
Sweden
Telephone: 08 764–8000

3895. Sweden Socialstyrelsen
S-103 Stockholm 13
Sweden
Telephone: 08 700–1300

3896. Sweden Statens Psykologisk-Pedagogiska Bibliotek
PO Box 50063
Frescati Hagvag 10
S-104 05 Stockholm
Sweden
Telephone: 08 151–820

3897. Sweden Statens Vag- och Trafikinstitut
Information and Documentation Section
S-581 01 Linkoping
Sweden
Telephone: 013 204–000
Fax: 013 141–436
Telex/E-mail: 50125 VTISGI S

3898. Sweden Tullverket
Box 2267
S-103 17 Stockholm
Sweden
Telephone: 08 789–7300

3899. Swedish Center for Technical Terminology
Kiell Westerberg
Vastra Vagen 9C
S-171 46 Solna
Sweden
Telephone: 08 735–8525
Fax: 08 273–286

3900. Swedish Council for Information on Alcohol and Other Drugs
Documentation Center
PO Box 27302
10254 Stockholm
Sweden
Telephone: 08 67 97 20
Fax: 08 661 64 84

3901. Swedish Institute of Building Documentation
Halsingegatan 49
113 31 Stockholm
Sweden
Telephone: 46 (8) 34 01 70
Fax: 46 (8) 32 48 59
Telex/E-mail: 12563 BYGGDOK S

3902. Swedish National Chemicals Inspectorate
PO Box 1384
171 27 Solna
Sweden
Telephone: 46 (8) 730 57 00
Fax: 46 (8) 735 76 98
Telex/E-mail: 10460 AMS S

3903. Swedish National Institute of Occupational Health
Library
171 84 Solna
Sweden
Telephone: 46 (8) 730 91 00
Fax: 46 (8) 730 19 67
Telex/E-mail: 15816 ARBSKY S

3904. Swedish Post Office
Skeppargen 90
Stockholm 11530
Sweden
Telephone: 46 8 664 6665

3905. Swedish Statens Naturvardsverk
Library and Documentation Section
Box 1302
S-171 25 Solna
Sweden
Telephone: 08 799–1000
Telex/E-mail: 11131 ENVIRON S

3906. Sweet & Maxwell Ltd
Anthony Kinakan Homa Wyatt
South Quay Plaza
183 Marsh Wall
London
E14 9FT
UK
Telephone: 071 538–8686
Fax: 071 538–9508

3907. Sweet's Group McGraw Hill Inc
T J Cardenas
1221 Avenue of the Americas
18th Floor
New York
NY 10020
USA
Telephone: (212) 512–1000;
(800) 848–9002
Fax: (212) 512 2908

3908. Swiss PTT
P. Boesiger
Viktoriastrasse 21
3030 Bern
Switzerland

3909. UN Advisory Committee for the Coordination of Information Systems
Palais des Nations
CH-1211 Geneva 10
Switzerland
Telephone: 022 988–591
Fax: 022 7401–1269
Telex/E-mail: 412912 CH; 289696 CH

3910. Sydjysk Universitets
Edith Clausen
Sydjysk Universitetscenter Biblioteket
Glentevej 7
6705 Esberg Oe
Denmark
Telephone: 45 (75) 140011

3911. Sydney Conservatorium Software Development Centre
Dennis Patterson
Macquarie Street
Sydney
NSW 2000
Australia
Telephone: 61–2–230–1222
Fax: 61–2–252–1243

3912. Sydney Stock Exchange
Research Department
20 Bond Street, 20th Floor
Sydney
NSW 2000
Australia
Telephone: 61 (2) 231–0066
Telex/E-mail: 20630 AA

3913. Syracuse Language Systems Inc.
719 East Genesee St.
Syracuse
NY 13210
USA
Telephone: (315) 478–6729
Fax: (315) 478–6902

3914. Syracuse Research Corporation
Life and Environmental Sciences Division
Merrill Lane
Syracuse
NY 13210
USA
Telephone: (315) 425–5100
Fax: (315) 425–1339

3915. Systemas Logicos (SilverPlatter Agent)
Fernando Rodriquez
Canales & Co
2019 Jefferson Street
Laredo TX 78040
USA
Telephone: (525) 254–5052

3916. Systems Educational Associates Inc
616 Enterprise Drive
Oak Brook
IL 60521
USA
Telephone: (312) 832–3838

3917. SZ – Saarbruecker Zeitung
Gutenbergstrasse 11–23
W-6600 Saarbruecken
Germany
Telephone: +49 681–5020
NUA: Available on application

3918. Taft Group, The
12300 Twinbrook Parkway
Suite 450
Rockville
MD 20852
USA
Telephone: (301) 816–0210

3919. Take 1 Productions
Leon Klinkers
Ganseweide 167
6413 GD Heerlen
Netherlands
Telephone: +31 45 225783
Fax: +31 45 212263

3920. Tandem Computers Inc
European Headquarters
CD-ROM Enquiries
Van Heuven Goedhartiann 935
1181 LD Amstelveen
Netherlands
Telephone: +31 20 54 4911
Fax: +31 20 643 6698

3921. Tandem Computers
Kim Taddeo
19333 Vallco Parkway
Cupertino
CA 95014–2599
USA
Telephone: (408) 285 6000

3922. Tandy Corporation
1800 One Tandy Center
Fort Worth
TX 76102
USA
Telephone: (817) 390–3700
Fax: (817) 390–2774

3923. Tanner Dokuments
Siegfried Minke; Catrin Eifert
Bregenzer Strasse 11–13
8990 Lindau (B)
Germany
Telephone: +49 8382 25084
Fax: +49 8382 25024

3924. TASS English Language News Service
50 Rockefeller Plaza
New York
NY 10020
USA
Telephone: (212) 245–4250

3925. TASS News Agency
Tverskoy bul 10
Moscow
Russia
Telephone: 095 229–8053

3926. TASS Press Agency
c/o Pergamon Press Limited
Headington Hill Hall
Oxford
OX3 0BW
UK
Telephone: 44 (865) 64881
Fax: 44 (865) 60285
Telex/E-mail: 83117 G

3927. Tate & Lyle
PO Box 68
Whiteknights
Reading
Berkshire
RG6 2BX
UK
Telephone: 44 (734) 861361
Fax: 44 (734) 867767
Telex/E-mail: 847915 G

3928. Tate Telex and Continuous Stationery Limited
47 Burners Lane South
Kiln Farm
Milton Keynes
Buckinghamshire
MK11 3HD
UK
Telephone: 44 (908) 567687
Fax: 44 (908) 564622
Telex/E-mail: 826932 G

3929. Tax Analysts
Ellie Kasten
6830 N Fairfax Drive
Arlington
VA 22213
USA
Telephone: (703) 532–1850;
(800) 336–0439

3930. Tax Management Inc
A subsidiary of the Bureau of National Affairs Inc
1231 25th Street, NW
Washington
DC 20037
USA
Telephone: (202) 452–4132

3931. TB – Telebroker
Luis Garcia Alonso
Venezuela 8
I-Izda
E-28014 Madrid
Spain
Telephone: +34 1–5228685
Fax: +34 1–5229032
NUA: Available on application

3932. TBD Time Sharing
Telematica e Bancos de Dados lda
Mrs Manuela Sola Castro
Rua Almeida Brandeo, 24 A
PT-1200 Lisbon
Portugal
Telephone: +351 1–603181
Telex/E-mail: 15823
NUA: 2680060100313

3933. TBS-Britannica Company Ltd
Hiroko Tabata
28–1 Sanbancho
Chiyoda-ku
Tokyo 102
Japan
Telephone: +81 3 3238 5836
Fax: +81 3 3238 5810

3934. TD-Finans
PO Box 140 Sentrum
N-0102 Oslo 1
Norway
Telephone: 02 33 43 90
Fax: 02 41 34 84

3935. Technical Advisory Service Inc
1166 DeKalb Pike
Blue Bell
PA 19422
USA
Telephone: (215) 275–8272;
(800) 523–2319
Fax: (215) 643–5557

3936. Technical Data Global Markets Group
A division of Thomson Financial Networks
11 Farnsworth Street
Boston
MA 02210
USA
Telephone: (617) 345–2400
Fax: (617) 426–3957

Addresses

3937. Technical Data Resources
5700 Executive Center Drive, Suite 200
Charlotte
NC 28212
USA
Telephone: (704) 568–5854

3938. Technical Database Services Inc
10 Columbus Circle
Suite 2300
New York
NY 10019
USA
Telephone: (212) 245–0044
Fax: (212) 247–0587
Telex/E-mail: 6714962

3939. Technical Indexes Ltd
Willoughby Road
Bracknell
Berkshire
RG12 4DW
UK
Telephone: 0344 426311
Fax: 0344 424971

3940. Technical Insights Inc
PO Box 1304
Fort Lee
NJ 07024–9967
USA
Telephone: (201) 568–4744
Fax: (201) 568–8247
Telex/E-mail: 425900 SWIFT UI

3941. Technical Research Centre of Finland (VTT)
Information Service
PO Box 42
SF-02151 Espoo
Finland
Telephone: +358 0 43561
Fax: +358 0 4554073
Telex/E-mail: 125175

3942. Technical Services Associates Inc (TSA)
Jim Brasleman; Dave Wilson
2 Market Plaza Way
Mechanicsburg
PA 17055
USA
Telephone: (717) 691 5691
Fax: (717) 691 5690

3943. Technion Research & Development Foundation Ltd
Senate House
Technion City
32000 Haifa
Israel
Telephone: 04 292–917
Fax: 04 221–581

3944. Technische Universitaet Berlin
Institut für Krankenhausbau
Dokumentation Krankenhauswesen
Strasse des 17. Juni 135
1000 Berlin 12
Germany
Telephone: 49 (30) 3 14 23 905
Fax: 49 (30) 3 14 23 222
Telex/E-mail: 184262 TUBLN D

3945. Technologie-Centrum Hannover GmbH
CS China-Service GmbH
Vahrenwalder Strasse 7
3000 Hannover 1
Germany
Telephone: 49 (511) 4 82 02
Fax: 49 (511) 356–3100

3946. Technology Access
7 Mount Lassen Drive
Suite D251
San Rafael
CA 94903
USA
Telephone: (415) 507–0190;
(800) 733–1516
Fax: (415) 507–0661
Telex/E-mail: 76236,1330 (CompuServe Information Service); 369–9038 (MCI Mail)

3947. Technology Resources Inc
PO Box H
Yardly
PA 19067
USA
Telephone: (215) 428–1060

3948. Technomic Information Service Inc
Sun Building, 7 Tomizawacho 8
Nihonbashi
Tokyo 103
Japan
Telephone: 81 (3) 666–2952
Fax: 81 (3) 666–2730
Telex/E-mail: 2524851 J

3949. Tecnobyte Studio
Ing P Spinoglio
Via Aladino Govoni 16
00136 Rome
Italy
Telephone: +39 6 3453442
Fax: +39 6 343121

3950. Tecnologias e Servicos de Telecomunicacoes sa
Rua Joao de Barros 265
4100 Porto
Portugal
Telephone: 02 610–1400
Fax: 02 610–1420
Telex/E-mail: 24793 SOTEIN P

3951. TECNON (UK) Ltd
12 Calico House
Plantation Wharf
York Place
Battersea
London
SW11 3TN
UK
Telephone: 071 924–3955
Fax: 071 978–5307
Telex/E-mail: 28521 TECNON G

3952. Teenage Research Unlimited
601 Skokie Boulevard
Northbrook
IL 60062
USA
Telephone: (708) 564–3440
Fax: (708) 564–3641

3953. Teikoku Databank Ltd
5–20 Minami Aoyama 2–Chome
Minato-ku
Tokyo 107
Japan
Telephone: 03 3404–4311

3954. Tekniikan Sanastokeskus ry
Soernaisten rantatie 25
SF-00500 Helsinki
Finland
Telephone: 08 731–5206
Fax: 08 731–9583

3955. Teknillinen Korkeakoulu
Laskentakeskus
Otakaari 1
SF-02150 Espoo
Finland
Telephone: 0 451–4340
Fax: 0 465–077
Telex/E-mail: 121591 TKK SF

3956. Teknillisen Korkeakoulun Kirjasto
Otaniementie 9
SF-02150 Espoo
Finland
Telephone: 0 451–4112
Fax: 0 451–4132
Telex/E-mail: 121591 TKK SF

3957. Tekniska Nomenklaturcentralen
Vastra Vagen 9C
S-171 46 Solna
Sweden
Telephone: 08 7358525

3958. Tekron Publications Limited
Tekron House
Small Business Industrial Estate
Hall Lane
Walton-on-Naze
Essex
CO14 8HT
UK
Telephone: 44 (255) 677868

3959. Tel Aviv University
The Dayan Center for Middle Eastern and African Studies
Shiloah Institute
Ramat-Aviv
Tel Aviv 69978
Israel
Telephone: 972 (3) 545–9993
Telex/E-mail: 342171 VERSY IL

3960. TELDAN Advanced Systems Limited
Asher Sofrin Dan Karmi
7 Derekh Hashalom
Tel Aviv 67892
Israel
Telephone: 972 3 9650 073
Fax: 972 3 9656 359
Telex/E-mail: 361579 CODE IL

3961. Tele Atlas Nederland BV
D.H.M. van Rijn
Postbus 420
Stationsplein 27
's-Hertogenbosch
Netherlands
Telephone: (+31) 073–125000

3962. Télé Consulte
Bernard Desolneux
44 rue du Four
75006 Paris
France
Telephone: 33 (1) 43 20 15 60
Fax: 33 (1) 42 84 11 08
Telex/E-mail: 021850 F

3963. Tele-Direct Publications Inc
A subsidiary of Bell Canada
Peter Dolan
55 Town Centre Street CTR CT
Scarborough
Ontario
M1P 4X5
Canada
Telephone: +1 416 296 4429
Fax: +1 416 296 5506

3964. Tele-Info Verlag GmbH
Rolf Cotthardt
Carl Zeiss Strasse 27
3008 Garbsen 4
Germany
Telephone: +49 5131 7000 17
Fax: +49 5131 7000 15

3965. Tele-tech Services
PO Box 757
McAfee
NJ 07428
USA
Telephone: (201) 827–4421;
(800) 443–6181
Fax: (201) 827–2908

3966. Tele/Scope Networks Inc
227 W 29th Street
5th Floor
New York
NY 10001
USA
Telephone: (212) 714–1300;
(800) 827–2673
Fax: (212) 714–9521
Telex/E-mail: 668298;
14062 (DIALMAIL)

3967. Telebase Systems Inc
763 W Lancaster Avenue
Bryn Mawr
PA 19010–9934
USA
Telephone: (215) 526–2800;
(800) 421–7616
Fax: (215) 527–1956

3968. Telebroker SA
Luis Garcia Alonso
Calle Valenzuela 8, 1–Izda
28014 Madrid
Spain
Telephone: 01 522–8685
Fax: 01 522–9032
Telex/E-mail: 45480 E

3969. Telecity CD-I NV
Mr Bochoce
Maastrichterstraat 63
3500 Hasselt
Belgium
Telephone: +32 11 24 21 67
Fax: +32 11 24 21 68

3970. Telecom Gold
60–68 St. Thomas Street
London
SE1 3QU
UK
Telephone: 071 403–6777
Telex/E-mail: 894001 TLGOLD G
NUA: 23421920100479

3971. Telecom Gold
42 Weston Street
London
SE1 3QD
UK
Telephone: 071 403–6777
Telex/E-mail: 894001 TLGOLD G
NUA: 23421920100479

3972. Telecom Publishing Group
A division of Capitol Publications Inc
1101 King Street, Suite 444
Alexandria
VA 22314
USA
Telephone: (703) 683–4100
Fax: (703) 739–6490
Telex/E-mail: 62928442

3973. Telecommunications Association
Yarakucho
Chiyoda-ku
Tokyo 100
Japan
Telephone: 81 (3) 215–5727

3974. Telecommunications Cooperative Network
505 8th Avenue
Suite 1805
New York
NY 10018
USA
Telephone: (212) 714–9780

3975. Telecommunications Reports
1333 H Street NW
11th Floor
West Tower
Washington
DC 20005
USA
Telephone: (202) 842–3006
Fax: (202) 842–3047

3976. Telecue Systems
62 Knollwood Road
Huntington
NY 11743
USA
Telephone: (516) 549–5911

3977. Teledata Srl Database Group
Paolo Scafati; Fulvio Duse
Via Cavour 33
00040 Pomexia
Italy
Telephone: +39 6 9108259
Fax: +39 6 9125275

3978. Teledata
Netdivisionen, NVT
Noerregade 21
1199 Koebenhavn K
Denmark
Telephone: 45 (38) 993970

3979. Teleflora Technologies
Teleflora Plaza
12233 Olympic Boulevard
Los Angeles
CA 90064
USA
Telephone: (800) 321–2654

3980. Telekurs (North America) Inc
3 River Bend Center
Stamford
CT 06907
USA
Telephone: (203) 353–8100
Fax: (203) 353–8152

3981. Telekurs AG
Hardturmstraße 201
CH-8021 Zurich
Switzerland
Telephone: 01 279–2111
Fax: 01 271–8010
Telex/E-mail: 823548 CH

3982. Telekurs
Cityfax
London
UK
Telephone: 071 256–6143

3983. Telemaco srl
SEAT Divisione STET SpA
Viale del Policlinico 147
I-00161 Rome
Italy
Telephone: 06 84941
Fax: 06 849–4421
Telex/E-mail: 212248 I

3984. Telematica e Bancos de Dados, LDA
Rua Almeida Brandao 24 A
1200 Lisbon
Portugal
Telephone: 351 (1) 60 81 56
Fax: 351 (1) 66 70 12

3985. Telematique Services et Logiciels
37 rue du Moulin
F-94210 St Maur
France
Telephone: 1 48 83 49 26

3986. Telephassa
Tilburg University Library
Mrs. Ellie Vermeer
PO Box 90153
5000 LE Tilburg
Netherlands
Fax: 31 13 662996

3987. Telerate Systems Inc
Harboreside Financial Center
600 Plaza Two
Jersey City
NJ 07311
USA
Telephone: (201) 860–4000

3988. Telescan Inc
2900 Wilcrest
Suite 400
Houston
TX 77042
USA
Telephone: (713) 952–1060

3989. Teleset Ltd
Charlton House
Chester Road
Old Trafford
Manchester
M16 0GW
UK
Telephone: 061 873 8282
Fax: 061 873 8416

3990. Teletel
Direction des Affaires Commerciales et Telematiques
20 avenue de Segur
F-75005 Paris
France
Telephone: 1 45 64 22 22

3991. Televerket
Torsten Olofson
Kryddgrand 6
Hokarangen
S-12386 Farsta
Sweden
Telephone: 46–8–713–7185

3992. Telex-Verlag Jaeger + Waldmann GmbH
Hans J Driess (CD-ROM Project Manager)
PO Box 111454
6100 Darmstadt 11
Germany
Telephone: 06151 33020
Fax: 06151 330–250;
06151 391–200
Telex/E-mail: 419548 DAV D

3993. Telmar Communications Limited
87 Jermyn Street
London
SW1Y 6JD
UK
Telephone: 071 930–6487

Addresses

3994. Telmar Group Inc
902 Broadway
New York
NY 10010
USA
Telephone: (212) 460–9000
Fax: (212) 460–9796

3995. Telmed
Claudine Magnin-Leuthold
rue Pedro-Meylan 7
Case Postale 260
1211 Geneva 17
Switzerland
Telephone: 41–1–432–04–67
Fax: 41–1–432–45–25

3996. Termfact Limited
447 Berwick Avenue
Mont-Royal
PQ H3R 1Z8
Canada

3997. TerraLogics Inc
Matthew Goldworm
114 Daniel Webster Highway South
Suite 256
Nashua
NH 03060
USA
Telephone: (603) 889 1800
Fax: (603) 880 2022

3998. Terry Biener
53 Brook Road
Valley Stream
NY 11581
USA

3999. Tescor Inc
Scott Buchanan
105B Douglas Court
Sterling
VA 22091
USA
Telephone: (703) 318 7064
Fax: (703) 318 7319

4000. Teton Data Systems
John Eastman
235 East Broadway
PO 3082
Jackson
WY 83001
USA
Telephone: (307) 733 5494
Fax: (307) 733 9258

4001. Tetragon Systems
Charles DeMartigny
5455 Pare Suite 102–2
Montreal
PQ H4P 1R1
Canada
Telephone: (514) 737–3550;
(800) 363–2372

4002. Texas A & M University
Sterling C Evans Library
Reference Division
College Station
TX 77843
USA
Telephone: (409) 845–5741

4003. Texas A & M University
Thermodynamics Research Center
Texas Engineering Experiment Station
College Station
TX 77843–3111
USA
Telephone: (409) 845–4940
Telex/E-mail: KNM5936 TAMSIGMA
(BITNET)

4004. Texas Caviar
Richard Smith
3933 Spicewood Springs Road
Suite E-100
Austin
Texas
TX 78759
USA
Telephone: (512) 346–7887
Fax: (512) 346–1393

4005. Texas Student Publications
University of Texas
PO Box D
Austin
TX 73713–7209
USA
Telephone: (515) 471–1865

4006. TFPL
22 Peter's Lane
London
EC1M 6DS
UK
Telephone: 071 251–5522
Fax: 071 251–8318

4008. Thermo Calc
Bo Sundman
Thermo Calc Gruppen Institutionen foer
Metallografi
Division of Physical Metallurgy
Royal Institute of Technology
10044 Stockholm
Sweden
Telephone: 46 (8) 787–9140
NUA: 240200101926

4009. Thermodata Association
THERMODATA
Mr Daniel
BP 66
F-38402 St Martin d'Heres Cedex
France
Telephone: 76 42 76 90
Telex/E-mail: RCHEYNET FRGEN81
(BITNET)
NUA: 208038020100; 208038020101

**4010. Thesaurus Linguae Graecae
(TLG)**
Betsy Shanor; T Brunner
TLG Project
University of California
Irvine
CA 92717
USA
Telephone: (714) 856–7031
Fax: (714) 856–8434

**4011. Thiede & Thiede
Mittelständische
Systemberatung GmbH**
Bereich Verlag
Kurfürstendamm 72
D-1000 Berlin 31
Germany
Telephone: 030 324–2096

4012. Thieme Verlag
Post Office 104853
Stuttgart 7000
Germany
Telephone: 49–711–89–310
Fax: 49–711–893–12–98

4013. Thomas Nelson Publishers
Nelson Place at Elm Hill Pike
PO Box 141000
Nashville
TN 37214–1000
USA
Telephone: (615) 889–9000

4014. Thomas Publishing Company
Gary Craig
One Penn Plaza
250 W 34th Street
New York
NY 10119
USA
Telephone: (212) 290–7291
Fax: (212) 290–7362
Telex/E-mail: 14016 (DIALMAIL)

4015. Thompson Henry Ltd
London Road
Sunningdale
Berkshire
SL5 0EP
UK
Telephone: 0344 24615
Fax: 0344 26120

4016. Thomson & Thomson
500 Victory Road
North Quincy
MA 02171–1545
USA
Telephone: (617) 479–1600;
(800) 692–8833;
(800) 338–1867
(in Canada)
Fax: (617) 786–8273;
(800) 543–1983
Telex/E-mail: 6971430;
11541 (DIALMAIL)

**4017. Thomson Financial Networks
Inc**
11 Farnsworth Street
Boston
MA 02210
USA
Telephone: (617) 330–7878
Fax: (617) 350–5011;
(617) 426–3957
Telex/E-mail: 466199

4018. Thorn EMI
Hugh Simmons
Highfield House
Foundation Park
8 Roxborough Way
Maidenhead
Berks.
SL6 3TZ
UK
Telephone: 0628 822181
Fax: 0628 822865

4019. Thorn EMI
8601 Dunwoody Place
Atlanta
GA 30338
USA
Telephone: (404) 587–0017

**4020. Three Sigma Research Center
Inc**
219 E 42nd Street
New York
NY 10017
USA
Telephone: (212) 867–1414

**4021. Throgmorton 85 (Publishing)
Ltd**
38 Ravenna Road
London
SW15 6AW
UK
Telephone: 071 785–6272

4022. Tidningarnas Telegrambyra AB
Kungsholmstorg 5
S-105 12 Stockholm
Sweden
Telephone: 08 13 26 00
Telex/E-mail: 19168 TTSTH S

4023. Tieteellisten Kirjastojen ATK-yksikko
Automation Unit of Finnish Research
  Libraries
PO Box 312
SF-00171 Helsinki
Finland
Telephone: 0 708–4298
Fax: 0 753–9514
Telex/E-mail: 122785 TSK SF

4024. Tietotehdas Oy
Nihtisillantie 1
PO Box 33
SF-02631 Espoo
Finland
Telephone: 0 5261
Fax: 0 526–2488
Telex/E-mail: 121712 SF

4025. Tiger Media Europe
Patrick Gibbins
PO Box 481
London
SW12 8LU
UK
Telephone: +44 71 702 4524
Fax: +44 71 702 4507

4026. Tiger Media
Ann Lediaev
5801 East Slauson
Suite 200
Los Angeles
CA 90040
USA
Telephone: (213) 721 8282
Fax: (213) 721 8336

4027. Tiger Publications
PO Box 8759
Amarillo
TX 79114
USA
Telephone: (806) 655–2009

4028. Tijl Data BV
Blaloweg 20
NL-8041 AH Zwolle
Netherlands
Telephone: 038 27 56 01;
        038 27 52 75
Fax: 038 21 37 32
Telex/E-mail: 42123 NL

4029. Tilburg University Library
Excerpta Informatica Documentation
  Centre
PO Box 90153
NL-5000 LE Tilburg
Netherlands
Telephone: 013 662–637
Fax: 013 662–996
Telex/E-mail: 52426 KHT NL

4030. Time Inc
Time-Life Building
New York
NY 10020
USA
Telephone: (212) 522–1212;
        (212) 522–5196;
        (212) 522–4944

4031. Time-Sharing SA
Direccao de Valor Acrescentado
Rua Castilho 39–13A
1200 Lisbon
Portugal
Telephone: 01 573–522
Fax: 01 578–361

4032. Timefame Epnitex plc
PO Box 107
Billinghay
Lincoln
LN4 4AW
UK

4033. Timeplace Inc
460 Totten Pond Road
Waltham
MA 02154
USA
Telephone: (617) 890–4636;
        (800) 544–4023
Fax: (617) 890–7274

4034. Times Magazine Development Group
David McGowan; Anne Newgarden
Time & Life Building, Room 2725
1271 Avenue of the Americas
New York
NY 10020
USA
Telephone: (212) 522 4944

4035. Times Mirror Company
Times Mirror Square
Los Angeles
CA 90012
USA
Telephone: (213) 237–5000

4036. Times Network Systems
Richard Gray
Priory House
St. John's Lane
London
EC1M 4BX
UK
Telephone: 071 782–7143
Fax: 071 782–7111

4037. Times Newspapers Limited
News International
1 Virginia Street
London
E1
UK
Telephone: 071 481–4100

4038. Times Publishing Company
Times Square
12th and Sassafrass Streets
Erie
PA 16534
USA
Telephone: (814) 456–8531

4039. Times Publishing Company
490 First Avenue S
St Petersburg
FL 33701
USA
Telephone: (813) 893–8111

4040. Times-Picayune Publishing Corporation
3800 Howard Avenue
New Orleans
LA 70140
USA
Telephone: (504) 826–3275

4041. Titus Software Corporation
Louis Beatty
28 ter Avenue de Versailles
93220 Gagny
France
Telephone: +33 1 43 32 10 92
Fax: +33 1 43 32 11 52

4042. Titus Software corporation
Michael Vupillat, CEO
20432 Corisco Street
Chatsworth
CA 91311
USA
Telephone: (818) 709 3692
Fax: (818) 709 6537

4043. TMM Inc
Total Multimedia
Daniel Shields
299 West Hillcrest Drive
Suite 106
Thousand Oaks
CA 91360
USA
Telephone: (805) 371 0500
Fax: (805) 371 0505

4044. TMS Inc
Leisa Wert; Todd Hagan
110 West 3rd Street
PO Box 1358
Stillwater
OK 74076
USA
Telephone: (405) 377 0880
Fax: (405) 372 9288

4045. TMS Teilemarkt Informationssystem GmbH
Dr P Feller; Hr. Eggers
Friedrich-Ebert-Damm 204
2000 Hamburg 70
Germany
Telephone: +49 40 66 96 33
Fax: +49 40 66 96 3401

4046. TNO Centre for Information and Documentation
Mr. A. Van Galen
PO Box 214
2600 AE Delft
Netherlands
Telephone: 31 (15) 5697283;
        31 (15) 69 68 00
Fax: 31 (15) 56 08 25
Telex/E-mail: 38071 ZPTNO NL
NUA: 204117302400

4047. TNO, Technical Scientific Services
Schoemakerstraat 97
Delft
Netherlands
Telephone: 31 (15) 69 72 83
Fax: 31 (15) 56 48 00
Telex/E-mail: 38071 ZPTNO NL

4048. Tobacco Merchants Association of the United States
231 Clarkville Road
PO Box 8019
Princeton
NJ 08543–8019
USA
Telephone: (609) 275–4900

4049. Toeristiek BV
Piet van der Lelig; Willem Bloem
Oostwouder Dorpsstraat 16
1679 HE Oostwoud
Netherlands
Telephone: +31 2291 2241
Fax: +31 2291 1987

4050. Tokyo Shoko Research Ltd
Data Bank Service Division
Tokeó Sugasawa
Shinichi Building
1–9–6 Shinbashi
Minato-ku
Tokyo 105
Japan
Telephone: 03 3574–2265;
        03 3574–2211
Fax: 03 3575–0376

4051. Top Business System Co Ltd
65–7 Kokufuchiba
Okayama-shi
Okayama-ken
Japan
Telephone: +81 862 75 5004
Fax: +81 862 75 4363

4052. Top Class Technology Ltd
Geoff Glossop
Suite 4E, 4th Floor
East Mill
Bridgefoot
Belper
Derbyshire
DE5 1XQ
UK
Telephone: 0773 820011
Fax: 0773 820206

4053. Toppan Printing Co Ltd
1 Kanda Izumi-cho
Chiyoda-ku
Tokyo 101
Japan
Telephone: 81–3–835–6751
Fax: 81–3–835–6867

4054. Torf Fulton Associates
1275 Sunnycrest Avenue
Ventura
CA 93003
USA
Telephone: (805) 642–7838
Telex/E-mail: 73310,2746 (CompuServe
    Information Service)

4055. Toronto Star Newspapers Ltd
1 Yonge Street
Toronto
ON M5E 1E6
Canada
Telephone: (416) 367–2000

4056. Toronto Stock Exchange
Electronic Information Products
Exchange Tower
2 First Canadian Place
Toronto
ON M5X 1J2
Canada
Telephone: (416) 947–4700
Fax: (416) 947–4494; (416) 947–4727
Telex/E-mail: 06217759

**4057. Toshiba America Information
    Systems Inc**
Disks Products Division
9740 Irvine Blvd
PO Box 19724
Irvine
CA 92713–9724
USA
Telephone: (714) 583 3000
Fax: (714) 583 3133

4058. Toshiba Europa (I›E) GmbH
Disk Product Division
Gordon Logan
Hammfeddamm 8
4040 Neuss 1
Germany
Telephone: +49 2101 158370
Fax: +49 2101 158583

**4059. Toshokan Ryutsu Centre Co
    Ltd**
CD-ROM Enquiries
3–4–7 Otsuka
Bunkyo-ku
Tokyo
Japan
Telephone: +81 3 3943 2221
Fax: +81 3 3943 3507

4060. TOTAL-NET
S.G.M. Computacion S.A.
Talcahuano 38 Piso 4
1013 Buenos Aires
Argentina
Telephone: 54 (1) 37–7644
Telex/E-mail: 823340 SGM UF AR

**4061. Tower Consultants
    International Inc**
642 Ridgewood Avenue
Oradell
NJ 07649
USA
Telephone: (201) 262–5938

4062. Towers Data Systems
8033 Herb Farm Drive
Bethesda
MD 20817
USA
Telephone: (301) 469–6699
Fax: (301) 469–6714

4063. Towers Data Systems
8033 Herb Farm Drive
Bethesda
MD 20817
USA
Telephone: (301) 469–6699
Fax: (301) 469–6714

4064. Toyo Keizai America Inc
Yoichi Sato
380 Lexington Avenue
Room 4505
New York
NY 10168
USA
Telephone: (212) 949 6737
Fax: (212) 949 6648

4065. Toyo Keizai Inc
S Nakagawa
1–2–1, Nihonbashi-Hongokucho
Chuo-ku
Tokyo 103
Japan
Telephone: +81 3 3246 5580
Fax: +81 3 3242 4067

**4066. Trace Research and
    Development Center**
Kelly Ford; Christine Thompson
S-151 Waisman Center
1500 Highland Avenue
Madison
WI 53705
USA
Telephone: (608) 262 6966
Fax: (608) 262 8848

4067. Track Data Corporation
95 Rockwell Place
Brooklyn
NY 11217
USA
Telephone: (718) 522–0222

4068. Trade Data Reports Inc
6 West 37th Street
New York
NY 10018
USA
Telephone: (212) 563–2772

4069. Trade*Plus Inc
480 California Avenue
Suite 301
Palo Alto
CA 94306
USA
Telephone: (415) 324–4554;
        (800) 952–9900;
        (800) 972–9900 (in CA)

**4070. Trans Union Credit Information
    Company**
Litigation Division, 8th Floor
95–25 Queens Blvd
Rego Park
NY 11374
USA
Telephone: (718) 830–5352
Fax: (718) 830–5329

**4071. TransAmerica Information
    Management Services**
Darryl De Bond
601 University Avenue
Suite 255
Sacramento
CA 95825
USA
Telephone: (916) 921 6629
Fax: (916 921 6781

4072. Transdata
CTT e TLP em Consorcio
Avenue Fontes Pereira de Melo 38, 9
1089 Lisbon Codex
Portugal
Telephone: 01 54 00 20
Telex/E-mail: 64200 TDATA P

4073. Transinove International
c/o INPI
26 bis, rue de Leningrad
F-75800 Paris Cedex 8
France
Telephone: 1 42 94 52 50
Telex/E-mail: 290368 INPI PARIS F

4074. Transport Canada
Library and Information Centre
Jacques Cadieux
2nd Floor
Tower C
Place de Ville
Ottawa
ON K1A 0N5
Canada
Telephone: (613) 998–5127
Fax: (613) 954–4731
Telex/E-mail: 0533130 MOT OTT

4075. Transportation News Ticker
A Knight-Ridder Business Information
    Service
One Exchange Plaza
55 Broadway, Suite 200
New York
NY 10006
USA
Telephone: (212) 269–1110
Fax: (212) 422–2717

**4076. Transportation Research
    Board**
National Academy of Sciences
2101 Constitution Avenue, NW
Washington
DC 20418
USA
Telephone: (202) 334–3250
Telex/E-mail: NARECO

4077. Transpotel BV
PO Box 30006
NL-3001 DA Rotterdam
Netherlands
Telephone: 010 405 67 00
Fax: 010 405 73 51

4078. Travei Scan Videotex Ltd
5 Penn Plaza
New York
NY 10001
USA
Telephone: (212) 695–5492

4079. Travelset Oy
Sinikalliontie 10
SF-02630 Espoo
Finland
Telephone: 0 502–2233
Fax: 0 502–2244

4080. TravelVision
A division of General Drafting Company
    Inc
PO Box 161
Convent Station
NJ 07961
USA
Telephone: (201) 538–7600;
           (800) 367–6277

4081. Treehouse Publishing Ltd
6440 Wiscasset Road
Bethesda
MD 20816
USA
Telephone: (301) 229–8889

4082. Trend Magazines Inc
PO Box 611
St Petersburg
FL 33731–0611
USA
Telephone: (602) 230–1117

4083. Trend Monitor
Jan Wyllie
UK
Telephone: +44 (0)705 864 714

4084. Trends-Tendances
Carine Brochier (Information Manager)
Research Park Zellik
De Haak
1731 Zellik (Brussels)
Belgium
Telephone: 02/467 59 00
Fax: 02/467 57 59

4085. Trendvest Corporation
Box 44115
Pittsburgh
PA 15205
USA
Telephone: (412) 921–6900;
           (800) 255–1148
Telex/E-mail: 6711649 NAICO UW;
    TRENDVEST (DELPHI)

4086. Tri-Star Publishing
Samuel Hardman; Spencer Nickel
275 Gibraltar Road
Horsham
PA 19044
USA
Telephone: (215) 641–6200;
           (800) 292–4253
Fax: (215) 441–6490

4087. Tri-Star Publishing
475 Virginia Drive
Fort Washington
PA 19034
USA
Telephone: (800) 872–2828;
           (800) 292–4253;
           (215) 476–8000
Fax: (215) 441–6490

4088. Triad Systems Corporation
Richard Ross
3055 Triad Drive
Livermore
CA 94550–9559
USA
Telephone: (800) 33–TRIAD;
           (415) 449–0606
Fax: (415) 449–8954

4089. Tribune Company
7505 Warwick Boulevard
PO Box 746
Newport News
VA 23607
USA
Telephone: (804) 247–4600

4090. Tribune, The
143 S Main Street
Salt Lake City
UT 84110
USA
Telephone: (801) 237–2800

4091. Tribun
Bertrand Retaillieu; Jacques Klossa
166 Bd de Montparnasse
75014 Paris
France
Telephone: 1 43 35 06 06
Fax: 1 43 22 03 41

4092. Trillium Computer Resources
450 Phillip Street
Unit A-4
Waterloo
ON N2L 5J2
Canada
Telephone: (519) 886–4404

4093. Trinet America Inc
9 Campus Drive
Parsippany
NJ 07054
USA
Telephone: (201) 267–3600;
           (800) 874–6381;
           (800) 367–3282
Fax: (201) 993–8287
Telex/E-mail: 703636

4094. Tritech Corporation nv
Patrick de Maeyer
Roekhout 45
1720 Groot-Bijgaarden
Belgium
Telephone: 02 466 75 35
Fax: 02 466 78 75

4095. TRW Business Credit Division
500 City Parkway W
Suite 200
Orange
CA 92668
USA
Telephone: (714) 385–7700

**4096. TRW Information Services
    Division**
Real Estate Information Services
2 City Parkway East, Suite 193
PO Box 6230
Orange
CA 92667
USA
Telephone: (714) 385–3550

4097. TRW Information Services
505 City Parkway W
Suite 200
Orange
CA 92668
USA
Telephone: (714) 385–7000

4098. TRW Information Services
2000 S Anaheim Boulevard
Suite 100
Anaheim
CA 92805
USA
Telephone: (714) 385–2100;
           (800) 527–9663
Fax: (714) 385–2197

4099. TRW Property Data
3610 Central Avenue
Riverside
CA 92506
USA
Telephone: (714) 276–3649

4100. TSINTICHIMNEFTEMASH
c/o International Center for Scientific
    and Technical Information
Ulita Kuusinena 21b
125252 Moscow
Russia
Telephone: 095 198–7460
Fax: 095 943–0089
Telex/E-mail: 411925 MCNTI SU

4101. TSNIIEIUGOL
c/o International Center for Scientific
    and Technical Information
Ulitsa Kuusinena 21b
125252 Moscow
Russia
Telephone: 095 198–7460
Fax: 095 943–0089
Telex/E-mail: 411925 MCNTI SU

4102. TSNIITSVETMET
c/o International Center for Scientific
    and Technical Information
Ulitsa Kuusinena 21b
125252 Moscow
Russia
Telephone: 095 198–7460
Fax: 095 943–0089
Telex/E-mail: 411925 MCNTI SU

4103. Tsunami Press
Gloria Farrell
275 Route 18
East Brunswick
NJ 08816
USA
Telephone: (908) 613–0509;
           (908) 613–0904
Fax: (908) 238 3053

4104. Tucson Citizen
Box 26767
Tucson
AZ 85726
USA
Telephone: (602) 573–4561

4105. Tulsa Tribune Company
315 S. Boulder Avenue
Tulsa
OK 74103
USA
Telephone: (918) 581–8800

4106. Turing Institute
George House
36 North Hanover Street
Glasgow
G1 2AD
Scotland, UK
Telephone: 44 (41) 552–6400

4107. Turner Broadcasting System
1 CNN Plaza
Atlanta
GA 30348
USA
Telephone: (404) 827–1700

**4108. Twente Technology Transfer
    (3T Educatie)**
R Muès
Institutenweg 1
Postbus 3639
7500 DP Enschede
Netherlands
Telephone: +31 53 336633
Fax: +31 53 336869

Addresses

4109. Twin Circle Publishing Company
12700 Ventura Blvd, Suite 200
Studio City
CA 91604
USA
Telephone: (818) 766–2270

4110. Twix Equipment AG
R Reichlin
Gewerbestrasse 12
8132 Egg
Switzerland
Telephone: 1 750 11 10;
            1 984 22 11
Fax: 1 984 33 37

4111. Tyoterveyslaitoksen Kirjasto
Topeliuksenkatu 41 a A
SF-00250 Helsinki
Finland
Telephone: 0 474–7383
Fax: 0 414–634
Telex/E-mail: 125070 TYO SF

4112. Ubisoft
8/10 Rue de Valmy
93100 Montreuil sous Bois
France

4113. UCC Systems Management Ltd
Bromley Data Centre
18 Elmfield Road
Bromley
Kent
BR1 1LR
UK
Telephone: 081 313–0813

4114. UCCEL Corporation
1930 Hiline Drive
Dallas
TX 75207
USA
Telephone: (214) 655–8694

4115. Udenrigsministeriet
Departementet for Udenrigsoekonomi
Lone Soendergaard
Asiatisk Plads 2
1448 Koebenhavn K
Denmark
Telephone: 45 (33) 920000

4116. Udviklingscenter for folkeoplysning og voksenundervisning
Tordenskjoldsgade 27
1055 Copenhagen K
Denmark

4117. UK Atomic Energy Authority
Safety and Reliability Directorate
Wigshaw Lane
Culcheth
Warrington
Cheshire
WA3 4NE
UK
Telephone: 0925 254–486
Fax: 0925 766–681
Telex/E-mail: 629301 ATOMRY G

4118. UK Atomic Energy Authority
Waste Management Information Bureau
Building 7,12
Harwell Laboratory
Didcot
Oxfordshire
OX11 0RA
UK
Telephone: 0235 821–111
Fax: 0235 432–854

4119. UK Atomic Energy Authority
Heat Transfer & Fluid Flow Service
Harwell Laboratory
Didcot
Oxfordshire
OX11 0RA
UK
Telephone: 0235 432–862
Fax: 0235 831–981
Telex/E-mail: 83135 ATOMHA G

4120. UK CD-ROM User Group
Paul Fletcher
PO Box 1
Kidwelly
Dyfed
SA17 4QY
UK

4121. Ulkoasiainministerio
Oikeudellinen Osasto
PO Box 176
SF-00161 Helsinki
Finland
Telephone: 0 1341–51
Fax: 0 1341–5755

4122. UMI (University Microfilms International)
Information Publications International
Susan M Orchard; Andrew Garnham
White Swan House
Godstone
Surrey
RH9 8LW
UK
Telephone: +44 883 744123
Fax: +44 883 744024
Telex/E-mail: 95212 IPI G

4123. UMI (University Microfilms International)
Carol Bamford; Marth Ewald; Sean Devine
300 N Zeeb Road
Ann Arbor
MI 48106
USA
Telephone: (313) 761–4700;
           (800) 521–0600 (in USA);
           (800) 343–5299 (in Canada)
Fax: (313) 761–1204;
     (313) 973–1540
Telex/E-mail: 314597; 14042
     (DIALMAIL); 0235569

4124. UMI/Data Courier
Rae Helton
620 S 3rd Street
Louisville
KY 40202–2475
USA
Telephone: (502) 583–4111;
           (800) 626–2823
Fax: (502) 589–5572
Telex/E-mail: 204235; 11491
     (DIALMAIL)

4125. Umweltbundesamt
Informations- und Dokumentations-
     system Umwelt
Bismarckplatz 1
D-1000 Berlin 33
Germany
Telephone: 030 8903–2291
Fax: 030 8903–2285
Telex/E-mail: 183756 D

4126. UN – CELADE
Mr. A.M. Conning
PO Box 91
ECLAC Casilla 179–D
Santiago
Chile
Telephone: 56–2–485051
Fax: 56–2–480252

4127. UN – UNCTAD
Division for Data Management
Mr. D. Zandee
Palais des Nations
Geneva 22 CH-1211
Switzerland
Telephone: 41–22–734–6011
Fax: 41–22–733–9879

4128. UN Department of International Economic and Social Affairs
Population Division, Estimates and
     Projection Section
New York
NY 10017
USA
Telephone: (212) 754–3217

4129. UN Department of Public Information
Development Business
Ms D del Rosario-Ugay
United Nations
United Nations Plaza
Room DC1–559
New York
NY 10017
USA
Telephone: (212) 963 1515
Fax: (212) 963 4116
Telex/E-mail: 422311

4130. UN Development Business/ Development Forum
1 United Nations Plaza
Room DC1–559
GCPO Box 5850
New York
NY 10163–5850
USA
Telephone: (212) 963–1515

4131. UN Disaster Relief Organisation
New York Office, Room S2935A
United Nations
New York
NY 10017
USA
Telephone: (212) 963–5704

4132. UN Economic Commission for Latin America and the Caribbean
Casilla 179–D
Santiago
Chile
Telephone: 56 (2) 485051
Fax: 56 (2) 480252

4133. UN Economic Commission for Latin America and the Caribbean
Subregional Headquarters for the
     Caribbean
22 St Vincent Street
PO Box 1113
Port of Spain
Trinidad and Tobago
Telephone: 623–7308
Fax: 623–8485
Telex/E-mail: 22394 ECLAC WG; TCN
     4015 (Dialcom); UN.ECLAC.
     PORTOFSPAIN (Telemail)

4134. UN Food and Agriculture Organization (FAO)
R Pepe (Fishery Information Officer)
Via delle Terme di Caracalla
I-00100 Rome
Italy
Telephone: 06 57971
Fax: 06 5797–3152; 06 578–2610
Telex/E-mail: 610181 FAO I; FAO.FIDI
     (Omnet, Inc.'s SCIENCEnet)

4135. UN Industrial Development Organisation (UNIDO)
Mr P Pembleton
Vienna International Centre
PO Box 300
Vienna 1400
Austria
Telephone: 43–222–26310
Fax: 43–222–32156

4136. UN International Labour Organisation
International Occupational Safety and Health Information Centre
Mr J Takala
4 route des Morillons
CP 500
CH-1211 Geneva 22
Switzerland
Telephone: 022 799 86 76;
022 799 61 11;
022 799 67 40
Fax: 022 798 86 85;
022 798 62 53;
022 798 86 85
Telex/E-mail: 415647 ILO CH; 22271 BIT CH

4137. UN International Telecommunication Union (See International Telecommunications Union)

4138. UN Office for Ocean Affairs and the Law of the Sea
Dottisie Sutherland
DC2 0440 United Nations Plaza
New York
NY 10017
USA
Telephone: (212) 963 3926
Fax: (212) 963 5847

4139. UN REPIDISCA Manager
Casilla 4337 – Lima 100
Los Pinos 259
Lima 3
Peru
Telephone: 51–14–35–4135

4140. UN Statistical Office
Room DC2–1620
New York
NY 10017
USA
Telephone: (212) 754–5252;
(212) 963–4996
Fax: (212) 963–4116

4141. UNESCO
CD-ROM Enquiries
7 Place de Fontenoy
75700 Paris
France
Telephone: 1 45 68 1000
Fax: 1 43 06 1640

4142. UNI-C
Vermundsgade 5
DK-2100 Copenhagen
Denmark
Telephone: 01 82 83 55; 01 83 95 11
Fax: 01 83 79 49

4143. UNI-COLL Corporation
3401 Market Street
Philadelphia
PA 19104
USA
Telephone: (215) 387–3890

4144. UNICEF
UNICEF House
3 United Nations Plaza
New York
NY 10017
USA
Telephone: (212) 326–7000
Fax: (212) 888–7465
Telex/E-mail: 02307607848 UNICF UC; 41:UNC021 (Dialcom); 41:UNC001 (Dialcom)

4145. UniDisc Inc
Chris Andrews
4401 Capitola Road
Suite 4
Capitola
CA 95010
USA
Telephone: (408) 464–0707
Fax: (408) 464–0187

4146. Unified Management Corporation
429 Pennsylvania Street
Indianapolis
IN 46204–1897
USA
Telephone: (317) 634–3300;
(800) 862–7283
Fax: (317) 634–3300 x8999

4147. UNILINC Ltd
CLANN Limited (formerly)
Rona Wade
349 Riley Street
Level 4
Surry Hills
NSW 2010
Australia
Telephone: 61 (2) 212–4444
Fax: 61 (2) 212–6495

4148. Uninet Japan Limited
Marunouchi Mitsu Building 1F
2–2–2 Marunouchi
Chiyoda-ku
Tokyo 100
Japan
Telex/E-mail: 24700 KDDSALES J

4149. Union des Caisses Centrales de Mutualite Agricole
8 rue d'Astorg
Paris
France

4150. Union des Groupements Artisanaux
Centre Technique d'Application et d'Innovation de l'Artisana
18 rue de Timken
PO Box 428
F-68007 Colmar Cedex
France
Telephone: 89 23 65 65

4151. Union Français des Annuaires Professionels
13 avenue Vladimir Komarov
F-78190 Trappes Cedex
France
Telephone: 30 50 61 48

4152. Union-Tribune Publishing Company
PO Box 191
San Diego
CA 92112
USA
Telephone: (619) 299–3131
Fax: (619) 293–2333

4153. Uniphoto Picture Agency
Micahel Pettypool
3205 Grace Street NW
Washington
DC 20007
USA
Telephone: (202) 333–0500;
(800) 345–0546
Fax: (202) 338 5578

4154. United Communications Group
Oil Price Information Service
4550 Montgomery Avenue
Suite 700N
Bethesda
MD 20814
USA
Telephone: (301) 961–8700
Fax: (301) 961–8666

4155. United Communications Group
11300 Rockville Pike
Suite 1100
Rockville
MD 20852
USA
Telephone: (301) 816–8950;
(800) 526–5307
Fax: (301) 961–8666

4156. United Directory Systems
Noel C Bailey
Level 7
91 Phillip St
Paramatta 2150 NSW
Australia
Telephone: +61 2 891 0017
Fax: +61 2 891 1771

4157. United Methodist Communications
PO Box 320
810 12th Avenue S
Nashville
TN 37202
USA
Telephone: (615) 742–5444

4158. United Nations (See UN)

4159. United Nations University
UNU
Toho Seimei Building (29th Floor)
15–1 Shibuya 2–chome
Shibuya-ku
Tokyo 150
Japan
Telephone: +81 3/499 2811
Fax: +81 3/499 2828
Telex/E-mail: J25442

4160. United Press International
5 Penn Plaza
461 8th Avenue
New York
NY 10001
USA
Telephone: (212) 560–1100

4161. Unitex Communications Network
1013 Bloomfield Street, 2nd Floor
Hoboken
NJ 07030
USA
Telephone: (201) 653–2806
Fax: (212) 787–1726

4162. Universal News Services
Communications House
Gough Square
Fleet Street
London
EC4P 4DP
UK
Telephone: 071 353–5200

Addresses

4163. Universal Serials and Book Exchange Inc
2969 W 25th Street
Cleveland
OH 44113
USA
Telephone: (216) 241–6960

4164. Universal Weather and Aviation Inc
8787 Tallyho
Houston
TX 77061
USA
Telephone: (713) 944–1440;
           (800) 366–8648
Fax: (713) 943–4651
Telex/E-mail: 1794388

4165. Universidad Complutense de Madrid
Facultad de Ciencias de la Informacion
Ciudad Universitaria
28040 Madrid
Spain
Telephone: 34 (1) 449 67 30

4166. Universidad de Colima
Direccion Gral. de Intercambio
   Academico y Desarrollo Bibliotecar
Lourdes Feria
edenida Universidad 333
Ap Postal 134
28000 Colima
Mexico
Telephone: +52 331 433 81
Fax: +52 331 430 06;
     +52 331 275 81

4168. Universidad de Valencia
Centro de Documentación e Informatica
   Biomedica (CEDIB)
Luz Terrada (Manager)
Avenida Blasco Ibanez 17
46010 Valencia 10
Spain
Telephone: 096 361 03 73
Fax: 096 361 39 75

4169. Universidad Nacional Autónoma de México
Centro de Información Científica y
   Humanistica
Apartado Postal 70–392
04510 Mexico City DF
Mexico
Telephone: 05 548 08 58;
           05 505 52 15
Telex/E-mail: 1774523 UNAM ME

4170. Universidad Nacional Autónoma de México
Facultad de Medicina Veterinaria y
   Zootecnia
Banco de Información BIVE-Biblioteca
Ciudad Universitaria
Circuito Exterior
04510 Mexico City DF
Mexico
Telephone: 05 50 52 15 x4992
Telex/E-mail: 1774523 UNAM ME

4171. Universidad Nacional Autónoma de México
Servicio de Consulta a Bancos de
   Información
Ciudad Universitaria
Circuito Exterior
04510 Mexico City DF
Mexico
Telephone: 05 50 52 15 x4992
Telex/E-mail: 1774523 UNAM ME

4172. Università degli Studi di Milano
Dipartimento di Scienze
   dell'Informazione – Biblioteca
   Informatica
Gian Carlo Dalto
Via Comelieo 39/41
20135 Milan
Italy
Telephone: +39 2 55006371

4174. Università di Roma
Centro di Calcolo Interfacolta
Piazzale Aldo Moro 5
Rome
Italy
Telephone: 06 49 12 42
Telex/E-mail: 613255 I

4175. Università di Siena
Dipartimento di Archeologia e Storia
   delle Arti
Via ES Piccolomini 1–3
I-53100 Siena
Italy
Telephone: 0577 28 02 45

4176. Universität Bonn
Institute of Inorganic Chemistry
Gerhard-Domagk-Straße 1
D-5300 Bonn 1
Germany
Telephone: 0228 732–657
Telex/E-mail: UNC412 DBNRHRZ1
   (BITNET)

4177. Universität Karlsruhe
Kaiserstrasse 12
7500 Karlsruhe 1
Germany
Telephone: 49 (721) 608 42 78
Fax: 49 (721) 608 42 90

4178. Universität Karlsruhe
Forschungsstelle für
   Brandschutztechnik
Abteilung Dokumentation
Hertzstraße 16
D-7500 Karlsruhe 21
Germany
Telephone: 0721 608 44 73

4179. Universität Oldenburg
Fachbereich Biologie
Postfach 2503
D-2900 Oldenburg
Germany
Telephone: 0441 798–3374
Fax: 0441 798–3000

4180. Universität Regensburg
Lehrstuhl Psychologie VI
Universitätstraße 31
D-8400 Regensburg
Germany
Telephone: 0941 943 21 44

4181. Universitätsbibliothek und TIB
Welfengarten 1 B
D-3000 Hannover 1
Germany
Telephone: 0511 762 22 68
Fax: 0511 71 59 36
Telex/E-mail: 922168 TIBHN D

4182. Universitatsbibliothek Bielefeld
Wolfgang Binder
PO Box 8620
Universitatsstrasse 25
Bielefeld 1
D-4800
Germany
Telephone: +49 521 106 6126;
           +49 521 106 4051
Fax: +49 521 106 4052

4183. Université d'Aix-Marseille II
Bibliotheque Interuniversitaire
Medecine Nord
Chemin des Bourrely
F-13326 Marseille Cedex 15
France
Telephone: 91 51 20 13

4184. Université d'Aix-Marseille II
Institut de Geographie CTIG
29 avenue Robert Schumann
F-13621 Aix en Provence Cedex
France
Telephone: 42 20 37 77

4185. Université de Bordeaux III
Lasic-Gresic
MSHA – Domaine universitaire
33405 Talence Cedex
France
Telephone: 33 (56) 80 77 20

4186. Université de Lille II
Faculte de Chirurgie Dentaire
Place de Verdun
59005 Lille Cedex
France
Telephone: 33 (20) 52 45 03

4187. Université de Lille III
Centre de Recherches et de
   Documentation Bibliographique pour
   l'Antiquite Classique
BP 149
F-59653 Villeneuve d'Ascq Cedex
France
Telephone: 20 91 64 99

4188. Université de Lyon I
Institut d'Evolution Moleculaire
43 boulevard du 11 novembre 1918
F-69622 Villeurbanne
France

4189. Université de Lyon II
Maison de l'Orient Mediterraneen,
   IRMAC
1 rue Raulin
F-69365 Lyon Cedex 07
France
Telephone: 78 72 02 53

4190. Université de Lyon
Bibliotheque Interuniversitaire
Section Sante
8 avenue Rockefeller
F-69373 Lyon Cedex 08
France
Telephone: 78 74 19 54

4191. Université de Montpellier I
Institute de Recherches et d'Etudes et
   Traitement de l'Information Juridique
Faculte de Droit et des Sciences
   Economiques
39 rue de l'Université
F-34060 Montpellier Cedex
France
Telephone: 67 60 45 55
Fax: 67 60 42 31

4192. Université de Montpellier
Bibliotheque Interuniversitaire
Section Medecine – Nimes
avenue Kennedy
F-30300 Nimes
France
Telephone: 66 64 35 63

4193. Université de Montréal
Groupe d'Analyse des Recherches
    en Didactique et Acquisition du
    Français
Departement de Didactique
CP 6128 succarsale A
Montreal
PQ H3C 3J7
Canada
Telephone: (514) 343–6692
Fax: (514) 343–2283

4194. Université de Montréal
Faculty of Dental Medicine
2900 boulevard Edouard-Montpetit
CP 6128 succarsale A
Montreal
PQ H3C 3J7
Canada
Telephone: (514) 343–6111

4195. Université de Nantes
Service Formation Continue
Pascal Quinaou George Fargeas
Centre Multimédia
Chemin de la Sensive du Tertre
44072 Nantes Cedex 03
France
Telephone: (33) 40 74 01 11;
            (33) 40 37 31 66
Fax: (33) 40 35 19 03

4196. Université de Nice
Laboratoire d'Oceanographie Biologique
28 avenue de Valrose
F-06034 Nice Cedex
France
Telephone: 93 84 91 91
Fax: 93 52 99 19
Telex/E-mail: 970281 UNICE F

4197. Université de Paris II
Centre de Documentation des Droits
    Antiques
12 place du Pantheon
F-75005 Paris Cedex
France
Telephone: 1 46 34 98 27

4198. Université de Paris V
ERGODATA
45 rue des Saint-Peres
75270 Paris Cedex 06
France
Telephone: 33 (1) 42 86 20 38
Fax: 33 (1) 42 61 53 80
Telex/E-mail: 240540 F

4199. Université de Paris V
Laboratoire d'Anthropologie Applique et
    d'Ecologie Humaine
45 rue des Saint-Peres
75270 Paris Cedex 06
France
Telephone: 33 (1) 42 60 37 20 x4015;
            33 (1) 42 60 37 20 x4268

4200. Université de Paris V
Centre Interuniversitaire de Traitement
    de l'Information
45 rue des Saints-Peres
F-75270 Paris Cedex 6
France
Telephone: 1 42 96 24 89
Fax: 1 42 96 34 97

4201. Université de Paris-Nanterre
Groupe d'Analyse Macroeconomique
    Appliquee
200 avenue de la Republique
F-92001 Nanterre
France
Telephone: 1 47 21 46 89
Telex/E-mail: 638898 UPX NANT F

4202. Université de Paris-Sud
Laboratoire de Physique des Gaz et des
    Plasmas
GAPHYOR Online Service
Building 212
F-91405 Orsay Cedex
France
Telephone: 1 69 41 72 50
Fax: 1 69 41 78 44
Telex/E-mail: UPPO004 FRORS31
    (BITNET)

4204. Université de Rennes
Faculte de Medecine
Laboratoire de Biophysique RMN
Avenue du Professeur Leon Bernard
35048 Rennes Cedex
France
Telephone: 33 (99) 59 20 20 x370;
            33 (99) 59 16 04 x755

**4205. Université des sciences
        sociales de Grenoble**
Ecole Superieure des Affaires
Reseau d'information en gestion des
    entreprises
B.P. 47X
38040 Grenoble Cedex
France
Telephone: 33 (76) 82 54 82

**4206. Université des sciences
        sociales de Grenoble**
Reseau d'information en economie
    generale
B.P. 47X
38040 Grenoble Cedex
France
Telephone: 33 (76) 54 81 78

4207. Université du Quebec
2875 boulevard Laurier
Sainte-Foy
PQ G1V 2M3
Canada
Telephone: (418) 657–3551

4208. Université Louis Pasteur
Rue de l'Universite 7
67000 Strasbourg
France

4209. Universitetet i Trondheim
Norges Tekniske Hogskole
Norges Tekniske Universitetsbibliotek
N-7034 Trondheim NTH
Norway
Telephone: 07 595–110
Fax: 07 595–103
Telex/E-mail: 55186 NTHHB N

**4210. Universitetets Sentrale
        EDB-Tjeneste**
PO Box 1059 Blindern
0316 Oslo 3
Norway
Telephone: 47 (2) 45 57 29

**4211. Universitets- och
        Hoegskoleaembetet**
PO Box 4550
104 30 Stockholm
Sweden

4212. Universitetsbiblioteket 2.afd.
Jytte Halling
Noerre Allee 49
2200 Koebenhavn N
Denmark
Telephone: 45 (31) 396523

4213. Universitetsbiblioteket i Oslo
Drammensveien 42
N-0255 Oslo 2
Norway
Telephone: 02 55 36 30

**4214. University Microfilms
        International (See UMI)**

4215. University of Alberta
University Computing Services, SPIRES
    System
352 General Services Building
Edmonton
AB T6G 2H1
Canada
Telephone: (403) 492–5212
Telex/E-mail: ABOMBAK UALTAVM
    (BITNET)

4216. University of Alberta
Department of Chemistry
Edmonton
AB T6G 2G2
Canada
Telephone: (403) 492–3254

4217. University of Alberta
Health Law Institute
Faculty of Law
Edmonton
AB T2G 2H5
Canada

4218. University of Alberta
John A Weir Memorial Law Library
Law Centre
Edmonton
AB T6G 2H5
Canada
Telephone: (403) 492–1449

4219. University of Arizona
College of Pharmacy
Tucson
AZ 85721
USA
Telephone: (602) 626–6400

4220. University of Arkansas Press
Fayetteville
AK 72701
USA

4221. University of British Columbia
Library
1956 Main Hall
Vancouver
BC V6T 1Y3
Canada
Telephone: (604) 228–6465
Fax: (604) 228–6465
Telex/E-mail: patscan (Envoy 100)

4222. University of Brussels
Institute of Phonetics
Max Wajskop (Professor, Director of the
    Institute)
CP 110
50 avenue F Roosevelt
1050 Brussels
Belgium
Telephone: 02 650 20 10
Fax: 02 650 35 95

**4223. University of California,
        Berkeley**
Chicano Studies Library
Lillian Costillo-Speed
3404 Dwinelle Hall
Berkeley
CA 94720
USA
Telephone: (415) 642–3859

Addresses

4224. University of California, Berkeley
Graduate School of Business
National Center for Research in
  Vocational Education
1995 University Avenue
Suite 375
Berkeley
CA 94704
USA
Telephone: (510) 642–4004

4225. University of California, Los Angeles ORION User Services
University Research Library
Room 11617
405 Hilgard Avenue
Los Angeles
CA 90024–1575
USA
Telephone: (213) 825–7557

4226. University of California
Division of Library Automation
300 Lakeside Drive
8th Floor
Oakland
CA 94612–3550
USA
Telephone: (415) 987–0522
Fax: (415) 839–3573

4227. University of Cambridge
Institute of Biotechnology
Microbial Strain Data Network
307 Huntingdon Road
Cambridge
CB3 0JX
UK
Telephone: 0223 276–622
Fax: 0223 277–605
Telex/E-mail: 81240 CAMSPL G
  75:DBI0001 (Dialcom);
  MSDN PHX.CAM.AC.UK. (JANET)

4228. University of Cambridge
Crystallographic Data Centre
University Chemical Laboratory
Lensfield Road
Cambridge
CB2 1EW
UK
Telephone: 0223 336408
Fax: 0223 312 288
Telex/E-mail: UK.AC.CAM.CHEMCRYS
  (JANET)

4229. University of Cambridge
Scott Polar Research Institute Library
William Mills
Lensfield Road
Cambridge
CB2 1ER
UK
Telephone: 0223 336–552
Fax: 0223 336–549
Telex/E-mail: 81240 CAMSPL G;
  WJM13 UK.AC.CAM.PHX (JANET)

4230. University of Chicago
Computation Center
5737 University Avenue
Chicago
IL 60637
USA
Telephone: (312) 962–6092

4231. University of Chicago
Department of Romance Languages
  and Literatures
1010 E 59th Street
Chicago
IL 60637
USA
Telephone: (312) 702–8488
Telex/E-mail: ARTFL ARTFL.
  UCHICAGO.EDU (InterNet)

4232. University of Colorado
Laboratory for Atmospheric and Space
  Physics
Randy Davis
Campus Box 590
Boulder
CO 80309
USA
Telephone: (303) 492–6867;
  (303) 492–7666
Fax: (303) 492–6444

4233. University of Durham
Unit 3P
Mountjoy Research Centre
Durham
DH1 3SW
UK
Telephone: 091 374–2468
Fax: 091 374–3741
Telex/E-mail: 537351 G;
  NOMIS.TEAM UK.AC.CHEVIOT
  (JANET)

4234. University of Florida
Ted Britton
Knowledge Utilisation Project
258 Norman Hall
Gainesville
FL 23601
USA
Telephone: (914) 392–0761
Fax: (904) 392–7159

4235. University of Gifu
Curriculum Research and Development
  Center
1–1 Yanagido
Gifu-shi
Gifu-ken 501–11
Japan
Telephone: 81 (582) 30–1111

4236. University of Glasgow
Department of Mechanical Engineering
Control Information Database
  Manager
James Watt South Building
University of Glasgow
Glasgow
G12 8QQ
Scotland, UK
Telephone: 041 339 8855 x5187
Fax: 041 330 4343
Telex/E-mail: D.Ballance uk.ac.glasgow;
  cid uk.ac.glasgow.eng.control

4237. University of Guam
Micronesian Area Research Center
UOG Station
Mangilao
Guam 96923
Guam
Telephone: (671) 734–4473

4238. University of Guelph Library
Library Administration Office
Larry Porter
Gordon Street
Guelph
ON N1G 2W1
Canada
Telephone: (519) 824–4120 x2159
Fax: (519) 824–6931
Telex/E-mail: GUELPH.MAIL (ENVOY
  100)

4239. University of Illinois at Chicago
College of Pharmacy
Program for Collaborative Research in
  the Pharmaceutical Sciences
Box 6998
Chicago
IL 60680
USA
Telephone: (312) 996–2246
Telex/E-mail: 206243

4240. University of Iowa
College of Pharmacy, Iowa Drug
  Information Service
Oakdale Hall
Oakdale
IA 52319
USA
Telephone: (319) 335–4800
Fax: (319) 335–4077
Telex/E-mail: 62008097

4241. University of Kentucky
Center for Business and Economic
  Research
College of Business and Economics
302 Matthews Building
Lexington
KY 40506–0047
USA
Telephone: (606) 257–7675
Telex/E-mail: UKCC OBD123 (BITNET)

4242. University of Leeds
Brotherton Library
Leeds
West Yorkshire
LS2 9JT
UK
Telephone: 0532 431751;
  0532 335524
Telex/E-mail: 556473 UNILDS G

4243. University of London Library
Library Resources Coordinating
  Committee
Senate House
Malet Street
London
WC1E 7HU
UK
Telephone: 071 636–8000

4244. University of London
Department of Phonetics & Linguistics
Kate Jones, Project Officer
SAM (Speech Assessment Methods)
ESPRIT Project 2589
Wolfson House
Stephenson Way
London
NW1 2HE
UK
Telephone: 071 380–7406
Fax: 071 383–0752

4245. University of London
Imperial College of Science and
  Technology
Rock Mechanics Information Service
Royal School of Mines
Prince Consort Road
London
SW7 2BP
UK
Telephone: 071 589–5111
Fax: 071 589–6806
Telex/E-mail: 929484 IMPCOL G

4246. University of Michigan
Inter-University Consortium for
Political and Social Research
(See Inter-University
Consortium for Political and
Social Research)

4247. University of Minnesota
College of Pharmacy, Drug Information
  Services
3-160 Health Sciences Center
Unit F
308 Harvard Street SE
Minneapolis
MN 55455
USA
Telephone: (612) 624-6492

4248. University of Nebraska,
Lincoln
Buros Institute of Mental Measurements
135 Bancroft Hall
Lincoln
NE 68588-0348
USA
Telephone: (402) 472-6203

4249. University of New Mexico
Latin American Institute
801 Yale NE
Albuquerque
NM 87131
USA
Telephone: (505) 277-2961
Fax: (505) 277-5989
Telex/E-mail: LADBAC UNMB (BITNET)

4250. University of North Carolina
Carolina Population Center
University Square 300A
Chapel Hill
NC 27514
USA
Telephone: (919) 962-8411;
            (919) 962-3081

4251. University of Notre Dame
Radiation Chemistry Data Center
Radiation Laboratory
Notre Dame
IN 46556
USA
Telephone: (219) 239-6527;
            (219) 239-6528
Telex/E-mail: 469669; RCDC
  NDRADLAB (BITNET)

4252. University of Oklahoma
Department of Botany and Microbiology
770 Van Vleet Oval
Room 135
Norman
OK 73019
USA
Telephone: (405) 325-3174;
            (405) 325-4321

4253. University of Osaka
1-1 Yamadaoka
Suita-shi
Osaka 565
Japan
Telephone: 81 (6) 877-5111

4254. University of Oslo
University Library
Planning Department
N-0242 Oslo 2
Norway
Telephone: 02 553-630

4255. University of Pittsburgh
Health Instrument File
354 Victoria Building
Pittsburgh
PA 15261
USA
Telephone: (412) 624-3554

4256. University of Rochester
Medical Center
Pharmacology and Toxicology
601 Elmwood Avenue
Rochester
NY 14642
USA

4257. University of Rochester
Computing Center
Taylor Hall
Rochester
NY 14627
USA
Telephone: (716) 275-4181

4258. University of Sherbrooke
Informatheque-PRAUS
Sherbrooke
PQ J1K 2R1
Canada
Telephone: (819) 821-7566
Fax: (819) 821-7824

4259. University of Sydney
BISA
NSW 2006
Australia
Telephone: 61 (2) 692-2222
Fax: 61 (2) 692-4203
Telex/E-mail: 20056 AA

4260. University of Tampere
PL 607
SF-33101 Tampere 10
Finland
Telephone: 031 156 111
Fax: 358 (31) 156 162
Telex/E-mail: 22263 TAYK SF

4261. University of Toronto Press
10 St Mary Street
Suite 700
Toronto
ON M4Y 2W8
Canada
Telephone: (416) 978-8651

4262. University of Tsukuba
Science Information Processing Center
1-1-1 Tenno-dai
Tsukuba-shi
Ibaraki-ken 305
Japan
Telephone: 0298 532-450
Telex/E-mail: 3652580 UNTUKU J

4263. University of Vermont
Albert Joy
Bailey/Howe Library
Burlington
VT 05405
USA
Telephone: (802) 656 8350
Fax: (802) 656 4038

4264. University of Victoria
Diana M Priestly Law Library
PO Box 2300
Victoria
BC V8W 3B1
Canada
Telephone: (604) 721-8566

4265. University of Washington
Department of Atmospheric Sciences
Dr Clifford F Mass
Mailstop AK-40
Seattle
WA 98195
USA
Telephone: (206) 685-0910
Fax: (206) 543-0308

4266. University of Waterloo Library
C. Presser
Waterloo
ON N2L 3G1
Canada
Telephone: (519) 885-1211

4267. University of Waterloo
Faculty of Human Kinetics and Leisure
  Studies
Specialized Information Retrieval and
  Library Services
Waterloo
ON N2L 3G1
Canada
Telephone: (519) 885-1211

4268. University of Western Ontario
Social Science Computing Laboratory,
  Information Services
Karen Stafford
London
ON N6A 5C2
Canada
Telephone: (519) 661-2152
Fax: (519) 661-3868
Telex/E-mail: REGISTER UWOVAX
  (BITNET)

4269. University of Western Ontario
Graduate School of Journalism
Centre for Mass Media Studies
London
ON N6A 5B7
Canada
Telephone: (519) 661-3383
Fax: (519) 661-3848

4270. University of Wisconsin,
Madison
Department of Psychiatry, Lithium
  Information Center
600 Highland Avenue
Madison
WI 53792
USA
Telephone: (608) 263-6171

4271. University of Wollongong
Department of Legal Studies
PO Box 1144
Wollongong
NSW 2500
Australia
Telephone: 042 270-730

4272. University Publications of
America
4520 East-West Highway
Bethesda
MD 20814-2289
USA
Telephone: (800) 692-6300

4273. Unternehmensberatung für
Informationsverarbeitung
Elisabethenstrasse 18
6368 Bad Vilbel 1
Germany
Telephone: 49 (6101) 81 13

Addresses

4274. Updata Publications
1736 Westwood Blvd.
Los Angeles
CA 90024
USA
Telephone: (310) 474–5900
Fax: (310) 474–4095

4275. Upplysnings Centralen AB
PO Box 5035
S-102 41 Stockholm
Sweden
Telephone: 46–8/663–1030
Fax: 46–8–800–470

4276. Uppsala Universitet
Institutionenen for Lararutbildning
Seminariegaten 1
Uppsala
Sweden
Telephone: 46–18–18–25–00

4277. Urbamet Reseau
Department of Urbanism
64 Rue de la Federation
Paris 75015
France
Telephone: 33–1–4567–3536
Fax: 33–1–4567–1220

4278. Urban Decision Systems Inc
PO Box 25953
2040 Armacost Avenue
Los Angeles
CA 90025
USA
Telephone: (213) 820–8931;
(800) 633–9568
Fax: (213) 207–0234; (213) 826–0933

4279. US Agency for International Development
USA
Telephone: (703) 351 4006
Fax: (703) 351 4039

4280. US Air Force
Air Force System Command, Electronic
Systems Division
Alan Drachan
Building 1704, Room 206
Hanscom AFB
MA 01731–5000
USA
Telephone: (617) 377–2105
Fax: (617) 377–2477

4281. US Army Corps of Engineers
Cold Regions Research and
Engineering Laboratory
Nancy Liston
72 Lyme Road
Hanover
NH 03755–1290
USA
Telephone: (603) 646–4221;
(603) 646–4238
Fax: (603) 646 4278

4282. US Army Corps of Engineers
Waterways Experiment Station
Environmental Laboratory
PO Box 631
Vicksburg
MS 39180
USA
Telephone: (601) 634–3774

4283. US Army Corps of Engineers
Ron Kerchival
20 Massachusetts Ave, NW
CEIM-SP, Rm 5121C
Washington
DC 20314–1000
USA
Telephone: (202) 475 9033

4284. US Army Publications and Printing Command
Leo F Pozo
2461 Eisenhower Ave
Alexandria
VA 22331–0302
USA
Telephone: (703) 325 6262
Fax: (703) 325 6260

4285. US Bureau of Economic Analysis
BE-53
Washington
DC 20230
USA
Telephone: (202) 523–0777

4286. US Bureau of the Census
Customer Services
Gary M Young
Public Information Office
Room 2705
Federal Office Building 3
Washington
DC 20233
USA
Telephone: (301) 763–4100;
(301) 763–4051
Fax: (301) 763–4794

4287. US Bureau of the Census
Data User Services Division
Mary Jane McCoy
Washington Plaza Room 321
Washington
DC 20233
USA
Telephone: (301) 763–4100;
(301) 763–2074
Fax: (301) 763–4794

4288. US Bureau of the Census
Foreign Trade Division
Washington
DC 20233
USA
Telephone: (301) 763–7662

4289. US Centers for Disease Control
Center for Chronic Disease Prevention
& Health Promotion
Chris Fralish
Technical Information Services Branch,
OD
1699 Clifton Road, Building 1 South,
SSB-249
Atlanta
GA 30333
USA
Telephone: (404) 629–3492
Fax: (404) 639–1552

4290. US Centers for Disease Control
Office on Smoking and Health
Technical Information Center
Rhodes Building
Mailstop K12
1600 Clifton Road NE
Atlanta
GA 30333
USA
Telephone: (404) 488–5080
Fax: (301) 443–1194

4291. US Central Intelligence Agency (CIA)
Washington
DC 20505
USA
Telephone: (703) 351 1100

4292. US Coast Guard
G-MTH-1
2100 2nd Street SW
Washington
DC 20593–0001
USA
Telephone: (202) 267–1577;
(202) 441–2669

4293. US Coast Guard
Office of Marine Safety, Security and
Environmental Protection
Marine Environmental Protection
Division
G-MEP-2
2100 2nd Street SW
Washington
DC 20590
USA
Telephone: (202) 267–2611
Fax: (202) 267–4816

4294. US Defense General Supply Center
Russell H Van Allen (Supervisory
Chemical Engineer)
Attn: DGSC-SSH
Richmond
VA 23297–5000
USA
Telephone: (804) 275–3104
Fax: (804) 275–4149

4295. US Defense Logistics Agency
Hazardous Materials Technical Center
Room 3A150 Cameron Station
Alexandria
VA 22304–6100
USA
Telephone: (202) 274–6000

4296. US Defense Mapping Agency
Lynn Martin (Contract Specialist)
DMA AQAI
8613 Lee Highway
Fairfax
VA 22031–2137
USA
Telephone: (703) 285–9220
Fax: (703) 285–9050

4297. US Defense Mapping Agency
US Naval Observatory
Building 56
Washington
DC 20305–3000
USA
Telephone: (202) 653–1375

4299. US Defense Technical Information Center
MATRIS Office
DTIC-DMA
San Diego
CA 92152–6800
USA
Telephone: (619) 553–7000

4300. US Defense Technical Information Center
Defense RDT&E OnLine System
(DROLS)
Cameron Station
Building 5
Alexandria
VA 22304–6145
USA
Telephone: (703) 274–7709;
(800) 841–9553
Fax: (703) 274–9274

4301. US Department of Agriculture
Agricultural Research Service
Office of Cooperative Interactions
Room 404
Building 005
BARC-West
Beltsville
MD 20705
USA
Telephone: (301) 344–4045

4302. US Department of Agriculture
Cooperative State Research Service
Current Research Information System
(CRIS)
5th Floor
National Agricultural Library Building
Beltsville
MD 20705
USA
Telephone: (301) 344–3850;
(301) 344–3846

4303. US Department of Agriculture
Office of Public Affairs
Information Technology Management
Staff
14th & Independence Avenue SW
Washington
DC 20250
USA
Telephone: (202) 447–7454;
(202) 447–5505
Fax: (202) 447–5340; (202) 245–5165
Telex/E-mail: AGR205 (Dialcom)

4304. US Department of Agriculture
Human Nutrition Information Service
6505 Belcrest Road
Hyattsville
MD 20708
USA
Telephone: (301) 436–8457

4305. US Department of Agriculture
Agricultural Statistics Board
14th Street & Independence Avenue,
SW
Washington
DC 20250
USA
Telephone: (202) 447–7017

**4306. US Department of Commerce
(See also US National
Technical Information Center)**

4307. US Department of Commerce
Office of Business Analysis
Paul Christy
Herbert C Hoover Building
Room 4885
14th & Constitution Avenue NW
Washington
DC 20230
USA
Telephone: (202) 377–0123;
(202) 377–1431
Fax: (202) 377–4985

4308. US Department of Commerce
Bureau of Economic Analysis
1401 K Street, NW
Washington
DC 20230
USA
Telephone: (202) 523–0777

4309. US Department of Commerce
Commerce Business Daily
Attn: H2852
Washington
DC 20230
USA
Telephone: (202) 377–0632

4310. US Department of Commerce
14th Street
Between Constitution Avenue & E
Street NW
Washington
DC 20230
USA
Telephone: (202) 377–2000

4311. US Department of Commerce
International Trade Administration
EPS/Information Management Division
14th & Constitution Avenue NW
Room 1322
Washington
DC 20230
USA
Telephone: (202) 377–4203

4312. US Department of Defense
Index of Specifications & Standards
(DODISS)
The Pentagon
Washington
DC 20230
USA
Telephone: (202) 545 6700

4313. US Department of Defense
Federal Aviation Administration
AFML/MLSF
Wright-Patterson Air Force Base
Dayton
OH 45433–6533
USA
Telephone: (513) 255–5128

4314. US Department of Education
National Institute on Disability and
Rehabilitation Research
Mailstop 2305
400 Maryland Avenue, SW
Washington
DC 20202
USA
Telephone: (202) 732–1192

4315. US Department of Education
Educational Resources Information
Center (ERIC)
555 New Jersey Avenue NW
Washington
DC 20208
USA
Telephone: (202) 219–1289;
(800) 424–1616
Fax: (202) 219–1859

4316. US Department of Education
Educational Resources Information
Center (ERIC)
ERIC Processing and Reference Facility
2440 Research Blvd, Suite 550
Rockville
MD 20850
USA
Telephone: (301) 656–9723

4317. US Department of Education
Office of Educational Research and
Improvement
Information Services
555 New Jersey Avenue NW
Washington
DC 20208–5725
USA
Telephone: (202) 357–6547;
(202) 357–6526;
(800) 222–4922;
(800) 424–1616;
(202) 357–6289
Telex/E-mail: 76077,1641 (CompuServe
Information Service); 41:ALA1693
(Dialcom)

4318. US Department of Energy
1000 Independence Avenue SW
Washington
DC 20585
USA
Telephone: (202) 252–2363

4319. US Department of Energy
Bartlesville Project Office
PO Box 1398
Bartlesville
OK 74005
USA
Telephone: (918) 336–2400

4320. US Department of Energy
Energy Information Administration
1000 Independence Avenue SW
Mail Stop EI421
Washington
DC 20585
USA
Telephone: (202) 252–1155

4321. US Department of Energy
Energy Library
AD-234.2
Washington
DC 20585
USA
Telephone: (202) 586–9534

4322. US Department of Energy
Idaho National Engineering Laboratory
550 2nd Street
Idaho Falls
ID 83401
USA

4323. US Department of Energy
Office of Oil Imports
PO Box 19267
Washington
DC 20036
USA
Telephone: (202) 653–3445

4324. US Department of Energy
Office of Scientific and Technical
Information
PO Box 62
Oak Ridge
TN 37831
USA
Telephone: (615) 576–6299;
(615) 576–1222
Fax: (615) 576–2865; (615) 576–1189

4325. US Department of Energy
Office of Building Technologies
George James
CE-421 Conservation & Renewable
Energy
Washington
DC 20585
USA
Telephone: (202) 252 1155

**4326. US Department of Health and
Human Services**
Health Care Financing Administration
200 Independence Avenue SW
Washington
DC 20201
USA
Telephone: (202) 245–6113

4327. US Department of Health and Human Services
Office of Disease Prevention and Health Promotion
Mary E Switzer Building
Room 21232
330 C Street NW
Washington
DC 20201
USA
Telephone: (202) 245–7611

4328. US Department of Housing and Urban Development
Duncan MacRae
Office of Public Affairs
451 7th Street
Washington
DC 20410
USA
Telephone: (202) 755–6980;
          (202) 755–5600

4329. US Department of Housing and Urban Development
Government National Mortgage Association
451 7th Street SW
Washington
DC 20410
USA
Telephone: (202) 708–0926

4330. US Department of Housing and Urban Development
Office of Policy Development and Research
PO Box 6091
Rockville
MD 20850
USA
Telephone: (301) 245–2691;
          (800) 245–2691

4331. US Department of Justice
Immigration and Naturalization Service
425 I Street NW
Room 5028
Washington
DC 20536
USA
Telephone: (202) 633–3059

4332. US Department of Justice
Justice Management Division
Chester Arthur Building
Room 129
425 I Street NW
Washington
DC 20530
USA
Telephone: (202) 633–1386

4333. US Department of Justice
National Institute of Justice
Martin Lively
633 Indiana Avenue
Washington
DC 20531
USA
Telephone: (202) 307–2942
Fax: (202) 307 6394

4334. US Department of Justice
Immigration and Naturalization Service
Office of Information Systems
Elizabeth Chase MacRae
425 I Street NW
Room 6112
Washington
DC 20536
USA
Telephone: (202) 633–2547
Fax: (202) 633–3296

4335. US Department of Labor
Bureau of Labor Statistics
James McCall
441 G Street NW
Washington
DC 20212
USA
Telephone: (202) 523–1364;
          (202) 523–1092
Fax: (202) 523–8763

4336. US Department of Labor
Office of Federal Contract Compliance Programs
200 Constitution Avenue NW, Room C-3325
Washington
DC 20210
USA
Telephone: (202) 523–9475

4337. US Department of State
2201 C Street NW
Washington
DC 20520
USA
Telephone: (202) 632–5225

4338. US Department of State
Citizens Emergency Center
2201 C Street NW
Washington
DC 20520
USA
Telephone: (202) 647–5225

4339. US Department of the Army
Army Reserve
The Pentagon
Room 1D 434
Washington
DC 20310
USA
Telephone: (202) 695–3001;
          (202) 696–3962

4340. US Department of the Army
Office of the Chief of Public Affairs
The Pentagon
Room 2E 626
Washington
DC 20310
USA
Telephone: (202) 695–3001
Fax: (202) 697–2159

4341. US Department of the Army
White Sands Missile Range
White Sands
NM 88002
USA

4342. US Department of the Interior
Fish and Wildlife Service
Division of Biological Sciences
National Ecology Center
Creekside One Building
2627 Redwing Road
Fort Collins
CO 80526
USA
Telephone: (303) 226–9323

4343. US Department of the Interior
Office of Public Affairs
Room 7221
Department of the Interior Building
Washington
DC 20240
USA
Telephone: (202) 343–6416

4344. US Department of the Treasury
Office of Thrift Supervision
1700 G Street, NW, 3rd Floor
Washington
DC 20552
USA
Telephone: (202) 906–6677

4345. US Department of Transportation
Data Administration Division
DIA-20, Room 4123
Office of Aviation Information Management, RSPA, DOT
400 7th Street, SW
Washington
DC 20590
USA

4346. US Department of Transportation
Center for Transportation Information
Kendall Square
Cambridge
MA 02142
USA
Telephone: (617) 494–2450

4347. US Department of Transportation
Office of Public Affairs
400 7th Street, SW
Washington
DC 20590
USA
Telephone: (202) 426–4000

4348. US Department of Transportation
Research and Special Programs Administration
Office of Aviation Information Management
400 7th Street SW
Washington
DC 20590
USA
Telephone: (202) 366–4381

4349. US Environmental Protection Agency
CIS Project
PM-218
401 M Street, SW
Washington
DC 20460
USA

4350. US Environmental Protection Agency
Emergency Response Division
OS210
401 M Street SW
Washington
DC 20460
USA
Telephone: (202) 382–2190;
          (202) 479–2449;
          (800) 535–0202

4351. US Environmental Protection Agency
Library Services Office
Air Pollution Technical Information Center
MD-35
Research Triangle Park
NC 27711
USA
Telephone: (919) 541–2777
Fax: (919) 541–1405

4352. US Environmental Protection Agency
Office of Pesticides and Toxic
  Substances
Gerry Brown
Public Data Branch
401 M Street
MS-TS799
Washington
DC 20460
USA
Telephone: (202) 382–3546;
         (202) 554–1404
Fax: (202) 382–4655
Telex/E-mail: 892758

4353. US Environmental Protection Agency
Office of Public Affairs
401 M Street, SW
Washington
DC 20460
USA
Telephone: (202) 387–2090;
         (800) 535–0202

4354. US Federal Deposit Insurance Corporation
Division of Accounting and Corporate
  Services
Management Information Services
  Branch
550 17th Street NW
F450
Washington
DC 20429
USA
Telephone: (202) 377–6000;
         (202) 898–7090

4355. US Federal Deposit Insurance Corporation
500 C Street, SW
Washington
DC 20424
USA
Telephone: (202) 382–0711

4356. US Federal Energy Regulatory Commission
Information Management Division
941 N Capitol Street NE
Washington
DC 20426
USA
Telephone: (202) 208–2474

4357. US Federal Reserve System
Board of Governors
Room MS-138
Washington
DC 20551
USA
Telephone: (202) 452–3244

4358. US Food and Drug Administration
Stuart Carlow
1901 Chapman Avenue
Rockville
MD 20857
USA
Telephone: (301) 443–1895
Fax: (301) 443 2017

4359. US General Services Administration
Federal Domestic Assistance Catalog
  Staff
300 7th Street SW
Ground Floor
Washington
DC 20407
USA
Telephone: (202) 453–4126
Fax: (202) 453–5576

4360. US Geological Institute
Kay Yost
4220 King Street
Alexandria
VA 22302
USA
Telephone: (703) 379–2480
Fax: (703) 379–7563

4361. US Geological Survey
Water Resources Division National
  Water Data Exchange
421 National Center
Reston
VA 22092
Telephone: (703) 648–6848

4362. US Geological Survey
Earth Science Data Directory
801 National Center
Reston
VA 22092
USA
Telephone: (703) 648–7112

4363. US Geological Survey
EROS Data Center
John Jones
804 National Centre
Reston
VA 22092–9998
USA
Telephone: (703) 648–4138;
         (605) 594–6507

4364. US Geological Survey
Geologic Division, Branch of
  Geochemistry
Box 25046
MS 973
Denver
CO 80225
USA
Telephone: (303) 236–5518
Fax: (303) 236–3200

4365. US Geological Survey
Water Resources Division, Office of
  Water Data Coordination
417 National Center
Reston
VA 22092
USA
Telephone: (703) 648–5014

4366. US Geological Survey
EROS Data Center Customer Services
Sioux Falls
SD 57198
USA
Telephone: (605) 594–6151
Fax: (605) 594–6589

4367. US Geological Survey
Water Resources Scientific Information
  Center
Raymond A Jensen
425 National Center
Reston
VA 22092
USA
Telephone: (703) 648–6820
Fax: (703) 648–5704

4368. US Geological Survey
National Mapping Division
John Jones
804 National Centre
Reston
VA 22092–9998
USA
Telephone: (703) 648–4138

4369. US Geological Survey
National Earthquake Information Center
Madelene Zirbes
Denver Federal Center
Box 25046
Mail Stop 967
Denver
CO 80225
USA
Telephone: (303) 236–1506
Fax: (303) 235–1519

4370. US Geological Survey
Water Resources Division
804 National Center
Reston
VA 22092–9998
USA
Telephone: (703) 648–4000

4371. US Geological Survey
Joint Office for Mapping Research
Millington Lockwood
915 National Center
Reston
VA 22092–9998
USA
Telephone: (703) 648–6525

4372. US Geological Survey
Jane Weaver
12201 Sunrise Valley Drive
Reston
VA 22092–9998
USA
Telephone: (703) 648–4460

4373. US Geological Survey
Bob Wybranies
509 National Center
Reston
VA 22092
USA
Telephone: (703) 648–5905
Fax: (703) 648–5939

4374. US Government Printing Office
5236 Eisenhower Avenue
Alexandria
VA 22304
USA
Telephone: (703) 557–2145

4375. US Government Printing Office
Information Dissemination
Judith C Russell; J Christian
  Sweterlitsch
Attn Customer Service Room C836
N Capitol & H Streets NW
Washington
DC 20401
USA
Telephone: (202) 512–1265;
         (202) 783–3238;
         (202) 512–1257
Fax: (202) 512–1434

4376. US Government Printing Office
Superintendent of Documents
Washington
DC 20402
USA
Telephone: (202) 783–3283
Telex/E-mail: 710 822 9413

4377. US Information Services
45 N Gaston Avenue
Suite 3C
Summerville
NJ 08876
USA
Telephone: (908) 685–1900
Fax: (908) 685–1662

4378. US Internal Revenue Service
Publishing Services Branch
1111 Constitution Avenue NW
Room 1552
Mail Stop HR:F:P
Washington
DC 20224
USA
Telephone: (202) 566–3053

4379. US Maritime Administration
Maritime Technical Information Facility
Kings Point
NY 11024–1699
USA
Telephone: (516) 773–5577

**4380. US National Agricultural
Library**
Gary K McCone
10301 Baltimore Boulevard
5th Floor
Beltsville
MD 20705
USA
Telephone: (301) 344–3813
Fax: (301) 344–3675; (301) 344–5473
Telex/E-mail: ALA 1029 (ALANET);
AGS3086 (Dialcom)

**4381. US National AIDS Information
Clearinghouse**
AIDS Clinical Trials Information Service
PO Box 6421
Rockville
MD 20850
USA
Telephone: (800) 874–2572

**4382. US National AIDS Information
Clearinghouse**
PO Box 6003
Rockville
MD 20850–6003
USA
Telephone: (301) 251–5730;
(800) 458–5231

**4383. US National Center on Child
Abuse and Neglect**
Clearinghouse on Child Abuse and
Neglect Information
PO Box 1182
Washington
DC 20013
USA
Telephone: (703) 821–2086

**4384. US National Environmental,
Satellite, Data and Information
Service**
Assessment and Information Services
Center
National Environmental Data Referral
Service
1825 Connecticut Avenue NW
Washington
DC 20235
USA
Telephone: (202) 606–4548
Fax: (202) 673–5586
Telex/E-mail: G.BARTON (OMNET);
NODC:BARTON (NASA/SPAN)

**4385. US National Institute for
Occupational Safety and
Health**
Standards Development and
Technology Transfer Division
Technical Information Branch
4676 Columbia Parkway
Cincinnati
OH 45226
USA
Telephone: (513) 533–8326

**4386. US National Institute of Dental
Research**
Research Information Management and
Analysis Information Section
Office of Planning, Evaluation and
Communications
Westwood Building
Room 537
5333 Westbard Avenue
Bethesda
MD 20892
USA
Telephone: (301) 496–7220;
(301) 496–7843
Fax: (301) 496–9241

4387. US National Institute of Justice
PO Box 6000
Rockville
MD 20850
USA
Telephone: (301) 251–5500;
(800) 851–4320
Fax: (301) 251–5212

**4388. US National Institute of
Standards and Technology**
Crystal and Electron Diffraction Data
Center
Materials Science and Engineering
Laboratory
Building 223
Room A215
Gaithersburg
MD 20899
USA
Telephone: (301) 975–6255
Fax: (301) 975–2128

**4389. US National Institute of
Standards and Technology**
Center for Fire Research
Building 224
Room A252
Gaithersburg
MD 20899
USA
Telephone: (301) 975–6862
Fax: (301) 975–4052

**4390. US National Institute of
Standards and Technology**
Chemical Thermodynamics Data Center
Chemistry Building
Room A158
Gaithersburg
MD 20899
USA
Telephone: (301) 975–2526

**4391. US National Institute of
Standards and Technology**
Crystal Data Center
Building 223
Room B222
Gaithersburg
MD 20899
USA
Telephone: (301) 975–6255

**4392. US National Institute of
Standards and Technology**
Office of Standard Reference Data
A323 Physics Building
Gaithersburg
MD 20899
USA
Telephone: (301) 975–2208

**4393. US National Institute on
Alcohol Abuse and Alcoholism**
Office of Scientific Affairs
5600 Fishers Lane
Room 16C-14
Rockville
MD 20857
USA
Telephone: (202) 443–3860

4394. US National Institutes of Health
PO Box NDIC
Bethesda
MD 20892
USA
Telephone: (301) 496–2162
Fax: (301) 770–5164

4395. US National Institutes of Health
National Cancer Institute
Bonnie Harding
International Cancer Information Center
9030 Old Georgetown Road
Building 82, Room 103
Bethesda
MD 20892
USA
Telephone: (301) 496–7403
Fax: (301) 480–8105
Telex/E-mail: 89422

4396. US National Institutes of Health
National Eye Institute
Building 31, Room 6A32
Bethesda
MD 20892
USA
Telephone: (301) 496–5248

4397. US National Institutes of Health
Division of Research Grants
Research Documentation Section
Westwood Building
Room 148
5333 Westbard Avenue
Bethesda
MD 20892
USA
Telephone: (301) 496–7543

**4398. US National Oceanic and
Atmospheric Administration**
Aeronautical Charting Division
David M Dudish
6010 Executive Boulevard
Room 1022
N/CG3x22 Rockville
MD 20852
USA
Telephone: (301) 443 8323
Fax: (301) 443 5071

**4399. US National Oceanic and
Atmospheric Administration**
National Weather Service
8060 13th Street
Silver Spring
MD 20910
USA
Telephone: (301) 427–7737

**4400. US National Oceanic and
Atmospheric Administration**
National Environmental Data Referral
Service
1825 Connecticut Avenue NW
Washington
DC 20235
USA
Telephone: (202) 673–5548
Fax: (202) 673–5586

4401. US Naval Observatory
Time Service Department
34th Street & Massachusetts Avenue
NW
Washington
DC 20392
USA
Telephone: (202) 653–1546

4402. US Naval Sea Systems Command
CEL-E, Room 11 S14
2531 Jefferson Davis Highway
Arlington
VA 22202
USA
Telephone: (202) 692–1150

4403. US Navy
Naval Fleet Analysis Center
Government-Industry Data Exchange
   Program
GIDEP Operations Center
Corona
CA 91720
USA
Telephone: (714) 736–4677

4404. US News and World Report Inc
2400 N Street NW
Washington
DC 20037
USA
Telephone: (202) 955–2000

4405. US Patent and Trademark Office
Office of Patent Depository Library
   Programs
Jane S Myers
Crystal Mall
Building 2, Room 304
Washington
DC 20231
USA
Telephone: (703) 557–5652;
               (703) 557–9686;
               (703) 557–0400;
               (703) 557–6154
Fax: (703) 557–0668

4406. US Postal Service
475 l'Enfant Plaza
Washington
DC 20260
USA
Telephone: (202) 268–2000

4407. US Public Health Service
Office of the Surgeon General
5600 Fishers Lane, Room 1866
Rockville
MD 20857
USA
Telephone: (301) 443–6496

4408. US Small Business Administration
Office of Procurement Assistance
1441 L Street NW
Room 600
Washington
DC 20416
USA
Telephone: (202) 653–6635

4409. US Social Security Administration
Office of Information
Baltimore
MD 21235
USA
Telephone: (301) 965–3970

4410. US Statistics Inc
Warren G Glimpse
PO Box 816
1101 King Street
Suite 601
Alexandria
VA 22314
USA
Telephone: (703) 979–9699
Fax: (703) 548–4585

4411. US Telecom Inc
315 Greenwich Street
New York
NY 10013
USA
Telephone: (212) 925–0667
Fax: (212) 925–1276
Telex/E-mail: 6501746064;
   Irobertberger (ATT&T Mail);
   174–6064 (MCI Mail)

4412. US Videotel Inc
Marathon Oil Tower
555 San Felipe
Suite 1200
Houston
TX 77056
USA
Telephone: (713) 840–9777

4413. US West Communications
1801 California Street
Room 1260
Denver
CO 80202
USA
Telephone: (303) 896–7111

4414. US West Optical Publishing
90 Madison Street
Suite 200
Denver
CO 80206
USA
Telephone: (303) 370–1465

4416. USA Information Systems, Inc
Steve Murdock
1092 Laskin Road
Suite 208
Virginia Beach
VA 23451
USA
Telephone: (804) 491 7525
Fax: (804) 491 7811

4417. USA TODAY Sports Center
Four Seasons Executive Center
Building 9
Terrace Way
Greensboro
NC 27403
USA
Telephone: (919) 855–3491;
               (800) 826–9688

4418. Usaco Corporation (SilverPlatter Agent)
Yuji Matsuyama
13–12 Shimbashi 1–Chome
Minato-Ku
Tokyo 105
Japan
Telephone: +81 3502 6471
Fax: +81 3593 2709

4419. USNI Military Database
1745 Jefferson Davis Highway
Crystal Square 4, Suite 501
Arlington
VA 22202
USA
Telephone: (703) 553–0208;
               (800) 443–7216
Fax: (703) 521–7447

4420. UTET Spa
Dr Fornaro
Corso Raffaello 28
10125 Torino
Italy
Telephone: +39 11 652 91
Fax: +39 11 6529240

4421. Utility Data Institute Inc
1700 K Street NW
Suite 400
Washington
DC 20006
USA
Telephone: (202) 466–3660
Fax: (800) 486–3660; (202) 466–3667

4422. Utlas International Canada
Robert Eastman
80 Bloor Street E
2nd Floor
Toronto
ON M5S 2V1
Canada
Telephone: (416) 923–0890;
               (800) 268–9882
Fax: (416) 923–0935
Telex/E-mail: 065 24479

4423. Utlas International Inc
8300 College Boulevard
Overland Park
KS 66210
USA
Telephone: (913) 451–3111;
               (800) 338–8527

4424. Valkieser Group B.V.
E Spin
's-Gravelandseweg 80A
1217 EW Hilversum
Netherlands
Telephone: +31 35 234858
Fax: +31 35 232711

4425. Valorinform SA
14 rue des Cordiers
PO Box 476
CH-1211 Geneva 6
Switzerland
Telephone: 022 786 32 33
Fax: 022 786 35 28
Telex/E-mail: 289587 VAL CH

4426. Valtion Tietokonekeskus
Finnish State Computer Centre
PO Box 40
SF-02101 Espoo
Finland
Telephone: 0 4571
Fax: 0 457–3756
Telex/E-mail: 125833 VTKK SF

4427. Value Line Inc
Renny Ponvert
711 3rd Avenue
4th Floor
New York
NY 10017
USA
Telephone: (212) 687–3965
Fax: (212) 661–2807;
       (212) 986–3243
Telex/E-mail: 9863243

4428. Van Dale Lexicografie, bv
M.A. Moerland
Mariaplaats 21 c
PO Box 19232
3511 LK Utrecht
Netherlands
Telephone: (31) 030–331484

4429. Vance Publishing Corporation
7950 College Boulevard
Overland Park
KS 66210
USA
Telephone: (913) 451–2200;
      (800) 255–5113
Fax: (913) 451–5821
Telex/E-mail: 4941149

4430. VCH Verlagsgesellschaft
Postfach 1260/1280
D-6940 Weinheim
Germany

4431. VDI-Verlag GmbH
Heinrichstraße 24
D-4000 Dusseldorf 1
Germany
Telephone: 0211 62141;
      0211 61880
Fax: 0211 618–8112
Telex/E-mail: 6 587 743 VDI V;
  08586525 D

4432. VE-data
Per Nielsen; Kirsten Kjaer Anderson
Fibigerstreede 2
DK-9220 Aalborg O
Denmark
Telephone: 09 815–8066

4433. VEB
Datenverarbeitungszentrum Statistik
Hnas-Beimler-Straße 70–72
Postschließfach 31
D-1020 Berlin
Germany

**4434. Vejdirektoratets
    Vejdatalaboratorium**
Jan Froelich; Erich Thor Straten
Stationsalleen 42
DK-2730 Herlev
Denmark
Telephone: 042 919–633
Fax: 042 916–141

4435. Vektor Ltd
Ian Robertson
Technology House
Lissadel Street
Salford
Manchester
M6 6AP
UK
Telephone: +44 61 745 9888
Fax: +44 61 745 8077

4436. Venture Economics Inc
75 2nd Avenue
Suite 700
Needham
MA 02158
USA
Telephone: (617) 449–2100
Fax: (617) 449–7660
Telex/E-mail: 948637 VENTICON WELL

4437. VERALEX Inc
One Graves Street
PO Box 92824
Rochester
NY 14692
USA
Telephone: (716) 546–7111;
      (800) 828–6373;
      (800) 462–6807 (in NY)
Fax: (716) 546–1097

**4438. Verband der Vereine
    Creditreform eV**
Herr Stenmans; Werner Strahler
Creditreform-Datenbank-Dienste
Postfach 10 15 52
Hellersbergstraße 12
D-4040 Neuss 1
Germany
Telephone: 02101 109–140;
      02101 1090
Fax: 02101 109–140
Telex/E-mail: 8517544 VVC D

4439. Verbum Magazine
Jeanne Juneau; Michael Gosney
670 7th Ave
2nd Floor
San Diego
CA 92101
USA
Telephone: (619) 233–9977
Fax: (619) 233–9976

**4440. Verein Deutscher
    Eisenhuttenleute**
Sohnstrasse 65
Postfach 8209
Dusseldorf 1
W-4000
Germany
Telephone: 42–211–67–07–310

**4441. Verein Textildokumentation
    und information**
Cromforder Allee 22
4030 Rattingen
Germany
Telephone: 49 (2102) 2 70 51

4443. Verlag Dr Otto Schmidt KG
Rolf-Dieter Humbert
Unter den Ulmen 96 – 98
5000 Cologne 51
Germany
Telephone: +49 2 21 34980
Fax: +49 2 21 3498181

4444. Verlag Dr. Josef Raabe KG
Rotebuehlstrasse 77
Postfach 599
7000 Stuttgart
Germany
Telephone: 49 (711) 6 67 22 – 71
Telex/E-mail: 722232 D

4445. Verlag H Schäfer GmbH, Die
Mr Vollrath (Manager)
Postfach 2243
6380 Bad Homburg 1
Germany
Telephone: 6172 7011
Fax: 6172 71288

**4446. Verlag Information &
    Kommunikation**
Saalburgstraße 157
D-6380 Bad Homburg
Germany
Telephone: 06172 32007
Fax: 06172 304–178

4447. Verlag Ingrid Czwalina
Prof Dr Clemens Czwalina (General
  Manager)
Reesenbüttier Redder 75
2070 Ahrensburg
Germany
Telephone: 4102 59190
Fax: 4102 50992

4448. Verlag W Sachon GmbH & Co
Schloß Mindelburg
Postfach
8948 Mindelheim
Germany
Telephone: +49 8261 9990
Fax: +49 8261 999132

4449. Verlagshaus Riedmuhle GmbH
Oberer Erlenbach 9
Alheim
W-6445
Germany
Telephone: 05664–7028
Fax: 05664–6055

4450. Vestek Systems Inc
388 Market Street
Suite 700
San Francisco
CA 94111
USA
Telephone: (415) 398–6340
Fax: (415) 392–6831

4451. Vestlandsforsking
Parkvegen 5
PB 142
5801 Sogndal
Norway
Telephone: (47) 593 21 00

4452. Vestlash Group Inc
627 E Street NW
Suite 300
Washington
DC 20004
USA
Telephone: (202) 347–6973
Fax: (202) 628–1133

**4453. Veterinary Information
    Company Inc, The**
Suite 108–110
Langmuir Laboratory
Cornell Industry Research Park
Brown Road
Ithaca
NY 14850
USA
Telephone: (607) 257–4303
Fax: (607) 257–2445
Telex/E-mail: 43:LSR001 (Dialcom)

4454. VGL & Associates
43 Emerick Street
Ashland
OR 97520
USA
Telephone: (503) 482–3194

**4455. Vickers Stock Research
    Corporation**
226 New York Avenue
Huntington
NY 11743
USA
Telephone: (516) 423–7710;
      (800) 645–5043;
      (800) 832–5280 (in NY)
Fax: (516) 423–7715

4456. Victoria Ministry of Education
Planning and Policy Branch, Schools
  Division Library
Helen Hargreaves
Level 7
Rialto Towers
525 Collins Street
Melbourne
VIC 3000
Australia
Telephone: 03 628–2464
Fax: 03 614–5068

4457. Victoria University of Technology
Footscray Institute of Technology
Dr Neil Shaw
Centre for Research & Development
Technology Based Training Group
PO Box 64
Footscray
Victoria 3011
Australia
Telephone: +61 3 688 4706
Fax: +61 3 687 2089

4458. Victorian Institute of Marine Sciences
14 Parliament Place
Melbourne
VIC 3002
Australia

4459. Vidmar Communications Inc
A subsidiary of Phillips Publishing Inc
1680 N. Vine Street, Suite 820
Hollywood
CA 90028
USA
Telephone: (213) 462–6350
Fax: (213) 467–0314

4460. Vierbergen NV
Hugo Vierbergen
Mechelse Steenweg 301
2830 Willebroek
Belgium
Telephone: +32 3 886 95 81
Fax: +32 3 886 75 45

4461. VIFI / Munksgaard
Tom Ornstrup Madsen
Norre Sogade 35
DK 1370 Copenhagen
Denmark
Telephone: 45 1 12 70 30

4462. VININFO SA
12 place de la Bourse
F-33076 Bordeaux Cedex
France
Telephone: 56 79 50 86
Fax: 56 81 80 45

4463. VINITI
All-Union Institute for Scientific and Technical Information
c/o International Center for Scientific and Technical Information
Ulllitsa Kuusinena 21b
125252 Moscow
Russia
Telephone: 095 198–7460
Fax: 095 943–0089
Telex/E-mail: 411925 MCNTI SU

4464. Violette Wine Cellars
1776 Massachusetts Avenue
Cambridge
MA 02140
USA
Telephone: (617) 876–4125

4465. Virgin Games Inc
Lyle J Hall II
18061 Fitch Avenue
Irvine
CA 92714
USA
Telephone: (714) 833 8710
Fax: (714) 833 8717

4466. Virgin Games
Catherine Spratt; Steve Clark
338A Ladbroke Grove
London
W10 5AH
UK
Telephone: 081 960–2055
Fax: 081 960–9900

4467. Virgin Mastertronic
16 Portland Road
London
W11 4LA
UK

4468. Virgin Mastertronic
18001 Cowan Street A7B
Irvine
CA 92714
USA

4469. Virginia Cooperative Extension – USDA
Mary Miller
Extension Information Systems
Virginia Tech
Plaza 1, Building D
Blacksburg
VA 24061–0524
USA
Telephone: (703) 961–7244

4470. Virginia Polytechnic Institute and State University
Department of Computer Science
Dr Edward A Fox
562 McBryde Hall
Blacksburg
VA 24061–0106
USA
Telephone: (703) 231 5113
Fax: (703) 231 6075

4471. Visa Advisors Inc
1930 18th Street NW
Suite 22
Washington
DC 20009
USA
Telephone: (202) 797–7976
Fax: (202) 667–6708

4472. Vision Information Inc
295 Greenwich Street
10th Floor
New York
NY 10007
USA
Telephone: (212) 840–6557
Fax: (212) 619–2724

4473. VLS – Video Laser Systems
5215–11 Monroe Street
Toledo
OH 43623
USA
Telephone: (419) 536–5820

4474. VNIIPM Research Institute
c/o International Center for Scientific and Technical Information
Ulitsa Kuusinena 21b
125252 Moscow
Russia
Telephone: 095 198–7460
Fax: 095 943–0089
Telex/E-mail: 411925 MCNTI SU

4475. VNU Business Publications BV
PO Box 9194
1006 CC Amsterdam
Netherlands
Telephone: 31 (20) 51 02 911

4476. VNU Business Publications BV
Margaret McPhee
VNU House
32–34 Broadwick Street
London
W1A 2HG
UK
Telephone: 071 439–4242
Fax: 071 437–9638

4477. Vocational Technologies Ltd
J. Twining
32 Castle Street
Guildford
Surrey
GU1 3UW
UK
Telephone: 44 483 579 472
Fax: 44 483 574 277

4478. Voight Industries Inc
PO Box 200
Lubec
ME 04652
USA
Telephone: (207) 733–5593

4479. Volkswagen AG
EI-Fachinformation und bibliothek
Postfach
3180 Wolfsburg 1
Germany
Telephone: 49 (5361) 92 46 39
Fax: 49 (5361) 92 82 82
Telex/E-mail: 95860 VWW D

4480. Volunteer Centre UK, The
29 Lower King's Road
Berkhamsted
Hertfordshire
HP4 2AB
UK
Telephone: 0442 873–311

4481. Vortex Interactive
R L Currier
1866 Laurel Road
Oceanside
CA 92054
USA
Telephone: (619) 439 1079
Fax: (619) 439 1079

4007. Voyager Company
Aleen Stein; Brenda Zozaya
1351 Pacific Coast Highway
Santa Monica
CA 90401
USA
Telephone: (213) 451 1383
Fax: (213) 394 2156

4482. VRC Consulting Group Inc
289 S San Antonio Road
Los Altos
CA 94022
USA
Telephone: (415) 948–1513
Fax: (415) 948–1339

4483. VSMI/PhotoNet
4200 Aurora Street
Suite N
Coral Gables
FL 33146–1850
USA
Telephone: (305) 444–0144;
                (800) 368–6638
Telex/E-mail: 42: 1200 (Dialcom)

4484. VU/TEXT Information Services
325 Chestnut Street
Suite 1300
Philadelphia
PA 19106
USA
Telephone: (215) 574–4400;
(215) 574–4421;
(800) 258–8080;
(800) 323–2940
Fax: (215) 627–0194

4485. Vuxenutbildarcentrum
Kaserngatan 34
582 28 Linkoeping
Sweden

4486. VVO Licensintorg
Oy LISTECH Ltd
Hameentie 103
PO Box 16
SF-00550 Helsinki
Finland
Telephone: 0 701–4544
Fax: 0 701–4151
Telex/E-mail: 121860 LISTE SF

4487. VWD
Niederurseler Alllee 8–10
Postfach 6105
D-6236 Eschborn 1
Germany
Telephone: 06196 405–205
Fax: 06196 482–007
Telex/E-mail: 4072895 D

4488. W-Two Publications Ltd
202 The Commons
Suite 401
Ithaca
NY 14850
USA
Telephone: (607) 277–0934

4489. Wakeman/Walworth Inc
300 N Washington Street
Suite 204
Alexandria
VA 22314
USA
Telephone: (703) 549–8606
Fax: (703) 549–1372

4490. Wall Street Transcript
99 Wall Street
New York
NY 10005
USA
Telephone: (212) 747–9500
Telex/E-mail: 127894

4491. Walnut Creek CD-ROM
1547 Palos Verdes Mall
Suite 260
Walnut Creek
CA 94596
USA
Telephone: (800) 786–9907

4492. Walters Lexikon
Goran Walter
Box 119
161 26 Bromma
Sweden
Telephone: +46 8261470
Fax: +46 8273286

4493. Walton
Françoise Verebelyi
4 rue de Ventadour
75001 Paris
France
Telephone: 1 45 35 22 03
Fax: 1 46 36 64 02

4494. Ward's Communications Inc
28 W Adams
Detroit
MI 48226
USA
Telephone: (313) 962–4433

4495. Warner Computer Systems Inc
17–01 Pollitt Drive
Fair Lawn
NJ 07410
USA
Telephone: (201) 794–2870

4496. Warner New Media
Linda Rich; Kim Sudhalter
3500 W Olive Avenue
Suite 1050
Burbank
CA 91505
USA
Telephone: (818) 955–9999
Fax: (818) 955–6499

4497. Warren Publishing Inc
2115 Ward Court NW
Washington
DC 20037
USA
Telephone: (202) 872–9200
Fax: (202) 293–3435
Telex/E-mail: 6502173616 Via WUI

4498. Washington Business Information Inc
1117 N 19th Street
Suite 200
Arlington
VA 22209
USA
Telephone: (703) 247–3434
Fax: (703) 247–3421

4499. Washington Center for Central American Studies
PO Box 7248
Silver Springs
MD 20907
USA
Telephone: (301) 270–9577

4500. Washington Monitor Inc, The
Suite 1000
1301 Pennsylvania Avenue NW
Washington
DC 20004
USA
Telephone: (202) 347–7757

4501. Washington On-Line
4200 Wilson, 10th Floor
Arlington
VA 22003
USA
Telephone: (202) 543–9101

4502. Washington Post Company
CD-ROM Enquiries
1150 15th Street NW
Washington
DC 20071
USA
Telephone: (202) 334–7341
Telex/E-mail: 89522 WSHA WASHPOST

4503. Washington Regulatory Reporting Associates
PO Box 2220
Springfield
VA 22152
USA
Telephone: (703) 451–4575;
(703) 690–8240

4504. Washington Research Associates
2103 North Lincoln Street
Arlington
VA 22207
USA
Telephone: (703) 276–8260

4505. Washington Researchers Ltd
2612 P Street NW
Washington
DC 20007–3062
USA
Telephone: (202) 333–3499
Fax: (202) 625–0656

4506. Washington Times, The
3600 New York Avenue NE
Washington
DC 20002
USA
Telephone: (202) 636–3028

4507. Waste Management Information Bureau
United Kingom Atomic Energy Authority
Building 46J
Harwell Laboratory
Harwell
Oxfordshire
OX11 0RB
UK
Telephone: 44 (235) 24141

4508. Water Research Centre
Stevenage Laboratory
Elder Way
Stevenage
Hertfordshire
SG1 1TH
UK
Telephone: 44 (438) 312444
Fax: 44 (438) 315694
Telex/E-mail: 826168 G

4509. Waterlow Information Service
Waterlow Signature
Michael Harrington; Kasia Rafalat
Paulton House
8 Shepherdess Walk
London
N1 7LB
UK
Telephone: 071 490–0049;
0800 181377
Fax: 071 490–2979
NUA: 234284400162

4510. Waters Information Services Inc
PO Box 2248
Binghamton
NY 13902
USA
Telephone: (607) 772–8086;
(607) 770–8535
Fax: (607) 798–1692; (607) 723–7151
Telex/E-mail: MTR (MCI Mail)

4511. Wayzata Technology
Mark Engelhardt
PO Box 807
Grand Rapids
MN 55744
USA
Telephone: (218) 326 0597;
(800) 735 7321
Fax: (218) 326 0598

4512. Weatherdisc Associates, Inc
Dr Clifford F Mass
4584 NE 89th
Seattle
WA 98115
USA
Telephone: (206) 524 4314
Fax: (206) 543 0308

4513. WEFA Benelux SA
Avenue des Arts 52
1040 Brussels
Belgium
Telephone: 32 (2) 511 11 44

4514. WEFA Canada Inc
777 Bay Street
Suite 2020
PO Box 143
Toronto
ON M5G 2C8
Canada
Telephone: (416) 599–5700

4515. WEFA CEIS
Wharton Consulting and Economic
    Information Services
Mr Lisse
25 rue de Ponthieu
75008 Paris
France
Telephone: 1 45 63 19 10
Telex/E-mail: 260710 F
NUA: 234212300110; 20809318012030
    (Comext Only)

4516. WEFA GmbH
Reuterweg 47
6000 Frankfurt am Main 1
Germany
Telephone: 49 (69) 72 87 97

4517. WEFA Group, The
401 City Avenue
Suite 300
Bala Cynwyd
PA 19004
USA
Telephone: (215) 667–6000;
            (800) 322–9332
Fax: (215) 660–6477; (215) 668–9524
Telex/E-mail: 831609

4518. WEFA Limited
Edbury Gate, 23
Lower Belgrave
London
SW1W 0NW
UK
Telephone: 071 730–8171

4519. WEFA-CEIS Srl
Via Montenapoleone 12
20121 Milan
Italy
Telephone: 39 (2) 70 10 07

4520. WEFA-CEIS Srl
Via Toscana, 10–int.8
00187 Rome
Italy
Telephone: 39 (6) 46 00 80

4521. Weiss Research Inc
2200 N Florida Mango Road
West Palm Beach
FL 33409
USA
Telephone: (407) 684–8100

4522. Welding Institute, The
Abington Hall
Abington
Cambridge
CB1 6AL
UK
Telephone: 0223 891–162
Fax: -223 892–588
Telex/E-mail: 81183 WELDEX G

**4523. Wer Liefert Was (Germany)
    (See Bezugsquellennachweis
    für den Einkauf)**

**4524. Wer Liefert Was? / Who
    Supplies What? Austria**
Marco Oliva; Stephan Preziger
Dannebergplatz 16
A-1030 Vienna
Austria
Telephone: 01 712 1074
Fax: 01 713 8948

**4525. Werbe- und
    Vertriebsgesellschaft
    Deutscher Apotheker mbH**
Dr Dorothee Helmecke
Beethovenplatz 1–3
Postfach 97 01 08
D-6000 Frankfurt am Main 97
Germany
Telephone: +49 69 75 44 1
Fax: +49 69 74 92 68

4526. Werbung Gert Richter
Bismarckstrasse 84
1000 Berlin 12
Germany
Telephone: 49 (30) 31 77 22

**4527. Werner Söderström
    Osakeyhtiö – WSOY**
Petri Arpo
Bulevardi 12
PO Box 222
SF-00121 Helsinki
Finland
Telephone: 0 61681
Fax: 0 6168510

4528. Wescom Corporation
333 Jericho Turnpike
Jericho
NY 11753
USA
Telephone: (516) 433–3770;
            (800) 634–6997
Telex/E-mail: 910 380 9088; 62900472
    ESL (EasyLink)

4529. West Publishing Company
Rahndy Jadinak
50 W Kellogg Boulevard
PO Box 64526
St Paul
MN 55164–0526
USA
Telephone: (612) 228–2500;
            (800) 328–0109;
            (800) 888–9907
Fax: (612) 228 2863

**4530. West Wales Training
    Information Service**
Mike Morgan
34a King Street
Carmarthen
SA31 1BS
Wales, UK
Telephone: 0800 515821

**4531. Western Australia Fire
    Brigades Board**
B Curtin L Higgins
480 Hay Street
Perth 6001
Australia
Telephone: +61 93239300
Fax: +61 92211935

4532. Western Legal Publications Ltd
1 Alexander Street
Suite 301
Vancouver
BC V6A 1B2
Canada
Telephone: (604) 687–5671;
            (800) 663–0422 (in Canada)
Fax: (604) 687–3012

4533. Western Library Network
Rushton Brandis
PO Box 3888
4224 6th Avenue SE
Building 3
Lacey
WA 98503
USA
Telephone: (206) 459–6518
Fax: (206) 459–6341
Telex/E-mail: (800) 342–5956; 510 101
    2449

4534. Western Union Corporation
1 Lake Street
Upper Saddle River
NJ 07458
USA
Telephone: (201) 825–5000;
            (800) 527–5184
Telex/E-mail: 642491

**4535. Western Union InfoMaster (See
    Western Union Corporation)**

**4536. Westgate Publishing Company
    Inc**
751 Main Street
PO Box 9079
Waltham
MA 02254
USA
Telephone: (617) 899–1271

4537. WGE Publishing
Forest Road
Hancock
NH 03449–0278
USA
Telephone: (603) 525–4201
Fax: (603) 525–4423

4538. Wheeler Arts
Stephen Wheeler
66 Lake Park
Champaign
IL 61821–7101
USA
Telephone: (217) 359 6816
Fax: (217) 359 8716

4539. Whig-Standard, The
306 King Street E
Kingston
ON K7L 4Z7
Canada
Telephone: (613) 544–5000

**4540. White Horse Technical
    Services**
Paul Fletcher
Meiro Hall
Kidwelly
Dyfed
SA17 5DE
Wales, UK

4541. Whitehall Press Limited
Earl House
Earl Street
Maidstone
Kent
ME14 1PE
UK
Telephone: 44 (622) 59841

**4542. Whitman, Requardt and
Associates**
2315 St Paul Street
Baltimore
MD 21218
USA
Telephone: (301) 235–3450

**4543. Wichita Eagle-Beacon
Publishing Company Inc**
825 E Douglas
Box 820
Wichita
KS 67202
USA
Telephone: (316) 268–6000
Fax: (316) 268–6604

**4544. Wiener Institut für
Internationale
Wirtschaftsvergleiche**
Postfach 87
A-1103 Vienna
Austria
Telephone: 0222 7826 0179;
0222 7825 674 79
Fax: 0222 78 71 20

4545. Wila-Verlag Wilhelm Lampl KG
Landsberger Straße 191 A
D-8000 Munich 21
Germany
Telephone: 089 579–5235;
089 579–5220
Fax: 089 570–6693

4546. William S Hein & Company Inc
Daniel P Rosati
1285 Main Street
Buffalo
NY 14209–1987
USA
Telephone: (716) 882 8600
Fax: (716) 883 8100

4547. Williams and Wilkins
Debbie Moody
428 East Preston Street
Baltimore
MD 21202
USA
Telephone: (301) 528 4118
Fax: (301) 528 4312

4548. Willow Tree Press Inc
PO Box 249
Monsey
NY 10952
USA
Telephone: (914) 354–9139
Fax: (201) 648–1275

4549. Wilshire Associates
1299 Ocean Avenue
Santa Monica
CA 90401
USA
Telephone: (213) 451–3051

4550. Window Book Inc
Marketing Department
61 Howard Street
Cambridge
MA 02139
USA
Telephone: (617) 661 9515
Fax: (617) 354 3961

4551. Windows Users Group
Tim Bunning
UK
Telephone: 0909 501351
Fax: 0909 501511

**4552. Windsor Systems Development
Inc**
11 W 42nd Street
New York
NY 10036
USA
Telephone: (212) 789–3555
Fax: (212) 789–3577

4553. Wine On Line International
J Walmar
400 E 59th Street
Suite 9F
New York
NY 10022
USA
Telephone: (212) 755–4363
Fax: (212) 755–4365
Telex/E-mail: PUNCH IN (DELPHI)

4554. Wing Aviation Press
1–14–5 Ginza
Chuo-ku
Tokyo 104
Japan
Telephone: 81 (3) 561–8305

4555. WIS – Wright Investors Service
10 Middle Street
Bridgeport
CT 06604
USA
Telephone: (203) 333–6666

**4556. Wisconsin State Library
Agency**
Department of Public Instruction
Mary Clark
2109 South Storeton Road
Madison
WI 53716
USA
Telephone: (608) 221 2166
Fax: (608) 221 6178

4557. WNET Learning Link
356 W 58th Street
New York
NY 10019
USA
Telephone: (212) 560–6613

4558. Wolters-Noordhoff BV
J D Dijkstra
Damsport 157
9700 MB Groningen
Netherlands
Telephone: +31 50 226922
Fax: +31 50 264866

4559. Woods & Poole Economics Inc
1794 Columbia Road NW
Washington
DC 20009
USA
Telephone: (202) 332–7111

4560. Woodside Research Ltd
PO Box 6359
Station D
Calgary
AB T2P 2C9
Canada
Telephone: (403) 269–6003

**4561. Worcester Telegram & Gazette
Inc**
20 Franklin Street
Worcester
MA 01613–0666
USA
Telephone: (617) 793–9100

**4562. Workers' Compensation
Appeals Tribunal**
Information Department
505 University Avenue
7th Floor
Toronto
ON M5G 1X4
USA
Telephone: (416) 598–4638
Fax: (416) 965–3558

4563. World 'Vest-Base
1335 N Dearborn Parkway
Chicago
IL 60610
USA
Telephone: (312) 266–0575

4564. World Bank, The
International Economics Department
1818 H Street NW
Washington
DC 20433
USA
Telephone: (202) 473–2939;
(202) 473–3800
Fax: (202) 473–8456

**4565. World Book – Childcraft
International**
Michael J Brown
World Book House
7 Mount Ephraim
Tunbridge Wells
Kent
TN4 8AZ
UK
Telephone: +44 892 547811
Fax: +44 892 24702

4566. World Book – Childcraft
Merchandise Mart Plaza
Chicago
IL 60654
USA
Telephone: (312) 245 3090

**4567. World Book Educational
Products of Canada**
James Mohler
5805 Whittle Road
Suite 106
Mississauga
Ontario
L4Z 2J1
Canada
Telephone: (416) 568 0105
Fax: (416) 568 0113

**4568. World Book Educational
Products**
Paul E Rafferty
101 Northwest Point Boulevard
Elk Grove Village
IL 60007
USA
Telephone: (708) 290 5300
Fax: (708) 290 5403

4569. World Book Publishing
A. Richard Harmet
525 West Monroe Street
Chicago
IL 60606
USA
Telephone: (312) 258–3700

4570. World Economic Intelligence Center
4-1-35 Mita
Suite 1006
Minato-ku
Tokyo 108
Japan
Telephone: 03 3769–0246
Fax: 03 3769–0248

4571. World Health Organisation
WHO
20 avenue Appia
1211 GENEVA 27
Switzerland
Telephone: +41 22/791 21 11
Fax: +41 22/791 07 46
Telex/E-mail: 27821 oms

4572. World Information Systems
PO Box 535
Harvard Square Station
Cambridge
MA 02238
USA
Telephone: (617) 491–5100
Fax: (617) 492–3312

4573. World Intellectual Property Organisation
Paul Claus
34 chemin des Colombettes
CH-1211 Geneva 20
Switzerland
Telephone: 022 730–9111;
022 730–9146
Fax: 022 733–5428
Telex/E-mail: 412912 OMPI CH

4574. World Library Inc
William A Hustwit CEO
12914 Haster Street
Garden Grove
CA 92640
USA
Telephone: (714) 748 7197
Fax: (714) 748 7198

4575. World Publishing Company
315 S Boulder Avenue
PO Box 1770
Tulsa
OK 74103
USA
Telephone: (918) 583–2161;
(918) 581–8400;
(918) 581–8300;
(800) 642–2525

4576. World Times Inc
210 World Trade Center
Boston
MA 02210
USA
Telephone: (617) 439–5400

4577. World Trade Center
1 Avenida do Brasil
1700 Lisbon
Portugal
Telephone: 351 (1) 73 35 71;
351 (1) 73 27 08
Fax: 351 (1) 76 84 36
Telex/E-mail: 12326 WTCLIS P

4578. World Trade Centers Association Inc
1 World Trade Center
Suite 55 East
New York
NY 10048
USA
Telephone: (212) 466–7196;
(800) 937–8886
Fax: (212) 321–3305
Telex/E-mail: 285472 WTNY UR

4579. Worldscope/Disclosure Partners
CD-Enquiries
Wright International Financial Center
1000 Lafayette Boulevard
Bridgeport
CT 06604
USA
Telephone: (212) 581 1414
Fax: (212) 765 8486

4580. Worldspan LP
PO Box 901555
7310 Tiffany Springs Parkway
Kansas City
MO 64153
USA
Telephone: (816) 891–5300
Fax: (816) 891–5320; (816) 891–6170

4581. Worldwide Exchange
1344 Pacific Avenue, Suite 103
Santa Cruz
CA 95060
USA
Telephone: (408) 425–0531
Telex/E-mail: 6503493973

4582. Worldwide Videotex
PO Box 138
Babson Park Branch
Boston
MA 02157
USA
Telephone: (617) 449–1603

4583. WRC plc
Library and Information Services
WRC Medmenham Laboratory
PO Box 16
Marlow
Buckinghamshire
SL7 2HD
UK
Telephone: 0491 571–531
Fax: 0491 579–094
Telex/E-mail: 848632

4584. Wright Enterprises
Hudson Road
Temple
NH 03804
USA

4585. Wright Investors' Service
Harold Sands
85–87 Jermyn Street
London
SW1Y 6JD
UK
Telephone: 0441 930–4734

4586. Wright Investors' Service
Jim Ford
Wright International Financial Center
1000 Lafayette Boulevard
Bridgeport
CT 06604
USA
Telephone: (203) 333–6666;
(800) 232–0013
Fax: (203) 579–0424
Telex/E-mail: 7104531048

4587. WSI Corporation
4 Federal Street
Billerica
MA 01821
USA
Telephone: (508) 670–5000
Telex/E-mail: 951184

4588. WSM Publishing Company
PO Box 466
Merrifield
VA 22116
USA
Telephone: (703) 255–3093
Telex/E-mail: 197652 T REP WASHDC

4589. X/Open
Phil Holmes
UK
Telephone: +44 (0)734 508311

4590. Xebec Multimedia Solutions
Peter Howell; Chris Horseman
Smith House
1–3 George Street
Nailsworth
Gloucestershire
GL6 0AG
UK
Telephone: 0453 835482
Fax: 0453 832241

4591. Xebec
2055 Gateway Place
Suite 600
San Jose
CA 95110
USA
Telephone: 408–287–7000

4592. Xinhua (New China) News Agency
United Nations Bureau
155 W 66th Street
New York
NY 10023
USA
Telephone: (212) 722–7493

4593. XIPHIAS
Susan Black
Helms Hall
8758 Venice Road
Los Angeles
CA 90034
USA
Telephone: (213) 841 2790
Fax: (213) 841 2559

4594. XMA Ltd
Wilford Industrial Estate
Ruddington Lane
Nottingham
NG11 7EP
UK
Telephone: 0602 8182222

4595. Xploratorium
Anglia Polytechnic
UK
Telephone: 0277 211363

4596. Yacht Exchange Inc, The
1661 SE 10th Terrace
Fort Lauderdale
FL 33316
USA
Telephone: (305) 467–1701
Fax: (305) 467–7252
Telex/E-mail: (800) 327–2515

4597. Yakugyo Jihoo Sha
Ro Midorikawa
2–36 Kanda-Jimbo-cho
Chiyoda-ku
Tokyo 103
Japan
Telephone: +81 3 3261 8527
Fax: +81 3 3261 8527

4598. Yearbook Medical Publishers
200 North La Salle
Chicago
IL 60601
USA
Telephone: (312) 726–9733;
(800) 861–9262

4599. Yomiuri Shimbunsha
Information Research Department,
Database Bunshitsu
7–1 Otemachi
1 Chome
Chiyoda-ku
Tokyo 100–55
Japan
Telephone: 03 3242–1111;
03 3217–8215

4600. Young Minds Inc
Thomas Stapleton
308 West State Street
Suite 2B
Redlands
CA 92373
USA
Telephone: (714) 335 1350
Fax: (714) 798 0488

4601. Youngstown Free-Net
Youngstown State University
Computer Center
Youngstown
OH 44555
USA
Telephone: (216) 742–3072
Telex/E-mail: AA001 YFN.YSU.EDU
(Internet)

4602. Yves Balbure
49 avenue de Colmar
F-92500 Rueil-Malmaison
France
Telephone: 1 47 51 84 31

4603. Zacks Investment Research Inc
155 N Wacker Drive
Chicago
IL 60601
USA
Telephone: (312) 630–9880

4604. Zagat Survey
45 W 45th Street
New York
NY 10036
USA
Telephone: (212) 302–0505

4605. Zanichelli Editore SpA
Via Irnerio 34
40126 Bologna
Italy
Telephone: +39 51 293219;
+39 51 293111
Fax: +39 51 249782;
+39 51 293224

4606. ZAP Optical
Alasdair Scott
B5R, Metropolitan Wharf
Wapping Wall
London
E11 9SS
UK
Telephone: 071 702–4524
Fax: 071 702–4507

4607. ZapoDel Inc
PO Box 1049
Del Mar
CA 92014
USA
Telephone: (619) 481–7337
Telex/E-mail: CALKOBRIN (GEnie
Mail); ZAPODEL (Delphi Mail)

4608. Zedtronics Pty Ltd.
4 Collingwood St.
Osborne Park
Western Australia 6005
Australia
Telephone: 61–9–244–3011

**4609. Zentrale Dokumentationsstelle
der Freien Wohlfahrtspflege für**
Flüchtlinge
Hans-Boeckler-Straße 3
D-5300 Bonn 3
Germany
Telephone: 0228 462–047;
0228 462–048
Fax: 0228 464–704

**4610. Zentralstelle für
Agrardokumentation und
-information (ZADI)**
Dr E König
Villichgasse 17
Postfach 20 14 15
D-5300 Bonn 2
Germany
Telephone: 0228 35 70 97
Fax: 0228 35 81 26

**4611. Zentralstelle für
Psychologische Information
und Dokumentation**
Universität Trier
Postfach 3825
D-5500 Trier
Germany
Telephone: 49 (651) 2 01 28 77
Fax: 49 (651) 25135
Telex/E-mail: 472680 UNITR D

**4612. Zentralverband der Elektro-
technischen Industrie eV**
Stresemannallee 19
D-6000 Frankfurt am Main 70
Germany
Telephone: 069 630–2277
Telex/E-mail: 411035 ZVEI D

4613. Ziff Communications Company
Computer Library
Paul O'Brien
1 Park Avenue
New York
NY 10016
USA
Telephone: (212) 503–4400
Fax: (212) 503–4414

**4614. Ziff Davis Technical
Information Company**
Angee Baker
80 Blanchard Road
Burlington
MA 01803
USA
Telephone: (617) 273 5500
Fax: (800) 227 1209

4615. Zondervan Corporation
1514 Lake Drive, SE
Grand Rapids
MI 49506
USA
Telephone: (616) 698–6900

**4616. Zweite Medizinische Klinik
rechts der Isar**
Toxikologische Abteilung
Ismaninger Straße 22
D-8000 Munich 80
Germany
Telephone: 089 4140–2240
Fax: 089 4140–2467
Telex/E-mail: 524404 D

INDEXES

HOST INDEX

(CNRS/INIST)   7:69, 7:150, 7:151,
7:152, 7:231, 7:232
CISTI MEDLARS   7:38, 7:282
CISTI, Canadian Online Enquiry Service
CAN/OLE   7:344
Compact Cambridge   7:53, 7:187,
7:261, 7:325
CompuServe Information Service   7:4,
7:11, 7:49, 7:110, 7:163, 7:166,
7:225, 7:247, 7:284, 7:345
Consejo Superior de Investigaciones
Científicas de España (CSIC)   7:176,
7:239
CORIS (Thomson Financial
Network)   7:275
COSTI   7:120
DAFA Data AB   7:217
Data-Star   7:5, 7:22, 7:50, 7:87, 7:121,
7:248, 7:283, 7:302, 7:312, 7:322,
7:346
DIALOG   7:6, 7:12, 7:31, 7:88, 7:122,
7:130, 7:138, 7:185, 7:193, 7:205,
7:226, 7:289, 7:303, 7:313
DIALOG OnDisc   7:125
DIALOG, Knowledge Index   7:51,
7:249, 7:259, 7:319, 7:326, 7:344
DIMDI   7:39, 7:92, 7:93, 7:94, 7:144,
7:160, 7:250, 7:266, 7:267, 7:270,
7:284, 7:304, 7:324, 7:336, 7:338,
7:340, 7:342
EBSCO   7:126, 7:202, 7:294
Epic Interactive Media   7:215
ESA-IRS   7:62, 7:133, 7:173, 7:227,
7:228, 7:229, 7:234
Européenne de Données   7:148, 7:154,
7:155, 7:278
Executive Telecom System
International, Human Resource
Information Network
(ETSI/HRIN)   7:139, 7:220, 7:241
Ferntree Computer Corporation Ltd,
AUSINET   7:196
FIZ Technik   7:27
FOA   7:142
G.CAM Serveur   7:278
GBI   7:45, 7:145, 7:333
HCI Service   7:168, 7:169
HELECON   7:181
Human Relations Area Files
Inc   7:76–7:77
HW Wilson Company   7:294, 7:296
Information Access Company
(IAC)   7:1, 7:7, 7:134, 7:158, 7:199
Information Ventures   7:116, 7:117
Institute for Scientific Information   7:89,
7:95, 7:96, 7:97, 7:98, 7:99, 7:211,
7:306, 7:307, 7:308, 7:309, 7:310
Japan Information Center of Science
and Technology (JICST)   7:174
Jouve   7:29
Mead Data Central (as a NEXIS
database)   7:243
MIC/Karolinska Institute Library and
Information Center (MIC KIBIC)   7:63
Micronet   7:82
Minitel   7:153, 7:233
National Council on Family
Relations   7:140
National Library of Medicine   7:40,
7:41, 7:285, 7:286
OCLC EPIC   7:251, 7:325
OCLC EPIC; OCLC FirstSearch   7:123,
7:292
OCLC FirstSearch   7:252, 7:331
ORBIT   7:64, 7:101, 7:118
PsyComNet   7:264
Questel   7:65, 7:149, 7:156, 7:157,
7:230
Scottish HCI Centre   7:71
SilverPlatter   7:13, 7:54, 7:55, 7:73,
7:75, 7:77, 7:79, 7:81, 7:112, 7:113,
7:127, 7:128, 7:194, 7:222, 7:255,

7:256, 7:257, 7:262, 7:268, 7:316,
7:327, 7:328, 7:349
Sociological Abstracts Inc   7:329
Statistika Centralbyrån (SCB)   7:318
STN   7:146, 7:186, 7:334
Swedish Council for Information on
Alcohol and Other Drugs   7:103
Tech Data   7:253, 7:348
Työterveyslaitoksen kirjasto
(TTL)   7:182
UN International Labour Organisation –
International Occupational Safety and
Health Information Centre   7:57,
7:58, 7:66
UNI-C, Denmark   7:237
University Microfilms
International   7:295
University of Tsukuba   7:254, 7:305
US Department of Education   7:129
US National Institute of Justice   7:213
Verlag Ingrid Czwalina   7:341
VTKK   7:179
WilsonLine   7:293

Dentistry

Australian MEDLINE Network   8:17,
8:37, 8:79
BLAISE-LINK   8:4, 8:18, 8:38, 8:80
BRS, Morning Search,
BRS/Colleague   8:25, 8:39
CD Plus   8:46
CDTV Publishing   8:33
CISTI MEDLARS   8:5, 8:19, 8:40, 8:81
Compact Cambridge   8:47
CompuServe Information Service   8:41,
8:57
Data-Star   8:42, 8:82
DIALOG OnDisc   8:55
DIALOG, Knowledge Index   8:43
DIMDI   8:20, 8:26, 8:44, 8:65, 8:83
EBSCO   8:48
FIZ Technik   8:66
Hoechst   8:67
Institute for Scientific Information   8:15,
8:27, 8:28, 8:29, 8:63
LifeART   8:61
MIC/Karolinska Institute Library and
Information Center (MIC KIBIC)   8:87
National Library of Medicine   8:6, 8:7,
8:21, 8:22, 8:45, 8:51, 8:69, 8:84,
8:85
NewsNet Inc   8:74
Services Documentaires Multimedia Inc
(SDM)   8:77
SilverPlatter   8:49, 8:50
SIS International   8:72
SUNIST   8:2, 8:11
University of Montreal, Faculty of Dental
Medicine   8:31
US National Institute of Dental
Research (NIDR), Office of Planning,
Evaluation and Communications,
Research Information Management
and Analysis Information
Section   8:70
VTKK   8:59
World Health Organisation – Division of
Noncommunicable Diseases   8:35
Youngstown Free-Net   8:89

Nutrition/Dietetics/Food Science

ACT Computer Services Ltd   9:66
Analyste-Conseil Systeme Informatique
Ltd   9:67
ASAS   9:15
BIOSIS Life Science Network   9:253
BIS   9:4, 9:34

BLAISE-LINK (as a part of
TOXNET)   9:254
BRS   9:176, 9:187
BRS, Morning Search,
BRS/Colleague   9:5, 9:6, 9:35, 9:52,
9:53
CAB International   9:51
Canada Systems Group   9:68
Canadian Centre for Occupational
Health and Safety (CCOHS)   9:264
CCINFOline   9:255
Centre National de la Recherche
Scientifique, Institut de l'Information
Scientifique et Technique, Science
Humaines et Sociales
(CNRS/INIST)   9:231, 9:232
Chemical Information Systems Inc
(CIS)   9:256
CISTI MEDLARS (as a part of
TOXNET)   9:257
CISTI, Canadian Online Enquiry Service
CAN/OLE   9:36, 9:85, 9:161
Compact Cambridge   9:126, 9:203,
9:242, 9:244
CompuServe Information Service   9:95,
9:181, 9:183, 9:188, 9:225, 9:286
Conference Board of Canada   9:69
CSIRO Australis   9:109, 9:268
Data Resources Inc (DRI)   9:70
Data-Star   9:37, 9:54, 9:55, 9:78, 9:86,
9:116, 9:159, 9:162, 9:189, 9:206,
9:211, 9:247, 9:258, 9:280
DIALOG   9:16, 9:79, 9:87, 9:100,
9:105, 9:129, 9:155, 9:190, 9:207,
9:226, 9:248, 9:249, 9:259
DIALOG, Knowledge Index   9:7, 9:8,
9:13, 9:38, 9:39, 9:56, 9:96, 9:163,
9:172
DIMDI   9:2, 9:9, 9:17, 9:18, 9:40, 9:57,
9:58, 9:59, 9:60, 9:124, 9:164, 9:260
Dimensions   9:71
Dow Jones News/Retrieval   9:250
EBSCO   9:197, 9:236
ESA-IRS   9:19, 9:23, 9:41, 9:42, 9:43,
9:61, 9:80, 9:88, 9:165, 9:208, 9:227,
9:228, 9:229, 9:234, 9:294
Executive Telecom System
International, Human Resource
Information Network
(ETSI/HRIN)   9:221
Fachinformationszentrum Technik (FIZ
Technik)   9:81, 9:209, 9:251 9:281
Food and Agriculture Organization of
the United Nations (FAO)   9:22
Food and Agriculture Organization of
the United Nations (FAO) Economic
and Social Policy Department Food
Policy and Nutrition Divisi on   9:132
FT Profile   9:210, 9:295
Gesellschaft für Elektronische Medien –
GEM   9:166
Hoechst   9:82
Hopkins Technology   9:149, 9:151,
9:271
Houghton-Mifflin   9:292
HW Wilson Company   9:178, 9:179,
9:288
Industrielle-Services Techniques
Inc   9:65
Information Access Company
(IAC)   9:191, 9:192, 9:194
Information Plus   9:72
INFORMIT (RMIT-INFORMIT)   9:269
International Atomic Energy Agency
(IAEA)   9:20
International Food Information Service
GmbH (IFIS)   9:171, 9:173
IP Sharp   9:73
Japan Information Center of Science
and Technology (JICST)   9:44, 9:167
Jouve   9:32

Health hazards and pollution

Forensic science

Hospital administration

Nursing

EBSCO 17:59, 17:72
Ellis Enterprises 17:68, 17:76
Healthcare Information Services
Inc 17:12
Knowledge Access 17:73
Mead Data Central (as a NEXIS
database) 17:17
MIC/Karolinska Institute Library and
Information Center (MIC
KIBIC) 17:91
National Library of Medicine 17:8,
17:9, 17:24, 17:25, 17:56, 17:62,
17:88, 17:89
NewsNet Inc 17:80
SilverPlatter 17:34, 17:35, 17:60,
17:61

Medical devices

Aldrich Chemical Co Inc 18:8, 18:10
Aries Systems Corporation 18:109
BIOSIS 18:25, 18:57, 18:64
BIOSIS Life Science Network 18:18
BRS 18:2, 18:5, 18:19, 18:100,
18:121, 18:147, 18:212, 18:213,
18:214, 18:225
BRS, BRS/Colleague 18:164
BRS, Morning Search,
BRS/Colleague 18:37, 18:38, 18:39,
18:69, 18:91, 18:145
CD Plus 18:73
CISTI, Canadian Online Enquiry Service
CAN/OLE 18:20, 18:40, 18:41,
18:42, 18:58
CMC ReSearch 18:205
Compact Cambridge 18:74
CompuServe Information
Service 18:43, 18:70, 18:101,
18:132, 18:139, 18:165, 18:215,
18:216, 18:217, 18:226
CORIS (Thomson Financial
Network) 18:163, 18:231
Corporate Technology Information
Services 18:89
Council of Scientific Research 18:44
Data Resources Inc (DRI) 18:107
Data-Star 18:3, 18:21, 18:35, 18:45,
18:46, 18:47, 18:59, 18:71, 18:87,
18:102, 18:122, 18:130, 18:148,
18:149, 18:166, 18:167, 18:168,
18:179, 18:218, 18:219, 18:220,
18:221, 18:232
Dialcom Inc 18:116
DIALOG 18:12, 18:22, 18:48, 18:49,
18:60, 18:103, 18:123, 18:140,
18:143, 18:157, 18:169, 18:180,
18:222, 18:223, 18:227,
18:233–18:234, 18:247, 18:248
DIALOG OnDisc 18:141, 18:153
DIALOG, Knowledge Index 18:72
DIMDI 18:29, 18:50, 18:51, 18:92,
18:199
DNAStar 18:250
Dom Optiki 18:208
Dow Jones 18:170, 18:235
ESA-IRS 18:23, 18:52, 18:61, 18:158
Fachhochschule Hamburg 18:78
FD Inc 18:118, 18:191
FIZ Technik 18:16, 18:200, 18:236
FIZ Technik (gateway) 18:171, 18:172,
18:173
FT Profile 18:80, 18:1744
General Electric Information Services
Company 18:114
General Videotex Corporation,
Delphi 18:155
Hamburg Educational
Partnership 18:134
Hoechst 18:201
IMS America Ltd 18:185

Informatievoorziening Gehandicapten
NL stichting 18:244, 18:245
Information Access Company
(IAC) 18:178
Informpribor 18:193, 18:236
Institute for Scientific
Information 18:31, 18:93, 18:94,
18:95, 18:187
International Institute of
Refrigeration 18:128
Japan Information Center of Science
and Technology (JICST) 18:53
Mead Data Central (as a NEXIS
database) 18:124, 18:125, 18:175
MIC/Karolinska Institute Library and
Information Center
(MIC-KIBIC) 18:240
MoldNIINTI 18:162
National Standards Association
Inc 18:14
NewsNet Inc 18:81, 18:83, 18:150,
18:176
NPO 18:210
NPO Rubin 18:105
OCLC EPIC; OCLC FirstSearch 18:54
ORBIT 18:88, 18:228
Preston Publications 18:67
REHADAT 18:234
Siemens AG 18:238
SilverPlatter 18:62, 18:63, 18:75,
18:76, 18:82, 18:111
SIS International 18:84
Socialstyrelsens
Läkemedelsavdelning 18:242
SOURCE, The 18:177
STN 18:24, 18:27, 18:55, 18:97,
18:159, 18:160, 18:229
Trace Research and Development
Center, Newington Children's
Hospital 18:6
University Microfilms International/Data
Courier Inc 18:230
University of Tsukuba 18:56

Veterinary medicine

ArmNIINTI 19:195
ASAS 19:35
BIOSIS 19:62
BIOSIS Life Science Network 19:55,
19:181
BIS 19:16, 19:72
BLAISE-LINK 19:250, 19:251
BLAISE-LINK (as a part of
TOXNET) 19:149
BRS 19:2, 19:56, 19:103, 19:221,
19:222, 19:223, 19:234
BRS, Morning Search,
BRS/Colleague 19:17, 19:18, 19:73,
19:90, 19:116, 19:117, 19:121,
19:252, 19:253
CAB International 19:89
Cambridge Scientific Abstracts 19:185,
19:186, 19:187, 19:188
Centre National de la Recherche
Scientifique, Institut de l'Information
Scientifique et Technique, Science
Humaines et Sociales
(CNRS/INIST) 19:213, 19:214
CISTI MEDLARS (as a part of
TOXNET) 19:150
CISTI, Canadian Online Enquiry Service
CAN/OLE 19:57, 19:74
Compact Cambridge 19:184
CompuKennel Information Service
Inc 19:106
CompuServe Information
Service 19:207, 19:224, 19:225,
19:226, 19:254
CSIRO Australis 19:114

Danmarks Veterinaer og
Jordbrugsbibliotek 19:168
Data-Star 19:3, 19:58, 19:75, 19:91,
19:118, 19:141, 19:227, 19:228,
19:229, 19:232, 19:235, 19:255,
19:256, 19:257, 19:258, 19:259
Datacentralen 19:12
DC Host Centre 19:128
DIALOG 19:27, 19:59, 19:108, 19:119,
19:182, 19:208, 19:230, 19:231,
19:239
DIALOG, Knowledge Index 19:19,
19:20, 19:25, 19:76, 19:77, 19:92,
19:260
DIMDI 19:10, 19:13, 19:21, 19:28,
19:29, 19:51, 19:78, 19:93, 19:94,
19:95, 19:96, 19:97, 19:122,
19:123, 19:147, 19:249, 19:261,
19:262
DTB 19:129
ESA-IRS 19:30, 19:34, 19:60, 19:79,
19:80, 19:81, 19:98, 19:209, 19:210,
19:211, 19:216
Food and Agriculture Organization of
the United Nations (FAO) 19:33
Forskningsbibliotekernes EDB
Kontor 19:130
GE Information Services (GEIS) 19:41
George Marinescu Hospital 19:203
Gosudarstwennaja Biblioteka SSSR im.
W. I. Lenina 19:143, 19:191
GPNTB SSSR 19:160
IIF 19:205, 19:247
IKONA Srl 19:8
IMS America Ltd 19:145
Institut eksperimentalnoj
Meteorologie 19:135
Institut obchej Genetiki 19:237
Institut Problem Kriobiologii i
Kriomedizinij 19:112
Institute for Scientific
Information 19:120, 19:124, 19:125,
19:126
International Atomic Energy Agency
(IAEA) 19:31
Japan Information Center of Science
and Technology (JICST) 19:82,
19:263, 19:264
Johan Bela Orszagos
Kozegeszsegugyi 19:45, 19:272
Knowledge Access 19:197
Minitel 19:215
Moskowskii Institut
Tjeplotechniki 19:133
MTA – SOTE Egyesitett
Kutatasi 19:201
National Information Services
Corporation (NISC) 19:155
National Library of Medicine 19:265,
19:266, 19:267, 19:268
National Library of Medicine (as a part
of TOXNET) 19:151
NIFTY Corporation,
NIFTY-Serve 19:70
NPO Wjesojusnaja knishnaja
Palata 19:137
OCLC EPIC; OCLC FirstSearch
19:64
OEMF 19:154
OHVI 19:177, 19:241
ORBIT 19:274, 19:275
Orszagos Kardiologiai Intezet 19:173,
19:175
Orszagos Sugarbiologiai es 19:162
Quanta 19:22, 19:23
Questel 19:212
Rijks Computer Centrum 19:199
SilverPlatter 19:24, 19:32, 19:85,
19:86, 19:87, 19:88, 19:99, 19:100,
19:109
Statens Husdyrbrugsforsoeg
Biblioteket 19:245

Host Index

MEDIUM INDEX

14:688, 14:690, 14:698,
14:701–14:705, 14:707, 14:708,
14:710, 14:713, 14:715, 14:717,
14:719, 14:720, 14:724–14:726,
14:728, 14:736, 14:739,
14:748–14:753, 14:757, 14:771,
14:772, 14:776–14:779–14:790,
14:792, 14:794, 14:795,
14:798–14:802, 14:807, 14:808,
14:810, 14:811, 14:813–14:819,
14:821, 14:826, 14:827, 14:829,
14:831, 14:835, 14:843, 14:845,
14:858, 14:862, 14:865–14:869,
14:872–14:880, 14:885, 14:887,
14:889–14:893, 14:898, 14:913,
14:916, 14:918, 14:920–14:923,
14:931, 14:932, 14:936, 14:941,
14:945, 14:947, 14:951, 14:953,
14:958–14:962, 14:969–14:986,
14:1008, 14:1009
Tape   14:48, 14:116, 14:144, 14:151,
14:194, 14:205, 14:268, 14:269,
14:271, 14:288, 14:292, 14:317,
14:345, 14:399, 14:468, 14:489,
14:508, 14:528, 14:581, 14:653,
14:655–14:660, 14:681, 14:755,
14:803, 14:805, 14:846, 14:870,
14:884, 14:964, 14:987, 14:988,
14:1018, 14:1019
Videotex   14:469, 14:470, 14:756

Forensic science

CD-ROM   15:13, 15:16, 15:20,
15:37–15:40, 15:52, 15:72–15:74,
15:82, 15:94, 15:104, 15:124, 15:130,
15:135, 15:141, 15:142, 15:162,
15:171, 15:173
CD-ROM 8cm   15:105
Diskette   15:22, 15:41
Online   15:2–15:4, 15:6, 15:9–15:12,
15:14, 15:19, 15:24–15:36,
15:42–15:51, 15:55, 15:58–15:71,
15:79, 15:84–15:87, 15:90, 15:92,
15:93, 15:97, 15:100–15:102, 15:107,
15:108, 15:110, 15:111, 15:114,
15:116, 15:117, 15:119,
15:121–15:123, 15:137–15:140,
15:143–15:158, 15:160, 15:161,
15:163–15:166, 15:169
Tape   15:125–15:127
Videodisc   15:133

Hospital administration

CD-ROM   16:7, 16:27–16:29, 16:35,
16:36, 16:60, 16:96–16:99, 16:112,
16:116
Diskette   16:49, 16:83
Fixed disk   16:30, 16:100
Online   16:2, 16:4–16:6, 16:10, 16:12,
16:14, 16:16–16:18, 16:23–16:26,
16:32, 16:38, 16:39, 16:41, 16:43,
16:45, 16:47, 16:51–16:55, 16:58,
16:59, 16:64, 16:65, 16:67, 16:69,
16:71, 16:73, 16:74, 16:80, 16:81,
16:85, 16:87–16:95, 16:105, 16:107,
16:110, 16:114, 16:118, 16:119,
16:122, 16:125, 16:128, 16:130,
16:132, 16:135, 16:138, 16:142,
16:146, 16:148–16:151, 16:154,

16:156–16:160, 16:162, 16:164,
16:166
Tape   16:19, 16:61, 16:101, 16:152
Videotex   16:62, 16:63

Nursing

CD-ROM   17:3, 17:12, 17:32–17:34,
17:57–17:60, 17:68, 17:72, 17:73,
17:76
Fixed disk   17:35, 17:61
Online   17:2, 17:6–17:8, 17:15, 17:17,
17:20–17:24, 17:28–17:31, 17:37,
17:38, 17:40, 17:42, 17:44, 17:46,
17:48–17:56, 17:66, 17:78, 17:80,
17:83–17:88, 17:91
Tape   17:9, 17:25, 17:62, 17:89

Medical devices

CD-ROM   18:6, 18:8, 18:10, 18:14,
18:31, 18:62, 18:63, 18:67,
18:73–18:75, 18:78, 18:82, 18:89,
18:109, 18:111, 18:118, 18:134,
18:141, 18:153, 18:178, 18:187,
18:191, 18:205, 18:234, 18:238,
18:244, 18:250
Diskette   18:93, 18:94, 18:105, 18:162,
18:208, 18:210, 18:236, 18:245
Fixed disk   18:76
Online   18:2, 18:3, 18:12, 18:16,
18:18–18:24, 18:27, 18:29, 18:35,
18:37–18:56, 18:58–18:61,
18:69–18:72, 18:80, 18:81, 18:83,
18:87, 18:88, 18:91, 18:92, 18:97,
18:100–18:103, 18:107, 18:114,
18:116, 18:121–18:125, 18:128,
18:130, 18:132, 18:139, 18:140,
18:143, 18:145, 18:147–18:150,
18:155, 18:157–18:159,
18:164–18:177, 18:179, 18:180,
18:185, 18:199–18:201,
18:212–18:223, 18:225–18:229,
18:232–18:236, 18:240, 18:242,
18:247, 18:248
Tape   18:25, 18:57, 18:64, 18:95,
18:160, 18:230
Videodisc   18:78

Veterinary medicine

CD-ROM   19:8, 19:22–19:24, 19:32,
19:49, 19:66, 19:85–19:88, 19:99,
19:100, 19:109, 19:154, 19:155,
19:184, 19:197, 19:213, 19:279
Diskette   19:43, 19:68, 19:89, 19:112,
19:124, 19:125, 19:133, 19:135,
19:158, 19:193, 19:195, 19:219,
19:237
Online   19:2, 19:3, 19:6, 19:10, 19:12,
19:13, 19:16–19:21, 19:25,
19:27–19:31, 19:34, 19:35, 19:38,
19:41, 19:45, 19:47, 19:51, 19:53,
19:55–19:61, 19:64, 19:65, 19:70,
19:72–19:84, 19:90–19:98, 19:103,
19:106, 19:108, 19:114,
19:116–19:119, 19:121–19:123,
19:128–19:130, 19:141, 19:145,
19:147, 19:149–19:151, 19:162,
19:168, 19:169, 19:173, 19:175,

19:177, 19:179, 19:181–19:183,
19:199, 19:201, 19:205,
19:207–19:212, 19:216,
19:221–19:232, 19:234, 19:235,
19:239, 19:241, 19:243, 19:245,
19:247, 19:249–19:266, 19:272,
19:274, 19:275, 19:277
Tape   19:33, 19:62, 19:120, 19:126,
19:185–19:188, 19:214, 19:267,
19:268
Videotex   19:215

Other topics

CD-I   20:498, 20:510
CD-ROM   20:7, 20:12, 20:25, 20:29,
20:33, 20:37, 20:41, 20:44, 20:47,
20:60, 20:63, 20:77, 20:88, 20:89,
20:91, 20:93, 20:98, 20:100, 20:114,
20:136–20:138, 20:140,
20:146–20:151, 20:156, 20:179,
20:182, 20:183, 20:195, 20:212,
20:227, 20:234, 20:273, 20:284,
20:293, 20:308, 20:312, 20:317,
20:326, 20:330, 20:340, 20:346,
20:351, 20:352, 20:354, 20:363,
20:366–20:376, 20:407, 20:410,
20:415, 20:421, 20:437, 20:441,
20:442, 20:463, 20:475, 20:489,
20:502, 20:508, 20:514, 20:515,
20:519, 20:522, 20:524
CD-ROM 8cm   20:236, 20:332
CDTV   20:203, 20:223
Diskette   20:22, 20:112, 20:153,
20:175, 20:177, 20:205, 20:229,
20:244, 20:246, 20:248, 20:250,
20:252, 20:254, 20:278, 20:328,
20:423, 20:448
DVI   20:197, 20:355
Online   20:4, 20:5, 20:11, 20:14, 20:16,
20:19, 20:24, 20:28, 20:32, 20:36,
20:40, 20:43, 20:46, 20:55, 20:58,
20:66–20:69, 20:75, 20:81, 20:84,
20:85, 20:103–20:107, 20:109,
20:116, 20:118, 20:122,
20:126–20:134, 20:142, 20:143,
20:145, 20:159, 20:164, 20:171,
20:173, 20:181, 20:186, 20:187,
20:189, 20:199, 20:201, 20:207,
20:209, 20:211, 20:214,
20:216–20:219, 20:232, 20:242,
20:256, 20:257, 20:261–20:263,
20:268, 20:269, 20:276, 20:280,
20:282, 20:286–20:292, 20:295,
20:297, 20:298, 20:300, 20:302,
20:310, 20:314, 20:315, 20:321,
20:323, 20:324, 20:334, 20:335,
20:342, 20:344, 20:345, 20:349,
20:350, 20:357, 20:358, 20:361,
20:378, 20:380, 20:381, 20:384,
20:386, 20:389–20:395,
20:398–20:400, 20:402, 20:403,
20:405, 20:409, 20:413, 20:427,
20:428, 20:432, 20:433, 20:440,
20:446, 20:450, 20:452,
20:457–20:461, 20:465, 20:467,
20:473, 20:477, 20:481, 20:483,
20:488, 20:512
Printout   20:124
Tape   20:185, 20:264, 20:294,
20:336–20:338, 20:347
Videotex   20:494

PRODUCER INDEX

Specific illnesses

Dentistry

CINAHL   18:68, 18:69, 18:70, 18:71,
   18:72, 18:73, 18:74, 18:75, 18:76
CMC ReSearch   18:204, 18:205
COMLINE Business Data Inc   18:79,
   18:80, 18:81, 18:82, 18:83
Commission of the European
   Communities (CEC)   18:77, 18:78
Corporate Technology Information
   Services   18:86, 18:87, 18:88, 18:89
Data Resources Inc (DRI)   18:106,
   18:107
DECHEMA Deutsche Gesellschaft für
   Chemisches Apparatewesen   18:96,
   18:97
DIALOG   18:152, 18:153
Diogenes   18:1, 18:2, 18:3, 18:99,
   18:100, 18:101, 18:102, 18:103
DNAStar   18:249, 18:250
Dom Optiki   18:207, 18:208
ECRI   18:138, 18:139, 18:140, 18:141,
   18:142, 18:143, 18:152, 18:153
Elsevier Advanced Technology
   Publications   18:32, 18:196
Elsevier Science Publishers   18:110,
   18:111, 18:204, 18:205, 18:246,
   18:247, 18:248
Fachinformationszentrum Technik (FIZ
   Technik)   18:15, 18:16, 18:198,
   18:199, 18:200, 18:201
FD Inc   18:117, 18:118, 18:190, 18:191
FDC Reports Inc   18:120, 18:121,
   18:122, 18:123, 18:124, 18:125,
   18:146, 18:147, 18:148, 18:149,
   18:150
FOI Services   18:99, 18:100, 18:101,
   18:102, 18:103
Fortia Marketing Consultants Ltd   18:98
Frost & Sullivan Inc   18:129, 18:130
Georgia Griffith   18:131, 18:132
Hamburg Educational
   Partnership   18:77, 18:78, 18:133,
   18:134
IMS America Ltd,
   Hospital/Laboratory/Veterinary
   Database Division   18:184, 18:185
Informatievoorziening Gehandicapten
   NL stichting   18:243, 18:244, 18:245
Informationzentrum für Biologie am
   Forschungsinstitut
   Senckenberg   18:28, 18:29
Informpribor   18:192, 18:193, 18:235,
   18:236
Institut der Deutschen
   Wirtschaft   18:233, 18:234
Institute for Scientific
   Information   18:30, 18:31, 18:90,
   18:91, 18:92, 18:93, 18:94, 18:95,
   18:186, 18:187
International Institute of Refrigeration
   (IIR)   18:127, 18:128
JA Micropublishing Inc   18:144, 18:145
Market Intelligence Research Company
   (MIRC)   18:194
MoldNIINTI   18:161, 18:162
National Standards Association
   Inc   18:13, 18:14
Newington Children's Hospital, Adaptive
   Equipment Center   18:5, 18:6
Newmedia International Japan   18:182
NPO Optika   18:209, 18:210
NPO Rubin   18:104, 18:105
Pharmaprojects PJB Publications
   Ltd   18:211, 18:212, 18:213, 18:214,
   18:215, 18:216, 18:217, 18:218,
   18:219, 18:220, 18:221, 18:222,
   18:223
Planning and Rationalization Institute for
   the Health and Social
   Services   18:239, 18:240
Predicasts International
   Inc   18:231–18:236
Preston Publications   18:66, 18:67

Robert Colbert   18:154, 18:155
Shirley Institute   18:246, 18:247,
   18:248
Siemens AG   18:237, 18:238
Socialstyrelsens
   Lääkemedelsavdelning   18:241,
   18:242
Spri Bibliotek och utredningsbanken
   Stiftelsen Stockholms läna
   Äldrecentrum   18:239, 18:240
Thomson Financial Networks
   Inc   18:163, 18:164, 18:165, 18:166,
   18:167, 18:168, 18:169, 18:170,
   18:171, 18:172, 18:173, 18:174,
   18:175, 18:176, 18:177, 18:178,
   18:179, 18:180
UCLA School of Medicine   18:108,
   18:109
United Communications Group   18:202
University Microfilms International/Data
   Courier Inc   18:224, 18:225, 18:227,
   18:228, 18:229, 18:230
US Food and Drug
   Administration   18:115, 18:116,
   18:117, 18:118, 18:188, 18:190,
   18:191
Washington Business Information
   Inc   18:99, 18:100, 18:101, 18:102,
   18:103

Veterinary medicine

ArmNIINTI   19:67, 19:68, 19:194,
   19:195
Bibliotheque Interuniversitaire Section
   Medecine   19:5, 19:6
BIOSIS   19:54, 19:55, 19:56, 19:57,
   19:58, 19:59, 19:60, 19:61, 19:62
BioWorld   19:69, 19:70
Bundesgesundheitsamt – BGA   19:50,
   19:51
CAB International   19:71, 19:72, 19:73,
   19:74, 19:75, 19:76, 19:77, 19:78,
   19:79, 19:80, 19:81, 19:82, 19:83,
   19:84, 19:85, 19:86, 19:87, 19:88,
   19:89, 19:90, 19:91, 19:92, 19:93,
   19:94, 19:95, 19:96, 19:97, 19:98,
   19:99, 19:100
Cambridge Scientific Abstracts   19:102,
   19:103, 19:180, 19:181, 19:182,
   19:183, 19:184, 19:185, 19:186,
   19:187
CD Systems   19:153, 19:154
Centre National de la Recherche
   Scientifique, Institut de l'Information
   Scientifique et Technique, Science
   Humaines et Sociales
   (CNRS/INIST)   19:206, 19:207,
   19:208, 19:209, 19:210, 19:211,
   19:212, 19:213, 19:214, 19:215,
   19:216
Commission of the European
   Communities (CEC)   19:11, 19:12,
   19:13
Commonwealth Scientific Industrial
   Research Organization   19:113,
   19:114
CompuKennel Information Service
   Inc   19:105, 19:106
Danmarks Veterinaer og
   Jordbrugsbibliotek   19:127, 19:128,
   19:129, 19:130, 19:167, 19:168,
   19:169
Derwent Publications Ltd   19:273,
   19:274, 19:275
Diogenes   19:1, 19:2, 19:3
ETi SpA   19:7, 19:8
Food and Agriculture Organization of
   the United Nations (FAO)   19:26,
   19:27, 19:28, 19:29, 19:30, 19:31,
   19:32, 19:33, 19:34, 19:35

Gale Research   19:238, 19:239
George Marinescu Hospital   19:202,
   19:203
Gosudarstwennaja Biblioteka SSSR im.
   W. I. Lenina   19:142, 19:143, 19:190,
   19:191
GPNTB SSSR   19:159, 19:160
HW Wilson Company   19:63, 19:64,
   19:65, 19:66
IKONA Srl   19:7, 19:8
IMS America Ltd,
   Hospital/Laboratory/Veterinary
   Database Division   19:144, 19:145
Information and Research Center on
   Health Services   19:37, 19:38
Institut eksperimentalnoj
   Meteorologie   19:134, 19:135
Institut obchej Genetiki   19:236, 19:237
Institut Problem Kriobiologii i
   Kriomedizinij   19:111, 19:112
Institute for Scientific
   Information   19:115, 19:116, 19:117,
   19:118, 19:119, 19:120, 19:121,
   19:122, 19:123, 19:124, 19:125,
   19:126
IS Datacentralen   19:127, 19:128,
   19:129, 19:130
Johan Bela Orszagos K zegeszseg
   gyi   19:44, 19:45, 19:254, 19:255
Müszi Rt., Budapest   19:246, 19:247
Merck Sharp & Dôhme   19:196, 19:197
Moskowskii Institut
   Tjeplotechniki   19:132, 19:133
MTA – SOTE Egyesitett
   Kutatasi   19:200, 19:201
National Information Services
   Corporation (NISC)   19:155
National Library of
   Medicine   19:248–19:268, 19:270
Netherlands Ministry of Welfare, Health
   and Cultural Affairs   19:198, 19:199
Nimbus Records Ltd   19:278, 19:279
NPO Wjesojusnaja knishnaja
   Palata   19:136, 19:137
Oak Ridge National Laboratory,
   Environmental Teratology Information
   Centre   19:148, 19:149, 19:150,
   19:151
OEMF   19:153, 19:154
Orszagos Haematologiai es   19:176,
   19:177, 19:240, 19:241
Orszagos Kardiologiai Intezet   19:172,
   19:173, 19:174, 19:175
Orszagos Munkavedelmi
   Tudomanyos   19:204, 19:205
Orszagos Sugarbiologiai es   19:161,
   19:162
Pacific Veterinary Services   19:40,
   19:41
Pharmaprojects PJB Publications
   Ltd   19:220, 19:221, 19:222, 19:223,
   19:224, 19:225, 19:226, 19:227,
   19:228, 19:229, 19:230, 19:231,
   19:232, 19:233, 19:234, 19:235
Research Knowledge Access   19:196,
   19:197
Statens Husdyrbrugsforsoeg
   Biblioteket   19:244, 19:245
Sveriges Lantbruksuniversitets Bibliotek
   (SLUB)   19:178, 19:179, 19:242,
   19:243
UK Departments of Health and Social
   Security Library   19:140, 19:141
Universidad de Colima, Director
   General de International Academy
   Des Biblio   19:48, 19:49
Universidad Nacional Autonoma de
   Mexico, Facultad de Medicina
   Veterraria-y-Zootecnica   19:46,
   19:47
US Department of Agriculture,

Other topics

DATABASE TYPE INDEX

General medical

Addresses/Telephone directory   1:92
Bibliographic   1:1, 1:3, 1:5, 1:7, 1:11,
   1:29, 1:36, 1:39, 1:41, 1:45, 1:47,
   1:52, 1:74, 1:76, 1:78, 1:81, 1:83,
   1:85, 1:89, 1:94, 1:96, 1:99, 1:102,
   1:104, 1:112, 1:115, 1:123, 1:126,
   1:128, 1:129, 1:135, 1:137, 1:145,
   1:152, 1:159, 1:163, 1:165, 1:178,
   1:195, 1:223, 1:225, 1:227, 1:243,
   1:247, 1:249, 1:262, 1:271, 1:273,
   1:276, 1:282, 1:288, 1:290, 1:292,
   1:298, 1:302, 1:304, 1:309, 1:311,
   1:314, 1:316, 1:327, 1:329, 1:332,
   1:345, 1:347, 1:353, 1:360, 1:365,
   1:368, 1:370, 1:430, 1:438, 1:440,
   1:449, 1:451, 1:454, 1:485, 1:487,
   1:508, 1:515, 1:518, 1:526, 1:528,
   1:530, 1:532, 1:534, 1:535, 1:540,
   1:542, 1:566, 1:570, 1:572, 1:574,
   1:584, 1:593, 1:595, 1:597, 1:599,
   1:605, 1:607, 1:611, 1:613, 1:614,
   1:617, 1:619, 1:628, 1:632
Catalogue   1:145
Chemical structures   1:117
Citation   1:304, 1:541
Clip sounds   1:176
Computer software   1:182, 1:589
Courseware   1:271, 1:456, 1:458,
   1:460
Dictionary   1:172, 1:174, 1:192, 1:251,
   1:271, 1:294, 1:349, 1:472, 1:537,
   1:589, 1:603, 1:622
Directory   1:17, 1:41, 1:43, 1:52, 1:56,
   1:58, 1:62, 1:66, 1:70, 1:112, 1:117,
   1:133, 1:147, 1:157, 1:178, 1:180,
   1:182, 1:186, 1:190, 1:236, 1:238,
   1:247, 1:255, 1:273, 1:338, 1:365,
   1:432, 1:510, 1:566, 1:568, 1:572,
   1:609
Encyclopedia   1:257, 1:284, 1:343,
   1:622
Factual   1:20, 1:22, 1:36, 1:41, 1:52,
   1:56, 1:58, 1:62, 1:66, 1:70, 1:78,
   1:89, 1:96, 1:147, 1:184, 1:188,
   1:253, 1:259, 1:266, 1:271, 1:273,
   1:286, 1:300, 1:309, 1:318, 1:320,
   1:329, 1:338, 1:341, 1:356, 1:365,
   1:432, 1:440, 1:443, 1:462, 1:476,
   1:479, 1:482, 1:572, 1:624, 1:626,
   1:630
Gazeteer   1:41
Image   1:7, 1:257, 1:338, 1:353, 1:358,
   1:456, 1:458, 1:460, 1:582, 1:599,
   1:603
Library catalogue/cataloguing
   aids   1:11, 1:47, 1:76, 1:83, 1:85,
   1:104, 1:112, 1:115, 1:159, 1:163,
   1:446, 1:485, 1:508, 1:574, 1:601,
   1:611, 1:613, 1:614, 1:617, 1:619
Multimedia   1:174, 1:176, 1:336, 1:341,
   1:456, 1:458, 1:460, 1:603
Numeric   1:52, 1:147, 1:286, 1:443
Organisational/Biographical   1:56, 1:58,
   1:62, 1:66, 1:70, 1:190, 1:253, 1:572
Reference   1:112, 1:230
Statistical   1:365
Textual   1:11, 1:15, 1:17, 1:22, 1:25,
   1:29, 1:30, 1:34, 1:36, 1:39, 1:41,
   1:45, 1:54, 1:78, 1:89, 1:94, 1:96,
   1:131, 1:135, 1:139, 1:147, 1:172,
   1:253, 1:257, 1:259, 1:264, 1:266,
   1:271, 1:282, 1:286, 1:288, 1:296,
   1:300, 1:306, 1:314, 1:316, 1:320,
   1:329, 1:332, 1:338, 1:341, 1:343,
   1:349, 1:351, 1:353, 1:358, 1:432,
   1:440, 1:456, 1:458, 1:460, 1:462,
   1:472, 1:474, 1:476, 1:479, 1:482,
   1:510, 1:512, 1:520, 1:526, 1:528,
   1:539, 1:564, 1:572, 1:582, 1:599,
   1:603, 1:605
Thesaurus   1:432
Various data formats included   1:436

Specific illnesses

Addresses/Telephone directory   2:47
Bibliographic   2:1, 2:3, 2:5, 2:7, 2:11,
   2:19, 2:26, 2:32, 2:47, 2:57, 2:59,
   2:67, 2:69, 2:80, 2:100, 2:105, 2:125,
   2:128, 2:130, 2:136, 2:140, 2:146,
   2:148, 2:149, 2:160, 2:166, 2:168,
   2:170, 2:181, 2:185, 2:193, 2:195,
   2:203, 2:207, 2:213, 2:221, 2:224,
   2:226, 2:228, 2:230, 2:232, 2:236,
   2:239, 2:243, 2:263, 2:265, 2:267,
   2:269, 2:283, 2:292, 2:300, 2:302,
   2:307, 2:332, 2:334, 2:347, 2:358,
   2:365, 2:368, 2:376
Computer software   2:158
Courseware   2:138, 2:162, 2:239
Dictionary   2:239, 2:300
Directory   2:9, 2:29, 2:47, 2:50, 2:128,
   2:130, 2:158, 2:168, 2:181, 2:211,
   2:243, 2:300, 2:307, 2:332, 2:376
Encyclopedia   2:300
Factual   2:15, 2:53, 2:55, 2:62, 2:82,
   2:86, 2:88, 2:90, 2:93, 2:102, 2:128,
   2:130, 2:134, 2:136, 2:138, 2:140,
   2:157, 2:168, 2:183, 2:205, 2:207,
   2:209, 2:239, 2:245, 2:248, 2:254,
   2:260, 2:281, 2:292, 2:302, 2:355,
   2:362, 2:365, 2:368, 2:376
Image   2:183, 2:250, 2:356
Library catalogue/cataloguing
   aids   2:146
Multimedia   2:132, 2:138, 2:164, 2:241,
   2:248, 2:250, 2:378
Numeric   2:55, 2:376
Patents   2:193, 2:368
Statistical   2:296
Textual   2:1, 2:7, 2:11, 2:15, 2:17, 2:19,
   2:21, 2:50, 2:53, 2:57, 2:59, 2:62,
   2:65, 2:67, 2:86, 2:90, 2:93, 2:96,
   2:102, 2:128, 2:130, 2:134, 2:136,
   2:146, 2:149, 2:157, 2:158, 2:160,
   2:164, 2:168, 2:170, 2:172, 2:181,
   2:183, 2:203, 2:205, 2:207, 2:211,
   2:221, 2:228, 2:230, 2:232, 2:239,
   2:243, 2:245, 2:250, 2:252, 2:254,
   2:256, 2:260, 2:279, 2:281, 2:296,
   2:298, 2:300, 2:302, 2:304, 2:307,
   2:332, 2:341, 2:356, 2:360, 2:362,
   2:365, 2:376, 2:378
Textual (book reviews)   2:47

Reproduction/Child care

Bibliographic   3:14, 3:17, 3:23, 3:25,
   3:38, 3:44, 3:46, 3:48, 3:56, 3:58,
   3:60, 3:62, 3:66, 3:68, 3:71, 3:74,
   3:77, 3:81, 3:83, 3:88, 3:93, 3:106,
   3:108, 3:112, 3:114, 3:116, 3:120,
   3:129, 3:134, 3:138, 3:148, 3:155,
   3:161, 3:166, 3:172, 3:177, 3:181,
   3:183, 3:185, 3:187, 3:189, 3:191,
   3:193, 3:195, 3:197
Computer software   3:53
Courseware   3:36
Directory   3:53, 3:88, 3:106, 3:134,
   3:146, 3:191, 3:207
Factual   3:5, 3:20, 3:50, 3:74, 3:86,
   3:104, 3:118, 3:131, 3:136, 3:140,
   3:142, 3:164, 3:168, 3:187, 3:191,
   3:195, 3:205
Image   3:131, 3:136, 3:140, 3:142,
   3:170
Library catalogue/cataloguing
   aids   3:71
Multimedia   3:36, 3:125, 3:199
Numeric   3:44, 3:108, 3:114, 3:158,
   3:191, 3:195, 3:209
Organisational/Biographical   3:88
Patents   3:62
Statistical   3:66, 3:134, 3:207
Textual   3:1, 3:3, 3:5, 3:9, 3:14, 3:20,
   3:40, 3:42, 3:50, 3:53, 3:58, 3:60,
   3:64, 3:74, 3:79, 3:93, 3:102, 3:104,
   3:106, 3:110, 3:116, 3:118, 3:127,
   3:131, 3:134, 3:136, 3:140, 3:142,
   3:146, 3:155, 3:164, 3:170, 3:172,
   3:187, 3:189, 3:191, 3:199, 3:201,
   3:203, 3:205, 3:207

Handicapped/Social medicine

Bibliographic   4:8, 4:10, 4:22, 4:24,
   4:33, 4:48, 4:50, 4:62, 4:64, 4:68,
   4:82, 4:85, 4:90, 4:92, 4:106, 4:110,
   4:123, 4:125, 4:127, 4:131, 4:133,
   4:139, 4:141, 4:146, 4:148, 4:150,
   4:153, 4:155, 4:157, 4:159, 4:162,
   4:164, 4:171, 4:174, 4:176, 4:179
Catalogue   4:3
Citation   4:10
Computer software   4:3
Courseware   4:20
Directory   4:1, 4:85, 4:100, 4:119,
   4:150, 4:157
Encyclopedia   4:12, 4:157
Factual   4:18, 4:20, 4:57, 4:104, 4:108,
   4:117, 4:139, 4:141, 4:153, 4:159,
   4:55
Library catalogue/cataloguing
   aids   4:50
Multimedia   4:20, 4:191
Numeric   4:60
Organisational/Biographical   4:85
Reference   4:188
Statistical   4:102, 4:135
Textual   4:3, 4:6, 4:12, 4:14, 4:16, 4:18,
   4:53, 4:55, 4:62, 4:90, 4:104, 4:108,
   4:110, 4:117, 4:119, 4:121, 4:125,
   4:135, 4:137, 4:143, 4:153, 4:157,
   4:159, 4:162, 4:171, 4:193

Gerontology

Bibliographic   5:1, 5:6, 5:9, 5:13, 5:16,
   5:28, 5:32, 5:38, 5:49, 5:56, 5:60,
   5:66, 5:69, 5:71
Computer software   5:25

Health hazards and pollution

Genetics

MASTER INDEX

Master Index

Master Index